The Companion to Specialist Surgical Practice

Series edited by

O. James Garden and Simon Paterson-Brown

The content of all eight volumes of the Fifth Edition of the **Companion to Specialist Surgical Practice** is now available both in print and as part of an electronic library. Your purchase of this book allows you to download the fully searchable contents to your desktop, laptop, tablet or smartphone.

Your **Companion to Specialist Surgical Practice eLibrary** is portable: the titles in the series download to your device or you can access online so they are with you whenever you need them.

Your eBook is much more than just 'pictures of pages':

- customize your page views
- search in single books that you have purchased or across any volumes in the series in your collection
- highlight and take searchable notes, and even print and copy-and-paste with bibliographic sup~~~~
- utilize reference lis~~~~   authors, title, source, and often~~~~   electronic full-text availability.

To purchase other eB~~~~   **actice eLibrary** please visit~~~~

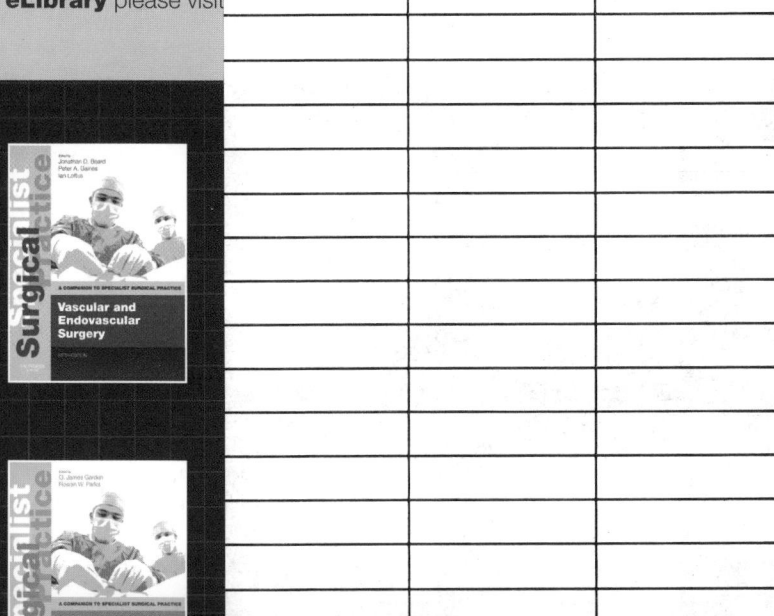

Vascular and Endovascular Surgery

Colorectal Surgery

Hepatobiliary and Pancreatic Surgery

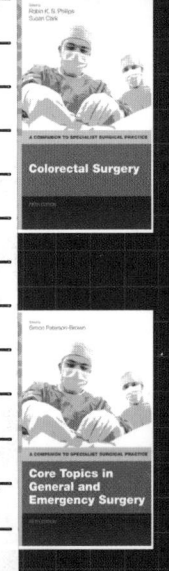

Core Topics in General and Emergency Surgery

A COMPANION TO SPECIALIST SURGICAL PRACTICE

Series Editors
O. James Garden
Simon Paterson-Brown

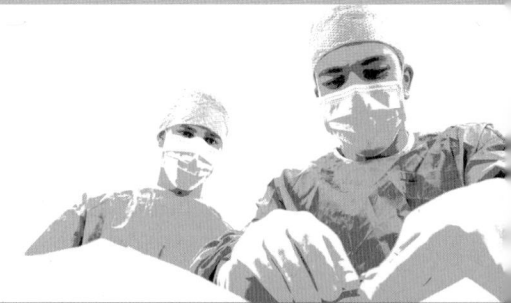

Breast Surgery

FIFTH EDITION

Edited by

J. Michael Dixon
OBE BSc(Hons) MBChB MD FRCS FRCSEd FRCPEd(Hon)
Professor of Surgery, University of Edinburgh;
Clinical Director, Edinburgh Breakthrough Unit;
Consultant Surgeon, NHS Lothian Edinburgh Breast Unit,
Western General Hospital, Edinburgh, UK

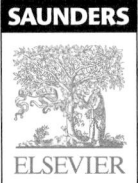

SAUNDERS

ELSEVIER

Edinburgh London New York Oxford Philadelphia St Louis Sydney Toronto 2014

SAUNDERS
ELSEVIER

First edition 1997
Second edition 2001
Third edition 2005
Fourth edition 2009
Fifth edition 2014
  Reprinted 2014 (twice)

ISBN 978-0-7020-4959-0
e-ISBN 978-0-7020-4967-5

British Library Cataloguing in Publication Data
A catalogue record for this book is available from the British Library

Library of Congress Cataloging in Publication Data
A catalog record for this book is available from the Library of Congress

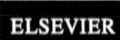 your source for books,
journals and multimedia
in the health sciences
www.elsevierhealth.com

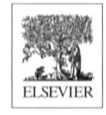 Working together
to grow libraries in
developing countries

The Publisher's policy is to use paper manufactured from sustainable forests

www.elsevier.com • www.bookaid.org

Printed in China

Commissioning Editor: Laurence Hunter
Development Editor: Lynn Watt
Project Manager: Vinod Kumar Iyyappan
Designer/Design Direction: Miles Hitchen
Illustration Manager: Jennifer Rose
Illustrator: Antbits Ltd

Contents

Contents

Contributors

Douglas J.A. Adamson, MBChB, MD, PhD, FRCP (Edin), FRCR
Consultant Clinical Oncologist and Honorary Senior Lecturer, Tayside Cancer Centre, Ninewells Hospital, Dundee, UK

Andrew D. Baildam, MD, FRCS
Professor of Breast and Oncoplastic Surgery, Queen Mary, University of London, London, UK

Nicola L.P. Barnes, MD, FRCS
Specialist Registrar Breast Surgery, South Manchester University Hospital, Manchester, UK

Tom Bates, FRCS
Honorary Professor of Surgery, Centre for Professional Practice, University of Kent, Canterbury, UK

Nigel J. Bundred, MD, FRCS
Professor in Surgical Oncology, University of Manchester; Consultant Surgeon, University Hospital of South Manchester NHS Foundation Trust, Manchester, UK

Anees B. Chagpar, MD, MSc, MPH, MA
Associate Professor, Department of Surgery Director, The Breast Center – Smilow Cancer Hospital at Yale; Yale Comprehensive Cancer Center – Diversity/Disparities Program Director, Yale Interdisciplinary Breast Fellowship, Yale University School of Medicine, New Haven, CT, USA

Daniel Xavier Choi, MD
United States Air Force, Air Mobility Command, 60th Surgical Operations Squadron, Travis Air Force Base, Fairfield, California, USA

Krishna B. Clough, MD
Chief of Surgery, Paris Breast Center, Paris, France

Tim Davidson, ChM, MRCP, FRCS
Consultant Breast Surgeon, University Department of Surgery, Royal Free Hospital, London, UK

John A. Dewar, MA, FRCR, FRCP
Consultant Clinical Oncologist and Honorary Professor of Clinical Oncology, Ninewells Hospital and Medical School, Dundee, UK

J. Michael Dixon, *OBE* BSc(Hons), MBChB, MD, FRCS, FRCSEd, FRCPEd(Hon)
Professor of Surgery, University of Edinburgh; Clinical Director, Edinburgh Breakthrough Unit; Consultant Surgeon, NHS Lothian, Edinburgh Breast Unit, Western General Hospital, Edinburgh, UK

Ian O. Ellis, BMBS, BMedSc, FRCPath
Professor of Cancer Pathology and Honorary Consultant Pathologist, University of Nottingham, School of Medicine, City Hospital, Nottingham, UK

D.Gareth R. Evans, MD, FRCP
Honorary Professor of Medical Genetics and Cancer Epidemiology, The University of Manchester; Consultant in Medical Genetics and Cancer Epidemiology, Central Manchester Hospitals NHS Foundation Trust and The Christie NHS Foundation Trust, Saint Mary's Hospital, Manchester, UK

Lesley Fallowfield, BSc, DPhil, FMedSci
Professor in Psycho-oncology and Director, Sussex Health Outcomes Research and Education in Cancer (SHORE-C), Brighton and Sussex Medical School, University of Sussex, Brighton, UK

Rosalie Fisher, MBChB, FRACP
The Breast Unit, Royal Marsden Hospital, London, UK

Gerald Gui, MS, FRCS, FRCS(Ed)
Academic Surgery (Breast Unit), Royal Marsden NHS Trust, London, UK

Valerie Jenkins, BSc, DPhil
Sussex Health Outcomes Research and Education in Cancer (SHORE-C), Brighton and Sussex Medical School, University of Sussex, Brighton, UK

Contributors

Gabriel J. Kaufman, MD
Department of breast cancer and reconstructive surgery, Paris Breast Center, Paris, France

Ian Kunkler, MA, MB, BCHIR, FRCR, FRCPE
Professor of Clinical Oncology, University of Edinburgh; Consultant in Clinical Oncology, Western General Hospital, Edinburgh, UK

Ava Kwong, MBBS(Lon), BSc(St Andrews), FRCS, FRCS (Edin), FCSHK, FHKAM (surgery)
Clinical Associate Professor, Chief of Division of Breast Surgery, The University of Hong Kong, Hong Kong, China

Pamela Levack, MBChB, BMedBiol, MRCGP, FRCP
Consultant in Palliative Medicine, Ninewells Hospital; Honorary Senior Lecturer in Surgery and Molecular Oncology, University of Dundee, Dundee, UK

R. Douglas Macmillan, MBChB, MD, FRCS
Oncoplastic Breast Surgeon, Associate Clinical Director, Nottingham Breast Institute, Nottingham City Hospital, Nottingham, UK

Monica Morrow, MD, FACS
Chief, Breast Service, Department of Surgery; Anne Burnett Windfohr Chair of Clinical Oncology, Memorial Sloan-Kettering Cancer Center; Professor of Surgery, Weill Medical College of Cornell University, New York, NY, UK

Claude Nos, MD
Department of breast cancer and reconstructive surgery, Paris Breast Center, Paris, France

Cameron Raine, MBChB, MD, FRCS(plastics)
Department of Plastic Surgery, St John's Hospital at Howden, Livingston, UK

Richard M. Rainsbury, MBBS, BSc, MS, FRCS
Consultant Oncoplastic Breast Surgeon, Royal Hampshire County Hospital, Winchester, UK

Emad A. Rakha, MB BCh, PhD, FRCPath
Clinical Associate Professor and Honorary Consultant Pathologist University of Nottingham, School of Medicine, City Hospital, Nottingham, UK

Rajendra S. Rampaul, MBChB, MD, FRCS
Consultant Oncoplastic Breast Surgeon, The Breast Centre, Woodbrook, Trinidad and Tobago

John F.R. Robertson, MBChB, FRCS
Professor of Surgery, University of Nottingham; Consultant Surgeon, City Hospital, Nottingham, UK

Mark Schaverien, MBChB, MD, MSc, MEd, FRCS(Plast)
Specialist Registrar, Department of Plastic Surgery, Ninewells Hospital, Dundee, UK

Ian Smith, MD, FRCP, FRCPE
Professor of Cancer Medicine; Head, The Breast Unit, Royal Marsden Hospital, London, UK

Sarah Tang, MBBS, MA, MRCS
Specialist Registrar in Breast Surgery, Breast Unit, Royal Marsden Hospital, London, UK

Alastair M. Thompson, BSc(Hons), MBChB, MD, FRCSEd
Professor of Surgical Oncology, Dundee Cancer Centre, University of Dundee, Dundee, UK

Steven Thrush, MBBS, FRCS(Gen Surg)
Consultant Surgeon, Worcester Breast Unit, Worcestershire Royal Hospital, Worcester, UK

A. Robin M. Wilson, MBChB, FRCR, FRCP(E)
Consultant Radiologist, Clinical Radiology, The Royal Marsden, London, UK

Series Editors' preface

It is now some 17 years since the first edition of the *Companion to Specialist Surgical Practice* series was published. We set ourselves the task of meeting the educational needs of surgeons in the later years of specialist surgical training, as well as consultant surgeons in independent practice who wished for contemporary, evidence-based information on the subspecialist areas relevant to their general surgical practice. The series was never intended to replace the large reference surgical textbooks which, although valuable in their own way, struggle to keep pace with changing surgical practice. This Fifth Edition has also had to take due account of the increasing specialisation in 'general' surgery. The rise of minimal access surgery and therapy, and the desire of some subspecialties such as breast and vascular surgery to separate away from 'general surgery', may have proved challenging in some countries, but has also served to emphasise the importance of all surgeons being aware of current developments in their surgical field. As in previous editions, there has been increasing emphasis on evidence-based practice and contributors have endeavoured to provide key recommendations within each chapter. The eBook versions of the textbook have also allowed the technophile improved access to key data and content within each chapter.

We remain indebted to the volume editors and all the contributors of this Fifth Edition. We have endeavoured where possible to bring in new blood to freshen content. We are impressed by the enthusiasm, commitment and hard work that our contributors and editorial team have shown and this has ensured a short turnover between editions while maintaining as accurate and up-to-date content as is possible. We remain grateful for the support and encouragement of Laurence Hunter and Lynn Watt at Elsevier Ltd. We trust that our original vision of delivering an up-to-date affordable text has been met and that readers, whether in training or independent practice, will find this Fifth Edition an invaluable resource.

O. James Garden, BSc, MBChB, MD, FRCS(Glas), FRCS(Ed), FRCP(Ed), FRACS(Hon), FRCSC(Hon), FRSE
Regius Professor of Clinical Surgery, Clinical Surgery School of Clinical Sciences, The University of Edinburgh and Honorary Consultant Surgeon, Royal Infirmary of Edinburgh

Simon Paterson-Brown, MBBS, MPhil, MS, FRCS(Ed), FRCS(Engl), FCS(HK)
Honorary Senior Lecturer, Clinical Surgery School of Clinical Sciences, The University of Edinburgh and Consultant General and Upper Gastrointestinal Surgeon, Royal Infirmary of Edinburgh

Editor's preface

I wrote in the last edition of how writing or editing a book is like running a marathon. At the outset when planning to run a marathon or to edit a book, you set out a program and timetable and to achieve a good outcome all you have to do is to follow carefully the schedule you spent so much time perfecting. But anyone who has run a marathon or who has edited a multi-author text knows that it is never that simple. There are competing demands on time as well as unexpected problems to deal with. Getting all the authors to deliver according to the carefully designed schedule is never easy, often through no fault of their own. The last few chapters, like the last few miles of a marathon, are the most difficult. The Fifth Edition has now run its course and despite ups and downs and a variety of problems, it is now here before you. Just as there is pride in finishing a marathon so I have pride in the efforts of the many who have contributed so much to bring you the best edition yet of the Breast section of the Companion Series. Although the target audience is trainee and consultant surgeons with a special interest in breast disease, I believe this book will be valuable to many more groups. Nurses working in breast clinics and operating departments and any doctor involved in breast clinics or the oncological management of breast cancer should find it of great value.

Breast diseases and breast cancer are fortunate in having a high public profile and being well supported financially. This irritates some colleagues working in other areas but what is impressive in breast cancer are the huge strides and advances in our understanding and treatment that this investment has produced. This means that for many women breast cancer is a treatable condition rather than the death sentence it once was. Despite these advances, there remains huge anxiety amongst women about breast cancer and it remains women's number one fear. Reducing the level of fear can only be achieved through education about the advances that have been achieved. These new advances are all here in this Fifth Edition, which provides all the necessary information for doctors and nurses involved in the care of patients with breast conditions. The chapters on imaging, including breast screening and pathology, have been revised and updated. More has been added on the controversies surrounding breast screening. Critics of screening express concern at the numbers of potentially unnecessary interventions and the potential over-treatment of cancers that would not have caused problems in the patient's lifetime. This is all addressed in the new revamped chapter. Benign disease is more common than breast cancer yet is often covered superficially in many texts. The chapter on benign conditions has been expanded to include a number of benign conditions which are not common but will not be diagnosed unless there is knowledge of them. A more detailed discussion of the management of nipple discharge including ductoscopy is included in a completely new chapter by new authors.

The chapters dealing with breast-conserving surgery and oncoplastic surgery have been revamped. Written by recognised experts in their fields, these chapters represent the current state of the art in breast-conserving surgery. In the last edition, a chapter on mastectomy was added. Far too many mastectomies are performed through incisions that leave a poor cosmetic outcome and this excellent chapter has been reworked. It is essential reading for all breast surgeons and now includes Goldilocks mastectomy. The chapter on uncommon cancers provides new and important information in an area that is not well covered in many texts. One area where practice continues to evolve and there have been dramatic changes since the Fourth Edition has been the management of the axilla. The Z0011 trial has divided opinion on the two sides of the Atlantic. A new transatlantic author presents a balanced view of how the Z0011 trial should be interpreted and how it has changed management of the axilla. Not everyone has been keen to reduce the number of axillary clearances and new trials in the UK and the USA are planned, but what do we do in the meantime? Read the chapter to find out.

There continue to be advances in our knowledge of the genetics of breast cancer. A rewritten chapter with the addition of a new author presents the latest knowledge, not only on genetics but also on how to manage such patients surgically. In the USA more women than ever are choosing mastectomy in preference to breast conservation, with these women often choosing bilateral mastectomy in part because of the increasing availability of good quality breast reconstruction. A brand new chapter with new authors covers the advances in breast reconstruction. There have been extensive revisions to the chapter on ductal carcinoma in situ. Building on the success of splitting the chapters on systemic therapy into early, locally advanced and metastatic therapy, all three chapters have been rewritten or revised. The chapter on the role of systemic therapy in early breast cancer is authoritative as well as comprehensive and would sit well in any major text on oncology. Partial breast radiotherapy after breast-conserving surgery has gained increasing popularity in the USA. Whether all older patients need radiotherapy after breast-conserving surgery continues to be debated. Controversy as to which patients benefit from postoperative chest wall radiotherapy after mastectomy abounds. There are new ongoing trials in these areas and a new chapter by an author who is leading some of these trials shows that the Fifth Edition is not merely a rewrite but a new book. The chapter on psychosocial issues provides excellent information and advice and reflects the expertise of the authors and is an important part of the book. Medical negligence cases continue to increase and so the book finishes with some sound advice and vignettes of what to watch out for to avoid negligence claims. Another chapter written by people at the top of their game and a must-read.

The content of this book has evolved over many years. Various authors over this time have been kind enough to share their knowledge, clinical expertise and understanding because they all want to do better for patients and this continues to be the main motivation behind this book. It has been reassuring to see people carrying, reading and quoting from the Fourth Edition. I hope and trust the Fifth Edition will be as well received. Seeing the editions evolve over time brings its own rewards. Ultimately it will be you, the reader, who will judge whether the efforts of the very many to get this book to the finish line have been worthwhile. Your feedback is always welcome. If there are topics we should have covered which have been omitted, or this text fails to meet your expectations, please let me know. If you enjoy this book, please tell your friends and colleagues.

Acknowledgements

I would like to say a big thank you to all those who have contributed to this Fifth Edition. The various authors past and present have been enormously cooperative and have produced consistently high-quality work. I would specifically like to thank Monica McGill, who has coordinated each chapter with the authors and made the numerous changes to the text as well as coping with the late addition of numerous new figures which, I believe, have added to the book's utility. I would also like to thank Lynn Watt, Development Editor, for her keen eye and endless patience with me. There are a number of people who have influenced me over my career who deserve special mention. I first became aware of the complexities of the breast by working with Professor David Page, a pathologist from Nashville. Professor Page spent a sabbatical in Edinburgh during the year I did pathology and his enthusiasm for his topic infected me. There are a number of surgeons who have been my heroes and who have taught me that success only comes through hard work and dedication and these include the late John Bostwick III, who worked in Atlanta, and my friend and contemporary, Krishna Clough from Paris. Professor Patrick Forrest in Edinburgh taught me that the patient is the focus and is paramount. I am fortunate to have been taught and known other great individuals, too many to mention. I hope they know who they are and I thank them. I would like to pay a special tribute to the many patients who have placed their faith and trust in me. They continue to inspire me and are the reason that we all need to try harder, learn more and do better for them. Finally, I would like to thank my family for their support. Writing and editing takes time away from those who are there when everyone has left. Pam, my wife, has been the rock on whom I have been able to build many projects including this, the Fifth Edition. Oliver and Jonathan, my sons, have helped by understanding that medicine is not just a profession.

Michael Dixon
Edinburgh

Evidence-based practice in surgery

Critical appraisal for developing evidence-based practice can be obtained from a number of sources, the most reliable being randomised controlled clinical trials, systematic literature reviews, meta-analyses and observational studies. For practical purposes three grades of evidence can be used, analogous to the levels of 'proof' required in a court of law:

1. **Beyond all reasonable doubt.** Such evidence is likely to have arisen from high-quality randomised controlled trials, systematic reviews or high-quality synthesised evidence such as decision analysis, cost-effectiveness analysis or large observational datasets. The studies need to be directly applicable to the population of concern and have clear results. The grade is analogous to burden of proof within a criminal court and may be thought of as corresponding to the usual standard of 'proof' within the medical literature (i.e. $P<0.05$).

2. **On the balance of probabilities.** In many cases a high-quality review of literature may fail to reach firm conclusions due to conflicting or inconclusive results, trials of poor methodological quality or the lack of evidence in the population to which the guidelines apply. In such cases it may still be possible to make a statement as to the best treatment on the 'balance of probabilities'. This is analogous to the decision in a civil court where all the available evidence will be weighed up and the verdict will depend upon the balance of probabilities.

3. **Not proven.** Insufficient evidence upon which to base a decision, or contradictory evidence.

Depending on the information available, three grades of recommendation can be used:

a. Strong recommendation, which should be followed unless there are compelling reasons to act otherwise.

b. A recommendation based on evidence of effectiveness, but where there may be other factors to take into account in decision-making, for example the user of the guidelines may be expected to take into account patient preferences, local facilities, local audit results or available resources.

c. A recommendation made where there is no adequate evidence as to the most effective practice, although there may be reasons for making a recommendation in order to minimise cost or reduce the chance of error through a locally agreed protocol.

✓✓ Evidence where a conclusion can be reached **'beyond all reasonable doubt'** and therefore where a **strong recommendation** can be given.
  This will normally be based on evidence levels:
- Ia. Meta-analysis of randomised controlled trials
- Ib. Evidence from at least one randomised controlled trial
- IIa. Evidence from at least one controlled study without randomisation
- IIb. Evidence from at least one other type of quasi-experimental study.

✓ Evidence where a conclusion might be reached **'on the balance of probabilities'** and where there may be other factors involved which influence the recommendation given. This will normally be based on less conclusive evidence than that represented by the double tick icons:
- III. Evidence from non-experimental descriptive studies, such as comparative studies and case–control studies
- IV. Evidence from expert committee reports or opinions or clinical experience of respected authorities, or both.

Evidence which is associated with either a **strong recommendation** or **expert opinion** is highlighted in the text in panels such as those shown above, and is distinguished by either a double or single tick icon, respectively. The references associated with double-tick evidence are highlighted in the reference lists at the end of each chapter along with a short summary of the paper's conclusions where applicable.

The reader is referred to Chapter 1, 'Evidence-based practice in surgery' in the volume, *Core Topics in General and Emergency Surgery* of this series, for a more detailed description of this topic.

The role of imaging in breast diagnosis including screening and excision of impalpable lesions

A. Robin M. Wilson
R. Douglas Macmillan

Introduction

Breast cancer is a major health problem. Worldwide it has an increasing incidence, with over 1 million newly diagnosed cases each year, and is the commonest cancer to affect women and the commonest cause of cancer death in women. Breast cancer mortality in the UK is among the highest in the world, with approximately 28 deaths per 100 000 women per annum. This equates to around 48 000 new breast cancers diagnosed and 11 500 deaths attributable to breast cancer each year. Approximately 1 in 9 women in the UK will develop breast cancer at some time during their life.[1]

Strategies for diagnosing and managing breast cancer are based on our current understanding of breast disease epidemiology. Around 5% of breast cancer is hereditary, mainly associated with the *BRCA1* and *BRCA2* gene defects. This type of breast cancer tends to occur in younger women. The remaining 95% of breast cancer is sporadic and its incidence increases with age. Breast cancer is rare under the age of 35 years and over 80% of breast cancer occurs in women over the age of 50. The main causes of sporadic breast cancer are believed to be environmental factors. Recognised risk factors include early menarche, late menopause, nulliparity, and long-term use of the contraceptive pill and hormone replacement therapy (HRT).

As there is a poor understanding of the causes of breast cancer, primary prevention is currently not a realistic or achievable option. It is known that earlier diagnosis of breast cancer is more likely to result in a favourable outcome. Tumour size at diagnosis, grade and lymph node stage are the best predictors of outcome. Regardless of tumour type or grade, the smaller a breast cancer is at the time of diagnosis, the more likely it is that it has not spread beyond the breast. As a result the current strategy for reducing breast cancer mortality is to seek diagnosis as early as possible.

Early detection and improvements in treatment have led to a 30% reduction in breast cancer mortality in the UK in all age groups over the past 30 years.[2]

Early diagnosis is achieved by encouraging women to present as soon as possible to breast clinics when they develop breast symptoms and through regular breast cancer screening. Breast imaging is fundamental to both.

Imaging in symptomatic breast practice

Based on mortality statistics from the 1980s and 1990s, although the UK did not have the highest incidence of breast cancer it did have the highest death rate.

✓✓ Recognising that breast cancer diagnosis and treatment required significant improvement, in 1995 the UK Department of Health published guidelines for improving outcomes in breast cancer. These guidelines were updated in 2002 and 2010 by the National Institute for Clinical Excellence (NICE).[3] The guidelines emphasise the following three key issues in breast cancer care:

- accurate and timely diagnosis;
- appropriate treatment decided by accurate staging of disease;
- appropriate follow-up of patients undergoing treatment.

Imaging is required at all three stages of this process, and mammography and ultrasound have a pivotal role to play. About 60% of breast cancer is diagnosed in symptomatic breast referral clinics. These clinics follow protocols that define the triple test, the combination of clinical assessment, imaging (mammography and ultrasound) and core biopsy or needle cytology, as the required standard.[4] 'One-stop' clinics are recommended at which all the necessary tests required to make a diagnosis, including needle biopsy, are performed at one clinic visit. In order to achieve the earliest possible diagnosis of symptomatic breast cancer, women are encouraged through a variety of health promotion methods to present to these clinics as soon as they develop any change in their breasts. The clinical and imaging assessments in these clinics should be performed by appropriately trained and experienced staff. All such staff do not need to be doctors but they need to be able to give an independent opinion and be trained to an appropriate level.

Breast imaging techniques

Mammography

X-ray mammography has been the basis of breast imaging for more than 30 years. The sensitivity of mammography for breast cancer is age dependent. The denser the breast, the less effective this method is for detecting early signs of breast cancer. Breast density tends to be higher in younger women and increased density obscures early signs of breast cancer. The sensitivity of mammography for breast cancer in women over 60 years of age approaches 95%, while mammography can be expected to detect less than 50% of breast cancers in women under 40 years of age.[5]

Mammography uses ionising radiation to obtain an image and therefore should only be used where there is likely to be a clinical benefit. Consensus is that the benefits of mammography in women over the age of 40 years are likely to far outweigh any oncogenic effects of repeated exposure. Screening of women over the age of 40 by mammography is accepted practice. However, in symptomatic practice, there is rarely an indication for performing mammography in women under the age of 35 unless there is a strong clinical suspicion of malignancy. In many centres, all women over the age of 35 presenting to breast clinics undergo mammography as a routine. Practice is changing and ultrasound alone is being used increasingly for the assessment of women with focal breast symptoms in women under 40 years of age and even in some women aged 40–50. Mammography is routine in all women in the screening age group attending symptomatic clinics who have not had a screening mammogram in the past year.

Most mammography in the UK is now carried out using digital image acquisition.[6–9] There are major benefits from acquiring mammograms in direct digital format.[9] Compared with conventional film/screen mammography, the benefits of full-field digital mammography include better imaging of the dense breast, the application of computer-aided detection and a number of logistical advantages providing potential for more efficient mammography services.[10,11] The much wider dynamic range of digital mammography means that visualisation of the entire breast density range on a single image is easily achievable. In the clinical setting, comparative studies have shown that digital mammography performs in general as well as film/screen mammography but is better in younger women and in women with dense breasts.[6,7]

Mammography is the basis of stereotactic breast biopsy, which can be carried out using a dedicated prone biopsy table or by using an add-on device to a conventional upright mammography unit. Stereotaxis is used to biopsy impalpable lesions that are not clearly visible on ultrasound (e.g. microcalcifications).

Ultrasound

High-frequency (≥10 MHz) ultrasound is a very effective diagnostic tool for the investigation of focal breast symptoms.[12] Ultrasound does not involve ionising radiation and is a very safe imaging technique. It has a high sensitivity for breast pathology and also a very high negative predictive value.[13]

> ✅ High-resolution ultrasound easily distinguishes between most solid and cystic lesions and can differentiate benign from malignant lesions with a high degree of accuracy. However, in most circumstances, solid lesions seen on ultrasound require needle sampling for accurate diagnosis.

Ultrasound is the technique of choice for the further investigation of focal symptomatic breast problems at all ages. Under 40 years of age, when the risk of breast cancer is very low, it is usually the only imaging technique required. Over 40, when the risk of breast cancer begins to increase, it is often used in conjunction with mammography. Ultrasound is less sensitive than mammography for the early signs of breast cancer and is therefore not used for population screening. However, ultrasound does increase the detection of small breast cancers in women who have a dense background pattern on mammography.[5] In the screening setting there is clear evidence that the addition of ultrasound improves small cancer detection rates, particularly in women with dense breasts, but there is currently insufficient evidence of any mortality benefit and insufficient resources to allow for routine ultrasound screening of women with dense breasts on mammography. Adding ultrasound to mammography or magnetic resonance imaging (MRI) screening does increase cancer detection but also significantly increases the false-positive rate. Ultrasound is the technique of first choice for biopsy of both palpable and impalpable breast lesions visible on scanning.

Ultrasound is now used routinely to assess the axilla in women with breast cancer in most units. Axillary nodes that show abnormal morphology can be sampled accurately by fine-needle aspiration (FNA) or needle core biopsy.[16,17] Discussion of the role of axillary ultrasound and FNA and core biopsy can be found in Chapter 7.

> ✅✅ Up to 50% of patients with axillary metastatic disease can be diagnosed by ultrasound combined with FNA or core biopsy, which may avoid the need for sentinel node biopsy in some women with pathologically proven nodal involvement.[14,15]

Doppler ultrasound adds little to breast diagnosis and is not widely used. Three-dimensional ultrasound of the breast is said to increase the accuracy of biopsy and the detection of multifocal disease but is not widely available. Elastography is a new application of ultrasound technology that allows the accurate assessment of the stiffness of breast tissue. It is being evaluated at present and may prove to be a useful tool in excluding significant abnormalities, for instance in assessment of asymptomatic abnormalities detected by ultrasound screening.

Magnetic resonance mammography (MRM)

MRM is now widely available. In order to image the breast the patient is scanned prone and injection of intravenous contrast is required. MRM is the most sensitive technique for detection of breast cancer, approaching 100% for invasive cancer and up to 92% for ductal carcinoma in situ (DCIS), but it has a high false-positive rate.[18,19,20] Rapid acquisition of images facilitates assessment of signal enhancement curves that can be helpful in distinguishing benign from malignant disease. Significant overlap in the enhancement patterns is seen, so needle sampling of the lesions detected is often required. Magnetic resonance-guided breast biopsy is available in a few centres but most breast lesions seen on MRM that are larger than 5 mm can be seen on ultrasound if they are clinically significant.

> ✅ MRM is the best method for screening younger women (under 40 years) at increased risk of breast cancer but, because of cost, it is unlikely to be used for general population screening.[21–24]

MRM is the best technique for imaging women with breast implants. It is also of benefit in identifying recurrent disease where conventional imaging and biopsy have failed to exclude recurrence. Provided it is carried out more than 18 months after surgery, MRI will accurately distinguish between scarring and tumour recurrence. MRI is recommended to detect multifocality prior to conservation surgery for women with lobular cancers and those with occult cancer on mammography or with a significant discrepancy of size on conventional imaging. However, it should not be used routinely and a randomised trial (COMICE) showed no benefit in reducing re-excision rates but did increase significantly the mastectomy rates for those who had MRI. Breast MRI is of value in assessing response of large or locally advanced breast cancers to neoadjuvant chemotherapy. MRI of the axilla can demonstrate axillary metastatic disease but its sensitivity is not sufficient to replace surgical staging of the axilla. For advanced breast cancer, MRI is the technique of choice for assessing spinal metastatic disease.

Computed tomography

Computed tomography (CT) has no current proven role in primary imaging of the breast. but dedicated low-dose breast CT is being introduced; its clinical efficacy has yet to be determined. CT is used to diagnose and stage systemic spread of breast cancer and to assess response of metastatic disease to treatment, particularly lung, pleural and liver metastases. Some patients with breast cancer do have their cancers diagnosed incidentally during a routine CT scan.

Isotope imaging

Breast scintigraphy is not widely used because of its lack of sensitivity compared with other techniques. It is used in a few centres to stage the breast prior to surgery and to assess response to treatment. Scintigraphy is widely used to diagnose and assess the presence of skeletal metastatic disease. It is now often combined with a low-resolution non-contrast CT scan.

Positron emission scintigraphy, particularly when combined with CT, is a technology that may have a role in future in staging breast cancer and monitoring response to treatment. It is widely used in the USA but elsewhere, at present, it continues to be regarded as a research tool and its specific uses and indications in assessing breast disease are still being defined.

Breast cancer screening

Aim

The aim of breast screening is to reduce mortality through early detection. Randomised controlled trials and case–control studies carried out between the 1960s and 1980s have demonstrated that population screening by mammography can be expected to

reduce overall breast cancer mortality by around 25% and by 35–40% in those who participate.

✔✔ The validity of these trials was questioned in 2000–2002 but subsequent reviews by the Swedish combined trials group and a World Health Organisation International Agency for Research on Cancer committee of experts have reaffirmed the mortality benefit of mammographic screening and determined that criticisms of the mammographic screening trials were unjustified.[25–30]

The mortality benefit of screening is greatest in women aged 55–70 years.[27,28] The mortality benefit of screening women aged between 40 and 55 is approximately 20%. Screening women under the age of 40 has not been shown to provide any mortality benefit.[27,28]

Population screening

Breast screening has been introduced in many countries over the past 25 years. In most countries, screening is recommended in all women aged 40 and over but in countries that provide population-based screening, women of 50 and over are specifically targeted. Breast cancer screening was introduced in the UK in 1987 and provides screening by invitation, free at the point of delivery, to all women between the ages of 50 and 70.[1] Women over 70 can attend but are not invited. Over 70% of the invited population need to attend for a significant overall mortality benefit to be achieved. Women under the age of 50 are not offered screening in the UK unless they are at increased risk. A randomised trial of extending the screening invitation to the age range 47–73 years was started in 2010. The results of this trial will not be available until after 2020. From 2010 screening with annual MRI in addition to mammography has been offered to women at very high risk of breast cancer, including *BRCA1* and *BRCA2* gene carrriers.

Method and frequency

✔✔ The optimum screening method is two-view mammography; clinical examination of the breast and breast self-examination have not been shown to contribute to mortality reduction through early detection and so are not recommended.[9,31,32]

Women aged 50–70 in the UK are invited for mammography every 3 years. There has been some concern that this screening interval is too long. Mammography can be expected to detect breast cancer approximately 2 years before it becomes clinically apparent. The frequency of mammographic screening is determined by the lead-time of breast cancer. Based on the average growth time of breast cancer in different ages, this means that mammographic screening should ideally be carried out yearly in women aged 40–50, every 2 years in women aged 50–60 and every 3 years thereafter. However, the UK breast screening frequency trial completed in 1995 did not show any predicted benefit for women aged 50–64 screened every year compared with those screened every 3 years.[33] Screening once every 3 years can be expected to detect approximately two-thirds of all breast cancers that will arise during the 3-year screening interval.

One-third of breast cancers present in the interval between screens and are called interval cancers. Half of these present in the third year after screening.

Factors affecting the effectiveness of screening

HRT increases breast density and in a proportion of women this reduces the sensitivity of mammography for breast cancer.[9,32–40] Up to 25% of women taking combined oestrogen/progestogen preparations continuously show increased density on mammography. This effect is significantly less with other HRT preparations. As well as reducing sensitivity HRT also reduces the specificity of mammographic screening. HRT also increases the risk of developing breast cancer.[34]

Quality assurance

Breast screening programmes should have inbuilt quality assurance; the UK NHS Breast Screening Programme is subject to comprehensive quality assessment and all 100 screening units across the country have to comply with nationally defined standard guidelines. There are national targets for screening set by a central Department of Health Advisory Committee (Table 1.1).

The screening process

Women invited for screening attend either a static or mobile screening unit where two-view mammography is performed. The images are then double read within a few days. The vast majority of women (95%) are informed by letter within 2 weeks of attendance that their mammograms show no evidence of breast cancer. Those women in the appropriate age range will be invited for screening 3 years later. They are advised to contact their general practitioner as soon as possible if they become aware of any change in their breasts in the meantime.

The screening process includes a fully integrated multidisciplinary assessment process for all screen-detected mammographic abnormalities; screening programmes should ideally retain responsibility through to definitive diagnosis. Approximately 5% of women screened are recalled for further assessment of a problem identified at screening. Some women are recalled for further assessment of a clinical sign or symptom identified at the time of screening but the vast majority of women are recalled because of a mammographic abnormality.

> ✔ The most important cancers detected at screening are high-grade DCIS, as most cases of this type will progress to grade 2 or 3 invasive breast cancer within the following 3 years, and grade 2 and 3 invasive breast cancers under 10 mm in diameter, as at this size these tumours are much less likely to have metastasised.[41,42]

The common types of mammographic abnormality and their positive predictive value for cancer are shown in Table 1.2. Well-defined masses are almost always benign and do not require recall, whereas ill-defined masses and spiculated lesions always require further assessment (**Figs 1.1** and **1.2**). Clustered microcalcifications account for a high proportion of recalls that result in needle biopsy. More than 20% of screen-detected breast cancer is DCIS, mostly high or intermediate grade, and most of this type of cancer is detected by the presence of clustered microcalcifications (**Fig. 1.3**). Invasive cancer is usually represented on mammography by either an ill-defined or spiculated mass. It is essential to detect these lesions at small size as they more commonly represent grade 2 or 3 invasive cancer.

Three-quarters of women recalled undergo further imaging (mammography and/or ultrasound) and clinical assessment before being reassured and

Table 1.1 • NHS Breast Screening Programme: screening targets, June 2005

Objective	Criteria	Minimum standard	Target
To maximise the number of eligible women who attend for screening	Percentage of eligible women who attend for screening	• ≥70% of invited women to attend for screening	• 80%
To maximise the number of cancers detected	(a) Rate of invasive cancers detected in eligible women	• Prevalent screen ≥2.7 per 1000 • Incident screen ≥3.1 per 1000	• Prevalent screen >3.6 per 1000 • Incident screen ≥4.2 per 1000
	(b) Rate of cancers detected that are in situ carcinoma	• Prevalent screen ≥0.4 per 1000 • Incident screen ≥0.5 per 1000	
	(c) Standardised detection ratio	• ≥0.85	• ≥1.0
To maximise the number of small invasive cancers	Rate of invasive cancers less than 15 mm in diameter detected in eligible women invited and screened	• Prevalent screen ≥1.7 per 1000	• Prevalent screen ≥2.3 per 1000
		• Incident screen ≥1.7 per 1000	• Incident screen ≥2.5 per 1000
To achieve optimum image quality	(a) High-contrast spatial resolution	• ≥12 lp/mm	
	(b) Minimal detectable contrast:		
	5–6 mm detail	• ≤1.2%	• ≤0.8%
	0.5 mm detail	• ≤5%	• ≤3%
	0.25 mm detail	• ≤8%	• ≤5%
	(c) Aim film density	• 1.5–1.9	
To limit radiation dose	Mean glandular dose per film for a standard breast at clinical settings	• ≤2.5 mGy	
To minimise the number of women undergoing repeat examinations	Number of repeat examinations	• ≤3% of total examinations	• <2% of total examinations
To minimise the number of women screened who are referred for further tests*	(a) Percentage of women who are referred for assessment	• Prevalent screen <10% • Incident screen <7%	• Prevalent screen <7% • Incident screen <5%
	(b) Percentage of women screened who are placed on early recall	• <0.5%	• ≤0.25%
To ensure that the majority of cancers, both palpable and impalpable, receive a non-operative tissue diagnosis of cancer	Percentage of women who have a non-operative diagnosis of cancer by cytology or needle histology after a maximum of two visits	• ≥80%	• >90%
To minimise the number of unnecessary operative procedures	Rate of benign biopsies	• Prevalent screen <3.6 per 1000	• Prevalent screen <1.8 per 1000

Table 1.1 • (cont.) NHS Breast Screening Programme: screening targets, June 2005

Objective	Criteria	Minimum standard	Target
To minimise the number of cancers in the women screened presenting between screening episodes	Rate of cancers presenting in screened women:	• Incident screen <2.0 per 1000 *Expected standard*	• Incident screen <1.0 per 1000
	(a) In the 2 years following a normal screening episode	• 1.2 per 1000 women screened in the first 2 years	
	(b) In the third year following a normal screening episode	• 1.4 per 1000 women screened in the third year	
To ensure that women are recalled for screening at appropriate intervals	Percentage of eligible women whose first offered appointment is within 36 months of their previous screen	• >90%	• 100%
To minimise anxiety for women awaiting the results of screening	Percentage of women who are sent their result within 2 weeks	• >90%	• 100%
To minimise the interval from the screening mammogram to assessment	Percentage of women who attend an assessment centre within 3 weeks of attendance for the screening mammogram	• >90%	• 100%
To minimise diagnostic delay for women who are diagnosed non-operatively	Proportion of women for whom the time interval between non-operative biopsy and result is 1 week or less	• ≥90%	• 100%
To minimise the delay for women who require surgical assessment	Proportion of women for whom the time interval between the decision to refer to a surgeon and surgical assessment is 1 week or less	• ≥90%	• 100%
To minimise any delay for women who require treatment for screen-detected breast cancer	Percentage of women who are admitted for treatment within 2 months of their first assessment visit	• >90%	• 100%

Table 1.2 • Positive predictive value (PPV) for malignancy of mammographic signs

Sign	PPV (%)
Well-defined mass	<1
Ill-defined mass	35–50
Spiculated mass	50–90
Architectural distortion	20–40
Asymmetric density	<2
Clustered microcalcifications	15

discharged. The remaining 25% proceed to needle biopsy and this results in a diagnosis of around six cancers per 1000 women screened. Interval follow-up of uncertain mammographic findings is discouraged; the emphasis is on obtaining a definitive diagnosis by the use of image-guided breast biopsy. Over 90% of breast cancers should be diagnosed prior to first surgery. Despite advances in breast needle biopsy techniques, a small proportion of women still require open surgical biopsy for diagnosis (up to 0.25% of women screened).

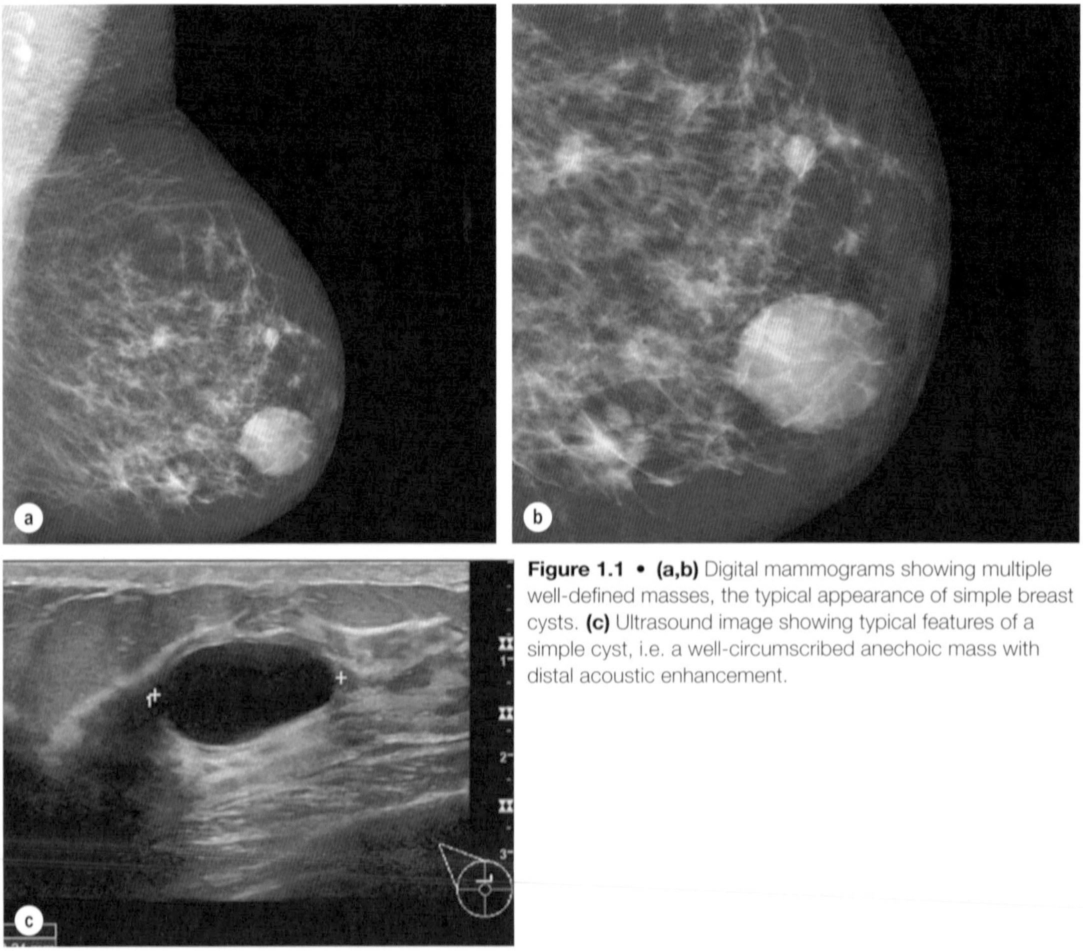

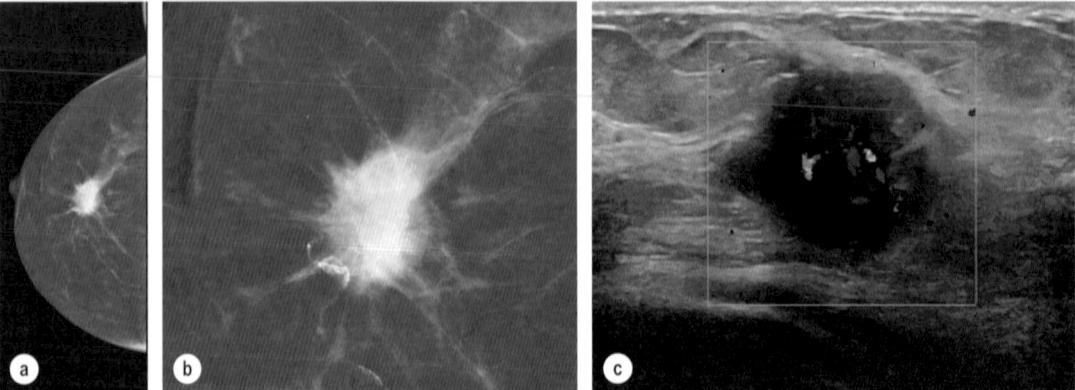

Figure 1.1 • (a,b) Digital mammograms showing multiple well-defined masses, the typical appearance of simple breast cysts. **(c)** Ultrasound image showing typical features of a simple cyst, i.e. a well-circumscribed anechoic mass with distal acoustic enhancement.

Figure 1.2 • (a,b) Digital mammograms showing a spiculated mass in the right breast. The appearances are typical of an invasive carcinoma. The mass contains microcalcifications and there is evidence of skin tether. **(c)** Doppler ultrasound image showing the typical features of an invasive carcinoma with an irregular mass containing abnormal central vessels.

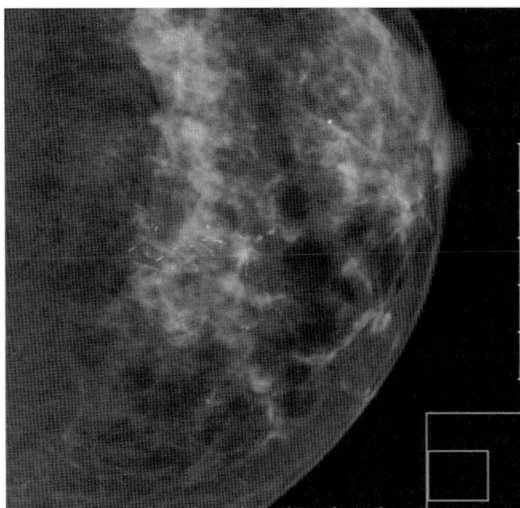

Figure 1.3 • Digital mammograms showing a cluster of casting microcalcifications in the left breast. The appearances are typical of high-grade ductal carcinoma in situ.

The performance of the NHS Breast Screening Programme in 2010 is shown in Table 1.3. The screening programme was predicted to produce a 25% reduction in mortality (1750 cancers per year) directly attributable to early detection through screening by the year 2010.

Adverse effects

Receiving an invitation for screening and attending for mammography are not associated with any significant anxiety. However, recall for further assessment does cause measurable anxiety, although this has largely subsided by 3 months.

The numbers of women who undergo open surgical biopsy for what proves to be benign disease should be kept to a minimum. Considerable training and investment in equipment has resulted in a fourfold decline in benign surgical biopsies generated through the screening programme, although rates of benign biopsy vary from unit to unit. False-positive recall and benign surgical biopsy are both more likely in younger women.

Overdiagnosis refers to the detection by screening of breast cancers that require treatment but that would never have threatened the life of the woman. This is inevitable in screening and there continues to be considerable debate about what proportion of screen-detected breast cancers fall into this category. It is likely that most low-grade DCIS and some special low-grade invasive cancers represent overdiagnosis, and detection of these cancers results in unnecessary treatment and unnecessary morbidity associated with knowledge of the diagnosis of cancer. The consensus view is that overdiagnosis applies to no more than 10% of screen-detected breast cancer and that at this level this does not negate the overall mortality benefit of breast screening. Women attending for screening must be informed fully about both the likely positive and negative effects of screening. Efforts continue to reduce the morbidity of screening and to understand better the natural history of cancers so that potential over-treatment is minimised. Even the most ardent critics of breast

Table 1.3 • NHS Breast Screening Programme: results 2010

	2008/2009	2009/2010
Total number of women invited (50–70)	2 642 511	2 662 298
Acceptance rate	73.8%	73.5%
Number of women screened (invited)	1947.424	1 954 815
Number of women screened (self-referral)	44,070	43 410
Total number of women screened	1 991 494	1 998 225
Number of women recalled for assessment	87,400	82 650
Percentage of women recalled for assessment	4.4%	4.1%
Number of benign surgical biopsies	1644	1519
Number of cancers detected	15 673	15 517
Number of in situ cancers detected	3253	3064
Number of cancers less than 15 mm	6460	6544
Standardised detection ratio (invited only)	1.45	1.44

From NHS Breast Screening Programme Annual Review 2011. Available at http://www.cancerscreening.nhs.uk.

screening believe screening should continue but they argue it needs to be refined. This is accepted by those who organise and run screening programmes.

Screening women at increased risk

Women at increased risk of developing breast cancer due to a proven inherited predisposing genetic mutation, family history (with no proven genetic mutation), previous radiotherapy (e.g. mantle radiotherapy for Hodgkin's lymphoma) or benign risk lesions (atypical hyperplasia, lobular intraepithelial neoplasia) may be selected for screening at young age. Whether it is possible to identify other substantially increased risk groups by summating various other epidemiological factors (e.g. age at menarche, body mass index, age at first pregnancy, alcohol intake) continues to be debated. The cut-off point at which clinical management of a woman is altered is often referred to as moderate risk. Those individuals likely or proven to be carriers of a predisposing genetic mutation are termed high risk.

✔ NICE guidelines have been produced (latest version 2006) to classify risk groups and guide care.[43] They state that women at or near population risk should be managed in primary care (defined as <3% risk for women aged 40–49). Women at moderate risk are those with a 10-year risk of 3–8% between 40 and 49 years or a lifetime risk >17%, and those at high risk are defined as those with a 10-year risk of >8% between 40 and 49 years or a lifetime risk >30%.

Such cut-offs are useful as guidelines for specialist referral, but most risk factors require clinical interpretation before risk management is discussed with the individual.

Unfortunately, the problem with screening young women at increased risk of breast cancer is that no screening test has as yet been shown to reduce mortality in such women. Screening in this group is therefore a management option for which an exact benefit cannot be quoted for an individual woman. Screening should not be offered to those who fall below the moderate-risk cut-off.

Methods of screening young women at increased risk: mammography

A national evaluation study of mammographic screening for young women with a family history of breast cancer has been conducted (FH01 study). The study compared screening in women aged 40–44 who were at moderate or high risk with the control arm of the age trial (population-based trial of screening women in their forties in which the control arm was not screened); this showed a non-significant mortality benefit for screening. It demonstrated that screening was likely to reduce deaths from breast cancer. The FH02 study is currently looking at the effectiveness of screening women aged 35–39.

✔✔ Mammography has a greater positive predictive value in young women at high risk when compared with age-matched controls but lacks sensitivity. This may be a particular problem in women with BRCA1 mutations.[24,44–47]

BRCA1-related breast cancer is usually high grade and often has a 'pushing' margin. It rarely presents with associated DCIS. The mammographic features are therefore usually of a mass lesion with no associated microcalcification and no architectural distortion (Fig. 1.4a). Such cancers often present symptomatically as interval cases. BRCA2-related cancers are more similar to sporadic cases and may be more likely to be detected by mammography. Ultrasound screening significantly improves sensitivity when there is a dense mammographic background pattern but has a lower positive predictive value and has not been shown to be a useful screening modality. Ultrasound features of BRCA1 cancers are often benign or indeterminate (Fig. 1.4b). If mammographic screening is performed, it should be repeated annually in women under age 50.

Methods of screening young women at high risk: MRI

MRI is the most sensitive method of imaging young women but has significant resource implications.[44,48] The specificity of MRI has been a concern, although with second-look recall (after which many potentially abnormal findings may resolve), targeted ultrasound and the slowly increasing availability of MRI-guided biopsy, this may be less of a problem than initially thought. The MARIBS study evaluating MRI in addition to mammography and several other studies have shown that MRI is the most sensitive screening test for young high-risk women, but it is arguable whether the cancers detected are sufficient to change the outcome of these young women.[49] On the basis of its better performance compared with

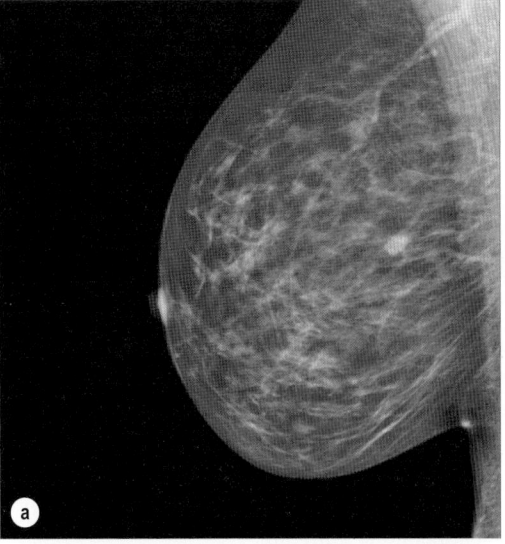
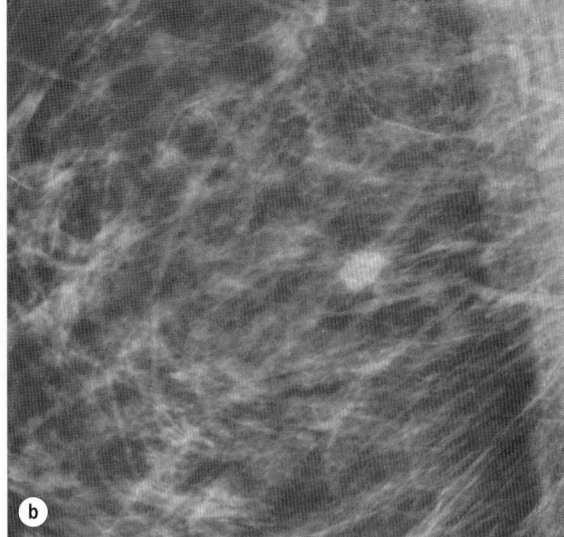
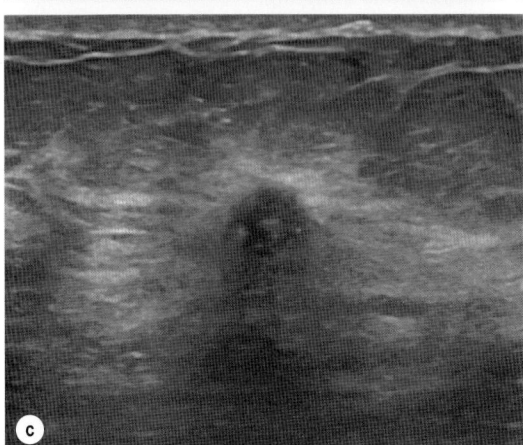

Figure 1.4 • (a,b) Digital mammograms showing a small circumscribed but ill-defined mass in the upper outer right breast. **(c)** Ultrasound image of the same mass. Core biopsy showed grade 3 invasive ductal carcinoma.

mammography in increasing sensitivity, NICE has recommended annual MRI surveillance for women aged 30–39 years with a 10-year risk of >8% and women aged 40–49 years with a 10-year risk >20%.[43] MRI is also recommended for high-risk women with a dense mammographic background pattern.

Age to start screening in young women at increased risk

The age for starting screening should be based on risk rather than the age of affected relatives. For women at moderate risk, screening should start at age 40. This can seem paradoxical if the reason moderate risk has been established is because there is one first-degree relative affected in their thirties. However, if this is the only relative affected then the individual is only at moderate risk and the emphasis of management should be on reassurance rather than screening. For women at high risk, screening may be started at age 30. Such high-risk women should ideally be managed in a specialist setting where experience with MRI screening is available. In the UK such women may be best managed within the NHS Breast Screening Programme. Women must be advised about the limitations of screening at young age. This is particularly relevant to known mutation carriers for whom there is no evidence that screening improves survival (cf. risk-reducing surgery).

Image-guided breast biopsy

Needle biopsy is highly accurate in determining the nature of most breast lesions.[50–53] Patients with benign conditions avoid unnecessary surgery; carrying out open surgical biopsy for diagnosis should be regarded as a failure of the diagnostic process. For patients who are proven to have breast cancer, needle biopsy provides accurate understanding of the type and extent of disease so ensuring that patients, and the doctors treating them, are able to make informed treatment choices. Needle biopsy not only provides accurate information on the nature of malignant disease, such as histological type and grade, but also facilitates pretreatment assessment of tumour biology.

Which biopsy technique?

The current methods available for breast tissue diagnosis are FNA cytology, needle core biopsy, vacuum-assisted biopsy (VAB) and open surgical biopsy.

FNA versus needle core biopsy

There has been much debate about the comparative benefits of FNA and core biopsy,[50-53] but 14 G 22-mm automated core biopsy provides significantly greater sensitivity, specificity and positive predictive value than FNA. Results with core biopsy are particularly superior to FNA in stereotactic biopsy of microcalcifications and architectural distortions.

The overall better performance achievable with core biopsy compared with FNA is illustrated in the performance of the NHS Breast Screening Programme in the UK. In 1994, using FNA as the primary diagnostic technique, fewer than 10% of 90 units were able to achieve the target of 70% preoperative diagnosis rate for cancer. By 2003, most units had converted to automated core biopsy and all units achieved the minimum standard and the majority exceeded the expected standard of 90% preoperative diagnosis rate.[1]

Vacuum-assisted biopsy (VAB)

The predominant reasons for not achieving an accurate diagnosis by needle biopsy are sampling error (missing the target) and failure to retrieve sufficient representative material. These problems have been largely addressed by the development of larger directional core techniques that yield significantly greater volumes of tissue.[54-56]

VAB is a very successful method for improving the diagnostic accuracy of borderline breast lesions and lesions at sites in the breast difficult to biopsy using other techniques. VAB has been shown to understage both in situ and invasive cancer approximately half as often as conventional core biopsy (typically 10% vs. 20%).[57,58] The VAB technique has a higher sensitivity because it allows sampling of lesions at sites that are difficult to biopsy using either FNA or core biopsy and because the amount of tissue harvested is at least five times greater per core specimen.

The indications for VAB include:

- very small mass lesions;
- architectural distortions;
- failed 'conventional' core biopsy;
- small clusters of microcalcifications;
- papillary and mucocele-like lesions;
- diffuse non-specific abnormality;
- excision of benign lesions;
- sentinel node sampling.

Core biopsy and VAB are now the recommended techniques for sampling calcifications and mammographic architectural distortions.[59,60] For calcifications it is imperative that there is proof of representative sampling with specimen radiography. If calcification is not demonstrated on the specimen radiograph and the histology is benign, then management cannot be based on this result as there is a high risk of sampling error; the procedure must either be repeated or open surgical biopsy carried out.

Guidance techniques for breast needle biopsy

✔✔ Ultrasound guidance is the technique of choice for biopsy of both palpable and impalpable breast lesions; it is less costly, easy to perform and more accurate than freehand or other image-guided techniques.[50]

Ultrasound provides real-time visualisation of the biopsy procedure and visual confirmation of adequate sampling. Between 80% and 90% of breast abnormalities will be clearly visible on ultrasound and amenable to biopsy using this technique. For impalpable abnormalities not visible on ultrasound, stereotactic X-ray-guided biopsy is required. A few lesions are only visible on MRI and require magnetic resonance-guided biopsy.[61] A number of different approaches have been developed for this procedure using both closed and open magnets. VAB is the biopsy technique recommended for magnetic resonance-guided sampling.

The negative predictive value of combined normal mammography and ultrasound is extremely high; where there is a clinically palpable abnormality and mammography and ultrasound are entirely normal, the likelihood of malignancy is low (<1%). However, in these circumstances it remains prudent in the presence of a localised clinical abnormality to carry out freehand needle biopsy to exclude the occasional diffuse malignant process, such as classical invasive lobular carcinoma or low-grade DCIS, that may be occult on both mammography and ultrasound.

For stereotactic procedures it is prudent to mark the biopsy site for future reference. Gel pellets or cellulose combined with a metallic marker are preferred and can be placed during the procedure to mark the biopsy site. These markers have the advantage of being visible on ultrasound so that repeat biopsy or localisation for surgery can be subsequently performed under ultrasound rather than X-ray guidance. These markers dissolve and are reabsorbed in a few weeks, leaving a small metal marker in case delayed X-ray identification of the biopsy site is required.

Number of samples

A simple rule for satisfactory sampling using needle techniques is to obtain sufficient material to achieve a diagnosis.[59,60,62] For ultrasound-guided core biopsy, a diagnosis may be possible on a single core. Showing on ultrasound that the needle has passed through the centre of the abnormality and by examining the sample with the naked eye, it is usually, but not always, possible to confirm whether a satisfactory sample has been obtained. Because of this and the knowledge that some lesions are heterogeneous, more extensive sampling of a lesion increases sensitivity. The number of core specimens obtained should reflect the nature of the abnormality being sampled. For ultrasound-guided biopsy where there is a suspicion of carcinoma, it is recommended that multiple core specimens are obtained.

As stereotactic biopsy is used for abnormalities that are difficult to define on ultrasound and are therefore more difficult to sample, a minimum of five core specimens should be obtained. Ensuring that calcification is present in at least three separate cores and/or five separate flecks of calcification are

retrieved from the area of suspicion is essential to ensure an accurate diagnosis. For calcifications many prefer VAB, although some units perform 14-gauge core biopsy as their initial biopsy technique.

When there is diagnostic uncertainty after core, VAB can be used to obtain larger tissue volumes (a 7-gauge VAB probe will retrieve approximately 300 mg per core). Ten- to seven-gauge mammotomy probes can be used and are preferred for therapeutic removal of breast lesions such as fibroadenomas.

Biopsy results

It is important that the results of FNA and/or core needle breast biopsy are always correlated with the clinical and imaging findings before clinical management is discussed with the patient. This is best achieved by reviewing each case prior to any surgical or other therapeutic procedure at multidisciplinary meetings.[50]

Surgery for clinically occult breast lesions

Wire-guided excision

The number of impalpable, clinically occult breast lesions detected by screening is increasing. Accurate localisation techniques are required to facilitate their surgical excision. The hooked wire is the most commonly employed technique and has proved very reliable but does have inherent associated problems. There are various designs of localisation wire in common use. All have some form of anchoring device such as a hook with a splayed or barbed tip. The wire is deployed under stereotactic or ultrasound guidance within a rigid over-sheath cannula, which is then removed once positioning is satisfactory (**Fig. 1.5**). The patient is then transferred to the operating theatre with the wire in situ. Most wires are very flexible and when the cannula is removed the wire may assume a quite circuitous course, especially after stereotactic insertion when the breast is released from compression. In a very fatty breast in which there is no solid lesion or the wire has not transfixed the lesion, care must be taken to avoid displacing the wire. A cosmetically considered incision is placed near to the tip of the wire and an excision performed. Accurate wire placement is essential and ideally the shortest possible length of

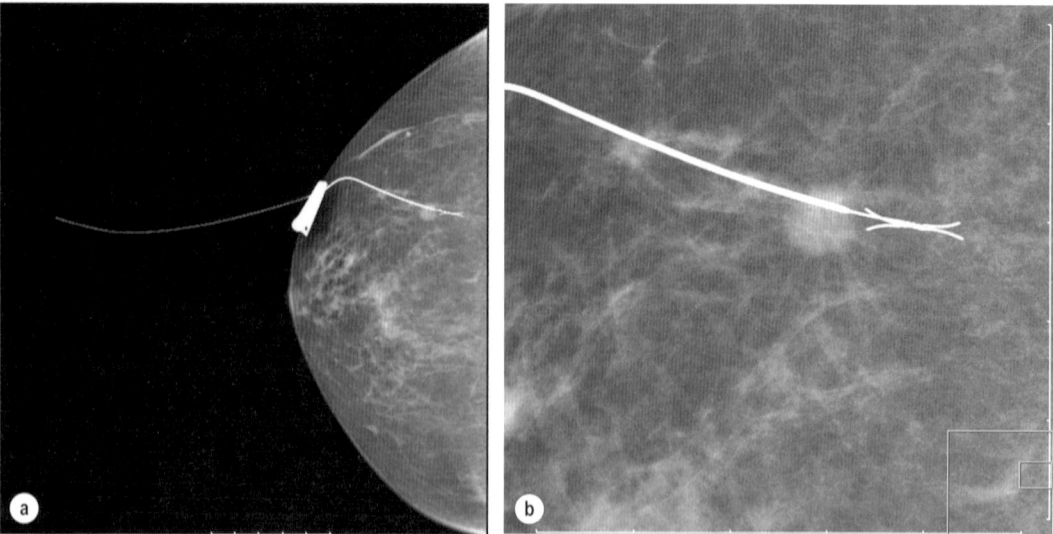

Figure 1.5 • Digital mammogram showing a Reidy localisation wire placed under ultrasound guidance transfixing and marking an impalpable mass to facilitate surgical wide local excision (as shown in Fig. 1.4).

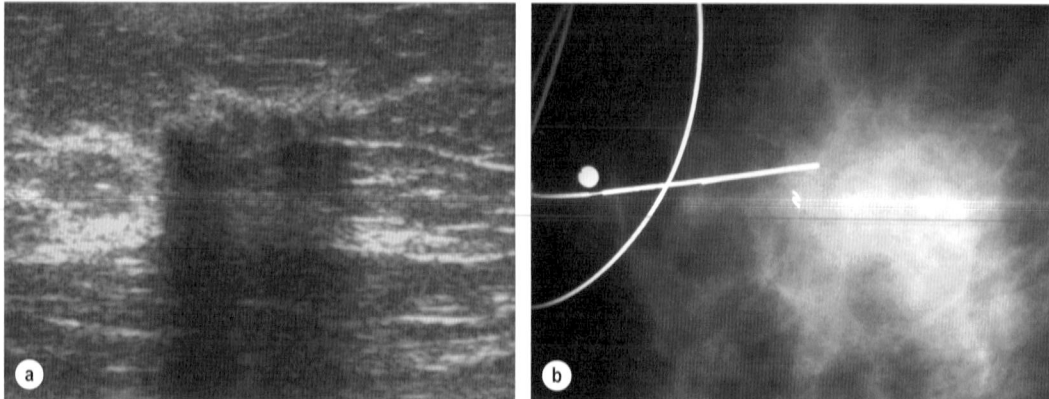

Figure 1.6 • **(a)** Ultrasound showing a cluster of gel pellets placed at the site of a previous stereotactic biopsy. The clear visibility of the pellets facilitates ultrasound localisation for surgery of abnormalities that would normally require X-ray localisation. **(b)** Mammogram after ultrasound localisation in the same case showing accurate placement of the marker wire.

wire should be within the breast. In recent practice this has been greatly facilitated by the use of radio-opaque and ultrasound visible markers placed at the time of initial stereotactic biopsy such that wire localisation can be performed under ultrasound guidance (**Fig. 1.6**). In addition, for superficial lesions a skin marker may be more appropriate.

Although lesions may be clinically occult prior to surgery, most mass lesions will be palpable intra-operatively. Procedures that can be surgically more challenging are wide local excisions for DCIS with no mass lesion. In such cases, where the distribution of disease is often more eccentric, careful excision

planning is necessary. Inserting more than one wire and bracketing the lesion with three or four wires can be useful.

If the procedure is being performed to establish a diagnosis, a representative portion of the lesion is excised through a small incision, so leaving a satisfactory cosmetic result if the lesion proves to be benign (the European surgical quality assurance guidelines require such diagnostic surgical excision specimens to weigh less than 30 g). For diagnostic excisions of very small lesions, a therapeutic wide excision may (after discussion with the patient) be considered appropriate, as the resulting cosmetic effect of removing an extra rim of normal surrounding tissue may be insignificant. Protocols vary for therapeutic excisions, but in general the lesion should be excised with a 10-mm macroscopic margin of normal tissue. Intraoperative specimen radiography is essential, both to check that the lesion has been removed and, if cancer has been diagnosed, to ensure that adequate wide local excision has been achieved.

Some surgeons experienced in this imaging technique have also used intraoperative ultrasound. Not only can excision be guided but the margins of a wide local excision specimen can also be assessed intraoperatively using ultrasound.

Radioisotope occult lesion localisation

Radioisotope occult lesion localisation (ROLL) has been advocated as an alternative to the hooked-wire technique.[63] ROLL was first described by the Milan group using ^{99m}Tc-labelled human macroaggregate albumin, using scintigraphy and a hand-held gamma probe to guide surgical excision. The Nottingham method has modified the Milan technique and uses radio-opaque contrast injected with the radiolabel and immediate check mammography (**Fig. 1.7**). Subsequently some centres have combined ROLL with sentinel node biopsy. ROLL uses essentially the same equipment as sentinel node biopsy. It has been described using macroaggregate (which does not migrate from the injection site) or low-molecular-weight colloid (which does migrate and is normally used for sentinel node biopsy). In both situations it is radiolabelled with ^{99m}Tc and injected directly into the lesion. The threshold of the signal processor on the gamma detector is then adjusted so that an audible signal is heard only when the probe is directly over the lesion. The probe then directs excision intraoperatively.

In a randomised trial of ROLL versus wire localisation, 2% of ROLL patients had a failed

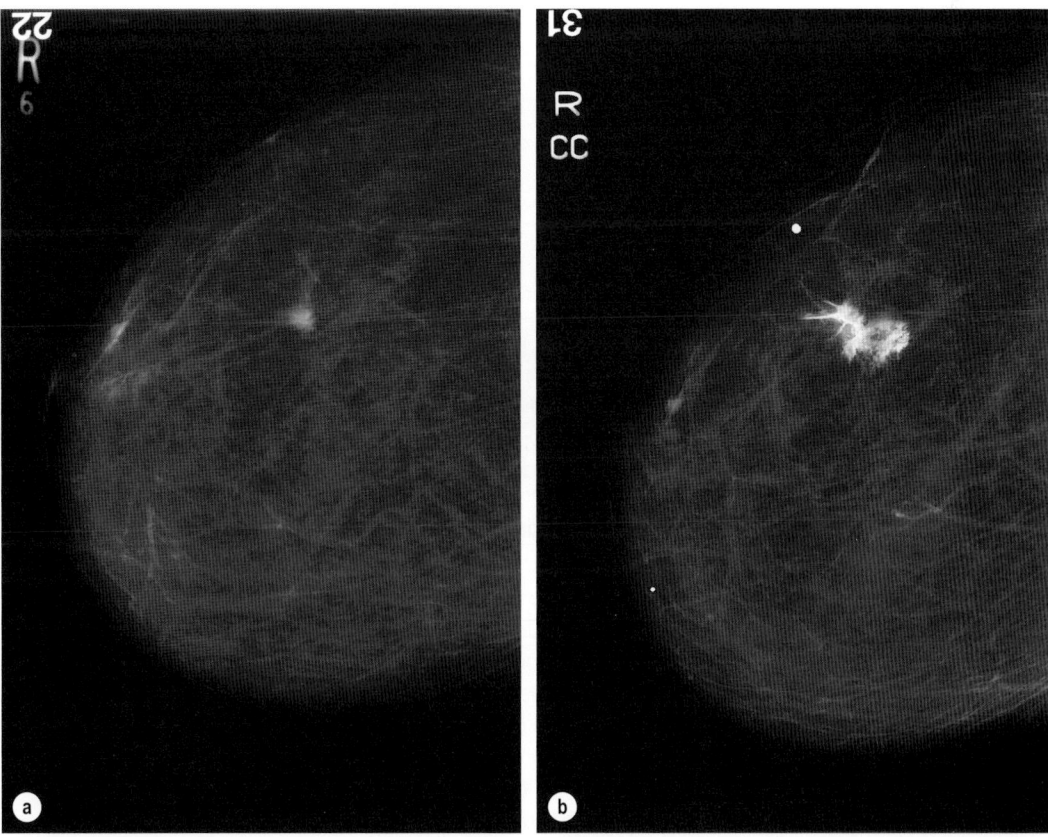

Figure 1.7 • (a) Mammogram of the right breast showing a small impalpable cancer. **(b)** Mammogram after injection of radionuclide mixed with X-ray contrast confirming satisfactory localisation (ROLL).

technique due to intraductal injection of radiolabelled colloid and dye that gave a ductogram appearance on check mammography in both cases.[64,65] As the radio-opaque dye is absorbed rapidly, both cases were successfully converted to wire localisation. The main differences between ROLL and wire guidance were that both surgeons and radiologists found ROLL easier to perform overall and patients found ROLL less painful. There has been no significant difference in accuracy of marking, operating time, mean specimen weight, intraoperative re-excision or second therapeutic operation in the majority of reports, although a recent European trial reported greater volumes of tissue were excised using ROLL than standard wire localisation. Some studies have suggested that obtaining clear margins may be significantly easier with ROLL. In reality there is little to choose between ROLL and wire localisation. ROLL may be a more suitable technique in the localisation of non-mass lesions (e.g. DCIS), although even for these lesions when multiple wires are placed any advantage is small.

There are various methods described for combining ROLL with sentinel node biopsy.[66–68] Low-molecular-weight colloid can be injected at a different site, at the same site with a different radiolabel, or into the tumour. With intratumoral injection of ^{99m}Tc nanocolloid, only one injection is required and high success rates have been reported. Combined with radio-opaque contrast, this modification of the Nottingham method has proved simple and successful.

Oncoplastic considerations for screen-detected lesions

Oncoplastic surgery aims to provide optimum effectiveness of surgical treatment for breast cancer with minimum effect on quality of life. As the 10-year survival of screen-detected disease is estimated at 87%, women do live a long time with the effects of breast cancer surgery on body image, quality of life and self-esteem. The degree to which these outcomes are affected is strongly related to the cosmetic outcome of surgery.

When assessing a woman for surgery for screen-detected cancer, there should be a strong emphasis towards the aesthetic outcome. Women should be offered the full range of oncoplastic procedures available to achieve a good outcome, including where appropriate the quality-of-life benefits from breast reduction. In addition, consideration should be given to whether such procedures which reduce re-operation rates may be desirable to achieve an excellent cosmetic outcome. The latter consideration may be particularly relevant for DCIS, for which over 30% require further surgery following an initial attempt at breast-conserving surgery that fails because of involved excision margins. For women with larger areas of DCIS, therapeutic mammoplasty may be the only option for achieving complete excision and a satisfactory cosmetic outcome. Such procedures should be available to all women.

Key points

- Breast imaging is an essential part of modern multidisciplinary breast diagnosis.
- Mammography is the technique of choice for population breast screening.
- Screening is targeted at women aged 50–70 years and can be expected to reduce mortality through early detection by approximately 25%.
- The aim should be to achieve as near as possible 100% non-operative diagnosis of breast problems.
- Both palpable and impalpable breast lesions are best sampled under image guidance.
- Automated core biopsy is the sampling technique of first choice.
- Ultrasound is the guidance technique of first choice.
- Digital stereotactic core biopsy should be reserved for sampling lesions not visible on ultrasound.
- A 14-gauge core biopsy can provide a definitive diagnosis in more than 90% of cases and should be the preferred method.
- Mammotomy can provide the diagnosis in most of the remainder.
- Stereo-guided vacuum-assisted biopsy is particularly effective for small clusters of indeterminate microcalcifications and calcifications in sites difficult to access with core biopsy.

- VAB is an effective and well-tolerated sampling technique for breast diagnosis and can also be used to completely excise benign lesions.
- All breast needle biopsy results should be discussed at prospective multidisciplinary meetings where the pathology results are correlated with the clinical and imaging findings.
- Accurate image-guided localisation and skills in wide local excision are required for the surgical treatment of impalpable breast lesions.
- The aim of surgery is to excise the cancer completely and produce an excellent cosmetic outcome.
- Oncoplastic surgery and therapeutic mammoplasty in appropriately selected women increases the rate of excellent cosmetic outcomes.

References

1. Office of National Statistics. Available from: http://www.ons.gov.uk/ons/rel/cancer-unit/cancer-incidence-and-mortality/2008-2010/stb-cancer-incidence-and-mortality-in-the-united-kindom--2008-2010.html; 2012.

2. Blanks RG, Moss SM, McGahan CE, et al. Effects of NHS breast screening programme on mortality from breast cancer in England and Wales, 1990–8: comparison of observed with predicted mortality. Br Med J 2000;321:665–9.

3. National Institute for Health and Clinical Excellence. NICE Clinical Guideline 80: Early and locally advanced breast cancer. 2009. Available from http://guidance.nice.org.uk/CG80/NICEGuidance/pdf/English;[accessed 23.07.12].

4. Willett AM, Michell MJ, Lee MJR. Available from Best Practice Guideline for Patients Presenting with Breast Symptoms. 2010. [accessed 23.07.12] http://www.associationofbreastsurgery.org.uk/media/4585/best_practice_diagnostic_guidelines_for_patients_presenting_with_breast_symptoms.pdf

5. Kolb TM, Lichy J, Newhouse JH. Comparison of the performance of screening mammography, physical examination, and breast US and evaluation of factors that influence them: an analysis of 27,825 patient evaluations. Radiology 2002;225:165–75.

6. Skaane P, Young K, Skjennald A. Comparison of film-screen mammography and full-field mammography with soft-copy reading in a population-based screening program: the Oslo II study. Radiology 2002;225:267.

7. Pisano ED, Gatsonis C, Hendrick E, et al. Diagnostic performance of digital versus film mammography for breast cancer screening. N Engl J Med 2005;353:1773–83.

8. James JJ. The current status of digital mammography. Clin Radiol 2004;59:1–10.

9. Committee on Technologies for the Early Detection of Breast Cancer. Mammography and beyond: developing technologies for the early detection of breast cancer. Washington, DC: National Academy Press; 2001.

10. Legood R, Gray A. NHSBSP Equipment Report 0403. A cost comparison of full-field digital mammography with film-screen mammography in breast cancer screening. Sheffield: NHS Breast Screening Programme Publications; 2004.

11. Gur D, Sumkin JH, Rockette HE, et al. Changes in breast cancer detection and mammography recall rates after the introduction of a computer-aided detection system. J Natl Cancer Inst 2004;96:185–90.

12. Wilson ARM, Teh W. Mini symposium: Imaging of the breast. Ultrasound of the breast. Imaging 1998;9:169–85.

13. Lister D, Evans AJ, Burrell HC, et al. The accuracy of breast ultrasound in the evaluation of clinically benign discrete breast lumps. Clin Radiol 1998;53:490–2.

14. Berg WA, Blume JD, Cormack JD, et al. ACRIN 6666 Investigators. Combined screening with ultrasound and mammography vs mammography alone in women at elevated risk of breast cancer. JAMA 2008;299:2151–63.

15. Berg WA, Zhang Z, Lehrer D, et al. Detection of breast cancer with addition of annual screening ultrasound or a single screening MRI to mammography in women with elevated breast cancer risk. JAMA 2012;307:1394–404.

16. Damera A, Evans AJ, Cornford EJ, et al. Diagnosis of axillary nodal metastases by ultrasound guided core biopsy in primary operable breast cancer. Br J Cancer 2003;89:1310–3.

17. Houssami N, Ciatto S, Turner R, et al. Preoperative ultrasound-needle biopsy of axillary nodes in invasive breast cancer: meta-analysis of its accuracy and utility in staging the axilla. Ann Surg 2011;254:243–51.

18. Kuhl C. The current status of breast MR imaging. Part 2. Clinical applications. Radiology 2007;244:672–91.

19. Sardanelli F, Boetes C, Borisch B, et al. Magnetic resonance imaging of the breast: recommendations of the EUSOMA working group. Eur J Cancer 2010;46:1296–316.

20. Kuhl CK, Schrading S, Bieling HB, et al. MRI for diagnosis of pure ductal carcinoma in situ: a prospective observational study. Lancet 2007;370:485–92.

21. Kuhl CK, Schmutzler RK, Leutner CC, et al. Mammography, breast ultrasound and magnetic resonance imaging for surveillance of women at high familial risk for breast cancer. J Clin Oncol 2005;23:8469–76.

22. Warner E, Plewes DB, Shumak RS, et al. Comparison of breast magnetic resonance imaging, mammography, and ultrasound for surveillance of women at high risk for hereditary breast cancer. J Clin Oncol 2001;19:3524–31.

23. Stoutjesdijk MJ, Boetes C, Jager GJ, et al. Magnetic resonance imaging and mammography in women with a hereditary risk of breast cancer. J Natl Cancer Inst 2001;93:1095–102.

24. Brekelmans CTM, Seynaeve C, Bartels CCM, et al. Effectiveness of breast cancer surveillance in BRCA1/2 gene mutation carriers and women with high familial risk. J Clin Oncol 2001;19:924–30.

25. Olsen O, Gotzsche PC. Cochrane review on screening for breast cancer with mammography. Lancet 2001;358:1340–2.

26. Olsen O, Gotzsche PC. Systematic review of screening for breast cancer with mammography. Available at http://image.thelancet.com/extras/fullreport.pdf

27. WHO handbook on cancer prevention. 7th ed Lyons: IARC Press; 2002.
   A comprehensive review of all the available data on the effectiveness of breast cancer screening in reducing breast cancer mortality.

28. Nystrom L, Andersson I, Bjurstam N, et al. Long-term effects of mammographic screening: update overview of the Swedish randomised trials. Lancet 2002;359:909–19.
   Long-term follow-up of the combined Swedish trials showing significant mortality benefit after more than 20 years.

29. Tabar L, Vitak B, Tony HH, et al. Beyond randomised controlled trials: organised mammographic screening substantially reduces breast carcinoma mortality. Cancer 2001;91:1724–31.

30. Duffy S, Tabar L, Chen HH, et al. The impact of organised mammographic screening on breast carcinoma mortality in seven Swedish counties. Cancer 2002;95:458–69.

31. Hackshaw AK, Paul EA. Breast self-examination and death from breast cancer: a meta-analysis. Br J Cancer 2003;88:1047–53.

32. Smith RA, Saslow D, Sawyer KA, et al. American Cancer Society guidelines for breast cancer screening: update 2003. CA Cancer J Clin 2003;53:141–69.

33. Breast Screening Frequency Trial Group. The frequency of breast cancer screening: results from the UKCCCR randomized trial. Eur J Cancer 2002;38:1458–64.

34. Million Women Study Collaborators. Breast cancer and hormone replacement therapy in the Million Women Study. Lancet 2003;362:419–27.
   Report of significantly increased risk of breast cancer in women taking HRT in the UK.

35. Perrson I, Thurfjell E, Holmberg I. Effect of estrogen and estrogen–progestin replacement regimes on mammographic breast parenchymal density. J Clin Oncol 1997;15:3201–7.

36. Sendag F, Cosan Terek M, Ozsener S, et al. mammographic density changes during different postmenopausal hormone replacement therapies. Fertil Steril 2001;76:445–50.

37. Evans A. Hormone replacement therapy and mammographic screening. Clin Radiol 2002;57:563–4.

38. Litherland JC, Stallard S, Hole D, et al. The effect of hormone replacement therapy on the sensitivity of screening mammograms. Clin Radiol 1999;54:285–8.

39. Kavanagh AM, Mitchell H, Giles GG. Hormone replacement therapy and accuracy of mammographic screening. Lancet 2000;355:270–4.

40. Litherland JC, Evans AJ, Wilson ARM. The effect of hormone replacement therapy on recall rate in the National Health Breast Screening Programme. Clin Radiol 1997;52:276–9.

41. Evans AJ, Pinder SE, Ellis IO, et al. Screen detected ductal carcinoma in situ (DCIS): over-diagnosis or obligate precursor of invasive disease? J Med Screen 2001;8:149–51.

42. Evans AJ, Burrell HE, Pinder SE, et al. Detecting which invasive cancers at mammographic screening saves lives? J Med Screen 2001;8:86–90.

43. National Institute for Clinical Excellence. Guidance on cancer services. Familial breast cancer. London: National Institute for Clinical Excellence; 2006. Available from http://www.nice.org.uk;[accessed 30.10.12].

44. Robson M. Breast cancer surveillance in women with hereditary risk due to BRCA1 or BRCA2 mutations. Clin Breast Cancer 2004;5:260–8.

45. Tilanus-Linthorst M, Verhoog L, Obdeijn I-M, et al. A BRCA1/2 mutation, high breast density and prominent pushing margins of a tumour independently contribute to a frequent false-negative mammography. Int J Cancer 2002;102:91–5.

46. Warner E, Plewes DB, Hill KA, et al. Surveillance of BRCA1 and BRCA2 mutation carriers with magnetic resonance imaging, ultrasound, mammography, and clinical breast examination. JAMA 2004;292:1317–25.

47. Hamilton LJ, Evans AJ, Wilson ARM, et al. Breast imaging findings in women with BRCA1- and BRCA2-associated breast cancer. Clin Radiol 2004;59:895–902.

48. Kriege M, Brekelmans CTM, Boetes C, et al. Efficacy of MRI and mammography for breast

cancer screening in women with a familial or genetic predisposition. N Engl J Med 2004;351:427–37.

49. Leach MO, Boggis CR, Dixon AK, et al. Screening with magnetic resonance imaging and mammography of a UK population at high familial risk of breast cancer: a prospective multicentre cohort study (MARIBS). Lancet 2005;365:1769–78.

50. Teh W, Wilson ARM. Definitive non-surgical breast diagnosis: the role of the radiologist. Clin Radiol 1998;53:81–4.

51. Britton PD. Fine needle aspiration or core biopsy. Breast 1999;8:1–4.

52. Britton PD, McCann J. Needle biopsy in the NHS Breast Screening Programme 1996/7: how much and how accurate? Breast 1999;8:5–11.

53. Vargas HI, Agbunag RV, Khaikhali I. State of the art of minimally invasive breast biopsy: principles and practice. Breast Cancer 2000;7:370–9.

54. Heywang-Kobrunner SH, Schaumloffel U, Viehweg P, et al. Minimally invasive stereotaxic vacuum core breast biopsy. Eur Radiol 1998;8:377–85.

55. Brem RF, Schoonjans JM, Sanow L, et al. Reliability of histologic diagnosis of breast cancer with stereotactic vacuum-assisted biopsy. Am Surg 2001;67:388–92.

56. Parker SH, Klaus AJ, McWey PJ, et al. Sonographically guided directional vacuum-assisted breast biopsy using a handheld device. AJR Am J Roentgenol 2001;177:405–8.

57. Kettritz U, Rotter K, Murauer M, et al. Stereotactic vacuum biopsy in 2874 patients: a multicenter study. Cancer 2004;100:245–51.

58. Brenner RJ, Bassett LW, Fajardo LL, et al. Stereotactic core needle breast biopsy: a multi-institutional prospective trial. Radiology 2001;218:866–72.

59. Wilson ARM. Therapeutic applications of vacuum biopsy. Breast Cancer Res 2008;4:31.

60. Wilson R, Kavia S. Comparison of large-core vacuum-assisted breast biopsy and excision systems. Recent Results Cancer Res 2009;173:23–41.

61. Kuhl CK, Morakkabati N, Leutner CC, et al. MR imaging-guided large-core (14-gauge) needle biopsy of small lesions visible at breast MR imaging alone. Radiology 2001;220:31–9.

62. Fishman JE, Milikowski C, Ramsinghani R, et al. US-guided core-needle biopsy of the breast: how many specimens are necessary? Radiology 2003;226:779–82.

63. Luini A, Zurrida S, Paganelli G, et al. Comparison of radioguided excision with wire localisation of occult breast lesions. Br J Surg 1999;86:522–5.

64. Rampaul RS, Bagnall M, Burrell H, et al. Radioisotope for occult lesion localisation: results from a prospective randomised trial of ROLL versus wire guidance in occult lesions of the breast. Br J Surg 2004;91:1575–7.

65. Rampaul RS, Macmillan RD, Evans AJ. Intraductal injection of the breast: a potential pitfall of radioisotope occult lesion localisation. Br J Radiol 2003;76:425–6.

66. Patel A, Pain SJ, Britton P, et al. Radioguided occult lesion localisation (ROLL) and sentinel node biopsy for impalpable invasive breast cancer. Eur J Surg Oncol 2004;30:918–23.

67. Tanis PJ, Deurloo EE, Valdes Olmos RA. Single intralesional tracer dose for radio-guided excision of clinically occult breast cancer and sentinel node. Ann Surg Oncol 2001;8:850–5.

68. Gray RJ, Giuliano R, Dauway EL, et al. Radioguidance for nonpalpable primary lesions and sentinel lymph node(s). Am J Surg 2001;182:404–6.

2

Pathology and biology of breast cancer

Rajendra S. Rampaul
Emad A. Rakha
John F.R. Robertson
Ian O. Ellis

Introduction

Management of women with breast carcinoma has undergone significant changes over the past 20 years. The pathology and biology of breast cancer influences diagnosis, selection of primary and adjuvant treatment, formulation of follow-up protocols, prognosis and provision of counselling and reassurance. Screening and public education have accounted for a major shift in the number and type of the breast carcinomas detected today. Cancers are now of smaller size and more often lymph node negative. There is an increasing need to discriminate accurately the risk of recurrence and select appropriate adjuvant systemic therapies. Modern clinical practice employs a significant input from histopathological data to assist in the decision-making process for selecting treatments. This can be achieved by identifying accurate prognostic and predictive factors. A prognostic factor is defined as any patient or tumour characteristic that is predictive of the patient's outcome. Outcome is usually measured in terms of cancer-specific survival or disease-free survival. A predictive factor is defined as any patient or tumour characteristic that is predictive of the patient's response (outcome) to a specified treatment. The factors currently employed in breast cancer prognostication and prediction each possess independent prognostic information and predictive power and may be combined into an index, making

it more 'user friendly', informative and reproducible. A prognostic index is defined as quantitative set of values based on results of a prognostic model. There are several reasons for the use of such prognostic indices in breast cancer, which include the ability:

1. to separate patients into groups with significantly differing survival probabilities;
2. to separate patients into groups that include a 'cured' group and a group with poor survival;
3. to place a sufficient percentage of cases into each group;
4. to be applicable for all operable breast cancers – small, screen detected as well as symptomatic and young age;
5. to be prospectively validated;
6. to be capable of use in all units and to be inexpensive.

In this chapter common pathological features of breast cancer are reviewed and their role in guiding patients' management considered.

Traditional factors

Lymph node stage

Involvement of local and regional lymph nodes by metastatic carcinoma is one of the most important prognostic factors in breast cancer. The revised

TNM staging system for breast cancer has confirmed that the absolute number of axillary lymph nodes involved in metastatic cancer ('positive lymph nodes') is one of the most important prognostic factors in breast cancer.[1] Lymph node stage has been used consistently as a guide for therapy. However, lymph node stage is considered as a time-dependent factor; the longer the tumour has been growing the more likely it is that lymph nodes are involved by spread. It has also been reported that, when taken alone, lymph node stage is incapable of defining either a cured group or one with close to 100% mortality from breast cancer.

The clinical assessment of nodal status (as in TNM classification) is unreliable.[2,3] Palpable nodes may be enlarged because they show benign reactive changes whilst nodes bearing tumour deposits can be impalpable. Although axillary sonography is a moderately sensitive and fairly specific technique in the diagnosis of axillary metastatic involvement,[4] histological examination of the lymph nodes from the axilla should be carried out in all patients with primary operable invasive breast cancer. It is well known that patients who have histologically confirmed lymph node involvement have a significantly poorer prognosis than those without nodal metastases. The 10-year survival is reduced from 85% for patients with no nodal involvement to 40% for those with involvement of multiple nodes. Prognosis worsens the greater the number of nodes involved, and the level of nodal involvement can provide useful information; metastasis to the higher level nodes (level II or III) in the axilla and particularly those at the apex (level III) carries a worse prognosis (**Fig. 2.1**).

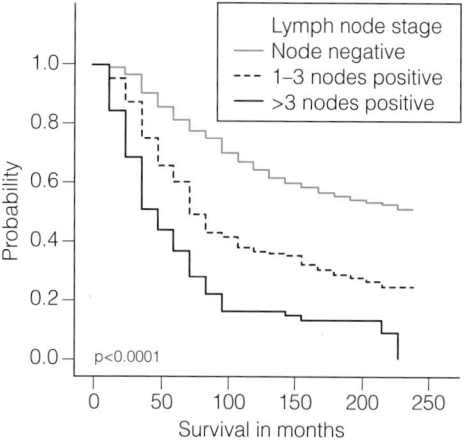

Figure 2.1 • Overall survival for patients in the NTPBCS according to lymph node stage (*P* < 0.0001).

✔✔ Studies show that overall survival is decreased as the number of nodes that are involved increases.[5–7]

Optimal management of the axilla is discussed in Chapter 9.

✔✔ Sentinel node biopsy or blue dye directed axillary sampling has been shown to provide accurate prognostic information and has an extremely low rate of lymphoedema.[2] Of 1275 patients undergoing axillary sampling, only 0.04% suffered symptomatic complaints of arm swelling and lymphoedema.

A refinement of lymph node sampling is provided by the technique of sentinel lymph node (SLN) biopsy. There have been several studies to examine the validity of this technique. The ALMANAC trial provides level I evidence for UK-based practice.[3]

From a pathological perspective, there are unresolved questions about how to optimally assess the sentinel node. Studies have shown that the mean number of sentinel nodes is close to 3. As the number of nodes removed during SLN biopsy is fewer, pathologists are now challenged to process these few nodes optimally. Several methods have been studied: routine paraffin histology; intraoperative frozen section; immunohistochemistry and more intensive methods such as serial sectioning and molecular methods including polymerase chain reaction (PCR) and reverse transcription–PCR (RT–PCR).

At present there is no consensus for the optimal handling of the SLN in the laboratory. Most centres have developed their own 'in-house' protocols, which are invariably tied to the institution's research ambitions. This ad hoc approach can influence interpretation of results, as the amount of material assessed between centres is not uniform. In a number of large studies, using different histopathological techniques, the SLN false-negative rate (defined as how often the SLN is negative for malignancy when cancer is present in the rest of the axilla) varies between 0% and 11%.

In Nottingham the MRC ALMANAC protocol is employed to assess all sentinel node biopsies.

These nodes are cut into slices about 3 mm thick, taken perpendicular to the long axis of the node to maximise the assessment of the marginal sinus, with one node per cassette. The majority of nodes can be completely embedded in one cassette. Larger nodes have alternate slices embedded and may require more than one cassette. Large, obviously involved nodes have one section taken.

Intraoperative frozen sections or imprint cytology of axillary lymph nodes have been advocated by some authors. Conventional frozen sections have a high false-negative rate of between 10% and 30%. More intensive intraoperative assessment with serial sections and immunohistochemistry has been described,[8] but is time consuming and labour intensive. Frozen section is best applied to selected cases; for example, if the node is macroscopically abnormal and this is confirmed histologically to be metastatic carcinoma, further axillary surgery can be performed immediately. Some studies have found low false-negative rates of 2–3% with intraoperative imprint cytology,[9] but not all have been able to achieve this level of accuracy. Lymph node status can be assessed peroperatively using ultrasound combined with FNA or core biopsy, and this reduces the need for preoperative frozen section and imprint cytology to assess axillary nodes intraoperatively.

RT–PCR is more sensitive than immunohistochemistry at detecting metastatic tumour in axillary nodes. Two types of methods have been used to detect tumour cells with molecular techniques. First, a genetic defect such as chromosomal rearrangement or mutation can be used. The problem with this is that no single genetic defect is seen in all breast carcinomas. The second method is to use a molecular marker that is present in tumour cells but not in the adjacent tissue. To identify a marker that has this specificity and is expressed in the majority of tumours is difficult. It may be necessary to use a panel of markers. A major problem with PCR is the potentially high false-positive rate due to the sensitivity of the method and potential for contamination. In addition, it is not possible with PCR to determine whether the DNA comes from cells that are viable. An advantage of haematoxylin/eosin sections and immunohistochemistry is that the morphology of the cells can be examined and malignancy confirmed. A major unresolved question is whether carcinoma detected only by PCR or RT–PCR has the same prognostic significance as haematoxylin/eosin positivity.

The detection rate of micrometastases in axillary lymph nodes has been reported to range from 9% to 46%.[10] Studies have used serial sectioning with or without immunohistochemical stains to detect micrometastatic foci and these methods have increased detection rates.

The European Working Group for Breast Screening Pathology[11] has formulated working guidelines for the assessment and pathological work-up of SLNs in breast cancer. From a literature review available at that time, the committee concluded that it was not possible to determine the significance of micrometastasis or isolated tumour cells. They noted that approximately 18% of cases are associated with other nodal (non-sentinel node) metastases. False-negative rates are most often determined via immunohistochemistry (IHC). However, at present it is recommended that an intensive work-up is not justified on a population level. The committee did suggest multilevel assessment and, where resources permit, intraoperative assessment, although the results of Z0011 (see Chapter 7) suggest that some node-positive patients may not require axillary dissection and this brings the whole issue of intraoperative assessment into question. The current view is that IHC should not be used routinely to assess axillary lymph nodes.

Tumour size

Tumour size is one of the most powerful predictors of prognostic factor in breast cancer.[12,13] The frequency of nodal metastases in patients with tumours <10 mm is 10–20%,[13] and node-negative patients with tumours <10 mm have a 10-year disease-free survival rate of greater than 90%.[14] Tumour size is a time-dependent prognostic factor that depends on the period between tumour development and detection, and on the balance between tumour cell proliferation and death (tumour growth rate). It is well known that the association between increasing tumour size and increasing number of positive lymph nodes and worse outcome is highly statistically significant.[13] Therefore, the main aim of population screening with mammography is to detect smaller tumours that are

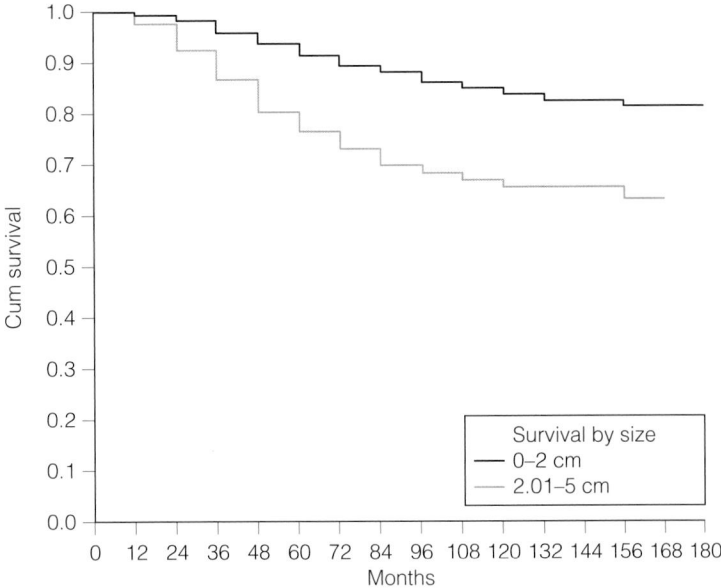

Figure 2.2 • Overall survival according to size.

likely to have a better outcome than those that present symptomatically (of a larger size). Patients with smaller tumours have a better long-term survival than those with larger tumours (**Fig. 2.2**). Estimation of tumour size has assumed particular importance since the introduction of population screening. In most studies the frequency of axillary lymph node metastasis in small <15 mm (so-called minimally invasive carcinoma (MIC)) invasive carcinomas is 15–20%,[15–17] compared with over 40% in tumours measuring 15 mm or more.[18] During the prevalent round of breast screening even more favourable results are obtained, with the frequency of axillary lymph node metastasis ranging from 0% to 15%.[19–22] The Nottingham Tenovus Primary Breast Cancer Study (NTPBCS) has generated data that suggest the cut-off point of 10 mm is not the best discriminator for MIC. Life-table analysis of survival curves found no difference between tumours measuring up to 9 mm and those measuring 10–14 mm. This indicates that <15 mm may be a more realistic watershed in defining small, invasive, carcinomas of good prognosis. It is clear that pathological tumour size is a valuable prognostic factor and it has become an important quality assurance measure for breast screening.[21,23–26] It is also used in part to judge the ability of radiologists to detect small impalpable invasive carcinomas.

Differentiation

Modern pathologists have recognised that invasive carcinomas can be divided according to their degree of differentiation. There are two ways to achieve this: (i) by allocating a histological type according to the architectural pattern of the tumour; (ii) by assigning a grade of differentiation based on semi-quantitative evaluation of structural characteristics.

Certain histological types of invasive carcinoma carry a favourable prognosis. Tubular, mucinous, invasive cribriform, medullary and tubulolobular types, together with rare tumour types such as adenoid cystic carcinoma, adenomyoepithelioma and low-grade and squamous carcinoma, have all been reported to have a more favourable outcome than invasive carcinoma of no special type (ductal NST). Undoubtedly, assessment of histological type provides prognostic information in breast cancer. However, this effect is relatively small in multivariate analysis[27] when compared with the prognostic value of histological grade; histological type may prove to be more useful in increasing our understanding of the biology of breast cancers.[28]

Invasive lobular carcinoma (ILC) is of particular importance. It comprises approximately 5–15% of breast cancers and appears to have a distinct biology. It is less common than invasive carcinoma of no special type, also called invasive ductal carcinoma (IDC).

✅✅ Recently, Rakha et al.[29] examined a large group of 5680 breast tumours (415 patients (8%) with pure ILC and 2901 (55.7%) with IDC (no special type)) and demonstrated that, compared to IDC, patients with ILC tended to be older and have tumours that were more frequently of lower grade (typically grade 2; 84%), hormone-receptor positive (86% compared to 61% in IDC), of larger size and with absence of vascular invasion. More patients with ILC compared with IDC were placed in the good Nottingham Prognostic Index group (40% compared to 21% in IDC). ILC showed indolent but progressive behavioural characteristics with nearly linear survival curves that crossed those of IDC after approximately 10 years of follow-up, thus eventually exhibiting a worse long-term outcome. Interestingly, ILC showed a better response to adjuvant hormonal therapy (HT), with improvement in survival in patients who received HT compared with matched patients with IDC.

Tumour grade

The Nottingham method (Elston and Ellis) is a modification and improvement of previously existing morphological grading systems and is able to provide greater objectivity of grade.[30]

In brief, assessment of grade considers three tumour characteristics: tubule formation, nuclear pleomorphism and mitotic counts. A numerical scoring system of 1–3 is used for each factor individually. The three scores are added together to produce scores of 3–9 on which an overall tumour grade is assigned:

- Grade 1 – well differentiated = score 3–5 points.
- Grade 2 – moderately differentiated = score 6–7 points.
- Grade 3 – poorly differentiated = score 8–9 points.

It should be noted that grade is valuable irrespective of histological type.

There is a highly significant correlation between tumour grade with long-term prognosis (**Fig. 2.3**); patients with grade 1 tumours have a 93% chance of surviving 10 years after diagnosis, whereas in patients with grade 3 tumours this is reduced to 70%. It has now been shown conclusively that the Nottingham method, with its more objective criteria, has excellent reproducibility when used by experienced pathologists.

Interestingly, grade is not included in the recent revision of the TNM staging system of breast cancer as its value is questioned in certain settings such as lobular type.

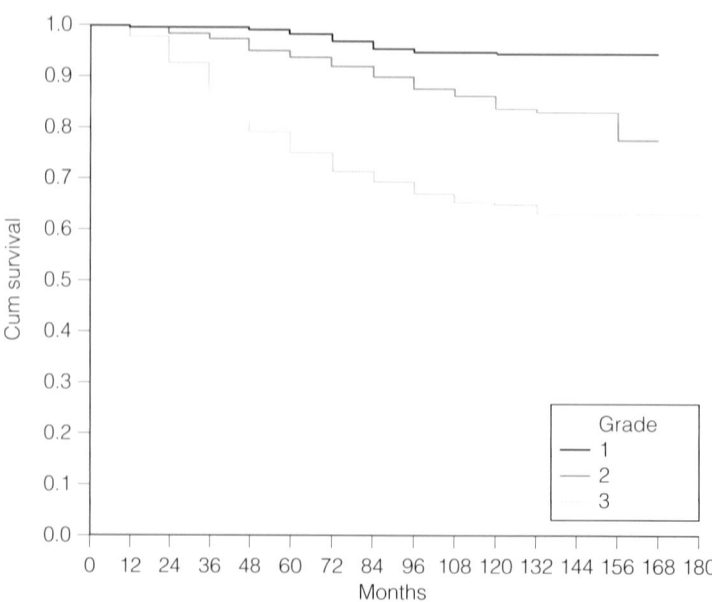

Figure 2.3 • Overall survival according to grade.

✅✅ The value of grade was addressed by Rakha et al.[31] in a large study of grade and overall survival in a large and well-characterised consecutive series of operable breast cancer (*n* = 2219 cases), with a long-term follow-up (median 111 months) using the Nottingham histological grading system. Histological grade was strongly associated with both breast cancer-specific survival (BCSS) and disease-free survival (DFS) in the whole series as well as in different subgroups based on tumour size (pT1a, pT1b, pT1c and pT2) and lymph node (LN) stages (pN0 and pN1 and pN2). The authors were able to demonstrate differences in survival between different individual grades (1, 2 and 3). In multivariate analyses histological grade was an independent predictor of both BCSS and DFS.

✅✅ Additionally, the usefulness of routinely assessing grade in invasive lobular cancer was examined by this group in 4987 patients,[32] of whom 517 were pure ILC cases. The majority of ILC was of classical type or mixed lobular variants (89%). Most ILC cases were moderately differentiated (grade 2) tumours (76%), while a small proportion of tumours were either grade 1 or 3 tumours (12% each). There were significant associations between histological grade and other clinicopathological variables of poor prognosis such as larger tumour size, positive lymph node status, vascular invasion, oestrogen receptor and androgen receptor negativity, and p53 positivity. Multivariate analyses showed that histological grade was an independent predictor of BCSS and disease-free interval.

Vascular invasion

The presence of tumour emboli in vascular and lymphatic spaces has emerged as an important prognostic factor. Several studies have now shown that the presence of vascular invasion correlates closely with local and regional lymph node involvement.[33,34] It has been suggested that it can provide prognostic information as powerful as lymph node stage. Reproducibility is the limiting factor in its widespread adoption and routine clinical assessment. In a Nottingham study of assessing vascular invasion, the issue of reproducibility was addressed specifically. Of 1704 cases, a subset of 400 cases was examined by two or more pathologists. There was a 77% overall inter-observer agreement on histological features and an 85.8% overall agreement in the classification of vascular invasion. Other studies have reported a similarly high concurrence between pathologists.[35,36] The assessment of vascular invasion is subjective but there is good evidence that a high rate of concurrence

can be obtained as long as strict criteria are used. Lymphatic and vascular invasion is considered to be a valuable surrogate for lymph node stage in cases where nodes have not been removed for examination. In patients whose axillary nodes are tumour free on histological examination there is a correlation between the presence of lymphovascular invasion (LVI) and early recurrence.

✅✅ Recently, Lee et al.[37] assessed the prognostic value of LVI in a group of 2760 patients with node-negative breast cancer with long-term follow-up (median 13 years). This study demonstrated a strong association between poor histological grade and younger age with LVI-positive cancers. LVI was prognostically significant and was independent of grade, size and type for overall survival (see **Fig. 2.4**).

Molecular/predictive factors

Despite the overall association between molecular markers with prognosis and outcome, they are limited in their ability to capture the nuances of the complex cascade of events that drive the clinical behaviour of breast cancer. Morphological factors are unable to predict response to systemic treatments, and tumours of apparently homogeneous morphological characteristics still vary in response to therapy and have distinct outcomes. The use of strategies ranging from hormone therapy to chemotherapy and recently to novel receptor-directed therapies and vaccines relies on the expression of predictive factors by the cancer, either individually (e.g. oestrogen receptors (ERs), progesterone receptors (PRs), human epidermal growth factor receptor (HER-2)

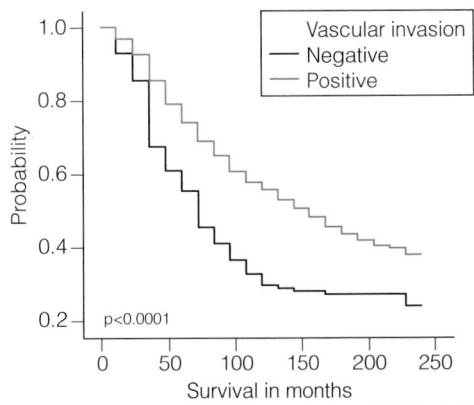

Figure 2.4 • LVI and breast cancer-specific survival.

and epidermal growth factor receptor (EGFR)) or globally (e.g. high-throughput gene expression assays). These molecular markers are used not only to guide treatments but are also being used to monitor response and detect relapse. It is envisaged that molecular predictive markers may form the basis of tailoring an individual's adjuvant therapy based on the genetic fingerprint of their cancer.

Oestrogen receptors (ERs)/ progesterone receptors (PRs)

Knowledge of the expression of hormone receptors and their subcellular regulatory pathways is one of the classic examples of the use of translational medicine in breast cancer to further diagnosis and treatment of this disease. The degree of ER expression is used to predict an individual's response to hormone therapy. Both ERs and PRs are steroid receptors that are located in the cell nucleus. Oestrogen and progesterone are considered to diffuse into cells, or be transported to the nucleus. Genes, regulated by steroid receptors, are involved in controlling cell growth, and it is currently believed that these effects are the most relevant to ERs and that ER expression influences the behaviour and treatment of breast cancer.[38] Elucidation of downstream effect on genes that are known to be influenced by hormones has led to the inclusion of these ER-regulated genes in high-density oligonucleotide array panels.[39] This may better define those pathways that are endocrine responsive and may lead to improved therapies with reduced side-effects and a greater potential for cure.[40]

In unselected patients, approximately 30% will respond to endocrine therapy. A tumour with both ER and PR expression has a 78% chance of responding to hormone therapy while those cancers that are ER/PR negative respond rarely, if ever.[41–43] Due to their close relationship with histological grade, ERs are not of independent prognostic significance.[43]

Methods of measuring ERs and PRs

There are a multitude of methods available; however, in clinical practice most are based on two distinct strategies. The first is an older method based on ligand-binding methods, i.e. radiolabelled steroid ligand is used to detect the receptor. The second relies on the recognition of the receptor protein by specific antibodies. Several studies examined the correlation between assay and outcome/response and studies have suggested that IHC analyses have a number of advantages.[42] IHC is currently the most commonly used method because it can be performed on paraffin-embedded material and allows assessment of the expression specifically in either invasive or in situ cancer.

Interpretation of assays

The optimal way to score IHC for ERs and PRs remains controversial. One method is to use an 'H' score (histo score), which takes into account the frequency of positive cells as well as intensity of staining and multiplies the two. The Allred score categorises the percentage of cells (scored from 0 to 5) with the intensity (scored from 0 to 3) and adds these two scores to give a numerical score from 0 to 8. Others simply estimate the percentage of positively stained tumour nuclei. It is important to appreciate that all methods are subjective and, at best, semiquantitative. ER/PR status in the histopathological report has a clearly defined role as a predictive factor for the response of systemic endocrine therapy. ERs and PRs should be assessed on all breast tumour specimens. As these assays have become simpler, and less costly, they are now available for all patients. Progress still needs to be made in standardisation of assay technique, objectivity and reproducibility.

Type 1 growth factor receptors

Activation of growth factor receptors was first found to be important in human cancers by identifying the homology between the viral oncogene v-*erbB* and EGFR. Sequence similarity between the *erbB-1* gene that encodes EGFR resulted in the isolation of a second growth factor receptor, the human ortholog *neu*, HER-2 (*erbB-2*). Screening of genomic DNA and messenger RNAs with probes allowed isolation of two additional relatives of the human *ERB1* gene. They were subsequently named *erbB-3* (HER-3) and *erbB-4* (HER-4).

To date there are four known receptors that belong to this growth factor receptor family, HER-1–4, and ligands for some of these have been identified. The family works in a co-receptor dimerisation type activation pathway.

The first two members of this family have been studied extensively in breast cancer. There are limited data on the role of HER-3 and HER-4 as well as their ligands. This family of signalling molecules is currently of immense clinical interest as the first two members are targets against which novel bio-receptor agents have been developed, including Iressa®, Tarveca® and Herceptin®.

EGFR

EGFR expression has been well studied in breast cancer. Consequent on major differences in study designs, the EGFR assay used and confounding factors such as adjuvant therapy, there is no consensus on its prognostic value. With the development of tyrosine kinase inhibitor (TKI)- and EGFR-directed biotherapies, there is now a growing impetus to not only standardise assays for detecting EGFR but also to delineate accurately its prognostic and predictive potential.

Methods of testing

Several techniques directed at DNA, RNA, protein (and functionally active (activated) as well) or serum can be employed to identify EGFR expression in breast cancer.

Of all such methods, IHC is the most practical. The advantages of IHC in EGFR as in HER-2 testing include reproducibility, ease of interpretation and the low cost compared to other techniques. It can also be employed on archival tissue. Protein levels can be quantified by Western analysis or enzyme immunoassay; however, architecture of tissue is lost in these procedures and there may be contamination by normal tissue cells or ductal carcinoma in situ. Serum EGFR levels have been examined in breast carcinoma; however, few data are available.[44,45] Due to the paucity of relevant data, it is difficult to draw conclusions on the current value of measuring EGFR in the serum of patients.

Prognostic and predictive value

The prognostic value of EGFR in breast cancer has been examined in several large studies. There remains no consensus on its prognostic value. The lack of a clear picture has been attributed to several factors: lack of a standard assay (monoclonal vs. polyclonal), lack of a cut-off for positivity and great variation in study designs (size, follow-up and influence of adjuvant therapy). Klijn et al.[46] reviewed data from over 5000 patients where EGFR had been assessed. Findings from this review demonstrated a great heterogeneity of study design, levels of cut-offs for positive and negative, and, not surprisingly, differences in its prognostic value in these various studies.

Recently, Tsutsui et al.[47] reported on a large series of 1029 patients (with adjuvant therapy) and found EGFR to be of independent prognostic value irrespective of nodal status. In contrast, studies by Rampaul et al.[48] and Ferrero et al.[49] (without adjuvant therapy) showed EGFR to be of no prognostic value (these latter series also incorporated grade and had longer follow-up).

The predictive value of this marker for hormone resistance or responsiveness is better defined. EGFR tumours are considered more resistant to endocrine therapy, and there exists an inverse relationship with EGFR-negative cancers (they are more likely ER positive), being more often sensitive to endocrine manipulation. Though some studies have been able to demonstrate that EGFR status is a predictor of tamoxifen failure and even response rates,[50] there are conflicting data from well-designed level II studies[51] that have shown no value of EGFR in predicting the efficacy of tamoxifen in high-risk postmenopausal women.

Perhaps the most exciting use of EGFR status and indeed the driving impetus for clinicians and scientist to measure it accurately is its putative role in defining those who should respond to novel EGFR-directed therapies.

HER-2

HER-2 is an important target in the development of a variety of new cancer therapies, which include monoclonal antibody (mAb)-based therapy, small-molecule drugs directed at the internal tyrosine kinase portion of the HER-2 oncoprotein, and vaccines. The most widely known HER-2-directed therapy is trastuzumab (Herceptin; Genentech, South San Francisco, CA, USA). Trastuzumab is a humanised recombinant mAb that specifically targets the HER-2 extracellular domain. There are a variety of techniques available to determine HER-2 status in breast cancer, some of which are employed for research purposes only. In diagnostic pathology laboratories HER-2 status is assessed routinely either by IHC, which assesses expression of the HER-2 oncoprotein, and fluorescence in situ hybridisation (FISH), which measures the number of *HER2* gene copies per chromosome 17 or gene amplification. Modifications of ISH using colorimetric detection are being developed, including chromogenic in situ hybridisation (CISH) and silver-enhanced in situ hybridisation (SISH).

Methods of HER-2 testing

Current guidelines for HER-2 testing[52] specify the methods that are suitable to detect either the HER-2 protein (by IHC) or gene amplification (using FISH or other in situ methods). Guidelines stress the need for stringent, reproducible and consistent criteria for testing.

Immunohistochemistry for HER-2 testing

Among the methods in use for determining HER-2 status, IHC is the most widely used. In studies employing various commercially available antibodies, a wide variety of sensitivity and specificity in fixed paraffin-embedded tissues is seen.[53,54] Antigen retrieval techniques are currently not standardised and they introduce the potential for false-positive staining. Nonetheless, IHC possesses many advantages to support its widespread adoption: (i) it allows for the preservation of tissue architecture and so can be used to identify local areas of overexpression within a heterogeneous sample, and can distinguish between HER-2 positivity in in-situ and invasive cancer; (ii) it is applicable to routine patient samples, facilitating use as a diagnostic test, and this allows prospective and retrospective research studies of HER-2 status to be undertaken.

Two Food and Drug Administration (FDA)-approved IHC tests for determining HER-2 status are available: HercepTest (DAKO, Carpeteria, CA, USA), based upon a polyclonal antibody; and CB11 (Pathway, Ventana Medical Systems, Tucson, AZ, USA), based upon a monoclonal antibody. The National Comprehensive Cancer Network guidelines[55] classify an IHC score of 0 or 1+ as representing HER-2-negative status, 3+ as positive, while 2+ is equivocal. Positive staining is defined as strong, continuous membranous expression of HER-2 in at least 10% of tumour cells. However, a joint report from the American Society of Clinical Oncology (ASCO) and the College of American Pathologists (CAP)[52] specified a threshold of >30% strong circumferential membrane staining for a positive result. If both uniformity and a homogeneous, dark circumferential pattern are seen, resultant cases are likely to be amplified by FISH as well as positive for HER-2 protein expression. The equivocal range for IHC (score 2+), which may include up to 23% of samples, is defined as complete membrane staining that is either non-uniform or weak in intensity but with obvious circumferential distribution in at least 10% of cells.

Equivocal or inconclusive results should be tested by FISH. Consistent with previous guidelines, a negative HER-2 test is defined as either an IHC result of 0 or 1+ for cellular membrane protein expression (no staining or weak, incomplete membrane staining in any proportion of tumour cells), though up to 5% of 1+ on IHC may be FISH positive.

In situ hybridisation for HER-2 testing

FISH and CISH measure directly the number of HER2 genes per chromosome 17, and when there is a chromosome centromeric enumeration probe (CEP) included, the copy number of chromosome 17 gene amplification is defined as an increase in HER-2/CEP17 ratio above 2.0. ISH results are semiquantitative, counting the number of signals in non-overlapping interphase nuclei of the lesion using either single-colour (HER-2 probe only, e.g. Ventana Inform) or dual-colour hybridisation (using HER-2 and chromosome 17 centromere probes simultaneously (e.g. Abbott, Chicago, USA, DAKO, Copenhagen, Denmark, etc.), the latter making it easier to distinguish true HER-2 amplification from chromosomal aneuploidy. ISH allows simultaneous morphological assessment, where evaluation of gene amplification can be restricted to invasive carcinoma cells. Many studies have compared FISH and IHC in the evaluation of HER-2 and have demonstrated concordance between the two techniques of up to 91%. Two studies have shown that FISH predicts more accurately HER-2 positivity than IHC when applied to molecularly characterised breast cancers.[56,57]

Three FISH tests are FDA approved for selecting patients for treatment with trastuzumab. The Path Vysion (Vysis Inc., Downers Grove, IL, USA) and PharmDx (Dako) tests require a ratio (HER-2 to CEP17) of 2.2 or greater for the sample to be considered amplified and both include an HER2 gene probe and a chromosome 17 probe. The INFORM test (Ventana Medical Systems) requires that at least 5.0 gene copies of HER2 be present if a sample is to be considered amplified as this kit uses a single HER2 gene probe without a chromosome 17 probe.

Recommended guidelines for HER-2 assessment in the UK have recently been updated and the reader is referred to these guidelines for further details.[58]

In brief, a two-phase testing algorithm based on IHC assay as the primary screen with FISH being reserved for equivocal cases is currently recommended.

This is based on evidence showing very good concordance between IHC and FISH results on breast carcinomas from 37 laboratories when tested in experienced reference centres.[59]

Chromogenic in situ hybridisation (CISH/SISH)

CISH and SISH are colorimetric methods to detect gene amplification that can be viewed using a standard light microscope. Concordance between FISH and SISH, for the validation of *HER2* gene status, is about 96% (kappa = 0.754).

Prognostic significance and association with other prognostic factors

The seminal work by Slamon et al.[60] in 1987 showed that *HER2* gene amplification independently predicted overall survival (OS) and disease-free survival (DFS) in a multivariate analysis in node-positive patients. Since then most large studies have confirmed this relationship in multivariate analysis. It is now well established that there is a significant correlation between HER-2 overexpression/amplification and poor prognosis for patients with nodal metastasis. There was until recently no consensus on the prognostic value of HER-2 in node-negative breast cancer patients, a group most often diagnosed through screening and representing a subgroup that could potentially benefit from appropriate adjuvant therapy. More recent studies have, however, shown a consistently poorer prognosis when comparing HER-2-positive versus -negative small node-negative breast cancers.

Rilke et al.[61] reported on the prognostic significance of HER-2 expression and its relationship with other prognostic factors. Using specimens from 1210 consecutive patients treated between 1968 and 1971 at a single institution (National Cancer Institute of Milan), with no systemic adjuvant therapy and 20-year follow-up, they found overexpression of HER-2 in 23% and showed a negative impact on survival of node-positive but not node-negative patients. Analysis of HER-2 in relation to the presence of lymphoplasmacytic infiltrate (LPI; favourable prognosis) and nodal status demonstrated that in node-negative, LPI-negative patients, HER-2 overexpression showed the same level of correlation with poor prognosis as with those patients with nodal metastasis. However, in the patients with node-negative disease and LPI positivity, HER-2 overexpression correlated with good prognosis. Some

studies have reported a prognostic value for HER-2 in node-negative patients in selected subgroups,[62–64] whereas others have shown no correlation.[65,66]

Mirza et al.[66] have published a systematic review of prognostic factors in node-negative disease. Data for HER-2 showed a lack of standardisation of assays and no association with survival. However, HER-2 status was shown to be of independent prognostic significance in several large studies with long-term follow-up, with worsened prognosis for those node-negative patients with HER-2-positive signalling.[67,68,69]

There is at present no agreement on the association between HER-2 and other prognostic factors. Several studies have shown a lack of association between HER-2 status and tumour size,[60,70,71] although some do report a correlation.[61,66,72–76]

Prediction of response to therapy: hormonal therapy

Transfection of normal breast cancer cells with the *HER2* gene has been shown to result in acquisition of oestrogen-independent growth that is insensitive to tamoxifen.[77,78]

A number of clinical studies, using various end-points such as time to relapse, more rapid spread to other sites, and DFS or OS, have reported an association between HER-2 positivity and resistance to hormonal therapy.[79–83] Some reports have described specific resistance to tamoxifen in HER-2-overexpressing tumours.[81,82] The 20-year update of the Naples GUN Trial[81] found that HER-2 overexpression not only predicted resistance to tamoxifen, but that HER-2-positive patients had a worse outcome on tamoxifen therapy compared with those who were untreated.

Several studies have also shown a reduction in response rates to hormonal therapy. Metastatic breast cancer that overexpressed HER-2, measured by high plasma levels of extracellular domain, demonstrated a substantial reduction in response rate to hormonal therapy.[84] Other studies have failed to find an association or even a trend between HER-2 status and response to hormonal therapy.[85–87] Elledge et al.[87] examined the response to tamoxifen in 205 tumours with ER-positive disease. In HER-2-positive compared to HER-2-negative patients, they found no significant evidence for a poorer response, time to treatment failure or survival. In a more recent study, the relationship between HER-2 overexpression and response to tamoxifen was examined in the adjuvant setting in 741 (650 ER positive, 91 ER negative/PR positive) of the total of 1572 patients in the CALGB 8541 Trial who had HER-2 measured.[88] Tamoxifen significantly improved response, DFS and OS, irrespective of HER-2 status. However, tamoxifen was not randomised within this trial and all patients received one of three regimens of doxorubicin. Thus these data on tamoxifen resistance have limitations to their interpretation.

With regards to HER-2 and prognosis, not only is there clinical value in its positive expression but also in its absence – in so-called 'triple-negative phenotype' cancers (TNP), i.e. cancers that are HER-2, ER and PR negative. It also denotes a biologically different subgroup. The recognition of basal phenotype in these triple-negative cancers is of growing importance, with several lines of evidence supporting the view that triple-negative tumours and basal phenotype are not interchangeable but rather distinct entities. Ninety-one per cent of TNP tumours display a significant association with the basal-like centroid and about 20% of non-TNP tumours cluster together with TNP tumours in the 'basal-like' cluster; these data support the view that the majority of, but not all, TNP tumours have a basal-like phenotype and that the majority of, but not all, basal-like tumours have a TNP phenotype.[89] Triple-negative breast cancers have a relapse pattern that is very different from hormone-positive breast cancers: the risk of relapse is much higher for the first 3–5 years but drops sharply and substantially below that of hormone-positive breast cancers after that. This relapse pattern has been recognised for all types of triple-negative cancers for which sufficient data exist, although the absolute relapse and survival rates differ across subtypes.

Previous studies have shown that the expression of 'basal markers' (i.e. CK5/6, CK14, CK17 and/or EGFR) is associated with a poor prognosis, regardless of hormone receptor expression. The expression of basal markers (basal cytokeratins and EGFR) in TNP tumours (core basal phenotype) also correlates with a worse prognosis and identifies a clinically distinct subgroup within the TNP group. Moreover, it should be noted that identification of a subgroup of tumours solely based on the lack of expression of immunohistochemistry (for example, TNP) risks misassignment based on technical artefacts.[89]

An in-depth discussion of these issues is beyond the scope of this work and the reader is directed to detailed reviews by Rakha et al.[89]

Histopathology of patients with *BRCA1* and *BRCA2* mutations

The cancers that develop in patients with a genetic predisposition to breast cancer as a result of mutations in the breast cancer susceptibility genes *BRCA1* and *BRCA2* are of great clinical interest. Identification of histological features that could indicate a genetic predisposition would be useful in providing an insight into the function of these genes and may aid in identifying those in whom screening for genetic mutations would be useful. There is a general agreement that *BRCA1*-related cancers are more frequently 'medullary-like' carcinomas and high grade compared to those in patients without this genetic alteration. Cancers associated with *BRCA1* mutations have a significantly higher mitotic rate, a larger proportion of tumour with a continuous pushing margin and more lymphocytic infiltration than sporadic breast cancers.[90,91] These are also likely to be less positive for ERs and PRs and are more often aneuploid, have a high S-phase fraction, show greater accumulation of p52 protein and expression of basal cytokeratins (CK5/6, CK14 and CK17) than do sporadic breast cancers.[92–97] However, none of these features alone or in combination can be used to identify a cancer as being from a *BRCA1* gene mutation carrier. Pathological features reported in *BRCA2*-related breast cancer have been less consistent. Marcus et al.[92] noted a significantly higher proportion of tubulolobular cancers in *BRCA2* mutation carriers than in other patients. However, it has been reported in another study that tubular carcinomas are less common in *BRCA2* mutation carriers.[94] Armes et al.[97] investigated the histological phenotypes of breast carcinoma in women under 40 years of age with and without *BRCA1* and *BRCA2* germline mutations. It was found that the pleomorphic variant of invasive lobular carcinoma was more common in patients with *BRCA2* mutations. Others have reported that *BRCA2*-related cancers tend to be of high histological grade,[94,98] whereas others have not noted any significant difference in grade between *BRCA2*-related cancers and controls.[99]

High-throughput molecular techniques as prognostic and predictive tools in breast cancer

Genomics

Mechanisms of genetic aberrations

The sequencing of the entire human genome has permitted the introduction of high-throughput technologies that allow survey of thousands of genes and their products in a single assay. Together with powerful analytical tools this has opened new avenues for classifying breast cancer into biologically and clinically distinct groups based on DNA copy number alterations and gene expression patterns.

Cancer development is driven by the accumulation of DNA changes within the genome. DNA repair defects lead to a genome-wide genetic instability and this can drive further cancer progression. **Genomics** (*the study of the human genome*), **transcriptomics** (*the study of the transcriptome* (mRNAs)) and **proteomics** (*the analysis of the protein complement of the genome*) are the three branches of molecular biology that are being explored in an effort to improve understanding, diagnosis, prognostication and provision of new therapeutic targets for the treatment of breast cancer.

The genetic fingerprint provides information on normal cellular processes and morphological/phenotypic expression. When this message is altered, it forms the nidus for the development and progression of cancer. These alterations can be caused by DNA mutations, chromosomal aberrations, epigenetic modification and protein interactions. DNA mutations can lead to a change in gene function. These mutations are often due to base substitutions that may directly cause a stop codon. As a result the gene is only partly transcribed and any functional protein production terminated. Chromosomal instability can be due to DNA modification, mutation or viral genome integration. Changes in chromosome numbers are also seen and cancers can be aneuploid (60–90 chromosomes) or near diploid (46 chromosomes). In solid tumours virtually all chromosomal rearrangements are unbalanced, the net result being loss or gain in certain parts of the chromosome. By screening the genome, current losses and gains can be identified. This information can be used to investigate regions of overlap to reveal the genes that are involved in malignant transformation and cancer progression. In some situations, the DNA copy number and code remain intact but the accessibility of this DNA for transcription is affected by epigenetic modifications. This process can occur through DNA methylation. It directly silences genes and interferes with the binding of transcription factors by changing the chromatin structure around the gene. Global hypomethylation is a characteristic feature of the genome of a cancer cell. However, some sequences can be hypermethylated, such as CpG islands, which tend to lie around the transcription start sites of approximately half of all human genes. DNA hypomethylation has been shown to correlate with chromosome instability. Chromatin architecture remodelling is essential for gene transcription; thus the prognostic significance of quantitative chromatin changes.[100,101]

Assessment of genomic status in breast cancer

Several high-throughput molecular techniques have been developed to assess the status of the genome in a given cell population, in terms of copy number, DNA sequencing and structure. Large-scale DNA or gene copy number alterations can be assessed using loss of heterozygosity (LOH) and comparative genomic hybridisation (CGH) studies as well as other techniques. LOH can be used to identify chromosomal regions where allelic losses are more frequent. In one study,[102] a panel of 150 polymorphic microsatellite markers from throughout the whole genome was used to identify such regions. These data were correlated with clinicopathological features and showed four specific loci that correlated with lymph node metastasis (11q23–24, 13q12, 17p13.3 and 22q13). Microsatellites can also be used to check the ability of cells to repair DNA replication errors. Microsatellite instability (MSI) can be employed to identify both genetic and epigenetic modification. It has been shown that both genetic and epigenetic alterations of *hMSH2* and *hMLH1* contribute to genomic instability and tumour progression in sporadic breast cancer.

Chromosome-based CGH can be used to identify the loss of one or both copies of a given gene, as well as regions of amplification. In addition, the technique provides information on the number of copies of any part of each chromosome throughout the whole genome. There have been several studies using CGH in breast carcinoma,[103,104] and those with clinical follow-up have led to the identification of genetic changes related to prognosis. However, the resolution of every chromosome-based CGH technique was limited to approximately 10 million base pairs (Mbp). This limitation makes it difficult to link copy number changes to the genes involved. Another limitation to this technique is the need to perform karyotyping for target identification in every experiment.

Therefore, array CGH has been developed to overcome the problems of chromosome-based CGH. Array CGH does not require a normal metaphase spread but rather an array of DNA fragments (100 bp to 100 kb) and their precise chromosomal locus. This approach can provide resolutions up to 1 Mb. Albertson et al. utilised this technique to map the recurrent breast cancer amplicon at chromosome 20q12.3. They were able to demonstrate that what was previously described as a single amplicon is in fact two distinct amplicons (ZNF217 and CYP24). A novel amplicon at 17q21.3 that is implicated in the amplification and overexpression of the *HOXB7* gene in breast cancer has also been recently characterised using array CGH.[105]

Assessment of gene expression in breast cancer

In gene expression profiling, each gene is usually represented by a single element (created with a complementary DNA (cDNA) or oligonucleotide for the gene studied) and with high-density oligonucleotide cDNA microarray technology many thousands of gene-specific mRNAs can be measured in parallel in a single tissue sample. The principle of gene expression cDNA array is comparable to array CGH, other than that it uses cDNA generated from mRNA. Similar to the two main types of expression microarrays (cDNA microarrays and oligonucleotide microarrays), serial analysis of gene expression (SAGE) can provide profiling of the transcriptome by taking a raw count of sequence tags, each representing a transcript in an RNA population with each one representing one gene.

Broadly speaking, molecular profiling of breast cancers by gene expression microarrays can be performed in one of two ways: unsupervised or supervised analysis. Unsupervised analysis is used mainly for partitioning tumour samples into groups or classes on the basis of gene expression profiles regardless of other features. The main objective of this approach is to determine whether discrete subsets of cancers can be defined on the basis of gene expression profiles, and whether new classes can be identified (class discovery) that may have clinical significance and to develop a new molecular taxonomy. Supervised analysis, on the other hand, is used to allocate tumours to specific groups based on clinical or pathological features (e.g. clinical outcome or response to therapy). There are two main types of supervised analysis: class comparison and class prediction. The former aims to identify the transcriptomic differences between two classes of tumours, whereas the development of a 'gene signature' is the ultimate goal of the latter.

In breast cancer, the class discovery studies were pioneered by the Stanford group,[106] which proved the principle that breast cancer could be classified into molecularly distinct groups based upon gene expression profiles and their similarity to normal cell counterparts. Multiple independent studies have confirmed and expanded the original results. According to these studies, breast cancer was classified into two main classes (ER-positive and ER-negative tumours) and each one can be classified into multiple molecularly distinct subclasses. For example, the ER-negative tumours encompass three subgroups, one overexpressing HER-2, one with tumours expressing genes characteristic of basal/myoepithelial cells (basal-like cancer), and one with a gene expression profile similar to normal breast tissue. cDNAs have also been used to distinguish cancers with *BRCA1/BRCA2* mutations[107,108] and to determine ER status,[109] lymph nodes status[110,111] and prognostic subgroups in node-negative breast cancer.[112] These recent studies demonstrate the ability of cDNA to have a direct translational use in clinical practice.

Proteomics

The genetic code does not inform on which proteins are expressed by a cancer, or whether they are functional, if expressed. Post-translational modifications such as glycosylations or phosphorylation of proteins affect their expression and function at the protein level, which cannot be detected by assessing the status of the genome or transcriptome in a given cell population. Therefore, proteomics aims to assess changes at the protein level in which the proteome is displayed. Proteomics is quickly evolving to provide supportive and critical information to data generated through genomic approaches in high-throughput formats. This can be achieved by using different techniques such as two-dimensional polyacrylamide gel electrophoresis, isotope-coded affinity tagging, surface-enhanced laser desorption ionisation and matrix-associated laser desorption ionisation–time of flight.

These global expression profiling approaches yield candidate proteins and related genes that require verification through application of other techniques. Tissue microarrays (TMAs) provide a method for high-throughput protein expression analysis of large cohorts of archival samples that can be readily linked to clinicopathological and long-term follow-up databases. TMAs have expedited the validation of the prognostic and predictive significance of several candidate biomarkers. The technique allows for a composite slide of up to 1000 cores of tissue to be constructed into one paraffin block. The advantages are obvious in screening for novel protein expression. There are concerns on the validity of the cores as being representative samples and indeed this aspect has not been well studied, with only one study examining a large sample size with correlation to corresponding larger histology sections.[103] This technology and its application have been extensively reviewed.[113]

Clinical use of the high-throughput molecular techniques

It is envisaged that gene expression profiles may be able to guide decisions on the choice of hormonal, chemotherapeutic or targeted agents for each individual in the future. Presently, one of the best examples of the use of genomics and proteomics in clinical practice is the use of HER-2 expression/amplification to select patients for trastuzumab. Such profiles are useful to identify prognostically significant genes, which studies have demonstrated can perform better than traditional markers.[104,114] In metastatic disease, expression patterns can be used to establish the origin of the metastatic lesion in patients with more than one primary. Transcription profiling has also been shown to differentiate accurately breast cancers with germ-line mutations in *BRCA1/BRCA2* from those without such mutations. Such findings, if validated in other

studies, open the way for molecular phenotyping in high-risk families. In addition, gene expression profiling has been used to develop expression predictors (class prediction studies) that can be used for many types of clinical management decisions, including risk assessment, diagnostic testing, prognostic stratification and treatment selection. There are two types of class prediction studies in breast cancer: prognostic and predictive class prediction. Prognostic class prediction includes (i) poor-prognosis gene signatures that can discriminate between a good and a poor outcome by comparison between highly aggressive and less aggressive primary tumours, and (ii) recurrence score gene signatures that define tumours based on the risk of disease relapse. The predictive class prediction includes predictors of response to therapy.[115,116]

An example of a prognostic class prediction study is that reported by van't Veer et al. Expression profiles of 117 primary breast cancers were compared with known prognostic factors and matched with 5 years of follow-up data. Twenty-five thousand genes were used to generate expression profiles, which separated the tumours into two groups. Group 1 developed distant metastasis in 34% and in group 2 70% developed distant metastases. From the 25000-gene set, 70 genes had great accuracy in predicting recurrent disease. Multivariate analysis with grade, size, LVI, age and ER showed the poor-prognosis microarray profile to be an independent predictor of recurrent disease. This approach was further tested in 295 patients and again the use of gene profiling was able to accurately identify a poor-prognosis group.[101,109] MammaPrint® assay, which is based on the Amsterdam 70-gene gene signature, is currently used as a molecular diagnostic test for breast cancer prognostication and prediction. Another predictor calculates a recurrence score on the basis of the expression of 21 known genes, with the use of RT–PCR in formalin-fixed, paraffin-embedded tissue. The 'Oncotype DX assay' has been developed by researchers at Genomic Health. Oncotype DX is currently used as a diagnostic test to quantify the likelihood of disease recurrence in women with early-stage breast cancer and assesses the likely benefit from tamoxifen and certain types of chemotherapy. Oncotype DX employs a mathematical algorithm called the recurrence score (range 1–100) to calculate continuous risk for relapse and death for patients receiving adjuvant tamoxifen, and has recently been shown in a large population-based case–control study to be an effective predictive test for ER-positive, node-negative breast cancer patients treated or untreated with tamoxifen and no chemotherapy.[117] In addition, a number of microarray studies have been published which identified other prognostic signatures with clinical significance. For example, Change et al.[118] have used a 'wound-response gene expression signature' to stratify breast cancer patients based on the hypothesis that features of the molecular programme of normal wound healing might play an important role in cancer metastasis. They found that this gene signature can improve the risk stratification of early breast cancer over that provided by standard clinicopathological features. A gene expression signature of hypoxia response, derived from studies of cultured mammary epithelial cells' 'hypoxia gene signature', showed a strong predictor of clinical outcomes in breast cancer.[119]

Although proteomics has a long history that predates profiling at the RNA level, difficulties in protein identification and the lack of reproducibility of several assay platforms have limited the utility of such profiling systems. In breast cancer research, however, proteomics has begun to take on a role in the monitoring of response, prediction of resistance and relapse in patients treated with novel bio-directed therapies.[120]

Clinical use of prognostic factors in patient management

Prognosis in breast cancer depends on the presence of spread of disease and on the inherent aggressiveness of the tumour. The latter depends on a number of intrinsic biological characteristics, some of which have already been evaluated, such as morphological features, growth rate and hormone responsiveness. Accurate prognostication is now required on an individual patient basis and this can only be achieved by using a Prognostic Index that includes both time-dependent and biological factors. The best way to obtain such an index is to take potential factors that have been shown to have some value in univariate analysis and submit them to multivariate analysis. This has been the approach in deriving the

Nottingham Prognostic Index (NPI), which is based on three factors using the following formula:

$$NPI = \text{Pathological tumour size(cm)} \times 0.2$$
$$+ \text{Lymph node stage}(1, 2 \text{ or } 3)$$
$$+ \text{Histological grade}(1, 2 \text{ or } 3)$$

Arbitrary cut-off points of 3.4 and 5.4 are used to divide patients into six prognostic groups: excellent (EPG), good (GPG), moderate (MPG) I and II, poor (PPG) and very poor (VPG) (Tables 2.1–2.3, **Figs 2.5** and **2.6**).

The NPI provides extremely powerful prognostic information within the NTPBCS and was able to demonstrate its utility and reproducibility in studies from other centres. In this respect Henson et al.,[18] in a retrospective analysis of prognostic data in over 22 000 women from the SEER Programme of the National Cancer Institute in the USA, confirmed that a

Table 2.1 • NPI showing percentage in each prognostic group

| | Percentage in prognostic group | |
	1980–86	1990–99
EPG	12	14
GPG	19	21
MPG I	29	28
MPG II	24	22
PPG	11	11
VPPG	5	4

Prognostic groups: EPG, excellent prognosis; GPG, good prognosis; MPG, moderate prognosis; PPG, poor prognosis; VPG, very poor prognosis.

Table 2.2 • Differences in 10-year survival for each prognostic group

	10-year survival (%)	±95% CL	P (log rank)
EPG	96	2	
GPG	93	4	0.14
MPG I	82	4	<0.0001
MPG II	75	4	0.0007
PPG	53	8	<0.0001
VPG	39	12	0.003
All	80	2	

Prognostic groups: EPG, excellent prognosis; GPG, good prognosis; MPG, moderate prognosis; PPG, poor prognosis; VPG, very poor prognosis.
CL, confidence limit.

Table 2.3 • Relative risk reduction by NPI

	1980–86	±95% CL	1990–99	±95% CL	RRR (death)	% ARR (death)
EPG	88	6	96	2	0.67	8
GPG	72	8	93	4	0.75	21
MPG I	61	6	82	4	0.54	21
MPG II	42	6	75	4	0.57	35
PPG	14	8	53	8	0.45	39
VPG	12	10	39	12	0.31	27
All	55		80		0.56	25

Prognostic groups: EPG, excellent prognosis; GPG, good prognosis; MPG, moderate prognosis; PPG, poor prognosis; VPG, very poor prognosis.
ARR, absolute risk reduction; CL, confidence limit; RRR, relative risk reduction.

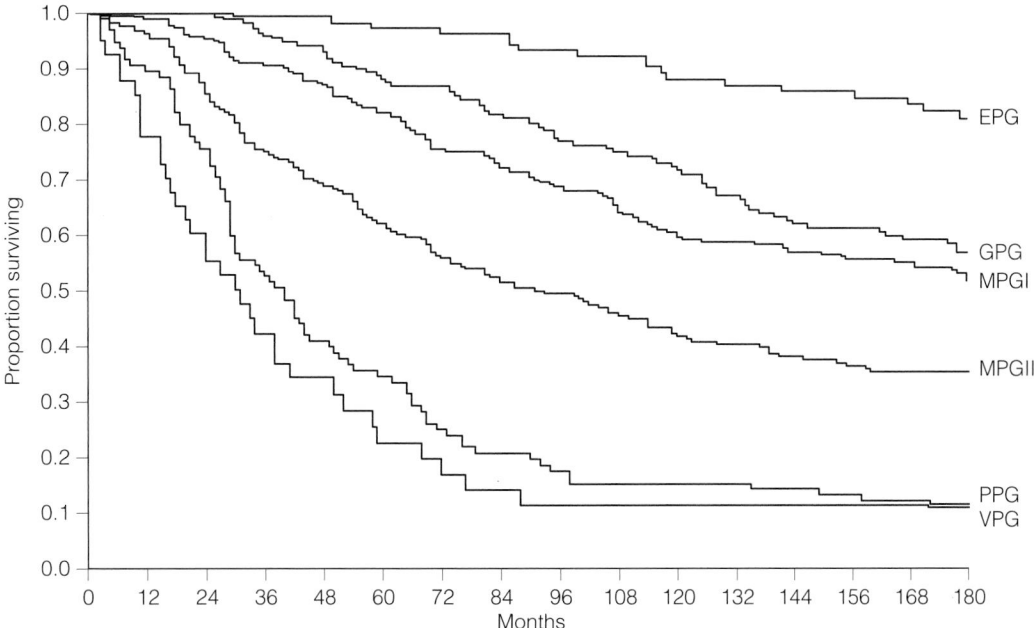

Figure 2.5 • Survival by NPI (1980–86).

combination of lymph node stage and histological grade improved prediction of prognosis. In a similar way to the NTPBCS, Chevallier et al.[121] have identified 'young' age, tumour size and histological grade as factors to be added to lymph node stage in the prediction of recurrence; these factors were used to divide lymph node-negative patients into three prognostic groups.

One of the strengths of the NPI is the fact that it has been verified prospectively in the NTPBCS. Further confirmation of its value has been provided by its validation in two large multicentre studies involving nearly 11 000 patients in total.[122,123] Such

studies demonstrate the inherent power of the pathological factors used in the NPI, which has become the most widely used index for the management of patients with breast cancer, certainly in the UK.

Other pathology-based prognostic indices used in breast cancer include Adjuvant!Online (AO)[124] and the St Gallen criteria,[125] and more recently Predict (a new UK prognostic model that predicts survival following surgery for invasive breast cancer).[126] This tool is a population-based validation of the prognostic model PREDICT for early breast cancer.

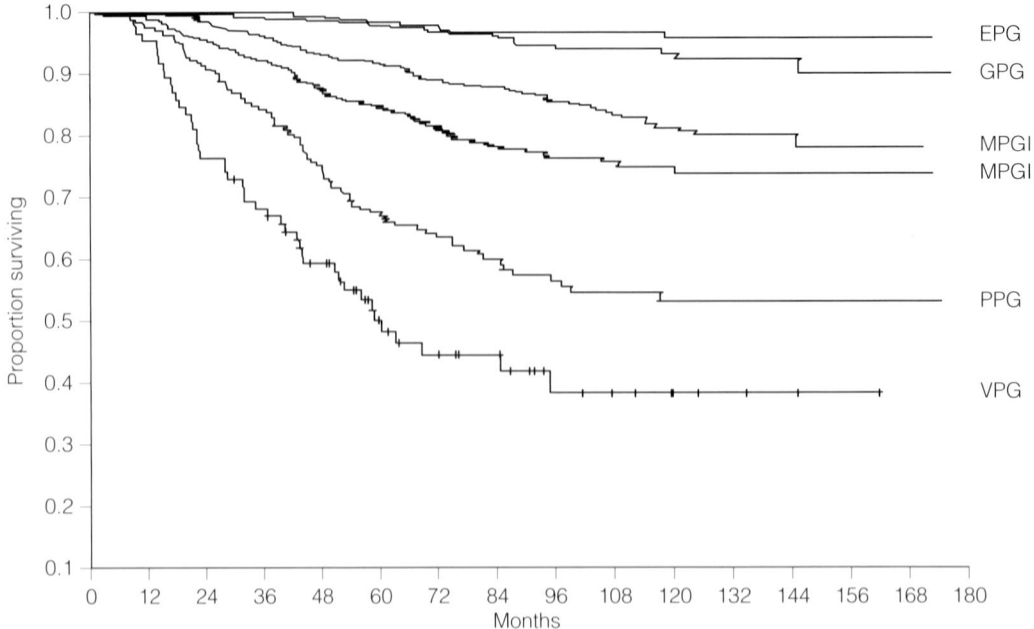

Figure 2.6 • Survival by NPI (1990–99).

Adjuvant!Online (http://www.adjuvantonline.com) was developed in the USA and published in 2001; users can input information on a patient's age, ER status, tumour grade, tumour size and number of positive nodes, and obtain predictions of 10-year OS (the likelihood of being alive 10 years after the diagnosis of breast cancer was first carried out), BCSS (the likelihood of not dying of breast cancer within 10 years of diagnosis) and event-free survival (EFS; the likelihood of surviving 10 years without recurrence (local, regional or distant), a second primary breast cancer, or death from breast cancer), both with and without any proposed adjuvant therapy. The performance of AO has been evaluated in cohorts of patients in Germany, Canada and the UK. It has an advantage over the NPI in that it integrates treatment, and for this reason AO is the programme most commonly used by oncologists.

The current St Gallen-derived algorithm for selection of adjuvant systemic therapy for early breast cancer patients includes tumour size and grade, nodal status, menopausal status, peritumoral vessel invasion, endocrine status and HER-2 status. Predict, which is similar in concept to AO but is based on UK patients, has been developed at the University of Cambridge. This tool is an alternative

updated method of assessing probability of survival for UK patients.

All of the above discussion applies to primary operable breast cancer. Prognostic factors have also been explored in locally advanced and metastatic breast cancer, albeit not to the same extent. In a small study of locally advanced pancreatic cancer patients ($n = 60$) treated with either tamoxifen or radiation therapy and with crossover upon failure, response to therapy correlated significantly with histological grade ($P = 0.02$), ER ($P = 0.02$), PR status ($P = 0.02$), mitotic index ($P = 0.01$) and tumour ploidy ($P = 0.04$). Survival from initial therapy correlated significantly with ER ($P = 0.01$) and PR status ($P = 0.04$).[127] In these patients, histological grade, mitotic index, tumour ploidy, and ER and PR status of the primary tumour may predict response and prognosis.

These authors also explored the prognostic value of certain factors as a composite index to guide decision-making in metastatic disease.[128] The advanced breast cancer (ABC) index comprises the grade, ER status, site of initial metastasis and disease-free interval. This index was tested both retrospectively and prospectively and shown to separate groups where the survival between each was highly significant ($P < 0.001$).

Breast cancer histopathology minimum dataset.

Surname.......................Forenames..........................Date of birth............

Sex...... Hospital............ Hospital No............ NHS No............

Date of receipt...................... Date of reporting .... Report No.....................

Side: [ ] Right [ ] Left   Pathologist.................   Surgeon ....

Specimen type: [ ] Diagnostic localisation biopsy   [ ] Diagnostic open biopsy

[ ] Therapeutic excision   [ ] Mastectomy

Specimen weight ....g

Axillary procedure: [ ] Lymph node sample [ ] Axillary clearance [ ] Sentinel node biopsy

----

Non-invasive malignant lesion [ ] Not present

[ ] Ductal,high grade   [ ] Ductal,intermediate grade   [ ] Ductal,low grade

Growth pattern(s): [ ] Solid   [ ] Cribriform [ ] Micropapillary [ ] Papillary

[ ] Apocrine   [ ] Flat/ clinging   [ ] Other

Size (pure DCIS only)..........................mm

[ ] Paget's disease of the nipple

[ ] Lobular neoplasia

Microinvasion: [ ] Not present [ ] Present [ ] Possible

Invasive carcinoma   [ ] Not present

Grade: [ ] I   [ ]II [ ]III [ ] Not assessable

[ ] Ductal / no specific type (NST)   [ ] Tubular carcinoma   [ ] Lobular carcinoma

[ ] Mucinous carcinoma   [ ] Medullary type carcinoma

[ ] Mixed (please tick component types present)   [ ] Not assessable

[ ] Other primary carcinoma (please specify)..

[ ] Other malignant tumour (please specify)..

Maximum diameter of invasive tumour ....mm

Whole size of tumour (to include DCIS extending >1mm beyond invasive area)...........mm

Vascular invasion (blood or lymphatic) [ ] Present   [ ] Possible   [ ] Not seen

----

For DCIS and invasive carcinoma

Excision margins: [ ] Reaches margin [ ] Uncertain   [ ] Does not reach margin

Nearest (surgically relevant) margin ....mm

Axillary nodes received: [ ] Yes [ ] No Number positive........... Total number...........

Other nodes received: [ ] Yes [ ] No Number positive........... Total number...........

Site of the nodes..

Oestrogen receptor status: [ ] Positive   [ ] Negative   [ ] Not known

Figure 2.7 • Breast cancer histopathology minimum dataset. DCIS, ductal carcinoma in situ.

Conclusion

Modern management of breast cancer requires a multifaceted understanding of both the clinico-pathological features and the molecular portraits of the cancer. Emerging evidence is suggesting that genomic approaches to prognosticating patients can be complementary to standard prognostic tools. Existing combinations of such factors are either largely clinical (e.g. NPI) or purely molecular (e.g. Oncotype DX), but a hybridised index is likely to yield more information. Updating the traditional NPI and incorporating well-established prognostic factors such as grade, stage and tumour size with biological factors have produced NPI+. This new tool, which combines updated methods for assessment of histological grade and tumour stage with biological class determination, has recently been shown to provide significant prediction of outcome in all biological classes.[129]

The need to accurately prognosticate each patient continues to drive research efforts to unravel the 'perfect' prognostic index. This information will allow us to use adjuvant therapies to influence and improve such prognosis for a better outcome and hopefully cure.

Contents of the final surgical pathology report: the minimum dataset

The Royal College of Pathologists' minimum dataset for breast cancer was originally developed in recognition that certain histopathological features of both in situ and invasive carcinoma are directly related to clinical outcome and may therefore be important in deciding the most appropriate treatment, including extent of surgery and use of and choice of adjuvant therapy. In addition, histopathological features can be used to monitor breast screening programmes, the success of which is reflected by more favourable prognostic features of the cancers detected and also changing patterns of disease, particularly identified by cancer registries.

The minimum set of data should be used by pathologists reporting all breast cancers, both screen detected and those presenting symptomatically.

The Royal College of Pathologists minimum dataset has been approved by the NHS Breast Screening Programme and the European Commission Working Group, the British Association of Surgical Oncologists, the British Breast Group and the United Kingdom Association of Cancer Registries (**Fig. 2.7**).

Key points

- Histopathological features such as size, grade and lymph node stage are key to prognosticating and guiding adjuvant therapy in breast cancer patients.
- The type 1 growth factor family (e.g. EGFR and HER-2) are becoming key molecular features in the design of novel biologically targeted therapies.
- The combination of standard pathological features and each cancer's genetic fingerprint will enable us in the future to individually tailor each patient's therapy.

References

1. Singletary SE, Allred C, Ashley P, et al. Revision of the American Joint Committee on Cancer staging system for breast cancer. J Clin Oncol 2002;20:3628–36.

2. Rampaul RS, Mullinger K, Macmillan RD, et al. Incidence of clinically significant lymphoedema as a complication following surgery for primary operable breast cancer. Eur J Cancer 2003;39(15):2165–7.

3. Mansel RE, Fallowfield L, Kissin M, et al. Randomized multicenter trial of sentinel node biopsy versus standard axillary treatment in operable breast cancer: the ALMANAC Trial. J Natl Cancer Inst 2006;98(9):599–609.

4. Alvarez S, Anorbe E, Alcorta P, et al. Role of sonography in the diagnosis of axillary lymph node metastases in breast cancer: a systematic review. Am J Roentgenol 2006;186:1342–8.

5. Rampaul RS, Evans AJ, Ellis IO, et al. Long term regional recurrence and survival after axillary nodal sampling for breast cancer. Eur J Cancer 2003;1(4):23(abstr.).

6. Shukla HS, Melhuish J, Mansel RE, et al. Does local therapy affect survival rats in breast cancer? Ann Surg Oncol 1999;6(5):455–60.

7. Macmillan RD, Rampaul RS, Lewis S, et al. Preoperative ultrasound-guided node biopsy and sentinel node augmented node sample is best practice. Eur J Cancer 2004;40(2):176–8.

8. Veronesi U, Galimberti V, Zurrida S, et al. Sentinel lymph node biopsy as an indicator for axillary dissection in early breast cancer. Eur J Cancer 2001;37(4):454–8.

9. Veronesi U, Paganelli G, Viale G, et al. Sentinel lymph node biopsy and axillary dissection in breast cancer: results in a large series. J Natl Cancer Inst 1999;91(4):368–73.

10. Schwartz GF, Guiliano AE, Veronesi U; Consensus Conference Committee. Proceeding of the consensus conference of the role of sentinel lymph node biopsy in carcinoma or the breast April 19–22, 2001, Philadelphia, PA, USA. Breast J 2002;8(3):124–38.

11. Cserni G, Amendoeira I, Apostolikas N, et al. Discrepancies in current practice of pathological evaluation of sentinel lymph nodes in breast cancer. Results of a questionnaire based survey by the European Working Group for Breast Screening Pathology. J Clin Pathol 2004;57(7):695–701.

12. Fisher ER, Fisher B, Sass R, et al. Pathologic findings from the National Surgical Adjuvant Breast Project (Protocol No. 4). XI. Bilateral breast cancer. Cancer 1984;54:3002–11.

13. Carter CL, Allen C, Henson DE. Relation of tumor size, lymph node status, and survival in 24,740 breast cancer cases. Cancer 1989;63:181–7.

14. Bennett RL, Evans AJ, Kutt E, et al. Pathological and mammographic prognostic factors for screen detected cancers in a multi-centre randomised, controlled trial of mammographic screening in women from age 40 to 48 years. Breast 2011;20(6):525–8.

15. Foulkes WD, Grainge MJ, Rakha EA, et al. Tumor size is an unreliable predictor of prognosis in basal-like breast cancers and does not correlate closely with lymph node status. Breast Cancer Res Treat 2009;117(1):199–204.

16. O'Dwyer PJ. Editorial. Axillary dissection in primary breast cancer; the benefits of node clearance warrant reappraisal. Br Med J 1992;302:360–1.

17. Blamey RW. Clinical aspects of malignant disease. In: Elston CW, Ellis IO, editors. Systemic pathology. The Breast. 3rd ed. London: Churchill Livingstone; 1998. p. 501–13.

18. Henson DE, Ries L, Freedman LS, et al. Relationship among outcome stage of disease and histologic grade for 22,616 cases of breast cancer. Br Cancer Res Treat 1991;68:2142–49.

19. Kutianawala MA, Sayed M, Stotter A, et al. Staging the axilla in breast cancer: an audit of lymph-node retrieval in one UK regional centre. Eur J Surg Oncol 1998;24:280–2.

20. Steele RJC, Forrest APM, Gibson T. The efficacy of lower axillary sampling in obtaining lymph node status in breast cancer: a controlled randomized trial. Br J Surg 1985;72:368–9.

21. Dixon JM, Dillon P, Anderson TJ, et al. Axillary sampling in breast cancer: an assessment of its efficacy. Breast 1998;7:206–8.

22. Cabanas RM. An approach for the treatment of penile carcinoma. Cancer 1977;39:456–66.

23. Royal College of Radiologists. Quality assurance guidelines for radiologists. 1990 NHS BSP Publications no. 15.

24. Royal College of Radiologists. Quality assurance guidelines for radiologists. 1997 NHS BSP Publications no. 15. January.

25. European Commission. European guidelines for quality assurance in mammography screening. 2nd ed Luxembourg: Office for Official Publications of the European Communities; 1996.

26. Mansel RE, Goyal A, Newcombe RG. ALMANAC Trialists Group. Internal mammary node drainage and its role in sentinel lymph node biopsy: the initial ALMANAC experience. Clin Breast Cancer 2004;5(4):279–84.

27. Rosen PP, Groshen S, Saigo S, et al. Pathological prognostic factors in stage I (TIN0M0) and stage II (TINIM0) breast carcinoma: a study of 644 patients with median follow-up of 18 years. J Clin Oncol 1989;7:1239–51.

28. Parker C, Rampaul RS, Pinder SE, et al. E-Cadherin as a prognostic indicator in primary breast cancer. Br J Cancer 2001;85:1958–63.

29. Rakha EA, El-Sayed ME, Powe DG, et al. Invasive lobular carcinoma of the breast: response to hormonal therapy and outcomes. Eur J Cancer 2008;44(1):73–83.

30. Elston CW, Ellis IO. Pathological prognostic factors in breast cancer I. The value of histological grade in breast cancer: experience from a large study with long-term follow-up. Histopathology 2002;41(3A):154–61.

31. Rakha EA, El-Sayed ME, Lee AH, et al. Prognostic significance of Nottingham histologic grade in invasive breast carcinoma. J Clin Oncol 2008;26(19):3153–8.

32. Rakha EA, El-Sayed ME, Menon S, et al. Histologic grading is an independent prognostic factor in invasive lobular carcinoma of the breast. Breast Cancer Res Treat 2008;111(1):121–7.

33. Pinder SE, Ellis IO, Galea M, et al. Pathological prognostic factors in breast cancer III. Vascular invasion: relationship with recurrence and survival in a large study with long-term follow-up. Histopathology 1994;24(1):41–7.

34. Truong PT, Yong CM, Abnousi F, et al. Lymphovascular invasion is associated with reduced locoregional control and survival in women with node-negative breast cancer treated with mastectomy and systemic therapy. J Am Coll Surg 2005;200(6):912–21.

35. Haybittle JL, Blamey RW, Elston CW, et al. A prognostic index in primary breast cancer. Br J Cancer 1982;45:361–6.

36. Ellis IO, Bell J, Todd J, et al. Evaluation of immunoreactivity with monoclonal antibody NCRC-II in breast carcinoma. Br J Cancer 1987;56:295–9.

37. Lee AH, Pinder SE, Macmillan RD, et al. Prognostic value of lymphovascular invasion in women with lymph node negative invasive breast carcinoma. Eur J Cancer 2006;42(3):357–62.

38. Gee JM, Eloranta JJ, Ibbitt JC, et al. Overexpression of TFAP2C in invasive breast cancer correlates with a poorer response to anti-hormone therapy and reduced patient survival. J Pathol 2009;217(1):32–41.

39. Sarwar N, Kim JS, Jiang J, et al. Phosphorylation of ERalpha at serine 118 in primary breast cancer and in tamoxifen-resistant tumours is indicative of a complex role for ERalpha phosphorylation in breast cancer progression. Endocr Relat Cancer 2006;13(3):851–61.

40. Gee JM, Shaw VE, Hiscox SE, et al. Deciphering antihormone-induced compensatory mechanisms in breast cancer and their therapeutic implications. Endocr Relat Cancer 2006;13(Suppl. 1):S77–88.

41. Dowle CS, Owainati A, Robins A, et al. The prognostic significance of the DNA content of human breast cancer. Br J Surg 1987;74:133–6.

42. Putti TC, El-Rehim DM, Rakha EA, et al. Estrogen receptor-negative breast carcinomas: a review of morphology and immunophenotypical analysis. Mod Pathol 2005;18(1):26–35.

43. Dowsett M, Allred C, Knox J, et al. Relationship between quantitative estrogen and progesterone receptor expression and human epidermal growth factor receptor 2 (HER-2) status with recurrence in the Arimidex, Tamoxifen, Alone or in Combination trial. J Clin Oncol 2008;26(7):1059–65.

44. Kumar RR, Meenakshi A, Sivakumar N. Enzyme immunoassay of human epidermal growth factor (hEGFR). Hum Antibodies 2001;10:143–7.

45. Eberhard DA, Huntzicker E, et al. Epidermal Growth Factor receptor immunohistochemistry: assay selection and amplification to breast cancers. ASCO 2002;no. 1791 (Abstr.).

46. Klijn JGM, Berns PMJ, Schmitz PI, et al. The clinical significance of epidermal growth factor receptor in human breast cancer: a review of 5232 patients. Endocr Rev 1992;13:3–17.

47. Tsutsui S, Ohno S, Murakami S, et al. Prognostic value of epidermal growth factor and its relationship to the ER status of 1029 patients with breast cancer. Breast Cancer Res Treat 2002;71:67–75.

48. Rampaul RS, Pinder SE, Robertson JF, et al. EGFR expression in operable breast cancer: is it of prognostic significance? Clin Cancer Res 2004;10(7):2578.

49. Ferrero JM, Ramaioli A, Largillier R, et al. Epidermal growth factor receptor expression in 780 breast cancer patients: a reappraisal of the prognostic value based on an eight-year median follow-up. Ann Oncol 2001;12(6):835–41.

50. Nicholson RI, McCelland RA, Gee JMW, et al. Epidermal growth factor receptor expression in breast cancer. Association with response to endocrine therapy. Breast Cancer Res Treat 1994;29:117–25.

51. Knoop A, Bentzen SM, Nielsen MM, et al. Value of epidermal growth factor receptor, HER-2, p53 and steroid receptors in predicting the efficacy of Tamoxifen in high risk postmenopausal breast cancer patients. J Clin Oncol 2001;19:3376–84.

52. Wolff AC, Hammond ME, Schwartz JN, et al. American Society of Clinical Oncology/College of American Pathologists guideline recommendations for human epidermal growth factor receptor 2 testing in breast cancer. J Clin Oncol 2007;25:118–45.

53. Ratcliffe N, Wells W, Wheeler K, et al. The combination of in situ hybridization and immunohistochemical analysis: an evaluation of Her2/neu expression in paraffin-embedded breast carcinomas and adjacent normal-appearing breast epithelium. Mod Pathol 1997;10:1247–52.

54. Busmanis I, Feleppa F, Jones A, et al. Analysis of cerbB2 expression using a panel of 6 commercially available antibodies. Pathology 1994;26:261–7.

55. Carlson RW, Moench SJ, Hammond ME, et al. HER2 testing in breast cancer: NCCN Task Force report and recommendations. J Natl Compr Canc Netw 2006;4(Suppl. 3):S1–24.

56. Bartlett JM, Going JJ, Mallon EA, et al. Evaluating HER2 amplification and overexpression in breast cancer. J Pathol 2001;195:422–8.

57. Press MF, Slamon DJ, Flom KJ, et al. Evaluation of HER-2/neu gene amplification and overexpression: comparison of frequently used assay methods in a molecularly characterized cohort of breast cancer specimens. J Clin Oncol 2002;20:3095–105.

58. Walker RA, Bartlett JM, Dowsett M, et al. HER2 testing in the UK: further update to recommendations. J Clin Pathol 2008;61(7):818–24.

59. Dowsett M, Bartlett J, Ellis IO, et al. Correlation between immunohistochemistry (HercepTest) and fluorescence in situ hybridization (FISH) for HER-2 in 426 breast carcinomas from 37 centres. J Pathol 2003;199:418–23.

60. Slamon DJ, Clark GM, Wong SG, et al. Human breast cancer: correlation of relapse and survival with amplification of the HER-2/neu oncogene. Science 1987;235(4785):177–82.

61. Rilke F, Colnaghi MI, Cascinelli N, et al. Prognostic significance of HER-2/neu expression in breast cancer and its relationship to other prognostic factors. Int J Cancer 1991;49(1):44–9.

62. Viani GA, Afonso SL, Stefano EJ, et al. Adjuvant trastuzumab in the treatment of her-2-positive early breast cancer: a meta-analysis of published randomized trials. BMC Cancer 2007;7:153.

63. Carter P, Presta L, Gorman CM, et al. Humanization of an anti-p185HER2 antibody for human cancer therapy. Proc Natl Acad Sci U S A 1992;89:4285–9.

64. Disis ML, Knutson KL, Schiffman K, et al. Pre-existent immunity to the HER-2/neu oncogenic protein in patients with HER-2/neu overexpressing breast and ovarian cancer. Breast Cancer Res Treat 2000;62:245–52.

65. Ward RL, Hawkins NJ, Coomber D, et al. Antibody immunity to the HER-2/neu oncogenic protein in patients with colorectal cancer. Hum Immunol 1999;60:510–5.

66. Mirza AN, Mirza NQ, Vlastos G, et al. Prognostic factors in node-negative breast cancer: a review of studies with sample size more than 200 and follow-up more than 5 years. Ann Surg 2002;235(1):10–26.

67. Bernards R, Destree A, McKenzie S, et al. Effective tumor immunotherapy directed against an oncogene-encoded product using a vaccinia virus vector. Proc Natl Acad Sci U S A 1987;84:6854–8.

68. Amar S, McCullough AE, Tan W, et al. Prognosis and outcome of small (≤1 cm), node-negative breast cancer on the basis of hormonal and HER-2 status. Oncologist 2010;15(10):1043–9.

69. Chia S, Norris B, Speers C, et al. Human epidermal growth factor receptor 2 overexpression as a prognostic factor in a large tissue microarray series of node-negative breast cancers. J Clin Oncol 2008;26:5697–704.

70. Kraus MH, Popescu NC, Amsbaugh SC, et al. Overexpression of the EGF receptor-related proto-oncogene erbB-2 in human mammary tumor cell lines by different molecular mechanisms. EMBO J 1987;6:605–10.

71. Ring CJ, Blouin P, Martin LA, et al. Use of transcriptional regulatory elements of the MUC1 and ERBB2 genes to drive tumour-selective expression of a pro-drug activating enzyme. Gene Ther 1997;4:1045–52.

72. Yu DH, Hung MC. Expression of activated rat neu oncogene is sufficient to induce experimental metastasis in 3T3 cells. Oncogene 1991;6:1991–6.

73. Bria E, Cuppone F, Fornier M, et al. Cardiotoxicity and incidence of brain metastases after adjuvant trastuzumab for early breast cancer: the dark side of the moon? A meta-analysis of the randomized trials. Breast Cancer Res Treat 2008;109(2):231–9.

74. Chang H, Riese 2nd DJ, Gilbert W, et al. Ligands for ErbB-family receptors encoded by a neuregulin-like gene. Nature 1997;387:509–12.

75. Juhl H, Downing SG, Wellstein A, et al. HER-2/neu is rate-limiting for ovarian cancer growth. Conditional depletion of HER-2/neu by ribozyme targeting. J Biol Chem 1997;272:29482–6.

76. Deshane J, Siegal GP, Wang M, et al. Transductional efficacy and safety of an intraperitoneally delivered adenovirus encoding an anti-erbB-2 intracellular single-chain antibody for ovarian cancer gene therapy. Gynecol Oncol 1997;64:378–85.

77. Schmidt M, Hynes NE, Groner B, et al. A bivalent single-chain antibody-toxin specific for ErbB-2 and the EGF receptor. Int J Cancer 1996;65:538–46.

78. Park JW, Hong K, Carter P, et al. Development of anti-p185HER2 immunoliposomes for cancer therapy. Proc Natl Acad Sci U S A 1995;92:1327–31.

79. Chen SY, Yang AG, Chen JD, et al. Potent antitumour activity of a new class of tumour-specific killer cells. Nature 1997;385:78–80.

80. Newby JC, Johnston SRD, Smith I, et al. Expression of epidermal growth factor and C-erb-2 during the development of tamoxifen resistance in human breast cancer. Clin Cancer Res 1997;3:1643–51.

81. Nicholson RI, McCelland RA, Finlay P, et al. Relationship between EGF-R, C-erb-2 protein expression and Ki67 immunostaining in breast cancer and hormone sensitivity. Eur J Cancer 1993;29A:1018–23.

82. Giai M, Roagna R, Ponzone R, et al. Prognostic and predictive relevance of C-erb-2 and ras expression in node positive and negative breast cancer. Anticancer Res 1994;14:1441–50.

83. Archer SG, Eliopoulos SA, Spandidos D, et al. Expression of ras p21, p53 and C-erb-2 in advanced breast cancer and response to first line hormonal therapy. Br J Cancer 1995;72:1259–66.

84. Pegram MD, Konecny GE, O'Callaghan C, et al. Rational combinations of trastuzumab with chemotherapeutic drugs used in the treatment of breast cancer. J Natl Cancer Inst 2004;96(10):739–49.

85. Muss H, Berry D, Thor A, et al. Lack of interaction of tamoxifen (T) use and ErbB-2/HER-2/neu (H) expression in CALGB 8541: a randomized adjuvant trial of three different doses of cyclophosphamide, doxorubicin and fluorouracil (CAF) in node-positive primary breast cancer (BC). Proc Am Soc Clin Oncol 1999;18:68a.

86. Paik S, Bryant J, Park C, et al. ErbB-2 and response to doxorubicin in patients with axillary lymph node positive, hormone receptor-negative breast cancer. J Natl Cancer Inst 1998;90:1361–70.

87. Elledge RM, Green S, Ciocca D, et al. HER-2 expression and response to tamoxifen in estrogen receptor-positive breast cancer: a Southwest Oncology Group Study. Clin Cancer Res 1998;4(1):7–12.

88. Ravin PM, Green S, Albain V, et al. Initial report of the SWOG biological correlative study of CerbB-2 expression as a predictor of outcome in a trial comparing adjuvant CAF with tamoxifen (T) alone. Proc Am Soc Clin Oncol 1998;17:97a.

89. Rakha EA, Reis-Filho JS, Ellis IO. Basal-like breast cancer: a critical review. J Clin Oncol 2008;26(15):2568–81.

90. Johannsson OT, Idvall I, Anderson C, et al. Tumour biological features of BRCA1-induced breast and ovarian cancer. Eur J Cancer 1997;33:362–71.

91. Chappuis PO, Nethercot V, Foulkes WD. Clinicopathological characteristics of BRCA1- and BRCA2-related breast cancer. Semin Surg Oncol 2000;18:287–95.

92. Marcus JN, Watson P, Page DL. Hereditary breast cancer. Pathobiology, prognosis and BRCA 1 and BRCA 2 linkage. Cancer 1996;77:697–709.

93. Marcus JN, Page DL, Watson P, et al. BRCA 1 and BRCA 2 hereditary breast cancer phenotypes. Cancer 1997;80:543.

94. Breast Cancer Linkage Consortium. Pathology of familial breast cancer: differences between breast cancer in carriers of BRCA 1 or BRCA 2 mutational and sporadic cases. Lancet 1997;349:1505.

95. Robson M, Gilewski T, Haas B, et al. BRCA-associated breast cancer in young women. J Clin Oncol 1998;16:1642–9.

96. Karp SE, Tonin PN, Bégin LR, et al. Influence of BRCA 1 mutations on nuclear grade and oestrogen receptor status of breast carcinoma in Ashkenazi Jewish women. Cancer 1997;80:435–41.

97. Armes JE, Egan AJM, Southey MC, et al. The histologic phenotypes of breast carcinoma occurring before age 40 in women with and without BRCA 1 or BRCA 2 germline mutations. Cancer 1998;83:2335–45.

98. Agnarsson BA, Jonasson JG, Björnsdottir IB, et al. Inherited BRCA 2 mutation associated with high grade breast cancer. Breast Cancer Res Treat 1998;47:121–7.

99. Marcus JN, Watson P, Page DL, et al. BRCA 2 hereditary breast cancer phenotype. Breast Cancer Res Treat 1997;44:275–7.

100. Baak JP, Colpaert CG, van Diest PJ, et al. Multivariate prognostic evaluation of the mitotic activity index and fibrotic focus in node-negative invasive breast cancers. Eur J Cancer 2005;41(14):2093–101.

101. Baak JPA, Vooiji GP, Brugal G. Nuclear image cytometry: quantitation of chromatin pattern, steroid receptor content and Ki-67. In: Baale JPA, editor. Manual of quantitative pathology in cancer diagnosis and prognosis. Heidelberg: Springer-Verlag; 1991. p. 232–43.

102. Palcic B, Garner DM, MacAulay CE. Image cytometry and chemoprevention in cervical cancer. J Cell Biochem 1995;23(Suppl.):43–54.

103. Nagahata T, Hirano A, Utada Y, et al. Correlation of allelic losses and clinicopathologic factors in 504 primary breast cancers. Breast Cancer 2002;9:208–15.

104. Hermsen M.A.J.A., Baak JPA, Weiss J, et al. Genetic analysis of 513 lymph node negative breast carcinomas by CGH and relation to clinical, pathologic, morphometric and DNA cytometric prognostic factors. J Pathol 1998;186:356–62.

105. Janssen EAM, Baak JPA, Guervos MA, et al. In lymph node-negative breast cancer, specific chromosomal aberrations are strongly associated with high mitotic activity and predict outcome more accurately than grade, tumour diameter, and oestrogen receptor. J Pathol 2003;201(4):555–61.

106. Hyman E, Kauraniemi P, Hautaniemi S, et al. Impact of DNA amplification on gene expression patterns in breast cancer. Cancer Res 2002;62:6240–5.

107. Hu Z, Fan C, Oh DS, et al. The molecular portraits of breast tumors are conserved across microarray platforms. BMC Genomics 2006;7:96.

108. Hedenfalk I, Duggan D, Chen Y, et al. Gene expression profiles in hereditary breast cancer. N Eng J Med 2001;344:539–48.

109. van't Veer LJ, Dai H, van de Vijer MJ, et al. Expression profiling predicts outcomes in breast cancer. Breast Cancer Res 2002;5:57–8.

110. Gruvberger S, Ringner M, Chen Y, et al. Oestrogen receptor status in breast cancer is associated with remarkably distinct gene expression profiles. Cancer Res 2001;61:5979–84.

111. West M, Blanchette C, Dressman H, et al. Predicting the clinical status of human breast cancer by using gene expression profiles. Proc Natl Acad Sci U S A 2001;98:11462–7.

112. Ahr A, Kam T, Solbach S, et al. Identification of high risk breast cancer by gene expression profiling. Lancet 2002;359:131–2.

113. van de Vijver MJ, He YD, van't Veer LJ. A gene expression signature as a predictor of survival in breast cancer. N Engl J Med 2002;347:1999–2009.

114. Leong A.S.-Y., Zhuang Z. The changing role of pathology in breast cancer diagnosis and treatment. Pathobiology 2011;78(2):99–114.

115. Bertucci F, Viens P, Hingamp P, et al. Breast cancer revisited using DNA array-based gene expression profiling. Int J Cancer 2003;103(5):565–71.

116. Perou CM, Sorlie T, Eisen MB, et al. Molecular portraits of human breast tumours. Nature 2000;406:747–52.

117. Habel LA, Shak S, Jacobs MK, et al. A population-based study of tumor gene expression and risk of breast cancer death among lymph node-negative patients. Breast Cancer Res 2006;8:R25.

118. Chang HY, Nuyten DS, Sneddon JB, et al. Robustness, scalability, and integration of a wound-response gene expression signature in predicting breast cancer survival. Proc Natl Acad Sci U S A 2005;102:3738–43.

119. Chi JT, Wang Z, Nuyten DS, et al. Gene expression programmes in response to hypoxia: cell type specificity and prognostic significance in human cancers. PLoS Med 2006;3:e47.

120. McCelland CM, Gullick WJ. Identification of surrogate markers for determining drug activity using proteomics. Biochem Soc Trans 2003;31(6):1488–90.

121. Chevallier B, Mossen V, Dauce JP, et al. A prognostic score in histological node negative breast cancer. Br J Cancer 1990;61:436–40.

122. Brown JM, Benson EA, Jones M. Confirmation of a long term prognostic index in breast cancer. Breast 1993;2:144–7.

123. Balslev I, Axesson CK, Zedelev K, et al. The Nottingham Prognostic Index applied to 9,149 patients from the studies of the Danish Breast Cancer Cooperative Group (DBCG). Br Cancer Res Treat 1994;32:281–90.

124. Ravdin PM, Siminoff LA, Davis GJ, et al. Computer programme to assist in making decisions about adjuvant therapy for women with early breast cancer. J Clin Oncol 2001;19:980–91.

125. Goldhirsch A, Glick JH, Gelber RD, et al. Meeting highlights: international expert consensus on the primary therapy of early breast cancer 2005. Ann Oncol 2005;16:1569–83.

126. Wishart GC, Azzato EM, Greenberg DC, et al. PREDICT: a new UK prognostic model that predicts survival following surgery for invasive breast cancer. Breast Cancer Res 2010;12(1):R1.

127. Robertson JF, Ellis IO, Pearson D, et al. Biological factors of prognostic significance in locally advanced breast cancer. Breast Cancer Res Treat 1994;29(3):259–64.

128. Robertson JF, Dixon AR, Nicholson RI, et al. Confirmation of a prognostic index for patients with metastatic breast cancer treated by endocrine therapy. Breast Cancer Res Treat 1992;22(3):221–7.

129. Ellis IO, et al. Improvement of the Nottingham Prognostic Index (NPI +). Cancer Res (In Press).

3

Nipple discharge and the role of ductoscopy in breast diseases

Sarah Tang
Gerald Gui

Introduction

After breast lumps and mastalgia, spontaneous nipple discharge forms the next most common symptom, comprising 3–8% of referrals to symptomatic breast clinics.[1,2] The majority of nipple discharge is benign, with up to 20% being associated with an underlying malignancy.[3] Conventional methods of investigating nipple discharge include mammography, ultrasound and smear cytology, each of which have recognised limitations. Standard operations such as microdochectomy and major duct excision are undirected procedures that carry a risk of leaving undiagnosed pathology in the breast.

Mammary ductoscopy allows direct visualisation of the duct epithelium to locate the lesion precisely and to map the three-dimensional anatomy. Endoscopic instruments for diagnostic biopsy and therapeutic excision are available. The ability to visualise normal or benign ductal structures may facilitate conservative management of symptomatic nipple discharge and enable targeted excision of visualised lesions or indeterminate areas.

Causes of nipple discharge

The causes of nipple discharge are wide ranging. The majority of discharge is physiological, hormone related or results from benign breast change. A recent meta-analysis that included over 3000 women with nipple discharge demonstrated an overall incidence of underlying breast malignancy of 18.7%,[3] which is higher than the figure reported in many individual series.

Bilateral multiduct discharge can be stimulated by nipple manipulation in the majority of premenopausal women. The production of such physiological fluid is exploited by researchers of the intraductal approach for cytological, molecular and protein-based studies. This fluid is more likely to be released from the ducts if the nipples are repeatedly stimulated by chafing against clothing and during physical activities such as jogging. Squeezing of the nipples to elicit such discharge perpetuates symptoms. This is because the nipple ducts are plugged by keratin and repeated stimulation or squeezing removes the keratin plugs and allows the fluid that is normally present in the ductal tree to leak on to the surface of the nipple. The fluid in physiological discharge ranges from clear to white to yellow to green to black.

The most common physiological nipple discharge is lactation. Ongoing milky discharge may occur up to 2 years following a pregnancy and is a normal phenomenon. Galactorrhoea can also result from prolactin-secreting pituitary adenomas, medication that influences the oestrogen, progesterone or prolactin pathways, hypothyroidism and recreational drugs such as marijuana. Commonly prescribed medical drugs that may cause nipple discharge are summarised in Table 3.1.

Table 3.1 • Common drugs that mimic galactorrhea and the likely underlying mechanisms of action

Mechanism of action	Medication
Dopamine receptor blockade	**Antidepressants:** Selective serotonin reuptake inhibitors (citalopram, fluoxetine, paroxetine, sertraline) Tricyclic antidepressants **Antipsychotics:** Risperidone Butyrophenones (haloperidol) Phenothiazines (chlorpromazine) Thioxanthenes (chlorprothixene, flupenthixol) **Anti-emetics:** Metoclopromide Domperidone
Dopamine depletion	Methyldopa Reserpine Monoamine oxidase inhibitors
Inhibition of dopamine release	Codeine Heroin Morphine
Histamine receptor blockade	Cimetidine Famotidine Ranitidine
Stimulation of breast tissue and lactotrophs	Oral contraceptives
Mechanism unknown	Verapamil

Duct ectasia and benign breast change are common causes of multiduct discharge. In duct ectasia, the breast ducts become tortuous and dilated, predisposing to fluid accumulation. This fluid may discharge spontaneously or upon manipulation when the sphincters distal to the lactiferous sinuses relax and the keratin plugs are displaced. Common situations that may trigger loss of these keratin plugs and sphincter relaxation include massage and warm comfortable environments such as in a bath or under bedsheets. Cysts do not usually communicate directly with breast ducts. It has been suggested that inflammation related to a cyst may result in erosion into a duct system but this is unproven. The colour of nipple discharge associated with duct ectasia and fibrocystic change can vary from clear to white, yellow, grey, green, brown or black. This is the same colour range seen in physiological discharge. Nipple discharge arising in relation to inflammation and irritation of the lining of the ducts may be blood stained and contain acute inflammatory cells.

Persistent spontaneous discharge from a single nipple orifice is usually indicative of specific pathology involving that duct. Benign intraductal papillomas account for about 80% of single-duct bloodstained nipple discharges.[2,4,5] Papillomas give rise to nipple discharge of varying colour but as these structures can bleed intermittently, papillomas are often associated with blood staining. Recent bleeding may manifest as frank blood, but stagnant bloodstained fluid can be dark red, brown or black.

Periductal mastitis is a chronic and recurrent inflammatory condition associated with smoking in younger women. Purulent nipple discharge can be seen in later stages when the duct ruptures and an abscess or mammary duct fistula has developed.

Invasive breast cancer is an uncommon cause of spontaneous nipple discharge as the proliferating mass usually obliterates the duct lumen. Ductal carcinoma in situ or an extensive area of in situ disease in association with an invasive breast cancer may predispose to bloodstained nipple discharge. Bloodstained nipple discharge should be distinguished from bleeding from the nipple surface that may occur with Paget's disease.

Assessment

A thorough breast problem orientated history is taken including a drug history, and a complete clinical examination should also be performed.

✔✔ Pathological nipple discharge is considered to be discharge arising from a single duct that is persistent (defined as more than twice per week). At age over 50 years, the presence of blood in the discharge and the presence of a clinical lump increase significantly the risk of associated malignancy,[3,6] and it is recommended that these patients are fully investigated by conventional imaging techniques. Normal imaging should direct further investigation as appropriate and consideration of diagnostic surgical excision.

Bilateral physiological multiduct discharge aggravated by manipulation in younger patients usually resolves when the triggering factors are removed. Bilateral and profuse milky discharge in the younger population should be investigated by measuring serum prolactin and if elevated, supplemented by magnetic resonance imaging (MRI) of the pituitary gland. Thyroid function tests may be indicated if there are appropriate clinical features.

The colour of nipple discharge is not a reliable method of distinguishing between physiological, benign or malignant aetiologies.

✓✓ However, a recent meta-analysis found a higher incidence of underlying malignancy in patients with bloodstained nipple discharge compared to those with non-bloody discharge (of any colour description; odds ratio (OR) = 2.27, 95% confidence interval (CI) = 1.32–3.89) or when compared to those with serous discharge alone (OR = 2.49, 95% CI = 1.25–4.93).[3] It is therefore recommended that all patients with bloodstained nipple discharge are investigated fully.

Mammography is indicated in women over the age of 35 years and may demonstrate a mass or microcalcification in association with nipple discharge of malignant aetiology. Even in younger women with bloodstained discharge, mammography can demonstrate calcification in women with widespread ductal carcinoma in situ (DCIS). Other mammographic features may also be evident in patients with benign nipple discharge. Duct ectasia may occasionally be visible on mammography. The sensitivity of mammography in detecting pathology in nipple discharge is 57.1% (positive predictive value (PPV) of 16.7% and negative predictive value (NPV) of 91.4%).[7] In a study of 306 patients with nipple discharge who had normal mammography and ultrasound, 10% were subsequently found to have underlying malignancy.[7]

Ultrasound can reliably diagnose duct ectasia and can identify discrete intraductal lesions. Papillomas below a threshold size of 1–2 mm may not be visible on ultrasound imaging. Ultrasound-guided core biopsy can be used to obtain a tissue diagnosis of any lesions visualised but papillary lesions are often assessed as an indeterminate B3 lesion and so usually still require excision for a definitive tissue diagnosis. A vacuum-assisted ultrasound-guided mammotome biopsy can be both diagnostic and therapeutic. Fine-needle aspiration of papillary lesions is usually unhelpful as cytology rarely resolves diagnostic uncertainty.

Ductography is less widely used but is an investigation that gives clear delineation of the breast anatomy. A small amount of radio-opaque contrast is instilled into a cannulated nipple duct. Accurate detection of small filling defect(s) caused by papillomas and duct narrowing or obstruction from malignant change can be recognised. However, ductography does not provide a tissue diagnosis and the precise position of the area of interest within the breast is not usually available to the surgeon, although it is possible to target the area of abnormality with a wire localisation procedure. The use of MRI to evaluate the ductal tree is gaining interest but is not a standard investigation of nipple discharge. In a comparative study of 163 patients with nipple discharge who had normal mammography and ultrasound, ductography was found to have a PPV of 19% and an NPV of 63%. MRI was performed in 52 patients and found to have a PPV of 56% and an NPV of 87%.[7]

Smear cytology of nipple discharge may show the presence of malignant cells, papillary cells, red blood cells, benign duct epithelium or foam cells of macrophage origin. The available literature demonstrates sensitivities of smear cytology ranging from 11.1% to 16.7%[8,9] and specificities ranging from 66.1% to 96.3%. In Simmons et al.'s study of 108 pathological specimens for nipple discharge, the PPV of smear cytology was 50% and the NPV was 76.5%.[8] These data arise from an era before mammary ductoscopy when surgery providing the pathology used as the gold standard could not be targeted, so some of the pathologies present may have been missed at surgery, hence lowering the PPV of cytology. A further limitation arises when insufficient epithelial cells are available for a reliable diagnosis. This may be overcome by enhanced techniques of obtaining nipple fluid such as ductal lavage to increase the cell yield, which can improve the performance of cytological assessment.

Conventional surgery

The indications for surgical intervention are persistent (defined as >2 per week) single-duct discharge in a woman over the age of 50 years, guided further by the results of abnormal investigations. Pressure over a discrete lesion such as a symptomatic papilloma often results in duct-specific discharge. The target lesion may be skin marked or wire localised if impalpable, to ensure excision of the target lesion.

Current surgery for pathological nipple discharge consists of major duct excision and microdochectomy.

Major duct excision in the absence of an imaging abnormality is an undirected operation where a disc or wedge of retroareolar tissue is excised. The amount of breast tissue that is excised is at the discretion of the surgeon's clinical judgment but often includes a considerable amount of tissue that does not need to be resected for a benign process. The greater the amount of tissue resected, the higher the risk of surgical complications including altered sensation, haemoseromas, poor aesthetic outcome from volume loss and nipple ischaemia. Microdochectomy aims to resect a single duct guided by passing a lacrimal probe down the offending duct system. The branching system of the ductal tree makes this procedure imprecise and the surgeon is blind throughout the operation as to the location, depth and number of lesions that form the target of the resection. The risk of perforating the cannulated duct with the probe is high and if the surgeon performs a wide resection around the probe then it in effect becomes a much bigger procedure. Proximal lesions further than 3 cm from the nipple base are likely to be missed by these undirected techniques.

Despite the limitations, these operations do form the current standard surgical practice. Surgery to the breast ducts should be avoided in women of childbearing age who wish to breast feed, as surgical injury or scarring are likely to lead to restricted or failed lactation.

Mammary ductoscopy and nipple discharge

Spontaneous nipple discharge lends itself well to mammary ductoscopy (MD) as the ductal orifice is readily identified and coexisting duct ectasia can aid scope passage. Positive endoscopic findings can be used to guide surgery resulting in targeted excision. Visualisation of remaining ducts can rule out coexisting pathology and avoid unnecessary resection of normal parenchyma. MD is not widely available and its role as an established procedure remains to be defined.

MD by an experienced endoscopist can be more accurate than mammography in identifying extensive in situ disease (65% vs. 50%).[10] Ling et al. found that MD-guided intraductal biopsy had a significantly higher papilloma detection rate than undirected miocrodochectomy (92.6% vs. 40.7%, $P<0.05$).[11] Normal findings at MD may endorse a

conservative approach or alternatively facilitate a recommendation for duct transaction alone to manage symptomatic nipple discharge.

History and technology

Microendoscopic technology has advanced and earlier limitations of poor optical resolution and problems with access because of the large calibre of scopes have been overcome. The development of working channels within microendoscopes has made it possible to biopsy lesions under direct vision using cytology brushes and microbiopsy forceps. Accessories for localisation, such as self-retaining hookwires or rhomboids that are immobilised by expansion within the duct, can be passed down the working channel to demarcate the area of interest for open therapeutic excision.

Current scopes can be flexible or rigid, with diameters that range from 0.7 to 1.2 mm (**Fig. 3.1**). Microendoscopes magnify up to 60 times to produce high-quality images with saline for insufflation and irrigation of the ducts. More recent developments include autofluorescence technology,[12] which may help to distinguish between benign, premalignant and malignant lesions.

Technical considerations

The duct orifices are identified by nipple fluid expression by warming, massage or gentle pressure. The orifice may be dilated and some systems require a working shaft to be inserted, through which the scope is passed.

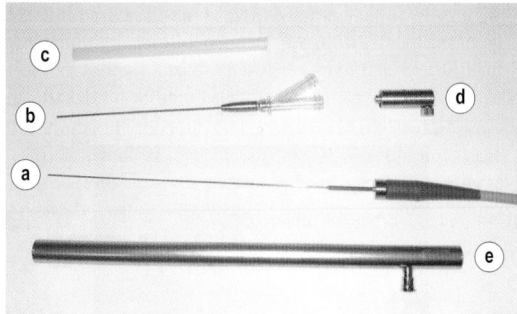

Figure 3.1 • The dissembled components of a 0.9-mm LaDuscope® (PolyDiagnost GmbH, Pfaffenhofen, Germany) comprising the fibreoptic scope **(a)**, disposable two-port cannula **(b)**, cannula sheath **(c)**, shifter **(d)** and protective metal sheath for the fibreoptic for use during sterilisation **(e)**.

MD, when associated with a standard surgical procedure, is often performed under general anaesthetic. Diagnostic MD can be performed as an outpatient procedure with topical local anaesthetic applied to the nipple, followed by periareolar infiltration and/or infusion down the cannulated duct, the latter facilitating relaxation of the muscle sphincters.[13,14] Methylene blue dye, marking wires, clips and transillumination[15] may be used for orientation, to localise lesions, guide surgical excision and facilitate pathological assessment.[15-17]

Complications of MD are uncommon and include pain, inflammation and infection. Duct perforation by the scope creates a false passage that can be recognised by the yellow cavernous honeycomb appearance of adipose tissue.

Intraduct appearances

There is general consensus on the intraductal appearances of common lesions from studies that have used histological correlation (**Figs 3.2** and **3.3**). Malignant lesions are more likely to display haemorrhagic characteristics, streaking, fissuring and irregularity of the ductal walls or present with a luminal mass that might obstruct the duct. In contrast, benign non-papillomatous lesions have a smooth, level surface without haemorrhagic features.[4,18-21]

MD sensitivity at detecting papillomas is high at 96–97%[11,19] with a PPV of 73%.[21] Benign duct strictures may on occasion limit MD access.[21] Sensitivity for detecting DCIS and invasive disease is lower, with reports ranging from 41% to 81%.[19,22] The presence of an extensive non-invasive component associated with an invasive cancer increases significantly the likelihood of abnormal ductoscopic findings (71% vs. 16%).[23]

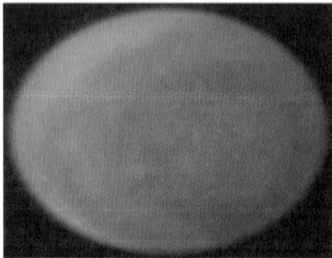

Figure 3.2 • A still image from mammary ductoscopy showing a large papilloma within a duct with otherwise normal epithelium.

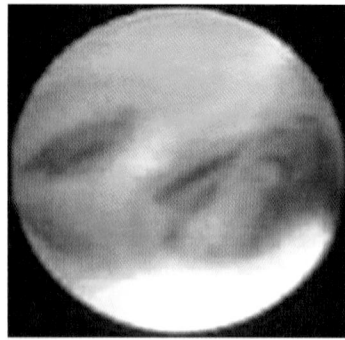

Figure 3.3 • A still image from mammary ductoscopy showing DCIS and invasive disease in branching ducts.

Pathological considerations

The diagnostic sensitivity of MD can be improved by incorporating ductal lavage cytology,[24] which generates information from the proximal ducts that may be out of reach of the ductoscope. In a study of 415 women, the PPV of 80% of MD alone in detecting DCIS was improved to 100% by the addition of lavage cytology.[25] The cell count can be further enhanced using fine brushes passed down the working channel to exfoliate intraluminal lesions under direct vision, yielding up to 33 000 cells.[26,27] A cell-rich endoscopy specimen allows better discrimination between benign cells, mild to severe atypia and malignant cells. A normal duct on MD is infrequently associated with abnormal cytology.[14]

Reliable methods of intraductal biopsy are essential if MD is to achieve a histological diagnosis without surgical excision. Various techniques have been developed using vacuum-assisted biopsy systems, endobaskets and grasping clips.[11,23,28] The intraductal breast biopsy (IDBB) system pioneered by Hunerbein and Matsunaga consists of a 0.7-mm gradient index endoscope covered by an external metal sheath containing a side opening aperture near its tip.[23,28] This technique yields diagnostic material in 89–92% of cases with a sensitivity of 76.2% and a specificity of 100% for papillomas.[10,23] Using biopsy clips, Ling et al. were able to produce diagnostic samples in 90% of patients.[11] Biopsy techniques can be extended to perform therapeutic endoscopic papillomectomy.[29,30] In two studies, IDBB stopped symptomatic nipple discharge with therapeutic efficacies of 77.6% and 95.4%.[28,29] Carcinomas are associated with a lower diagnostic biopsy yield (58.3%).[28] It is postulated that carcinomas are generally located more peripherally in the terminal ducts and can be difficult to access by MD.[28]

Limitations

In the context of nipple discharge, the majority of lesions are found within 5 cm of the nipple but up to 37% may be proximal and therefore out of the reach of a 6-cm ductoscope.[15,21] Unlike other applications for microendoscopy such as the salivary gland, where there is a sizeable single-duct orifice, breast ducts open via multiple tiny orifices at or just below the nipple surface. There is variability in the number of duct systems, with one anatomy study demonstrating 29 ducts arising from 15 orifices.[31] This study also found that some ducts branch within the nipple itself and may not be accessed readily by lavage cannulae or MD.

Ductoscopy and breast cancer

MD as an adjunct to breast conservation surgery for cancer is technically feasible, with high rates of tumour visualisation.[13] In a subsequent publication, Dooley successfully identified the malignant lesion on MD in 150 out of 201 patients (74.6%), found additional lesions outside the planned excision site in 83 cases (41%) and decreased the positive margin rate from 23.5% to 5%.[32] Louie et al. reported lower tumour visualisation rates in 6 of 14 (43%) patients and did not show any benefit of MD in reducing positive margin rates.[22] The role of duct endoscopy in breast cancer management is currently limited outside clinical trials.

Key points

- Nipple discharge is the third most common presenting symptom to breast clinics.
- More than 80% of nipple discharge is benign.
- Mammography and ultrasound have a low sensitivity and specificity for diagnosing the cause of nipple discharge.
- Nipple smear cytology has a low sensitivity and positive predictive value.
- The risk of an underlying malignancy is increased if the nipple discharge is spontaneous, single duct, persistent (occurs more than twice per week), bloody, age >50 years and associated with a palpable abnormality.
- Mammary ductoscopy allows direct visualisation of the ductal epithelium and can be used to direct surgical resection of target lesions while limiting resection of normal breast tissue.
- The development of microbiopsy forceps, cytology brushes and intraductal localisation wires has enhanced the role of mammary ductoscopy as an interventional diagnostic and therapeutic procedure.

References

1. Baitchez G, Gortchev G, Todorova A, et al. Intraductal aspiration cytology and galactography for nipple discharge. Int Surg 2003;88:83–6.

2. Okazaki A, Hirata K, Okazaki M, et al. Nipple discharge disorders: current diagnostic management and the role of fibre-ductoscopy. Eur Radiol 1999;9:583–90.

3. Chen L, Zhou WB, Zhao Y, et al. Bloody nipple discharge is a predictor of breast cancer risk: a meta-analysis. Breast Cancer Res Treat 2012;132(1):9–14. This is the first meta-analysis of bloodstained nipple discharge in relation to breast cancer incidence. It showed a significant association between bloodstained nipple discharge and underlying malignancy when compared to serous or coloured discharge.

4. Kapenhas-Valdes E, Feldman SM, Cohen J-M, et al. Mammary ductoscopy for evaluation of nipple discharge. Ann Surg Oncol 2008;15:2720–7.

5. Khan SA, Mangat A, Rivers A, et al. Office ductoscopy for surgical selection in women with pathologic nipple discharge. Ann Surg Oncol 2011;18:3785–90.

6. Dolan RT, Butler JS, Kell MR, et al. Nipple discharge and the efficacy of cytology in evaluating breast cancer risk. Surgeon 2010;8:252–8. This retrospective study of 313 patients with nipple discharge found that duct cytology was diagnostic of only 50% of underlying breast carcinoma but identified four risk factors as having a significant association with breast carcinoma: (a) age >50 years (P<0.0001); (b) bloody nipple discharge (P<0.008); (c) presence of a breast lump (P<0.0001); and (d) single-duct discharge (P<0.006). This provides evidence in line with current expert opinion and contributes to the strong recommendation made in conjunction with Ref. 3.

7. Morrogh M, Morris EA, Liberman L, et al. The predictive value of ductography and magnetic resonance imaging in the management of nipple discharge. Ann Surg Oncol 2007;14:3369–77.

8. Simmons R, Adamovich T, Brennan M, et al. Nonsurgical evaluation of pathologic nipple discharge. Ann Surg Oncol 2003;10:113–6.

9. Kooistra BW, Wauters C, van de Ven S, et al. The diagnostic value of nipple discharge cytology in 618 consecutive patients. Eur J Surg Oncol 2009;35:573–7.

10. Dobowy A, Raubach M, Topalidis T, et al. Breast duct endoscopy: ductosocpy from a diagnostic to an interventional procedure and its future perspective. Acta Chir Belg 2011;111:142–5.

11. Ling H, Liu GY, Lu JS, et al. Fiberoptic ductoscopy-guided intraductal biopsy improve the diagnosis of nipple discharge. Breast J 2009;15:168–75.

12. Jacobs VR, Paepke S, Schaaf H, et al. Autofluorescence ductoscopy: a new imaging technique for intraductal breast endoscopy. Clin Breast Cancer 2007;8:619–23.

13. Dooley WC. Endoscopic visualization of breast tumors. JAMA 2000;284:1518.

14. Dooley W, Francescatti D, Clark L, et al. Office-based breast ductoscopy for diagnosis. Am J Surg 2004;188:415–8.

15. Dooley WC. Routine operative breast endoscopy for bloody nipple discharge. Ann Surg Oncol 2002;9:920–3.

16. Escobar PF, Baynes D, Crowe JP. Ductoscopy-assisted microdochectomy. Int J Fertil Womens Med 2004;49:222–4.

17. Zhu X, Xing C, Jin T, et al. A randomized controlled study of selective microdochectomy guided by ductoscopic wire marking or methylene blue injection. Am J Surg 2011;201:221–5.

18. Shen KW, Wu K, Lu JS, et al. Fiberoptic ductoscopy for patients with nipple discharge. Cancer 2000;89:1512–9.

19. Matsunaga T, Ohta D, Misak T, et al. Mammary ductoscopy for diagnosis and treatment of intraductal lesions of the breast. Breast Cancer 2001;8:213–21.

20. Rose C, Bojahr B, Grunwald S, et al. Ductoscopy-based descriptors of intraductal lesions and their histopathologic correlates. Onkologie 2010;33:307–12.

21. Moncrief RM, Nayar R, Diaz L, et al. A comparison of ductoscopy-guided and conventional surgical excision in women with spontaneous nipple discharge. Ann Surg 2005;241:575–81.

22. Louie LD, Crowe JP, Dawson AE, et al. Identification of breast cancer in patients with pathologic nipple discharge: does ductoscopy predict malignancy? Am J Surg 2006;192:530–3.

23. Hunerbein M, Dubowy A, Raubach M, et al. Gradient index ductoscopy and intraductal biopsy of intraductal breast lesions. Am J Surg 2007;194:511–4.

24. Denewer A, El-Etribi K, Nada N, et al. The role and limitations of mammary ductoscopy in management of pathologic nipple discharge. Breast J 2008;14:442–9.

25. Shen KW, Wu J, Lu JS, et al. Fiberoptic ductoscopy for breast cancer patients with nipple discharge. Surg Endosc 2001;15:1340–5.

26. Khan SA, Baird C, Staradub VL, et al. Ductal lavage and ductoscopy: the opportunities and the limitations. Clin Breast Cancer 2002;3:185–91.

27. Johnson-Maddux A, Ashfaq R, Cler L, et al. Reproducibility of cytologic atypia in repeat nipple duct lavage. Cancer 2005;103:1129–36.

28. Matsunaga T, Kawakami R, Namba K, et al. Intraductal biopsy for diagnosis and treatment of intraductal lesions of the breast. Cancer 2004;101:2164–69.

29. Bender O, Balci F, Yuney E, et al. Scarless endoscopic papillectomy of the breast. Onkologie 2009;32:94–8.

30. Kamali S, Bendoer O, Aydin MT, et al. Ductoscopy in the evaluation and management of nipple discharge. Ann Surg Oncol 2010;17:778–83.

31. Rusby JE, Brachtel EF, Michaelson JS, et al. Breast duct anatomy in the human nipple: three dimensional patterns and clinical applications. Breast Cancer Res Treat 2007;106:171–9.

32. Dooley WC. Routine operative breast endoscopy during lumpectomy. Ann Surg Oncol 2003;10:38–42.

4

Breast-conserving surgery: the balance between good cosmesis and local control

J. Michael Dixon

Introduction

The aim of local treatment of breast cancer is to achieve long-term local disease control with the minimum of local morbidity. The majority of women presenting symptomatically to breast clinics and those who are diagnosed through screening programmes have small breast cancers, which are suitable for breast-conserving surgery.

✅✅ The major advantages of breast-conserving treatment are as follows:

- breast-conserving treatment produces an acceptable cosmetic appearance in the majority of women with breast cancer;[1]
- breast-conserving treatment results in lower levels of psychological morbidity, with less anxiety and depression and improved body image, sexuality and self-esteem, compared with mastectomy;[2,3]
- two systematic reviews have shown equivalence in terms of disease outcome for breast-conserving treatment and mastectomy.[4,5]

One of these reviews (search date 1995) analysed data from six randomised controlled trials that compared breast conservation treatment with mastectomy.[4] A meta-analysis of data from five of these six trials involving 3006 women found no significant difference in the risk of death at 10 years (odds ratio 0.91, 95% confidence interval (CI) 0.78–1.05). The sixth randomised trial used different protocols. In the second systematic review, nine randomised controlled trials involving 4981 women

randomised to mastectomy or breast-conserving treatment were included in the analysis.[5] A meta-analysis of these nine trials found no significant difference in the risk of death over 10 years: the relative risk reduction for breast-conserving surgery compared with mastectomy was 0.02 (95% CI −0.05 to +0.09).[5] There was also no difference in the rates of local recurrence in the six randomised controlled trials involving 3006 women where data were available: the relative risk reduction for mastectomy versus breast-conserving surgery was 0.04 (95% CI −0.04 to +0.12).[4]

✅ Originally it was thought that local therapy had little influence on overall survival but it is clear that local failure is responsible, at least in part, for some patients developing metastatic disease.[6,7]

It is thus important in patients selected for breast-conserving surgery to minimise local recurrence while at the same time achieving a good cosmetic outcome.

Selection of patients for breast conservation

Traditionally, single cancers clinically measuring 4 cm or less, without signs of local advancement, have been managed by breast-conserving treatment (Box 4.1). Different units have different size criteria and many units have a tumour size cut-off for breast-conserving surgery of 3 cm or less clinically.

Box 4.1 • Indications and contraindications for breast-conserving surgery

Indications

- T1, T2 (<4 cm), N0, N1, M0
- T2 >4 cm in large breasts
- Single clinical and mammographic lesion

Relative contraindications*

- T4, N2 or M1
- Patients who prefer mastectomy†
- Clinically or radiologically evident multifocal/multicentric disease
- Collagen vascular disease
- Large or central tumours in small breasts
- Women with a strong family history of breast cancer or who are proven BRCA1 and BRCA2 mutation carriers

*None of these are absolute contraindications.
†Following a fully informed discussion of the pros and cons of breast-conserving surgery vs mastectomy.

✔ Increasing tumour size does not equate with increasing local recurrence rates and limiting breast-conserving surgery to cancers below a certain size is illogical.

Clinical tumour size overestimates actual tumour size. There is a much better correlation between pathological tumour size and the size measured on imaging, with ultrasound assessment being more accurate than mammographic measurements.[8] Magnetic resonance imaging (MRI) appears better than ultrasound in assessing disease extent, particularly in invasive lobular carcinoma.[9] The problem with MRI is that it has a low specificity and a low positive predictive value in that only two-thirds of lesions identified by MRI as suspicious of malignancy are subsequently confirmed as malignant.[10] The role of MRI in assessing patients for breast-conserving surgery has been investigated in a randomised study and the conclusions of this study were that routine use of MRI is not worthwhile.[8,11] MRI did not reduce the rate of incomplete excisions and was not associated with a reduction in short-term local recurrence but did significantly increase the mastectomy rate in patients who were otherwise considered good candidates for breast-conserving surgery. It is the balance between tumour size as assessed by imaging and breast volume that determines whether

a patient is suitable for breast-conserving surgery rather than tumour size per se. Options for patients with tumours considered too large, relative to the size of the breast, for breast-conserving treatment include neoadjuvant systemic therapy to shrink the tumour, an oncoplastic procedure (see Chapter 6) involving either transfer of tissue into the breast or remodelling of the breast with surgery to the opposite breast to obtain symmetry (see Chapter 6).[12,13] In a patient with small breasts, excision of even a small tumour may produce an unacceptable cosmetic result.

Patients with multiple tumours in the same breast have not previously been considered good candidates for breast-conserving treatment because they were reported to have a high reported incidence of in-breast recurrence[14,15] and so have usually been treated by mastectomy, combined in appropriate patients with immediate reconstruction. Recent evidence has, however, demonstrated similar rates of local recurrence for both patients with unifocal and with multifocal and even multicentric disease.[16,17] If it is feasible to excise the separate cancers in different parts of the breast and produce an acceptable cosmetic outcome then such patients should no longer be treated routinely by mastectomy. Satisfactory rates of local control following breast-conserving treatment for multifocal or multicentric cancers are achieved providing all disease is excised to clear margins.[16,17] Early studies on multifocal and multicentric cancers often failed to achieve clear margins and this explains the high rates of local recurrence reported in these early series.[15] Patients with bilateral cancers can also be treated by bilateral breast conservation. The rates of breast-conserving surgery vary significantly between countries and within countries. These rates are clearly influenced as much by the views of the surgeon treating the patient as the availability of radiotherapy locally. Failure to offer breast-conserving surgery to suitable and appropriate patients has become a medico-legal issue. If a patient who fulfils the criteria for breast-conserving surgery is treated by mastectomy then the exact reasons for the decision to proceed to mastectomy should be recorded legibly in the patient's notes. Some patients choose mastectomy in preference to breast-conserving surgery but do so based on an inadequate understanding that outcomes for the two treatments are identical. In one series of patients choosing mastectomy rather than breast-conserving surgery, over half of patients did not know that mastectomy and breast-conserving surgery produces identical rates of survival.[18]

A range of clinical and pathological factors have influenced surgeons selecting patients for breast-conserving surgery because of their perceived impact on local recurrence. These include young age (under 35–39 years), the presence of an extensive in situ component associated with an invasive tumour, grade 3 histology and widespread lymphatic/vascular invasion. These are considered in detail below.

Breast-conserving surgery

Two surgical procedures have been studied extensively: quadrantectomy and wide local excision. Quadrantectomy was based on the belief that the breast is organised into segments, with each segment draining into its own major duct, and that invasive cancer spreads down the duct system towards the nipple.[19] Both of these premises are incorrect.

✔ A single major subareolar duct does not drain a localised segment of tissue but can drain widespread areas of the breast.

The effectiveness of quadrantectomy relates to the large amount of tissue excised around the tumour rather than to the removal of a cancer and its draining duct. In an early randomised study of lumpectomy or quadrantectomy, a significantly greater number of patients who had lumpectomy had incomplete local excisions.[20] Not surprisingly, therefore, local recurrence was more common after lumpectomy than after quadrantectomy, although survival was no different.[20] Other non-randomised studies have shown similar rates of local recurrence for both quadrantectomy and wide local excision, providing margins of excision are clear.[21] Quadrantectomy or segmental excisions are no longer appropriate breast-conserving options because they produce identical rates of local recurrence to wide excision but produce a significantly poorer cosmetic outcome compared with wide excision.[22]

✔ Patients having breast-conserving surgery are adequately treated by wide local excision and do not require either a segmental or quadrantic excision.[23,24]

Special technical details: wide local excision

The aim of wide local excision is to remove all invasive and any ductal carcinoma in situ with a margin of normal surrounding breast tissue. Controversy has surrounded which incisions give the best cosmetic results. The predominant orientation of collagen fibres in the skin was described by Langer[25] and these skin crease lines around the breast are essentially circular (**Fig. 4.1**). Subsequent work by Kraissl[26] demonstrated that the lines of maximum resting skin tension run in a more transverse orientation across the breast (Fig. 4.1). In general, scars that are parallel both to the lines of maximum resting skin tension and to the orientation of collagen fibres are quickest to heal and produce the best cosmetic outcomes, with the lowest rates of scar hypertrophy and keloid formation.

✔ Incisions that follow the lines of maximum resting skin tension produce the most cosmetically acceptable scars.

A knowledge of Langer's lines and Kraissl's lines thus allows a surgeon to make incisions that enhance the cosmetic outcome of breast-conserving surgery. It has been tradition to place an incision to excise a cancer directly over the lesion, but this can result in an unsightly scar, particularly if the cancer is high and medial. In such instances plac-

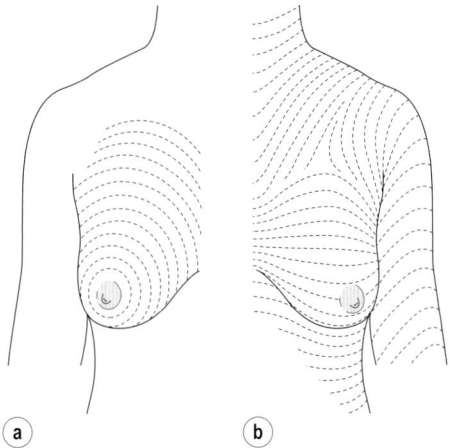

Figure 4.1 • The direction of Langer's lines **(a)** and lines of maximum resting skin tension in the breast **(b)** (so-called dynamic lines of Kraissl).

ing the scar some distance below in the skin crease lines and tunnelling up to the lesion produces a better cosmetic result. Cancers close to the nipple and even those some distance away in the upper half of the breast can be excised through circumareolar incisions. A cancer low in the breast close to the inframammary fold can similarly be excised through an incision placed in the fold. A cancer in the upper outer quadrant can be excised easily through an axillary incision. Excising skin directly overlying a cancer is only necessary if the skin is involved. It is not necessary to remove dimpled or tethered skin. The cosmetic result after breast-conserving surgery is influenced by the amount of skin excised, with poor results being obtained in those patients who have most skin removed. In patients with direct skin involvement, the aim should be to minimise the skin excised and to remove only enough skin to get microscopically clear margins.

✔ Routine excision of skin when performing a wide excision cannot be justified.[23]

Limiting the length of incision is also important, as longer incisions produce significantly poorer cosmetic outcomes. A knowledge of the depth of the cancer within the breast provided by preoperative or intraoperative breast ultrasound can be valuable when planning the extent of excision. For instance, if a cancer is 2 cm deep within the breast, then at least 1 cm of fat and subcutaneous tissue can be left on the skin flaps; leaving this tissue improves the cosmetic outcome. Whatever incision is used, it is important to have discussed the position of all scars with the patient prior to surgery.

Having made the skin incision, the skin and subcutaneous fat are dissected off the breast tissue. Care should be taken when elevating skin not to remove subcutaneous fat unnecessarily as thin skin flaps give a poor postoperative cosmetic result. Where the cancer is close to the skin, hydrodissection infiltrating 1 in 400 000 adrenaline in saline can help to separate the skin and subcutaneous fat from the breast tissue and breast fat, and facilitates skin elevation over the cancer. Skin flaps beyond the edge of the cancer for at least 1–2 cm are mobilised. This allows the fingers of the non-dominant hand to be placed over the palpable cancer. The breast tissue is then divided beyond the fingertips. The line of incision through the breast should be approximately

1 cm beyond the limit of the palpable mass. Having incised through the breast tissue, dissection continues under the cancer. In the majority of patients it is necessary to divide the whole thickness of breast tissue down to the pectoral fascia, to ensure that there is an adequate margin of tissue removed deep to the cancer. If the lesion is superficial, and there is a significant amount of breast tissue deep to the cancer, it may not be necessary to remove full thickness of breast tissue. Likewise if the lesion is deep, more tissue can be left superficially on the skin flaps. Having reached the deep margin, which is usually the pectoral fascia, the breast tissue and cancer are lifted from this fascia. It is not necessary to excise pectoral fascia unless it is tethered to the tumour or the tumour is involving it. If a carcinoma is infiltrating one of the chest wall muscles, then a portion of the affected muscle should be excised beneath the tumour, the aim being to remove sufficient muscle to get beyond the limits of the cancer. Having dissected under the cancer, the cancer and surrounding tissue are grasped between the finger and thumb of the non-dominant hand and excision of the cancer at the other margins is completed. The specimen should be orientated immediately following excision with Liga-clips, sutures or metal markers, prior to specimen radiography and submission to the pathologist.[27] Metal markers or Liga-clips are preferred because they can be seen on specimen radiography. Routine X-ray of orientated specimens is recommended because it has been shown to help the surgeon confirm the target lesion has been excised and allows assessment of completeness of excision at the radial margins.[27] If the specimen radiograph shows the cancer or any associated microcalcification is close to a particular margin, then further tissue can and should be removed from the margin of concern, before being orientated and sent to pathology.

A number of studies have evaluated the use of cavity shavings and bed biopsies, but few have compared these with standard assessment of margins. A minority of surgeons continue to take cavity shavings and bed biopsies routinely. Neither has been shown to be reliable indicators of local recurrence. A major concern of taking cavity shavings routinely is that significant amounts of extra breast tissue can be removed, particularly if the whole cavity is shaved; this unfortunately can adversely affect cosmetic outcome. Most importantly, however, centres who do not use these techniques report excellent local control rates, which have continued to fall over time.[28,29] Wide excision with standard examination of margins thus provides sufficient information on margin status for clinical use. Bed biopsies or cavity shavings are only of value and warranted where there is concern at operation that one particular margin is involved.

New devices that use ultrasound or rely on the electrical properties of the tissue are in trials and are being used to assess whether they can detect margin involvement and facilitate increased rates of complete excision at the first operation.

Having excised the cancer from the breast, suturing the defect in the breast without mobilisation of the breast tissue usually results in distortion of the breast contour. Defects in the breast are best closed by mobilising surrounding breast tissue from the overlying skin and subcutaneous tissue and in some patients mobilisation from the underlying chest wall is required. Large defects (>10% breast volume) that are left open fill with seroma, which often absorbs later, following which scar tissue develops and contracts and can result in an ugly distorted breast. Following large-volume excisions, after mobilisation it is usually possible to close the defect in the breast tissue by a series of interrupted absorbable sutures. Given the success of lipofilling or lipomodelling for improving some patients with poor cosmetic outcomes following breast-conserving surgery and radiotherapy, a number of surgeons are exploring whether immediate lipofilling after wide local excision can improve outcomes, particularly for women with small breasts. Very large defects require oncoplastic breast reshaping (see Chapter 6) or a latissimus dorsi miniflap.[12,13] Drains are not necessary after wide local excision and should not be used routinely. They do not protect against haematoma formation and increase infection rates. Breast skin wounds should be closed in layers with absorbable sutures, finishing with a subcuticular suture.

✅ Staples and interrupted sutures do not produce satisfactory results and are not an acceptable method of wound closure in the breast.

Complications of wide excision include haematoma, infection, incomplete excision, seroma and poor cosmetic results. Haematoma requiring evacuation is uncommon but occurs in approximately 2% of patients. Infection requiring treatment affects 5–10% and is more common when combined with an axillary dissection. Incomplete excision rates should be in the range 10–25%. The most common problem following surgery by wide local excision is a poor cosmetic result. Factors influencing cosmetic outcome and methods of avoiding this are considered in detail below.

Excising impalpable cancers

Impalpable lesions can be localised prior to surgery using one of a number of different techniques, including skin marking, injection of blue dye, carbon or radioisotope, insertion of a hooked wire, or intraoperative ultrasound. Although excising an impalpable cancer is easier if the skin incision is made directly over the cancer, remote incisions produce the best cosmetic results. Most impalpable small cancers should thus be approached through a cosmetically placed incision. The location of the lesion can be determined in a number of ways: (i) the surgeon can calculate the position of the breast lesion from the mammogram taken after wire insertion; (ii) the radiologist or the surgeon can mark the skin overlying the lesion using ultrasound; or (iii) if radioactivity has been injected to localise the cancer, the surgeon can use a gamma probe to localise the area of maximum radioactivity. After making an appropriately sized and cosmetically placed skin incision, this is deepened. If a wire is in place, then dissection continues towards the wire in the plane between the breast and subcutaneous fat so that the wire can be located some distance before it enters the lesion. For instance, if a mammographic abnormality has been localised in the craniocaudal position, then it helps to identify the wire superiorly before it enters the cancer. Wires that are marked with beads or that change in diameter, or have a guide that can be placed over the wire, help the surgeon to determine exactly how far along the wire the lesion is situated. Ideally the hook of the wire should be 1 cm through the lesion rather than within its centre. The direction of the wire on the preoperative mammogram is not always a reliable guide to the course of the wire through the breast. Once the wire is in place standard mammographic views are not always possible and thus a lesion that is apparently lateral to the entry point of the wire may not be lateral on the check craniocaudal film once the compression from the breast has been released. The aim is to remove the mammographic lesion with a 1-cm clear radiological margin and in most women to excise tissue up to subcutaneous fat and down to pectoral fascia.

As for palpable lesions, all specimens should be orientated with Liga-clips or metal markers, or secured to an orientated grid so that an orientated specimen radiography can be performed. Radiography is best performed in an X-ray machine designed specifically to X-ray specimens, such as a Bioptics® machine. There have been conflicting reports about whether compressing the specimen affects the incidence of subsequent positive margins as reported by the pathologist. Orientated specimen radiography improves the rate of complete excision of impalpable cancers.[27] Cooperation between surgeon and pathologist is required so that the area of concern can be identified and assessed by the pathologist to ensure adequacy of excision.

The majority of wide excisions of palpable and impalpable cancers are performed under general anaesthesia, but it is possible to perform these procedures under local anaesthesia.

Factors affecting local recurrence after breast-conserving surgery

Until recently there was a reported large variation between different centres in recurrence rates following breast-conserving surgery combined with whole breast radiotherapy for invasive breast carcinoma. Over 80% of all local recurrences were reported to be located adjacent to the site of initial excision. This is no longer true and an increasing percentage of 'recurrences' in treated breasts are actually second primaries.[25] Megavoltage radiation therapy delivered to the whole breast in a dose of 4000–5000 cGy given over 3–5 weeks continues to be used in most patients after breast-conserving surgery because radiotherapy both reduces the rate of local recurrence and improves overall survival.[30] Studies continue to evaluate whether localised radiotherapy delivered either during or within a few days of surgery is as effective as whole-breast radiotherapy. As yet it has not been possible to identify groups of patients who do not require radiotherapy. However, there is likely

to be a group of older patients with low-risk cancers (completely excised, node negative and hormone receptor positive on hormone treatment) and women of any age whose cancers have an extremely good prognosis (small grade 1 or special type cancers that are completely excised, node negative and hormone receptor positive on hormone treatment) whose rates of local recurrence without radiotherapy are acceptable. Following whole-breast radiotherapy, it is possible to increase the local dose of radiotherapy by boosting the tumour bed. This reduces local recurrence rates, particularly in younger women, although there are cosmetic penalties associated with the use of boost.[31]

The rates of in-breast tumour recurrences continue to fall over time[28,29] (**Fig. 4.2**). Whereas a 1% annual rate of in-breast cancer events was formerly considered acceptable, rates are now less than 0.5% per annum. The rates of in-breast tumour events continue at a similar rate for at least 20 years. This needs to be borne in mind when considering surveillance programmes for such patients.

Patient-related factors

✔✔ Local recurrence following breast-conserving therapy is significantly more common in younger patients.[32–35]

In contrast, local recurrence is much less of a problem in older patients (>65 years).

Recurrence is less frequent in women with large breasts but whether this relates to the larger excisions

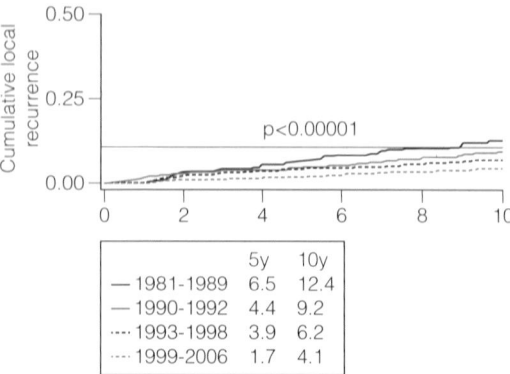

Figure 4.2 • Local recurrence rates in Edinburgh over four separate time periods showing a significant and continued fall in local recurrence rates over time. (Data unpublished, courtesy of Gill Kerr, Edinburgh Cancer Centre.)

that can be performed in these patients or to alterations in steroid metabolism (fat is known to be an important site of conversion of androgens to oestrogens) is uncertain.[36] A family history of breast cancer, particularly carriage of a mutation in one of the breast cancer genes, predisposes a patient to an increased rate of second primary cancers in both the treated and contralateral breast unless these women undergo a prophylactic oophorectomy, when local recurrence rates fall to levels similar to those of the general population.[37,38]

Tumour-related factors

Tumour location, tumour size, the presence of skin or nipple retraction, and the presence or absence of axillary node involvement have not been shown consistently to predict for local recurrence after breast-conserving surgery.[39–42] The hormone receptor status of a breast cancer does not seem to exert any influence on local control rates.[31–35,39–42] In-breast tumour recurrence has been reported to be more common in human epidermal growth factor receptor (HER2)-positive cancers.

Tumour size

Size is not significantly associated with local recurrence. Only 3 of 28 series that have examined the relationship of tumour size and occurrence have shown any significant association between tumour size in breast recurrence.[43,44] A large study from Boston[44] demonstrated that cancers over 4 cm in size that were treated by breast conservation surgery had a rate of recurrence similar to that of smaller cancers (Table 4.1).

Tumour grade

A number of reports have analysed the relationship between tumour grade and local recurrence.

Table 4.1 • Size of tumour related to local recurrence

Size (cm)	Local recurrence (%)
0–1	21
1.1–2	8
2.1–3	13
3.1–4	17
4.1–5	4

Data from Eberlein TG, Connolly JN, Schnitt JS et al. Predictors of local recurrence following conservative breast surgery and radiation therapy. The influence of tumour size. Arch Surg 1990; 125:771–9.

✔ The lowest rates of local recurrence are reported in grade 1 tumours.

Although some series report a higher recurrence rate in grade 3 compared with grade 2 cancers, this is by no means universal.[31–35,39–42] The relative risk of local recurrence between grade 1 and grade 2/3 cancer is approximately 1.5. The British Association of Surgical Oncology undertook a trial that randomised patients with node-negative grade 1 or special-type cancers to no further treatment, tamoxifen alone, radiotherapy alone or both radiotherapy and tamoxifen. A recent update of this study reported an exceedingly small rate of recurrence in patients randomised to radiotherapy and tamoxifen, and acceptably low rates of annual recurrence in patients treated with either tamoxifen alone or radiotherapy alone. Higher rates of recurrence were seen in patients who received neither radiotherapy nor tamoxifen. In these low-risk cancers treatment by radiotherapy alone or tamoxifen alone may therefore produce an acceptable rate of long-term control.

Histological type

There are few data relating histological tumour type to recurrence. Invasive lobular cancer has not been reported to be associated with a higher recurrence rate than so-called invasive 'ductal' carcinoma.[45–48] One study did suggest that patients with invasive lobular carcinoma who developed local recurrence were more likely to develop multifocal recurrence[42] but this has not been confirmed by others. Patients with invasive lobular cancer appear more likely than patients with no special-type tumours to have an incomplete excision. This is explained in part by the underestimation of tumour extent by mammography and ultrasound and the inability of surgeons to feel the extent of the cancer at operation. Patients with invasive lobular cancer on core biopsy should be warned of an increased likelihood of positive margins and where the extent of disease is not easy to assess on mammography and/or ultrasound, MRI may be valuable.[9]

Lymphatic/vascular invasion

Increased local failure rates have been reported in most, but not all, series in patients with histological evidence of lymphatic/vascular invasion (LVI).[31–35,39–42,45–48] Of concern, the percentage of tumours reported to have LVI varies widely between different series by up to a factor of 4.

✅ Carcinomas with LVI have approximately double the rate of local breast recurrence compared with tumours with no evidence of this feature.

LVI is more common in and around the cancer of younger women (<35 years) compared with cancers in older women (>50 years).

Extensive in situ component

The histological factor that was initially thought to be associated with an increased rate of local recurrence was the presence of an extensive in situ component (EIC) within and surrounding an invasive cancer. A tumour is defined as having EIC if 25% or more of the tumour mass is non-invasive and non-invasive carcinoma is also present in the breast tissue surrounding the invasive cancer.[48] EIC was considered not only a predictor of local recurrence but also of residual disease within the breast following an incomplete wide excision. Early reports indicated that local recurrence rates were three to four times higher in cancers with EIC.[31–35,39–42,45–48] The majority of these studies did not, however, take account of margins and the authors did not perform multivariate analysis. Providing clear margins are obtained, it is now known that there is no increased rate of local recurrence in patients with EIC.[49–51] There is an interaction between age and EIC, with younger women being more likely to have EIC. It has been suggested that the higher frequency of EIC in younger women might explain some of the increased rate of local recurrence seen in younger women.[42]

Multiple tumours

Patients with macroscopically multiple cancers were formerly considered to have an increased risk of local recurrence compared with a patient with a unifocal cancer but patient numbers in such early series on which this evidence is based were small.[14,15] If multifocality is identified by the pathologist or there are two cancers that are adjacent, then acceptable local recurrence rates can be obtained provided that all margins of excision are clear of disease. This led some to attempt breast-conserving surgery for patients with multiple separate tumours in the same breast. Provided that the cancers are excised completely and clear margins obtained then reports indicate a satisfactory rate of local control can be obtained with breast-conserving surgery in patients with both multifocal and multicentric cancers.[16,17]

✅✅ The most important surgical-related factor is completeness of excision. Current practice is to aim for at least microscopically disease-free margins. Ideally, there should be a clear rim of normal tissue (≥1 mm) around the carcinoma at all radial margins.[28,29]

Treatment-related factors

Controversy has surrounded how much extra tissue around a cancer needs to be removed and what constitutes an involved or positive margin. Some studies have defined a positive or involved margin as disease at the margin, others consider disease within 1 mm or even disease within 2 mm of the margins as involved. Conversely, negative margins or uninvolved margins have been variably defined as no tumour at the margin, or tumour within 1, 2, 5 and 10 mm of the margin. Whatever definition has been used, almost all studies have reported an increased rate of local recurrence in patients with positive, non-negative or involved margins. When comparing patients with involved margins to those with uninvolved or negative margins, the relative risk of local recurrence varies between 1.4- and 9-fold.[28,29,31–35,39–42,45–47,49–54] This is despite, in almost half of these series, patients with involved or close margins having received higher doses of radiotherapy than patients with clear margins. In the few studies which found that margins are not important predictors of local recurrence, the dose of radiotherapy delivered to the tumour bed ranged from 65 to 72 cGy, i.e. a dose range that is effective without surgery.[51–54] In one study, patients with involved margins who underwent re-excision to achieve a negative margin had a zero local recurrence rate; this compares with a 22% local recurrence rate in those patients who had re-excision but still had non-negative margins ($P=0.001$).[50] Surveys in the UK and USA have demonstrated that approximately 50% of surgeons aim for a margin of more than 2 mm, whereas 50% of surgeons are happy with a margin of 2 mm or less.[55] There is thus no consensus about what constitutes an adequate margin of excision for breast-conserving surgery. A systematic review of margins and local recurrence was conducted by Singletary, who reported that some of the lowest rates of local recurrence were in centres that had used narrow margins of excision (1 or 2 mm).[28]

Table 4.2 • Local recurrence rates (%) at 5 years in patients from Boston[48] and Stanford[50] subdivided by margin status and the presence (EIC+) or absence (EIC–) of an extensive in situ component

	Boston		Stanford	
Margins	**EIC+**	**EIC–**	**EIC+**	**EIC–**
Positive/non-negative	37	7	21	11
Close	0	5		
Negative	0	2	0	1

A recent large comprehensive meta-analysis of margins has confirmed that wider margins do not reduce local recurrence.[29] Wider margins remove more tissue and so impact on cosmetic outcomes. The meta-analysis confirmed an increased rate of local recurrence for both involved and close (<1 mm) margins.[29] Compared with no ink on cancer cells a 1-mm margin was associated with a significantly lower rate of local recurrence. Recent data from Edinburgh show there is no need to re-excise if anterior or posterior margins are <1 mm, providing full thickness of breast tissue has been excised and boost radiotherapy given. Unpublished data from Edinburgh show similar local recurrence rates whether the distance to the nearest margin was in the range 1–5 mm or 5–10 mm, confirming the results from the meta-analysis that narrow 1-mm margins are sufficient.

✓✓ A recent meta-analysis concluded that wider margins do not reduce rates of local recurrence. Incomplete excision, i.e. tumour at a margin, does, however, result in an unacceptable rate of local control.[28,29] A 1-mm margin is sufficient.

A recent large series of patients treated by breast-conserving surgery with a ≥1 mm margin reported rates of local recurrence of <0.5% per year (Fig. 4.2).[56] The majority of these so-called recurrences were in fact second primaries. In conclusion, a 1- or 2-mm margin is adequate and produces acceptable rates of long-term control. Any centre excising margins wider than 1 or 2 mm on breast-conserving excisions should consider their protocols.

Studies have looked at the presence of lobular carcinoma in situ[57] and atypical ductal hyperplasia[58] at the margins of excision. Neither of these features significantly increases local recurrence rates and so there is no need for re-excision if the pathologist reports these features alone at any of the margins of excision.

Age interacts with margins. Involved margins have their greatest impact on local recurrence in younger rather than in older women.[53]

There is a direct interaction between EIC and margins (Table 4.2). Patients with EIC and positive margins who proceeded to radiotherapy without re-excision had a 37% local recurrence rate in a series from Boston[48] and a 21% recurrence rate in a Stanford series.[50] In contrast, patients with EIC and negative margins, on primary or re-excision, had a zero local recurrence rate. These two studies demonstrate that patients with EIC do not have an increased rate of local recurrence providing the margins of excision are clear of invasive and in situ cancer.

Patients undergoing re-excision for close or involved margins have only a 30% incidence of residual cancer in re-excised tissue.[59] More than two foci of microscopic margin involvement in the original wide excision appears to be associated with a greater incidence of residual cancer (65%) compared with fewer than two foci, which had a much lower rate of residual cancer. If there was no residual disease at re-excision then there was a 4% local failure rate at 4.7 years compared with a 13% failure rate in patients who had residual disease at re-excision. Patients younger than age 50 in this study were also more likely to have disease in the re-excision specimen. The conclusion was that the majority of patients who undergo re-excision do not benefit from this procedure. Patients with lucent breasts and a well-defined lesion appear particularly unlikely to benefit from re-excision, if margins are close or focally positive, whereas younger women with dense breasts are much more likely to benefit from further surgery, as many of these women will have residual disease in the re-excision specimen.[59] Further studies in this area are required. If it were possible to identify a group of women who do not benefit from re-excision, this would have great clinical utility.

Adjuvant systemic therapy

Aromatase inhibitors, tamoxifen and chemotherapy, in the presence of radiotherapy, reduce local recurrence rates after breast-conserving surgery.[60,61] In the absence of radiotherapy, aromatase inhibitors, tamoxifen or chemotherapy alone do not produce satisfactory rates of local control apart from in low-grade, node-negative cancers.[62] The interval between surgery and radiotherapy may be important and there are suggestions that the rates of local recurrence increase if radiotherapy is delayed. The sequencing of radiotherapy and chemotherapy is the subject of ongoing trials but it appears that giving both synchronously rather than sequentially improves local recurrence.

Factors influencing cosmetic outcome after breast-conserving surgery

There is a great variation in different series in the number of patients with good to excellent cosmetic results after breast-conserving surgery (**Fig. 4.3**).

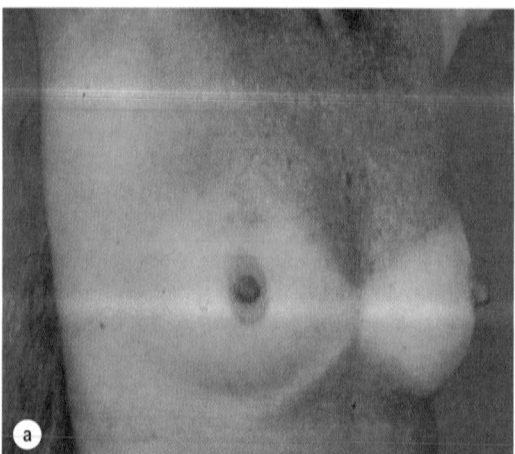

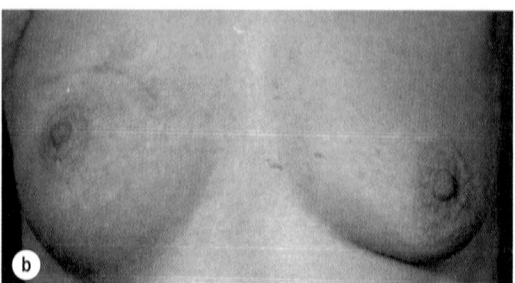

Figure 4.3 • Examples of excellent **(a)** and poor **(b)** cosmetic results from breast-conserving surgery and radiotherapy.

✅✅ The importance of a good cosmetic outcome is based on studies that have shown a significant correlation between poor cosmetic outcome and increased levels of anxiety, depression, poor body image, problems with sexuality and low self-esteem.[2]

Patient factors

There is conflicting evidence about whether age influences cosmetic outcome, with some studies claiming that older women have worse cosmetic results than younger women.[1] One problem in younger women is that as the patient ages the normal contralateral breast tends to increase in size, whereas the treated breast tends not to and some treated breasts shrink. A treated breast that is symmetrical immediately following treatment can thus become asymmetrical over time.

There is a trend towards increased fibrosis in larger breasts, which leads to poorer cosmetic results than seen in smaller breasts.[63] For this reason large-breasted women may be best treated by an operation that excises their cancer and at the same time reduces the volume of the breast (therapeutic mammaplasty). The best option to achieve symmetry in such women is to reduce both breasts through reduction-type incisions. Better cosmetic results following breast-conserving surgery and radiotherapy are obtained in medium- and moderate-sized breasts; achieving a good cosmetic outcome can often be a problem in small breasts.[1]

Tumour factors

Increasing tumour size means that increasingly large amounts of tissue have to be removed. The volume of tissue excised is the most important factor relating to cosmetic outcome and so not surprisingly patients with larger tumours tend to have worse cosmetic results than women with smaller cancers.[64,65] There are some data indicating that in surgery for small and impalpable cancers, a disproportionately large amount of normal surrounding breast tissue is removed to ensure that all the affected tissue is excised. The role of the surgeon is to excise the cancer completely in as small a volume as possible. Removing large volumes of tissue when excising small screen-detected cancers is not satisfactory surgical practice.

Location of tumour

Cosmetic outcomes tend to be better if the tumour is located in the upper outer quadrant.[66] Studies have shown that major downward displacement of the nipple occurs when surgery is performed on tumours located in the inferior half of the breast. This can be corrected at the time of initial surgery by de-epithelialising a crescentic portion of skin above the nipple to re-centre it on the new breast mound (see Chapter 6). If the tumour is central and the nipple–areola complex needs to be removed, then this can have a major effect on cosmetic outcomes.[1] This is why central tumours were at one time considered a relative contraindication to breast-conserving surgery. However, studies have suggested that excision of central cancers not directly involving the nipple–areola complex can be treated by wide excision and nipple preservation, without significantly increasing the rate of local recurrence compared with more peripherally situated cancers.[67] Good cosmetic outcomes are possible in some women with this approach (**Fig. 4.4**). In women with moderate-sized breasts who have cancers that directly involve, or are very close to the nipple, the nipple and/or areola can be excised in continuity with the cancer and the skin closed by a purse-string suture (**Fig. 4.5**). Another option is to rotate a dermoglandular local flap from the lower part of the breast to fill the defect (**Fig. 4.6**). This produces very satisfactory cosmetic outcomes.[68] In women with central superficial cancers in larger breasts, the nipple can be excised as part of a reduction-type procedure with direct closure, or the defect caused by excising the nipple and areola can be filled with a new island of skin developed on an inferior dermoglandular pedicle.

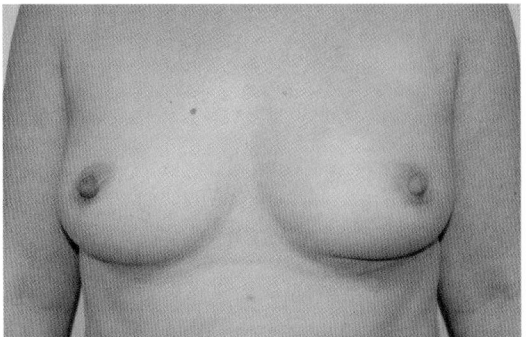

Figure 4.4 • Good cosmetic results from excision of a subareolar cancer left breast via a circumareolar incision.

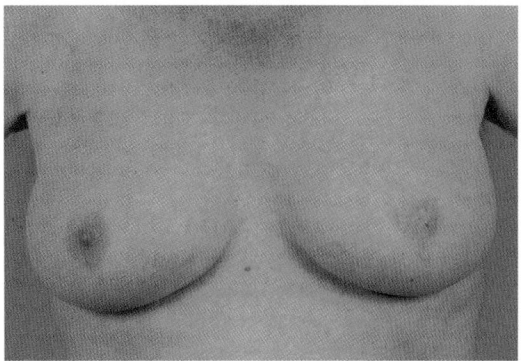

Figure 4.5 • Result after a central excision of a cancer and use of a purse-string suture to close the central defect.

This can only be performed if there is at least 9 cm of skin between the margin of skin excision and the inframammary fold (**Fig. 4.7**).

Surgical factors

✔✔ The extent of surgical excision or the volume of resected breast tissue is the most important factor affecting cosmesis.[1,64]

The poorer cosmetic results obtained with quadrantectomy, even in the most experienced hands, compared with wide excision are well documented and are related to the much larger volumes of tissue removed by quadrantectomy.[69]

Even more critical than the volume of tissue resected is the percentage volume of the breast excised. There is a highly statistical correlation between cosmetic outcome and percentage volume of the breast excised (**Fig. 4.8**), with excisions of less than 10% of breast volume generally being associated with a good cosmetic outcome, whereas excisions over 10% often produce a poor cosmetic result (**Fig. 4.9**). Where it is clear that more than 10% of breast volume needs to be excised in order to remove the cancer, then consideration should be given to one of a number of procedures that can improve the final cosmetic result. These include volume replacement with a myocutaneous or local lipocutaneous flap,[12,13] volume replacement using immediate lipofilling following the tumour excision, an oncoplastic reduction procedure (therapeutic mammoplasty), neoadjuvant drug therapy or a mastectomy with or without immediate reconstruction.

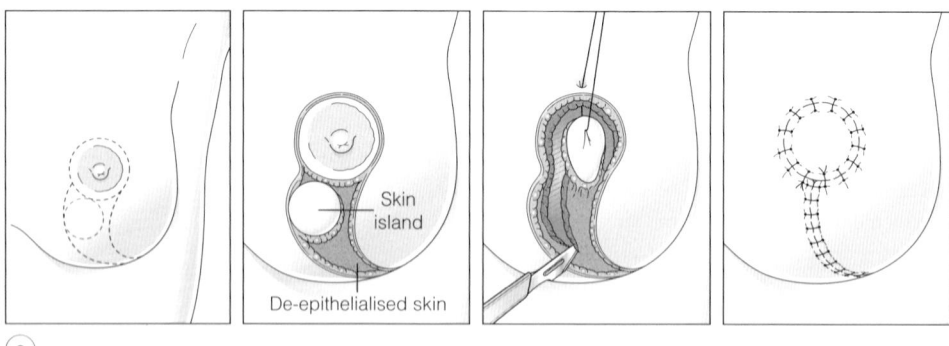

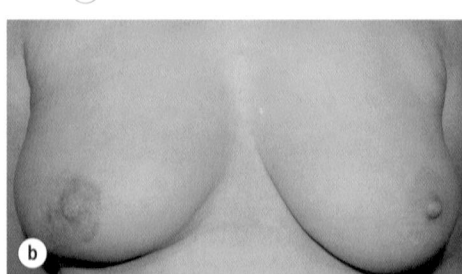

Figure 4.6 • (a) How to excise a central cancer under the nipple and produce a satisfactory cosmetic outcome without major breast distortion. This procedure has been called central quadrantectomy. The nipple–areola complex is excised and a portion of skin inferior is marked out. An incision around the circular skin island is made and the remaining skin around the island is de-epithelialised. A full-thickness incision is then made in the breast and the skin island is rotated to fill the central defect. Staples are useful to position the flap. When the flap is deemed to be in an optimal position, the staples are removed and the wound closed in two layers with absorbable sutures. **(b)** Final result from a right wide local excision Grissotti flap and nipple reconstruction.

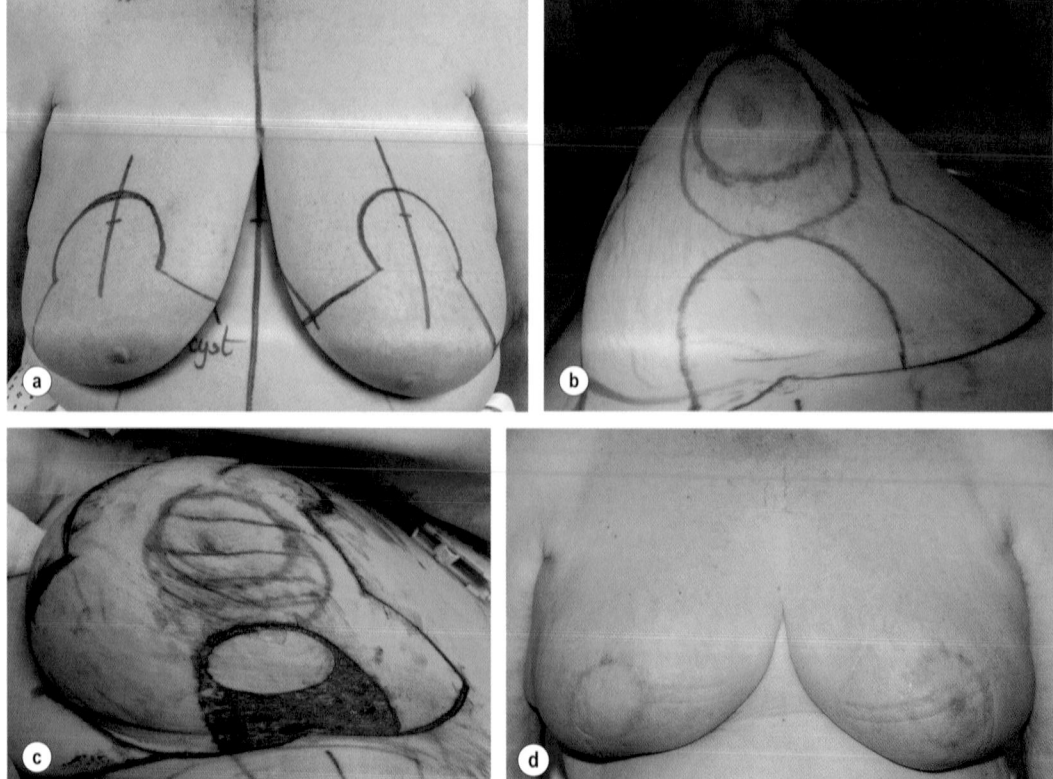

Figure 4.7 • (a) Patient prior to operation – cancer under right nipple evident by asymmetry with right nipple flatter and right nipple higher than left. **(b)** Preoperative markings showing the area around the nipple that will be excised. **(c)** Operative view of the island of skin that is mobilised on a de-epithelialised inferior dermoglandular flap. **(d)** Final result after radiotherapy prior to nipple reconstruction.

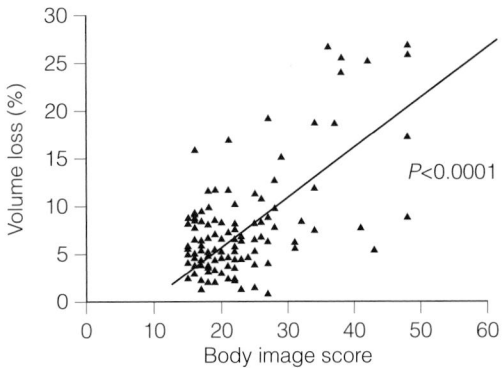

Figure 4.8 • Percentage of breast excised compared with body image score. Percentage of breast excised calculated by measuring total weight of excision and estimating breast volume (from initial diagnostic craniocaudal mammogram). Body image score based on patient-administered questionnaire of 15 questions (score runs from 15, the best possible score, to 60, the worst and highest possible score). Data from a series of 120 patients treated in the Edinburgh Breast Unit.

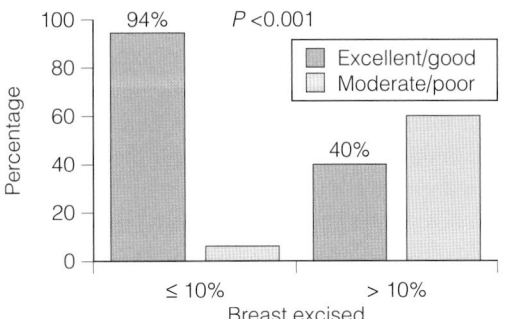

Figure 4.9 • Percentage of good/excellent results in patients subdivided according to whether 10% or less or more than 10% of breast volume was excised by breast-conserving surgery.

Re-excision and number of procedures

Re-excision of the tumour bed has a negative impact on cosmesis.[64] This is mainly as a consequence of the increased total volume of tissue excised from the breast. There is no limit to the number of re-excisions that a patient can have to achieve complete removal of all invasive and in situ disease,[70] but with the greater number of re-excisions more tissue is removed and so the likelihood of a good cosmetic result decreases. For patients who require multiple excisions to get clear margins then consideration should be given to correcting any volume deficit prior to delivery of radiotherapy or considering subsequent contralateral symmetrising surgery.

Axillary surgery

Axillary clearance does appear to be associated with a worse cosmetic outcome compared with sentinel node biopsy, primarily because of the volume of tissue removed, which results in an axillary deficit, but also because removing all nodes increases the risk of breast oedema.[63,64,71]

Postoperative complications

Development of a haematoma, seroma or postoperative infection tends to increase the chances of the patient getting a poor cosmetic result.[1]

Breast-conserving surgery after neoadjuvant therapy

Significant numbers of patients are diagnosed with large or locally advanced breast cancer, many of whom are treated initially by neoadjuvant chemotherapy or endocrine therapy. Up to a half of these patients will subsequently become candidates for breast-conserving surgery. To improve complete excision rates and minimise cosmetic deformity in these patients there are some guiding principles when performing breast conservation surgery after completion of neoadjuvant therapy. First, it is important to know the exact site of the tumour within the breast, as significant numbers of patients with HER2-positive and triple negative cancers will have a complete pathological response. All patients undergoing neoadjuvant chemotherapy who might be candidates for subsequent breast-conserving surgery should therefore have one or more tumour markers placed centrally prior to or early during treatment. The patterns of response to neoadjuvant chemotherapy and neoadjuvant endocrine therapy differ.[72] The most common form of pathological change in patients undergoing neoadjuvant endocrine therapy is central scar formation,[72] which results in concentric reduction in tumour size and tumour volume. Breast-conserving surgery following neoadjuvant endocrine therapy is therefore usually successful at excising all disease in one operation and few patients have involved margins. In contrast, a significant number of patients after neoadjuvant chemotherapy have a diffuse pattern of response to chemotherapy, with reduction in tumour cellularity but without significant shrinkage of volume. This diffuse tumour may be impalpable and more than 25% of patients undergoing

breast-conserving surgery after neoadjuvant chemotherapy will have incomplete excision of disease. All patients undergoing breast-conserving
surgery after neoadjuvant chemotherapy should be
warned of this rate of incomplete excision and the
possible need for a further operation.

> ✅ MRI following neoadjuvant chemotherapy is the
> best of the currently available imaging methods to
> assess extent of disease and is the best predictor of
> whether a cancer is suitable for breast-conserving
> surgery.[73]

Radiotherapy

Increasing doses of radiotherapy, particularly with
the addition of boost, have a detrimental effect on
cosmetic outcomes.[31,63,64] Long-term follow-up is
necessary to assess cosmetic outcome; 3 years after treatment, radiotherapy effects tend to stabilise.
Fibrosis is a late effect of radiotherapy and produces breast retraction and contour distortion. The
treated breast tends not to increase in size to the
same extent as the opposite untreated breast, so patients as they age can develop asymmetry even when
the initial cosmetic result was excellent. Boost has
a negative impact on cosmesis because it produces
intense fibrosis and unsightly skin changes, including telangiectasia.[31]

Other treatment effects

Tamoxifen and aromatase inhibitors have little if
any effect on cosmetic outcome, whereas some studies have suggested that chemotherapy has a negative
impact on the cosmetic outcome of breast-conserving
surgery.[1]

Treatment of poor cosmetic results after breast-conserving surgery

Prevention is better than treatment, so minimising volume, closing breast defects and immediate
lipofilling (**Fig. 4.10**) are much better options than
trying to correct asymmetry once it has developed.
Options for improving poor cosmetic outcomes include increasing the volume of one or both breasts

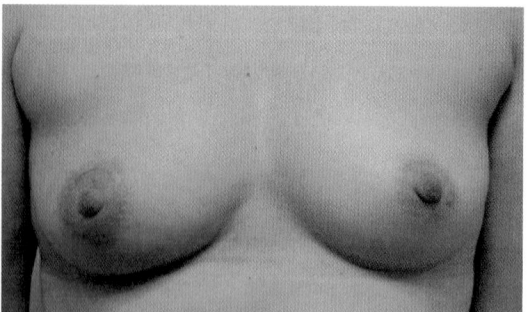

Figure 4.10 • Result from wide local excision right of
a cancer in the upper inner quadrant via a circumareola
incision with immediate lipofilling and postoperative
radiotherapy.

if the main problem is essentially loss of volume
rather than significant radiation fibrosis. While
placement of silicone prosthesis or prostheses has
been described, they are successful only for patients
with little or no deformity and absence of marked
skin changes.[74] Swelling following implant insertion
in a radiotherapy-treated breast is often marked and
takes many months to settle. Some patients develop
marked capsular contraction after implant placement following radiotherapy but there are no data
on whether this incidence is greater than in women
having augmentation with no prior radiotherapy.
The use of implants has been largely superseded
by lipofilling. Fat is aspirated from the abdomen
and thighs and centrifuged, washed or filtered.[75,76]
Having removed the oil and blood it is then injected
as microdroplets into the area of distortion and/or
asymmetry. Approximately 40% of the injected fat
survives. Multiple episodes of lipofilling combined
with scar release or scar excision are often required
to correct significant breast deformity and asymmetry (**Fig. 4.11**).[76] If the problem is simply one of
asymmetry and the treated breast is a satisfactory
shape but smaller than the normal contralateral
breast, then the contralateral breast can be reduced.
If the treated breast is shrunken, misshapen and
scarred, then another option is to excise part or
the whole of the treated breast and reconstruct either part of the breast or the whole breast. Pedicled
myocutaneous latissimus dorsi or transverse rectus
abdominis myocutaneous (TRAM) flaps offer an
opportunity to excise unsightly areas of skin and/
or breast distortion and scarring, and provide one
option to regain symmetry (**Fig. 4.12**).

Pre Lipofilling   **After Lipofilling**   **Scar Release + 2ⁿᵈ Fill**

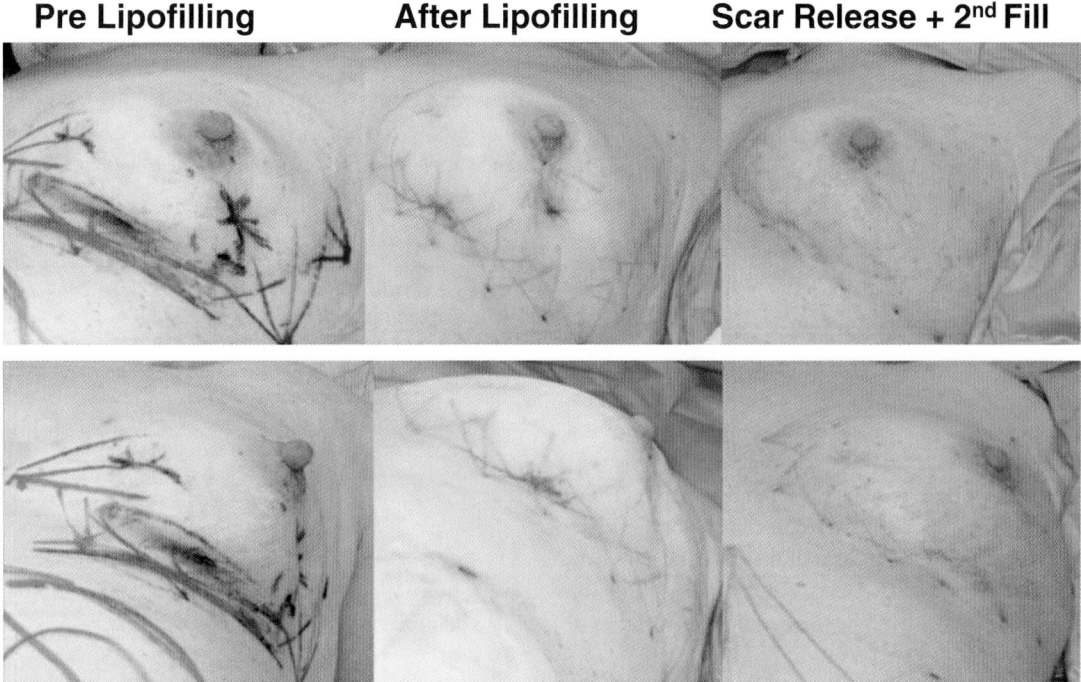

Figure 4.11 • Patient with a defect from a previous wide local excision and radiotherapy before and after lipofilling and then scar release and lipofilling of the left breast.

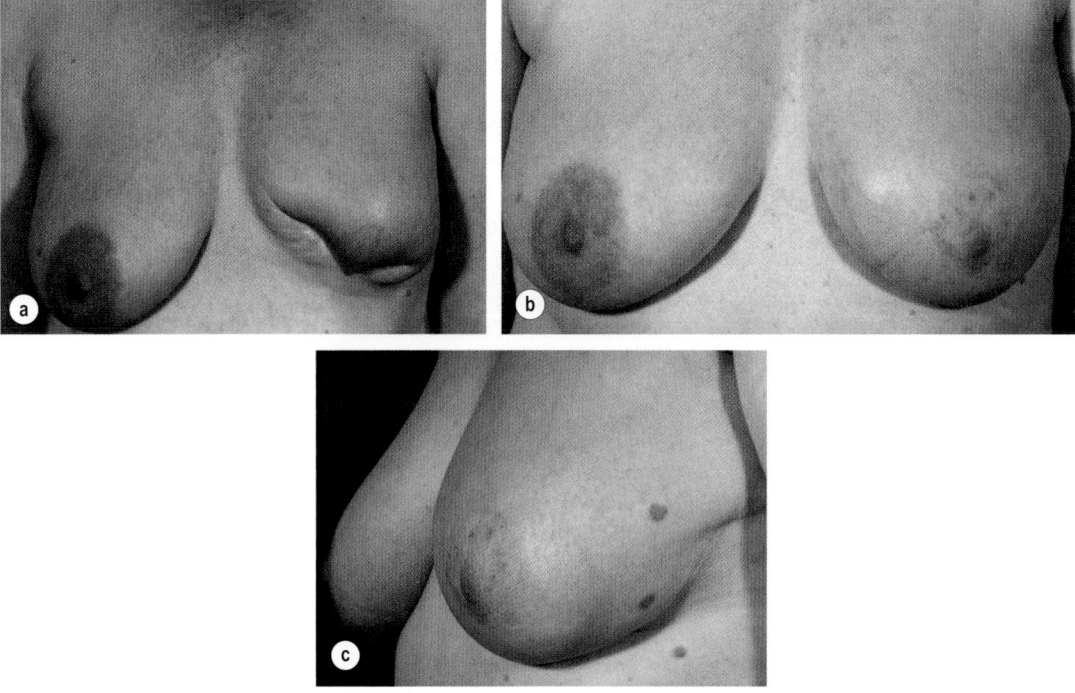

Figure 4.12 • Patient with a poor cosmetic result after breast-conserving surgery before **(a)** and after **(b,c)** partial breast reconstruction with a pedicled latissimus dorsi myocutaneous flap.

Significance and treatment of local recurrence

Local recurrence rates of 0.5% or less per year after breast-conserving treatment are now achievable.

✅✅ An isolated local breast recurrence does not appear to be a threat to survival, but breast recurrence is a predictor of distant disease,[7,77,78] and the aim of primary treatment is to avoid local recurrence if at all possible.

Isolated recurrences of the breast can be treated by re-excision or mastectomy.[77–79] Re-excision alone is associated with a high rate of subsequent local recurrence if the initial recurrence occurs within the first 5 years of treatment.[78] Until recently 80% of local recurrences in the conserved breast occurred at the site of the original breast cancer, with 90% of these local recurrences following breast-conserving surgery being invasive. This is no longer true and an increasing percentage of 'recurrences' in treated breasts are now second primary cancers. Local recurrence within the first 5 years is associated with a worse long-term outlook than recurrence thereafter.[7,77–79] The role of systemic therapy following mastectomy for an apparently localised breast recurrence appears to be of benefit.[79] Uncontrollable local recurrence is uncommon after breast conservation, but when it does occur it is difficult to treat.

✅✅ Extended hormonal treatment with letrozole following completion of 5 years of tamoxifen reduces' in breast. Local recurrence is reduced by letrozole compared with tamoxifen given as adjuvant therapy to postmenopausal women with ER positive breast cancer (Table 4.3). Extended recurrences by almost two-thirds and also reduces the rate of contralateral breast cancer development.[79]

Prolonging adjuvant hormonal therapy beyond 5 years has a significant impact on the rate of subsequent local relapse in postmenopausal patients with hormone receptor-positive breast cancer.

Table 4.3 • Efficacy end-points in 4922 patients enrolled into the BIG 1-98 trials

	Letrozole (*n* = 2463)		Tamoxifen (*n* = 2459)	
	No. of patients	%	No. of patients	%
Disease-free survival events	352	14.3	418	17.0
Local	19	0.8	38	1.6
Contralateral breast	14	0.6	26	1.1
Regional	13	0.5	11	0.5
Distant	182	7.4	212	8.6
Deaths without cancer	60	2.4	48	2.0
Deaths (overall survival events)	194	7.9	211	8.6
Systemic failures	331	13.4	374	15.2

Modified from Coates AS, Keshaviah A, Thurlimann B et al. Five years of letrozole compared with tamoxifen as initial adjuvant therapy for postmenopausal women with endocrine-responsive early breast cancer: update of study BIG 1–98. J Clin Oncol 2007; 25(5):486–92. Published by the American Society of Clinical Oncology.

Key points

- For patients with single breast cancers, survival outcomes from breast-conserving treatment are equivalent to that of mastectomy.
- Radiotherapy (after breast-conserving surgery) reduces the rate of local recurrence and improves overall survival. No subgroup of patients has yet been identified that can avoid radiotherapy.
- The major surgical factor influencing local recurrence is completeness of excision, and clear margins (≥1 mm) must be obtained when performing breast-conserving surgery.
- Wider margins (>5 mm) do not appear to achieve better local control rates than narrow margins (≥1 mm).
- Younger patients have an increased rate of local recurrence after breast-conserving surgery. Conversely, older patients have a lower rate of local recurrence.

- Tumour grade, EIC and LVI have a limited influence on the rate of local recurrence. Patients with these factors should not be denied breast-conserving surgery, providing the cancer can be excised to clear margins.
- There is a direct correlation between cosmetic outcome after breast-conserving surgery and psychological morbidity, with better cosmetic outcomes being associated with less anxiety and depression and better body image and self-esteem.
- The most important factor influencing cosmetic outcome after breast-conserving surgery is the percentage volume of breast excised. Removing more than 10% of the breast volume dramatically increases the number of women having a poor cosmetic outcome.
- Patients who develop local recurrence after breast-conserving surgery, particularly in the first 5 years, are at increased risk of having systemic relapse.
- Isolated local recurrences after breast-conserving surgery are usually treated by mastectomy, although re-excision is possible, particularly if the recurrence develops more than 5 years after treatment or the patient has not received radiotherapy to the breast.
- Prolonging hormonal therapy beyond 5 years in postmenopausal women with hormone receptor-positive breast cancer reduces the rate of subsequent 'in-breast recurrence' and the rate of contralateral breast cancer development.

References

1. Sharif K, Al-Ghazal SK, Blamey RW. Cosmetic assessment of breast-conserving surgery for primary breast cancer. Breast 1999;8:162–8.

2. Al-Ghazal SK, Fallowfield L, Blamey RW. Comparison of psychological aspects and patient satisfaction following breast conserving surgery, simple mastectomy and breast reconstruction. Eur J Cancer 2000;36:1938–43.

3. Shain WS, d'Angelo TM, Dunn ME, et al. Mastectomy versus conservative surgery and radiation therapy: psychological consequences. Cancer 1994;73:1221–8.

4. Early Breast Cancer Trialists' Collaborative Group. Effects of radiotherapy and surgery in early breast cancer: an overview of the randomised trials. N Engl J Med 1995;333:1444–55.
   This review analyses data on 10-year survival from six randomised controlled trails comparing breast conservation with mastectomy. Meta-analysis of data from five of the randomised trials (3006 women) found no difference in the risk of death at 10 years. Where more than half of node-positive patients in both the mastectomy and breast-conserving groups received adjuvant nodal radiotherapy, both groups had similar survival rates. In contrast, where less than half of node-positive women in both groups received adjuvant nodal radiotherapy, survival was better for the breast-conserving surgery group (overall risk vs. mastectomy 0.69, 95% CI 0.5, 90% 0.57). Level I evidence.

5. Morris AD, Morris RD, Wilson JF, et al. Breast conserving therapy versus mastectomy in early stage breast cancer: a meta-analysis of 10 year survival. Cancer J Sci Am 1997;3:6–12.
   In this review nine randomised controlled trials involving 4981 women potentially suitable for breast-conserving surgery were analysed. Meta-analysis found no significant difference in the risk of death over 10 years for patients treated by mastectomy or breast-conserving surgery. The authors also found no significant difference in the rates of local recurrence in the six trials where data were available. Level I evidence.

6. Fortin A, Larochelle M, Laverdière J, et al. Local failure is responsible for the decrease in survival for patients with breast cancer treated with conservative surgery and postoperative radiotherapy. J Clin Oncol 1999;17:101–9.

7. Fisher B, Anderson S, Fisher E, et al. Significance of ipsilateral breast tumour recurrence after lumpectomy. Lancet 1991;338:327–31.

8. Turnbull LW, Brown SR, Olivier C, et al. Multicentre randomized controlled trial examining the cost-effectiveness of contrast-enhanced high field magnetic resonance imaging in women with primary breast cancer scheduled for wide local excision (COMICE). Health Technol Assess 2010;14(1):1–182.

9. Mann RM, Hoogeveen YL, Blickman JG, et al. MRI compared to conventional diagnostic work-up in the decision and evaluation of invasive lobular carcinoma of the breast: a review of existing literature. Breast Cancer Res Treat 2008;107:1–14.

10. Houssami N, Ciatto S, Macaskill P, et al. Accuracy and surgical impact of MRI in breast cancer staging: systematic review and meta-analysis in detection of multifocal and multicentric cancer. J Clin Oncol 2008;26(19):3248–58.
    This is a review of the accuracy of MRI in breast cancer and shows that MRI has a high sensitivity but poor specificity.

11. Turnbull L, Brown S, Harvey J, et al. Comparative effectiveness of MRI in breast cancer (COMICE) trial: a randomized controlled trial. Lancet 2010; 375(9714):563–71.

This is the only randomised trial of MRI in breast-conserving surgery. This study shows that routine MRI in breast-conserving surgery is not indicated.

12. Dixon JM, Venizelos B, Chan P. Latissimus dorsi mini-flap: a technique for extending breast conservation. Breast 2002;11:58–65.

13. Raja MAK, Straker VF, Rainsbury RM. Extending the role of breast-conserving surgery by immediate volume replacement. Br J Surg 1997;84:101–5.

14. Fisher ER, Sass R, Fisher B, et al. Pathologic findings from the national surgical adjuvant breast project (protocol 6): relation of local breast recurrence to multicentricity. Cancer 1986;57: 1717–24.

15. Kurtz JM, Jacquemier G, Amalaric R, et al. Breast-conserving therapy for macroscopically multiple cancers. Ann Surg 1990;212:38–44.

16. Lim W, Park EH, Choi SL, et al. Breast conserving surgery for multifocal breast cancer. Ann Surg 2009;249(1):87–90.

17. Gentilini O, Botteri E, Rotmensz N, et al. Conservative surgery in patients with multifocal/multicentric breast cancer. Breast Cancer Res Treat 2009;113(3):577–83.

18. Ballinger S, Mayer KF, Lawrence G, et al. Patients' decision-making in a UK specialist centre with high mastectomy rates. The Breast 2008;17:574–9.

19. Holland DR, Connolly JL, Gelman R, et al. The presence of an extensive intraductal component (EIC) following a limited excision predicts for prominent residual disease in the remainder of the breast. J Clin Oncol 1990;8:113–8.

20. Veronesi U, Volterrani F, Luini A, et al. Quadrantectomy versus lumpectomy for small size breast cancer. Eur J Cancer 1990;26:671–3.

21. Ghossein NA, Alpert S, Barba J, et al. Importance of adequate surgical excision prior to radiotherapy in the local control of breast cancer in patients treated conservatively. Arch Surg 1992;127:411–5.

22. Sacchini V, Luini A, Tana S, et al. Quantitive and qualitative cosmetic evaluation after conservation treatment for breast cancer. Eur J Cancer 1991;27:1395–400.

23. NIH Consensus Conference. Treatment of early-stage breast cancer. JAMA 1991;265:391–5.

24. Fisher B, Wolmark N, Fisher ER, et al. Lumpectomy and axillary dissection for breast cancer: surgical, pathological and radiation considerations. World J Surg 1985;9:692–8.

25. Langer K. Zur anatomie und physiologie der Haut. Huber Die Spaltbarkiet Der Cutis. S-b-Akad Wiss Wein 1861;44:19–46.

26. Kraissl CJ. The selection of appropriate lines for elective surgical incisions. Plast Reconstr Surg (1946) 1951;8:1–28.

27. Nedelman R, Dixon JM. Marking of specimens in patients undergoing stereotactic wide local excision for breast cancer. Br J Surg 1992;79:55.

28. Singletary SE. Surgical margins in patients with early-stage breast cancer treated with breast conservation therapy. Am J Surg 2002;184:383–93.

Ten-year follow-up of a cohort of patients treated by breast conservation reporting patterns of local, regional and systemic recurrence. Study reports low annual rate of breast tumour recurrence with a ≥1 mm margin.

29. Houssami N, Macaskill P, Marinovich ML, et al. Meta-analysis of the impact of surgical margins on local recurrence in women with early-stage invasive breast cancer treated with breast-conserving therapy. Eur J Cancer 2010;46(18):3219–32.

A meta-analysis of margins that demonstrates that wide margins are unnecessary in breast-conserving surgery. It shows that both involved and close <1 mm margins are associated with a significant increase in local recurrence. This meta-analysis concludes that a 1-mm margin is sufficient.

30. Early Breast Cancer Trialists' Collaborative Group. Effect of radiotherapy after breast-conserving surgery on 10-year recurrence and 15-year breast cancer death: meta-analysis of individual patient data for 10 801 women in 17 randomised trials. Lancet 2011;378(9804):1707–16.

A meta-analysis demonstrating the value of radiotherapy after breast-conserving surgery in both reducing recurrence and improving overall survival.

31. Bartelink H, Horiot JC, Poortmans P, et al. Recurrence rates after treatment of breast cancer with standard radiotherapy with or without additional radiation. N Engl J Med 2001;345:1378–87.

32. Kurtz JM. Factors influencing the risk of local recurrence in the breast. Eur J Cancer 1992;28:660–6.

33. Mate TP, Carter D, Fischer DB, et al. A clinical and histopathological analysis of the results of conservation surgery and radiation therapy in stage I and stage II breast carcinoma. Cancer 1986;58:1995–2002.

34. Zafrani B, Viehl P, Fourqhet A, et al. Conservative treatment of early breast cancer: prognostic value of the ductal in situ component and other pathological variables on local control and survival. Long term results. Eur J Cancer Clin Oncol 1989;25:1645–50.

35. Ryoo MC, Kagan AR, Wollin M. Prognostic factors for recurrence and cosmesis in 393 patients after radiation therapy for early mammary carcinoma. Radiology 1989;172:555–9.

36. Chauvet B, Simon JM, Reynaud-Bougnoux A, et al. Récidives mammaires après traitement conservateur des cancers du sein: facteurs prédictifs et signification pronostique. Bull Cancer 1990;77:1193–205.

37. Pierce L, Levin A, Rebbeck T, et al. Ten-year outcome of breast-conserving surgery (BCS) and radiotherapy (RT) in women with breast cancer (BC) and germline BRCA 1/2 mutations: results from an international collaboration. Breast Cancer Res Treat 2003;82:S7.

38. Rebbeck TR, Lynch HT, Neuhausen SL, et al. Prophylactic oophorectomy in carriers of BRCA1 or BRCA2 mutations. N Engl J Med 2002;346(21):1616–22.

39. Fowble BL, Solin LJ, Schultz DJ, et al. 10 year results of conservative surgery and irradiation for stage I and II breast cancer. Int J Radiat Oncol Biol Phys 1991;21:269–77.

40. Haffty BG, Fischer D, Rose M, et al. Prognostic factors for local recurrence in the conservatively treated breast cancer patient: a cautious interpretation of the data. J Clin Oncol 1991;6:997–1003.

41. Locker AP, Ellis IO, Morgan DAL, et al. Factors influencing local recurrence after excision and radiotherapy for primary breast cancer. Br J Surg 1989;76:890–4.

42. Kurtz JM, Jacquemier G, Amalric R, et al. Risk factors for breast recurrence in premenopausal and postmenopausal patients with ductal cancers treated by conservation therapy. Cancer 1990;65:1867–78.

43. Asgiersson KS, McCulley SJ, Pinder SE, et al. Size of invasive breast cancer and risk of local recurrence after breast-conservation therapy. Eur J Cancer 2003;39:2462–9.

44. Eberlein TG, Connolly JN, Schnitt JS, et al. Predictors of local recurrence following conservative breast surgery and radiation therapy. The influence of tumour size. Arch Surg 1990;125:771–9.

45. Jacquemier RG, Kurtz JM, Amalric R, et al. An assessment of extensive intraductal component as a risk factor for local recurrence after breast-conserving surgery. Br J Cancer 1990;61:873–6.

46. Fourquet A, Campan F, Zafrani B, et al. Prognostic factors of breast recurrence in the conservative management of early breast cancer: a 25 year follow up. Int J Radiat Oncol Biol Phys 1989;17:719–25.

47. du Toit RS, Locker AP, Ellis IO, et al. An evaluation of differences in prognosis, recurrence patterns and receptor status between invasive lobular and other invasive carcinomas of the breast. Eur J Surg Oncol 1991;17:251–7.

48. Schnitt SJ, Connolly JL, Kettry U. Pathologic findings on re-excision of the primary site in breast cancer patients considered for treatment by primary radiation therapy. Cancer 1987;59:675–81.

49. Gage I, Schnitt SJ, Nixon AJ, et al. Pathologic margin involvement and the risk of recurrence in patients treated with breast-conserving therapy. Cancer 1996;78:1921–8.

50. Smitt MC, Nowels KW, Zdeblick MJ, et al. The importance of the lumpectomy surgical margin status in long term results of breast conservation. Cancer 1995;76:259–67.

51. Solin LJ, Fowble BL, Schultz DJ, et al. The significance of the pathology margins of the tumour excision on the outcome of patients treated with definitive irradiation for early stage breast cancer. Int J Radiat Oncol Biol Phys 1991;21:279–87.

52. Spivack B, Khanna MM, Tafra L, et al. Margin status and local recurrence after breast-conserving surgery. Arch Surg 1994;129:952–7.

53. Wazer DE, Jabro G, Ruthazer R, et al. Extent of margin positivity as a predictor for local recurrence after breast conserving irradiation. Radiat Oncol Investig 1999;7:111–7.

54. Schmidt-Ullrich R, Wazer DE, DiPetrillo T, et al. Breast conservation therapy for early stage breast carcinoma with outstanding ten year locoregional control rates: a case for aggressive therapy to the tumour bearing quadrant. Int J Radiat Oncol Biol Phys 1993;27:545–52.

55. Vallasiadou K, Young OE, Dixon JM. Current practices in breast conservation surgery: results of a questionnaire. Br J Surg 2003;90:44.

56. Montgomery DA, Krupa K, Jack WJL, et al. Changing pattern of the detection of locoregional relapse in breast cancer: the Edinburgh experience. Br J Cancer 2007;96:1802–7.

57. Abner AL, Connolly JL, Recht A, et al. The relation between the presence and extent of lobular carcinoma in situ and the risk of local recurrence for patients with infiltrating carcinoma of the breast treated with conservative surgery and radiation therapy. Cancer 2000;88:1072–7.

58. Fowble B, Hanlon AL, Patchefsky A, et al. The presence of proliferative breast disease with atypia does significantly influence outcome in early-stage invasive breast cancer treated with conservative surgery and radiation. Int J Radiat Oncol Biol Phys 1998;42:105–15.

59. Swanson GP, Rynearson K, Symmonds R. Significance of margins of excision on breast cancer recurrence. Am J Clin Oncol 2002;25:438–41.

60. Rose MA, Henderson IC, Gellman R, et al. Premenopausal breast cancer patients treated with conservative surgery, radiotherapy and adjuvant chemotherapy have a low risk of local failure. Int J Radiat Oncol Biol Phys 1989;17:711–17.

61. Goss PE, Ingle JN, Martino S, et al. A randomized trial of letrozole in postmenopausal women after five years of tamoxifen therapy for early-stage breast cancer. N Engl J Med 2003;349:1793–802.

62. Forrest P, Stewart HJ, Everington D, et al. Randomised controlled trial of conservative therapy for breast cancer: 6-year analysis of the Scottish trial. Lancet 1996;348:708–13.

63. Prosnitz LR, Goldenberg IS, Packard RA, et al. Radiation therapy as initial treatment for early stage cancer of the breast without mastectomy. Cancer 1977;39:917–23.

64. Wazer DE, DiPetrillo T, Schmidt-Ullrich R, et al. Factors influencing cosmetic outcome and complication risk after conservative surgery and radiotherapy for early-stage breast carcinoma. J Clin Oncol 1992;10:356–63.

65. Dewar JA, Benhamou S, Benhamou E, et al. Cosmetic results following lumpectomy, axillary dissection and radiotherapy for small breast cancers. Radiother Oncol 1988;12:273–80.

66. Liljegren G, Holmberg L, Westman G, et al. The cosmetic outcome in early breast cancer treated with sector resection with or without radiotherapy. Eur J Cancer 1993;29A:2083–9.

67. Haffty BG, Wilson LD, Smith R, et al. Subareolar breast cancer: long-term results with conservative surgery and radiation therapy. Int J Radiat Oncol Biol Phys 1995;33:53–7.

68. Petit JY, Garusi C, Greuse M, et al. One hundred and eleven cases of breast conservation treatment with simultaneous reconstruction at the European Institute of Oncology. Tumori 2002;88:41–7.

69. Amichetti M, Busana L, Caffo O. Long-term cosmetic outcome and toxicity in patients treated with quandrantectomy and radiation therapy for early-stage breast cancer. Oncology 1995;52:177–81.

70. Coopey S, Smith BL, Hanson S, et al. The safety of multiple re-excisions after lumpectomy for breast cancer. Ann Surg Oncol 2011;18(13):3797–801.

71. Sneeuw KA, Aaronson N, Yarnould J, et al. Cosmetic and functional outcomes of breast conserving treatment for early stage breast cancer. 1. Comparison of patients' ratings, observers' ratings and objective assessments. Radiother Oncol 1992;25:153–9.

72. Thomas JS, Julian HS, Green RV, et al. Histopathology of breast carcinoma following neoadjuvant systemic therapy: a common association between letrozole therapy and central scarring. Histopathology 2007;51:219–26.

73. Manton DJ, Chaturvedi A, Hubbard A, et al. Neoadjuvant chemotherapy in breast cancer: early response prediction with quantitative MR imaging and spectroscopy. Br J Cancer 2006;94:427–35.

74. Schaverien MV, Stutchfield BM, Raine C, et al. Implant-based augmentation mammaplasty following breast conservation surgery. Ann Plast Surg 2012; 69(3):240–43 Feb 21. Epub ahead of print.

75. Delay E, Garson S, Tousson G, et al. Fat injection to the breast: technique, results and indications based on 880 procedures over 10 years. Aesthetic Surg J 2009;29:360–76.

76. Rigotti G, Marchi A, Stringhini P, et al. Determining the oncological risk of autologous lipoaspirate grafting for post-mastectomy breast reconstruction. Aesthetic Plast Surg 2010;34:475–80.

77. Haffty BG, Fischer D, Beinfield M, et al. Prognosis following local recurrence in the conservatively treated breast cancer patient. Int J Radiat Oncol Biol Phys 1991;21:293–8.

78. Kurtz JM, Jacquemier G, Amalric R. Is breast conservation after local recurrence feasible. Eur J Cancer 1991;27:240–4.

79. Anderson EDC. Treatment of breast recurrence after breast conservation. In: Dixon JM, editor. Breast cancer: diagnosis and management. London: Elsevier; 2000. p. 1–5.

5

Techniques of mastectomy: tips and pitfalls

R. Douglas Macmillan

Introduction

Mastectomy is used to treat approximately 35% of all breast cancers. The procedure can be accomplished using one of a wide variety of techniques, depending on the clinical setting. Any mastectomy should be sensitive to the aims and principles of oncoplastic breast surgery, namely that optimal treatment of the malignancy should be achieved with minimal impact on quality of life.

Techniques of mastectomy are largely not evidence based. A few small trials exist but much of what is described in this chapter is based on reports of case series, expert opinion and personal preference. It is not intended to be prescriptive or dogmatic but merely a description of an approach to a commonly performed operation. Factors such as breast size, physical activities, preference for certain clothes (necklines) and expectations are all important discussion points that may influence choice of technique in many situations.

General considerations

The patient may have risk factors for poor wound healing, which include:

- smoking;
- obesity;
- diabetes;
- poor skin quality;
- previous radiotherapy;
- previous surgery to the breast;
- severe comorbidities.

Of these, smoking is the most commonly encountered factor that can be improved to optimise outcome within the timescale of the urgent case. This and other factors may affect technique selection.

Smoking

There are more than 4000 chemicals present in cigarette smoke, including nicotine and carbon monoxide.[1] One effect of nicotine is to cause vasoconstriction of the dermal–subcutaneous vascular plexus. This has important consequences, as mastectomy flaps rely on this plexus for survival.[2] As well as inducing a hypoxic state and causing vasoconstriction, smoking can lead to increased platelet aggregation, which results in the formation of tiny thromboses in capillaries. This is detrimental to wound healing, which relies heavily on blood flow in newly formed capillaries. Smokers have higher levels of fibrinogen and haemoglobin, which increase blood viscosity, which further increases the likelihood of blood clotting, and blood velocity can be reduced by up to 42% in smokers.[3] The combination of decreased oxygen delivery to tissues and the thrombogenic effects of smoking, together with increased viscosity and reduced velocity, explain why wound healing in smokers is significantly impaired.

The link between smoking and wound healing was first documented in the 1970s. One study of 425 patients undergoing mastectomy and breast-conserving surgery identified smoking as an independent predictor for wound infection and skin necrosis regardless of the number of cigarettes smoked.[4]

Another study of 716 patients having free transverse rectus abdominis myocutaneous (TRAM) flaps showed mastectomy flap necrosis, abdominal flap necrosis and abdominal hernias were significantly higher in smokers.[5] This study did demonstrate a dose effect with smokers who had a history of more than a pack a day for 10 years being at increased risk of developing problems compared with smokers who had smoked for a smaller number of pack years (55.8% vs. 23.8%). One observation in this study was that delayed breast reconstruction in smokers was associated with a significantly lower rate of wound complications compared with immediate breast reconstruction in smokers. The risk of wound complications in delayed reconstructions in smokers was similar to the rate in non-smokers. Complications were also less common in women who stopped smoking 4 or more weeks before surgery.

There was one small study of 108 patients investigating smoking cessation prior to surgery that was a randomised clinical trial with 40 patients in the control group and 68 patients in the interventional group.[6] Patients assigned to intervention were given counselling and nicotine replacement therapy. This study showed a significant reduction in complications in the intervention group, with a reduction in both wound-related complications and the need for secondary surgery.

In this study patients stopped smoking 6–8 weeks before surgery and did not smoke for 10 days after the operation. In the literature there is no consensus on the optimal duration of preoperative smoking cessation but there is evidence from a variety of studies that there are potential benefits from even a brief period of abstention. Part of the problem is that the majority of studies are retrospective and have inherent weaknesses in their design.

Considerations for simple mastectomy

In addition to general considerations, four questions should be answered:

1. Is it necessary/desirable to excise skin overlying the cancer?

In principle, skin only requires to be excised if the cancer is involving the skin or is so close that a clear margin cannot clearly be achieved around the cancer without skin resection.

2. Is there likely to be a lateral dog ear/redundant tissue?

The all too frequently seen but completely avoidable complication of mastectomy is redundant tissue, also known as a dog ear, which is unsightly, causes difficulty with bra fitting and often chafes on the prosthesis, arm or bra (**Fig. 5.1**).

3. Would the patient benefit from a contralateral breast reduction?

This is a simple and very effective option to enable women with a heavy breast to wear a lighter prosthesis and feel less unbalanced (**Fig. 5.2a**). In some cases a woman may choose a bilateral mastectomy to achieve better overall symmetry.

4. Is a delayed breast reconstruction planned?

The scar should be sympathetic to the method of delayed reconstruction planned. In most cases a low scar is best (as in Fig. 5.2a). It allows a flap-based reconstruction to be set at the inframammary fold, with the upper scar low enough to be hidden in low-neckline clothes (**Fig. 5.2b**).

Planning a mastectomy

- Examine the patient sitting up to assess lateral tissue and plan the likely lateral end of scar. The predicted lateral extent of the incision can be marked.
- The extent of the scar is important if radiotherapy is planned as the whole scar will be covered and can result in large volumes of tissue being treated if the scar extends a long distance posteriorly.

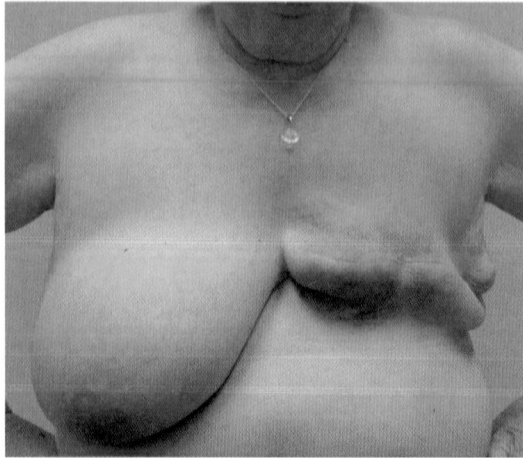

Figure 5.1 • Poor result from mastectomy.

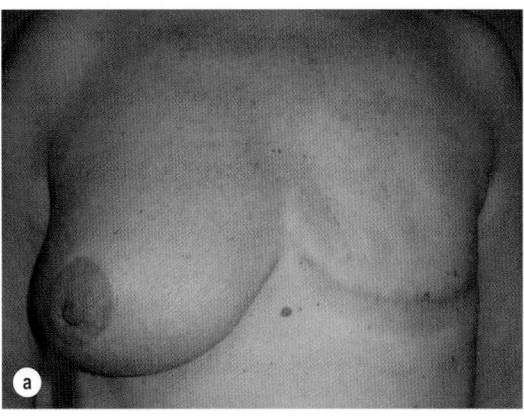 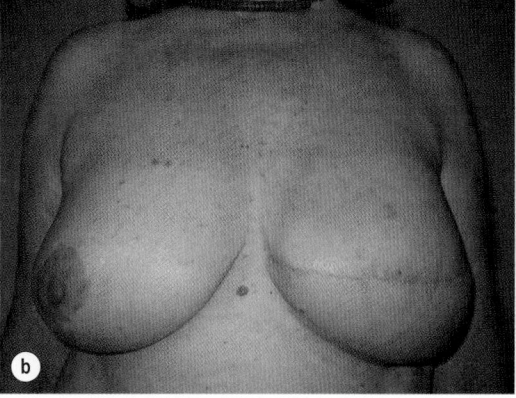

Figure 5.2 • **(a)** A low mastectomy scar with contralateral reduction. **(b)** Delayed reconstruction with LD flap.

- Mark any skin that needs to be removed over the cancer.
- Decide if a second incision is required for sentinel node biopsy (usually not necessary).

Technique

Most scars can be based around the inframammary fold (IMF). The incision pattern is drawn in theatre initially with a line at or just below the IMF (in women with any intertrigo the scar should be placed below this). Then with repeated upward and downward movement of the breast the planned transposition of this line on the breast skin can be marked (**Fig. 5.3**). In most cases the upper incision line passes a little above the areola. Attention should be paid to the degree of tension applied to the upward or downward breast movement as this represents the tension that will be exerted on the wound on closure. The upper and lower incision lines should be planned so that they meet comfortably but without excess laxity. Incisions should be planned to avoid any dog ear. To achieve this it is often best to continue the incision along the bra line laterally, curving up slightly until the upper and lower lines meet (**Fig. 5.4**) or, if there is doubt about how to fashion the lateral end, stop the incision at the lateral edge of the breast and fashion it once the mastectomy is complete, before closure (see comments regarding dog ear below). Transverse mastectomy scars are commonly used but rarely, if ever, can be closed without significant excess of tissue, particularly laterally. It is beholden on all surgeons to be familiar with a range of mastectomy incisions and given that there are always better alternatives, transverse mastectomy scars should be avoided.

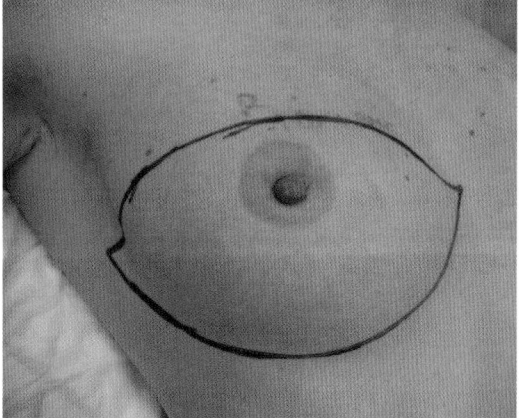

Figure 5.3 • Drawing of IMF-based incision.

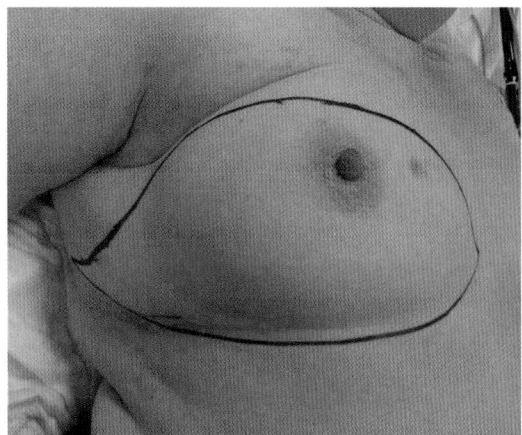

Figure 5.4 • IMF-based incision with lateral extension.

Inferior broad-based flaps can be designed to allow skin excisions in the upper pole. In breasts with a high nipple position or in cases where skin excision in the upper pole is desired, the lower incision line

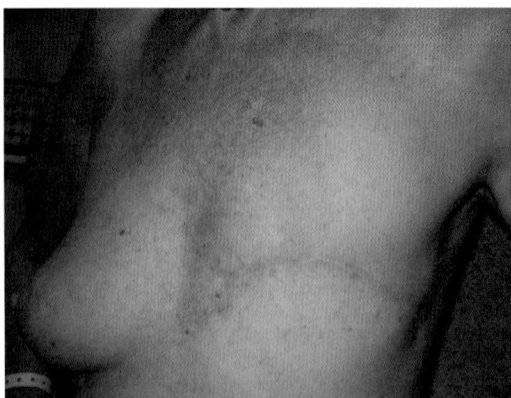

Figure 5.5 • Dome-type mastectomy scar to allow excision of upper pole skin.

can be adjusted to preserve skin on the lower flap. Such modifications to the inferior skin flap should be broad based. Other scar patterns to consider in such situations include the Wise pattern or dome-shaped scar (**Fig. 5.5**).

Lighting

A headlight is valuable and should be part of the equipment available for any breast operation.

Retraction

Care should be taken with the edges of the mastectomy flaps. Sharp hooks or tissue forceps applied to dermis cause less trauma to mastectomy flaps than blunt retractors.

Identifying the 'plane'

Some would contest its existence, but there is a readily identifiable plane between the breast and subcutaneous fat that defines the dissection. That is not to say that it is obvious in every case and it may be quite irregular. The thickness of fat on mastectomy flaps varies between patients and increases further the distance from the nipple. Importantly, however, the subcutaneous vessels (extensions of the intercostal perforators) lie superficial to this plane. The plane can be defined by hydrodissection infiltrating saline (I use 1 in 1 million – others use 1 in 500 000)/adrenaline using a spinal needle, Verres needle or blunt infiltration cannula attached to a 50-mL syringe or a pressure bag (100–150 mmHg) of saline/adrenaline solution. The plane is identified as a white line after performing a skin incision before the flaps are lifted and retracted. With opposing retraction on skin and breast and light initial dissection, tissues are seen to separate at the level of the plane. Dissection then chases this white line with continued opposing retraction (with skin hook retraction on the upper flap, skin kept as straight as possible), cutting on its superficial surface. This produces a flap of uniform thickness that will be thicker in fatter women and thinner in others.

Surgical tools

My preference is to use a hand-held diathermy on a fulgurate setting throughout. If using hydrodissection, scissors or a knife can be used as the plane is bloodless. Different surgeons have different preferences. Blood loss should be less than 100 mL if diathermy is used. Some prefer scissors or the knife because of concern of the 'burn' that results from diathermy dissection; blood loss is generally greater with scissors or the knife.

Preserving the intercostal perforators

These represent the main blood supply to the mastectomy flaps once the breast tissue is removed. Their preservation is important, not just for the prevention of flap necrosis and wound problems, but also to maximise the longer-term quality of the skin. The largest tend to originate at the second or third intercostal space. These are usually encountered early in the dissection just superior to the areola and can be seen (especially in thin women) and preserved during dissection upwards and medially.

Issues regarding posterior margin

Strong opinions are often expressed regarding whether or not to excise the pectoral fascia and when to excise some muscle. The posterior plane or breast plate is very well defined, certainly in the middle and upper part of the breast. In these areas there is no need and no clinical evidence to support removal of the pectoral fascia. For mastectomy, preservation of the fascia is only an issue if the cancer lies posterior in the breast. If this is the case and there is any doubt about adherence to muscle, then a portion of pectoral muscle can also be taken. In such situations a wide margin of muscle excision avoids the situation where a margin is reported as histologically involved or close (often due to its contraction following fixation), at no additional cost in terms of morbidity.

Inframammary fold

With a simple mastectomy this is normally excised, avoiding a ridge and producing a flat surface.

The anterior fat over the shoulder

This is often prominent and yet not part of the breast. If not contoured, it can produce a bulge in the upper outer aspect of the mastectomy site. Undermining the upper flap towards the shoulder often releases this fat pad so that it is more evenly distributed.

A flat surface

After mastectomy, before closure, the chest wall should be palpated with the flat of the hand to make sure there are no ridges or prominent irregularities. If so, these can be contoured prior to closure. There is some evidence that suturing the mastectomy flaps to the chest wall, so-called 'quilting', reduces seroma formation.

Suturing

Interrupted deep dermal sutures to approximate skin edges and gather any discrepancy between upper and lower flaps are advisable prior to a subcuticular suture. My preference is to use 3/0 absorbable suture throughout.

Managing the potential dog ear

Several techniques have been described for this. First and foremost, however, do not use incisions – such as a transverse mastectomy scar – which produces a 'dog ear' or 'angel wings' in the majority of patients in whom it is used. One approach to reduce 'dog ears' is as follows. If the patient is fairly thin, a flat lateral chest wall can be achieved by using an IMF scar as described above. In women with excess lateral tissue, it is often useful to complete the mastectomy with minimal extension of the scar laterally and then tidy this part of the scar. The easiest way to do this is to close the skin with temporary placement of skin staples. This then allows variations of lateral scar closure to be visualised before commitment to any particular one. The staples can be removed and replaced as many times as necessary to get the best and shortest scar. Final wound closure is with two layers of absorbable deep and superficial subcuticular absorbable sutures. Some lateral laxity can be accommodated by gathering the upper flap.

The three most useful techniques for lateral scar design in my experience are lateral extensions of the IMF scar, liposuction and the fishtail technique (**Fig. 5.6**). When performing fishtailing use staples to approximate the wound edges and take the lateral end of the transverse incision and move it and staple it medially to flatten out the lateral end of

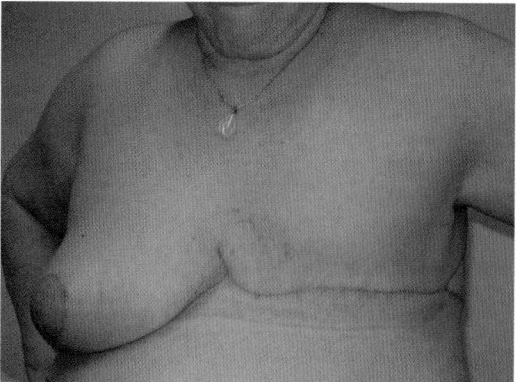

Figure 5.6 • Fishtail scar with contralateral reduction (correction of case in Fig. 5.1).

the wound to leave two smaller dog ears. Mark out incisions to excise these dog ears and then excise or de-epithelialise these (to preserve blood supply at the 'T' where the three wounds meet) to produce the fishtail pattern. Ensure that the wound is flat, if necessary by using liposuction. Liposuction is a useful adjunctive technique in many mastectomies.

Cases in which difficulty with the lateral tissue is predicted preoperatively can be performed either with the patient on their side (ideally) or with some degree of rotation. Women with excess lateral tissue can be challenging cases, and should be managed by those familiar with a range of flap-based surgery as well as liposuction, and be planned preoperatively. Glue provides a dressing that does not need to be changed, is waterproof (so patients can shower next day) and rarely produces skin reaction, so minimising further trauma to the skin surface around the flap edges.

Goldilocks mastectomy

Although it has been tradition to excise the excess skin over the breast during a mastectomy to leave a flat chest wall, other options may be considered. Skin that would normally be discarded may be de-epithelialised, shaped and buried to improve the cosmetic result. This may avoid the concave appearance that often results from mastectomy and in some cases can produce a small breast mound. Skin incisions are marked as normal but the skin between the upper and lower incisions is de-epithelialised. The de-epithelialised lower flap is then buried under the upper mastectomy flap. The amount of tissue that can be preserved and used in this way will vary considerably, depending on risk factors for tissue viability and the amount of skin required to be removed for oncological reasons. Care is required in wound closure to maintain the superficial vasculature (**Fig. 5.7a–c**).

Bilateral simple mastectomy

Ideally these should be symmetrical. Bilateral IMF-based scars work well. It is important to leave a skin bridge in the midline and not have a continuous scar across the chest.

Undesirable scar patterns

High transverse and most diagonal scars should be historical other than in salvage situations, likewise any scar that does not leave a flat surface with a contoured lateral chest wall. Transverse scars rarely leave a satisfactory result without fishtailing at the lateral end and are not recommended.

Considerations for mastectomy with immediate reconstruction

Of the general issues listed above, smoking is a particular concern and the major risk factor for flap necrosis and wound problems with skin-sparing mastectomy.[7] The following questions should be considered:

1. Is it necessary/desirable to excise skin overlying the cancer?

In general terms, the same principles apply as described above. However, immediate breast reconstruction is enhanced by preserving most (if not all) of the breast skin. Studies assessing the safety of this procedure relative to rates of local recurrence are summarised in Table 5.1. Although there are several that report acceptable recurrence rates, no large randomised trial data are available. It seems sensible to apply the same principles as one would for simple mastectomy. In other words, if the cancer is close to skin such that a healthy margin of normal tissue cannot easily be excised around it, then the overlying skin should be resected. An important

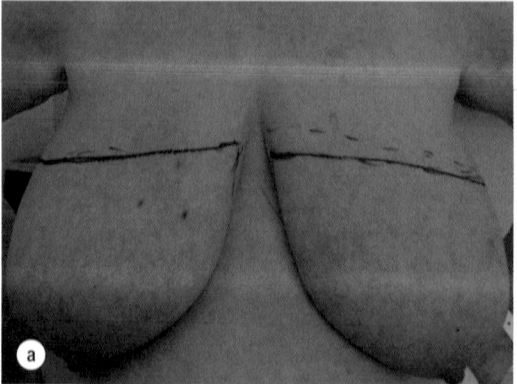
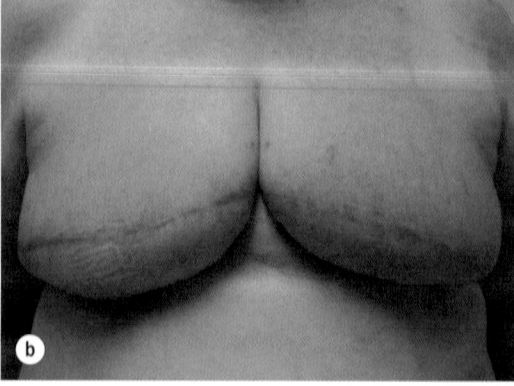
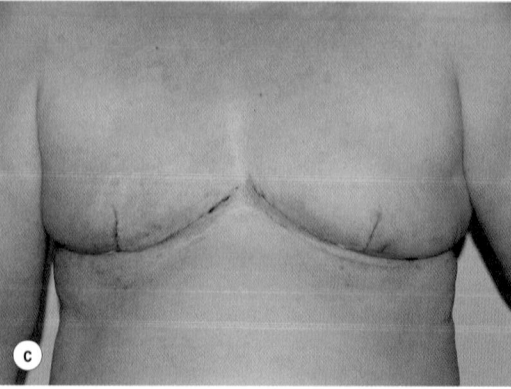

Figure 5.7 • Goldilocks mastectomy. **(a)** Preoperative markings. **(b)** Final outcome. **(c)** Bilateral Goldilocks mastectomy.

Table 5.1 • Case series of over 100 patients reporting local recurrence rates after skin-sparing mastectomy

Authors	Year of publication	Number of patients	Local recurrence rate/annum (%)	Follow-up (months)
Newman et al.[8]	1998	372	1.5	50
Kroll et al.[9]	1999	114	1.2	72
Medina-Franco et al.[10]	2002	173	0.7	73
Spiegel and Butler[11]	2003	221	0.5	118
Carlson et al.[12]	2003	565	1.0	65
Gerber et al.[13]	2003	112	1.0	65
Greenway et al.[14]	2005	225	0.4	49
Meretoja et al.[15]	2007	146	0.6	51
Petit et al.[16]	2009	1001	0.8	20

principle of oncoplastic surgery is that treatment must not be compromised for the sake of cosmesis. Different designs of skin-sparing mastectomy can allow skin excisions at any site.

2. Is overall reduction or augmentation planned?

This will obviously influence the scar pattern planned to facilitate the adjustment and obtain optimal symmetry of scars.

3. What scar design will give the optimum balance of access and aesthetic result?

Access to perform the mastectomy adequately cannot be compromised. Familiarity with a range of different options will enable the best outcome. Designs will vary according to method of reconstruction, as described below.

4. Is the nipple–areola complex to be excised?

This is increasingly considered an option in small breasts, particularly for prophylactic mastectomy but also in cancer cases.[8–16] Scar placement in this setting should allow good access to the breast and the nipple itself.

Planning a mastectomy with reconstruction

Examine and mark up with the patient standing. Different techniques are best described according to whether tissue-based or implant-based reconstruction is being performed.

Tissue-based reconstruction
Circumareolar

This is perhaps the most commonly employed technique. It gives excellent access to all but very large

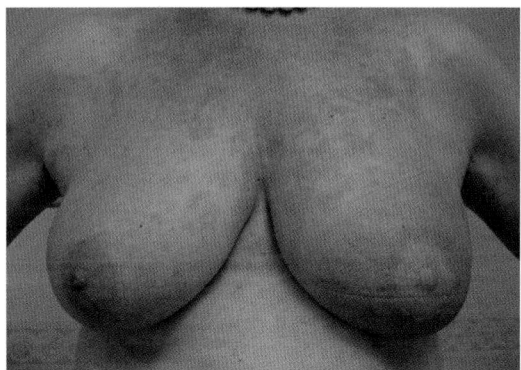

Figure 5.8 • Circumareolar mastectomy with immediate LD flap and nipple reconstruction.

breasts. It can be extended easily by a lateral or inferior extension or by widening the circular skin excision. The resulting defect is replaced with skin from the flap, often with nipple reconstruction at the same time (Fig. 5.8).

Wise pattern

This is another commonly employed technique that can be used for any ptotic breast. The design is more conservative than would be used for a standard breast reduction, and is often best planned as very conservative, with adjustment of the vertical limbs at the time of closure according to viability and tension. A vulnerable part of this design is the lateral part of the inverted 'T'. A recent modification is to de-epithelialise the lower mastectomy flap as for a 'Goldilocks' mastectomy so the vulnerable part of the T incision is placed directly over the de-epithelialised lower flap of the mastectomy scar. With division of the lateral thoracic vessels as part of the mastectomy, this often ends up as the most ischaemic part of the mastectomy flap. Designing an inverted 'V' component to

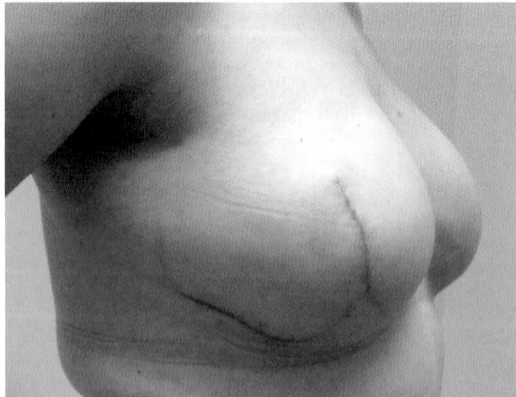

Figure 5.9 • Preservation of inverted 'V' on lower flap in Wise pattern mastectomy with implant reconstruction.

the lower incision that will release tension at the 'T' junction is often prudent (**Fig. 5.9**). Preservation of a larger section of lower flap skin until the time of closure enables the option of wider skin excision if viability is a concern or, as outlined above, de-epithelialisation and double-breasting of the scar.

Dome

This allows excision of an aesthetic unit of the breast of variable size. It also allows the flap to be inserted directly into the IMF. It is a very 'safe' design for higher risk cases.

Vertical

This is only really suitable for small breasts.

Implant reconstruction
Wise pattern

This is probably the best option for the large breast and possibly any breast with some ptosis. It gives excellent access to the breast. It is particularly useful when a lower de-epithelialised flap is being used to create a partial submuscular/partial subdermal pocket (**Fig. 5.10a,b**). This has become a standard approach when available. A de-epithelialised lower flap can also be combined with the use of a dermal matrix for breast reconstruction and can provide complete cover of the dermal matrix, particularly in the vulnerable area where all three scars meet.

Vertical

This is a good option in small breasts when a total submuscular pocket is planned. Shortening of the scar is rarely possible to any significant degree. This can sometimes be combined with a de-epithelialised

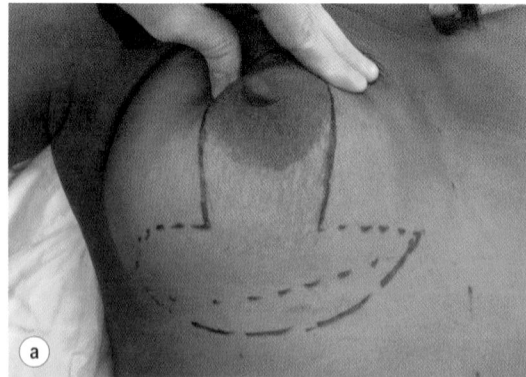

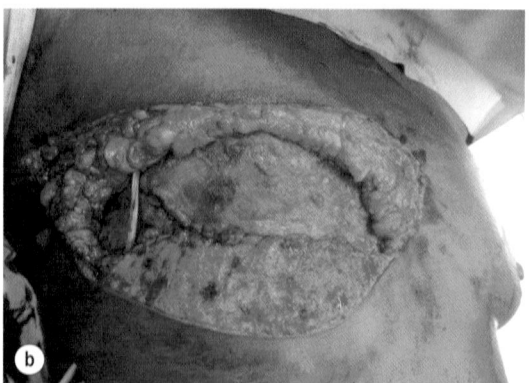

Figure 5.10 • **(a)** Drawing of a Wise pattern mastectomy. **(b)** Intraoperative demonstration of implant placed in a partial submuscular (pectoralis major and serratus anterior)/partial subdermal pocket before skin closure.

vertical mastopexy scar to allow repositioning of the nipple/areola.

IMF

A more technically demanding approach, but a scar based on the outer half/third of the IMF is very suited to one-stage implant reconstruction with subcutaneous mastectomy. This is similarly the case for the lateral skin crease or lateral breast curvature scar (**Fig. 5.11**).

Short transverse

This is sometimes a good option when a patient has a small areola that can be excised as a circumareolar incision but closed transversely.

Is a second incision required for sentinel lymph node biopsy?

This is often prudent with skin-sparing mastectomy to allow a timely search for blue nodes and limit

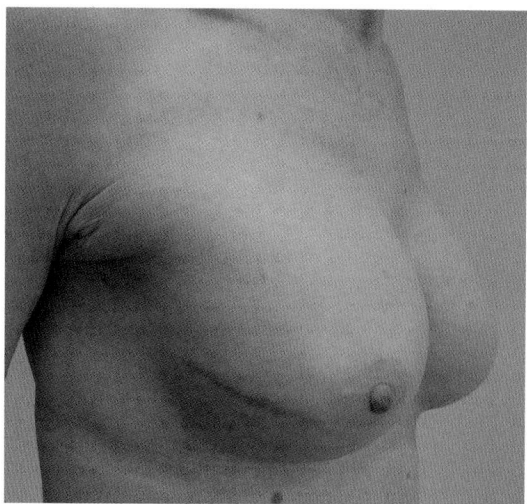

Figure 5.11 • Lateral skin crease scar.

the degree with which skin flaps are retracted, with small distal incisions to access the axilla. It can also be valuable if a latissimus dorsi flap is being used for the breast reconstruction.

Undesirable scar patterns

- **Hemicircumareoalar.** This allows very restricted and, in my opinion, difficult access to the breast in all but very small breasts and compromises nipple blood supply.
- **Any long transverse/oblique scar.** These really have no role in immediate reconstruction.
- **Purse-string.** This is intuitive, but creates ischaemia at the skin edge, can result in a central sinus, stretches to produce an unsightly scar, and results in a scar that presents difficulties for nipple reconstruction and tattooing.

Technique

Preoperative marking

Mark with the patient standing. Put a mark on the midline and draw a dashed line around the circumference of the breast. For the periphery above the IMF take the weight of the breast and move it towards each periphery to enable the edge of the breast to be seen and marked. In practice this becomes most useful when a mastectomy is performed with the patient on their side simultaneous to raising a latissimus dorsi (LD) flap.

Other markings will depend on the scar pattern to be used.

Circumareolar incisions can be marked pre- or intraoperatively. In women with a large areola some areola can be preserved.

For Wise and vertical patterns the breast meridian is drawn and patients marked up as for a reduction or mastopexy but with more conservative vertical incision lines (Fig. 5.10a). In Wise pattern mastectomy the vertical components are usually 10 cm in length from apex to horizontal incision. They often hug the areola margin. They can always be trimmed if necessary on closure and the 'T' junction modified as described above.

Dome-shaped incisions are based on the IMF. The base width can be varied. The apex of the dome is on the breast meridian and can be extended to the required height.

IMF incisions start medially at a line drawn vertically from the medial edge of the areola and extend laterally along the IMF/lateral breast curvature (usually 6–8 cm).

In a similar fashion to simple mastectomy, the plane is often best identified using opposing traction on the wound before skin hooks or similar retractors are applied. For incisions where access is limited, hydrodissection an adrenaline/saline solution injected using a blunt infiltration cannula is very useful. A bloodless field is essential to allow visualisation of the plane of dissection throughout and preservation of the perforators. If access is really felt to be compromising the dissection, then the incision should be extended. For IMF incisions the mastectomy is usually best achieved by dissecting the subcutaneous plane with half open scissors. This is quick, usually bloodless and avoids excess retraction. Once the subcutaneous plane is dissected, the submammary plane is dissected with cautery. The peripheral attachments can then be dissected under direct vision. For subcutaneous mastectomies, the nipple/areola is preserved by first bluntly dissecting the subareolar plane with scissors. The ducts are then divided close to the nipple base. With the nipple inverted any remaining ducts can be trimmed from the nipple 'core'.

Inframammary fold

This should be preserved.

Pectoral fascia

It is an advantage to preserve this if an implant reconstruction is being performed as it adds reinforcement to a submuscular pocket.

Wound closure

The use of deep dermal interrupted sutures before subcuticular closure maximises wound quality. Wound edges should be 'freshened', particularly if traumatised by retraction during operation. Often wounds can be double-breasted, with the small reinforcing de-epithelialised segment.

Skin stapler

This is particularly useful in Wise pattern mastectomy or any mastectomy where a skin-bearing flap is being inserted. The shape can be visualised and flaps trimmed as appropriate. Staples are always removed and wound closure should be with absorbable subcuticular sutures.

Glue

This produces a waterproof dressing that does not need re-dressing.

Over-dressing

If a support over-dressing (e.g. gauze and Elastoplast) is used this should be lightly applied so as not to compromise mastectomy flap blood flow. Steri-strips, if used, should be wide 0.5- or 1-inch and placed parallel to the wound, *not* at 90° to the skin incision, as they can cause blistering.

Flap necrosis

Using the principles and techniques described this should be a rarity (1% or 2% of cases). The main reasons for it are smoking, poor technique selection, poor execution of dissection, failure to preserve the intercostal perforators and too much tension of wound edges. In the circumstances where flap necrosis is encountered, early surgical debridement may allow direct re-closure and usually results in a satisfactory outcome (**Fig. 5.12a,b**). Occasionally a small skin graft is required.

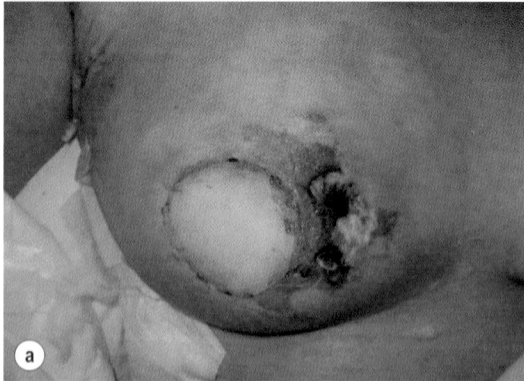

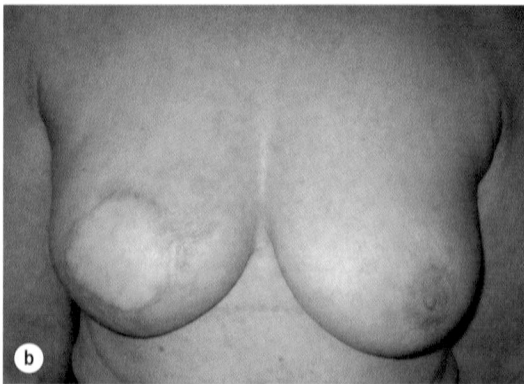

Figure 5.12 • (a) Skin necrosis after circumareolar mastectomy and LD flap in a heavy smoker. **(b)** Appearance a few weeks after early (next day) debridement and primary re-closure.

Radical mastectomy

This still has a role to control locally advanced disease. Formal removal of all of the pectoralis major muscle is, however, rarely required and partial excisions removing the area of muscle involved with a margin of normal muscle are usually sufficient. In escalating order, the following options for wound closure should be considered:

- abdominal advancement flap;
- split-skin graft;
- lateral chest wall perforator flap;
- LD flap;
- deep inferior epigastric perforator/transverse rectus abdominis myocutaneous flap.

All have a potential role depending on the size of defect, patient fitness and suitability of donor sites.

Key points

Mastectomy

- A flat, even chest wall should be achievable in all patients.
- The aim should be to avoid so-called 'dog ears' by using an incision that avoids these and in particular avoiding transverse incisions.
- The technique should be sympathetic to a delayed reconstruction if planned.

Mastectomy with reconstruction

- Many techniques are available.
- The technique should be appropriate to the method of reconstruction.
- The technique should not compromise on access or cancer excision.

References

1. Krueger JK, Rohrich RJ. Clearing the smoke: the scientific rationale for tobacco abstention with plastic surgery. Plast Reconstr Surg 2001;108(4):1063–73.

2. Chang LD, Buncke G, Slezak S, et al. Cigarette smoking, plastic surgery and microsurgery. J Reconstr Microsurg 1996;12(7):467–74.

3. Sarin CL, Austin JC, Nickel WO. Effects of smoking on digital blood flow velocity. JAMA 1974;229(10):1327.

4. Sorensen LT, Horby J, Friis E, et al. Smoking as a risk factor for wound healing and infection in breast cancer surgery. Eur J Surg Oncol 2002;28(8):815–20.

5. Chang DW, Reece GP, Wang B, et al. Effect of smoking on complications in patients undergoing free TRAM flap breast reconstruction. Plast Reconstr Surg 2000;105(7):2374–80.

6. Moller WM, Villebro N, Pederson T, et al. Effect of preoperative smoking intervention on postoperative complications: a randomised clinical trial. Lancet 2002;359(9301):114–7.

7. Woerdeman LAE, Hage JJ, Hofland MMI, et al. A prospective assessment of surgical risk factors in 400 cases of skin-sparing mastectomy and immediate breast reconstruction with implants to establish selection criteria. Plast Reconstr Surg 2007;119:455–63.

8. Newman LA, Kuerer HM, Hunt KK, et al. Presentation, treatment, and outcome of local recurrence after skin-sparing mastectomy and immediate breast reconstruction. Ann Surg Oncol 1998;5:620–6.

9. Kroll SS, Khoo A, Singletary SE, et al. Local recurrence risk after skin-sparing and conventional mastectomy: a 6-year follow-up. Plast Reconstr Surg 1999;104:421–5.

10. Medina-Franco H, Vasconez LO, Fix RJ, et al. Factors associated with local recurrence after skin-sparing mastectomy and immediate breast reconstruction for invasive breast cancer. Ann Surg 2002;235:814–9.

11. Spiegel AJ, Butler CE. Recurrence following treatment of ductal carcinoma in situ with skin-sparing mastectomy and immediate breast reconstruction. Plast Reconstr Surg 2003;111:706–11.

12. Carlson GW, Styblo TM, Lyles RH, et al. Local recurrence after skin-sparing mastectomy: tumor biology or surgical conservatism? Ann Surg Oncol 2003;10:108–12.

13. Gerber B, Krause A, Reimer T, et al. Skin-sparing mastectomy with conservation of the nipple–areola complex and autologous reconstruction is an oncologically safe procedure. Ann Surg 2003;238:120–7.

14. Greenway RM, Schlossberg L, Dooley WC. Fifteen-year series of skin-sparing mastectomy for stage 0 to 2 breast cancer. Am J Surg 2005;190:918–22.

15. Meretoja TJ, von Smitten KAJ, Leidenius MHK, et al. Local recurrence of stage 1 and 2 breast cancer after skin-sparing mastectomy and immediate breast reconstruction in a 15 year series. Eur J Surg Oncol 2007;33:1142–5.

16. Petit J-Y, Veronesi U, Orecchia R, et al. Nipple sparing mastectomy with nipple areola intraoperative radiotherapy: one thousand and one cases of a five years experience at the European Institute of Oncology of Milan (EIO). Breast Cancer Res Treat 2009;117:333–8.

6

Oncoplastic procedures to allow breast conservation and a satisfactory cosmetic outcome

Richard M. Rainsbury
Krishna B. Clough
Gabriel J. Kaufman
Claude Nos
J. Michael Dixon

Part 1
Volume replacement techniques to improve cosmetic outcomes after breast-conserving surgery

Richard M. Rainsbury

Introduction

Breast-conserving surgery (BCS) combined with radiotherapy has become the treatment of choice for the majority of women presenting with primary breast cancer over the last 20 years.

> ✔✔ A number of prospective randomised trials have compared BCS with mastectomy, showing a survival rate that is unrelated to the type of surgery performed,[1–4] although local recurrence (LR) rates may be higher when the breast is conserved.[1]

The risk of LR is related to a number of factors, including positive margins, tumour grade, extent of in situ component, lymphovascular invasion and age. Whole-breast section analysis techniques have been used to show the likelihood of complete excision of unicentric carcinomas using different margins of excision (see Chapters 4 and 15).

> ✔✔ Holland et al.[5] showed that a margin of 2 cm would eradicate all microscopic disease in about 60% of cases compared with a margin of 4 cm, which increases this figure to about 90%.

Local recurrence and cosmetic outcome

The margins of clearance and to a lesser degree the extent of local excision during BCS are strong predictors of subsequent LR.[6]

The extent of local excision remains a controversial issue in BCS. The wider the margin of clearance, the less the risk of incomplete excision and thus potentially of LR (Table 6.1), but the greater the amount of tissue removed, the higher the risk of visible deformity leading to an unacceptable cosmetic result. This clash of interests[8] is most evident when attempting BCS in patients with smaller breast–tumour ratios, for example when planning BCS for a 10-mm tumour in a 200-g breast or a 5-cm tumour in a 700-g breast.

The chances of a poor cosmetic outcome are increased still further when the tumour is in a central, medial or inferior location.[9,10] Cosmetic failure is more common than generally appreciated, occurring

Table 6.1 • Technique-related outcomes of breast-conserving surgery

	Quadrant-ectomy	Wide local excision
Margin (cm)	2–4	1–2
Clearance (%)*	<90	<58
Recurrence (%)[†]	2	7
Cosmesis	Fair	Good

*Holland et al.[5]
[†]Veronesi et al.[7]

in up to 50% of patients after BCS.[11–15] A number of factors are responsible, including volume loss of more than 10–20% leading to retraction and asymmetry, nipple–areola displacement or distortion, the use of ugly and inappropriate incisions, and the local effects of radiotherapy. Volume loss underlies many of the most visible and distressing examples of poor cosmetic outcome and the effects may be compounded by associated displacement of the nipple–areola complex (NAC). Poor surgical technique leading to postoperative haematoma, infection or breast tissue and fat necrosis will increase the amount of scarring and retraction, and add to the risks of deformity. Moreover, the use of suction drains, inappropriate incisions and en bloc resections can worsen the cosmetic result still further.

Role of oncoplastic surgery

The interrelationship between breast–tumour ratio, volume loss, cosmetic outcome and margins of clearance is complex, and the widespread popularity of BCS has focused attention on new oncoplastic techniques that can avoid unacceptable cosmetic results. Until now, surgical options have been limited to BCS or mastectomy, the choice depending on fairly well-defined indications and factors. Oncoplastic techniques provide a 'third option' that avoids the need for mastectomy in selected patients and can influence the outcome of BCS in three respects:

1. Oncoplastic techniques allow wider excision of breast cancers without risking major local deformity.
2. The use of oncoplastic techniques to prevent deformity can extend the scope of BCS to include patients with 3–5 cm tumours, without compromising the adequacy of resection or the cosmetic outcome.

3. Volume replacement can be used after previous BCS and radiotherapy to correct unacceptable deformity[16] and may prevent the need for mastectomy in some cases of local recurrence when further local excision would result in considerable volume loss.

Choice of oncoplastic technique

The choice of technique depends on a number of factors, including the extent of resection, position of the tumour, timing of surgery, experience of the surgeon and expectations of the patient. Reconstruction at the same time as resection (breast-sparing reconstruction) is gaining in popularity. As a general rule, it is much easier to prevent than to correct a deformity that has developed as the sequela of previous surgery. Immediate reconstruction at the time of mastectomy is associated with clear surgical,[17] financial[18,19] and psychological[20] benefits, and similar benefits are seen in patients undergoing immediate breast-sparing reconstruction after partial mastectomy.

Resection defects can be reconstructed in one of two ways: (i) by volume replacement, importing volume from elsewhere to replace the amount of tissue resected; or (ii) by volume displacement, recruiting and transposing local dermoglandular flaps into the resection site. Volume replacement techniques can restore the shape and size of the breast, achieving symmetry and excellent cosmetic results without the need for contralateral surgery. However, these techniques require additional theatre time and may be complicated by donor-site morbidity, flap loss and an extended convalescence. In contrast, volume displacement techniques require less extensive surgery, can limit scars on the breast and limit donor-site problems. These procedures may be complicated by necrosis of the dermoglandular flaps and contralateral surgery is usually required to restore symmetry as volume loss is inevitable (Table 6.2).

A number of factors need to be considered when making the choice between volume replacement and volume displacement. Volume replacement is particularly suitable for patients who wish to avoid volume loss and contralateral surgery after extensive local resections. They must be prepared to accept a donor-site scar and be made aware of the possibility

Table 6.2 • Comparison of techniques for breast-conserving reconstruction

	Volume replacement	Volume displacement
Symmetry	Good	Variable
Scars	Breast + back	Periareolar inverted-T
Problems	Donor scar Seroma flap loss	Parenchymal necrosis Nipple necrosis Volume loss
Theatre time (hours)	2–3	1–2 (per side)
Convalescence (weeks)	4–6	1–2
Timing	Immediate or delayed	Immediate > delayed
Mammographic surveillance	Possibly enhanced	Unaffected

of complications that may result in prolonged convalescence. Volume replacement is equally well suited to immediate and delayed reconstruction and is the method of choice for correcting severe deformity after previous breast irradiation.

Volume displacement techniques are particularly useful for patients with large ptotic breasts who gain benefit from a 'therapeutic' reduction mammaplasty that incorporates wide removal of the tumour. Volume displacement is less reliable in irradiated breasts, and patients need to be warned about the risk of asymmetry that may require simultaneous or subsequent contralateral surgery.

Volume replacement techniques

Several different approaches to volume replacement have been developed over the last 10 years, including myocutaneous, myosubcutaneous, perforator and adipose tissue flaps, lipomodelling and implants. Autologous latissimus dorsi (LD) flaps are the most popular option because of their versatility and reliability.

The myocutaneous LD flap carries a skin paddle that can be used to replace skin which has been resected at the time of BCS or as a result of contracture and scarring following previous resection and radiotherapy[16] (**Fig. 6.1**). Although the skin paddle adds to the replacement volume, it can lead to an ugly 'patch' effect because of the difference in colour between the donor skin and the skin of the native breast.

✔️ A myosubcutaneous LD miniflap[21] circumvents this problem by harvesting the flap in a plane deep to Scarpa's fascia. This produces a bulky flap without a skin island and includes a layer of fat on its superficial surface that is used to reconstruct defects following wide excision with preservation of the overlying skin (**Fig. 6.2**).

Transverse rectus abdominis myocutaneous (TRAM) and deep inferior epigastric perforator (DIEP) flaps are used much less frequently, as the greater risk of these procedures renders them a less attractive choice than LD flaps in this particular situation. Moreover, fat necrosis is a more common

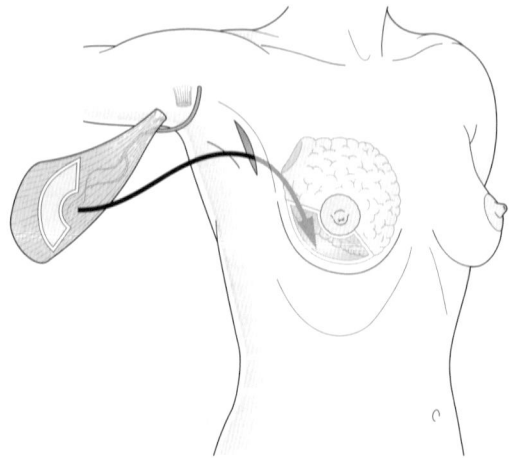
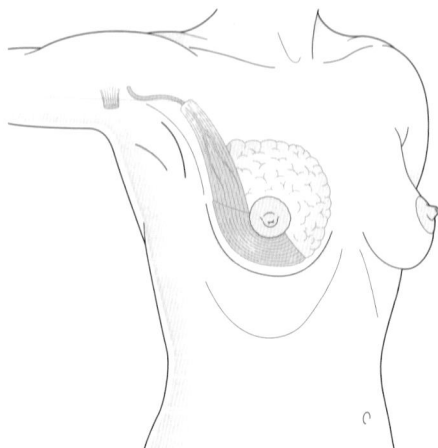

Figure 6.1 • Latissimus dorsi myocutaneous miniflap.

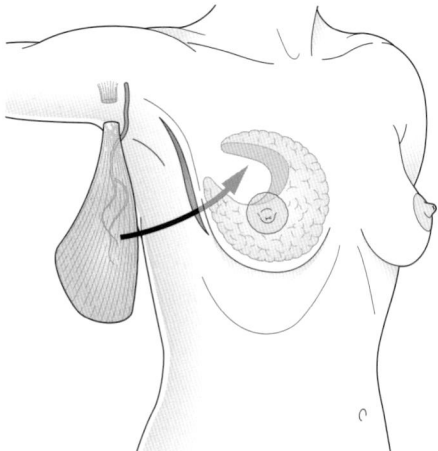
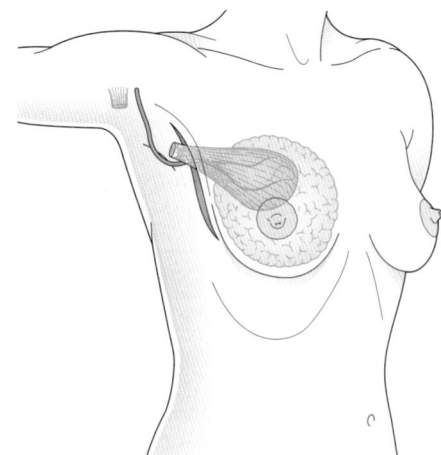
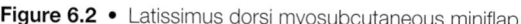

Figure 6.2 • Latissimus dorsi myosubcutaneous miniflap.

complication of abdominal flaps, creating the potential for diagnostic confusion on follow-up.

Perforator flaps[22,23] based on thoracodorsal artery perforators ('TDAP flaps') and lateral intercostal artery perforators ('LICAP flaps') are gaining popularity. They provide skin and subcutaneous fat for volume replacement, are relatively quick to perform, and appear to be associated with a faster recovery and less morbidity than LD flaps. As the LD is relatively undisturbed, the LD muscle can be used for breast reconstruction if a mastectomy is required for a subsequent local recurrence. TDAP flaps are most suitable for lateral and upper pole defects, while LICAP flaps can be used to reconstruct small to medium-sized lateral pole defects. Neither flap can be transposed sufficiently to reconstruct medial pole defects, which are more suitable for reconstruction by an LD miniflap that has been fully mobilised following divison of the tendon, all the serratus anterior branches of the vessels and all remaining fascial attachments to terres major. Other flaps, such as the lateral thoracic adipose tissue flap, have been described[24] but their clinical utility is unclear.

Lipomodelling techniques[25] have been used to correct rather than to prevent deformity after BCS.[26] Stem cells harvested from fat are injected around the defect, into underlying pectoralis muscle and overlying subcutaneous fat, avoiding the breast parenchyma. This helps to avoid the confusing mammographic images resulting from areas of calcified fat necrosis in the vicinity of the tumour bed. The theoretical risk of tumour induction by injected stem cells remains a concern, and has led to the somewhat cautious introduction of this innovative technique into clinical practice.[26] Some surgeons have started to use lipomodelling at the same time as wide local excision but no long-term results of this technique have yet been reported.

Non-autologous volume replacement with saline or silicone implants has been tried with mixed success.[27,28] Implants can be placed directly into the resection defect or under pectoralis major. They cannot be moulded to fit the resection defect and they form localised capsules, particularly in irradiated tissues. This may interfere with clinical examination and also mammographic surveillance, although there are techniques to allow mammaplasty in breasts with implants and magnetic resonance imaging (MRI) follow-up is an option in such patients. If using implants, low height and low projection implants placed low in the treated breast combined with lipomodelling gives the best results. If there is deformity and significant nipple deviation then a myocutaneous flap is preferred. Autologous tissue transfer is usually the best option for most patients and results in a lifelike breast of normal shape and size.

A number of innovative surgical procedures have evolved that facilitate volume replacement at the time of BCS or at a later date:

1. Resection through a radial incision and LD harvest through an axillary incision.[29]

> ✔ This was the original description by Noguchi et al. of the use of LD myocutaneous flaps to reconstruct resection defects during BCS in small-breasted Japanese patients. Radial incisions are not the incisions of choice.

2. Conventional LD myocutaneous flap harvest for correction of major resection defects.[16]
3. Resection through a circumferential incision and endoscopic LD flap harvest and reconstruction through an axillary incision.[30]
4. Resection, LD harvest and reconstruction through a single lateral incision.[21]

Indications for volume replacement

Volume replacement should always be considered when adequate local tumour excision leads to an unacceptable degree of local deformity in those patients who wish to avoid mastectomy or contralateral surgery.

✅ Resection of more than 20% of breast volume, particularly from central, medial or inferior locations, significantly increases the likelihood of a significant and unsightly local deformity,[31] which results in psychological morbidity.[32] In these patients, volume replacement can extend the role of BCS and avoid mastectomy when resecting up to 70% of the breast.

Breast conservation with or without reconstruction was formerly reserved for patients with unifocal tumours, but the much wider excision achieved in patients undergoing immediate volume replacement allows resection of multifocal disease with clear margins and excellent local control.[33] Volume replacement may be inappropriate in those with more widespread disease or locally advanced T4 tumours. Likewise, LD volume replacement is hazardous in patients with a history suggesting damage to the thoracodorsal pedicle or to the LD muscle, and alternative methods should be considered (Box 6.1). Patients should be informed that using LD for breast conservation precludes its subsequent use for later breast reconstruction. If a mastectomy is required to treat recurrent disease, the options include a variety of free flaps or subpectoral implant-based reconstruction.

Timing of procedures

Ideally, reconstruction of the partial mastectomy defect should be performed immediately or within

Box 6.1 • Selection of patients for volume replacement

Indications
Breast of any size
Resection of 10–50% breast volume
Specimen weight typically 150–350 g
Correcting deformity after breast-conserving surgery
When mastectomy declined
When full reconstruction declined
When contralateral surgery declined
When radiotherapy planned after mastectomy
Contraindications
Multicentric tumours
T4 tumours
Diffuse malignant microcalcification
Comorbidity
Previous division of vascular pedicle
Previous ipsilateral thoracotomy

a few weeks of the tumour resection in order to prevent deformity rather than to correct deformity months or years later. The emergence of the multiskilled 'oncoplastic' breast surgeon will in future help to circumvent the current problems encountered when organising a 'two-team' approach involving breast and plastic surgeons. Moreover, immediate reconstruction is associated with fewer technical problems and complications than delayed procedures. Delayed reconstruction may be compromised by previous radiotherapy, leading to reduced tissue viability and an increased risk of fat necrosis, infection and delayed wound healing.

Immediate reconstruction can be carried out as a one-stage procedure,[21,34] which involves simultaneous resection and correction of the resulting defect. This requires perioperative confirmation of complete tumour excision using frozen-section techniques. As an alternative, the procedure can be split into two steps.[35] The first step involves excising the cancer and performing a sentinel node biopsy if the nodes are clinically and radiologically normal and the second step includes axillary dissection if required, flap harvest and reconstruction, and is carried out a few days later after confirmation of clear tumour resection margins. Patients undergoing a one-stage procedure must be informed that a mastectomy with or without reconstruction may be required if subsequent histopathological analysis confirms incomplete tumour excision.

Volume replacement with latissimus dorsi miniflaps

There are many similarities between the different surgical approaches used in breast-conserving reconstruction and these can be best illustrated by summarising the main steps involved in LD miniflap reconstruction, which has been described in detail elsewhere.[36,37] This procedure involves the use of a myosubcutaneous flap of LD for immediate reconstruction of a partial mastectomy defect, most commonly in the central zone but also in the upper outer and upper inner quadrants of the breast. The term 'miniflap' is somewhat misleading, as the flap needs to be of sufficient volume to replace resection defects resulting from the excision of 150–350 g of breast tissue. Moreover, the miniflap needs to be bulky enough to allow for a small degree of postoperative flap atrophy.

When planning immediate volume replacement, the patient needs to be fully informed about the nature of the procedure and the possibility that a subsequent total mastectomy may be required if partial mastectomy results in incomplete excision. Careful preoperative mark-up of the tumour, the margins of resection and the line of incision are essential. The operation allows simultaneous partial mastectomy, axillary dissection, mobilisation of part of LD (the miniflap) and reconstruction of the resection defect through a single lateral incision. The procedure is greatly simplified by high-quality equipment, which is essential when developing the narrow optical spaces behind the breast and on the superficial and deep surfaces of the miniflap.

The operation involves tumour resection, axillary dissection, flap harvest and reconstruction. First, the tumour is resected in a subcutaneous plane by separating the skin envelope overlying the tumour-bearing quadrant from the underlying breast disc by sharp dissection, using the preoperative skin marks to determine the exact extent of dissection. By developing a mirror-image retromammary space deep to pectoralis fascia, the mobilised tumour-bearing quadrant is gripped firmly between fingers and thumb and resected with a generous margin of normal breast tissue. Four biopsies taken from opposite poles of the resection defect are sent for frozen-section analysis to allow intraoperative assessment of completeness of excision. The cavity wall is inked in situ with methylene blue to identify the inner surface, and then can be re-excised in its entirety if considered necessary. Further bed biopsies can also be examined after re-excising the cavity wall if frozen-section examination of the initial biopsies shows incomplete excision. A mastectomy is performed if these further bed biopsies fail to confirm complete excision. Next, appropriate axillary surgery (sentinel node or axillary dissection) is carried out and the vascular pedicle is prepared.

The third step involves mobilisation of the LD miniflap by developing superficial and deep perimuscular spaces that mirror each other. The myosubcutaneous flap carries a layer of fat on its superficial surface to increase its volume and this is achieved by developing the superficial pocket just deep to Scarpa's fascia. Division of the miniflap around the perimeter of the dissection pocket and division of the tendon of the LD near its insertion ensures unrestricted transposition of the miniflap into the resection defect. Finally, reconstruction of the resection defect is completed by careful use of sutures to model the flap, before fixing it to the cavity walls.

Perioperative outcomes

The time required for breast-conserving immediate reconstruction with a miniflap lies somewhere between BCS alone and total mastectomy combined with immediate LD reconstruction. Early postoperative complications include infection, flap necrosis, haematoma formation and transient brachial plexopathy,[34] although postoperative stay and disability are similar to other types of BCS. Breast oedema is common, particularly after extensive resection, but usually settles within 6–8 weeks. It may be caused by division of multiple afferent lymphatic pathways during retromammary dissection. Donor-site seroma formation occurs in almost all patients, and can be reduced by 'quilting' or delaying drain removal. Flap necrosis is rare, and can be avoided by gentle resection and handling of the pedicle and by taking care to prevent traction and twisting injuries during transposition and fixation of the flap after tendon division.

Late sequelae of volume replacement include lateral retraction of the flap, leading to distortion and hollowing of the resection site, and flap atrophy. Flap retraction can be avoided by division and fixation of the tendon and careful suture of the flap into the resection defect. Detectable flap atrophy occurs in a minority of patients followed for up to 10 years.[38] It can be counteracted by over-replacement of the resected volume with a fully innervated flap that has been harvested with a generous layer of subcutaneous fat, by using a myocutaneous flap or by later lipofilling.[16]

Frozen-section analysis of bed biopsies has been found to correlate closely with the adequacy of excision determined by formal histopathology.[33] Moreover, the use of LD miniflap reconstruction leads to a significant fall in the number of incomplete excisions compared with BCS alone[24] without compromising the cosmetic outcome. Sensory loss following miniflap reconstruction is minimal compared with the loss following total mastectomy.[39] The sensory innervation of the breast and NAC is largely intact, except over the resected quadrant. Finally, volume replacement preserves symmetry, avoiding the need for alterations to the contralateral breast in almost all patients (**Fig. 6.3**).

Mammographic surveillance

The mammographic appearance of the partially reconstructed breast compares favourably with the appearances after routine BCS. Symmetry is preserved and the fibres of the isodense flap may be detectable, often associated with a variable zone of radiolucency that corresponds to the layer of surface fat. Flaps may be indistinguishable from the surrounding breast tissue, and important radiological characteristics such as skin thickening, stellate lesions and microcalcifications are easily visualised

after flap transfer. Volume replacement does not compromise the early detection of LR,[40] which typically develops at the junctional zone between muscle and breast parenchyma. The appearance of miniflap on mammograms contrasts with the radiodense distorting stellate scars that are a common source of diagnostic confusion following conventional BCS. Lastly, very few patients develop clinically detectable flap atrophy, with the majority of flaps remaining bulky and functional throughout the period of follow-up.

Future prospects

The role of breast-conserving volume replacement is set to increase as more precise, image-guided resection of specific zones of breast tissue becomes possible. Increasingly sophisticated imaging techniques, such as high-frequency ultrasound and contrast-enhanced dynamic magnetic resonance imaging,[41] may in future enable exact delineation and excision of all malignant and premalignant changes. Endoscopically assisted techniques[42] may increase the ability to harvest more bulky myosubcutaneous flaps, allowing the reconstruction of more extensive resection defects. This will require the further development of novel techniques for endoscopic dissection,[30] including the use of balloon-assisted techniques[42,43] and carbon dioxide insufflation to maintain the epimuscular optical cavities. Current progress is hampered by the use of non-flexible straight endoscopes to carry out dissection over the rigid convex surface of the chest wall.

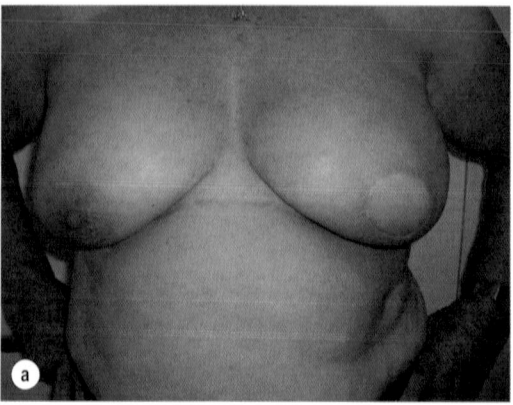 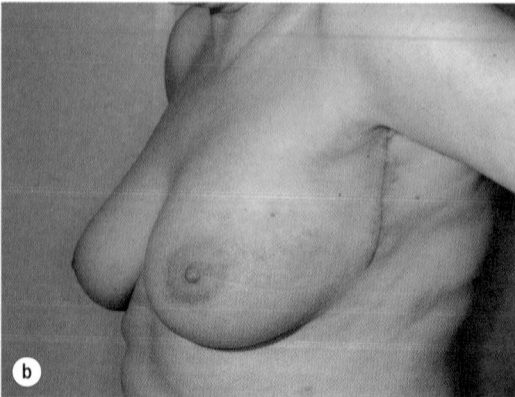

Figure 6.3 • **(a)** Latissimus dorsi myocutaneous miniflap. **(b)** Latissimus dorsi myosubcutaneous miniflap.

Deformities following breast-conserving surgery

Until recently, little attention has been paid to the cosmetic sequelae of BCS, as most patients are relieved not to lose their breast and many surgeons are unfamiliar with the plastic surgery techniques that can eliminate postoperative deformities. Moreover, there has been a tendency to recommend delayed reconstructive surgery some time after completion of radiotherapy. Although this is possible, partial reconstruction of the breast after surgery and radiotherapy is technically challenging and requires sophisticated techniques, with cosmetic results that are often disappointing.

In order to better assess the surgical approach for these patients, a classification of the cosmetic sequelae after BCS has been published by Clough et al.[44,45] This simple classification defines three groups of patients based on clinical examination (**Fig. 6.4**). The advantage of this classification is that it is a valuable guide for choosing the optimal reconstructive technique, but it is also a good predictor of the final cosmetic result after surgery.

- **✔** • Type I deformities: patients have a treated breast with a normal appearance but there is asymmetry between the two breasts.
  - Type II deformities: patients have a deformity of the treated breast. This deformity can be corrected by partial breast reconstruction and breast conservation, with the irradiated breast tissue being spared in the reconstruction.
  - Type III deformities: patients have a major distortion of the treated breast, or diffuse painful fibrosis. These sequelae are so severe that only a mastectomy can be considered.[44]

For type I deformities, a contralateral mammaplasty is performed to restore symmetry, avoiding any surgery on the irradiated breast. This is a simple and reliable approach, the irradiated breast serving as the model for a contralateral breast lift or breast reduction. Type II sequelae are almost always postoperative and are the most difficult to treat. A wide range of techniques can be used to repair these defects, from recentralisation of the nipple to the insetting of a flap to reconstruct a missing quadrant. Type III sequelae require treatment by

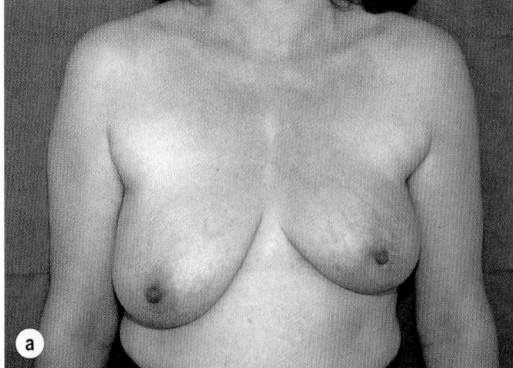

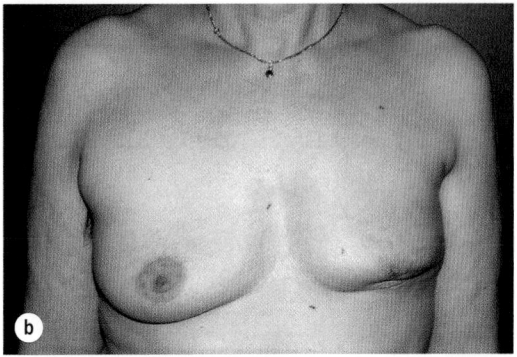

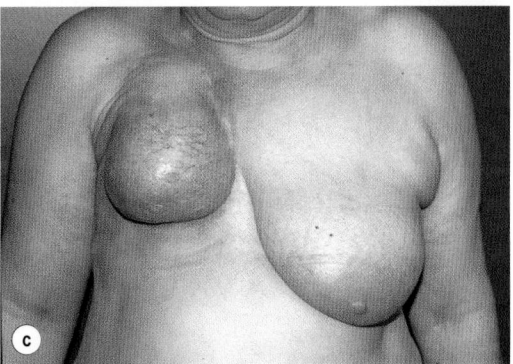

Figure 6.4 • Deformities after conservative treatment of breast cancer. **(a)** Type I: a symmetrical breast with no deformity of the treated breast. **(b)** Type II: deformity of the treated breast, compatible with partial reconstruction and breast conservation. **(c)** Type III: major deformity of the breast requiring mastectomy. Reproduced from Clough KB, Claude N, Fitoussi A et al. Oncoplastic conservative surgery for breast cancer. In: Operative techniques in plastic and reconstructive surgery. Philadelphia: WB Saunders, 1999; pp. 50–60. With permission from Elsevier.

mastectomy and immediate reconstruction with a myocutaneous flap.

Poor remodelling is one of the reasons for an ugly deformity after lumpectomy or quadrantectomy.[46,47] Some surgeons perform no remodelling at all, leaving an empty defect and relying on a postoperative haematoma to fill the dead space. This may produce acceptable results in the short term but breast retraction of larger defects invariably occurs with longer follow-up, leading to major deformities that are increased by postoperative radiotherapy.[10,44,48,49]

✅ Reshaping of the breast is required after any tumour excision in order to recreate a normal breast shape in one operative procedure. In most cases this can be achieved with a simple unilateral approach, mobilising glandular flaps to close the defect or by recentralising the NAC. In other cases, a bilateral approach incorporating a bilateral mammaplasty will be the only way to perform a wide excision with no deformity.[50] This graded approach to breast reshaping is discussed below.

Conclusion

Breast-conserving partial breast reconstruction extends the role of BCS by enabling complete excision of a greater range of tumours without compromising cosmesis, postoperative surveillance or symmetry. Volume replacement and displacement techniques are likely to become increasingly popular as an alternative to mastectomy in patients with small breast–tumour ratios and localised disease who wish to avoid more major surgery and the use of implants. Further experience of these techniques will lead to a better understanding of their role in the surgical management of primary breast cancer and in the management of local relapse and cosmetic deformity after previous breast-conserving procedures.

Key points

- Local recurrence following BCS is related to margin involvement that is less when wider excisions are performed.
- Deformity following wide local excision even for large cancers can be avoided by breast-sparing reconstruction using volume replacement or volume displacement.
- Volume replacement is most suitable for patients with small or medium-sized breasts who wish to avoid contralateral surgery. It can also be used for the correction of deformity following previous BCS.
- Breast-conserving reconstruction may be carried out as a one-stage or two-stage procedure.
- The type of breast-sparing reconstruction selected will be determined by the site and extent of resection, and by the patient's size, morphology and personal preference.

References

1. Fisher B, Redmond C, Posson R, et al. Eight-year results of a randomised clinical trial comparing total mastectomy and lumpectomy with or without irradiation in the treatment of breast cancer. N Engl J Med 1989;320:822–8.

   A seminal trial (NSABP B-06) showing equivalent overall survival in patients with breast cancer treated either by mastectomy or by lumpectomy and radiotherapy.

2. Veronesi U, Saccozzi R, Del Vecchio M, et al. Comparing radical mastectomy with quadrantectomy, axillary dissection and radiotherapy in patients with small cancers of the breast. N Engl J Med 1981;305:6–11.

   A seminal trial comparing the treatment of patients with breast cancer by radical mastectomy or quadrantectomy, showing equivalent overall survival in each group.

3. Veronesi U, Banfi A, Del Vecchio M, et al. Comparison of Halsted mastectomy with quadrantectomy, axillary dissection, and radiotherapy in early breast cancer: long-term results. Eur J Cancer Clin Oncol 1986;22:1085–9.

   A seminal trial comparing the treatment of patients with breast cancer by radical mastectomy or quadrantectomy, showing equivalent overall survival in each group after long-term follow-up.

4. Abrams J, Chen T, Giusti R. Survival after breast-sparing surgery versus mastectomy. J Natl Cancer Inst 1994;86:1672–3.

5. Holland R, Veling SH, Mravunac M, et al. Histologic multifocality of T_{IS}, T_{1-2} breast-carcinomas: implications for clinical trials of breast-conserving surgery. Cancer 1985;56:979–90.

   A detailed study using serial whole-breast sections to establish the distribution of breast malignancy in relation to the margin of the reference tumour.

6. Dixon J. Histological factors predicting breast recurrence following breast-conserving therapy. Breast 1993;2:197.

7. Veronesi U, Voltarrani F, Luini A, et al. Quadrantectomy versus lumpectomy for small size breast cancer. Eur J Cancer 1990;26:671–3.
   A seminal trial comparing very wide local excision (quadrantectomy) with limited excision of breast carcinoma (lumpectomy). Quadrantectomy was associated with significantly lower rates of local recurrence when compared with lumpectomy.

8. Audretsch WP. Reconstruction of the partial mastectomy defect: classification and method. In: Spear SL, editor. Surgery of the breast: principles and art. Philadelphia: Lippincott-Raven; 1998. p. 155–95.

9. Pearl RM, Wisnicki J. Breast reconstruction following lumpectomy and irradiation. Plast Reconstr Surg 1985;76:83–6.

10. Berrino P, Campora E, Sauti P. Postquadrantectomy breast deformities: classification and techniques of surgical correction. Plast Reconstr Surg 1987;79:567–72.

11. Borger JH, Keijser AH. Conservative breast cancer treatment: analysis of cosmetic role and the role of concomitant adjuvant chemotherapy. Int J Radiat Oncol Biol Phys 1987;13:1173–7.

12. Van Limbergen E, Rijnders A, van der Schueren E, et al. Cosmetic evaluation of conserving treatment for mammary cancer. 2. A quantitative analysis of the influence of radiation dose, fractionation schedules and surgical treatment techniques on cosmetic results. Radiother Oncol 1989;16:253–67.

13. Van Limbergen E, Van der Schueren E, Van Tongelen K. Cosmetic evaluation of breast conserving treatment for mammary cancer. 1. Proposal of quantitative scoring system. Radiother Oncol 1989;16:159–67.

14. Olivotto IA, Rose MA, Osteen RJ, et al. Late cosmetic outcome after conservative surgery and radiotherapy: analysis of causes of cosmetic failure. Int J Radiat Oncol Biol Phys 1989;17:747–53.

15. Ray GR, Fish BJ, Marmor JB, et al. Impact of adjuvant chemotherapy on cosmesis and complications in stages 1 and 2 carcinoma of the breast treated by biopsy and radiation therapy. Int J Radiat Oncol Biol Phys 1984;10:837–41.

16. Slavin SA, Love SM, Sadowsky NL. Reconstruction of the irradiated partial mastectomy defect with autogenous tissues. Plast Reconstr Surg 1992;90:854–65.

17. O'Brien W, Hasselgren P-O, Hummel RP, et al. Comparison of postoperative wound complications in early cancer recurrence between patients undergoing mastectomy with or without immediate breast reconstruction. Am J Surg 1993;166:1–5.

18. Eberlein TJ, Crespo LD, Smith BL, et al. Prospective evaluation of immediate reconstruction after mastectomy. Ann Surg 1993;218:29–36.

19. Elkowitz A, Colen S, Slavin S, et al. Various methods of breast reconstruction after mastectomy: an economic comparison. Plast Reconstr Surg 1993;92:77–83.

20. Dean C, Chetty U, Forrest APM. Effect of immediate breast reconstruction on psychosocial morbidity after mastectomy. Lancet 1983;i:459–62.

21. Raja MAK, Straker VF, Rainsbury RM. Extending the role of breast-conserving surgery by immediate volume replacement. Br J Surg 1997;84:101–5.

22. Hamdi M, Van Landuyt K, Hijjawi JB, et al. Surgical technique in pedicled thoracodorsal artery perforator flaps: a clinical experience with 99 patients. Plast Reconstr Surg 2008; 121:1632–41.

23. Hamdi M, Spano A, Van Landuyt K, et al. The lateral intercostal perforators: anatomical study and clinical application in breast surgery. Plast Reconstr Surg 2008;121:389–96.

24. Ohuchi N, Harada Y, Ishida T, et al. Breast-conserving surgery for primary breast cancer; immediate volume replacement using lateral tissue flap. Breast Cancer 1997;4:135–41.

25. Coleman SR, Saboeiro AP. Fat grafting for the breast revisited: safety and efficacy. Plast Reconstr Surg 2007;119:775–85.

26. Chan CW, McCulley SJ, Macmillan RD. Autologous fat transfer – a review of the literature with a focus on breast cancer surgery. J Plast Reconstr Aesthet Surg 2008;61:1438–48.

27. Schaverien MV, Stutchfield BM, Raine C, et al. Implant-based augmentation mammaplasty following breast conservation surgery. Ann Plast Surg 2012;69:(3):240–3 Feb 21. Epub ahead of print.

28. Elton C, Jones PA. Initial experience of intramammary prostheses in breast conserving surgery. Eur J Surg Oncol 1999;25:138–41.

29. Noguchi M, Taniya T, Miyasaki I, et al. Immediate transposition of a latissimus dorsi muscle for correcting a post quadrantectomy breast deformity in Japanese patients. Int Surg 1990;75:166–70.

30. Eaves FF, Bostwick J, Nahai F, et al. Endoscopic techniques in aesthetic breast surgery. Clin Plast Surg 1995;22:683–95.

31. Cochrane R, Valasiadou P, Wilson A, et al. Cosmesis and satisfaction after breast conserving surgery correlates with the percentage of breast volume excised. Br J Surg 2003;90:1505–9.

32. Al-Ghazal SK, Fallowfield L, Blamey RW. Does cosmetic outcome from treatment of pimary breast cancer influence psychological morbidity? Eur J Surg Oncol 1999;25:571–3.

33. Rusby J, Paramanathan N, Laws S, et al. Immediate miniflap volume replacement for partial mastectomy: use of intraoperative frozen sections to confirm negative margins. Am J Surg 2008;196:512–8.

34. Rainsbury RM, Paramanathan N. Recent progress with breast-conserving volume replacement using latissimus dorsi miniflaps in UK patients. Breast Cancer 1998;5:139–47.

35. Dixon JM, Venizelos B, Chan P. Latissimus dorsi miniflap: a technique for extending breast conservation. Breast 2002;11:58–65.

36. Rainsbury RM. Breast-sparing reconstruction with latissimus dorsi miniflaps. Eur J Surg Oncol 2002;28:891–5.

37. Rainsbury RM. The mini latissimus dorsi flap. In: Querci della Rovere G, Benson JR, Nava M, editors. Oncoplastic and reconstructive surgery of the breast. New York: Informa Healthcare; 2011. p. 96–104.

38. Laws SAM, Cheetham JE, Rainsbury RM. Temporal changes in breast volume after surgery for breast cancer and the implications for volume replacement with the latissimus dorsi miniflap. Eur J Surg Oncol 2001;27:790.

39. Gendy RK, Able JA, Rainsbury RM. Impact of skin-sparing mastectomy with immediate reconstruction and breast-sparing reconstruction with miniflaps on the outcomes of oncoplastic breast surgery. Br J Surg 2003;90:433–9.

40. Monticciolo DL, Ross D, Bostwick J, et al. Autogenous breast reconstruction with endoscopic latissimus dorsi with musculo-subcutaneous flaps in patients choosing breast-conserving therapy: mammographic appearance. Am J Radiol 1996;167:385–9.

41. Gilles R, Guinebretiere J-M. Magnetic resonance imaging. In: Silverstein MJ, editor. Ductal carcinoma in situ of the breast. Baltimore: Williams & Wilkins; 1997. p. 159–66.

42. Bass LS, Karp NS, Benacquista T, et al. Endoscopic harvest of the rectus abdominus free flap: balloon dissection in the fascial plain. Ann Plast Surg 1995;34:274–9.

43. Van Buskark ER, Krehnke RD, Montgomery RL, et al. Endoscopic harvest of the latissimus dorsi muscle using balloon dissection technique. Plast Reconstr Surg 1997;99:899–903.

44. Clough KB, Cuminet J, Fitoussi A, et al. Cosmetic sequelae after conservative treatment for breast cancer: classification and results of surgical correction. Ann Plast Surg 1998;41:471–81.
    The original classification of types of deformity following partial mastectomy and the use of therapeutic mammaplasty to avoid rather than correct deformity.

45. Clough KB, Thomas SS, Fitoussi AD, et al. Reconstruction after conservative treatment for breast cancer: cosmetic sequelae classification revisited. Plast Reconstr Surg 2004;114(7):1743–53.

46. Petit J-Y, Rigault L, Zekri A, et al. Poor esthetic results after conservative treatment of breast cancer. Techniques of partial breast reconstruction. Ann Chir Plast Esthet 1989;34:103–8.

47. Rose MA, Olivotto IA, Cady B, et al. Conservative surgery and radiation therapy for early breast cancer. Long-term cosmetic results. Arch Surg 1989;124:153–7.

48. Berrino P, Campora E, Leone S, et al. Correction of type II breast deformities following conservative cancer surgery. Plast Reconstr Surg 1992;90:846–53.

49. Petit J-Y, Rietjens M. Deformities following tumourectomy and partial mastectomy. In: Noone B, editor. Plastic and reconstruction surgery of the breast. Philadelphia: BC Decker; 1991.

50. Clough KB, Kroll S, Audretsch W. An approach to the repair of partial mastectomy defects. Plast Reconstr Surg 1999;104:409–20.
    Pooled experience of breast-conserving reconstruction from France, USA and Germany using volume replacement and volume displacement techniques.

Part 2

Breast displacement techniques to increase resection volumes for breast-conserving surgery

Krishna B. Clough
Gabriel J. Kaufman
Claude Nos
J. Michael Dixon

Introduction

Breast-conserving surgery (BCS) combined with postoperative radiotherapy has become the preferred locoregional treatment for the majority of patients with early-stage breast cancer, with equivalent survival to that of mastectomy and improved body image and lifestyle. The success of BCS for breast cancer is based on the tenet of complete removal of the cancer with adequate surgical margins while preserving the natural shape and appearance of the breast. Achieving both goals together in the same operation can be challenging, and BCS does not produce good cosmetic results in all patients. The limiting factor is the amount of tissue removed, not only in absolute volume, but also in relation to tumour location and relative size of breast. If either of these two goals is not achievable, mastectomy is often chosen as an alternative to BCS. The failure of classical BCS techniques to offer solutions for challenging scenarios has stimulated the growth and advancement of new techniques in breast surgery during the past decade. The dichotomy between extent of excision and cosmetic outcome has made it evident that new surgical techniques need to be developed to address the problems and shortfalls of BCS, and accommodate the expanding indications for BCS.

Oncoplastic surgery (OPS) has emerged as a new approach to allow wide excisions for BCS without compromising the natural shape of the breast. It is based upon integrating plastic surgery techniques with immediate reshaping of the breast together with oncological surgery to excise the breast cancer. The conceptual idea of OPS is not new and its oncological efficacy in terms of margin status and recurrence compares favourably to traditional BCS.[1,2]

The difference in the level of difficulty in performing various oncoplastic procedures has created a dichotomy in oncoplastic surgery. Oncoplastic techniques range from simple reshaping and mobilisation of breast tissue to more advanced mammaplasty techniques that allow resection of up to 50% of the breast volume. Variations in difficulty and the need for advanced training for some OPS techniques require a clear classification system of oncoplastic techniques, which provides a systematic approach that all breast surgeons can follow when undertaking BCS.

Oncoplastic considerations

Selection criteria for oncoplasty

There are three elements that are important in the identification of patients who would benefit from an oncoplastic approach. The two factors already recognised as major indications for OPS are excision volume and tumour location.[3] The third additional element is glandular density, a recently recognised factor in the determination of the safety of major breast reshaping. When considered together, these three major elements provide a sound basis for determining when and what type of OPS to perform and, more importantly, in reducing the guesswork when performing BCS.

Volume

> ✔ The first element is excision volume, which is the single most predictive factor for cosmetic surgical outcome and potential for breast deformity. Studies have suggested that once 10–20% of the breast volume is excised there is a clear risk of deformity[4] (see Chapter 4).

Excision volume compared to the total breast volume is estimated preoperatively. Through systematic correlation of specimen weights compared with tumour size, an accurate preoperative estimation of excision volume can be achieved, once the tumour size is known from preoperative imaging. The average specimen from BCS should weigh between 20 and 40 g, and as a general rule 80 g of breast tissue is the maximum weight that can be removed from a medium-sized breast without resulting in deformity (see Chapter 4).

OPS techniques allow for significantly greater excision volumes while preserving the natural breast shape. Reshaping of the breast is based upon rearrangement of the breast parenchyma to create a homogeneous redistribution of volume loss. This redistribution can be achieved easily though either the advancement or rotation of breast tissue into excision defects. Another option is to harvest a latissimus dorsi 'miniflap' to fill in the lumpectomy cavity (see Part 1 of this chapter).[3]

Tumour location

High-risk zones in the breast are more likely to be followed by deformity after BCS when compared to more forgiving locations.

> ✔ The upper outer quadrant of the breast is a favourable location for large-volume excisions. In this location, defects can readily be corrected by the mobilisation of adjacent tissue. Excision from less favourable locations such as the lower pole or upper inner quadrants of the breast often results in breast deformity.

One example is the 'bird's beak' deformity that is classically seen during excision of tumours from the lower pole of the breast (**Fig. 6.5a**). Other examples of difficult areas include excision of a central tumour (**Fig. 6.5b**) and removal of cancers from the upper inner quadrant (**Fig. 6.5c**). Therefore, it is important when planning the appropriate surgical approach to determine the tumour location and the likely level

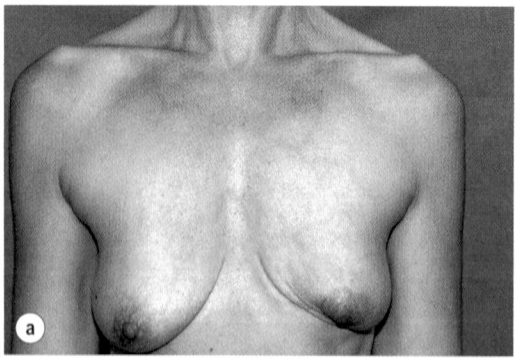

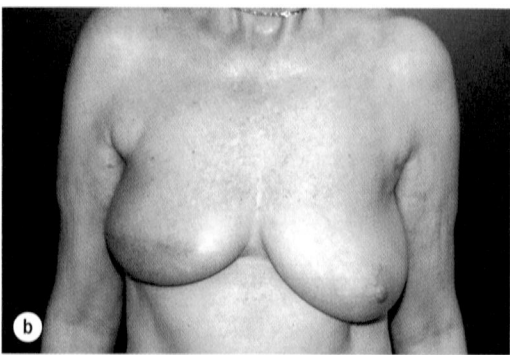

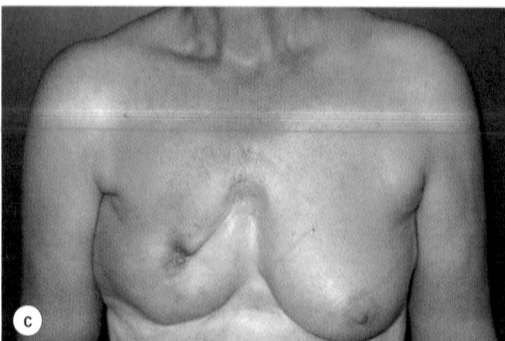

Figure 6.5 • Deformities after breast-conserving surgery. **(a)** Lower pole: bird's beak deformity. **(b)** Central tumour. **(c)** Upper inner quadrant.

for breast density determination. Breast density predicts the amount of fat in the breast and determines the ability to perform extensive breast undermining and reshaping without complications. Breast density can be classified into four categories based on the Breast Imaging Reporting and Data System (BI-RADS). The four categories comprise: (1) fatty; (2) scattered fibroglandular; (3) heterogeneously dense; or (4) extremely dense breast tissue.[5]

A dense glandular breast (BI-RADS 3/4) can be mobilised easily with undermining and advancement of breast tissue into the excision cavity without risk of necrosis. Low-density breast tissue with a major fatty component (BI-RADS 1/2) has a much higher risk of fat necrosis if extensive undermining is performed. Undermining the breast from both the skin and pectoralis fascia is a major requirement to perform level I OPS. A low breast density means that either the amount of undermining from the breast and skin during level I OPS should be limited, or a decision made to proceed with a level II option that requires limited skin undermining. Level II procedures that require extensive skin undermining such as the round-block technique are likewise not suitable for the patient with a predominantly fatty breast.

Classification system

Complexity of surgical procedure: a bi-level system

A new classification of OPS techniques has been proposed based upon the relative level of surgical difficulty. Level I techniques should be able to be performed by all breast surgeons without specific training in OPS. A level I approach includes skin and glandular undermining, including the nipple–areola complex (NAC), and NAC recentralisation if nipple deviation is anticipated. Level II techniques encompass more complex procedures that involve skin excision and glandular mobilisation to allow major volume resection. Level II techniques are derived from breast reduction techniques and require additional training.

The bi-level classification system lends itself to the creation of a practical guide to OPS and provides the necessary framework during surgical planning to correctly select the most appropriate surgical procedure for the patient (Table 6.3).

of associated deformity. An oncoplastic atlas of surgical techniques based on tumour location has been developed. The atlas provides a specific surgical technique for each possible tumour location in the breast.

Glandular characteristics and breast density

Glandular density is evaluated both clinically and radiographically. Although clinical examination provides reliable information on density, mammographic evaluation is a more reproducible approach

Table 6.3 • Oncoplastic decision guide

Criteria	Level I	Level II
Maximum excision volume ratio	20%	20–50%
Requirement of skin excision for reshaping	No	Yes
Specific training in reduction and mammaplasty techniques	No	Yes
Glandular characteristics	Dense	Dense or fatty

If less than 20% of the breast volume is excised then a level II approach is not usually required and a level I procedure is usually adequate. Anticipation that 20–50% of breast volume is to be excised or the cancer is in a specific location will require a level II procedure to produce a satisfactory cosmetic outcome. Large-volume excisions require concurrent skin excision to adequately reshape the skin envelope. If the breast parenchyma is fatty in composition, it may be risky to employ a level I technique if excising more than 10% of the breast volume. A superior outcome is likely to be obtained in such patients by selecting an appropriate level II procedure.

General considerations for all OPS techniques

The approach to OPS includes careful patient selection and starts with patient counselling. It is important to stress to the patient that although oncoplastic procedures can provide greater satisfaction with a better final breast shape and in some situations will avoid the need for mastectomy, outcomes do vary. During the consultation period patients need to be informed that OPS may result in longer and multiple scars. The position of each incision should be described in detail. The patient should also be made aware of the possible asymmetry that will follow from a level II OPS. Asymmetry in volume is expected, but necessary to limit breast distortion and deformity. The patient must be informed that, in such circumstances, to achieve symmetry an immediate reduction of the contralateral side can be performed either at the same time or later as a second-stage procedure.

All oncoplastic procedures begin with preoperative marking of the patient sitting upright or standing prior to the induction of anaesthesia. Once marked,

the patient is carefully centred on the operating room table and secured so that she can be moved from the supine to the upright position during the operation. The arms can be extended if any axillary surgery is planned, or secured by the side if no axillary surgery is required. Movement between these positions allows optimisation of contralateral breast symmetry and allows for optimal reshaping.

Level I oncoplastic techniques

The step-by-step approach for level I OPS

The driving force behind level I OPS is the ability of all surgeons to adopt the following steps into their surgical practice. There are six general steps for level I OPS that begin with the skin incision (1) followed by undermining of the skin (2) and NAC (3). After completion of undermining, a full-thickness glandular excision incorporating the cancer and a surrounding rim of normal breast tissue is performed from subcutaneous fat down to pectoralis fascia (4). The glandular defect is subsequently closed, following specimen X-ray to demonstrate complete radiological excision, with tissue re-approximation (5). If required, an area in the shape of a crescent bordering the areola is de-epithelialised to reposition the NAC (6). If this is not performed the NAC displaces towards the site of excision and is no longer positioned in the centre of the breast mound.

Incisions

The concepts of oncoplastic surgery are not based on minimising incision length. Short incision lengths limit mobilisation of the gland and do not allow creation of adequate glandular flaps to fill excision defects.

> ✔ Effective mobilisation of the gland is a key component in achieving a natural breast shape.

In our experience, OPS is not minimally invasive surgery. The location of the incision is at the discretion of the operating surgeon. In general, incisions should allow for both en bloc excision of the cancer, without causing fragmentation of the specimen, and also allow undermining of the surrounding breast tissue to facilitate reshaping. The general principle for placing incisions is to follow Kraissl's lines of maximum resting skin tension to limit visible scarring[6] (see Chapter 4). However, in many cases an incision away from the cancer is possible, such as along the areola border with radial extension towards the tumour in the axilla for upper outer quadrant lesions, or in the inframammary fold for cancers in the lower half of the breast.

Skin undermining

Extensive subcutaneous undermining ranging from one-half to two-thirds of the breast envelope may be required to facilitate glandular redistribution after removal of the tumour (**Fig. 6.6a**). Aggressive undermining can free an entire quadrant from the overlying skin envelope. In terms of technique, it is easier to undermine a large area of skin before excising the lesion. Skin undermining should be performed in the plane between the breast tissue and subcutaneous fat and definition of this plan is enhanced by the use of hydrodissection using saline containing 1 in 500,000 to 1 in a million adrenaline (see Chapter 5).

> ✅ Risk factors for vascular compromise should be evaluated prior to performing extensive undermining. Smoking, diabetes mellitus and connective tissue disease are recognised as risk factors to be taken into consideration prior to planning the surgery to be performed.

Although smoking does not prevent the completion of a safe level I oncoplasty, it decreases the total area of skin that can be undermined safely. Patients who smoke should be warned of the greater risk of complications and advised to reduce or stop smoking for as long as possible before and immediately after surgery (see Chapter 5).

The area of undermining should be inversely proportional to the number of risk factors present, but the final factor in determining the amount of undermining that is safe is the fat composition of the breast. Division of the chest wall perforating blood vessels in a fatty breast is much more of a problem, and to maintain tissue vascularity and reduce the risk of postoperative necrosis, a level II procedure, which involves direct glandular excision and less skin undermining, should be considered if extensive undermining is considered necessary to close the defect.

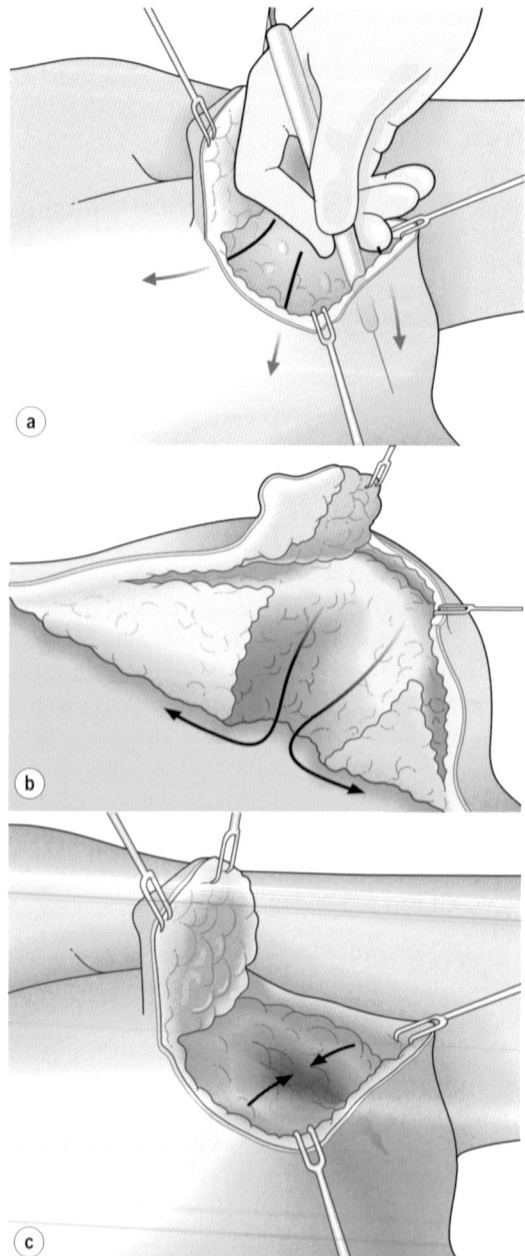

Figure 6.6 • Level I oncoplastic techniques: skin and NAC undermining. **(a)** Extensive skin undermining. **(b)** Wide excision from subcutaneous fat to muscle, then NAC undermining. **(c)** Glandular flap re-approximation.

Nipple–areola complex undermining

> ✅ Major NAC distortion is a common cause of breast deformity.

Fibrosis after surgery creates tension on adjacent tissue, which results in NAC deviation towards the area of excision. Fortunately, NAC repositioning can be performed easily with simple undermining and this is a key component of both level I and II OPS. The first step is to completely transect the terminal ducts under the nipple and separate the NAC from the underlying breast tissue. A width of 0.5–1 cm of glandular tissue is generally left attached to the nipple to ensure the integrity of its vascular supply. This amount of subareolar tissue prevents NAC necrosis and limits venous congestion. Even if the nipple is undermined and the ducts divided immediately under the skin in most women (>90%), the nipple will survive. The level of NAC sensitivity is reduced by extensive mobilisation and undermining and patients should be warned of this.[7]

Tissue excision

The standard approach is to perform a full-thickness excision from the subcutaneous fat underlying the skin down to the pectoral fascia.

✅ Full-thickness excision ensures free anterior and posterior margins, leaving only the lateral margins in question (**Fig. 6.6b**).

The breast parenchyma itself may be excised in a fusiform pattern oriented towards the NAC to facilitate re-approximation of the remaining gland, although this potentially increases the total volume of tissue excised. In general, excise only what is needed and use the remainder to help fill the defect. Before closing the defect, metal clips are placed on the lateral edges (superior, inferior, medial and lateral) of the tissue defect in the breast to guide future radiotherapy. For superficial or deep cancers in breasts with an anterior posterior distance of >4 cm then full-thickness excisions are not always required. Preoperative imaging is valuable in planning such excisions.

Re-approximation of the glandular defect

During BCS, breast tissue is either re-approximated or left open allowing for the eventual formation of a haematoma or seroma. Seroma formation, however, does not always result in predictable long-term cosmetic results for larger volume excisions. Once reabsorption of the seroma occurs, the seroma absorbs and the excision cavity contracts due to fibrosis and retraction of the surrounding tissue, creating a noticeable defect together with distortion, which then results in NAC displacement. For this reason, where there has been an extensive resection, redistribution of the remaining breast volume to redistribute the loss is required. Tissue mobilised from lateral portions of the remaining gland or recruited from the central part of the breast allows the creation of glandular flaps that can be sutured together to close the defect (**Fig. 6.6c**).

De-epithelialisation and NAC repositioning

A major source of patient dissatisfaction after BCS is the usatisfactory position of the NAC because it is deviated towards the excision site. This is likely to happen after any extensive volume resection. NAC repositioning is exceedingly difficult after radiotherapy, so immediate recentralisation is advised and the need to recentralise the NAC should be anticipated during the operation to resect the cancer and should be performed then.

Avoiding NAC displacement is a key element for both level I and II OPS. The NAC is repositioned to adjust for both the anticipated deviation of the nipple and the new shape of the breast. A crescentic area of periareolar skin opposite the excision defect is de-epithelialised (**Fig. 6.7a–c**). De-epithelialisation can be achieved using a scalpel blade or fine scissors. This technique is simple and safe and used systematically in aesthetic surgery of the breast. The vascular supply of the NAC after its separation from the gland and de-epithelialisation is based on the vasculature from the dermal plexus and this is not compromised by careful de-epithelialisation.[8]

Level II oncoplastic surgery

Introduction

The major consideration when choosing the oncoplastic technique to be used is the extent of excision volume. A level I approach is suitable for excision volumes less than 20% of the entire gland. The resulting glandular defect can usually be filled by advancement of adjacent tissue. Immediate lipofilling in

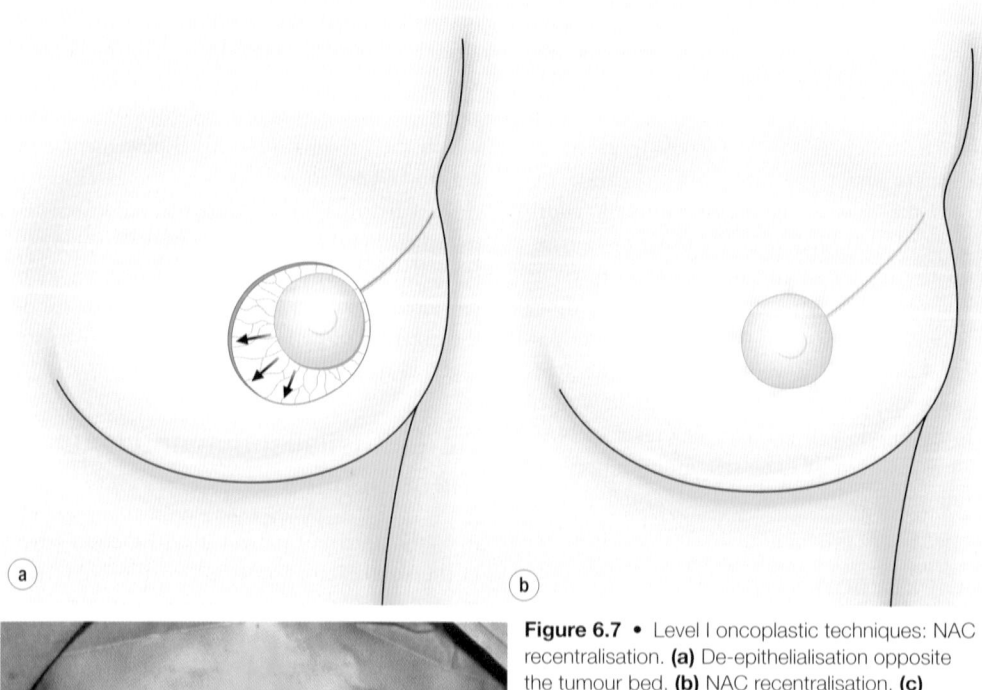

Figure 6.7 • Level I oncoplastic techniques: NAC recentralisation. **(a)** De-epithelialisation opposite the tumour bed. **(b)** NAC recentralisation. **(c)** Intraoperative result (upper outer quadrant resection).

addition to tissue advancement adds extra flexibility to the level I approach. Level II techniques are generally reserved for situations that require major volume excisions of between 20% and 50%.

To simplify the selection of a level II OPS technique, an atlas has been devised based on tumour location. This atlas does not contain an exhaustive list of options, but provides one or two options for each tumour location.

Atlas principles

The concept of the oncoplastic atlas is based primarily on tumour location. Initially used only for lower pole tumours, OPS has evolved to allow resection of breast lesions located almost anywhere in the breast. Different mammaplasty techniques have been adapted for specific locations in the breast.[9]

The superior pedicle reduction mammaplasty is a model for the description of all mammaplasty techniques. Schematically rotating the NAC on a pedicle based directly opposite the site of tumour excision allows the application of this technique for a variety of tumour locations. These procedures are listed in an anticlockwise direction and described for the left breast.

Level II OPS will generally result in a smaller breast that is rounder and higher on the chest wall than the contralateral breast, thus there is a need for a contralateral symmetrisation and the necessity to discuss this with the patient prior to the excision. Either immediate or delayed symmetrisation can be performed, depending on the amount of tissue resected and the desire of the patient. In a recent series of 175 women having an oncoplastic breast-conserving procedure, a contralateral breast reduction was performed in 25% of patients (19% during the initial operation and 6% as a secondary procedure). A higher rate of contralateral surgery was performed in patients who had an inverted-T mammaplasty (50% vs. 14% with other techniques; $P<0.001$).[10]

Lower pole location (4–7 o'clock)

General principles

The lower pole of the breast was the first location recognised to be at high risk of deformity following BCS.[1] Removal of tissue from the 6 o'clock position results in retraction of the skin and downward deviation of the NAC, producing what is known as the 'bird's beak' deformity, which results in a low level of patient satisfaction. A superior pedicle mammaplasty can permit large-volume excision of the lower pole without causing NAC deviation and has the added benefit of breast reshaping and elevation.

Techniques

'Standard' superior pedicle mammaplasty with inverted-T scar (Fig. 6.8a–e)

The superior pedicle mammaplasty technique that is in routine use involves using the inverted-T and peri-areolar scars as utilised in most breast reductions.[11] The procedure begins with the de-epithelialisation of the area surrounding the NAC. Once completed, the NAC is dissected away from the underlying breast tissue. A superior pedicle of dermoglandular tissue is preserved to provide the NAC with a blood supply.

The inframammary incision is then completed, followed by wide undermining of the breast tissue from the pectoral fascia, which can be preserved. The undermining starts inferiorly and proceeds superiorly beneath the tumour while encompassing the medial and lateral aspects of the breast as well as the NAC. The tumour is removed en bloc with a wide margin of normal breast tissue and overlying skin as determined by the preoperative marking.

As for all BCS, the goal of the excision is to obtain at least a 1-cm macroscopic margin of normal tissue in order to ensure free microscopic margins. Mobilisation

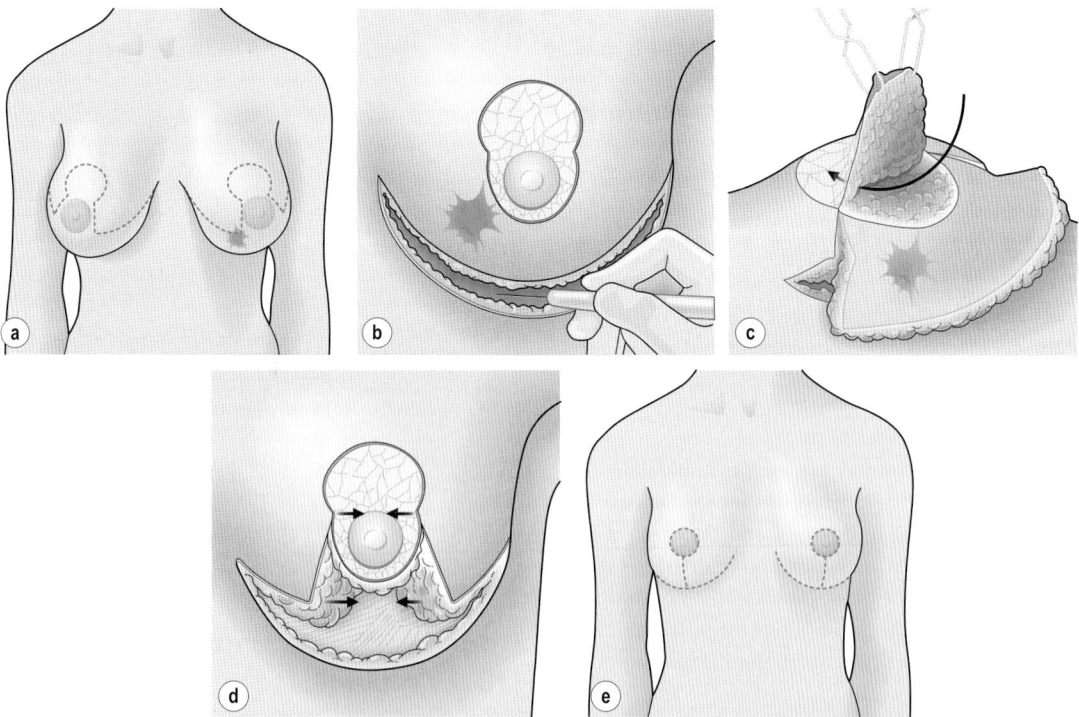

Figure 6.8 • Level II oncoplastic techniques for lower pole breast cancers: superior pedicle mammaplasty. **(a)** Treatment planning: superior pedicle mammaplasty and contralateral symmetrisation. **(b)** Superior pedicle de-epithelialised. Submammary fold incision. **(c)** Superior pedicle elevated. Wide excision of tumour and surrounding tissues. **(d)** Breast reshaping. **(e)** Result.

of the breast tissue from the pectoralis fascia allows for palpation of both the deep and superficial surfaces of the tumour, which improves the ability of the surgeon to obtain clear margins. The breast tissue is remodelled after the resection is completed. Remodelling incorporates the re-approximation of the medial and lateral glandular columns towards the midline to fill in the defect, followed by NAC recentralisation. All tissues excised should be weighed, as this provides a guide to the amount of tissue to be excised in any contralateral reduction procedure. As a general rule the resection of the cancer-bearing breast should be 10–20% less than excised from the opposite breast to allow for shrinkage of the treated breast following whole-breast radiotherapy. Results from excision of ductal carcinoma in situ at the lower pole of the left breast are shown in **Fig. 6.9a** and **b**. The result 2 years after operation is shown in **Fig. 6.9c**.

Vertical mammaplasty (Lejour/Lassus)

One modification to the technique to excise lower quadrant tumours is to use the vertical-scar mammaplasty described by Lejour[12] and Lassus.[13] The site and volume of excision are identical to the inverted-T scar, but this approach avoids the submammary scar. In general, T-shaped reductions work best in the largest breasts and vertical scar reductions in smaller breasts.

Lower inner quadrant (7–9 o'clock)

General principles

Standard superior pedicle mammaplasty described for tumours located at the 6 o'clock position can be extended to 7 o'clock. However, adaptation for tumours located more medially, between 7 and 8 o'clock, is more difficult and requires a novel level II technique.

Technique
V mammaplasty

This procedure involves excising a pyramidal section of skin and underlying breast tissue with the base located in the submammary fold and the apex at the border of the areola. This skin and underlying breast tissue are removed en bloc down to the pectoral fascia. An incision is then made along the inframammary fold and developed starting at the medial aspect of the base of resection moving towards the anterior axillary line and taken as far as necessary to perform adequate mobilisation of the breast tissue laterally. The lower pole of the breast is then mobilised off the pectoralis fascia medially and laterally for use as an

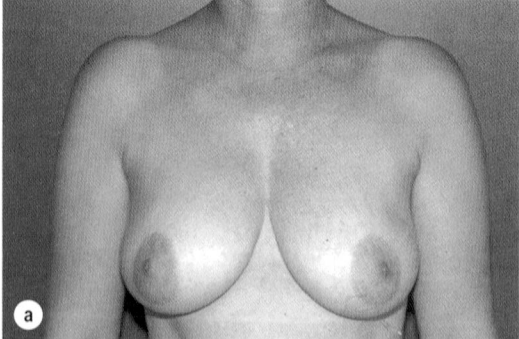
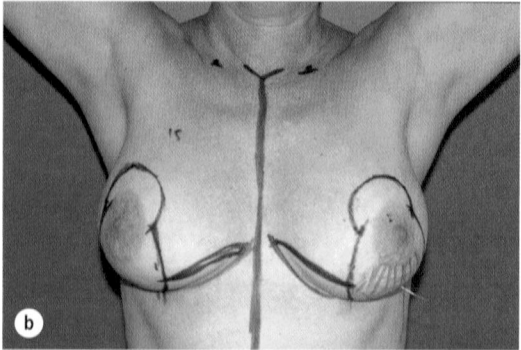
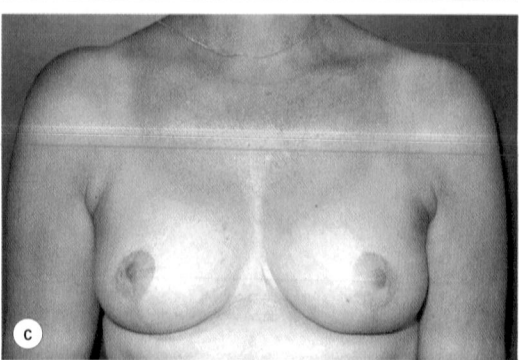

Figure 6.9 • Level II technique for a 6-cm ductal carcinoma in situ of the lower pole of the left breast. Wide excision and postoperative radiotherapy. **(a,b)** Preoperative. **(c)** Two years postoperation.

advancement flap to fill the defect. Volume replacement is thus achieved through the advancement of the gland from the remaining lower medial and lateral aspects of the breast. The NAC is then recentralised on a de-epithelialised superior lateral pedicle.[14]

Upper inner quadrant (10–11 o'clock)

General principles

Special caution is needed when considering BCS for lesions in the upper inner aspect of the breast.

A wide excision in this location can have a significant impact on the overall quality of the breast shape by distorting the visible breast line known as the 'décolleté'. This represents the visible area of the breast.

For moderate resections, level I techniques can be utilised safely and combined with immediate lipofilling to achieve a very smooth final contour. For more extensive excisions, the ability and likelihood of being able to preserve the natural breast shape should be discussed with the patient. Standard level II oncoplastic procedures that reliably address the specific limitations of BCS at this troublesome location are limited. Silverstein and colleagues have described an effective OPS procedure to address the upper inner quadrant. Their approach utilises a batwing excision pattern.[15] Silverstein et al.'s OPS solution is innovative but excises tissue in excess of that which is required, leaves a large scar and, as described, removes pectoral fascia as well as skin. Immediate lipofilling may offer the best solution at present to this difficult area, combined with mobilisation and closure of the defect.

Upper pole (11–1 o'clock)

General principles

Lesions located at the 12 o'clock position can be excised widely followed by volume redistribution of tissue from a central location. Access to lesions in this location of the breast is accomplished either using an inferior pedicle or round-block mammaplasty approach. The inferior pedicle mammaplasty is commonly performed in the USA as a breast reduction technique and utilises an inverted-T scar pattern.[16] A round-block approach, on the other hand, is more technically challenging when trying to achieve the desired breast shape. These two techniques are used extensively for breast reduction, with low complication rates and durable results. They can be applied for wide excision of upper pole tumours while preserving a patient's natural breast shape. There are dangers with this technique when trying to preserve breast tissue superior to the nipple to advance into the defect. So-called 'bottoming out' is a problem with inferior mammaplasty techniques.

Techniques

Inferior pedicle mammaplasty

The skin markings are identical to those described for the superior pedicle reduction. The resection,

however, is located in the upper pole, hence the vascular supply of the NAC is based on its inferior and posterior glandular attachments. The excision of the cancer is performed through an incision placed within the skin to be removed. Once the cancer has been excised and the specimen X-ray shows complete radiological excision, the inferior pedicle is de-epithelialised and advanced upwards towards the excision defect to achieve volume redistribution. Resection of the breast tissue is performed in the inner and outer lower quadrants to optimise the breast shape.

Round-block mammaplasty

The round-block mammaplasty utilises a periareolar incision and was originally described by Benelli.[17,18] The procedure starts by making two concentric periareolar incisions, followed by de-epithelialisation of the intervening skin. The outer edge of de-epithelialised skin is incised and the entire skin envelope can then be undermined to allow access to the tumour. The NAC remains vascularised through its posterior glandular base. Resection of the lesion from the subcutaneous tissue down to the pectoralis fascia is performed and this results in the formation of an external and internal glandular flap. The flaps are then mobilised off the pectoralis fascia and advanced towards each other to eliminate the excision defect. The two incisions are then approximated, resulting in a periareolar scar.

Although the round-block mammaplasty has been used mainly for upper pole tumours, it is a versatile technique that can be easily adapted for tumours in any location of the breast. The round-block technique is not a method of breast reduction favoured by most breast surgeons because it has limitations. In general, there are alternative options to the round-block technique so, although some surgeons use it widely, others use it rarely, if ever. Given its lack of universal favour, this suggests the technique has its limitations.

Upper outer quadrant (1–3 o'clock; Fig. 6.10a–c)

General principles

In the upper outer quadrant, large lesions can usually be excised with standard BCS without causing deformity. However, resection of greater than 20% of the breast volume will result in retraction of the overlying skin with NAC displacement towards the excision site. A result of a patient with a T3 cancer treated by neoadjuvant chemotherapy and wide

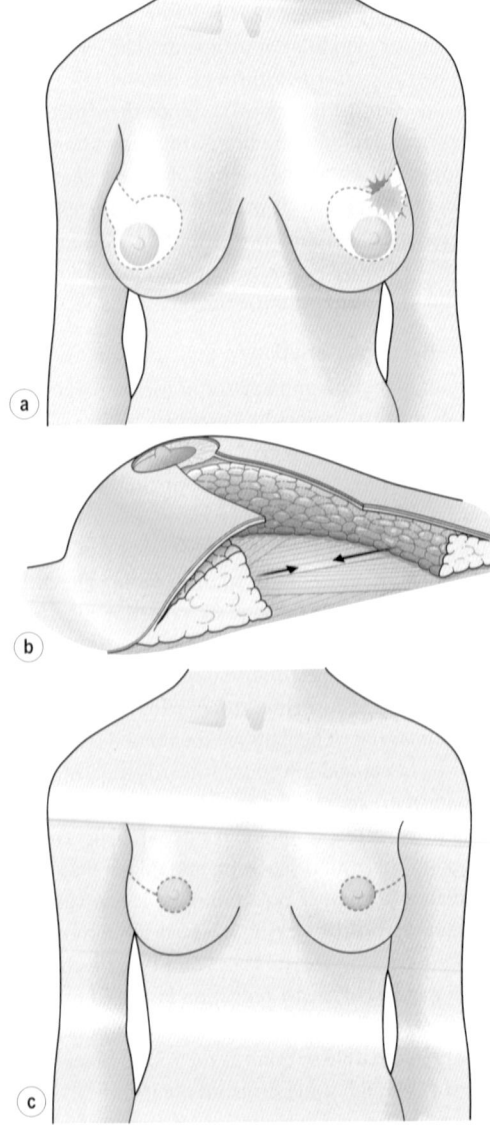

Figure 6.10 • Level II oncoplastic techniques for upper outer quadrant breast cancers. **(a)** Treatment planning: wide resection and NAC de-epithelialisation. **(b)** Resection. **(c)** Breast reshaping and contralateral symmetrisation.

excision with mammaplasty is shown in **Fig. 6.11a–d**. Level II OPS can be utilised to increase resection possibilities while limiting deformity risk in this forgiving region of the breast.

Techniques
Fusiform mammaplasty

A large portion of the upper outer quadrant can be excised utilising a fusiform skin excision pattern oriented in a radial direction from the NAC towards the axilla, similar to a quadrantectomy.[19,20] After wide excision, the reshaping is performed by mobilising the lateral and central gland into the cavity and suturing it together. Central gland advancement is accomplished easily following NAC undermining. Complete detachment of the retroareolar gland from the NAC enables the central part of the gland to be available for volume redistribution without compromise of NAC vascularity. Once the defect is eliminated, the NAC is placed in its optimal position, at the centre of the new breast mound. The area of glandular excision directly follows the skin excision. Additional glandular excision can be accomplished to remove almost the entire quadrant, depending on tumour size and the amount of tissue required to be removed to obtain clear margins.

Superior pedicled therapeutic mammaplasty

Given the increasing use of superomedial pedicles in breast reduction surgery, tissue that is normally removed from the lower breast can be kept alive on a superomedial pedicle and rotated into the upper outer quadrant. To be successful, care is needed to maintain a wide base to the pedicle and thus maintain a good blood supply to the whole of the tissue to be rotated.

Lower outer quadrant (4–5 o'clock)

General principles

A large-volume resection of the lower outer quadrant leaves a deformity similar to a bird's beak. As for lower inner pole lesions, the inverted-T mammaplasty does not always 'fit' well for excisions within this quadrant. One option is a J-type mammaplasty described by Gasperoni et al.[21]

Techniques
J mammaplasty (Gasperoni)

The first incision begins at the medial edge of the de-epithelialised periareolar area and then gently curves upwards with a concavity to the inframammary crease. The second incision starts at the lateral border of the de-epithelialised zone and follows a similar pattern. The parenchymal excision then follows the skin pattern in the shape of the letter J. The NAC remains vascularised on a de-epithelialised superior pedicle and is detached from the retroareolar gland. Lateral and central breast

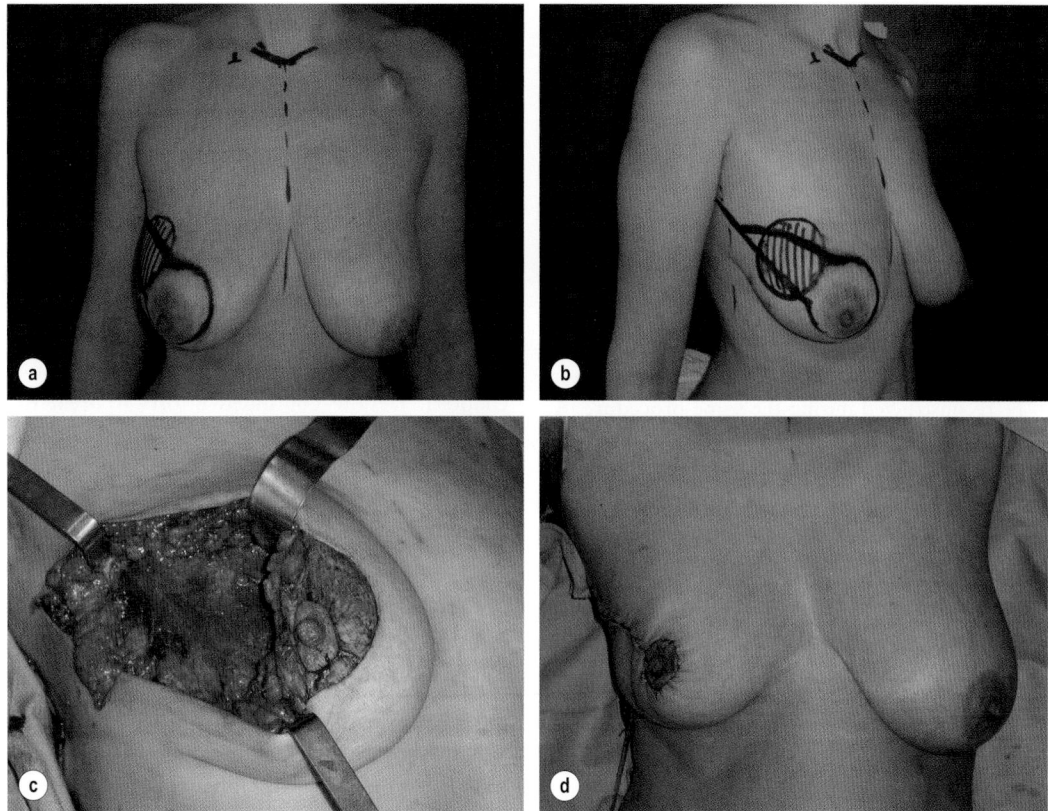

Figure 6.11 • Level II technique for a T3N0 cancer of the upper outer quadrant of the right breast. Preoperative chemotherapy: partial response. Wide excision and mammaplasty. **(a,b)** Preoperative. **(c)** Resection weight 215 g. **(d)** Result prior to contralateral symmetrisation.

tissue can then be recruited into the excision defect to achieve an equitable redistribution of remaining breast volume.

Secondary pedicles

An alternative is to excise the cancer, leaving the skin intact through the incision selected for reducing the breast – be that a T-shaped or vertical scar. The skin that would normally be removed, is de-epithelialised and using primary pedicles attached to the nipple–areola complex or secondary pedicles attached to the inframammary fold, the defect is closed.

Retroareolar location

General principles

Subareolar breast cancers are candidates for BCS. However, superficial subareolar tumours are associated with a risk of NAC involvement approaching 50%.[22] Such cases require en bloc removal of the NAC with the tumour. This results in a 'flattened breast' or 'shark-bite' deformity and poor cosmetic outcome unless techniques are used to avoid this. If the patient has a glandular breast that allows wide undermining for reshaping, a level I OPS is a reasonable option.

Level II mammaplasty techniques are reserved for patients with ptosis or fatty breasts or for patients for whom excision of more than 20% of the breast volume is required. There are a number of mammaplasty approaches that can be chosen for the centrally located lesion. They include the inverted-T mammaplasty with resection of the NAC, a modified Lejour or J pattern with NAC excision or a Grisotti flap (see Chapter 4). The latter offers the advantage of allowing for immediate NAC reconstruction through preservation of a skin island on an advancement flap.[23]

Technique

Modified inverted-T mammaplasty

Oncoplastic techniques for centrally located tumours have recently been outlined by Huemer et al.[24] An inverted-T incision is preferred, similar to that used in a superior pedicle mammaplasty. The only modification is that the two vertical incisions encompass the NAC, which is removed together with the tumour. The breast shape is reconstructed as already demonstrated for the superior pedicle approach. The NAC is usually reconstructed at a later stage, after completion of radiotherapy, although it can be reconstructed during the same procedure. A modification of this technique is to leave a circular island of skin or an inferior dermoglandular flap, which is relocated in the position of the new NAC and produces symmetry with the opposite NAC (see Chapter 4).

Discussion

General

Until recently, the breast surgeon has been able to provide only two options for patients with breast cancer: either a modified radical mastectomy or a wide local excision followed by radiation. BCS indications have expanded, but only moderate surgical advancements have been made since its introduction.

The integration of plastic surgery techniques at the time of tumour excision has delivered new alternatives, enabling surgeons to perform major resections involving more than 20% of breast volume without causing breast deformity. This new combination of oncological and reconstructive surgery is commonly referred to as oncoplastic surgery. This has allowed surgeons to extend the indications for BCS without compromising oncological goals or aesthetic outcomes. It is a logical extension of the quadrantectomy technique described by Veronesi et al.[19] The innovation of the quadrantectomy provided women with a safe oncological option for conserving their breasts.

✅✅ The recurrence rates of quadrantectomy compared favourably with those of lumpectomy, but cosmetic outcomes were unpredictable and were worse than a wide excision alone, so are no longer advocated.[25–27]

✅ With immediate reshaping employing OPS, resections of larger cancers can now be achieved with satisfactory cosmetic outcomes.

A major advantage of OPS is avoiding the need for secondary reconstruction by preventing major breast deformities.[28] Prior to the development of OPS, patients with major deformities were referred subsequently to plastic surgeons.[29] A classification system of these deformities has been described and reconstructive techniques for breast deformity after BCS have been developed[30,31] (see Part 1 of this chapter). Despite continued efforts to treat these deformities, the results of postoperative repair of BCS defects in irradiated tissue are poor, regardless of the surgical procedure or team.[32,33] Immediate reshaping of the breast will eliminate some of the need for these complex procedures.

Advances in OPS have been restricted by the diversity of techniques used, the lack of uniformity in classifying oncoplastic techniques and the limited guidelines of the optimum OPS procedures in the surgical literature. This has generated confusion and difficulty in patient and technique selection. The foundation of OPS starts with simple techniques that are easily incorporated into everyday practice (level I techniques), followed by acquiring the experience to perform the various mammaplasty techniques utilised for more extensive resections (level II techniques).

Indications for oncoplastic surgery

The main indication for OPS is the need to excise large lesions or a significant percentage of the breast, so permitting BCS for large lesions for which a standard excision with safe margins would be either impossible or lead to major deformity. Extensive ductal carcinoma in situ, invasive lobular carcinoma, multifocality, and partial or poor responses to neoadjuvant therapy are areas where there may be benefits for OPS intervention. Standard BCS with positive margins where re-excision is being considered is an additional category of patients for whom OPS is appropriate.[34]

Oncoplastic and oncological safety

Large randomised prospective clinical trials have not validated the efficacy and safety of oncoplastic techniques, but there is growing evidence, through prospective series, that the techniques offer patients safe and effective surgical treatment. Our prospective analysis of over 100 patients undergoing OPS at our institution demonstrated 5-year overall and disease-free survival rates of 95.7% and 82.8%, respectively.[11] Delay in adjuvant treatment was related to slow wound healing in only four patients, but all patients were able to receive appropriate postoperative radiotherapy and chemotherapy during the study. The cosmetic results at a median of 49 months in our most recent series of 175 pateints were favourable in 85% of patients.[10] Final cosmetic outcomes and complication rates are not altered in patients undergoing neoadjuvant chemotherapy. A more recent retrospective review of 298 patients treated with OPS demonstrated a 5-year recurrence-free rate of 93.7% and 94.6% overall survival. This larger review confirms the equivalent outcomes of OPS and standard BCS.[35] Rietjens et al. have reported long-term results from the European Institute of Oncology indicating no local relapse in the pT1 cohort. The pT2 and pT3 combined group had a 5-year local recurrence rate of 8% and a mortality rate of 15%. The overall local recurrence rate was determined to be 3%.[36]

Integration into multidisciplinary treatment

Clinical management is enhanced by OPS and does not change the need for or adherence to the guidelines for preoperative chemotherapy. Our surgical approach using OPS is fully integrated into the multidisciplinary environment. Radiation treatment is not disturbed by the extensive undermining during OPS and has complication rates comparable to BCS. There is no increase in treatment delays with the more extensive level II techniques, and the remodelling process does not affect continued screening and radiographic follow-up of patients.[37]

Complications of oncoplastic surgery

Mammaplasty techniques for cosmetic breast reduction have acceptable complication rates. Early common complications include seroma, haematoma, infection, and skin or NAC necrosis leading to delayed healing. Late complications during the postoperative course may involve fat necrosis, loss of nipple sensitivity and NAC necrosis.[38,39]

Extensive data are not available on complication rates for oncoplastic procedures. Our prospective evaluation of complications in an initial oncoplastic surgery series demonstrated low seroma rates (1%), but a higher overall incidence of delayed wound healing (9%). A delay in postoperative treatment was observed in only 4% of patients[11] in our first series, falling to 1.7% in our most recent publication.[10] This complication rate is not dissimilar to that for cosmetic mammaplasty despite the need for greater glandular undermining in OPS compared to cosmetic breast reduction to achieve volume redistribution to less favourable tumour locations.

Surgeons embarking on OPS should be aware of complications, their frequency and the factors that increase this risk. Glandular necrosis is the most challenging complication. Patient selection and careful surgical technique will avoid this.

> ✓ Aggressive undermining of the skin envelope and gland from the pectoralis fascia can lead to glandular necrosis if the breast is fatty, as such breasts have less vascularity compared to glandular breasts.

Areas of fat necrosis can become infected and cause wound dehiscence resulting in postoperative treatment delay. Our rates of delayed wound healing have been reduced considerably since we incorporated the third key element of breast density into our decision-making process. Our complication rate is now less than 5%, with no delay in postoperative treatment over the last 150 cases. If fat necrosis does occur, liposuction with lipofilling or lipomodelling can result in rapid resolution and good long-term results.

Limitations of oncoplastic surgery

We have identified four different reasons that limit the use of OPS: patient characteristics, tumour size, surgical level of difficulty and increased operative time.

Patient considerations including breast size and comorbidities are integrated into the initial evaluation. Although level I procedures can be applied to all patients, level II OPS is of limited value in women with small breast size, either A or smaller B cups. For these patients with small breasts who require excision of greater than 20% of the breast volume, immediate lipofilling, a latissimus dorsi miniflap or a total mastectomy with immediate reconstruction should be considered. Immediate lipofilling works best for excisions in areas where cosmetic outcomes can be poor (upper inner quadrant, lower half of the breast) in a patient with small breasts where the total volume of tissue excised is small but constitutes a significant percentage of the total breast volume. Comorbidities that increase the risk of tissue necrosis, such as history of smoking, diabetes and obesity, must also be considered during surgical planning.

Once an acceptable risk is established for the patient, then tumour characteristics are used to decide the appropriate procedure and the best approach. Excision of tumours too large to redistribute volume into the index quadrant may require a volume replacement procedure such as a latissimus dorsi miniflap.[3] Location of the tumour is also critical, as upper inner quadrant tumours have few volume redistribution solutions, so immediate lipofilling in this location is the current best option.

Difficulty in performing advanced level II techniques comprises another category of limitation. However, training for OPS can be acquired gradually and level I techniques do not require any advanced training. Another solution for the more complex cases is to incorporate a plastic surgeon in the multidisciplinary team. This may be the best option for most breast surgeons that do not wish to or do not have the time to invest in specific training for complex level II techniques. The big advantage of incorporating a plastic surgeon and an oncoplastic surgeon is that it allows simultaneous bilateral procedures, which reduce operating time. This can be difficult to arrange logistically, so dual training of breast surgeons is an alternative long-term solution.

Finally, can the additional time required for advanced procedures be justified? The increased length of the initial operation does translate into major benefits for both the patient and the surgeon. OPS leads to an overall reduction in operation time for many patients because it is more likely to achieve free margins in one procedure. The reduction in re-excision rates improves resource management for the whole cohort of patients. The greater amount of time utilised during the initial procedure also has the added benefit of reducing deformity rates, thus eliminating the need for repair of partial mastectomy defects. It also reduces the numbers who require mastectomy and breast reconstruction.

Oncoplastic evolution and revolution

As surgical practice guidelines continue to evolve in the field of breast surgery, the training of future breast surgeons should include OPS techniques and rely on the experience and methodology gained from the fields of both surgical oncology and plastic and reconstructive surgery. Growth and acceptance of OPS as an alternative to BCS have seen an active collaboration between the divisions of breast and plastic surgery in the UK and much of Western Europe.

The pathway for obtaining the necessary training differs throughout the surgical world. In the UK, a formal oncoplastic training programme has already been established. Participants in this programme obtain both plastic and reconstructive training, as well as experience in the surgical oncological management of breast cancer. France has also witnessed the creation of a formal certification programme for breast surgeons interested in OPS. The programme involves clinical mentoring, technical lectures and a standardised written examination. The interest in OPS continues to expand, with courses on offer at the major breast surgery conferences in the USA and Europe. These courses provide the necessary background to complete level I procedures, but do not allow for application of level II OPS.

Conclusions

The proliferation of oncoplastic publications in the surgical literature is a direct result of the awareness of the advantages of OPS.

> ✅ Oncoplastic surgery allows large resections of breast tissue with favourable cosmetic outcomes and integrates easily into the standard multidisciplinary approach for BCS.

The ultimate goal is to allow large-volume resections with free margins and fewer mastectomies than are currently obtainable with standard BCS.

OPS is best stratified into two levels. Three key factors have been defined – excision volume, tumour location and glandular density – and these form the basis of a cohesive set of surgical principles and teaching guidelines. The goal for developing an OPS classification and a quadrant-by-quadrant atlas is to improve communication between surgeons and their patients.

Key points

- Volume displacement is most suitable for patients with medium or large breasts who are willing to undergo breast reduction (often bilateral), avoiding more major reconstructive surgery.
- Volume displacement allows large-volume resection of tissue without cosmetic penalty.
- Volume displacement can be designed around modifications of the superior pedicle, inferior pedicle and round-block techniques.
- Immediate lipofilling performed at the same time as a wide local excision of the cancer is a new technique currently being evaluated to improve cosmetic outcomes in patients with smaller breasts where excision of even a small cancer would produce a poor cosmetic outcome.
- Specific training is required to be able to perform level II techniques but all surgeons doing breast surgery should be able to perform level I oncoplastic surgical techniques.
- Training in breast surgery should include training in oncoplastic surgery.

References

1. Clough KB, Nos C, Salmon RJ, et al. Conservative treatment of breast cancers by mammaplasty and irradiation: a new approach to lower quadrant tumours. Plast Reconstr Surg 1995;96(2):363–70.

2. Cothier-Savey I, Otmezquine Y, Calitchi E, et al. Value of reduction mammaplasty in the conservative treatment of breast neoplasm. Apropos of 70 cases. Ann Chir Plast Esthet 1996;41(4):346–53.

3. Rainsbury R. Surgery insight: oncoplastic breast-conserving reconstruction – indications, benefits, choices and outcomes. Nat Clin Pract Oncol 2007;4(11):657–64.

4. Bulstrode NW, Shortri S. Prediction of cosmetic outcome following conservative breast surgery using breast volume measurements. Breast 2001;10:124–6.

5. American College of Radiology. Breast imaging reporting and data systems (BI-RADS). Reston, VA: American College of Radiology; 2003.

6. Kraissl CJ. The selection of appropriate lines for elective surgical incisions. Plast Reconstr Surg (1946) 1951;8(1):1–28.

7. Schlenz I, Rigel S, Schemper M, et al. Alteration of nipple and areola sensitivity by reduction mammaplasty: a prospective comparison of five techniques. Plast Reconstr Surg 2005;115(3):743–51.

8. O'Dey D, Prescher A, Pallua N. Vascular reliability of the nipple–areola complex-bearing pedicles: an anatomical microdissection study. Plast Reconstr Surg 2007;119(4):1167–77.

9. Smith ML, Evans GR, Gurlek A, et al. Reduction mammaplasty: its role in breast conservation surgery for early-stage breast cancer. Ann Plast Surg 1998;41(3):234–9.

10. Clough KB, Ihrai T, Oden S, et al. Oncoplastic surgery for breast cancer based on tumour location and a quadrant-per-quadrant atlas. Br J Surg 2012; 99(10):1389–95.

11. Clough KB, Lewis J, Couturaud B, et al. Oncoplastic techniques allow extensive resections for breast-conserving therapy of breast carcinomas. Ann Surg 2003;237(1):26–34.

12. Lejour M. Reduction of mammaplasty scars: from a short inframammary scar to a vertical scar. Ann Chir Plast Esthet 1990;35(5):369–79.

13. Lassus C. A 30-year experience with vertical mammaplasty. Plast Reconstr Surg 1996;97(2):373–80.

14. Clough KB, Kroll S, Audretsch W. An approach to the repair of partial mastectomy defects. Plast Reconstr Surg 1999;104(2):409–20.

15. Anderson BO, Masetti R, Silverstein MJ. Oncoplastic approaches to partial mastectomy: an overview of volume-displacement techniques. Lancet Oncol 2005;6:145–57.

16. Spear SL, Pelletiere CV, Wolfe AJ, et al. Experience with reduction mammaplasty combined with breast conservation therapy in the treatment of cancer. Plast Reconstr Surg 2003;111(3):1102–9.

17. Benelli L. A new periareolar mammaplasty: the "round block" technique. Aesthetic Plast Surg 1990;14(2):93–100.

18. Hammon DC. Short scar periareolar inferior pedicle reduction (SPAIR) mammaplasty. Plast Reconstr Surg 1999;103(3):890–901.

19. Veronesi U, Banfi A, Saccozzi R, et al. Conservative treatment of breast cancer. A trial in progress at the cancer institute of Milan. Cancer 1977;39(6):2822–6.

20. Veronesi U, Banfi A, del Vecchio M, et al. Comparision of Halsted mastectomy with quadrantectomy, axillary dissection, and radiotherapy in early breast cancer: long term results. Eur J Cancer Clin Oncol 1986;22:1085–9.

21. Gasperoni C, Salgarello M, Gasperoni P. A personal technique: mammaplasty with J scar. Ann Plast Surg 2002;48(2):124–30.

22. Gerber B, Krause A, Reimer T, et al. Skin-sparing mastectomy with conservation of the nipple–areolar complex and autologous reconstruction is an oncologically safe procedure. Ann Surg 2003;238(1):120–7.

23. Galimberti V, Zurrida S, Grisotti A, et al. Central small size breast cancer: how to overcome the problem of nipple and areola involvement. Eur J Cancer 1993;29A(8):1093–6.

24. Huemer G, Schrenk P, Moser F, et al. Oncoplastic techniques allow breast-conserving treatment in centrally located breast cancers. Plast Reconstr Surg 2007;120(2):390–8.

25. Veronesi U, Luini A, Galimberti V, et al. Conservation approaches for the management of stage I/II carcinoma of the breast: Milan cancer institute trials. World J Surg 1994;18(1):70–5.

26. Mariani L, Salvadori B, Veronesi U, et al. Ten year results of a randomized trial comparing two conservative strategies for small size breast cancer. Eur J Cancer 1998;34(8):1156–62.

27. Amichetti M, Busana L, Caffo O. Long term cosmetic outcome and toxicity in patients treated with quadrantectomy and radiation therapy for early-stage breast cancer. Oncology 1995;52:177–81.

28. Dewar JA, Benhamou E, Arrigada R, et al. Cosmetic results following lumpectomy, axillary dissection and radiotherapy for small breast cancer. Radiother Oncol 1988;12(4):273–80.

29. Petit J-Y, Regault L, Zekri A, et al. Poor aesthetic results after conservative treatment of breast cancer. Techniques of partial breast reconstruction. Ann Chir Plast Esthet 1989;34:103–8.

30. Clough KB, Cuminet JC, Fitoussi A, et al. Cosmetic sequelae after conservative treatment for breast cancer: classification and results of surgical correction. Ann Plast Surg 1998;41(8):471–81.

31. Clough KB, Thomas S, Fitoussi A, et al. Reconstruction after conservative treatment for breast cancer. Cosmetic sequelae: classification revisited. Plast Reconstr Surg 2004;114(7):1743–53.

32. Berrino P, Campora E, Leone S, et al. Correction of type II breast deformities following conservative cancer surgery. Plast Reconstr Surg 1992;90: 846–53.

33. Bostwick J, Paletta C, Hartampf CR. Conservative treatment for breast cancer: complications requiring reconstructive surgery. Ann Surg 1986;203:481–90.

34. Schwartz GF, Veronesi U, Clough KB, et al. Proceedings of the consensus conference on breast conservation, April 28 to May 1, 2005, Milan, Italy. Cancer 2006;107(2):242–50.

35. Staub G, Fitoussi A, Falcou MC, et al. Breast cancer surgery: use of mammaplasty. Results from a series of 298 cases. Ann Chir Plast Esthet 2007;53(2):124–34.

36. Rietjens M, Urban CA, Petit JY, et al. Long-term oncologic results of breast conservation treatment with oncoplastic surgery. Breast 2007;16(4):387–95.

37. Brown FE, Sargernt SK, Cohen SR, et al. Mammographic changes following reduction mammaplasty. Plast Reconstr Surg 1987;80(5):691–8.

38. Spear SL, Evans KK. Complications and secondary corrections after breast reduction and mastopexy. Surg Breast 2006;2:1220–34.

39. Munhoz AM, Montag E, Arruda EG, et al. Critical analysis of reduction mammaplasty techniques in combination with conservative breast surgery for early breast cancer treatment. Plast Reconstr Surg 2006;117(4):1091–103.

7

The axilla: current management including sentinel node and lymphoedema

Anees B. Chagpar

Introduction

While there are aspects of breast surgical oncology that have moved towards a more radical approach, the management of the axilla has tended to become incrementally less invasive. Although it is clear that the status of the axillary lymph nodes continues to be the most significant prognostic marker in the management of breast cancer patients,[1] removal of lymph nodes carries no survival benefit.[2,3] As such, the purpose of axillary surgery in the context of breast cancer management is primarily for staging and local control.

The last several decades have witnessed a metamorphosis in terms of management of the axilla, with significant paradigm shifts occurring within the last several years. Historically, a complete axillary node dissection with removal of level I and II lymph nodes or even levels I–III was standard (**Fig. 7.1**), and while this operation provided excellent prognostication and local control, it was associated with significant morbidity in terms of lymphoedema and decreased range of movement of the shoulder. Through the pioneering efforts of Cabanas,[4] who first coined the term 'sentinel node' based on cadaveric studies of penile cancer, and the subsequent groundbreaking work of Donald Morton, who introduced this into the management paradigm in melanoma,[5] sentinel node biopsy has revolutionised breast cancer treatment.

The concept of sentinel node biopsy is that one can map the lymphatic drainage of a tumour to the first draining lymph nodes, and that these nodes will be representative of the lymphatic basin. David Krag and Armando Giuliano[6–8] introduced the technique into clinical practice for breast cancer. While initially considered an investigational procedure, large validation studies[9–11] have confirmed that sentinel node biopsy is a safe, reliable, minimally invasive procedure that accurately stages the axilla. Subsequent randomised controlled trials[12] have corroborated these findings (Table 7.1). The National Surgical Adjuvant Breast and Bowel Project B-32 trial found overall survival, disease-free survival and locoregional recurrence were equivalent between patients who were randomised to sentinel node biopsy followed by routine axillary dissection compared with sentinel node biopsy followed by axillary node dissection only in sentinel node-positive patients.[12] Given these trial data and those from numerous other studies, sentinel node biopsy is now considered the standard of care in the management of patients with clinically node negative breast cancer.

> ✔✔ Sentinel node biopsy has been validated in large cohort studies,[9–11] as well as randomised controlled trials (like the NSABP B-32 trial),[12] which demonstrated that the false-negative rate is low, and that survival is no different for node-negative patients who undergo sentinel node biopsy compared with axillary node dissection. Sentinel node biopsy is therefore a safe, accurate, and minimally invasive technique to stage the axilla in patients with breast cancer, and should be considered the standard of care.

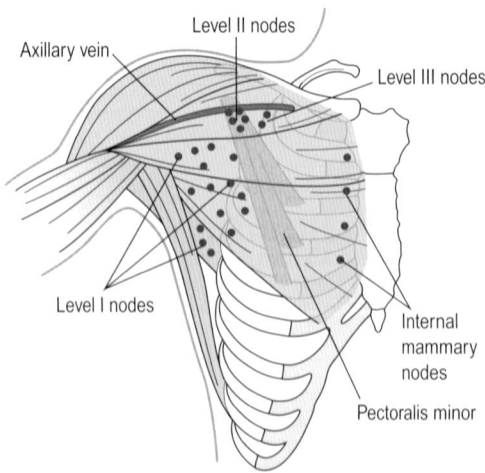

Level II nodes

Axillary vein

Level III nodes

Level I nodes

Internal mammary nodes

Pectoralis minor

Figure 7.1 • Anatomy of the axillary nodes and levels of axillary nodes related to the pectoralis minor. Level I nodes below and lateral, level II nodes under muscle and level III nodes medial to the muscle.

Sentinel lymph node biopsy: technique

Injection material/location

Considerable debate has surrounded the type of injection material used for sentinel node mapping. Some have advocated the use of blue dyes (such as patent blue V or Isosulphan blue) (**Fig. 7.2**) alone (severe hypersensitivity reactions with these drugs occur in approximately 1 in every 2000 patients), while others have preferred the use of radioactive tracers (such as technetium-99-labelled sulphur colloid or albumin). Still others have advocated the use of agents together. Numerous retrospective studies have found that while the false-negative rates are similar for the three techniques,[7,10,13–15] identification of

sentinel nodes is improved with the use of a combined technique.[16] A recent prospective trial found that identification rates were 99.1% when dual tracers were used, as opposed to 93.8–95.6% for blue dye and 96.0–96.2% for radioactive tracer.[17] An approach that uses radioisotope in all patients and adds blue dye only in those patients where radioisotope uptake into sentinel lymph nodes is not apparent has appeal in that it reduces the number who require blue dye.

While originally many practitioners injected tracers at the site of the tumour, the concept of subareolar injection is appealing, particularly for non-palpable and/or multiple tumours, given the embryologic origins of the lymphatics in Sappey's plexus. A number of authors have found that subareolar injection identifies the same sentinel node as a peritumoural technique,[18,19] has a high identification rate, and the same false-negative rate as other techniques.[17,20] Therefore, while the presence of multifocal/multicentric tumours had once been thought to be a relative contraindication to the use of sentinel node biopsy, more recent

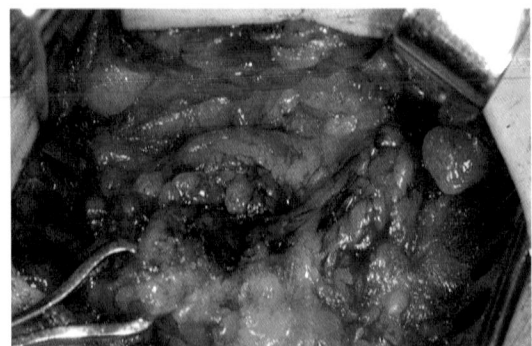

Figure 7.2 • Sentinel lymph node biopsy – blue-stained lymphatic leading to blue node.

Table 7.1 • Prospective randomised controlled trials validating sentinel lymph node biopsy

Study	Follow-up metric	ALND (95% CI)*	SLNB (95% CI)†
Zavagno et al.[85]	5-year DFS	89.9% (85.3–93.1%)	87.6% (83.3–90.9%)
	5-year OS	95.5% (92.2–97.5%)	94.8% (91.6–96.8%)
Krag et al.[12]	8-year DFS	82.4% (80.5–84.4%)	81.5% (79.6–83.4%)
	8-year OS	91.8% (90.4–93.3%)	90.3% (88.8–91.8%)
Veronesi et al.[86]	10-year DFS	88.8% (84.6–92.9%)	89.9% (85.9–93.9%)
	10-year OS	89.7% (85.5–93.8%)	93.5% (90.3–96.8%)

ALND, axillary lymph node; DFS, disease-free survival; OS, overall survival; SLNB, sentinel lymph node biopsy.
*Sentinel node biopsy followed by routine axillary node dissection.
†Sentinel node biopsy followed by axillary node dissection only in sentinel node-positive patients.

studies (many of which used a subareolar injection technique, although some utilised multiple peritumoural injections) have found the accuracy, identification and false-negative rates to be similar to smaller unifocal cancers.[21]

✅✅ Dual tracer technique is superior to use of blue dye or radioactive tracer alone in terms of sentinel node identification and false-negative rates, and is the technique of choice to identify sentinel nodes.[16,17] The subareolar injection technique has been found to be accurate in finding sentinel nodes in the setting of multifocal and multicentric breast cancer.[17]

Use of lymphoscintigraphy

Lymphoscintigraphy is often used in melanoma, where drainage patterns can vary widely; however, in breast cancer, where 98–99% of lymphatics drain to the ipsilateral axilla, (**Fig. 7.3**) lymphoscintigraphy has not been found to be of significant value (uptake of sentinel nodes of radioisotope takes minutes only, allowing injection of isotope after induction of anaesthesia).[22,23] In cases of recurrent breast cancer, however, particularly if 10 or more lymph nodes have previously been removed, alternative drainage pathways may be encountered and lymphoscintigraphy is recommended.[24] Even in patients who have had prior complete axillary node dissections, Kaur et al. have demonstrated that lymphoscintigraphy can identify drainage in 29% of patients and, of these, drainage may be non-axillary (contralateral and/or internal mammary) in 38% of cases.[25] Furthermore, of the non-axillary sentinel nodes biopsied in the recurrent setting, 40% were positive and thus may alter management plans.[25]

✅ Lymphoscintigraphy is of limited utility in routine sentinel node biopsy; however, it should be considered in the setting of recurrent breast cancer, where it may be able to demonstrate alternative drainage pathways.

Intraoperative evaluation

Sentinel nodes may be sent for intraoperative pathological evaluation so as to minimise the possibility of the need for a subsequent completion axillary node dissection in node-positive patients. A number of techniques have been evaluated for intraoperative

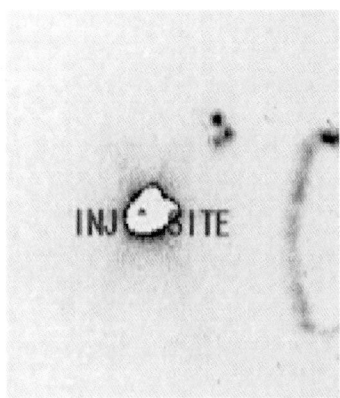

Figure 7.3 • Scintiscan showing drainage of technetium-99m human albumin colloid to show multiple sentinel axillary nodes.

evaluation – most commonly, frozen section and touch imprint cytology.

Frozen section is the most common technique used, and is associated with a specificity of 99–100% and a sensitivity of 57–74%.[26] The sensitivity is far better for macrometastases (84–92%) than micrometastases (17–61%),[26] and may be particularly difficult to interpret in patients with invasive lobular carcinomas who have cytologically bland cells and an infiltrative growth pattern. Nonetheless, the overall accuracy of this technique is 83–91%.[26]

Tew et al. conducted a meta-analysis of 31 studies of touch imprint cytology, and found that specificity and sensitivity of this technique were 94–100% and 34–95% respectively.[27] Pooled estimates from 11 studies comparing macro- and micrometastases found that the sensitivity for touch imprint cytology was significantly better for the larger deposits: 81% (95% confidence interval (CI) 74–86%) vs. 22% (95% CI 14–33%) for macro- and micrometastases, respectively.[27] On a more global level, the sensitivity of touch imprint cytology is lower than that of frozen section (62% (95% CI 53–70%) vs. 76% (95% CI 65–84%)), while specificity is comparable for both (99%).[27] Molecular techniques are available that detect cancer cells in sentinel nodes but these have not found widespread utility.

While intraoperative evaluation has long been advocated to avoid a second operative procedure, given that the majority of screen-detected breast cancer patients will be node negative, and that node-positive patients may not always require axillary node dissection (see

'Is axillary node dissection necessary in node-positive patients?' below), the value of intraoperative evaluation of sentinel nodes is under scrutiny.

Sentinel lymph node biopsy: controversial situations

While sentinel node biopsy is widely accepted as the standard of care for lymph node evaluation for patients with early stage clinically node negative invasive breast cancer, its use is less clear-cut in certain controversial situations.

Prophylactic mastectomy

For women at high risk who are undergoing prophylactic mastectomy, some have advocated sentinel node biopsy, as this avoids the need for subsequent axillary surgery if there is an occult breast cancer that is noted on final pathology, and the sentinel node is negative. Others, however, have argued that the risk of there being a cancer with associated lymph node metastasis is so low in the prophylactic setting that routine sentinel node biopsy, despite being of minimal additional morbidity, is not warranted. In a meta-analysis of six papers including 1251 patients who underwent 1343 prophylactic mastectomies, the rate of occult invasive cancer was 1.7% and the rate of positive sentinel nodes was 1.9%.[28] Patients with positive sentinel nodes in the prophylactic setting have often been found to have had a locally advanced breast cancer in the originally treated breast so, in these patients, sentinel node biopsy may be warranted when a prophylactic contralateral mastectomy is being performed.[28,29]

✅ Routine use of sentinel node biopsy in patients undergoing prophylactic mastectomy is not recommended, given that the finding of lymph node metastases in this setting is low. The risk of a positive sentinel node in the setting of contralateral prophylactic mastectomy is increased in patients who have had a mastectomy in the opposite breast for locally advanced breast cancer. Therefore, in such patients sentinel node biopsy should be considered.

Ductal carcinoma in situ (DCIS)

Some have argued that patients with DCIS who are at high risk of having concomitant invasive disease should have a sentinel node biopsy at the time of their excisional surgery to obviate the need to return to the operating room for a sentinel lymph node biopsy should an invasive focus be found on final pathology. The rate of DCIS on large core biopsy being upgraded to invasive disease on final pathology is reported to be up to 47%.[21,30–32] Fewer samples and the use of non-vacuum-assisted devices increase the rates of underestimation of invasive disease.[32] Further, clinical factors such as young age, a palpable mass, large tumour size by imaging, high grade, and comedo necrosis are also associated with an increased risk of concomitant invasive disease in patients with core biopsy diagnosis of DCIS.[33,34]

While some argue that such patients should have a sentinel lymph node biopsy, others prefer to confirm diagnosis of invasive disease before subjecting patients to a potentially unnecessary lymph node evaluation procedure. While sentinel node biopsy is minimally invasive and associated with few risks, it is not innocuous. It is well established that sentinel node biopsy can be performed after breast-conserving surgery has been performed. A recent meta-analysis comparing sentinel node identification and false-negative rates for patients who underwent surgical versus needle biopsy found that rates were comparable (sentinel node identification rates 91.3% vs. 92.8%; false-negative rates 12.3% vs. 9.9%).[35] Therefore, prior surgery does not affect the ability to perform this technique accurately and consensus guidelines have accepted that sentinel node biopsy should not be performed routinely in patients with DCIS undergoing breast-conserving surgery. It is accepted that for patients undergoing mastectomy for DCIS, a sentinel lymph node biopsy should be considered at the same time as the mastectomy,[36,37] as this technique cannot be performed once the breast is removed and an invasive focus is identified. In those with confirmed DCIS the node positivity rate is low at <1%.

✅✅ Sentinel node biopsy should be considered for patients undergoing mastectomy for DCIS.[36,37]

Neoadjuvant chemotherapy

Many patients with locally advanced or inflammatory breast cancers undergo neoadjuvant systemic therapy, and the use of preoperative chemotherapy is becoming increasingly popular even in patients with operable breast cancer, as a means to increase breast conservation rates as well as to evaluate in vivo tumour response to therapy. The burgeoning widespread use of neoadjuvant chemotherapy has led to a plethora of controversies regarding the accuracy and timing of sentinel node biopsy in this situation.

Some have argued that sentinel node biopsy should be performed prior to neoadjuvant systemic therapy. Studies have demonstrated a high identification (98–100%) and an exceedingly low false-negative rate (0%) in this situation.[38] Given that this technique is performed *prior* to any therapy, there can be no confounding of negative results as a result of therapy, which has resulted in false-negative rates as high as 39% in selected series[39] reported in patients who have a sentinel node biopsy following chemotherapy. Others, however, have argued that to do a sentinel node biopsy prior to chemotherapy eliminates the opportunity to spare the 2–35% of patients who have a pathologically complete response in the axilla the morbidity of an axillary dissection.[38] Furthermore, to evaluate sentinel nodes after neoadjuvant therapy, when surgery for the primary tumour is planned, may reduce the need for a second operative procedure.

A recent meta-analysis has demonstrated that sentinel node biopsy after neoadjuvant chemotherapy is associated with identification rates of between 71% and 100% (summary estimate 90.9%), false-negative rates between 0% and 39% (summary estimate 10.5%), and accuracy rates between 77% and 100% (summary estimate 94.4%).[40] Two groups have performed trials of sentinel lymph node biopsy (SLNB) in the neoadjuvant setting in women with node positive breast cancer whose nodes are cleared by chemotherapy. The issue these trials addressed is whether axillary dissection (AD) can be avoided in responding patients. The ACOSOG Z1071 trial was a single arm study of 756 women (T0-4, N1-2, M0) undergoing neoadjuvant chemotherapy (NAC) with axillary nodal involvement confirmed by ultrasound guided FNA or core biopsy.[41] Some patients had the involved nodes clipped. Following completion of NAC, SLNB was performed and there had to be at least 2 SLNs removed before proceeding to AD. The primary endpoint was to determine if the false negative rate (FNR) was <10% in women with N1 disease who had at least 2 sentinel nodes biopsied after NAC. Of 643 patients with a SN identified, 40.3% had a complete pathological response in the axilla. SLNB correctly identified nodal status after NAC in 84% of 695 patients. There was a 12.6% false negative rate (higher than the primary endpoint of 10%). The false negative rate (FNR) was significantly lower (10.8%) if dual tracer

with both radiolabelled colloid and blue dye was used, compared with blue dye (4/24 - 16.7%) or radioisotope alone (20/101 - 20%) (p=0.046). The FNR was lower if more than 2 nodes were examined, 9.8% for 3 sentinel nodes, 6.7% for 4 sentinel nodes, but 11% for 5 or more, p=0.004 for trend. Placement of a clip in the positive node at diagnosis also decreased the FNR to 7.4% vs 13.6% without clip placement. An apparent chemotherapy effect in the SNs removed as marked by greater fibrosis or other histopathological changes in the sentinel nodes was also associated with a lower FNR (10.8% vs 13.5% without). Avoiding a high rate of false negatives in patients with node positive disease is essential and the results of this study highlight that technical factors are important for accurate SLNB after NAC. Performance can be improved by the use of dual tracer, examination of a minimum of 2 sentinel lymph nodes and placement of clips in involved nodes at diagnosis. These are the requirements if this technique is to be used after NAC.

The German Breast Group addressed the issue of optimal timing for sentinel lymph node in the prospective German, multi-institutional SENTINA-trial.[42] Of 1737 patients entered, 1022 women were clinically node negative and underwent SLNB prior to NAC. The SLN detection rate in this group of women was 99.1 % (1013/1022). Among these, 360 patients had histologically involved nodes and these women underwent a second SLNB followed by AD after NAC. The SLN detection rate in these patients undergoing their second SLNB after NAC was 60.8% (219/360). 592 patients, who presented initially with suspicious axillary nodes converted to a cN0 status after NAC and underwent SLNB, combined with AD. The SLN detection rate in these women was 80.1% (474/592). The difference between the detection rates of these three groups was highly statistically significant (p < 0.001).

The false negative rate in patients who had a repeat SLNB after NAC was very high at 51.6% and so performing 2 SLNB before and after NAC cannot be recommended. In patients who were down-staged with NAC from positive to negative axillary status, the false negative rate was 14.2%. There are many aspects of the SENTINA study which are unclear. There was no use of clips in nodes. Many sentinel nodes were visualised on scans but not removed. No information has so far been presented on false negative rates related to the number of nodes removed. The results from these two studies are not that different. SLNB after NAC is a difficult procedure. While SLNB before NAC is accurate, patients with involved nodes at diagnosis require AD but many will have their nodes cleared by NAC. For this reason SLNB after chemotherapy has started to be incorporated into clinical practice in selected N1 patients whose primary cancer and nodes respond to NAC. It can however only be recommended when strict criteria are adhered to.

Isolated tumour cells and micrometastases

More thorough pathological evaluation of sentinel lymph nodes using serial sectioning and immunohistochemistry has allowed identification of occult metastases in up to 31% of previously 'node-negative' patients.[43] This stage migration, and the relevance of this previously undetected disease, has been a source of considerable controversy. The American Joint Committee on Cancer classifies sentinel node metastases into three categories: 'isolated tumour cells' for metastases <0.2 mm (which are considered node negative, pN0(i+); **Fig. 7.4**); 'micrometastases' for deposits between 0.2 and 2.0 mm (considered node positive, pN1mi; **Fig. 7.5**); and 'macrometastases', defined as deposits >2.0 mm (also considered node positive, pN1a; **Fig. 7.6**).[1] These somewhat arbitrary cut-offs have generated debate as to the true implications of both isolated tumour cells and micrometastases.

In a pooled analysis of 58 studies of patients with metastases <2 mm, de Boer et al. found that the presence of this small-volume disease in the axillary lymph node was associated with a reduction in survival, which was independent of other prognostic variables (hazard ratio (HR) = 1.44; 95% CI 1.29–1.62).[44] Data from the National Surgical Adjuvant Breast and Bowel Project

(NSABP) B-32 trial (**Fig. 7.7**) showed that any occult metastases were associated with a small increased risk of death (HR = 1.40; 95% CI 1.05–1.86), any outcome event (HR = 1.31; 95% CI 1.07–1.60) and distant disease (HR = 1.30; 95% CI 1.02–1.66).[45] On subgroup analysis, isolated tumour cells had a smaller increased risk of death, any outcome event and distant disease than micrometastases. The hazard ratios (95% CI) for these three outcomes were 1.27 (1.04–1.54), 1.18 (1.02–1.33) and 1.19 (1.00–1.41), respectively, for isolated tumour cells, and 1.60 (1.32–1.96), 1.38 (1.15–1.60) and 1.41 (1.19–1.68), respectively, for micrometastases.[45] The absolute differences in outcomes were, however, very small and the recommendations of the trial committee were that the differences were such that a search for occult metastases by immunohistochemistry on a routine basis when assessing sentinel lymph nodes could not be supported. The 'Micrometastases and Isolated Tumour Cells: Relevant and Robust, Or Rubbish' (MIRROR) Study also found that patients with both isolated tumour cells and those with micrometastases who did not receive systemic adjuvant therapy had a higher adjusted event rate than node-negative patients (HR = 1.50, 95% CI 1.15–1.94 and HR = 1.56, 95% CI 1.15–2.13, respectively).[46]

A number of authors have evaluated the significance of isolated tumour cells and micrometastases in terms of the likelihood of there being other non-sentinel node metastases (Table 7.2). Cserni et al., in a meta-analysis of 25 studies, reported that up to 57% of patients with isolated tumour cells or micrometastases had non-sentinel node involvement.[47] The pooled estimates for non-sentinel node involvement vary with tumour burden in the sentinel nodes, and are 20.2% (95% CI

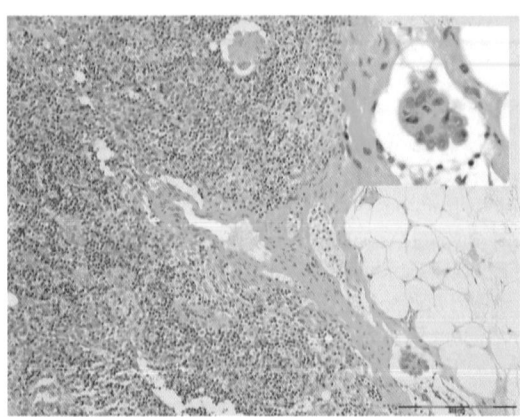

Figure 7.4 • Isolated tumour cells in an axillary lymph node.

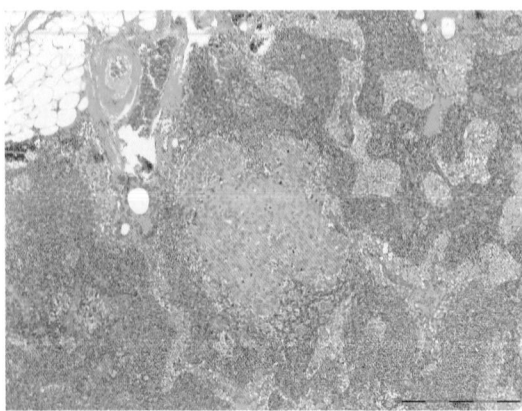

Figure 7.5 • Micrometastases in an axillary lymph node.

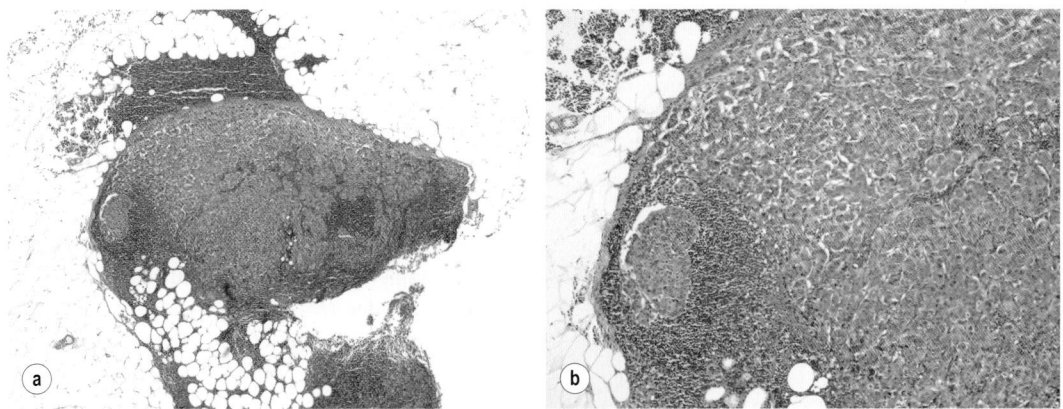

Figure 7.6 • Axillary lymph node with an obvious macrometastasis: (left) low power; (right) high power.

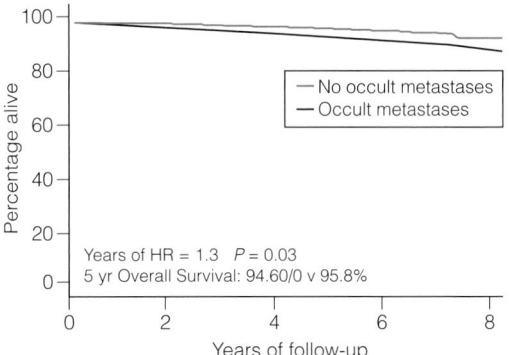

Figure 7.7 • Data from NSABP B32 trial comparing overall survival in patients with no metastases vs occult metastases demonstrated on immunohistochemistry.

15.5–24.9%) for micrometastases and 9.4% (95% CI 6.2–12.6%) for isolated tumour cells.[47] In keeping with these data, van Deurzen et al. found that 12.3% (95% CI 9.5–15.7%) of patients with isolated tumour cells or micrometastases had non-sentinel node involvement.[48]

Non-sentinel node metastases

Prediction models

Given that a significant proportion of patients with a positive sentinel node will have no further disease in their non-sentinel lymph nodes, a number of authors have

Table 7.2 • Non-sentinel node metastases in patients with isolated tumour cells and micrometastases

Study	N	Type of deposit	Non-SLN metastases
Nos et al.[87]	123	ITC/micrometastases	8 (6.5%)
	140	Macrometastases	55 (39.3%)
Viale et al.[88]	116	ITC	17 (15.8%)
	318	Micrometastases	68 (21.3%)
	794	Macrometastases	399 (50.3%)
Houvenaeghel et al.[89]	187	ITC	30 (16.0%)
	301	Micrometastases	43 (14.3%)
Gipponi et al.[90]	116	Micrometastases	16 (13.8%)
van Deurzen et al.[91]	23	ITC	3 (13.0%)
	101	Micrometastases	20 (19.8%)
	193	Macrometastases	93 (48.2%)
Chen et al.[56]	3	ITC	1 (33.3%)
	28	Micrometastases	6 (21.4%)
	128	Macrometastases	74 (57.8%)

SLN, sentinel lymph node.

developed nomograms and clinical prediction models in an effort to spare some patients with involved sentinel nodes the morbidity of axillary node dissection. Perhaps the best known of these is the Memorial Sloan-Kettering Nomogram developed by Kim van Zee and colleagues. This model predicts the probability of non-sentinel node status based on a number of factors, including pathological tumour size, grade, lymphovascular invasion, multifocality, oestrogen receptor status, the number of positive and negative sentinel lymph nodes, and the method used to identify sentinel lymph node metastases (either by immunohistochemistry, routine haematoxylin–eosin staining, serial sectioning with haematoxylin–eosin, or frozen section).[49] A number of other models have also been created, including the Cambridge nomogram,[50] the Mayo nomogram,[51] the Tenon model,[52] the MD Anderson score[53] and the Stanford nomogram.[54] All of these include some elements that are often available only after the sentinel nodes have been examined histologically, such as lymphovascular invasion and/or size of sentinel node metastases. These elements are clearly important in predicting non-sentinel node metastases, but in order to assist intraoperative decision-making, the Louisville clinical prediction model was developed as a simple clinical prediction model using variables that are available either pre- or intraoperatively, such as tumour size category, number of positive sentinel nodes and number of sentinel nodes removed.[55]

A recent study by Chen et al. evaluated all of these models in a small independent cohort of 81 patients.[56] All models were similar, with areas under the curve ranging from 0.54 (95% CI 0.45–0.63) for the Stanford model to 0.73 (95% CI 0.65–0.81) for the Cambridge. Aside from these two outliers, all other models had areas under the curve ranging from 60% to 68%. The false-negative rate for the prediction models ranged from 0% in the Louisville model to 19.8% in the Tenon model. There is a trade-off, however, between the false-negative rate and the number of patients who fall below the threshold for avoiding axillary dissection – so that models such as the Louisville model that had a very low false-negative rate often were more stringent and allowed fewer patients to avoid an axillary dissection.

Is axillary node dissection necessary in node-positive patients?

While nomograms and models can help to define a cohort of node-positive patients who are at low risk

of having non-sentinel node disease, the results of recent randomised controlled trials appear to have rendered such models irrelevant. The American College of Surgeons Oncology Group (ACOSOG) Z-0011 trial randomised 891 sentinel node-positive patients to complete axillary node dissection versus no axillary node dissection.[57] All patients received whole-breast tangential irradiation, which will have covered some of the lower two-thirds of the axilla, although no defined characteristics of the axillary radiation dose were specified in the trial and radiation fields used have yet to be reported. The median total number of nodes removed was 17 in the axillary lymph node dissection and two in the sentinel lymph node biopsy group alone. The median number of nodes with histologically demonstrated involvement was one in both groups; however, 27.3% of patients having a subsequent axillary dissection arm had non-sentinel node metastases.

With a median follow-up of 6.3 years, there was no significant difference in axillary recurrence between the patients who had a complete axillary node dissection (0.5%) and those who did not (0.9%). The adjusted hazard ratio for locoregional recurrence comparing complete dissection with sentinel node biopsy alone was 0.825 (95% CI 0.263–2.586, $P = 0.7411$).[55] Rates of locoregional recurrence did not differ between the two arms; local recurrence-free survival at 5 years was 96.7% (95% CI 94.7–98.6%) in the sentinel lymph node biopsy alone group, and 95.7% (95% CI 93.6–97.9%) in the axillary lymph node dissection group ($P = 0.28$). Disease-free survival did not differ significantly between the two treatment arms; the 5-year disease-free survival was 83.9% (95% CI 80.2–87.9%) for the sentinel lymph node biopsy alone group and 82.8% (95% CI 78.3–86.3%) for the axillary lymph node dissection group (**Fig. 7.8**). At a median follow-up of 6.3 years, there was no evidence that sentinel lymph node biopsy compared with axillary lymph node dissection resulted in a statistically significant inferior survival (Fig. 7.8). The unadjusted hazard ratio between the two groups was in favour of sentinel lymph node biopsy with a hazard ratio of 0.79 (90% CI 0.56–1.10). The hazard ratio for overall survival, adjusting for adjuvant therapy and age, was 0.87 (90% CI 0.63–1.23). The rates of wound infections, axillary seromas and paraesthesia were significantly higher for the axillary lymph node dissection group (70% vs. 25%, $P < 0.001$). Lymphoedema was also significantly more common in the axillary lymph node

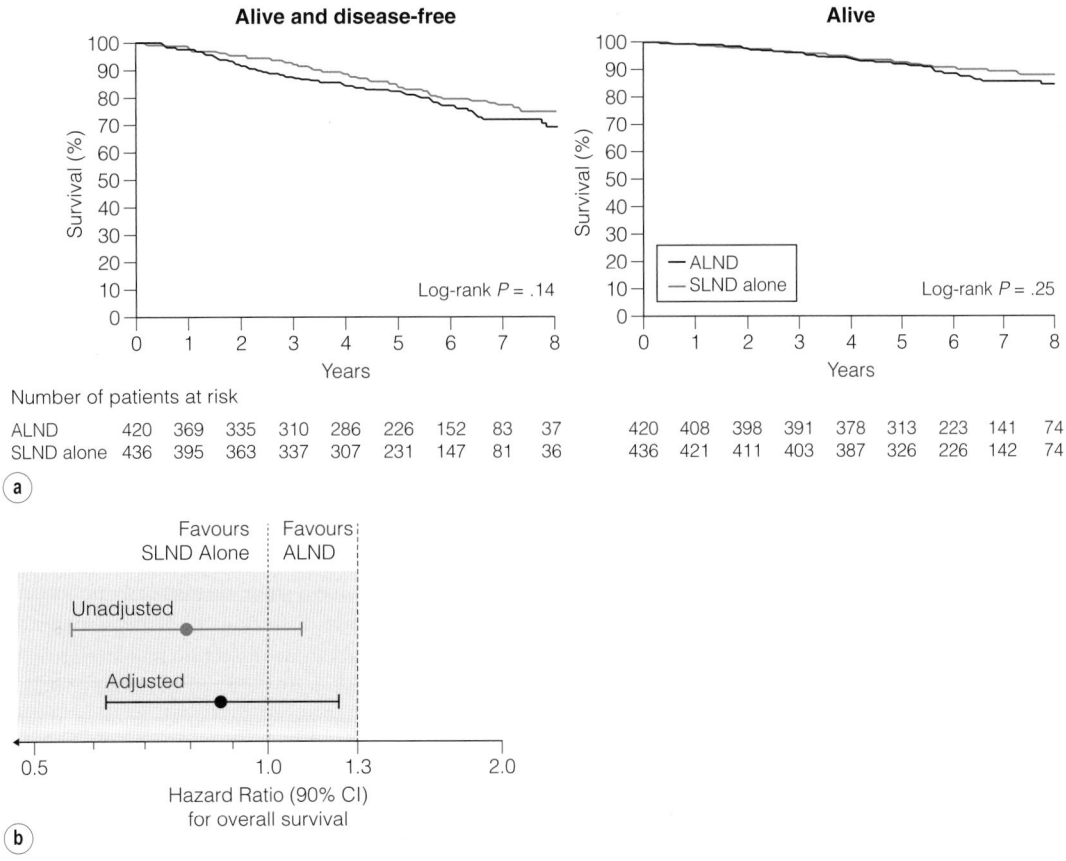

Figure 7.8 • Disease-free and overall survival from the Z-0011 study.

dissection group (*P*<0.001), in accordance with other comparisons of sentinel lymph node biopsy and axillary lymph node clearance.

For many surgeons, this trial has been practice changing and has questioned the need for routine axillary dissection in the setting of a positive sentinel node. It should be noted, however, that this study had several important exclusion criteria. Patients who had locally advanced disease or who underwent neoadjuvant chemotherapy were not candidates for the trial. Further, only patients with fewer than three positive nodes were eligible. Patients must have had breast-conserving surgery with whole-breast irradiation (accelerated partial breast irradiation or brachytherapy was an exclusion factor), and most had systemic adjuvant therapy. There are also some other concerns about the trial, specifically the amount of missing data, the inclusion of a number of ineligible patients, the selective nature of the patients entered into the study and the large numbers lost to follow-up. Despite the numbers lost to follow-up, data were complete on survival so the primary end-point does appear secure. Furthermore,

although the statistical end-point was achieved, it may be underpowered to show a small but potentially clinically significant effect on outcome. There are, however, large amounts of reassuring data on patients who have involved nodes treated by sentinel node biopsy alone, so the results of the Z-0011 study do not stand alone in indicating that it should no longer be routine practice to advise complete axillary dissection on all patients with a positive sentinel node.

The International Breast Cancer Study Group (IBCSG) 23-01 recently reported as yet unpublished results at the San Antonio Breast Cancer Symposium in December 2011. In this trial, 934 patients with sentinel nodes involved with micrometastases were randomised to complete axillary node dissection compared with no complete axillary node dissection.[58] Unlike the ACOSOG Z-0011 trial, only 75% of patients had breast-conserving surgery; 89% of patients in the group randomised to axillary node dissection received adjuvant breast or chest wall radiation therapy, and 92% of patients randomised to no complete axillary dissection received radiation. Five-year disease-free survival was 87.3% for the 464 patients who underwent axillary node dissection and 88.4% for the 467 patients who did not undergo this procedure, with low rates of axillary recurrence in both groups. Locoregional recurrences were seen in five patients (1.1%) of those having no axillary dissection: two in the axilla alone, one in the axilla together with internal mammary nodes, one in the breast and axilla, and one in the internal mammary nodes alone. There was only one patient in the axillary dissection group (0.2%) who developed locoregional recurrence and this was an isolated axillary recurrence. Overall survival was 98% at 5 years in both groups.

The European Organisation of Research and Treatment of Cancer (EORTC) 10981 'After Mapping of the Axilla, Radiotherapy or Surgery?' (AMAROS) trial aims to assess whether surgery or radiation to the axilla produce similar outcomes in sentinel node-positive patients. Between 2001 and 2005, 2000 sentinel node-positive patients were enrolled in the trial, and were randomised to either complete axillary node dissection or axillary radiotherapy, and the trial continues.[59] Long-term recurrence and survival data are as yet unpublished, but this trial should provide valuable information regarding the relative utility of dedicated axillary radiation and axillary dissection in providing locoregional control as well as the relative rates of lymphoedema.

> ✔✔ Axillary node dissection is not associated with improved survival in sentinel node-positive patients, and locoregional recurrence is low for patients receiving whole-breast irradiation and systemic therapy in patients with fewer than three positive sentinel nodes.[57] Consideration may be given to omitting axillary node dissection in such patients.

Complications of axillary surgery

Much of the significant effort that has gone into predicting non-sentinel node metastases and trials has been aimed at avoiding axillary dissection in the setting of a positive sentinel node and thus avoiding the complications associated with axillary surgery. While even sentinel node biopsy is not innocuous, because of the risk of anaphylaxis associated with blue dye,[60] the risks of numbness, lymphoedema and decreased range of motion are significantly less with sentinel node compared with full axillary dissection.[61-63] The 'Axillary Lymphatic Mapping

Against Nodal Axillary Clearance' (ALMANAC) trial demonstrated, in a multicentre randomised controlled trial, that patient-reported quality of life and arm function were significantly better with sentinel node biopsy than axillary node dissection.[64] In addition, using both subjective and objective criteria, they found that sentinel node biopsy was associated with less lymphoedema (relative risk (RR) = 0.37; 95% CI 0.23–0.60; 5% vs. 13%) and numbness (RR = 0.37; 95% CI 0.25–0.5; 11% vs. 31%) at 1 year than axillary dissection.[64]

Lymphoedema is one of the most dreaded complications of axillary surgery and/or radiation therapy. The rate of lymphoedema varies in part by the definition that is used, and can range from subclinical swelling that is detected by bioimpedence monitoring or perometer measurements to massive elephantiasis of the upper extremity. In general, however, up to 20% of patients may have some degree of lymphoedema after axillary node dissection. In a meta-analysis of 22 studies, axillary node dissection had a relative risk of 3.07 (95% CI 2.20–4.29) of developing lymphoedema compared to sentinel node biopsy alone.[65] Axillary radiation therapy was also associated with a relative risk of 2.97 (95% CI 2.06–4.28) of developing lymphoedema compared to no axillary radiation.[65]

Given the longevity of breast cancer survivors, the impact of axillary surgery on morbidity and quality of life long term is important. Even in patients undergoing a sentinel node biopsy alone, Liu et al., in a systematic review, demonstrated a prevalence of late morbidity that included pain (7.5–36%), decreased range of motion (0–31%), oedema (0–14%), weakness (11–19%) and sensory disorders (1–66%).[66] These effects decreased over time, and were more prevalent in young women.[66] Similar findings were noted in the NSABP B-32 trial, which found that while arm morbidity was less in the sentinel node biopsy group (as opposed to those who underwent axillary node dissection), less than 15% of patients in either group reported significant symptoms or limitations beyond 12 months.[67] Other prospective trials evaluating the morbidity of sentinel node biopsy compared with axillary node dissection have reported similar findings (Table 7.3).

> ✔✔ While sentinel node biopsy does cause morbidity, this is significantly less than for complete axillary node dissection.[64,67] Quality of life, as well as functional outcomes, are significantly better after sentinel node biopsy alone than after axillary dissection.[64,67]

Table 7.3 • Morbidity of sentinel node biopsy vs. axillary node dissection in prospective trials

| | OR (95% CI) for SLNB vs. ALND | | |
	Lymphoedema	Decreased range of motion	Numbness
Zavagno et al.[85]	0.48 (0.3–0.8)	0.55 (0.3–0.9)	0.51 (0.4–0.7)
Purushotham et al.[92]	0.30 (0.18–0.68)		0.32 (0.19–0.51)
Ashikaga et al.[93]	0.52 (0.43–0.65)	0.64 (0.53–0.79)	0.19 (0.15–0.23)
Mansel et al.[64]	0.37 (0.23–0.60)		0.37 (0.27–0.50)
Lucci et al.[94]	0.52 (0.26–1.06)		0.15 (0.06–0.37)

ALND, axillary lymph node; OR, odds ratio; SLNB, sentinel lymph node biopsy.

Some have attempted to reduce morbidity following sentinel node biopsy by adopting a technique in which the lymphatics of the arm are also mapped, and the nodes draining the upper extremity are avoided.[68,69] Some have argued that this 'axillary reverse mapping' or ARM technique does not reliably identify arm lymph nodes, and that the ARM nodes may harbour metastases or be the same nodes as those draining the breast in a minority of patients.[70] As yet, the true reduction in lymphoedema rates associated with this technique remains to be determined, and this procedure remains investigational.

Imaging techniques

A number of authors have investigated various imaging modalities as an alternative or adjunct to surgical staging of the axilla. The most well established of these is ultrasound, which is often combined with fine-needle aspiration for suspicious lymph nodes (Fig. 7.8); however, other techniques such as positron emission tomography and magnetic resonance imaging have also been described.

Ultrasound and fine-needle aspiration

Axillary ultrasound and fine-needle aspiration or core biopsy has been embraced as a means of staging the axilla to avoid sentinel node biopsy in node-positive patients, allowing them to proceed directly to axillary node dissection (**Fig. 7.9**). Given the findings from the Z-0011 trial, the value of this approach has been questioned as not all node-positive patients may need axillary dissection. Sentinel node biopsy in such patients

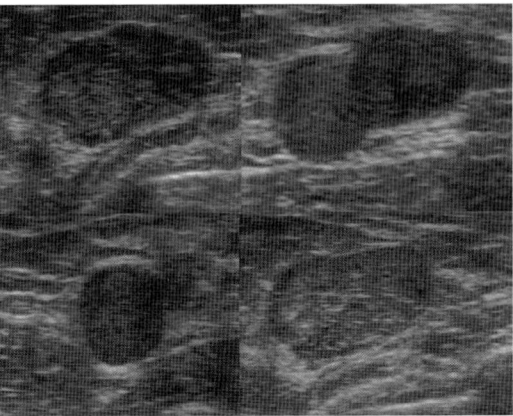

Figure 7.9 • Ultrasound images of involved axillary nodes in patients with breast cancer. All such nodes should have fine-needle aspiration or core to confirm whether the abnormal node is involved.

may still be valuable to determine whether less than three sentinel nodes are involved. A number of studies have found the sensitivity of ultrasound with fine-needle aspiration to range from 21% to 86%, with higher rates being found in patients with more extensive lymph node involvement.[71] A recent meta-analysis found the sensitivity and specificity of ultrasound in the detection of lymph node metastases to be 79.6% (95% CI 74.1–84.2) and 98.3% (95% CI 97.2–99.0), respectively.[72] Furthermore, the rate of ultrasound-guided needle biopsy yielding an insufficient sample was 4.1% (interquartile range 0–10.9%).[72] The role of ultrasound and fine-needle aspiration may therefore need to be redefined. While some may argue that patients who have a positive ultrasound-guided fine-needle aspiration should proceed directly to axillary node dissection given the propensity for extensive disease in this population, others have suggested that patients with limited nodal disease identified in this manner could be treated with sentinel node biopsy. This would give the option of avoiding axillary dissection in some, given the lack of survival benefit of removing lymph nodes, and the widespread use of adjuvant therapy, which may not change even as the number of positive nodes involved increases.

Positron emission tomography (PET)

PET has been explored as a potential means of detecting disease in the axilla, but to date results have been disappointing. In a meta-analysis of 26 studies, Cooper et al. found the sensitivity of PET to be 63% (range 20–100%; 95% CI 52–74%), with a specificity of 94% (range 75–100%; 95% CI 91–96%). The sensitivity was somewhat improved in studies evaluating PET-only (versus PET–computed tomography (CT); 66% vs. 56%, respectively); specificity, however, was improved by PET-CT (versus PET-only; 96% vs. 93%, respectively).[73] Sensitivity was 11% for micrometastases (based on five studies of 63 patients) and 57% for macrometastases (based on four studies of 111 patients).[73]

Magnetic resonance imaging (MRI)

MRI has become popular as a breast imaging technique and its utility in evaluating axillary lymph nodes has also been investigated. In a meta-analysis of nine studies, Harnan et al. found that the ranges of sensitivity and specificity of this technique were 65–100% and 54–100%, respectively.[74] Pooled estimates for sensitivity and specificity were 90% for each, but these varied significantly by technique. Ultra-small superparamagnetic iron oxide-enhanced MRI had the highest sensitivity and specificity (98% and 96%, respectively), gadolinium-enhanced MRI performed less well (with a sensitivity and specificity of 88% and 73%, respectively) and magnetic resonance spectroscopy (based on only one study) had sensitivity and specificity of 65% and 100%, respectively.[73] At the moment, imaging (whether by ultrasound, PET or MRI) has limited utility without histological confirmation of lymph node metastases.

Management of lymphoedema (see Box 7.1)

Given the need for histological confirmation of lymph node metastases, surgical evaluation of axillary nodes remains a major component of staging for patients with breast cancer. Such surgical excision of nodes, the vast majority of which are normal, carries with it the risk of lymphoedema (**Fig. 7.10**), albeit in a

Box 7.1 • Management of lymphoedema

There are four cornerstones of treatment:

- **Skin care** is required to maintain good skin condition and reduce the risk of infection.
- **Exercise** promotes lymph flow and maintains good limb function.
- **Manual lymphatic drainage** is a gentle skin massage that encourages lymph flow and is carried out by a trained therapist.
- **Support/compression** with multilayer lymphoedema bandaging is applied to reduce the size and improve the condition of the limb to allow fitting of elastic compression garments, which when fitted correctly control swelling and encourage lymph flow. Compression garments should be worn while the patient is exercising to reduce lymphatic filtration. Maintaining an adequate weight helps to prevent lymphoedema development, so dietary advice is important in all patients, but particularly in those who are overweight.

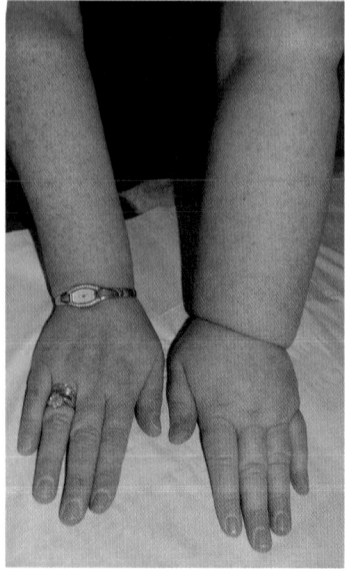

Figure 7.10 • Lymphoedema of the left arm and hand.

relatively small proportion of patients. When it does occur, however, there are several techniques for management of this upper extremity swelling.

Complete decongestive therapy

Often considered the primary modality for managing lymphoedema, complete decongestive therapy consists of manual lymph drainage, compression garments/bandaging, lymphatic/decongestive exercises and self-care education.[75] Intermittent pneumatic compression is often used as an adjunct to manual drainage.[76]

Pharmaceutical interventions

While pharmaceutical interventions with diuretics, benzopyrones and flavonoid derivatives have been investigated as potential therapies in the setting of lymphoedema, none have been found to be universally efficacious, and these modalities have been largely abandoned.[77]

Surgical therapies for lymphoedema

Historic operations, described by Sistrunk[78] and Thompson,[79] aimed to create a connection between the superficial and deep lymphatic collection systems by resecting subcutaneous soft tissue and deep fascia. While these procedures may have reduced the size of lymphoedematous extremities, they also caused extensive scarring and morbidity without any objective evidence that new lymphatic pathways were created. Hence, these procedures have been abandoned and are of historic interest only. Liposuction has also been proposed as a technique that could reduce the volume of lymphoedematous extremities;[80] however, given the risk of injury to residual lymphatics, this technique may actually exacerbate this condition. It is effective in arms with non-pitting swelling with significant excess of fat in the subcutaneous tissue.

Other procedures, aimed at draining excess lymphatic fluid into other lymphatic or venous vessels, have also been described. In particular, some have advocated placing greater omental flaps into the upper extremity while maintaining continuity with the ipsilateral gastroepiploic vessels through a subcutaneous tunnel in the chest.[81] The concept behind this procedure is that the omentum has more lymphatic vessels and that excess lymph fluid may be drained through the omental graft, although there is no objective evidence for this. Some have had success with lymphaticolymphatic bypass using lymphatic vessels of the medial thigh as a free composite graft to bypass routes between the upper arm and the supraclavicular region.[82] Others have similarly found significant prolonged improvement in lymphoedema using a lymphaticovenular bypass;[83] however, these procedures are still anecdotal and not widely adopted.

Finally, microvascular lymph node transfer in which inguinal lymph nodes are transplanted into the axilla as part of a composite soft tissue graft has been suggested.[84] Although the hypothesis is that this procedure would sprout new lymphatics that would allow improved lymphatic drainage, there are no data to demonstrate that lymphatics regenerate from these nodes. Therefore, surgical management of lymphoedema remains investigational.

> ✅ Complete decongestive therapy remains the initial treatment of choice for lymphoedema. Pharmacological and surgical therapies are investigational.

Conclusion

The management of the axilla has changed significantly in recent years. While lymph node status remains one of the most important prognostic factors in breast cancer patients, routine axillary node dissection should no longer be performed. Sentinel node biopsy has been validated as a simple, accurate and minimally invasive technique to stage the axilla. While this had often been followed by routine dissection in the setting of node-positive disease, recent trials have questioned the need for this practice in all patients, given the increased morbidity of complete dissection and the lack of survival benefit in removing additional nodes. There remain numerous controversies surrounding appropriate management of the axilla in breast cancer patients, and this continues to be a fertile area for further research.

Key points

- Sentinel node biopsy is a safe, accurate and minimally invasive means of staging the axilla in patients with breast cancer.
- Dual tracer has been shown to be superior to injection of either radioactive tracer or blue dye alone in terms of sentinel node identification rate.
- A subareolar injection technique can be used for sentinel node biopsy in patients with multifocal and multicentric breast cancer.
- Lymphoscintigraphy has limited utility for most cases of sentinel node mapping; however, this technique may be particularly useful in identifying alternative drainage pathways in cases of recurrent breast cancer.
- Intraoperative evaluation with frozen section and/or touch imprint cytology has a high specificity (99%); the sensitivity of frozen section is better than that of touch imprint cytology (76% vs. 62%). The use of routine intraoperative evaluation is now under question and many no longer use it.
- Sentinel node biopsy in the setting of prophylactic mastectomy is controversial. Patients with ipsilateral locally advanced breast cancer have an increased risk of a positive contralateral sentinel node.
- Sentinel node biopsy should be considered in patients undergoing mastectomy for DCIS.
- Sentinel node biopsy is feasible after neoadjuvant chemotherapy; however, its accuracy in this setting has been questioned, and this is the subject of ongoing randomised controlled trials.
- Micrometastases (defined as those measuring 0.2–2.0 mm) are classified as node positive, while isolated tumour cells (defined as those measuring <0.2 mm) are classified as node negative. The prognostic difference between these two groups remains somewhat controversial.
- A number of prediction models have been validated to predict non-sentinel node metastases, but none of them is perfect. Given the recent findings of the ACOSOG Z-0011 trial, which demonstrated no survival advantage of complete axillary node dissection and a low locoregional recurrence rate in sentinel node-positive patients who do not have further axillary surgery, such models now have limited utility.
- While the Z-0011 data suggest that some node-positive patients may safely omit axillary dissection, patients in this trial all had whole-breast irradiation therapy and only one or two positive nodes.
- Sentinel node biopsy is not without risk; however, it is associated with significantly less morbidity than axillary dissection. Techniques such as axillary reverse mapping remain intriguing, but still investigational.
- Given that not all node-positive patients require axillary dissection, the current role of ultrasound and fine-needle aspiration of suspicious axillary nodes may need revisiting. The utility of imaging techniques such as PET and MRI for evaluating lymph node metastases is limited in the absence of histological confirmation.
- The mainstay of management of lymphoedema is decompressive therapy; pharmacological and surgical therapies are still investigational.

References

1. American Joint Committee on Cancer. Breast. In: Edge SB, Byrd DR, Compton CC, Fritz AG, Greene FL, Trotti A, editors. AJCC cancer staging handbook. 7th ed. New York: Springer-Verlag; 2010. p. 417–60.

2. Fisher B, Jeong JH, Anderson S, et al. Twenty-five-year follow-up of a randomized trial comparing radical mastectomy, total mastectomy, and total mastectomy followed by irradiation. N Engl J Med 2002;347(8):567–75.

3. Veronesi U, Cascinelli N, Mariani L, et al. Twenty-year follow-up of a randomized study comparing breast-conserving surgery with radical mastectomy for early breast cancer. N Engl J Med 2002;347(16):1227–32.

4. Cabanas RM. An approach for the treatment of penile carcinoma. Cancer 1977;39(2):456–66.

5. Morton DL, Wen DR, Wong JH, et al. Technical details of intraoperative lymphatic mapping for early stage melanoma. Arch Surg 1992;127(4):392–9.

6. Krag DN, Weaver DL, Alex JC, et al. Surgical resection and radiolocalization of the sentinel lymph node in breast cancer using a gamma probe. Surg Oncol 1993;2(6):335–9.

7. Giuliano AE. Sentinel lymphadenectomy in primary breast carcinoma: an alternative to routine axillary dissection. J Surg Oncol 1996;62(2):75–7.

8. Giuliano AE, Kirgan DM, Guenther JM, et al. Lymphatic mapping and sentinel lymphadenectomy for breast cancer. Ann Surg 1994;220(3):391–8.

9. McMasters KM, Tuttle TM, Carlson DJ, et al. Sentinel lymph node biopsy for breast cancer: a suitable alternative to routine axillary dissection in multi-institutional practice when optimal technique is used. J Clin Oncol 2000;18(13):2560–6.
Multi-institutional, prospective validation of the sentinel node biopsy technique.

10. Krag D, Weaver D, Ashikaga T, et al. The sentinel node in breast cancer – a multicenter validation study. N Engl J Med 1998;339(14):941–6.
Multi-institutional, prospective validation of the sentinel node biopsy technique.

11. Veronesi U, Paganelli G, Galimberti V, et al. Sentinel-node biopsy to avoid axillary dissection in breast cancer with clinically negative lymph-nodes. Lancet 1997;349(9069):1864–7.
Multi-institutional, prospective validation of the sentinel node biopsy technique.

12. Krag DN, Anderson SJ, Julian TB, et al. Sentinel-lymph-node resection compared with conventional axillary-lymph-node dissection in clinically node-negative patients with breast cancer: overall survival findings from the NSABP B-32 randomised phase 3 trial. Lancet Oncol 2010;11(10):927–33.
The NSABP B-32 trial randomised patients to sentinel node biopsy followed by routine axillary dissection versus sentinel node biopsy followed by axillary node dissection in node-positive patients only.

13. Veronesi U, Paganelli G, Viale G, et al. Sentinel lymph node biopsy and axillary dissection in breast cancer: results in a large series. J Natl Cancer Inst 1999;91(4):368–73.

14. Tafra L, Lannin DR, Swanson MS, et al. Multicenter trial of sentinel node biopsy for breast cancer using both technetium sulfur colloid and isosulfan blue dye. Ann Surg 2001;233(1):51–9.

15. McMasters KM, Wong SL, Martin RC, et al. Dermal injection of radioactive colloid is superior to peritumoural injection for breast cancer sentinel lymph node biopsy: results of a multiinstitutional study. Ann Surg 2001;233(5):676–87.

16. Chagpar AB, Martin RC, Scoggins CR, et al. Factors predicting failure to identify a sentinel lymph node in breast cancer. Surgery 2005;138(1):56–63.
Large cohort study demonstrating that the dual injection technique was superior to either injection of radiotracer or blue dye alone in terms of identification rates.

17. Rodier JF, Velten M, Wilt M, et al. Prospective multicentric randomized study comparing periareolar and peritumoural injection of radiotracer and blue dye for the detection of sentinel lymph node in breast sparing procedures: FRANSENODE trial. J Clin Oncol 2007;25(24):3664–9.
Prospective randomised trial of periareolar vs. peritumoural injection using dual technique that validates the use of peri-areolar injection. Further, this study demonstrated that the overall identification rates (either blue or hot nodes) were higher than for either blue or hot nodes alone.

18. Tuttle TM, Colbert M, Christensen R, et al. Subareolar injection of ^{99m}Tc facilitates sentinel lymph node identification. Ann Surg Oncol 2002;9(1):77–81.

19. Klimberg VS, Rubio IT, Henry R, et al. Subareolar versus peritumoural injection for location of the sentinel lymph node. Ann Surg 1999;229(6):860–4.

20. Chagpar A, Martin III RC, Chao C, et al. Validation of subareolar and periareolar injection techniques for breast sentinel lymph node biopsy. Arch Surg 2004;139(6):614–8.

21. Spillane AJ, Brennan ME. Accuracy of sentinel lymph node biopsy in large and multifocal/multicentric breast carcinoma – a systematic review. Eur J Surg Oncol 2011;37(5):371–85.

22. McMasters KM, Wong SL, Tuttle TM, et al. Preoperative lymphoscintigraphy for breast cancer does not improve the ability to identify axillary sentinel lymph nodes. Ann Surg 2000;231(5):724–31.

23. Mathew MA, Saha AK, Saleem T, et al. Pre-operative lymphoscintigraphy before sentinel lymph node biopsy for breast cancer. Breast 2010;19(1):28–32.

24. Port ER, Garcia-Etienne CA, Park J, et al. Reoperative sentinel lymph node biopsy: a new frontier in the management of ipsilateral breast tumour recurrence. Ann Surg Oncol 2007;14(8):2209–14.

25. Kaur P, Kiluk JV, Meade T, et al. Sentinel lymph node biopsy in patients with previous ipsilateral complete axillary lymph node dissection. Ann Surg Oncol 2011;18(3):727–32.

26. Layfield DM, Agrawal A, Roche H, Cutress RI. Intraoperative assessment of sentinel lymph nodes in breast cancer. Br J Surg 2011;98(1):4–17.

27. Tew K, Irwig L, Matthews A, et al. Meta-analysis of sentinel node imprint cytology in breast cancer. Br J Surg 2005;92(9):1068–80.

28. Zhou WB, Liu XA, Dai JC, et al. Meta-analysis of sentinel lymph node biopsy at the time of prophylactic mastectomy of the breast. Can J Surg 2011;54(5):300–6.

29. Nasser SM, Smith SG, Chagpar AB. The role of sentinel node biopsy in women undergoing prophylactic mastectomy. J Surg Res 2010;164(2):188–92.

30. Dillon MF, McDermott EW, Quinn CM, et al. Predictors of invasive disease in breast cancer when core biopsy demonstrates DCIS only. J Surg Oncol 2006;93(7):559–63.

31. Goyal A, Douglas-Jones A, Monypenny I, et al. Is there a role of sentinel lymph node biopsy in ductal carcinoma in situ?: analysis of 587 cases. Breast Cancer Res Treat 2006;98(3):311–4.

32. Jackman RJ, Burbank F, Parker SH, et al. Stereotactic breast biopsy of nonpalpable lesions: determinants of ductal carcinoma in situ underestimation rates. Radiology 2001;218(2):497–502.

33. Yen TW, Hunt KK, Ross MI, et al. Predictors of invasive breast cancer in patients with an initial diagnosis of ductal carcinoma in situ: a guide to selective use of sentinel lymph node biopsy in management of ductal carcinoma in situ. J Am Coll Surg 2005;200(4):516–26.

34. Shapiro-Wright HM, Julian TB. Sentinel lymph node biopsy and management of the axilla in ductal carcinoma in situ. J Natl Cancer Inst Monogr 2010;2010(41):145–9.

35. Javan H, Gholami H, Assadi M, et al. The accuracy of sentinel node biopsy in breast cancer patients with the history of previous surgical biopsy of the primary lesion: systematic review and meta-analysis of the literature. Eur J Surg Oncol 2012;38(2):95–109.

36. Lyman GH, Giuliano AE, Somerfield MR, et al. American Society of Clinical Oncology guideline recommendations for sentinel lymph node biopsy in early-stage breast cancer. J Clin Oncol 2005;23(30):7703–20.
    ASCO guidelines for sentinel node biopsy.

37. Schwartz GF, Giuliano AE, Veronesi U. Proceedings of the consensus conference on the role of sentinel lymph node biopsy in carcinoma of the breast, April 19–22, 2001, Philadelphia, Pennsylvania. Cancer 2002;94(10):2542–51.
    International consensus conference for role of sentinel node biopsy.

38. Chung A, Giuliano A. Axillary staging in the neoadjuvant setting. Ann Surg Oncol 2010;17(9):2401–10.

39. Vigario A, Sapienza MT, Sampaio AP, et al. Primary chemotherapy effect in sentinel node detection in breast cancer. Clin Nucl Med 2003;28(7):553–7.

40. van Deurzen CH, Vriens BE, Tjan-Heijnen VC, et al. Accuracy of sentinel node biopsy after neoadjuvant chemotherapy in breast cancer patients: a systematic review. Eur J Cancer 2009;45(18):3124–30.

41. Boughey JC, Suman VJ, Mittendorf EA, et al. The role of sentinel lymph node surgery in patients presenting with node positive breast cancer (T0-T4, N1-2) who receive neoadjuvant chemotherapy – results from the ACOSOG Z1071 trial. Cancer Research: December 15, 2012;72(24):Supplement 3.

42. Kuehn T, Bauerfeind IGP, Fehm T, et al. Sentinel Lymph Node Biopsy Before or After Neoadjuvant Chemotherapy - Final Results from the Prospective German, multiinstitutional SENTINA-Trial. Cancer Research: December 15, 2012;72(24):Supplement 3.

43. Nasser IA, Lee AK, Bosari S, et al. Occult axillary lymph node metastases in "node-negative" breast carcinoma. Hum Pathol 1993;24(9):950–7.

44. de Boer M, van Dijck JA, Bult P, et al. Breast cancer prognosis and occult lymph node metastases, isolated tumour cells, and micrometastases. J Natl Cancer Inst 2010;102(6):410–25.

45. Weaver DL, Ashikaga T, Krag DN, et al. Effect of occult metastases on survival in node-negative breast cancer. N Engl J Med 2011;364(5):412–21.

46. de Boer M, van Deurzen CH, van Dijck JA, et al. Micrometastases or isolated tumour cells and the outcome of breast cancer. N Engl J Med 2009;361(7):653–63.

47. Cserni G, Gregori D, Merletti F, et al. Meta-analysis of non-sentinel node metastases associated with micrometastatic sentinel nodes in breast cancer. Br J Surg 2004;91(10):1245–52.

48. van Deurzen CH, de Boer M, Monninkhof EM, et al. Non-sentinel lymph node metastases associated with isolated breast cancer cells in the sentinel node. J Natl Cancer Inst 2008;100(22):1574–80.

49. Van Zee KJ, Manasseh DM, Bevilacqua JL, et al. A nomogram for predicting the likelihood of additional nodal metastases in breast cancer patients with a positive sentinel node biopsy. Ann Surg Oncol 2003;10(10):1140–51.

50. Pal A, Provenzano E, Duffy SW, et al. A model for predicting non-sentinel lymph node metastatic disease when the sentinel lymph node is positive. Br J Surg 2008;95(3):302–9.

51. Degnim AC, Reynolds C, Pantvaidya G, et al. Nonsentinel node metastasis in breast cancer patients: assessment of an existing and a new predictive nomogram. Am J Surg 2005;190(4):543–50.

52. Barranger E, Coutant C, Flahault A, et al. An axilla scoring system to predict non-sentinel lymph node status in breast cancer patients with sentinel lymph node involvement. Breast Cancer Res Treat 2005;91(2):113–9.

53. Hwang RF, Krishnamurthy S, Hunt KK, et al. Clinicopathologic factors predicting involvement of nonsentinel axillary nodes in women with breast cancer. Ann Surg Oncol 2003;10(3):248–54.

54. Kohrt HE, Olshen RA, Bermas HR, et al. New models and online calculator for predicting non-sentinel lymph node status in sentinel lymph node positive breast cancer patients. BMC Cancer 2008;8:66.

55. Chagpar AB, Scoggins CR, Martin RC, et al. Prediction of sentinel lymph node-only disease in women with invasive breast cancer. Am J Surg 2006;192(6):882–7.

56. Chen K, Zhu L, Jia W, et al. Validation and comparison of models to predict non-sentinel lymph node metastasis in breast cancer patients. Cancer Sci 2012;103(2):274–81.

57. Giuliano AE, McCall L, Beitsch P, et al. Locoregional recurrence after sentinel lymph node dissection with or without axillary dissection in patients with sentinel lymph node metastases: the American College of Surgeons Oncology Group Z0011 randomized trial. Ann Surg 2010;252(3):426–32.
    Findings of locoregional recurrence between the sentinel node biopsy alone vs. the axillary node dissection arms in the ACOSOG Z-0011 trial for sentinel node-positive patients.

58. Galimberti V, Cole B, Zurrida S, et al. Update of International Breast Cancer Study Group Trial 23-01 to compare axillary dissection versus no axillary dissection in patients with clinically node negative breast cancer and micrometastases in the sentinel node. Cancer Res 2012;71(Suppl. 24):102s.

59. Straver ME, Meijnen P, van Tienhoven G, et al. Sentinel node identification rate and nodal involvement in the EORTC 10981-22023 AMAROS trial. Ann Surg Oncol 2010;17(7):1854–61.

60. Bezu C, Coutant C, Salengro A, et al. Anaphylactic response to blue dye during sentinel lymph node biopsy. Surg Oncol 2011;20(1):e55–9.

61. Veronesi U, Paganelli G, Viale G, et al. A randomized comparison of sentinel-node biopsy with routine axillary dissection in breast cancer. N Engl J Med 2003;349(6):546–53.

62. Schijven MP, Vingerhoets AJ, Rutten HJ, et al. Comparison of morbidity between axillary lymph node dissection and sentinel node biopsy. Eur J Surg Oncol 2003;29(4):341–50.

63. Haid A, Koberle-Wuhrer R, Knauer M, et al. Morbidity of breast cancer patients following complete axillary dissection or sentinel node biopsy only: a comparative evaluation. Breast Cancer Res Treat 2002;73(1):31–6.

64. Mansel RE, Fallowfield L, Kissin M, et al. Randomized multicenter trial of sentinel node biopsy versus standard axillary treatment in operable breast cancer: the ALMANAC Trial. J Natl Cancer Inst 2006;98(9):599–609.
    Prospective randomised controlled trial demonstrating the lower morbidity associated with sentinel node biopsy compared to standard axillary node dissection.

65. Tsai RJ, Dennis LK, Lynch CF, et al. The risk of developing arm lymphoedema among breast cancer survivors: a meta-analysis of treatment factors. Ann Surg Oncol 2009;16(7):1959–72.

66. Liu CQ, Guo Y, Shi JY, et al. Late morbidity associated with a tumour-negative sentinel lymph node biopsy in primary breast cancer patients: a systematic review. Eur J Cancer 2009;45(9):1560–8.

67. Land SR, Kopec JA, Julian TB, et al. Patient-reported outcomes in sentinel node-negative adjuvant breast cancer patients receiving sentinel-node biopsy or axillary dissection: National Surgical Adjuvant Breast and Bowel Project Phase III Protocol B-32. J Clin Oncol 2010;28(25):3929–36.
    Patient-reported outcomes in the NSABP B-32 trial demonstrating that sentinel node biopsy is associated with less morbidity than axillary node dissection. Long-term morbidity (beyond 12 months), however, is shown to be minimal.

68. Nos C, Kaufmann G, Clough KB, et al. Combined axillary reverse mapping (ARM) technique for breast cancer patients requiring axillary dissection. Ann Surg Oncol 2008;15(9):2550–5.

69. Thompson M, Korourian S, Henry-Tillman R, et al. Axillary reverse mapping (ARM): a new concept to identify and enhance lymphatic preservation. Ann Surg Oncol 2007;14(6):1890–5.

70. Noguchi M. Axillary reverse mapping for breast cancer. Breast Cancer Res Treat 2010;119(3):529–35.

71. Mainiero MB. Regional lymph node staging in breast cancer: the increasing role of imaging and ultrasound-guided axillary lymph node fine needle aspiration. Radiol Clin North Am 2010;48(5):989–97.

72. Houssami N, Ciatto S, Turner RM, et al. Preoperative ultrasound-guided needle biopsy of axillary nodes in invasive breast cancer: meta-analysis of its accuracy and utility in staging the axilla. Ann Surg 2011;254(2):243–51.

73. Cooper KL, Harnan S, Meng Y, et al. Positron emission tomography (PET) for assessment of axillary lymph node status in early breast cancer: a systematic review and meta-analysis. Eur J Surg Oncol 2011;37(3):187–98.

74. Harnan SE, Cooper KL, Meng Y, et al. Magnetic resonance for assessment of axillary lymph node status in early breast cancer: a systematic review and meta-analysis. Eur J Surg Oncol 2011;37(11): 928–36.

75. Mondry TE, Riffenburgh RH, Johnstone PA. Prospective trial of complete decongestive therapy for upper extremity lymphedema after breast cancer therapy. Cancer J 2004;10(1):42–8.

76. Szolnoky G, Lakatos B, Keskeny T, et al. Intermittent pneumatic compression acts synergistically with manual lymphatic drainage in complex decongestive physiotherapy for breast cancer treatment-related lymphedema. Lymphology 2009;42(4):188–94.

77. Cormier JN, Askew RL, Armer JM. Lymphedema: a treatment sequelae. Advanced therapy of breast disease. Shelton, CT: People's Medical Publishing House, USA; 2012.

78. Sistrunk WE. Contribution to plastic surgery: removal of scars by stages; an open operation for extensive laceration of the anal sphincter; the Kondoleon operation for elephantiasis. Ann Surg 1927;85(2):185–93.

79. Thompson N. The surgical treatment of chronic lymphoedema of the extremities. Surg Clin North Am 1967;47(2):445–503.

80. O'Brien BM, Khazanchi RK, Kumar PA, et al. Liposuction in the treatment of lymphoedema; a preliminary report. Br J Plast Surg 1989;42(5):530–3.

81. Goldsmith HS, De los Santos R, Beattie Jr EJ. Relief of chronic lymphedema by omental transposition. Ann Surg 1967;166(4):573–85.

82. Baumeister RG, Siuda S. Treatment of lymphedemas by microsurgical lymphatic grafting: what is proved? Plast Reconstr Surg 1990;85(1):64–74.

83. Chang DW. Lymphaticovenular bypass for lymphedema management in breast cancer patients: a prospective study. Plast Reconstr Surg 2010;126(3):752–8.

84. Becker C, Assouad J, Riquet M, et al. Postmastectomy lymphedema: long-term results following microsurgical lymph node transplantation. Ann Surg 2006;243(3):313–5.

85. Zavagno G, De Salvo GL, Scalco G, et al. A randomized clinical trial on sentinel lymph node biopsy versus axillary lymph node dissection in breast cancer: results of the Sentinella/GIVOM trial. Ann Surg 2008;247(2):207–13.

86. Veronesi U, Viale G, Paganelli G, et al. Sentinel lymph node biopsy in breast cancer: ten-year results of a randomized controlled study. Ann Surg 2010;251(4):595–600.

87. Nos C, Harding-MacKean C, Freneaux P, et al. Prediction of tumour involvement in remaining axillary lymph nodes when the sentinel node in a woman with breast cancer contains metastases. Br J Surg 2003;90(11):1354–60.

88. Viale G, Maiorano E, Pruneri G, et al. Predicting the risk for additional axillary metastases in patients with breast carcinoma and positive sentinel lymph node biopsy. Ann Surg 2005;241(2):319–25.

89. Houvenaeghel G, Nos C, Mignotte H, et al. Micrometastases in sentinel lymph node in a multicentric study: predictive factors of nonsentinel lymph node involvement – Groupe des Chirurgiens de la Federation des Centres de Lutte Contre le Cancer. J Clin Oncol 2006;24(12):1814–22.

90. Gipponi M, Canavese G, Lionetto R, et al. The role of axillary lymph node dissection in breast cancer patients with sentinel lymph node micrometastases. Eur J Surg Oncol 2006;32(2):143–7.

91. van Deurzen CH, van Hillegersberg R, Hobbelink MG. Predictive value of tumour load in breast cancer sentinel lymph nodes for second echelon lymph node metastases. Cell Oncol 2007;29(6):497–505.

92. Purushotham AD, Upponi S, Klevesath MB, et al. Morbidity after sentinel lymph node biopsy in primary breast cancer: results from a randomized controlled trial. J Clin Oncol 2005;23(19):4312–21.

93. Ashikaga T, Krag DN, Land SR, et al. Morbidity results from the NSABP B-32 trial comparing sentinel lymph node dissection versus axillary dissection. J Surg Oncol 2010;102(2):111–8.

94. Lucci A, McCall LM, Beitsch PD, et al. Surgical complications associated with sentinel lymph node dissection (SLND) plus axillary lymph node dissection compared with SLND alone in the American College of Surgeons Oncology Group Trial Z0011. J Clin Oncol 2007;25(24):3657–63.

The genetics of breast cancer, risk-reducing surgery and prevention

D. Gareth R. Evans
Ava Kwong
Andrew D. Baildam

Introduction

The last 20 years have seen a substantial rise in our knowledge of inherited breast cancer. It is now possible to identify women at very high levels of risk of the disease. Whilst there are promising signs for reducing breast cancer risk using hormonal and other manipulations, the level of risk reduction still falls far short of that provided by surgical removal of breast tissue. Until another reliable risk-reducing measure is developed, risk-reducing surgery will remain a mainstay of management in women at very high risk who want to reduce substantially their chances of developing breast cancer.

Genetic predisposition

The presence of a significant family history is the strongest risk factor for the development of breast cancer. Even at extremes of age, the presence of a *BRCA1* mutation confers significant risks. A 25-year-old woman who carries a mutation in *BRCA1* has a greater risk of developing breast cancer in the following decade than a woman aged 70 years in the general population. About 4–5% of breast cancer is thought to be due to inheritance of a high-penetrance, autosomal-dominant, cancer-predisposing gene.[1,2]

✔✔ Inheritance of a germline mutation or deletion in a predisposing gene predisposes to early-onset, and frequently bilateral, breast cancer. Certain mutations also confer an increased susceptibility to other malignancies, such as ovary (*BRCA1/2*) and sarcomas (*TP53*)[3–5] (Table 8.1).

Multiple primary cancers in one individual or related early-onset cancers in a family pedigree are highly suggestive of a predisposing gene. It is thought that over 25% of breast cancers in women under 30 years of age are due to mutation in a dominant gene, compared with less than 1% in women who develop the disease over 70 years.[2] It has recently been found that at least 27% of breast cancers under 30 years of age are due to mutations in the known high-risk genes *BRCA1*, *BRCA2* and *TP53*. Nonetheless, risk is still largely based on family history and the detection rate for mutations in isolated breast cancer cases even at very young ages is considerably less than 10%,[6] although sporadic grade 3 triple-negative cancers have a little over a 10% chance of a *BRCA1* mutation in women under 40 years of age.[7]

There are few families where it is possible to be certain of a dominantly inherited susceptibility. However, the Breast Cancer Linkage Consortium (BCLC) data suggest that in families with four or more cases of early-onset or bilateral breast cancer, the risk of an unaffected woman inheriting a mutation in a predisposing gene is close to 50%.

Table 8.1 • Breast cancer genes: frequency and proportion of risk

Gene	Other tumour % of susceptibility	Population frequency	Proportion of breast cancer	Proportion of HPHBC	Proportion of familial breast cancer risk	Lifetime risk in women (RR)
BRCA1 AD	Ovary/prostate colorectal	0.1%	1.5%	40%	5–10%	60–85%
BRCA2 AD	Ovary/prostate Pancreas HoZ Fanconi (AR)	0.1%	1.5%	40%	5–10%	50–85%
TP53 LFSPD	Sarcoma, glioma Adrenal	0.0025%	0.02%	2%	0.1%	80–90%
PTEN Cowden's AD	Thyroid Colorectal	0.0005%	0.004%	0.3%	0.02%	25–50%
CHEK2	Colorectal, prostate	0.5%	0.5%	0%	2%	18–20% (2.0)
ATM AD and AR	HoZ (AR) Lymphoma, leukaemia	0.5%	0.5%	0%	2%	20%
STK11 AD	Colorectal	0.001%	0.001%	0.6%	0.04%	50%
BRIP1	HoZ Fanconi (AR)	0.1%	0.1%	0%	0.4%	20% (2.0)
PALB2	HoZ Fanconi (AR)	0.1%	0.1%	0%	0.4%	20% (2.0)
RAD51C	HoZ-Fanconi (AR)	0.1%	0.1%	0%	0.2%	14–20%
RAD51D	HoZ-Fanconi (AR)	0.1%	0.1%	0%	0.2%	14–20%
18 SNPs from GWA	FGFR2 TRCN9, MAP3K, LSP1, 8q128424800, etc.	30–46%	0.5–1%	0%	10%	11–13% (1.1–1.3)
Totals		80% for any	5%	83%	35%	

AD, autosomal dominant; AR, autosomal recessive; GWA, genome-wide association studies; HeZ, heterozygous; HoZ, homozygous; HPHBC, highly penetrant hereditary breast cancer (e.g. more than three affected relatives); LFS, Li–Fraumeni syndrome; RR, relative risk; SNP, single nucleotide polymorphism.

These studies have estimated that the majority of such families harbour mutations in *BRCA1* or *BRCA2*, especially when male breast cancer or ovarian cancer is present. In breast-only families, the frequency of *BRCA1/2* involvement falls to below 50% in four-case families.[8] Family and epidemiological studies have demonstrated that approximately 70–85% of *BRCA1* and *BRCA2* mutation carriers develop breast cancer in their lifetime, although the risk is a little lower for *BRCA2*.[8-11] The very low figures published on small numbers of families from population studies have now been addressed by a meta-analysis,[11] which gives risks to 70 years of age of around 70% for *BRCA1* and 55% for *BRCA2*.

The chances that a family with a history of breast and/or ovarian cancer harbours mutations in *BRCA1* or *BRCA2* can be assessed from computer models.[12-14] We have recently validated these models using a dataset of 258 patients and their samples tested for *BRCA1/2* mutations. We found that at the lower levels of likelihood for mutations, the computer models substantially overpredict the presence of mutations, particularly for *BRCA1*.[15] The Manchester manual model was much better at predicting a mutation in both genes and indeed was better than other manual models (Table 8.2). Further indicators for the presence of a *BRCA1* mutation within a family are grade and oestrogen receptor status. *BRCA1* tumours are more frequently grade 3 and oestrogen receptor negative or triple negative, and often have a medullary-like histology.[16] Further studies incorporating pathology information into risk models such as the BOADICEA have improved their prediction accuracy.[17] Ovarian cancers that develop in *BRCA1/2* families are nearly always non-mucinous epithelial cancers.[18]

Table 8.2 • Scoring system for identification of a pathogenic *BRCA1/2* mutation

	BRCA1	BRCA2
Female breast cancer <30 years	6	5
Female breast cancer 30–39 years	4	4
Female breast cancer 40–49 years	3	3
Female breast cancer 50–59 years	2	2
Female breast cancer >59 years	1	1
Male breast cancer <60 years	5 (if *BRCA2* tested)	8
Male breast cancer >59 years	5 (if *BRCA2* tested)	5
Ovarian cancer <60 years	8	5 (if *BRCA1* tested)
Ovarian cancer >59 years	5	5 (if *BRCA1* tested)
Pancreatic cancer	0	1
Prostate cancer <60 years	0	2
Prostate cancer >59 years	0	1

Scores for each cancer in a direct lineage are summed. A score of 10 is equivalent to a 10% chance of identifying a mutation in each gene.

The likelihood of identifying a *BRCA1/2* mutation should not be confused with the ability to detect a mutation if one is present in the family. No single technique is able to detect all mutations. Even by sequencing the entire gene (exons and intron/exon boundaries), the detection rate only equates to about 75%. If a strategy is added to detect large deletions or duplications in *BRCA1*, this can boost detection to around 95%.[19]

The proportion of breast/ovarian cancers attributable to *BRCA1* or *BRCA2* depends on the ethnic origin of families. Many countries or ethnic groups have particular founder mutations that are not seen in other populations. In countries with a small founder population, very few mutations may account for the vast majority of breast cancer families, such as in Iceland.

✔✔ The Ashkenazi Jewish population has three founder mutations: 185delAG and 5382insC in *BRCA1*, and 6174delT in *BRCA2*.[16] The three mutations are found in over 2% of the Ashkenazi Jewish population. One study showed that one of the three mutations was present in 59% of high-risk families.[20]

Populations that are more outbred, such as the UK, have larger numbers of mutations and founder mutations occur at lower frequencies. In the past, some laboratories concentrated on the large exons (exon 11 in both genes and exon 10 in *BRCA2*) and the smaller exons commonly reported to be involved, such as exons 2 and 20 in *BRCA1*. This cuts down the number of polymerase chain reactions using the

protein truncation test (PTT) to as little as five for *BRCA1* and four for *BRCA2*. However, this strategy reduces the sensitivity of identifying mutations down to as little as 50%.[19] With the great strides made in reducing cost and time of mutation searching using next generation sequencing these older strategies are now outdated.

Genetic testing

Once a mutation in a predisposing gene like *BRCA1* or *BRCA2* has been identified in a family, definitive genetic testing is possible. This can then more accurately inform women of their risks and give them an informed choice of different options, including risk-reducing surgery. Undertaking mutation analysis on an unaffected individual (without checking an affected relative), particularly in a breast cancer-only family, is problematic. Whilst identifying a pathogenic mutation will confirm a high risk, the absence of a mutation will not exclude the possibility that other genes or even a mutation refractory to the mutation screening techniques used are present. Although other genes are now being identified (see Table 8.1), many more remain to be found and screening for mutations is not clinically useful outside of *BRCA1/2* and in certain circumstances *TP53*. Nevertheless, the outcomes of genome-wide association studies indicate that all breast cancer cases will carry at least one risk allele.[21,22] Once all the lower risk alleles have been found a definitive genetic test can then be developed.

Breast cancer risk estimation

Where there is not a dominant family history or it is not possible to identify a mutation in *BRCA1/2*, risk estimation is based on large epidemiological studies, which give a 1.5- to 3-fold relative risk with a family history of a single affected relative.[1,2] Clinicians must be careful to differentiate between lifetime and age-specific risks. Some studies quote a ninefold or greater risk associated either with bilateral disease in a mother or with severe atypical hyperplasia. However, these risks are time limited and if these at-risk individuals are observed for many years, their relative risk is reduced over time.[23] Clearly, if one uses these risks and multiplies them against the lifetime incidence of 1 in 8–12 then some women will apparently have a greater than 100% chance of having the disease. Risks importantly do not multiply and may not even be additive. The best way to assess risk is to take the strongest risk factor, which in most cases is nearly always the family history. If risk is assessed on this alone, minor adjustments can then be made for other factors. It is arguable whether these other factors have any major effect on an 80% penetrant gene other than to speed up or delay the onset of breast cancer. Therefore, we can only really assume an effect on non-hereditary elements of risk. Although studies do point to an increase in risk in family history cases associated with certain factors, these may just represent an earlier age expression of the gene. Generally, therefore, non-mutant gene carriers will have risks somewhere between 40–45% and 8–10%, although lower risks are occasionally given. Higher risks are only applicable when a woman at 40–45% genetic risk is shown to have a germline mutation and to have inherited a high-risk allele or to have proliferative breast disease.

✅✅ Within Europe, risk estimation in the family history setting is based mainly on the Claus dataset.[2,24,25] However, within the USA, the Gail model of risk estimation is widely used.[26] As well as these datasets allowing estimation of risk, there are specific computer programs available, including Tyrer–Cuzick,[27] Cyrillic, BOADICEA and BRCAPRO.[14]

These programs take into consideration varying permutations of age of onset of diagnosis, number of affected and unaffected women, and hormonal factors;

as a consequence, different programs result in different risk estimations. The Gail model does not take into account age of relatives or second-degree relatives. A newer model, the Tyrer–Cuzick,[27] incorporates the majority of the currently known risk factors.

A major deficiency of current genetic models is the assumption that all inherited breast cancer is due to a single high-risk dominant gene or two genes (*BRCA1* and *BRCA2*). The problem this causes in a program like BRCAPRO is that in order to obtain an accurate assessment for identifying a *BRCA1* or *BRCA2* mutation in a family, all other potential genetic factors are overlooked. Therefore, while BRCAPRO provides reasonably accurate estimates for the presence of *BRCA1/2* mutations in high-risk families,[12] its ability to predict breast cancer incidence is substantially hampered in smaller aggregations of breast cancer. Variation in their value in different ethnicities has also been found.[28-30] We have recently found that BRCAPRO underestimates the risk of breast cancer in moderate/high-risk families by about 50%.[31] The most accurate computer model was the Tyrer–Cuzick model, although a manual model incorporating the Claus tables and data from the BCLC and adjustment for hormonal and reproductive factors was similarly accurate. A fuller explanation of the manual model[25,31] and a detailed review[32] are available elsewhere.[32]

Management options

Management options available to reduce the risks of developing breast cancer for women at high lifetime risk due to their family history or for those women known to be carrying a mutation in *BRCA1/2* are limited. Screening with mammography or magnetic resonance imaging (MRI) is one option but this detects cancer, it does not prevent it. Therefore, imaging surveillance can be combined with chemoprevention. However, many women consider or undergo risk-reducing mastectomy (RRM) if found to be at high risk, e.g. mutation carriers for *BRCA1* or *BRCA2*. The efficacy of surgical procedures for reducing the risk of breast cancer is controversial but of proven benefit,[33,34] although it would appear that the residual risk of breast cancer depends on the amount of residual breast tissue following the surgical procedure. It would be ideal to perform a prospective randomised clinical trial where women with the same risk were randomised to either intensive surveillance or prophylactic surgery, but it would be difficult to recruit women for this type of trial and so it is unlikely to happen. Recent work suggests that more women are considering RRM,[35,36] although uptake rates even for *BRCA* mutation carriers vary enormously, with a much lower uptake in Israel and southern Europe, almost certainly due to different cultural beliefs, protocols and availability.[36] Protocols should be in place to deal with requests for RRM at all cancer genetics and oncoplastic clinics. It has been suggested that surgery does increase life expectancy in *BRCA1* or *BRCA2* mutation carriers.[37]

✔✔ The first study to demonstrate that women with a high risk of breast cancer can significantly reduce their subsequent incidence of the disease with RRM was published in 1999.[38] This was followed by a Dutch study that confirmed risk reduction in those at highest risk (*BRCA1/BRCA2* carriers).[39] Current evidence would suggest that RRM is associated with an approximately 90–95% reduction in risk.[40,41]

Genetic counselling and the family history clinic

Breast cancer family history clinics started to be established in the UK in 1987,[42,43] and these clinics are now established across Europe, North America and are now also emerging in Asia.[44,45] Genetic counselling sessions and family history clinics are important not only to provide a means to select suitable individuals for genetic testing, but also to aid decision-making in individual women on surveillance and preventative measures. They are generally administered by consultants in medical oncology, clinical genetics and breast surgery, often with a multidisciplinary approach and with close involvement of radiologists and a psychiatrist/psychologist. At these clinics unaffected women at increased risk of breast cancer are assessed as to their lifetime and shorter-term risks of breast cancer development. After assessing risk, women are presented with a number of choices including regular surveillance, usually with a combination of clinical examination, mammography, ultrasonography and in some circumstances breast MRI[46] that commences between 20 and 40 years depending on the age of onset of cancers in the family and

the overall risk. Women are generally divided into three risk groups: average, moderate and high risk. It is only in the high-risk group that RRM should be considered. This usually equates to a lifetime risk of 1 in 4 (25%) or greater. As a rough guide, this equates to having a heterozygote risk of 1 in 4 with two relatives, including one first-degree relative, with breast cancer diagnosed below 50 years of age or three affected relatives under 60 years. All affected relatives should be first-degree relatives or related through a male.

In a survey of 10 European centres,[42] only three (Manchester, Edinburgh, Heidelberg/Dusseldorf) routinely mentioned the possibility of RRM to women with a lifetime risk of 1 in 4 or greater. This information is often only given as a statement of the availability of the procedure as an option for prevention of breast cancer. This allows women to extend the discussion if they wish to do so, or to state that they are not interested in surgery. Many centres only mention risk-reducing surgery to potential mutation carriers undertaking a genetic test. Indeed, there is a cultural shift across Europe from north to south, with RRM being less acceptable to both physician and patient as one moves southward.[47,48] In the USA, in centres where mastectomies for benign breast disease were commonplace in the 1970s and 1980s,[38] there appears to be less enthusiasm for mastectomy now even among gene mutation carriers.[49] What is absolutely clear is that adequate preparation of a woman contemplating RRM is essential.

The RRM protocol

Women who wish to consider RRM should be given time to consider the procedure thoroughly prior to making the decision. In Manchester, a protocol is in place for women who are assessed as at high risk who would be suitable for RRM despite not having certain knowledge of mutation status. For example, an individual's calculated lifetime risk may be 40%, but a recognised gene mutation may not have been identified in the family. This exact same protocol may not be offered in other centres but the general principles of counselling apply. In general, most centres will offer multiple sessions of discussion of available surgical procedures and counselling. Most women would be offered a further appointment at least 1 month later. This not only gives the women time to consider more fully all options but also allows time for them to discuss it with appropriate members of their family. The mean time interval from a personal genetic diagnosis to the date of surgery of RRM is approximately 9 months.[50] Usually the partner or a family member selected by the patient is encouraged to attend the clinic session to help decision-making. At the second appointment, with a geneticist or oncologist, a basic description of the surgery is provided, including the potential residual risk of different procedures. It is emphasised that a residual breast cancer risk and complication rates from surgery are still present after RRM and may be higher if the surgery preserves the nipple–areola complex (NAC). Options of simultaneous breast reconstruction can also be discussed. It is important to prepare the patient for the likely consequences of mastectomy including pain and any possible complications that, if they occur after breast reconstruction, may result in a poor cosmetic result, as well as considering the impact upon her personal life and family dynamics. Because of potential pitfalls such operations should only be undertaken by surgeons highly skilled in RRM and its possible complications, to optimise both oncological and aesthetic outcomes.

When possible, a living affected member should be the first to undertake genetic testing as this provides more information on the underlying genetic structure of the family.[25,51,52] A time scale for genetic testing is discussed, and the woman is asked to consider the potential impact of proceeding with surgery, particularly if she then undergoes genetic testing and finds that she does not in fact carry the causative mutation. It is also emphasised that the genetic risk of breast cancer decreases with age and that the remaining risk of breast cancer if the woman is older (>40 years) and has not developed breast cancer becomes lower than the lifetime risk.[25] Indeed, a mutation carrier for *BRCA1* may have no more than a 50% risk of breast cancer in her remaining lifetime if she has reached 50 years, but this is still a substantial personal risk. Psychological assessement and counselling should be arranged for women who are considering proceeding.

✔ Confirmation of breast cancers in the family must be sought proactively if this has not already been done. This ensures that risk assessment is as accurate as possible. The Manchester group

has previously reported the presence of factitious histories within some families where women have fabricated their family history in order to obtain surgery, or are implicated innocently as being at risk by another family member who has promoted an inaccurate family history.[53]

The whole process, from first consultation to the surgical procedure itself, usually takes between 6 and 12 months. This time delay is deliberate; in most centres the greatest delay is at the beginning of the protocol in order to allow women time for the decision-making process. If the protocol is run concurrently with a decision for predictive genetic testing, then the wait will generally be shorter. The full protocol of two sessions at the family history clinic, a session with a psychiatrist and sessions with the surgeon was established in 1993 in Manchester. The major difference between this protocol and that offered by some other centres both locally and internationally is that RRM in other centres is offered only when raised by the patient, and it is generally only offered in these centres when a woman is proven to be a *BRCA1/2* mutation carrier. Even with a proven mutation carrier no centre actively recommends surgery, but offers this as part of a range of choices. The incorporation of counselling during decision-making and treatment has been shown to improve psychological and social outcome.[54,55]

There are various approaches of surgery that could be recommended to the patient, including nipple–areola-sparing mastectomy with an option of breast reconstruction, depending on the centre, and the women's preference, as well as breast size and shape of the individual. Availability of appropriate surgeon expertise is paramount. There is no clear consensus in terms of the surgical procedure recommended in women who decide on surgery and a detailed surgical consultation should aid the woman's decision.

Surgical consultation

The aim of risk-reducing surgery is not only to reduce cancer risk and breast cancer mortality, but also to reduce the psychological distress and anxiety of an individual.[56] For unaffected mutation carriers RRM reduces lifetime risk of breast cancer to less than 5%.[57,58] However, any surgical procedure, particularly in a preventative setting, warrants a balanced discussion of its benefits and risks. Due to lack of level I evidence from randomised controlled clinical trials, recommendations are usually based on cohort studies of prophylactic surgery.[59,60] Moreover, to date, although risk of breast cancer is reduced there are still no data that show statistically significant improvement in survival after RRM. It is also important that when a women embarks on such a decision, a full understanding of the surgery involved is achieved and the woman understands that risk reduction of cancer is never 100%. Risk reduction surgery is not a minor cosmetic procedure but major surgery, and hence the nature and extent of the surgery and possible complications need to be considered. The expected cosmetic result, changes in the patient's breast sensation and also the impact of RRM on a patient's social life should be addressed. The whole range of evolving surgical techniques that can be offered should be discussed thoroughly before a decision is made for surgery.

In order to properly select suitable individuals for RRM, at least two detailed surgical consultations are needed to discuss the types of mastectomy and breast reconstruction procedures that are available. The techniques, limitations, outcomes and potential complications, and photographs of a range of aesthetic outcomes should be shown. It must be emphasised that there is still a small chance of getting cancer after RRM and that subjectively the breasts may look and feel different from the original breasts even if a successful surgical outcome is achieved. Time should be given for the women to digest this information. Consultations should involve a breast oncoplastic surgeon, plastic surgeon if appropriate and also a breast nurse specialist. More intimate issues including quality-of-life concerns, changes of body image and impact on sexual relationship with her partner may result in further questions following surgical consultation.[61] Before discussing details of options for surgery, during the consultation session it is important to identify any women where RRM may not be advisable. There are relative contraindications to RRM taking place (see Box 8.1).

The decision of which surgical option to choose will vary between individuals (see Box 8.2).[62] For some women a traditional total simple mastectomy without reconstruction may offer what she wants as it reduces risk and can be cosmetically acceptable if performed appropriately (see Chapter 5), whereas for others NAC-sparing mastectomy with

Box 8.1 • Absolute and relative contraindications to risk-reducing mastectomy

- Risk of breast cancer is not high or confirmed
- Genetic test has been performed but results are still unavailable
- Unreliable family history
- Munchausen syndrome (Factitious history)
- Risk of surgery outweighs its benefit

Psychosocial related
- Not personal choice but choice of family members and partner
- Unrealistic expectation of aesthetic result
- Psychiatric disorders

The ability to understand the procedure
- Choice of surgery is for cosmetic rather than oncological reasons
- Unrealistic expectation of the amount of risk reduction possible

Box 8.2 • Choice of surgical technique for risk-reducing mastectomy*

- Simple total mastectomy (STM)[†] with or without breast reconstruction
- Skin-sparing mastectomy (SSM)[‡] with or without breast reconstruction
- Nipple–areola complex-sparing mastectomy (NSM)[§] with or without breast reconstruction
- Areola-sparing mastectomy (ASM)[§] with or without breast reconstruction

*All of the above types of mastectomies involve the removal of breast tissue and vary with respect to the skin that is spared.
†Total mastectomy removes an ellipse of skin including the nipple–areola complex.
‡SSM preserves the majority of the skin but removes the nipple–areola complex.
§NSM and ASM preserve the nipple and areola respectively, and preserve more skin.
Reproduced from Guillem JG, Wood WC, Moley JF et al. ASCO/SSO review of current role of risk-reducing surgery in common hereditary cancer syndromes. J Clin Oncol 2006; 24(28):4642–60.

reconstruction is the only acceptable aesthetic outcome. Skin-sparing mastectomy (SSM) has already been shown to be as oncologically safe as total simple mastectomy on selected patients, but the data available are mainly from patients with existing breast cancer. There are no specific data for prophylactic surgery using SSM, but it does appear to be an acceptable approach oncologically.[63,64] Non-SSM, also known as subcutaneous mastectomy, evolved due to psychological studies that found that the feeling of mutilation is increased after removal of the NAC when performing mastectomy.[65] It is unsafe to compare directly data from women who have been treated for breast cancer with those who have not; however, there have been controversies behind the safety of saving the NAC, as occult tumour involvement behind the NAC in mastectomy specimens in cancer patients has been reported to occur in 0–50% of cases.[66–68] However, many of these studies were performed more than two decades ago when significant amounts of breast tissue were left behind the nipple and there are new data indicating that for selected individuals nipple-sparing mastectomy (NSM) is oncologically safe. Moreover, it is likely that, formerly, case selection was less well planned and with improvement of case selection of patients who are deemed more suitable for NSM, either by clinical presentation or after MRI with use of intraoperative frozen section to exclude patients with nipple involvement, it is likely that long-term results would be favourable.[69–71] There is a risk of nipple–areola complex necrosis of about 5–15% when performing NSM, which can be partial or complete, and this is more common in smokers (see Chapter 5). In general, partial necrosis usually heals without further surgical intervention. There is a proportion of women who suffer nipple sensation loss of 25%.[72–74] Loss of nipple projection and de-pigmentation of the areola skin are also common problems with NSM. The improvement of psychological outcome from NSM[65] makes this the option of choice for most women considering RRM.

Various techniques have been suggested as incisional options for NSM.[74]

Incisions for nipple-sparing mastectomy (Figs 8.1–8.6)

In a study by Esserman and colleagues, it was found that NAC necrosis was higher when an incision crossing the NAC was used (18%).[74] If the incision spanned less than one-third of the circumference of the areola the results were good. Those that cover more than one-third of the circumference are likely to compromise the blood supply of the nipple, which can result in loss of nipple–areola skin. Inframammary incisions were found to be more

suitable for women with small breasts, as this incision allows only limited exposure of the upper part of the breast, being particularly problematic if performed in women who have larger breasts. A radial incision in this study provided the best access for breast tissue removal and was most likely to maintain NAC viability, but can result in nipple deviation in the direction of the incision. If reconstruction is planned, then the choice of incision is even more important and should be based on the size of the breast and the degree of ptosis.

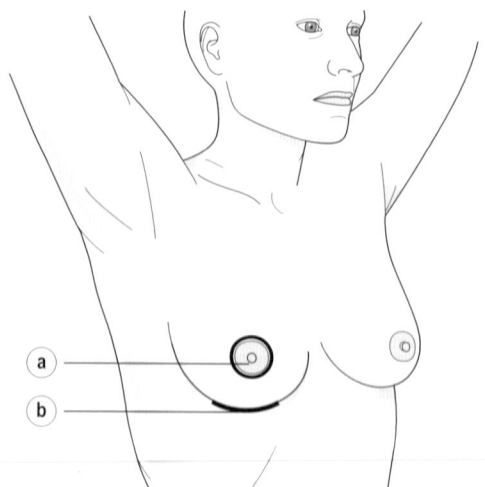

Figure 8.1 • (a) Skin-sparing dissection with removal of the nipple and areola skin and replacement of the nipple alone or the nipple–areola complex as a free graft. **(b)** Submammary/inframammary incision.

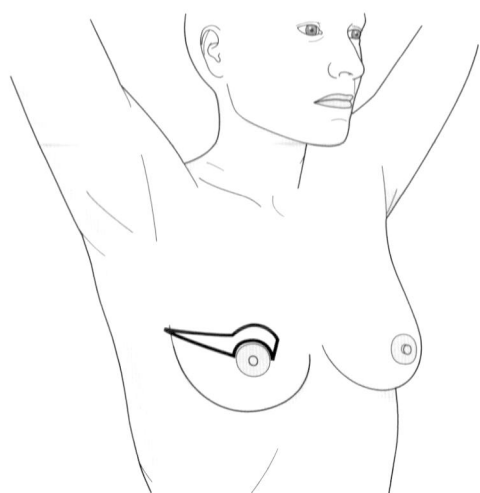

Figure 8.2 • Batwing incision to reduce the upper skin and elevate the nipple.

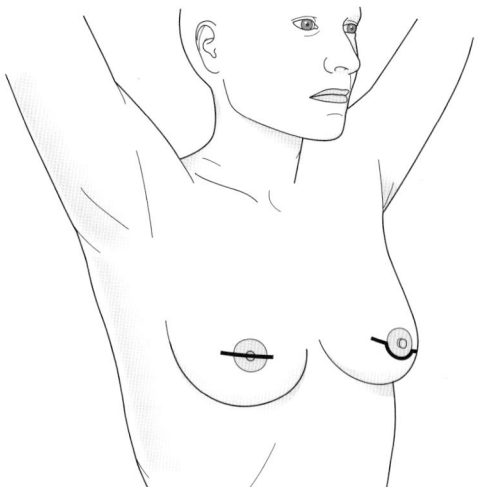

Figure 8.3 • Incisions across or below the nipple.

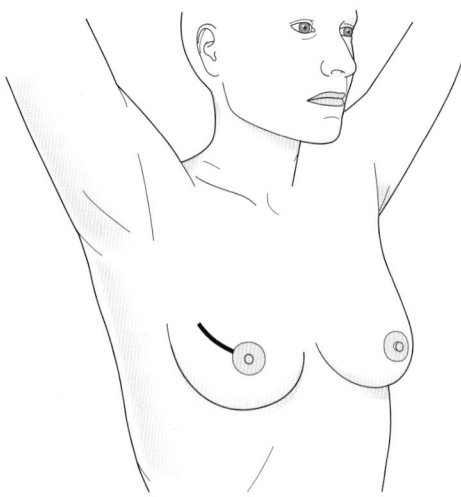

Figure 8.5 • Radial or skin crease incision.

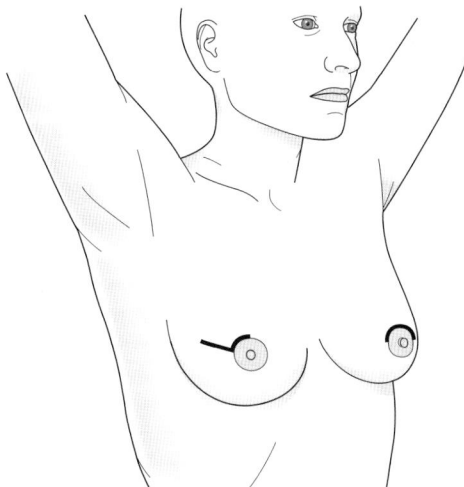

Figure 8.4 • Incisions above the nipple with or without skin crease lateral extension.

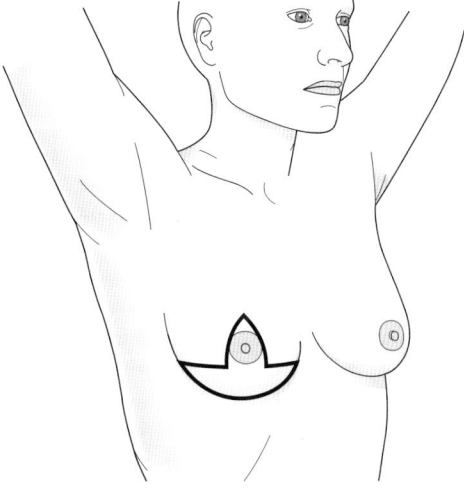

Figure 8.6 • Wise pattern risk-reducing mastectomy planning.

Areola-sparing mastectomy (ASM) has also been proposed as an option to NSM, as in theory it is the ducts that transverse the nipple that can harbour occult metastatis and not the areola disc, which is more similar to 'skin'.[34] Hence, over recent years this has also become an option for women who choose to have a mastectomy.

Risk-reducing surgery and breast reconstruction

Mastectomy can be a mutilating surgery for many women and so during the last century there has been increased use of reconstruction for women who opt for mastectomy. This is even more relevant for the group of high-risk women who opt for RRM, who have not themselves had breast cancer, and who need long-term reconstruction of functional and aesthetic excellence. The need for more and better breast reconstruction options after mastectomy has resulted in an increase in the number and types of different reconstructive techniques to achieve the best aesthetic outcomes with a more personalised approach based on a woman's breast size, desired outome and technical feasibility (see Box 8.3).

Box 8.3 • Options for women who choose to have RRM with reconstruction

Autologous myocutaneous flaps

Most commonly used:

- Transverse rectus abdominis flap (TRAM)
- Latissimus dorsi flap (LD)
- Rectus muscle-sparing deep inferior epigastric perforator flap (DIEP)

Less commonly used:

- Buttock flaps including inferior gluteal artery perforator and superior gluteal artery perforator flaps
- Gracilis-base thigh flaps

Myocutaneous flaps can be de-epithelialised if NSM or SSM techniques are used for mastectomy

Implants

- Permanent implants
- Expander/implants (Becker expander/implants)
- Expanders followed by implants

Combination of autologous flap with implant

- LD flap with implant

Reconstructions after RRM can be performed immediately or in a staged fashion. In general, unless contraindicated, immediate reconstruction should be performed as it avoids the woman having a period of time without a 'breast' and it allows skin to be spared, which improves the final cosmetic result (**Fig. 8.7**). Although most reconstructions produce satisfactory results, it is not uncommon for a patient to have expectations that there will be no visible scars. Moreover, providing patients with photographs of possible complications is an important part of informing the patient, as is providing a specialist nurse to liaise with the woman and to address further questions that the woman may have.

Sharing experience with others who have undergone the procedure may also help to better prepare an individual when deciding on RRM and breast reconstruction.

In women with large breasts, the skin envelope may need to be reduced when performing breast reconstruction (**Figs 8.8** and **8.9**). The placement of an acellular dermal matrix can also be used in addition to fat injection to achieve a better aesthetic result.[71] Autologous myocutaneous flaps use natural tissue, and give women the feeling that they are using living tissue and have a warm soft consistency that can be more realistic. Expertise in oncoplastic and plastic surgery is required to decrease complication rates when microvascular anastomoses are warranted.

The use of implant devices after RRM seems a simpler option compared with the transfer of myocutaneous flaps but complications are common and considerable skill and expertise is required to get good, consistent results. There are different types of prosthesis in relation to shape and contour. Prostheses can be permanent or allow expansion, with saline being injected gradually into the expandable chamber of the prosthesis until the desired volume is achieved. These help in providing a natural 'breast' projection and may result in better contour in the upper breast.[75] Anatomical expanders permit more rapid expansion and result in lower pressures within the implant, appear less likely to migrate and cause less chest deformity. Silicon gel implants are available in a range of specifications and gel types, to allow a more natural look and feel. Implants are usually placed under the chest wall muscle and, combined with well planned and carried out surgery, can give a good aesthetic outcome. Complications from such surgery include

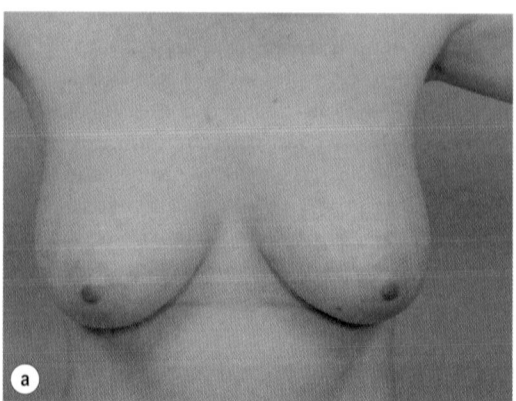
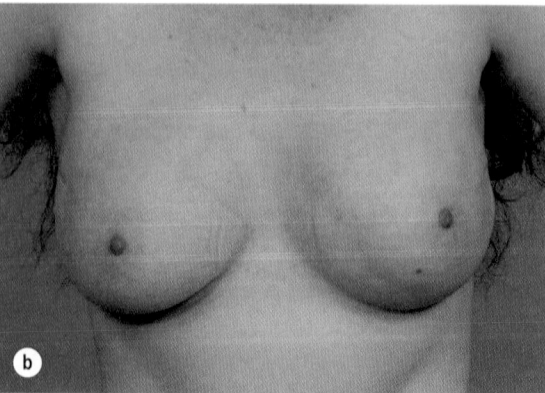

Figure 8.7 • Horizontal/oblique risk-reducing mastectomy (RRM) before **(a)** and after **(b)** operation.

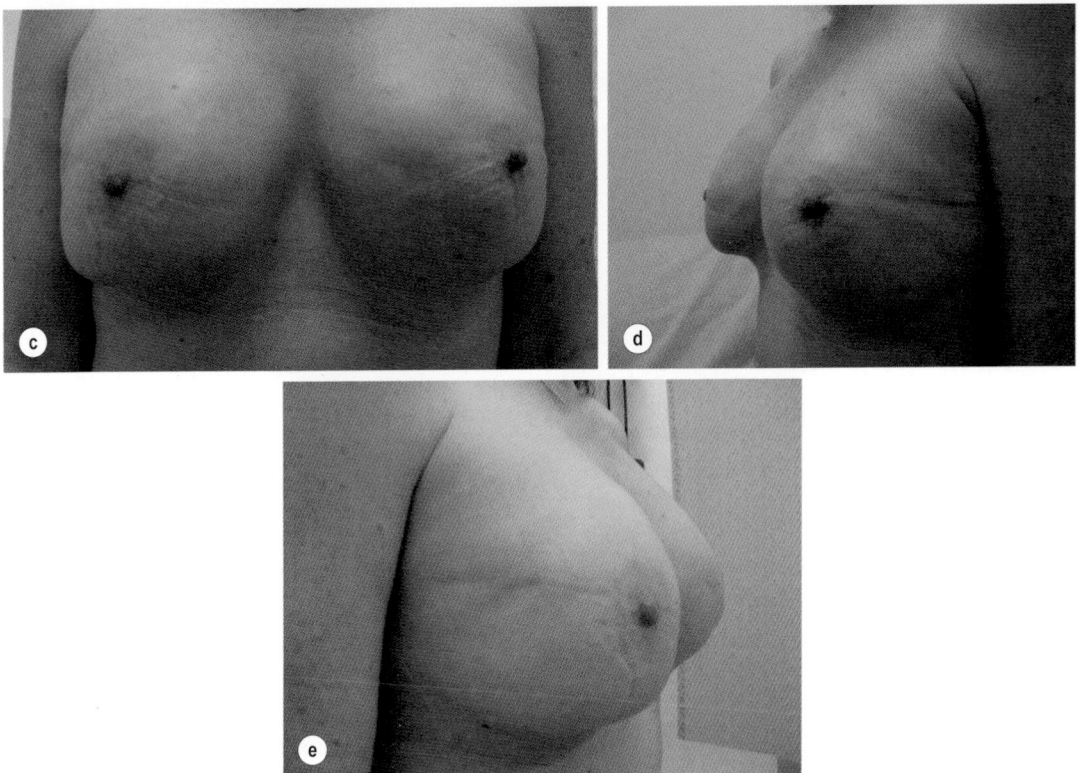

Figure 8.7, cont'd • (c–e) The same patient 15 years after RRM and implant reconstruction.

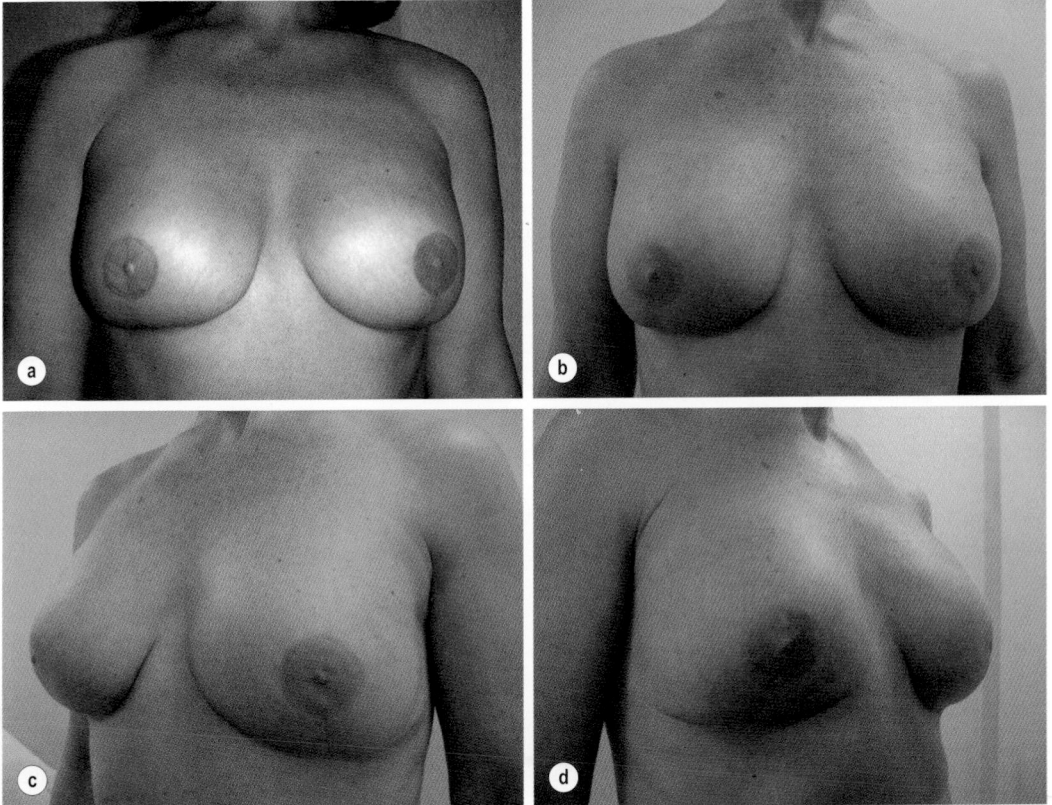

Figure 8.8 • (a) Wise pattern risk-reducing mastectomies with nipple reconstructions. **(b–d)** The same patient 10 years later, with left lateral view **(c)** and right lateral view **(d)**.

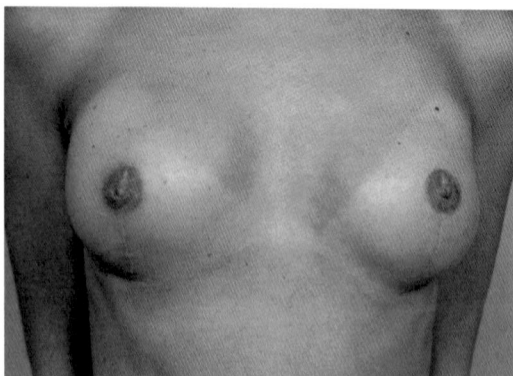

Figure 8.9 • Wise pattern risk-reducing mastectomy after nipple–areola reconstruction.

implant loss, haematoma, wound infection and skin flap necrosis, and the rate has been quoted as greater than 10%. For women who choose to have NSM, the use of expanders or Becker expander/prostheses allows gradual expansion to minimise skin tension and is associated with lower infection and implant loss compared with fixed-volume implants, particularly if the implants are of a volume greater than the original breast size.[74] Use of permanent expander prostheses with detachable valves is associated with low infection rates and good recovery in women who have RRM and reconstruction.[76] Alternative incisions have been proposed when performing RRM with reconstruction for high-risk women and these include the inverted drip incision.[77] Implants can also be combined with a myocutaneous flap and acellular dermal matrix. The overall complication rate using a direct-to-implant immediate breast reconstruction using human acellular dermal matrix (ADM) or ADM from porcine or bovine skin or bovine pericardium has been reported to be low, at 3.9% in some series (implant loss 1.3%, skin necrosis 1.1%, haematoma 1.1%, human acellular dermal matrix exposure 0.6 %, capsular contracture 0.4%, and infection 0.2%).[78] More recent reports using non-human acellular dermal matrices report an implant loss rate closer to 10%. There is a higher rate of seroma, infection and implant loss compared to when ADM is not used, but the aesthetic results are superior with ADM (see Chapter 9). RRM with breast reconstruction is considered a reasonably safe and acceptable procedure for risk reduction until other risk reduction methods become available.

If the NAC is removed during RRM, the NAC can be reconstructed with the areola tattooed. There has also been a description of nipple grafting, in particular if the areola is kept and the nipple is retransplanted to the reconstructed breast.[76]

Follow-up

After risk-reducing surgery, women should have a prolonged follow-up protocol and should be reviewed annually at a multidisciplinary clinic. Long-term aesthetic outcome should be assessed and, if necessary, surgical interventions offered to improve the costmetic outcome. Problems do arise and, when necessary other members of the team should be involved. Clinical examination by palpation of the breasts is considered to be adequate, as remaining breast tissue is very superficial in all types of surgical procedure.

> ✅ The mean expected rate of breast cancer for our cohort of high-risk women is 1% annually, reflecting a lifetime risk that ranges from 25% to 80%. To date, although RRM can reduce the risk of breast cancer, it has not been proven to have a survival benefit. It is unlikely there will be randomised trials and hence more cohort studies will be necessary to provide more data to support its use.

Uptake

Data from Manchester, UK[79] show that 6% of women who are at a 1 in 4 (31/902) lifetime risk or above seek further advice about RRM and 1.8% (16/902) have undergone surgery; this rises to 6% (49/798) in those at 40–45% lifetime risk. Although the uptake in *BRCA1/2* carriers tended to be early, there was a continued increase in uptake so that by 7 years the actuarial uptake for RRM for *BRCA1* carriers was 60% and for *BRCA2* carriers was 43%. Results from the Netherlands show a similarly high uptake (52%).[39] Thus far, 35 mutation carriers in our series and several in the Dutch series that initially opted not to have surgery have developed breast cancer, whereas only two of the operated cases have. Newer research including non-European/American cohorts from Asia have found that RRM is generally considered only in women who already have breast cancer and decide to opt for completion mastectomy and contralateral prophylactic mastectomy, although the uptake of prophylactic salpingo-oopherectomy is slightly higher. There is also a proportion of women who consider risk-reducing surgery after a period of intensive surveillance.[44]

Role of sentinel lymph node biopsy in RRM

It has been suggested that as occult cancers are found in 5% of prophylactic mastectomy specimens, to avoid a second operation sentinel lymph node biopsy (SLNB) should be performed when performing RRM. However, the latest research has found that although occult malignancy can be present in prophylactic mastectomy specimens, it is rare for the occult carcinoma to spread to the lymph nodes. A meta-analysis of available research studies found that the rate of occult invasive cancer was 1.7% and the rate of positive SLNB was 1.9%. Hence, it is concluded that SLNB should not be performed during RRM of women without cancer but may be considered if cancer is present (see chapter 7).[80]

Psychosocial consequences of RRM

✅ The majority of studies exploring the psychological impact of RRM have found that surgery is associated overall with fairly high levels of satisfaction, reduced anxiety and psychological morbidity amongst women who undergo this procedure.[81–88] This is particularly so when there is support from family and friends.[83] A number of studies suggest that provision of presurgical multidisciplinary support appears to have a bearing on outcome, particularly in those who have initial anxiety and negative psychological reactions. These negative effects are usually related to surgical complications and reduce with longer follow-up. A minority of women do express regrets and experience adverse psychosocial events following surgery, including adverse emotional stability, self-esteem and problems in sexual relationships.[87]

Surgery for high-risk women with established breast cancer

For women who are diagnosed with unilateral breast cancer, there is a 2–5% risk of having cancer in the contralateral breast. For BRCA mutation carriers, studies have found that if breast-conserving surgery is performed, the 10-year cumulative incidence of ipsilateral breast cancer recurrences is 27% for mutation carriers versus 4% for sporadic controls. The 10-year cumulative incidence of contralateral breast cancer is 25% in mutation carriers compared with 1% in sporadic controls.[89] Hence, it is most likely that women who are BRCA mutation carriers should consider mastectomy on the diseased breast and also consider contralateral prophylactic mastectomy (CPM). CPM can reduce contralateral cancer development by 90%, but its effectiveness in preventing breast cancer mortality is far from clear. Although most studies have found good psychological outcomes and also satisfaction in women who undergo CPM, the operation is not risk free and complications related to the surgical procedures, including breast reconstruction, do occur. These factors all need to be addressed when considering a decision on CPM. Any contralateral procedure can be delayed until treatment for the primary cancer is completed. The prognosis depends on the primary cancer tumour biology. A woman who is found to have substantial lymph node involvement is unlikely to benefit from CPM. Hence the management decision of this group of women should be decided at a multidisciplinary meeting and the aim must be to prioritise treatment of the primary malignancy.[90]

✅ These women are often young, and if their family history is attributable to a gene mutation, identified or not, their personal risk of local recurrence or development of a second primary cancer in the same breast is higher than in women with sporadic breast cancer; their risk of contralateral new primary malignancy is also high.[81–83]

Individual circumstances vary widely; the decision on how to proceed is individual to each patient. Rates of contralateral mastectomy are high in gene mutation carriers where the efficacy of contralateral mastectomy is now well established. Proof that this may save lives is now emerging.[91–98]

Bilateral risk-reducing salpingo-oophorectomy

Bilateral risk-reducing salpingo-oophorectomy is an option that can be undertaken in women with BRCA1/2 mutations in order to reduce the risk of ovarian cancer.

✅ In addition to reducing the risk of ovarian cancer, prophylactic salpingo-oophorectomy has also been shown to decrease the risk of breast cancer in women with a BRCA1/2 mutation by 46–56%.[99]

This can be seen from the risk of breast cancer in unaffected women and in the contralateral breast for those with breast cancer. Moreover, a recent study has shown that prophylactic salpingo-oophorectomy not only reduced the risk of breast and ovarian cancer but also lowered all-cause mortality, as well as breast cancer and ovarian cancer specific mortality.[57]

If salpingo-oophorectomy is performed at a pre-menopausal age, usually at about 40 years old, particularly in *BRCA1/2* mutation carriers, and if hysterectomy is performed at the same setting, the use of unopposed oestrogen as hormone replacement therapy (HRT) can ameliorate symptoms of surgical menopause and does not seem to increase the risk of breast cancer.[100,101] However, as long-term effects are still not known, the effects of an early menopause and doubts over long-term HRT use have to be considered if the primary purpose is breast cancer prevention.

Bilateral risk-reducing oophorectomy in high-risk women prior to the menopause will therefore decrease the risk of both breast and ovarian cancer.

Use of chemopreventive agents

Selective oestrogen receptor modulators (SERMs)

Four large trials with tamoxifen in high-risk women without breast cancer have been undertaken, and long-term follow-up information is now available. An overview of these trials has shown a 43% reduction in oestrogen receptor (ER)-positive invasive cancer, but no impact on ER-negative disease. Importantly, a reduced incidence has been seen in the period after active treatment was completed, with an additional 38% reduction in years 6–10. As side-effects were minimal in the post-treatment period, the risk–benefit ratio has improved with longer follow-up and an unanswered question is whether there is additional benefit after 10 years of follow-up. The effectiveness and side-effect profile of tamoxifen is now very well understood and it is currently considered the agent of choice for preventive therapy, especially in premeno-pausal high-risk women or those with atypical hyper-plasia or lobular carcinoma in situ (LCIS).

Another SERM, raloxifene, has been evaluated in three randomised trials. In two of these trials breast cancer was not the primary end-point but nevertheless the results showed a marked decrease in breast cancer inci-dence with raloxifene. Early reports suggested a greater benefit than tamoxifen. The most recent direct com-parison with tamoxifen in the STAR trial at 81 months indicated that the risk ratio of raloxifene:tamoxifen was 1.24 for invasive cancer and 1.22 for non-invasive disease. Adverse events were less common with raloxi-fene: relative risk 0.55 for endometrial cancer, 0.19 for endometrial hyperplasia and 0.75 for thromboembolic events. Raloxifene for postmenopausal women thus appears to have advantages compared with tamoxifen.

More recently, lasofoxifene and arzoxifene have been investigated in randomised trials where the pri-mary focus was on fracture prevention in osteoporotic women. Both trials have shown a significant decrease in ER-positive breast cancers with these agents.

None of the SERMs has demonstrated any impact on ER-negative tumours, so that other approaches are needed for this type of breast cancer.

Aromatase inhibitors

A reduction in contralateral breast cancer has been seen in all adjuvant trials comparing an aromatase inhibitor with tamoxifen or placebo, with an over-all reduction of 50% compared to tamoxifen, sug-gesting a potential 75% reduction overall. The use of aromatase inhibitors in the preventive setting is being tested in two randomised clinical trials in high-risk women without breast cancer but of course is limited to the postmenopausal setting – which for most women at high risk is past the age at which they are more likely to make preventive decisions.

> ✔ Tamoxifen reduces breast cancer incidence by 40–50%[93,102–105] and this is maintained in long-term follow-up after cessation of treatment.[105] However, this reduction is almost exclusively a reduction in oestrogen receptor-positive disease and whether this translates into a reduction in cancers related to *BRCA1* mutations remains unclear. The NSABP Study of Tamoxifen and Raloxifene (STAR) Trial has shown that raloxifene is nearly as effective as tamoxifen in reducing invasive breast cancer risk and has fewer adverse side-effects.[106] However, there are no data available on the efficacy of raloxifene for breast cancer risk reduction among *BRCA* gene mutation carriers.

Acknowledgement

Thanks to Dr Louis Kwong, Jr for supplying the original line drawings in this chapter.

Key points

- Gene testing can be useful but may not be possible for many women with a strong family history as no genetic mutation can be identified.
- Between 4% and 5% of breast cancer is due to high-penetrance cancer-susceptibility genes.
- *BRCA1* and *BRCA2* gene mutations result in breast cancer in young women, often bilateral.
- Familial breast cancer can be associated with ovarian and some other malignancies.
- Gail, Claus, Tyrer–Cuzick, BRCAPRO and BOADICEA models predict individual breast cancer risk.
- RRM decreases breast cancer incidence by over 90–95%.
- Common RRM approaches combine breast parenchymal removal with breast reconstruction.
- Breast reconstruction should be appropriate for individual breast morphology.
- RRM can produce profound relief of anxiety, but is major surgery and complications must be avoided wherever possible.
- RRM should be undertaken by multidisciplinary specialised teams working within a protocol.
- Follow-up should ensure that results and outcomes are audited.

References

1. Newman B, Austin MA, Lee M, et al. Inheritance of human breast cancer: evidence for autosomal dominant transmission in high-risk families. Proc Natl Acad Sci U S A 1988;85(9):3044–8.

2. Claus EB, Risch N, Thompson WD. Autosomal dominant inheritance of early-onset breast cancer. Implications for risk prediction. Cancer 1994;73(3):643–51.

3. Miki Y, Swensen J, Shattuck-Eidens D, et al. A strong candidate for the breast and ovarian cancer susceptibility gene BRCA1. Science 1994;266(5182):66–71.

4. Wooster R, Bignell G, Lancaster J, et al. Identification of the breast cancer susceptibility gene BRCA2. Nature 1995;378(6559):789–92.

5. Malkin D, Li FP, Strong LC, et al. Germ line p53 mutations in a familial syndrome of breast cancer, sarcomas, and other neoplasms. Science 1990;250(4985):1233–8.

6. Evans DG, Moran A, Hartley R, et al. Long-term outcomes of breast cancer in women aged 30 years or younger, based on family history, pathology and BRCA1/BRCA2/TP53 status. Br J Cancer 2010;102(7):1091–8.

7. Evans DG, Howell A, Ward D, et al. Prevalence of BRCA1 and BRCA2 mutations in triple negative breast cancer. J Med Genet 2011;48(8):520–2.

8. Ford D, Easton DF, Stratton M, et al. Genetic heterogeneity and penetrance analysis of the BRCA1 and BRCA2 genes in breast cancer families. The Breast Cancer Linkage Consortium. Am J Hum Genet 1998;62(3):676–89.

9. Ford D, Easton DF, Bishop DT, et al. Risks of cancer in BRCA1-mutation carriers. Breast Cancer Linkage Consortium. Lancet 1994; 343(8899):692–5.

10. Evans DG, Shenton A, Woodward E, et al. Penetrance estimates for BRCA1 and BRCA2 based on genetic testing in a Clinical Cancer Genetics service setting: risks of breast/ovarian cancer quoted should reflect the cancer burden in the family. BMC Cancer 2008;8:155.

11. Antoniou A, Pharoah PD, Narod S, et al. Average risks of breast and ovarian cancer associated with BRCA1 or BRCA2 mutations detected in case series unselected for family history: a combined analysis of 22 studies. Am J Hum Genet 2003;72(5):1117–30.

12. Parmigiani G, Berry DA, Aguilar O. Determining carrier probabilities for breast cancer-susceptibility genes BRCA1 and BRCA2. Am J Hum Genet 1998;62(1):145–58.

13. Berry DA, Iversen ES, Gudbjartsson DF, et al. BRCAPRO validation, sensitivity of genetic testing of BRCA1/BRCA2, and prevalence of other breast cancer susceptibility genes. J Clin Oncol 2002;20(11):2701–12.

14. Antoniou AC, Cunningham AP, Peto J, et al. The BOADICEA model of genetic susceptibility to breast and ovarian cancers: updates and extensions. Br J Cancer 2008;98(8):1457–66.

15. Evans DG, Eccles DM, Rahman N, et al. A new scoring system for the chances of identifying a BRCA1/2 mutation outperforms existing models including BRCAPRO. J Med Genet 2004;41(6):474–80.

16. Lakhani SR, Van De Vijver MJ, Jacquemier J, et al. The pathology of familial breast cancer: predictive value of immunohistochemical markers estrogen receptor, progesterone receptor, HER-2, and p53 in patients with mutations in BRCA1 and BRCA2. J Clin Oncol 2002;20(9):2310–8.

17. Mavaddat N, Rebbeck TR, Lakhani SR, et al. Incorporating tumour pathology information into breast cancer risk prediction algorithms. Breast Cancer Res 2010;12(3):R28.

18. Evans DG, Young K, Bulman M, et al. Probability of BRCA1/2 mutation varies with ovarian histology: results from screening 442 ovarian cancer families. Clin Genet 2008;73(4):338–45.

19. Evans DG, Bulman M, Young K, et al. Sensitivity of BRCA1/2 mutation testing in 466 breast/ovarian cancer families. J Med Genet 2003;40(9):e107.

20. Struewing JP, Hartge P, Wacholder S, et al. The risk of cancer associated with specific mutations of BRCA1 and BRCA2 among Ashkenazi Jews. N Engl J Med 1997;336(20):1401–8.

21. Easton DF, Pooley KA, Dunning AM, et al. Genome-wide association study identifies novel breast cancer susceptibility loci. Nature 2007;447(7148):1087–93.

22. Turnbull C, Ahmed S, Morrison J, et al. Genome-wide association study identifies five new breast cancer susceptibility loci. Nat Genet 2010;42(6):504–7.

23. Dupont WD, Page DL. Relative risk of breast cancer varies with time since diagnosis of atypical hyperplasia. Hum Pathol 1989;20(8):723–5.

24. Vasen HF, Haites NE, Evans DG, et al. Current policies for surveillance and management in women at risk of breast and ovarian cancer: a survey among 16 European family cancer clinics. European Familial Breast Cancer Collaborative Group. Eur J Cancer 1998;34(12):1922–6.

25. Evans DG, Lalloo F. Risk assessment and management of high risk familial breast cancer. J Med Genet 2002;39(12):865–71.

26. Gail MH, Brinton LA, Byar DP, et al. Projecting individualized probabilities of developing breast cancer for white females who are being examined annually. J Natl Cancer Inst 1989;81(24):1879–86.

27. Tyrer J, Duffy SW, Cuzick J. A breast cancer prediction model incorporating familial and personal risk factors. Stat Med 2004;23(7):1111–30. This model incorporates the majority of currently known breast cancer risk factors.

28. Kwong A, Wong CH, Suen DT, et al. Accuracy of BRCA1/2 mutation prediction models for different ethnicities and genders: experience in a Southern Chinese cohort. World J Surg 2012;36(4):702–13.

29. Kurian AW, Gong GD, Chun NM, et al. Performance of BRCA1/2 mutation prediction models in Asian Americans. J Clin Oncol 2008;26(29):4752–8.

30. Kurian AW, Gong GD, John EM, et al. Performance of prediction models for BRCA mutation carriage in three racial/ethnic groups: findings from the Northern California Breast Cancer Family Registry. Cancer Epidemiol Biomarkers Prev 2009;18(4):1084–91.

31. Amir E, Evans DG, Shenton A, et al. Evaluation of breast cancer risk assessment packages in the family history evaluation and screening programme. J Med Genet 2003;40(11):807–14.

32. Amir E, Freedman OC, Seruga B, et al. Assessing women at high risk of breast cancer: a review of risk assessment models. J Natl Cancer Inst 2010;102(10):680–91.

33. Goodnight JE, Quagliana JM, Morton DL. Failure of subcutaneous mastectomy to prevent the development of breast cancer. J Surg Oncol 1984;26(3):198–201.

34. Ziegler LD, Kroll SS. Primary breast cancer after prophylactic mastectomy. Am J Clin Oncol 1991;14(5):451–4.

35. Evans D, Lalloo F, Shenton A, et al. Uptake of screening and prevention in women at very high risk of breast cancer. Lancet 2001;358(9285):889–90.

36. Metcalfe KA, Birenbaum-Carmeli D, Lubinski J, et al. International variation in rates of uptake of preventive options in BRCA1 and BRCA2 mutation carriers. Int J Cancer 2008;122(9):2017–22.

37. Schrag D, Kuntz KM, Garber JE, et al. Decision analysis – effects of prophylactic mastectomy and oophorectomy on life expectancy among women with BRCA1 or BRCA2 mutations. N Engl J Med 1997;336(20):1465–71.

38. Hartmann LC, Schaid DJ, Woods JE, et al. Efficacy of bilateral prophylactic mastectomy in women with a family history of breast cancer. N Engl J Med 1999;340(2):77–84. This retrospective US cohort study examined the incidence of, and risk of death from, breast cancer after a median follow-up of 14 years among 639 women who had a family history of breast cancer and who had undergone bilateral subcutaneous or total prophylactic mastectomy. In the mastectomy group, women were divided into high-risk (n=214) or moderate-risk (n=425) subgroups, with most women in each subgroup having undergone subcutaneous mastectomy (89% and 90%, respectively). The study showed a reduction in the risk of breast cancer of 89.5% (P<0.001) in moderate-risk women who had undergone prophylactic mastectomy, and a reduction in risk of 90–94% in the high-risk women.

39. Meijers-Heijboer H, van Geel B, van Putten WLJ, et al. Breast cancer after prophylactic bilateral mastectomy in women with a BRCA1 or BRCA2 mutation. N Engl J Med 2001;345(3):159–64.

40. Evans DG, Baildam AD, Anderson E, et al. Risk reducing mastectomy: outcomes in 10 European centres. J Med Genet 2009;46(4):254–8.

41. Friebel TM, Domchek SM, Neuhausen SL, et al. Bilateral prophylactic oophorectomy and bilateral prophylactic mastectomy in a prospective cohort of unaffected BRCA1 and BRCA2 mutation carriers. Clin Breast Cancer 2007;7(11):875–82.

42. Evans DG, Cuzick J, Howell A. Cancer genetics clinics. Eur J Cancer 1996;32A(3):391–2.

43. Evans DG, Anderson E, Lalloo F, et al. Utilisation of prophylactic mastectomy in 10 European centres. Dis Markers 1999;15(1–3):148–51.

44. Kwong A, Wong CH, Shea C, et al. Choice of management of southern Chinese BRCA mutation carriers. World J Surg 2010;34(7):1416–26.

45. Han SA, Park SK, Ahn SH, et al. The Korean Hereditary Breast Cancer (KOHBRA) study: protocols and interim report. Clin Oncol (R Coll Radiol) 2011;23(7):434–41.

46. Pruthi S, Gostout BS, Lindor NM. Identification and management of women with BRCA mutations or hereditary predisposition for breast and ovarian cancer. Mayo Clin Proc 2010;85(12):1111–20.

47. Julian-Reynier C, Eisinger F, Moatti JP, et al. Physicians' attitudes towards mammography and prophylactic surgery for hereditary breast/ovarian cancer risk and subsequently published guidelines. Eur J Hum Genet 2000;8(3):204–8.

48. Julian-Reynier CM, Bouchard LJ, Evans DG, et al. Women's attitudes toward preventive strategies for hereditary breast or ovarian carcinoma differ from one country to another: differences among English, French, and Canadian women. Cancer 2001;92(4):959–68.

49. Evans DG, Howell A, Baildam A, et al. Re: risk-reduction mastectomy: clinical issues and research needs. J Natl Cancer Inst 2002;94(4):307–8.

50. Meijers-Heijboer H, Brekelmans CT, Menke-Pluymers M, et al. Use of genetic testing and prophylactic mastectomy and oophorectomy in women with breast or ovarian cancer from families with a BRCA1 or BRCA2 mutation. J Clin Oncol 2003;21(9):1675–81.

51. Eccles DM, Evans DG, Mackay J. Guidelines for a genetic risk based approach to advising women with a family history of breast cancer. UK Cancer Family Study Group (UKCFSG). J Med Genet 2000;37(3):203–9.

52. Eeles R. Testing for the breast cancer predisposition gene, BRCA1. Br Med J 1996;313(7057):572–3.

53. Evans DG, Kerr B, Cade D, et al. Fictitious breast cancer family history. Lancet 1996;348(9033):1034.

54. Wasteson E, Sandelin K, Brandberg Y, et al. High satisfaction rate ten years after bilateral prophylactic mastectomy – a longitudinal study. Eur J Cancer Care (Engl) 2011;20(4):508–13.

55. Brandberg Y, Sandelin K, Erikson S, et al. Psychological reactions, quality of life, and body image after bilateral prophylactic mastectomy in women at high risk for breast cancer: a prospective 1-year follow-up study. J Clin Oncol 2008;26(24):3943–9.

56. Roukos DH, Briasoulis E. Individualized preventive and therapeutic management of hereditary breast ovarian cancer syndrome. Nat Clin Pract Oncol 2007;4(10):578–90.

57. Domchek SM, Friebel TM, Singer CF, et al. Association of risk-reducing surgery in BRCA1 or BRCA2 mutation carriers with cancer risk and mortality. JAMA 2010;304(9):967–75.

58. Rebbeck TR, Friebel T, Lynch HT, et al. Bilateral prophylactic mastectomy reduces breast cancer risk in BRCA1 and BRCA2 mutation carriers: the PROSE Study Group. J Clin Oncol 2004;22(6):1055–62.

59. Fatouros M, Baltoyiannis G, Roukos DH. The predominant role of surgery in the prevention and new trends in the surgical treatment of women with BRCA1/2 mutations. Ann Surg Oncol 2008;15(1):21–33.

60. Klaren HM, van't Veer LJ, van Leeuwen FE, et al. Potential for bias in studies on efficacy of prophylactic surgery for BRCA1 and BRCA2 mutation. J Natl Cancer Inst 2003;95(13):941–7.

61. Tercyak KP, Peshkin BN, Brogan BM, et al. Quality of life after contralateral prophylactic mastectomy in newly diagnosed high-risk breast cancer patients who underwent BRCA1/2 gene testing. J Clin Oncol 2007;25(3):285–91.

62. Guillem JG, Wood WC, Moley JF, et al. ASCO/SSO review of current role of risk-reducing surgery in common hereditary cancer syndromes. J Clin Oncol 2006;24(28):4642–60.

63. Carlson GW, Bostwick J, Styblo TM, et al. Skin-sparing mastectomy. Oncologic and reconstructive considerations. Ann Surg 1997;225(5):570–8.

64. Newman B, Mu H, Butler LM, et al. Frequency of breast cancer attributable to BRCA1 in a population-based series of American women. JAMA 1998;279(12):915–21.

65. Didier F, Radice D, Gandini S, et al. Does nipple preservation in mastectomy improve satisfaction with cosmetic results, psychological adjustment, body image and sexuality? Breast Cancer Res Treat 2009;118(3):623–33.

66. Laronga C, Kemp B, Johnston D, et al. The incidence of occult nipple–areola complex involvement in breast cancer patients receiving a skin-sparing mastectomy. Ann Surg Oncol 1999;6(6):609–13.

67. Lakhani SR, Reis-Filho JS, Fulford L, et al. Prediction of BRCA1 status in patients with breast cancer using estrogen receptor and basal phenotype. Clin Cancer Res 2005;11(14):5175–80.

68. Wertheim U, Ozzello L. Neoplastic involvement of nipple and skin flap in carcinoma of the breast. Am J Surg Pathol 1980;4(6):543–9.

69. Petit JY, Veronesi U, Orecchia R, et al. Nipple sparing mastectomy with nipple areola intraoperative radiotherapy: one thousand and one cases of a five years experience at the European institute of oncology of Milan (EIO). Breast Cancer Res Treat 2009;117(2):333–8.

70. Sacchini V, Pinotti JA, Barros AC, et al. Nipple-sparing mastectomy for breast cancer and risk reduction: oncologic or technical problem? J Am Coll Surg 2006;203(5):704–14.

71. Maxwell GP, Storm-Dickerson T, Whitworth P, et al. Advances in nipple-sparing mastectomy: oncological safety and incision selection. Aesthet Surg J 2011;31(3):310–9.

72. Gerber B, Krause A, Dieterich M, et al. The on-cological safety of skin sparing mastectomy with conservation of the nipple–areola complex and autologous reconstruction: an extended follow-up study. Ann Surg 2009;249(3):461–8.

73. Crowe JP, Patrick RJ, Yetman RJ, et al. Nipple-sparing mastectomy update: one hundred forty-nine procedures and clinical outcomes. Arch Surg 2008;143(11):1106–10.

74. Wijayanayagam A, Kumar AS, Foster RD, et al. Optimizing the total skin-sparing mastectomy. Arch Surg 2008;143(1):38–45.

75. May JW, Attwood J, Bartlett S. Staged use of soft-tissue expansion and lower thoracic advancement flap in breast reconstruction. Plast Reconstr Surg 1987;79(2):272–7.

76. Wickman M, Sandelin K, Arver B. Technical aspects and outcome after prophylactic mastectomy and immediate breast reconstruction in 30 con-secutive high-risk patients. Plast Reconstr Surg 2003;111(3):1069–77.

77. Van Geel AN, Contant CM, Wai RT, et al. Mastectomy by inverted drip incision and immediate reconstruction: data from 510 cases. Ann Surg Oncol 2003;10(4):389–95.

78. Salzberg CA, Ashikari AY, Koch RM, et al. An 8-year experience of direct-to-implant immediate breast reconstruction using human acellular der-mal matrix (AlloDerm). Plast Reconstr Surg 2011;127(2):514–24.

79. Evans DG, Lalloo F, Ashcroft L, et al. Uptake of risk-reducing surgery in unaffected women at high risk of breast and ovarian cancer is risk, age, and time dependent. Cancer Epidemiol Biomarkers Prev 2009;18(8):2318–24.

80. Zhou WB, Liu XA, Dai JC, et al. Meta-analysis of sentinel lymph node biopsy at the time of pro-phylactic mastectomy of the breast. Can J Surg 2011;54(5):300–6.

81. Hatcher MB, Fallowfield L, A'Hern R. The psycho-social impact of bilateral prophylactic mastectomy: prospective study using questionnaires and semi-structured interviews. Br Med J 2001;322(7278):76.

82. Hopwood P, Lee A, Shenton A, et al. Clinical follow-up after bilateral risk reducing ('prophylac-tic') mastectomy: mental health and body image outcomes. Psychooncology 2000;9(6):462–72.

83. Stefanek ME, Helzlsouer KJ, Wilcox PM, et al. Predictors of and satisfaction with bilateral prophy-lactic mastectomy. Prev Med 1995;24(4):412–9.

84. Borgen PI, Hill AD, Tran KN, et al. Patient regrets after bilateral prophylactic mastectomy. Ann Surg Oncol 1998;5(7):603–6.

85. Lloyd SM, Watson M, Oaker G, et al. Understanding the experience of prophylactic bilat-eral mastectomy: a qualitative study of ten women. Psychooncology 2000;9(6):473–85.

86. Josephson U, Wickman M, Sandelin K. Initial experiences of women from hereditary breast cancer families after bilateral prophylactic mas-tectomy: a retrospective study. Eur J Surg Oncol 2000;26(4):351–6.

87. Frost MH, Schaid DJ, Sellers TA, et al. Long-term satisfaction and psychological and social function following bilateral prophylactic mastectomy. JAMA 2000;284(3):319–24.

88. Bresser PJ, Seynaeve C, Van Gool AR, et al. Satisfaction with prophylactic mastec-tomy and breast reconstruction in geneti-cally predisposed women. Plast Reconstr Surg 2006;117(6):1675–82.

89. Garcia-Etienne CA, Barile M, Gentilini OD, et al. Breast-conserving surgery in BRCA1/2 mutation carriers: are we approaching an answer? Ann Surg Oncol 2009;16(12):3380–7.

90. Tuttle T, Habermann E, Abraham A, et al. Contralateral prophylactic mastectomy for pa-tients with unilateral breast cancer. Expert Rev Anticancer Ther 2007;7(8):1117–22.

91. Eccles D, Simmonds P, Goddard J, et al. Familial breast cancer: an investigation into the outcome of treatment for early stage disease. Fam Cancer 2001;1(2):65–72.

92. Metcalfe K, Lynch HT, Ghadirian P, et al. Contralateral breast cancer in BRCA1 and BRCA2 mutation carri-ers. J Clin Oncol 2004;22(12):2328–35.

93. Narod SA, Brunet JS, Ghadirian P, et al. Tamoxifen and risk of contralateral breast cancer in BRCA1 and BRCA2 mutation carriers: a case–control study. Hereditary Breast Cancer Clinical Study Group. Lancet 2000;356(9245):1876–81.

94. Heemskerk-Gerritsen BA, Brekelmans CT, Menke-Pluymers MB, et al. Prophylactic mastectomy in BRCA1/2 mutation carriers and women at risk of hereditary breast cancer: long-term experiences at the Rotterdam Family Cancer Clinic. Ann Surg Oncol 2007;14(12):3335–44.

95. McDonnell SK, Schaid DJ, Myers JL, et al. Efficacy of contralateral prophylactic mastectomy in women with a personal and family history of breast cancer. J Clin Oncol 2001;19(19):3938–43.

96. Herrinton LJ, Barlow WE, Yu O, et al. Efficacy of prophylactic mastectomy in women with unilateral breast cancer: a cancer research network project. J Clin Oncol 2005;23(19):4275–86.

97. Bedrosian I, Hu CY, Chang GJ. Population-based study of contralateral prophylactic mastectomy and survival outcomes of breast cancer patients. J Natl Cancer Inst 2010;102(6):401–9.

98. Boughey JC, Hoskin TL, Degnim AC, et al. Contralateral prophylactic mastectomy is associ-ated with a survival advantage in high-risk women with a personal history of breast cancer. Ann Surg Oncol 2010;17(10):2702–9.

99. Rebbeck TR, Lynch HT, Neuhausen SL, et al. Prophylactic oophorectomy in carriers of BRCA1 or BRCA2 mutations. N Engl J Med 2002;346(21):1616–22.

100. Rebbeck TR, Friebel T, Wagner T, et al. Effect of short-term hormone replacement therapy on breast cancer risk reduction after bilateral prophylactic oophorectomy in BRCA1 and BRCA2 mutation carriers: the PROSE Study Group. J Clin Oncol 2005;23(31):7804–10.

101. Armstrong K, Schwartz JS, Randall T, et al. Hormone replacement therapy and life expectancy after prophylactic oophorectomy in women with BRCA1/2 mutations: a decision analysis. J Clin Oncol 2004;22(6):1045–54.

102. Beral V, Million Women Study Collaborators. Breast cancer and hormone-replacement therapy in the Million Women Study. Lancet 2003;362(9382): 419–27.

103. Fisher B, Costantino JP, Wickerham DL, et al. Tamoxifen for prevention of breast cancer: report of the National Surgical Adjuvant Breast and Bowel Project P-1 Study. J Natl Cancer Inst 1998;90(18):1371–88.

104. Cuzick J, Forbes J, Edwards R, et al. First results from the International Breast Cancer Intervention Study (IBIS-I): a randomised prevention trial. Lancet 2002;360(9336):817–24.

105. Cuzick J, Forbes JF, Sestak I, et al. Long-term results of tamoxifen prophylaxis for breast cancer – 96-month follow-up of the randomized IBIS-I trial. J Natl Cancer Inst 2007;99(4):272–82.

106. Vogel VG. The NSABP Study of Tamoxifen and Raloxifene (STAR) trial. Expert Rev Anticancer Ther 2009;9(1):51–60.

9

Breast reconstruction

Mark Schaverien
Cameron Raine

Introduction

Surgery for breast cancer is not finished until the reconstruction has been completed in those patients who choose to have it. Mastectomy for breast cancer can lead to negative psychological effects on the patient and breast reconstruction, whether immediate or delayed, can provide significant psychosocial benefits.[1–4] Even the most sophisticated breast reconstruction, however, will never fully replicate the breast that has been lost in terms of feel, movement, and erogenous sensation, although some spontaneous sensory recovery may occur.[5]

Women must be fully informed of all available options for breast reconstruction at the time of planning initial surgical treatment so that they can make informed decisions, even if it is their personal preference to have a delayed reconstruction or no reconstruction at all.[6,7] The ultimate goal of breast reconstruction is to produce a 'breast' that satisfies the patient's wishes and matches the contralateral breast, also improving the preoperative breast aesthetics if possible. Breast reconstruction may be either autologous, non-autologous, or a combination of the two, with the use of symmetrising mastopexy, reduction or augmentation surgery if necessary.[8] The decision regarding the timing and technique of breast reconstruction should be made by the patient and a multidisciplinary breast cancer team, which should include reconstructive surgeons who are able to provide the full range of commonly used reconstructive procedures.

Timing

The principal aim of breast cancer surgery is to provide safe and successful oncological treatment. The decision for delayed or immediate breast reconstruction and the reconstruction offered may be affected by the anticipated need for adjuvant therapy.[8]

Immediate breast reconstruction

The main advantage of immediate breast reconstruction is that the patient does not have to spend any time without a breast mound. It allows preservation of the native breast skin envelope and inframammary fold and therefore the reconstruction usually assumes a more natural shape when the breast volume is restored. The mastectomy skin flaps are pliable and unaffected by soft-tissue contracture and scar, and have not suffered the effects of radiotherapy. Skin-sparing and subcutaneous mastectomy techniques can lead to better cosmetic results, with a reduced need for contralateral symmetrisation surgery.[8–10]

The disadvantages of immediate reconstruction are the limited time for decision-making by the patient due to the need to perform the oncological surgery, increased operating time, and the difficulties of coordinating two surgical teams where different surgeons are required to perform the mastectomy and desired reconstruction. Immediate breast reconstruction does not compromise adjuvant treatment, although there is a potential in individual patients for complications to result in a delay in starting adjuvant treatment.[8,11,12]

The current indications for post-mastectomy radiotherapy lead many patients to receive radiotherapy as part of their breast reconstruction algorithm. The possibility of radiotherapy should be anticipated before proceeding with immediate breast reconstruction. Radiotherapy can have detrimental effects on breast reconstructions, but these can be reduced by choosing autologous reconstruction over implant-based procedures. With current radiotherapy delivery regimens good cosmetic outcomes can be expected in the majority of cases.[13,14] Delayed-immediate reconstruction is also an option in these circumstances. Whether the use of acellular dermal matrix confers any protective effect for implant reconstruction requiring radiotherapy is unclear at present.[15]

It is now well established that immediate breast reconstruction does not adversely affect breast cancer outcome.[13,16–18] Breast reconstruction may be indicated even in advanced disease to control locoregional disease and improve quality of remaining life.[8,19,20] There is also evidence to suggest that survival may be improved by removal of the primary tumour.[21]

Where the viability of parts of the mastectomy skin flap is uncertain, it may be necessary to delay implant reconstruction to avoid risk of exposure of the prosthesis. In the case of autologous reconstruction it may be prudent not to de-epithelialise the part of the flap skin paddle under the questionable part of the mastectomy skin flap until any area of necrosis has declared itself over the subsequent few days.

Delayed breast reconstruction

Delayed breast reconstruction allows the patient time for decision-making, psychological adjustment following their breast cancer diagnosis and mastectomy, and allows the full pathology to be available prior to reconstructive surgery. It avoids any potential delay of adjuvant treatment and also avoids any detrimental effects of adjuvant therapy on the reconstruction. In addition, the mastectomy skin flaps can be allowed to heal if necessary and any skin damaged by radiotherapy can be excised. The

Box 9.1 • Advantages and disadvantages of immediate and delayed breast reconstruction

Advantages of immediate breast reconstruction
- Potential for a single operation and one period of hospitalisation
- Maximum preservation of breast skin
- Preservation of the inframammary fold
- Good-quality skin flaps
- Better cosmetic results for skin-sparing mastectomy
- Reduced need for balancing surgery to the contralateral breast
- Lower costs than delayed reconstruction

Disadvantages of immediate reconstruction
- Limited time for decision-making by patient
- Increased single operating time
- Difficulties of coordinating two surgical teams when required
- Potential in individual patients for complications to result in delay of adjuvant treatment

Advantages of delayed breast reconstruction
- Allows unlimited time for decision-making by the patient
- Avoids any potential delay of adjuvant treatment
- Avoids detrimental effects of radiotherapy or chemotherapy on the reconstruction

Disadvantages of delayed breast reconstruction
- Requires replacement of a larger amount of breast skin
- Mastectomy flaps may be thin, scarred, contracted or irradiated
- Mastectomy scar may be poorly positioned
- May result in a less aesthetically pleasing outcome
- Requires separate episode of hospitalisation
- Increased treatment cost compared with immediate breast reconstruction

main disadvantage is that skin-sparing mastectomy techniques cannot be used due to the poor aesthetic outcomes of a contracted skin envelope, and therefore a much larger skin paddle is required. In addition, a second operation and episode of hospitalisation is required and treatment costs are increased compared with immediate reconstruction (see Box 9.1).[22]

Delayed-immediate breast reconstruction

Delayed-immediate breast reconstruction provides some of the benefits of both immediate and delayed breast reconstruction. A skin-sparing mastectomy and immediate reconstruction with a tissue expander is performed. Once the final pathology is available, patients who do not require adjuvant radiotherapy proceed to immediate breast reconstruction. Those who require radiotherapy have their expander fully deflated prior to radiotherapy to allow optimal delivery of the radiotherapy, following which the expander is serially re-expanded within a few weeks of completion of radiotherapy to prevent contraction of the skin envelope whilst awaiting delayed reconstruction.[23]

Contraindications

Contraindications to breast reconstruction include serious comorbidities, unresectable local chest wall disease, or rapidly progressive uncontrollable metastatic disease.

Techniques

Breast reconstruction involves the replacement of breast volume and may involve the replacement of breast skin and nipple–areola complex. Surgical options for reconstruction include the use of breast implants, tissue expanders or expander implants, and the use of autologous tissue with or without an implant. The most commonly used surgical techniques are tissue expansion, latissimus dorsi musculocutaneous flap with or without implant, or the use of a free lower abdominal tissue flap.

Implant-based techniques have the shortest operating time, inpatient stay and fastest recovery, but these initial advantages are offset by the finite lifespan of the prosthesis, requiring exchange in the future, and the deterioration of aesthetic appearance with time. The reconstructed breast will not behave similarly to a normal breast and the larger or more ptotic the contralateral breast is, the harder it will be to obtain symmetry unless the contralateral breast is augmented. This option may suit women who are simply seeking symmetry in a bra and do not wish to use an external prosthesis.

The aesthetics of autologous reconstruction do not deteriorate with time as with implant-based reconstruction, and are considered to be superior in terms of more natural appearance, feel and durability.[24] Autologous tissue can also better withstand radiotherapy.[25,26]

> ✔ The timing and type of reconstruction need to be individualised to the need for adjuvant treatment, risk factors for surgery, breast size, body habitus, skin quality and thickness, availability and quality of flap donor sites, the patient's general health and smoking habits, and the contralateral breast. Patients must be fully informed on the reconstructive options available so that they can make high-quality decisions regarding their care, and the reconstructive surgical team must be able to provide the full range of commonly used reconstructive options.[8,27]

Non-autologous reconstruction

Breast reconstruction by tissue expansion involves the serial expansion of chest-wall tissue to replace permanently the skin lost following mastectomy by repeated injections of saline into an inflatable silicone expander placed behind the pectoralis major muscle[28] (**Fig. 9.1**). This may either be followed by replacement with a definitive implant once expansion is complete, or in the case of a permanent expandable breast implant that consists of a silicone outer lumen and an expandable saline inner lumen, only the filling port may need removal if it is not integrated into the device.

The outcomes of the technique are dependent on careful patient and implant selection. The technique appears simple and is generally good for restoring volume (**Fig. 9.2**), but it is difficult to create ptosis, and therefore good symmetry with the unaffected breast and true symmetry with implant-based reconstruction is best achieved by bilateral procedures (**Fig. 9.3**).

Indications

This technique is most suitable for patients with small non-ptotic breasts, when performing bilateral reconstruction, or for women who are happy to accept a mastopexy or augmentation procedure on the opposite breast. It is ideal for patients who want minimal scarring and are unwilling or unfit to undergo autologous tissue reconstruction.[8,27]

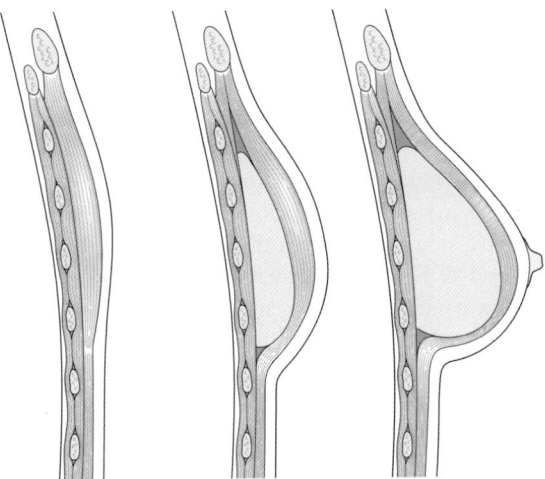

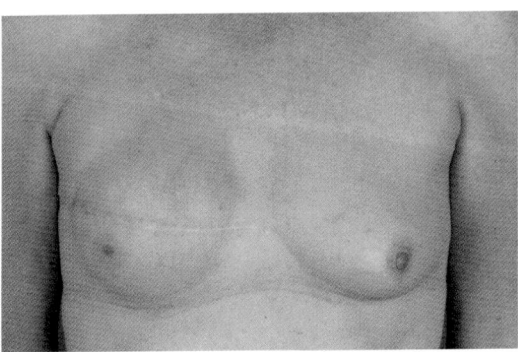

Figure 9.2 • Delayed breast reconstruction by tissue expansion. Courtesy of Eva M. Weiler-Mithoff.

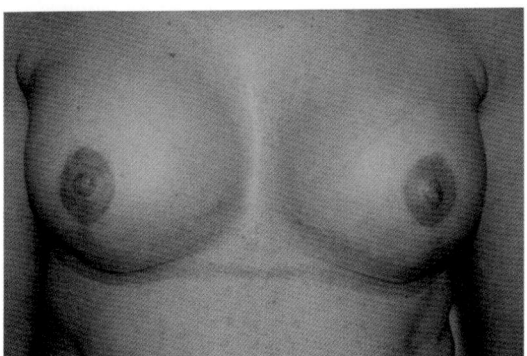

Figure 9.3 • Bilateral mastectomy with breast reconstruction with implants and nipple reconstructions.

Contraindications

Patients are unsuitable for implant reconstruction if the chest-wall tissues are very thin, if the mastectomy skins flaps are of uncertain viability, or if the pectoralis major muscle is absent, either congenitally or following radical mastectomy. Radiotherapy significantly increases the risk of complications and diminishes the aesthetic result of implant/expander breast reconstruction.[25,26] This may therefore not be the best method of reconstruction if adjuvant radiotherapy is planned or has already been given.

Surgical techniques

The inframammary fold is an important landmark for implant reconstruction that can be preserved safely during mastectomy and should be restored with sutures if it has been violated. Careful choice of the expander is important, and the size should take into account the base width, height and projection of the normal, intact breast.[29]

Tissue expanders are placed under the pectoralis major muscle and the inferolateral portion may be covered by serratus fascia, allo- or xenograft, or the serratus anterior and external oblique muscles in a submuscular plane to reduce palpability. There is growing popularity for using acellular dermal matrix, most commonly human (AlloDerm®) or porcine (Strattice®) skin derived, as well as bovine skin and pericardium, to cover the inferolateral portion of the implant (**Fig. 9.4**). This potentially allows a one-stage immediate implant reconstruction or shortens the time taken for expansion. This technique expands the indications for immediate implant-based reconstruction in women with large ptotic breasts; however, these advantages need to be offset against the costs of the product. In the setting of one- versus two-stage reconstruction, though, the initial increased costs may be offset overall. Acellular dermal matrices (ADM) do allow much better inframammary fold definition. They are not without complications. There is a higher rate of seroma, infection and reconstruction failure with the use of ADMs. The key is to try and place the mastectomy incision over muscle and not over the matrix when inserted and to ensure primary wound healing by refreshing the mastectomy wound. This is achieved by excising the traumatised skin edges at the end of the operation. A good alternative in immediate reconstruction of large ptotic breasts is to perform a skin-reducing mastectomy and use the deepithelialised lower skin flap sutured to the caudal edge of the pectoralis major muscle to cover the inferolateral portion of the prosthesis as a vascularised dermal flap, although a contralateral reduction procedure is usually necessary.

Tissue expansion can be used for immediate or delayed breast reconstruction (**Fig. 9.5**). The expander is only partially inflated at insertion to allow closure of overlying mastectomy skin flaps without tension. The actual expansion starts 2–4 weeks

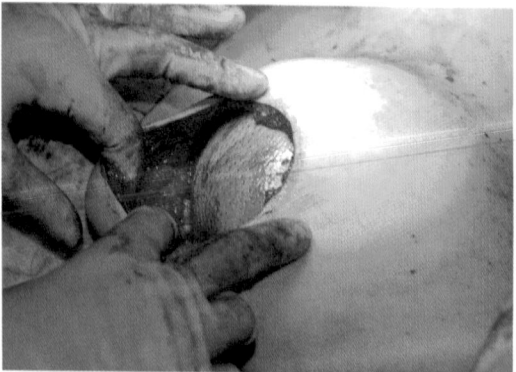

Figure 9.4 • One-stage reconstruction after mastectomy with Strattice sling visible covering lower half of implant.

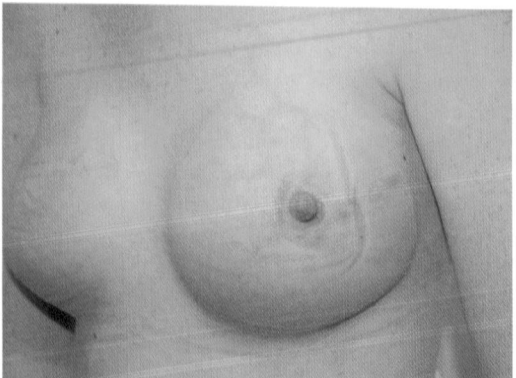

Figure 9.5 • Right delayed reconstruction with implant and Strattice. Left prophylactic mastectomy with immediate reconstruction with implant and Strattice.

postoperatively following an interval for healing and is usually performed at weekly intervals. The volume of expansion at each occasion should be guided by patient comfort. Overexpansion was a technique that was used to create a degree of ptosis to produce a more natural-looking breast, but this is unnecessary when anatomical devices are used. Once expansion is completed, the expander is left in place for 1–3 months to allow the skin envelope to maintain its stretch permanently. The expander is then removed, a capsulectomy or capsulotomy is performed, and a definitive implant is inserted based on the width and height of the pocket and the desired projection. Reconstruction of the breast mound can therefore take up to 6 months using tissue expansion. A slightly larger definitive prosthesis is often used following expansion with an anatomical device to reduce the risk of rotation, which can be problematic. Revisional procedures are often required to optimise the aesthetic appearance of the reconstructed breast, and over one-third of patients require further surgery within the first 5 years after implant-based breast reconstruction.[30] In addition mastopexy, reduction or augmentation of the contralateral breast and lipofilling are often required to improve symmetry. The long-term aesthetic results of implant-based reconstruction can be expected to decline with time, independent of the implant type or volume, due to gradual ptosis of the contralateral side and failure of the implanted side to undergo normal ptosis, leading to late asymmetry.[31] This procedure requires approximately 1 hour of operating time, a short period of hospitalisation and 2–4 weeks of recovery time.

Complications

Early complications include haematoma, infection, mastectomy skin flap necrosis and wound dehiscence, and late complications include implant rupture/deflation, capsular contracture, implant malposition/rotation, implant rippling, extrusion and asymmetry. Even with the latest prosthetic materials and modern radiation delivery techniques, the complication rate for implant-based breast reconstruction in patients undergoing post-mastectomy radiation therapy may be as high as 40%, and the extrusion rate is 15%.[32] The commonest and least predictable complication of implant reconstruction is capsular contracture, which may lead to firmness and visible distortion of the breast, as well as pain in advanced cases, and may warrant surgical revision. The risk of capsular contracture is significantly increased following radiotherapy.[33] There is some evidence that textured implants may reduce the risk of capsular contracture.[34] Lipofilling appears to improve capsular contracture and can help improve cosmetic outcomes. It is particularly valuable for implant rippling and achieving a greater degree of symmetry.

✅✅ Implant-based breast reconstruction is a suitable option for those unwilling or unfit to undergo autologous reconstruction. Patients do, however, need to be counselled that the results tend to deteriorate with time due to gradual ptosis of the contralateral side and failure of the implant side to undergo normal ptosis, leading to late asymmetry despite contralateral symmetrising surgery[31] **(Fig. 9.6)**. In addition an implant has a finite lifespan and may need replacement due to implant leakage or rupture or due to capsular contracture.

Autologous breast reconstruction

Background

Autologous breast reconstruction allows creation of a breast whose texture and appearance match more closely that which has been lost compared with an implant-based reconstruction. In addition, the aesthetic

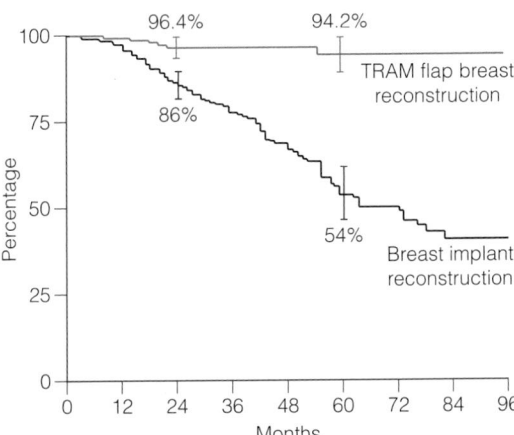

Figure 9.6 • The actuarial percentage cosmetic outcome for acceptable results for breast implant reconstruction (lower line) and TRAM flap breast reconstruction with estimates at 2 and 5 years. Adapted from Clough KB, O'Donoghue JM, Fitoussi AD et al. Prospective evaluation of late cosmetic results following breast reconstruction: implant reconstruction. Plast Reconstr Surg 2001; 107:1702–9, and Clough BC, O'Donoghue JM, Fitoussi AD et al. Prospective evaluation of late cosmetic results following breast reconstruction. II. TRAM flap reconstruction. Plast Reconstr Surg 2001; 107:1710–6.

result of autologous breast reconstruction tends to improve with time. While the latissimus dorsi (LD) and transverse rectus abdominis musculocutaneous (TRAM) flaps remain popular options for breast reconstruction, there is increasing popularity of the deep inferior epigastric artery (DIEP) flap due to its reduced abdominal donor-site morbidity.

Autologous reconstruction is indicated for immediate breast reconstruction when adjuvant radiotherapy is planned, in delayed breast reconstruction following adjuvant radiotherapy, in patients with large ptotic breasts, and in patients where previous implant reconstruction has failed. Abdominal flap reconstruction is ideal for those patients in whom an aesthetic abdominoplasty may be seen as an advantage.

Latissimus dorsi (LD) flap reconstruction

The LD flap may be used either as a muscle or musculocutaneous flap. With its excellent blood supply to the overlying skin it affords a variety of skin paddle designs that can be hidden within the bra strap lines **(Fig. 9.7)**. It is usually combined with an implant and reduces clinically evident capsular contracture and rippling of the prosthesis **(Fig. 9.8)**. The extended LD flap includes the subcutaneous fat overlying the muscle deep to the superficial fascia to increase volume and reduce the chance of needing an implant **(Fig. 9.9)**. Where volume is still deficient with this method, later lipofilling can be used to provide the necessary volume without the need for an implant.

The pedicled LD flap has the lowest flap failure rate of the autologous reconstructions available and may be indicated in patients who are higher risk for autologous reconstruction. The best indication is in cases where the abdomen is unsuitable as a donor site either due to insufficient tissue volume or the presence of multiple scars, or where the deep inferior epigastric pedicle has been previously ligated. Disadvantages include a scar on the back, possible shoulder stiffness and impairment of upper limb function. The functional deficit of the upper limb has been investigated in multiple studies, and although its absence is well compensated for by the teres major muscle, it is necessary to counsel patients who have high demands of their upper limb, in particular for activities involving shoulder extension and adduction such as climbing and swimming, that this option may result in some functional deficit. Additional physiotherapy may also be required to restore full shoulder mobility.[35]

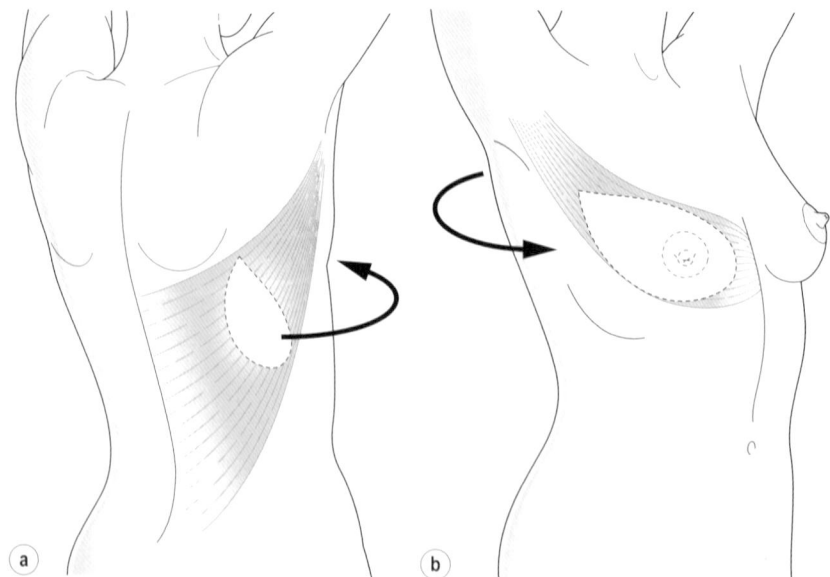

Figure 9.7 • Breast reconstruction using latissimus dorsi myocutaneous flap.

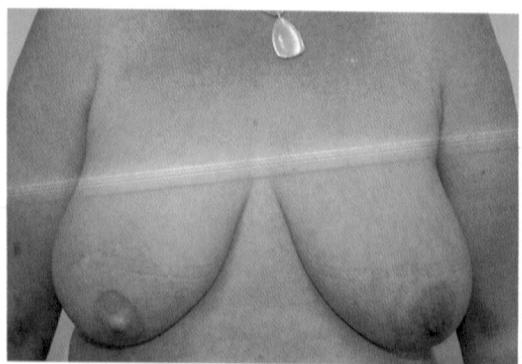

Figure 9.8 • Immediate right breast reconstruction with extended LD flap, a very small implant and nipple reconstruction.

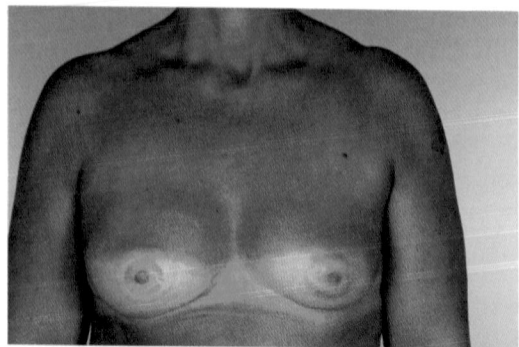

Figure 9.9 • Immediate right breast reconstruction by autologous latissimus dorsi flap after skin-sparing mastectomy. Courtesy of Eva M. Weiler-Mithoff.

The tissue from the back is thicker than that of the native chest skin and the colour match may be different, and this needs to be taken into consideration. The procedure generally requires 3–4 hours operating time, with an extended LD usually taking longer than an LD and implant, a hospital stay of 5–7 days and a recovery time of 4–8 weeks.

Indications

Indications for this technique include the reconstruction of large ptotic breasts, if the chest wall tissues are unsuitable for tissue expansion, or if additional skin needs to be imported following mastectomy. Additional indications include chest-wall reconstruction in locally advanced breast cancer, partial breast reconstruction after breast conservation surgery, or for salvage following loss of an abdominal tissue flap.

Contraindications

The LD flap is contraindicated where it is suspected that previous surgery has damaged the flap pedicle, such as a thoracotomy or extensive and radical axillary surgery, congenital absence of the LD muscle, and significant patient comorbidity. Immediate LD breast reconstruction, even in the setting of postoperative radiotherapy, yields satisfactory results.[36]

Flap options

The LD flap is most commonly used as a musculocutaneous flap with either an oblique or horizontally orientated skin paddle. A muscle-only flap can be used where no additional skin is required, and where only skin is required, a muscle-sparing or thoracodorsal artery perforator flap may be used.[37-40]

Preoperative planning

It is necessary to confirm the presence of the LD muscle prior to surgery by asking patients to push down onto their hips and palpate the anterior axillary fold for muscle contraction. This is also particularly important following previous axillary surgery to indicate that the pedicle is likely to be intact, as the nerve lies in close proximity. Next it is important to decide how much skin needs to be replaced and to test the amount of skin that can be taken from the back whilst allowing closure of the donor site, taking into account skin-fold thickness. This is usually between 6 and 9 cm in width, with a lesser amount of skin taken in high risk patients such as smokers to reduce the risk of wound breakdown, and approximately 20 to 25 cm in length. In our experience using the extended LD flap, the total volume in a lean back can be expected to be approximately 200 cc, an average back 400–700 cc, and a variable amount more can be harvested in larger backs.

Surgical technique

The patient is positioned in the lateral decubitus position and secured with well-padded table attachments with the arm supported with attachments at 90°. Infiltration of the incision lines is performed using local anaesthetic with adrenaline to reduce postoperative pain, induce haemostasis and facilitate location of Scarpa's fascia through tissue tumescence where an extended LD flap is planned. The plane of dissection in an extended flap is immediately deep to Scarpa's fascia to preserve the blood supply to the back skin and it can be difficult to locate in some patients. In this situation it is easiest to start with the caudal flap, where it is usually better defined. Additional areas of subcutaneous fat harvest including the parascapular area, fat anterior to the anterior border of the muscle and supra-iliac fat deposits are included in the extended flap.

The anterior border of the LD muscle is usually identified first. The muscle can then be raised from cephalad, posterior and inferior. Dissection then proceeds under the anterior border with care to avoid inadvertently including slips of serratus anterior muscle with the flap and the thoracodorsal neurovascular pedicle and the serratus branch, which can allow retrograde flap perfusion if the thoracodorsal pedicle has been

previously damaged, are identified and preserved. The posterior part of the tendon insertion into the intertubercular groove of the humerus may be divided to allow additional mobility to the flap if required. A high axillary tunnel is fashioned to allow transposition of the flap whilst avoiding the risk of lateralisation of the flap into the axilla. Flap haemostasis is checked prior to transfer anteriorly, and the flap is transferred to the mastectomy wound, with care not to twist the pedicle. It is also important to check that there is adequate room for the pedicle without risk of compression prior to transfer – four finger breadths is usually adequate. On occasions where additional reach is required, the humeral insertion can be divided fully or the serratus branch ligated. Some surgeons divide the thoracodorsal nerve routinely at the level of the pedicle by excising a segment to avoid postoperative muscle twitching and flap animation and although it was thought that denervation may decrease the flap bulk over time due to atrophy. Recent studies have shown no volume loss over time. Muscle twitching also tends to decrease with time in those where the nerve is preserved and is rarely a problem. The donor site may be quilted to reduce the tension on the closure and reduce the risk of seroma, drains are inserted, and the wound is then closed in three layers. The patient may then be repositioned in a supine position for flap inset. The flap is then sutured and shaped to create a breast mound, drains are inserted and the skin is closed in layers. The flap should be sutured to the base of the mastectomy flaps rather than the chest wall.

The patient is encouraged to wear a well-supporting brassiere for 6 weeks postoperatively. Physiotherapy may be instituted to help with shoulder rehabilitation.

Complications

Early postoperative complications include haematoma, infection, breast skin necrosis, partial or complete flap failure, or wound breakdown. Late complications include seroma, implant rupture and capsular contracture. Seroma formation may be reduced by quilting sutures at the donor site, and once established may be reduced by the use of intracavity steroid injections.[41,42]

✔✔ Several strategies have been suggested in order to reduce the incidence of postoperative seroma following LD harvest. The use of quilting sutures has been shown to reduce significantly the risk of seroma formation, and once established the use of intracavity steroid injections following aspiration has been shown to significantly reduce the risk of reaccumulation.[41,42]

✅ Ischaemic complications of the LD flap are rare due to its robust blood supply, with a complete failure rate of less than 1%, and it is therefore a useful technique for autologous reconstruction in higher risk patients.[37,43–46] The long-term aesthetic outcome of the LD flap in combination with an implant is between those of an implant reconstruction and a purely autologous reconstruction. The purely autologous LD flap may withstand adjuvant radiotherapy better than the LD flap with implant.[36,47–49]

The silicone issue

In the UK the Independent Review Group in 1998 concluded in an exhaustive report that silicone breast implants are safe, and no new contradictory evidence has arisen since the publication of the report.[50]

✅✅ The Independent Review Group considered immense amounts of complex evidence and reached a number of conclusions, including that there is no histopathological or conclusive immunological evidence for an abnormal immune response to silicone from breast implants in tissue, and that there is no epidemiological evidence for any link between silicone gel breast implants and any established connective tissue disease.[50]

Breast reconstruction with lower abdominal tissue

The lower abdominal pannus is usually an excellent source of tissue for autologous breast reconstruction and leaves an acceptable donor scar as well as serving as a simultaneous aesthetic abdominoplasty (**Fig. 9.10**). This technique achieves aesthetically stable results that are stable with time[24,51] (Fig. 9.2). It must be acknowledged, however, that there is a risk of donor-site bulge and hernia with any technique that transgresses the anterior rectus sheath.[52,53]

Indications

Lower abdominal tissue can be used for immediate or delayed breast reconstruction in any patient with sufficient tissue. For a microvascular procedure patients need to be surgically fit. Due to the versatility, resemblance to a normal breast and excellent long-term outcome, lower abdominal flaps have become the first choice for breast reconstruction for many surgeons.

Contraindications

The only absolute contraindications are previous ligation of the flap pedicle or previous abdominoplasty.

Multiple abdominal scars are a relative contraindication, as is previous abdominal liposuction, and imaging of the vascularity may be indicated in these cases. Midline abdominal scars may necessitate harvest of only a hemiflap, or use of a bipedicled flap in certain circumstances. The most predictable and safest outcomes after prior breast irradiation involve the use of autologous tissue, and where radiotherapy is anticipated to follow immediate breast reconstruction, autologous tissue is the current accepted standard due to its better tolerance of irradiation.[14,26]

Surgical techniques

The lower abdominal pannus receives its dominant blood supply from perforators of the deep inferior epigastric artery, a branch of the external iliac artery, through the rectus abdominis muscle. This vessel connects through reduced calibre vessels within the muscle with the deep superior epigastric artery, the terminal branch of the internal mammary artery, which is the blood supply to the pedicled flap, and this flap therefore necessitates inclusion of the muscle and the venous drainage is retrograde. The lower abdominal flap also receives a variable contribution from the superficial inferior epigastric artery (SIEA), which lies superficial to the anterior rectus sheath.

The triple blood supply to the lower abdominal tissue allows it to be used in a variety of techniques, including the pedicled TRAM flap, free TRAM flap, free deep inferior epigastric artery perforator (DIEP) flap and free SIEA flap.[54–59] The free TRAM and DIEP flaps utilise the dominant blood supply and are associated with a reduced risk of flap complications compared with the pedicled TRAM flap. In addition, the potential to completely or partially preserve the rectus muscle and its intercostal motor nerves leads to reduced donor-site morbidity. It is important, therefore, to take a careful history of the activities and hobbies of the patient when considering the most appropriate reconstruction. With any technique there may always be persistent absence of sensory recovery in a triangle between the new umbilicus position and the abdominal scar.

Pedicled TRAM flap

The pedicled TRAM flap relies on blood flow through the deep superior epigastric vessels within the substance of the rectus abdominis muscle. The flap is transferred onto the chest wall through a large epigastric subcutaneous tunnel that may be either ipsilateral or contralateral. The contralateral

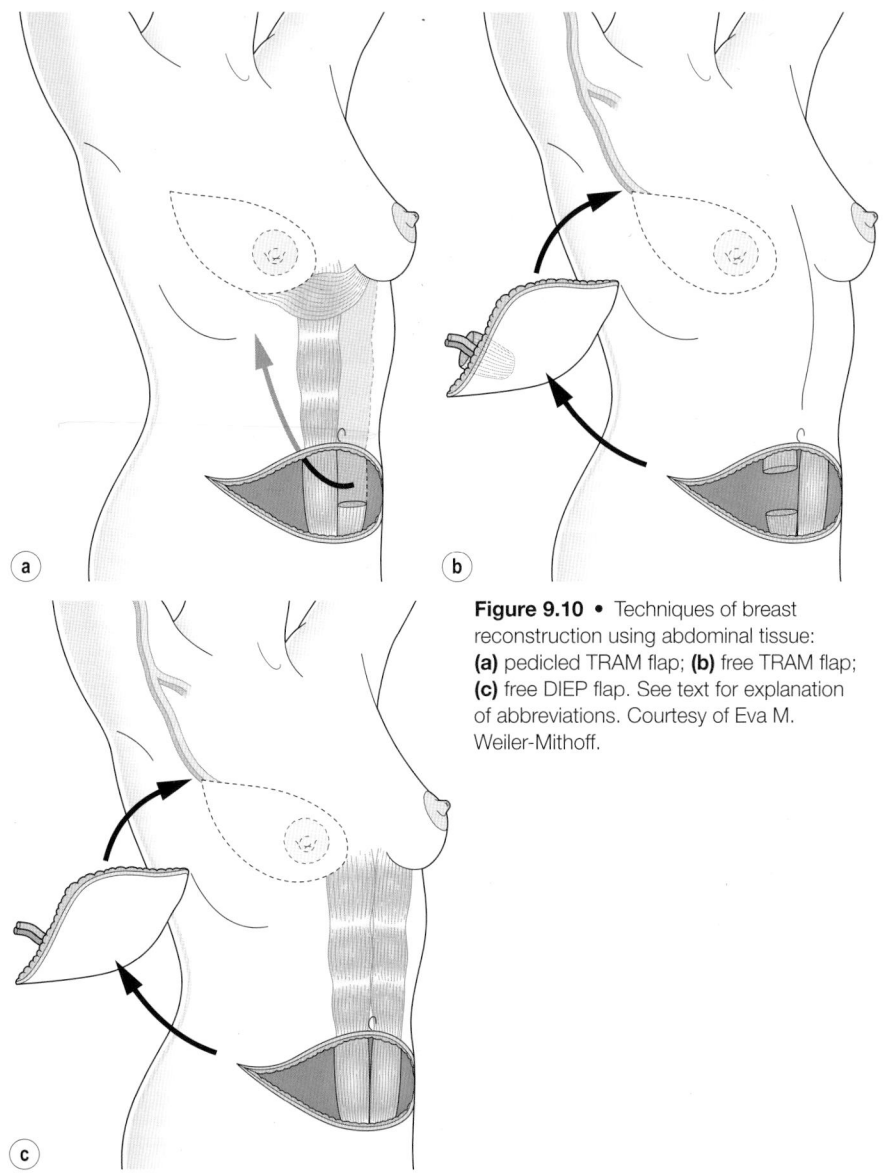

Figure 9.10 • Techniques of breast reconstruction using abdominal tissue: **(a)** pedicled TRAM flap; **(b)** free TRAM flap; **(c)** free DIEP flap. See text for explanation of abbreviations. Courtesy of Eva M. Weiler-Mithoff.

pedicle may produce superior aesthetic results because it reduces the bulge in the epigastrium and may avoid disruption of the ipsilateral inframammary fold.[56] The only absolute contraindication is previous ligation of the deep superior epigastric artery pedicle. The flap does not require microvascular skills; however, perfusion through the non-dominant blood supply leads to higher rates of complications than the free flap, including fat necrosis. For this reason some surgeons advocate

flap 'delay' by ligation of the ipsilateral deep and superficial inferior epigastric arteries before transfer, to allow augmentation of the remaining blood supply, especially in those considered high risk for flap necrosis, such as smokers and obese persons.

As the full muscle width is required, the donor site needs to be reconstructed with prosthetic material and the donor-site morbidity is higher than with free flap options.[56,60] Bilateral pedicled TRAM flaps may further increase donor-site morbidity.[61]

Free TRAM flap

In many centres free flaps from the lower abdominal wall are the first choice in breast reconstruction with autologous tissue (**Fig. 9.11**). The deep inferior epigastric vessels are the dominant blood supply for a free TRAM flap. The lower abdominal skin is transferred with a segment of rectus abdominis muscle and the deep inferior epigastric vessels, which are anastomosed to the recipient vessels of the subscapular axis or the internal mammary system. An ipsilateral pedicle will place the better vascularised tissue towards the midline. Muscle- and fascial-sparing techniques are now widely used to avoid the need for insertion of synthetic mesh at the donor site. Due to the improved blood supply the rate of fat necrosis is reduced and a larger flap can be safely transferred compared with the pedicled flap.[62] Muscle-sparing free TRAM flap techniques have demonstrated reduced donor-site morbidity.[63–65] Many large-volume centres are reporting total flap failure rates of around 1%.[53]

The operation typically requires 6–8 hours operating time, a hospital stay of 7–10 days and postoperative recovery of 2–3 months.

Deep inferior epigastric perforator (DIEP) flap

The DIEP flap spares the whole of the rectus abdominis muscle through meticulous dissection of deep inferior epigastric artery perforators within the rectus abdominis muscle and preservation of the intercostal motor nerves (**Fig. 9.12**). This reduces the donor-site morbidity when compared with the TRAM flap.[59,66,67] No muscle and little or no fascia is harvested and mesh is not usually required for donor-site closure.

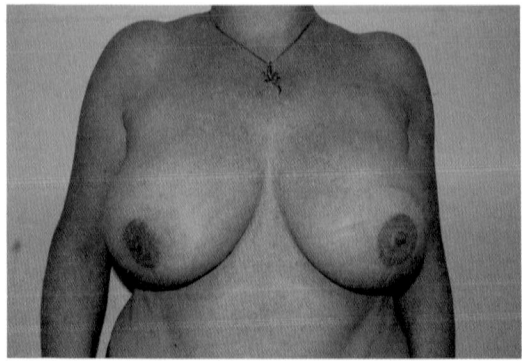

Figure 9.11 • Immediate left breast reconstruction with TRAM flap and with nipple reconstruction.

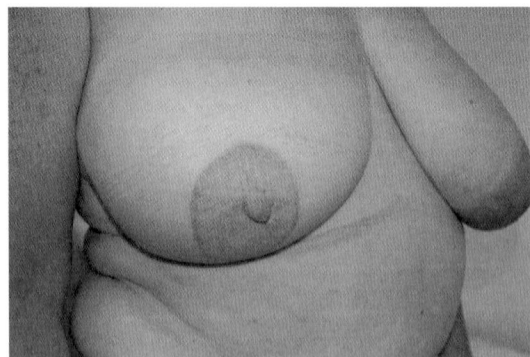

Figure 9.12 • Delayed DIEP flap and nipple reconstruction.

Superficial inferior epigastric artery (SIEA) flap

The SIEA flap is based on the superficial inferior epigastric artery and vein, which arise from the common femoral artery and saphenous bulb, respectively. Donor-site morbidity from SIEA flap harvest is minimal as the vessels are dissected at the level of Scarpa's fascia and the rectus fascia is left intact.[68] The main disadvantage of the SIEA flap is variability of the SIEA in presence, calibre and cutaneous territory. Vessels of at least 1 mm in diameter at the level of the inferior incision can be used safely for flap transfer. The vascular pedicle is short and therefore the internal mammary recipient vessels are preferred, and flap inset requires special consideration due to the peripheral location of the pedicle. Perfusion of the flap across the midline is unreliable, and thus its use is limited to where only a hemiflap is required and for bilateral procedures.[68–71]

Techniques

The flaps are harvested through standard abdominoplasty incisions extending laterally to the anterior superior iliac spines.[59,66] Dissection is from lateral to medial, taking care to identify the superficial inferior epigastric pedicle. If the artery is of sufficient size, then a SIEA flap can be harvested, otherwise the superficial inferior epigastric vein is dissected for a short distance for use in case of venous compromise later. The perforators are inspected and if one dominant perforator or two or three smaller suitable perforators in the same intramuscular septum can be harvested then a DIEP flap is harvested with careful intramuscular dissection of the perforators to the pedicle, which is located on the underside of the muscle. Where suitable perforators for DIEP flap harvest are not present, muscle is included (as much as is necessary to incorporate the perforators) and the dissection continues until a pedicle of sufficient length and calibre is obtained. Sensory nerves to the flap typically run with the perforators and may be connected to the lateral branch of the fourth intercostal nerve, although spontaneous recovery of sensation often occurs.[5]

A two-team approach with simultaneous preparation of the recipient site and harvest of the flap works well. The internal mammary vessels are often preferred and can be approached either through excision of a segment of the third costal cartilage or through the interspaces above or below this. The anastomosis is performed and the flap inset and drains inserted, with variable de-epithelialisation depending on the amount of native breast skin that has been preserved. Because of its often inadequate perfusion, the part of the flap furthest from the pedicle (zone IV) is often excised. The abdomen is closed in layers and the umbilicus retrieved as per an aesthetic abdominoplasty and drains inserted.

✔ The DIEP flap provides the optimal free flap breast reconstruction in many centres, although gaining expertise in its harvest requires a significant learning curve.[72] The SIEA flap has the lowest donor-site morbidity as the rectus sheath remains intact, but this flap is limited to a hemiflap and can only be used in selected cases when the vascular anatomy is suitable. An algorithm is usually employed where the vessels to the SIEA flap are inspected first, and if these are not of sufficient calibre for an SIEA flap then the superficial inferior epigastric vein is usually dissected for a short distance for harvest with the flap for secondary anastomosis should the flap develop venous congestion. Next the flap is harvested from lateral towards the midline and the perforators explored. If perforators of sufficient calibre are found to support a perforator flap, then a DIEP flap is harvested, and if not then a TRAM flap is harvested to include the perforators, with consideration of a muscle-sparing technique where this can be performed safely.[69]

Complications

Early complications include thrombosis of the arterial or venous anastomosis, haematoma, partial or total flap loss, fat necrosis, wound breakdown, and infection of prosthetic mesh if used. Late complications include donor-site bulge or hernia and reduced abdominal strength (Table 9.1). Overweight (body mass index 25–29) and obese (body mass index ≥30) patients have a significantly increased rate of flap and

Table 9.1 • Pooled complication rates for DIEP and free TRAM flap patients (%)

	DIEP flap	Free TRAM flap
Fat necrosis	10.1	4.9
Partial flap loss	2.5	1.8
Total flap loss	2.0	1.0
Abdominal bulge	3.1	5.9
Abdominal hernia	0.8	3.9

DIEP, deep inferior epigastric perforator; TRAM, transverse rectus abdominis myocutaneous.
Modified from Man LX, Selber JC, Serletti JM. Abdominal wall following free TRAM or DIEP flap reconstruction: a meta-analysis and critical review. Plast Reconstr Surg 2009; 124(3):752–64.

donor-site complications.[73] Smokers have a higher incidence of mastectomy flap necrosis and donor-site abdominal flap necrosis and hernia, although not thrombosis of the anastomosis or flap loss.[74]

Superior and inferior gluteal artery perforator flaps

A superior or inferior gluteal artery perforator (SGAP, IGAP) flap is indicated when the abdominal donor site is unavailable due to insufficient tissue or the presence of multiple abdominal scars or if the patient wants a more inconspicuous donor-site scar.[75–77] The flaps are limited to small-volume reconstructions and tissue is firmer and less able to create ptosis than that from the abdomen. The donor site, however, particularly with the IGAP flap, can be excellent in well-selected patients and recovery is shorter than with abdominal flaps. The internal mammary vessels are preferred for the anastomosis to aid inset, due to the relatively short pedicle.

Transverse upper gracilis flap

The transverse upper gracilis (TUG) flap utilises a transverse skin ellipse from the upper thigh, which is usually discarded in a traditional aesthetic medial thigh lift, based on musculocutaneous perforators through the gracilis muscle from the medial circumflex iliac artery. As with the gluteal artery perforator flaps the disadvantages include small volume and firmer tissue than from the abdomen, but the donor-site scar is very well hidden and there is good patient satisfaction.[78–80]

Alternative free flap donor sites

Alternative options of autologous tissue breast reconstruction in selected patients without other suitable donor sites include the anterolateral thigh flap, omentum and Rubens flap based on the deep circumflex iliac artery. The free contralateral LD flap may be used in selected cases of ipsilateral congenital absence.

Finishing touches

Further surgery may be necessary to the reconstructed breast, the contralateral breast or the donor site of the autologous reconstruction. Complete breast reconstruction including nipple–areola reconstruction requires on average 3.3 separate procedures.[81]

Surgery to the reconstructed breast

The reconstructed breast may require adjustment in size or shape by liposuction, excision of fat necrosis, mastopexy or augmentation. Lipomodelling transfers fat cells that have been harvested by liposuction into autologous breast reconstructions such as the autologous LD flap or the DIEP. This technique is particularly useful for contour irregularities or generalised volume loss after adjuvant radiotherapy. Lipomodelling may be used for adding volume to the reconstructed breast and smoothing out irregularities, and also for preparing the irradiated bed prior to implant breast reconstruction.[82–84] Further adjustments of the position of the breast on the chest wall, improvement of projection, adjustment of the inframammary fold or revisional surgery for capsular contracture may be necessary.

Surgery to the contralateral breast

Symmetrising surgery may be achieved by mastopexy, reduction or breast augmentation. Augmentation is particularly useful for gaining symmetry where implant breast reconstruction has been utilised. Some patients may want a contralateral risk-reducing mastectomy with reconstruction where they are deemed at high risk of contralateral breast cancer after a formal assessment of genetic risk.[85]

Surgery to the flap donor site

Scar revision, liposuction, lipofilling, treatment of persistent seroma, correction of dog ears or repair of an abdominal bulge or hernia may be necessary.

Nipple–areola reconstruction

The breast reconstruction is not complete until the nipple–areola complex (NAC) has been reconstructed, although some patients may be happy with a customised prosthetic nipple alone.[86] NAC reconstruction is usually the last step of the reconstruction as its position is difficult to alter. The aims of NAC reconstruction are to achieve symmetry with the contralateral NAC in terms of size, colour, texture, position and projection (see Figs 9.3, 9.8 and 9.11). The ideal NAC reconstruction technique has not yet been discovered, as evidenced by the number of techniques that have been described, mainly as a result of loss of projection with time.[87]

Nipple reconstruction techniques can be broadly catagorised as either composite grafts from the opposite breast or local flaps. Nipple-sharing is ideal for women with a large, ptotic contralateral nipple; however, this causes morbidity to the normal nipple, the graft may fail and there is poor long-term projection. Almost all local flaps suffer some loss of projection over time, usually at a rate inversely proportional to the thickness of the tissue used to create them, and for this reason overcorrection of flaps is usually performed. The use of autologous or prosthetic implants has also been described for placement within the local flap construct in an attempt to increase longevity of projection.

Areola reconstruction can be performed by full-thickness skin grafting or by tattooing. Grafts are usually obtained from the contralateral areola or the labia majora, with the aim to match the pigmentation and texture of the contralateral areolar as closely as possible. For this reason, where the contralateral areola is not suitable, tattooing is usually preferred. It is a quick and simple technique with minimal morbidity and very few complications apart from fading with time, and may be performed either before or after the nipple reconstruction.[88]

✔ Patients should be offered nipple–areola reconstruction as an integral part of their reconstruction. It completes the reconstructed breast, leads to increased satisfaction with the reconstruction, a sense of completeness and an enhanced sense of attractiveness, especially when the patient is unclothed.[86]

Complications of breast reconstruction

Mastectomy skin flap necrosis can be a common complication of immediate breast reconstruction. Management may be conservative with dressings if small, or the area can be excised and closed by advancement of the skin flap or autologous flap skin paddle, or by split skin grafting. Partial autologous flap failure usually requires debridement and management involves dressings, excision, and possibly skin grafting, but complete flap loss requires removal of the flap and either direct closure of the skin flaps, or placement of a tissue expander or implant, or immediate LD flap breast reconstruction, depending on the patient's wishes. Implant infection can sometimes be salvaged by washout and reinsertion of the implant, but severe infection or extrusion usually requires removal of the prosthesis (**Fig. 9.13**) and replacement at a later date once the tissues are healed and free from infection. Contour defects following fat necrosis, muscle atrophy or following radiotherapy may be corrected either by prosthetic augmentation or by lipomodelling.

Local recurrence

Salvage surgery for chest-wall recurrence is best dealt with in a multidisciplinary setting. The aims of surgery are local control of disease, palliation of symptoms and enhancement of the quality of remaining life. Chest-wall reconstruction may be required, and importation of well-vascularised non-irradiated flap tissues may allow for further radiotherapy. Reconstruction of the resultant defect often requires extensive surgery utilising local flaps

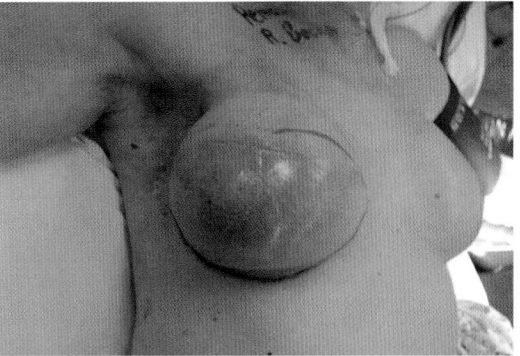

Figure 9.13 • Infected prosthesis after right breast reconstruction that required removal.

or abdominal advancement, regional flaps such as LD, pectoralis major and parascapular flaps, omental transposition, pedicled or free abdominal flaps, or a combination of these techniques.[19,20,89,90]

Summary

The aim of breast reconstruction is to recreate the natural breast as closely as possible following mastectomy. Decisions regarding breast reconstruction are best made by the fully informed patient within the setting of a multidisciplinary breast cancer team that can deliver the oncological surgery as well as the full range of commonly used breast reconstruction techniques. Breast reconstruction leads to a high degree of satisfaction but high levels of preoperative information and psychological support are necessary.[91] Close collaboration between oncological and reconstructive surgeons or management by an oncoplastic surgeon and careful patient selection and counselling can achieve excellent outcomes for breast reconstruction in the majority of patients.

Key points

- Breast reconstruction plays a significant role in the woman's physical, emotional and psychological recovery from breast cancer.
- Even the best reconstruction will not be able to replace the natural breast that has been lost.
- Surgical options for reconstruction include the use of tissue expanders or breast implants and the use of autologous tissue.
- The most commonly used surgical techniques are tissue expansion, LD musculocutaneous flap with or without implant, lower abdominal tissue and other free tissue transfers.
- Implant-based techniques require limited surgery initially but have limitations and are not always quick and trouble free. The quality of the long-term result is directly related to the tolerance of breast implants but is often disappointing unless performed after bilateral mastectomy.

- Further procedures are often required for complications and maintenance. Asymmetry may reoccur due to the effects of gravity on the contralateral breast and fluctuations in body weight.
- The aesthetic results from autologous reconstruction are superior to those of implant-based reconstruction due to their versatility, more natural appearance, consistency and durability.
- Autologous tissue can better withstand radiotherapy.
- The autologous LD flap is highly versatile and has acceptable donor-site morbidity.
- The skin and fat of the lower abdomen are ideal for autologous breast reconstruction but donor-site morbidity is being increasingly appreciated. Muscle-sparing techniques preserve abdominal wall function at the cost of a more complex procedure.
- Further surgery is often necessary following reconstruction to the reconstructed breast, the contralateral breast or the donor site of the breast reconstruction.
- Nipple–areola reconstruction leads to increased patient satisfaction with breast reconstruction.
- Salvage surgery may be required for complications of the reconstruction or for oncological reasons.
- It is important for any woman undergoing mastectomy to be able to make a fully informed decision about reconstruction, and information about different techniques and their advantages and disadvantages should be freely available.
- Due to the variable needs of individual patients, the reconstructive surgeon must be able to provide the full range of reconstructive options.

References

1. Harcourt DM, Rumsey NJ, Ambler NR, et al. The psychological effect of mastectomy with or without breast reconstruction: a prospective, multicenter study. Plast Reconstr Surg 2003;111:1060–8.

2. Elder EE, Brandberg Y, Bjorklund T, et al. Quality of life and patient satisfaction in breast cancer patients after immediate breast reconstruction: a prospective study. Breast 2005;14:201.

3. Atisha D, Alderman AK, Lowery JC, et al. Prospective analysis of long-term psychosocial outcomes in breast reconstruction: two-year postoperative results from the Michigan Breast Reconstruction Outcomes Study. Ann Surg 2008;247(6):1019–28.

4. Fourth annual report of the National Mastectomy and Breast Reconstruction Audit, www.ic.nhs.uk/services/national-clinical-audit-support-programme-ncasp/audit-reports/mastectomy-and-breast-reconstruction; 2011 [accessed 11.08.12].

5. Shridharani SM, Magarakis M, Stapleton SM, et al. Breast sensation after breast reconstruction: a systematic review. J Reconstr Microsurg 2010;26(5):303–10.

6. Alderman AK, Hawley ST, Waljee J, et al. Understanding the impact of breast reconstruction on the surgical decision-making process for breast cancer. Cancer 2008;112(3):489–94.

7. Second annual report of the National Mastectomy and Breast Reconstruction Audit, www.ic.nhs.uk/services/national-clinical-audit-support-programme-ncasp/audit-reports/mastectomy-and-breast-reconstruction; 2009 [accessed 11.08.12].

8. Baildam A, Bishop H, Boland G, et al. Oncoplastic breast surgery – A guide to good practice. Eur J Surg Oncol 2007;33(Suppl. 1):S1–23.

9. Yi M, Kronowitz SJ, Meric-Bernstam F, et al. Local, regional, and systemic recurrence rates in patients undergoing skin-sparing mastectomy compared with conventional mastectomy. Cancer 2011;117(5):916–24.

10. Kronowitz SJ. Immediate versus delayed reconstruction. Clin Plast Surg 2007;34(1):39–50.

11. Alderman AK, Collins ED, Schott A, et al. The impact of breast reconstruction on the delivery of chemotherapy. Cancer 2010;116(7):1791–800.

12. Wilson CR, Brown IM, Weiler-Mithoff EM, et al. Immediate breast reconstruction is not associated with a delay in the delivery of adjuvant chemotherapy. Eur J Surg Oncol 2004;30:624–27.
No statistically significant difference was found in the time between surgery and first dose of adjuvant chemotherapy in 285 patients undergoing wide local excision, simple mastectomy or mastectomy and immediate breast reconstruction with a variety of techniques.

13. Veronesi P, Ballardini B, De Lorenzi F, et al. Immediate breast reconstruction after mastectomy. Breast 2011;20(Suppl. 3):S104–7.

14. Barry M, Kell MR. Radiotherapy and breast reconstruction: a meta-analysis. Breast Cancer Res Treat 2011;127(1):15–22.

15. Spear SL, Parikh PM, Reisin E, et al. Acellular dermis-assisted breast reconstruction. Aesthet Plast Surg 2008;32:418–25.

16. Nedumpara T, Jonker L, Williams MR. Impact of immediate breast reconstruction on breast cancer recurrence and survival. Breast 2011;20(5):437–43.

17. Eriksen C, Frisell J, Wickman M, et al. Immediate reconstruction with implants in women with invasive breast cancer does not affect oncological safety in a matched cohort study. Breast Cancer Res Treat 2011;127(2):439–46.

18. Petit JY, Gentilini O, Rotmensz N, et al. Oncological results of immediate breast reconstruction: long term follow-up of a large series at a single institution. Breast Cancer Res Treat 2008;112(3):545–9.

19. Crisera CA, Chang EI, Da Lio AL, et al. Immediate free flap reconstruction for advanced-stage breast cancer: is it safe? Plast Reconstr Surg 2011;128(1):32–41.

20. Lim W, Ko BS, Kim HJ, et al. Oncological safety of skin sparing mastectomy followed by immediate reconstruction for locally advanced breast cancer. J Surg Oncol 2010;102(1):39–42.

21. Ruiterkamp J, Ernst MF, van de Poll-Franse LV, et al. Surgical resection of the primary tumour is associated with improved survival in patients with distant metastatic breast cancer at diagnosis. Eur J Surg Oncol 2009;35:1146–51.

22. Khoo A, Kroll SS, Reece GP, et al. A comparison of resource costs of immediate and delayed breast reconstruction. Plast Reconstr Surg 1998;101(4):964–8.

23. Kronowitz SJ, Lam C, Terefe W, et al. A multidisciplinary protocol for planned skin-preserving delayed breast reconstruction for patients with locally advanced breast cancer requiring postmastectomy radiation therapy: 3-year follow-up. Plast Reconstr Surg 2011;127(6):2154–66.

24. Hu ES, Pusic AL, Waljee JF, et al. Patient-reported aesthetic satisfaction with breast reconstruction during the long-term survivorship period. Plast Reconstr Surg 2009;124(1):1–8.

25. Chevray PM. Timing of breast reconstruction: immediate versus delayed. Cancer J 2008;14(4):223–9.

26. Jugenburg M, Disa JJ, Pusic AL, et al. Impact of radiotherapy on breast reconstruction. Clin Plast Surg 2007;34(1):29–37.

27. Bostwick III J. Plastic and reconstructive breast surgery. St Louis: Quality Medical Publishing; 1990.

28. Radovan C. Breast reconstruction after mastectomy using the temporary expander. Plast Reconstr Surg 1982;69:195–208.

29. Spear SL, Mesbahi AN. Implant-based reconstruction. Clin Plast Surg 2007;34(1):63–73.

30. Gabriel SE, Woods JE, O'Fallon WM, et al. Complications leading to surgery after breast implantation. N Engl J Med 1997;336:677–82.

31. Clough KB, O'Donoghue JM, Fitoussi AD, et al. Prospective evaluation of late cosmetic results following breast reconstruction: implant reconstruction. Plast Reconstr Surg 2001;107:1702–9.
Prospective evaluation of morbidity and cosmesis of 334 patients with unilateral implant reconstructions showed a significant deterioration of long-term results in a linear fashion, from an initial acceptable result of 86% 2 years after patients completed their reconstruction to only 54% at 5 years, despite a 92.5% rate of symmetry surgery. This deterioration was unrelated to the type of implant used, the volume of the implant, the age of the patient or the type of mastectomy incision employed, but after a retrospective photographic review the authors are of the opinion that it was related to late asymmetry produced by the failure of both breasts to undergo symmetrical ptosis with ageing.

32. Kronowitz SJ, Robb GL. Radiation therapy and breast reconstruction: a critical review of the literature. Plast Reconstr Surg 2009;124(2):395–408.

33. Cordeiro PG, Pusic AL, Disa JJ, et al. Irradiation after immediate tissue expander/implant breast reconstruction: outcomes, complications, aesthetic results, and satisfaction among 156 patients. Plast Reconstr Surg 2004;113(3):877–81.

34. Wickman M, Jurell G. Low capsular contraction rate after primary and secondary breast reconstruction with a textured expander prosthesis. Plast Reconstr Surg 1997;99(3):692–7.

35. Clough KB, Louis-Sylvestre C, Fitoussi A, et al. Donor site sequelae after autologous breast reconstruction with an extended latissimus dorsi flap. Plast Reconstr Surg 2002;109:1904–11.

36. McKeown DJ, Hogg FJ, Brown IM, et al. The timing of autologous latissimus dorsi breast reconstruction and effect of radiotherapy on outcome. J Plast Reconstr Aesthet Surg 2009;62(4):488–93.

37. Delay E, Gounot N, Bouillot A, et al. Autologous latissimus breast reconstruction: a 3 year clinical experience with 100 patients. Plast Reconstr Surg 1998;102:1461–78.

38. McCraw JB, Papp C, Edwards A, et al. The autogenous latissimus breast reconstruction. Clin Plast Surg 1994;21:279–88.

39. Germann G, Steinau HU. Breast reconstruction with the extended latissimus dorsi flap. Plast Reconstr Surg 1996;97:519–26.

40. Saint-Cyr M, Nagarkar P, Schaverien M, et al. The pedicled descending branch muscle-sparing latissimus dorsi flap for breast reconstruction. Plast Reconstr Surg 2009;123(1):13–24.

41. Dancey AL, Cheema M, Thomas SS. A prospective randomized trial of the efficacy of marginal quilting sutures and fibrin sealant in reducing the incidence of seromas in the extended latissimus dorsi donor site. Plast Reconstr Surg 2010;125(5):1309–17.
Prospective, double-blinded, clinical trial under a single surgeon involving 26 patients followed up for 6 months randomised to receive either quilting sutures only or a combination of fibrin sealant and marginal quilting sutures. The combination of fibrin sealant and marginal quilting sutures significantly reduced total drainage, hospital stay and seroma formation. The authors caution that potential, albeit small, risk of virus transmission and allergic reaction, however, needs to be taken into

consideration with the use of fibrin sealant, as with any blood transfusion product.

42. Taghizadeh R, Shoaib T, Hart AM, et al. Triamcinolone reduces seroma re-accumulation in the extended latissimus dorsi donor site. J Plast Reconstr Aesthet Surg 2008;61(6):636–42.
   This prospective study involved 52 extended LD breast reconstructions in 49 patients, with patients exhibiting seromas at their first postoperative visit randomised to receive either intracavity triamcinolone 80 mg or saline following seroma aspiration. Triamcinolone significantly reduced the need for any further aspiration, total number of aspirations, total volume aspirated and total time to dryness. Steroid injections were well tolerated and there were no infective complications.

43. Kroll SS, Baldwin B. A comparison of outcomes using three different methods of breast reconstruction. Plast Reconstr Surg 1992;90:455–62.

44. Roy MK, Shrotia S, Holcombe C, et al. Complications of latissimus dorsi myocutaneous flap breast reconstruction. Eur J Surg Oncol 1998;24:162–5.

45. Hardwicke JT, Prinsloo DJ. An analysis of 277 consecutive latissimus dorsi breast reconstructions: a focus on capsular contracture. Plast Reconstr Surg 2011;128(1):63–70.

46. Hammond DC. Latissimus dorsi flap breast reconstruction. Clin Plast Surg 2007;34(1):75–82.

47. Gui GPH, Tan SM, Faliakou EC. Immediate breast reconstruction using biodimensional anatomical permanent expander implants: a prospective analysis of outcome and patient satisfaction. Plast Reconstr Surg 2003;111:125–38.

48. Tarantino I, Banic A, Fisher T. Evaluation of late results in breast reconstruction by latissimus dorsi flap and prosthesis implantation. Plast Reconstr Surg 2006;117:1387–94.

49. Chang DW, Barnea Y, Robb GL. Effects of an autologous flap combined with an implant for breast reconstruction: an evaluation of 1000 consecutive reconstructions of previously irradiated breasts. Plast Reconstr Surg 2008;122(2):356–62.

50. Report of the Independent Review Group. Silicone gel breast implants. London: HMSO; 1998.
   The Independent Review Group considered immense amounts of complex evidence and reached a number of conclusions, including that there is no histopathological or conclusive immunological evidence for an abnormal immune response to silicone from breast implants in tissue, and that there is no epidemiological evidence for any link between silicone gel breast implants and any established connective tissue disease.

51. Clough BC, O'Donoghue JM, Fitoussi AD, et al. Prospective evaluation of late cosmetic results following breast reconstruction. II. TRAM flap reconstruction. Plast Reconstr Surg 2001;107:1710–6.
   Prospective study of 171 TRAM flap patients for 8 years showed aesthetically pleasing long-term results in 94.2%.

52. Yueh JH, Slavin SA, Adesiyun T, et al. Patient satisfaction in postmastectomy breast reconstruction: a comparative evaluation of DIEP, TRAM, latissimus flap, and implant techniques. Plast Reconstr Surg 2010;125(6):1585–95.

53. Man LX, Selber JC, Serletti JM. Abdominal wall following free TRAM or DIEP flap reconstruction: a meta-analysis and critical review. Plast Reconstr Surg 2009;124(3):752–64.

54. Robbins TH. Rectus abdominis myocutaneous flap for breast reconstruction. Aust N Z J Surg 1979;49:527–30.

55. Hartrampf CR. Breast reconstruction with a transverse abdominal island flap. Plast Reconstr Surg 1982;69:216–24.

56. Jones G. The pedicled TRAM flap in breast reconstruction. Clin Plast Surg 2007;34(1):83–104.

57. Holmstroem H. The free abdominoplasty flap and its use in breast reconstruction. Scand J Plast Reconstr Surg 1979;13:423–6.

58. Koshima I, Soeda S. Inferior epigastric artery skin flaps without rectus abdominis muscle. Br J Plast Surg 1989;42:645–8.

59. Allen RJ, Treece P. Deep inferior epigastric perforator flap for breast reconstruction. Ann Plast Surg 1994;32:32–8.

60. Atisha D, Alderman AK. A systematic review of abdominal wall function following abdominal flaps for postmastectomy breast reconstruction. Ann Plast Surg 2009;63(2):222–30.

61. Chun YS, Sinha I, Turko A, et al. Comparison of morbidity, functional outcome, and satisfaction following bilateral TRAM versus bilateral DIEP flap breast reconstruction. Plast Reconstr Surg 2010;126(4):1133–41.

62. Kroll SS, Gherardini G, Martin JE, et al. Fat necrosis in free and pedicled TRAM flaps. Plast Reconstr Surg 1998;102(5):1502–7.

63. Nelson JA, Guo Y, Sonnad SS, et al. A comparison between DIEP and muscle-sparing free TRAM flaps in breast reconstruction: a single surgeon's recent experience. Plast Reconstr Surg 2010;126(5):1428–35.

64. Wu LC, Bajaj A, Chang DW, et al. Comparison of donor-site morbidity of SIEA, DIEP, and muscle-sparing TRAM flaps for breast reconstruction. Plast Reconstr Surg 2008;122(3):702–9.

65. Bajaj AK, Chevray PM, Chang DW. Comparison of donor-site complications and functional outcomes in free muscle-sparing TRAM flap and free DIEP flap breast reconstruction. Plast Reconstr Surg 2006;117(3):737–46.

66. Granzow JW, Levine JL, Chiu ES, et al. Breast reconstruction using perforator flaps. J Surg Oncol 2006;94(6):441–54.

67. Futter CM, Webster MHC, Hagen S, et al. A retrospective comparison of abdominal muscle strength

following breast reconstruction with a free TRAM or DIEP flap. Br J Plast Surg 2000;53:578–83.

68. Grotting JC. The free abdominoplasty flap for immediate breast reconstruction. Ann Plast Surg 1991;27(4):351–4.

69. Chevray PM. Update on breast reconstruction using free TRAM, DIEP, and SIEA flaps. Semin Plast Surg 2004;18(2):97–104.

70. Lipa JE. Breast reconstruction with free flaps from the abdominal donor site: TRAM, DIEAP, and SIEA flaps. Clin Plast Surg 2007;34(1):105–21.

71. Selber JC, Samra F, Bristol M, et al. A head-to-head comparison between the muscle-sparing free TRAM and the SIEA flaps: is the rate of flap loss worth the gain in abdominal wall function? Plast Reconstr Surg 2008;122(2):348–55.

72. Busic V, Das-Gupta R, Mesic H, et al. The deep inferior epigastric perforator flap for breast reconstruction, the learning curve explored. J Plast Reconstr Aesthet Surg 2006;59(6):580–4.

73. Chang DW, Wang B, Robb GL, et al. Effect of obesity on flap and donor-site complications in free transverse rectus abdominis myocutaneous flap breast reconstruction. Plast Reconstr Surg 2000;105(5):1640–8.

74. Chang DW, Reece GP, Wang B, et al. Effect of smoking on complications in patients undergoing free TRAM flap breast reconstruction. Plast Reconstr Surg 2000;105(7):2374–80.

75. Allen RJ, Tucker Jr C. Superior gluteal artery perforator free flap for breast reconstruction. Plast Reconstr Surg 1995;95(7):1207–12.

76. Allen RJ, Levine JL, Granzow JW. The in-the-crease inferior gluteal artery perforator flap for breast reconstruction. Plast Reconstr Surg 2006;118(2):333–9.

77. LoTempio MM, Allen RJ. Breast reconstruction with SGAP and IGAP flaps. Plast Reconstr Surg 2010;126(2):393–401.

78. Arnez ZM, Pogorelec D, Planinsek F, et al. Breast reconstruction by the free transverse gracilis (TUG) flap. Br J Plast Surg 2004;57(1):20–6.

79. Schoeller T, Huemer GM, Wechselberger G. The transverse musculocutaneous gracilis flap for breast reconstruction: guidelines for flap and patient selection. Plast Reconstr Surg 2008;122(1):29–38.

80. Pülzl P, Schoeller T, Kleewein K, et al. Donor-site morbidity of the transverse musculocutaneous gracilis flap in autologous breast reconstruction: short-term and long-term results. Plast Reconstr Surg 2011;128(4):233e–42e.

81. Malyon AD, Husein M, Weiler-Mithoff EM. How many procedures to make a breast? Br J Plast Surg 2001;54:227–31.

82. Petit JY, Lohsiriwat V, Clough KB, et al. The oncologic outcome and immediate surgical complications of lipofilling in breast cancer patients: a multicenter study – Milan–Paris–Lyon experience of 646 lipofilling procedures. Plast Reconstr Surg 2011;128(2):341–6.

83. Sarfati I, Ihrai T, Kaufman G, et al. Adipose-tissue grafting to the post-mastectomy irradiated chest wall: preparing the ground for implant reconstruction. J Plast Reconstr Aesthet Surg 2011;64(9):1161–6.

84. Delay E, Garson S, Tousson G, et al. Fat injection to the breast: technique, results, and indications based on 880 procedures over 10 years. Aesthet Surg J 2009;29(5):360–76.

85. Sauven P. Guidelines for the management of women at increased familial risk of breast cancer. Eur J Cancer 2004;40:653–65.

86. Wellisch DK, Schain WS, Noone RB, et al. The psychological contribution of nipple addition in breast reconstruction. Plast Reconstr Surg 1987;80:699–704.

87. Henseler H, Cheong V, Weiler-Mithoff EM, et al. The use of Munsell colour charts in nipple areola tattooing. Br J Plast Surg 2001;54:338–40.

88. Farhadi J, Maksvytyte GK, Schaefer DJ, et al. Reconstruction of the nipple–areola complex: an update. J Plast Reconstr Aesthet Surg 2006;59(1):40–53.

89. Hathaway CL, Rand RP, Moe R, et al. Salvage surgery for locally advanced and locally recurrent breast cancer. Arch Surg 1994;129:582–7.

90. Munhoz AM, Montag E, Arruda E, et al. Immediate locally advanced breast cancer and chest wall reconstruction: surgical planning and reconstruction strategies with extended V-Y latissimus dorsi myocutaneous flap. Plast Reconstr Surg 2011;127(6):2186–97.

91. Damen TH, de Bekker-Grob EW, Mureau MA, et al. Patients' preferences for breast reconstruction: a discrete choice experiment. J Plast Reconstr Aesthet Surg 2011;64(1):75–83.

10

Breast cancer: treatment of uncommon diseases

Daniel Xavier Choi
Monica Morrow

Introduction

This chapter discusses uncommon diseases of the breast and treatments thereof. These include: (i) pregnancy-associated breast cancer; (ii) male breast cancer; (iii) Paget's disease of the breast; (iv) other breast malignancies, including melanoma, lymphoma, angiosarcoma and metastases.

Pregnancy-associated breast cancer

Pregnancy-associated breast cancer (PABC) includes breast cancer diagnosed during pregnancy, up to 1 year after delivery, or during lactation. PABC is rare; it constitutes 0.2–3.8% of all breast cancers, occurring in 1 in 10 000 to 1 in 3000 pregnancies.[1] Nonetheless, PABC is the second most common malignancy in pregnant women (cervical cancer is the most common). As more women delay childbearing, the incidence of PABC may increase.[2]

Age for age, compared to non-pregnant women with breast cancer, pregnant women with breast cancer tend to be diagnosed at later stages.[3] The aetiology of this phenomenon is unclear. One possible explanation is that PABC may have a more aggressive biology. Alternatively, the significant anatomical and physiological changes in the breast during pregnancy may delay diagnosis.

Pathology

Histologically, PABC and non-PABC are similar. Compared to non-PABC, PABC tends to be oestrogen- and progesterone-receptor negative, while data on expression of human epidermal growth factor receptor (HER-2)/neu are conflicting.[4,5] PABC stains strongly for Ki67 and p53; the clinical significance of these findings is undetermined.[6]

Clinical presentation

The majority of PABCs present as a palpable breast mass. Gravid breasts undergo significant ductal and lobular proliferation under the influence of elevated levels of oestrogen, progesterone, prolactin and chorionic gonadotrophin. Mammary blood flow increases by 180%; the breast may become nodular and double in weight and volume.[7] Therefore, clinical breast examinations may be difficult, and may contribute to a delay in diagnosis and consequential poorer prognosis. Moreover, the differential diagnosis of breast mass in pregnant women is broad, including lactating adenoma, fibroadenoma, cystic disease, lobular hyperplasia, galactocoele, abscess, lipoma, hamartoma and PABC; 70–80% of breast biopsies in pregnant women are benign.[8]

Because PABC is rare, detailed evaluations of risk factors for PABC development are lacking. One study of 383 patients, including 192 patients with PABC, found that patients with PABC were 300% more likely to have a family history of breast cancer than age-matched, non-pregnant, non-lactating counterparts.[3]

Diagnosis

As in all women, dominant breast masses in pregnant women should be investigated with imaging and biopsies. While screening mammography is not routine for pregnant women, diagnostic mammography may be useful and can be performed safely with the use of abdominal shielding. Despite the fact that women with PABC are young and have dense, proliferative breasts, diagnostic mammograms detect 78–90% of palpable PABCs.[9]

Ultrasound is a particularly attractive imaging modality in the setting of PABC. It does not harbour teratogenic potential, it distinguishes and characterises solid and cystic lesions, and if, clinically, a mass cannot be distinguished from the normal nodularity of the gravid breast, it may be useful in excluding the presence of a suspicious lesion.

As in non-PABC, core-needle biopsy is the preferred method of diagnosis in PABC and offers two specific advantages in the work-up of a breast mass. Because the gravid breast is proliferative, fine-needle aspiration (FNA) and cytological evaluation may result in false-positive diagnoses of atypia or carcinoma. Additionally, benign lesions, i.e. adenomas, cysts or fibroadenomas, may increase in size during pregnancy. Thus, a core-needle biopsy may offer definitive benign diagnosis and avoid excision.

However, core-needle biopsy is not without risk. In addition to bleeding, milk fistulas are known rare complications.[10] Therefore, core-needle biopsy ought to be used with caution for the diagnoses of centrally located lesions in lactating women.

Metastatic work-up for non-PABC and PABC are similar and are guided by clinical stage and constellation of symptoms. Chest radiography with abdominal shielding is safe. Computed tomography (CT) scans are generally discouraged due to high radiation exposure. While magnetic resonance imaging (MRI) does not utilise ionising radiation – and, in fact, has been utilised in foetal imaging in utero – gadolinium is known to cross the placenta and to affect foetuses

adversely in animals and is not recommended.[5,11] No studies have investigated the role of position emission tomography (PET) in pregnant patients; in fact, pregnancy is often an exclusion criterion. Bone scans using lower doses of radioisotope have been performed in pregnant women, but are not generally recommended.[11]

Treatment (Fig. 10.1)

Local therapy

In general, treatment should not be delayed by pregnancy and should be guided by a multidisciplinary team consisting of a surgical oncologist, a medical oncologist and a high-risk obstetrician.

A landmark report of 2565 patients demonstrated no differences in congenital abnormalities between pregnant women who did and did not undergo surgery.[12] However, surgery during pregnancy was associated with an increased rate of spontaneous abortion. The risk of spontaneous abortion is highest in the first trimester, and the patient and surgeon may choose to defer surgery until after the 12th week of pregnancy.

The surgical team must be aware of the physiological changes of pregnancy, including increased plasma volume, increased cardiac output, decreased systemic vascular resistance, hypercoagulable state, dilutional anaemia with associated decreased oxygen-carrying capacity, and delayed gastric emptying. Additionally, a pillow should be placed on the right side of the patient to keep the gravid uterus from pressing upon the inferior vena cava. The foetus should be monitored intraoperatively and postoperatively.

Surgery should be tailored according to the clinical stage of the PABC and the gestational age of the foetus. Mastectomy can be performed during any trimester, although immediate breast reconstruction is not usually recommended due to the increased operative time and the difficulty of achieving symmetry with the contralateral breast as it continues to change during and after pregnancy. The decision to undertake breast-conserving therapy in the pregnant woman is much more complex. Breast-conserving therapy is generally not recommended in the first trimester because of a need to delay radiotherapy until after delivery, increasing

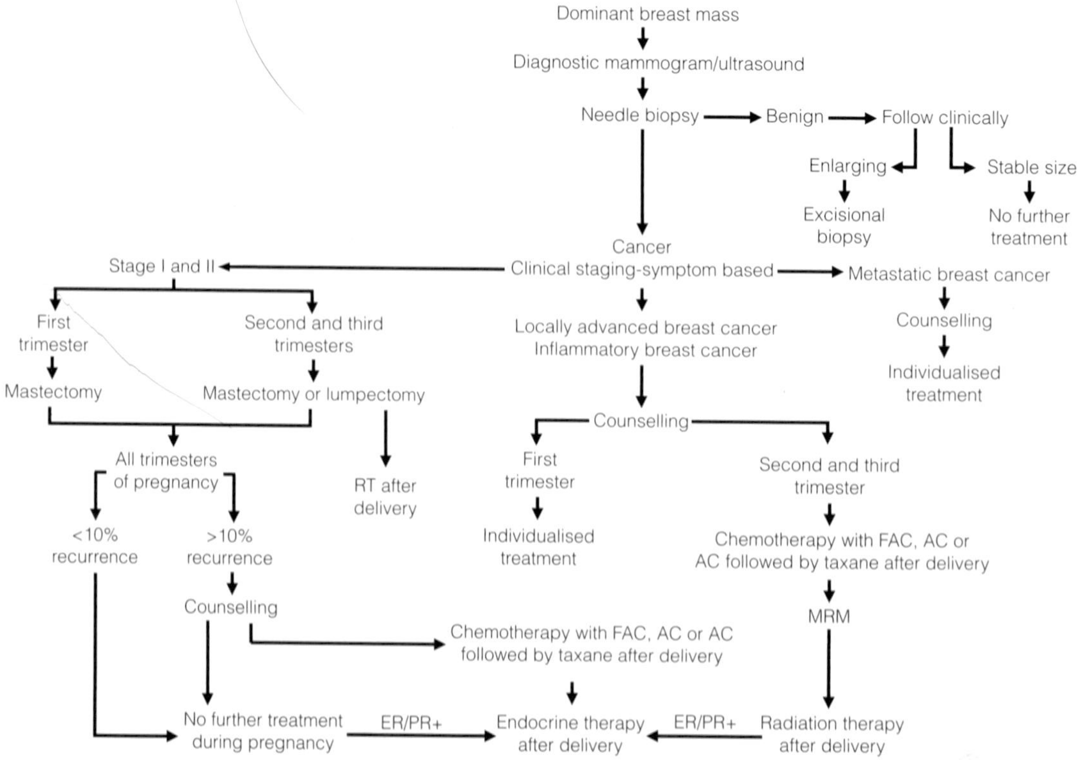

Figure 10.1 • Management algorithm for the pregnant woman with a dominant breast mass. ER/PR+, oestrogen and progesterone receptor positive; FAC, fluorouracil, doxorubicin and cyclophosphamide; MRM, Modified Radical Mastectomy.

the risk of local recurrence. However, for the patient who receives adjuvant chemotherapy, this delay is no longer than that of the non-pregnant patient. Breast-conserving therapy is feasible in the second and third trimesters.

Axillary staging

Previously, sentinel lymph node biopsy (SLNB) was not recommended in gravid or lactating women. Lymphazurin blue, patent blue V and methylene blue, the most commonly used dyes, have not been studied in pregnant women and their safety has not been established. Technetium-99m, the most commonly used radioactive tracer, involves low doses of radiation (1.85–3.7 MBq). Gentilini et al. found that sentinel lymph nodes were successfully identified in all patients, foetal radiation exposure was minimal and there were no adverse foetal outcomes.[13] Although there are no medical contraindications to lymphatic mapping with radioactivity during pregnancy, it remains to be seen if this procedure will be widely adopted.

Systemic therapy

In general, chemotherapy is contraindicated during the first trimester, for it exposes the foetus to an increased risk of abortion and malformation. In a small series, Ebert et al. noted that all the abortions that occurred in women during pregnancy were in those women who had received chemotherapy during the first trimester of pregnancy; while chemotherapy during the first trimester resulted in a 14–19% risk of foetal malformation, chemotherapy during the second trimester resulted in a 1.3% risk.[14] A prospective cohort study of 24 women, who received 5-fluorouracil, doxorubicin and cyclophosphamide during the second and third trimesters, found no congenital malformations, or short- or long-term complications in the infants; there were no stillbirths, miscarriages or perinatal deaths. Except for one child with Down's syndrome, the vast majority of infants demonstrated 'normal development' and eventually grew into functional school-aged children.[15,16]

During pregnancy, methotrexate should be avoided due to a risk of associated abnormalities. A review examining the use of taxanes, vinorelbine and trastuzumab demonstrated that taxanes and vinorelbine were safe for mother and offspring in the limited experience available, but trastuzumab was associated with anhydramnios in 50% of cases.[17] Endocrine therapy is not recommended during pregnancy. Tamoxifen has been associated with spontaneous abortions, teratogenicity and foetal demise.[18]

In general, for women with PABC with positive lymph nodes, chemotherapy is ideally administered after the first trimester, but within 6 weeks of surgery. For patients diagnosed early in the first trimester, this may be impossible. For women with PABC, negative lymph nodes and low-risk cancers (where the survival benefit of chemotherapy is 5% or less), treatment during pregnancy is usually avoided. For women with PABC also having negative lymph nodes and high-risk cancers, treatment decisions must be made on an individual basis. Chemotherapy ought to be stopped 3 weeks prior to delivery to avoid myelosuppression and septic complications in mothers and their offspring.[6]

Locally advanced and inflammatory breast cancers

The treatment of locally advanced and inflammatory breast cancers during pregnancy is problematic for women diagnosed during early pregnancy because of the foetal risks of chemotherapy. Three strategies exist: first, termination of pregnancy with prompt oncological treatment; second, administration of chemotherapy with acceptance of associated obstetric risks; third, delayed oncological treatment with acceptance of associated oncological risks. None of these is ideal, and deciding between them is difficult. As in non-pregnancy-associated inflammatory breast cancer, surgery as an initial approach to pregnancy-associated inflammatory breast cancer should be avoided.

Termination of and future pregnancy

Historically, the prognosis of PABC was considered so dismal that therapeutic abortion was advocated for all women. However, compared to women who terminated their pregnancies, women who continued their pregnancies did not demonstrate worsened overall or disease-free survivals.[1,5] There are currently no formal recommendations for therapeutic abortions in patients with PABC. However, as discussed, therapeutic abortion can simplify treatment in patients with locally advanced and inflammatory breast cancers. Women should be counselled that chemotherapy may adversely affect future fertility.

Though fertility may be hindered by patient age and chemotherapy, retrospective studies demonstrated that pregnancy after diagnosis and treatment of breast cancer was safe. Gemignani et al. reported that compared to patients treated for PABC who did not become pregnant, those who did had equivalent or better survival,[1] although this may be a result of selection bias. A population-based study conducted by the Danish Breast Cancer Cooperative Group found no difference in survival amongst 371 patients with PABC who became pregnant after treatment and 9865 patients with PABC who did not.[19]

Despite the fact that the rate of relapse is fairly constant for the first 10 years after treatment, some experts advocate waiting 2–5 years for future pregnancies,[6] contending that this affords a period during which recurrences can become manifest – up to 2 years for high-risk cancers, up to 5 years for low-risk cancers. However, a population-based report showed that for women with localised disease and good prognosis, conception 6 months after completion of treatment was unlikely to reduce survival.[20]

Prognosis

Because of the anatomical and physiological changes of the gravid and lactating breast, PABC tends to be diagnosed at a more advanced stage. In one study, fewer than 20% were diagnosed prior to delivery, median tumour size at diagnosis was 3.5 cm, and 62% of PABC patients had lymph-node metastases compared to 39% of matched controls.[1] Additionally, relative to non-PABC patients, PABC patients are more likely to have larger tumours, vascular invasion and distant metastasis.[4]

Historically, it was believed that, compared to non-PABC, PABC was intrinsically more aggressive and thereby carried a worse prognosis. However, recent studies have demonstrated this may not be correct. A review of 104 PABC and 564 non-PABC patients demonstrated that PABC had a more advanced T classification, N classification and stage.[21] Moreover, the two groups did not demonstrate any differences in locoregional recurrence, distant metastases or overall survival. For patients with PABC, the timing of diagnosis and treatment was the only factor associated with overall survival; those who had prompt diagnosis and treatment had better overall survival than those who had delayed diagnosis and treatment. In an older study, Gemignani et al. found that, for stage I and stage II disease, PABC and non-PABC patients had similar survivals.[1] However, compared to non-PABC, there was a trend towards a worse prognosis in stage III and stage IV PABC. Similarly, with negative lymph nodes, PABC patients had the same 5-year survival as non-PABC controls; however, for patients with positive lymph nodes, PABC and non-PABC patients had 5-year survivals of 47% and 59%, respectively.

Male breast cancer (Fig. 10.2)

In the 14th century, John of Arderne, an English surgeon, reported the first case of male breast cancer (MBC).[22] He cared for a priest who had progressive nipple–areolar ulceration. Almost certainly he died of this disease.

In the West, MBC accounts for less than 1% of all breast cancers and for 0.1% of cancer deaths in men.[23] These rates have remained stable in the second half of the 20th century.[24] However, rates of MBC have recently increased.[25] Though a complete explanation is elusive, this is likely due in part to an increase in the number of men diagnosed with ductal carcinoma in situ (DCIS) between 1973 and 2001.[26] Interestingly, there is an MBC 'belt' that extends from the Atlantic to the Indian Oceans in sub-Saharan Africa.[27] In Tanzania, 6% of breast cancers are diagnosed in men.

Pathology

Almost all pathological types of breast cancer found in women have been described in men. Ninety per cent of MBCs are invasive; of these, 80% are ductal, 5% are papillary and 1% are lobular.[28] The scarcity of lobular carcinoma probably reflects the paucity of terminal lobular units in male mammary tissue. Paget's disease of the breast and inflammatory breast cancer are as frequent in men as they are in women.[29] Less common subtypes, i.e. medullary, mucinous, squamous and tubular, have also been reported in men, but at lower frequencies than in women. Ten per cent of MBCs are non-invasive; almost all are DCIS,[28] and most are of the papillary subtype and of low or intermediate grade.[30] Lobular carcinoma in situ is rare.

When matched for age, stage and grade, men with breast cancer have a higher rate of oestrogen receptor positivity than women with breast cancer. A 25-year review of the Surveillance Epidemiology and End Results (SEER) database, which included 2357 MBCs, demonstrated oestrogen and progesterone positivity in 90% and 80% of breast cancers in men, and in 76% and 67% of breast cancers in women.[31] Data on the overexpression of erbB-2 or

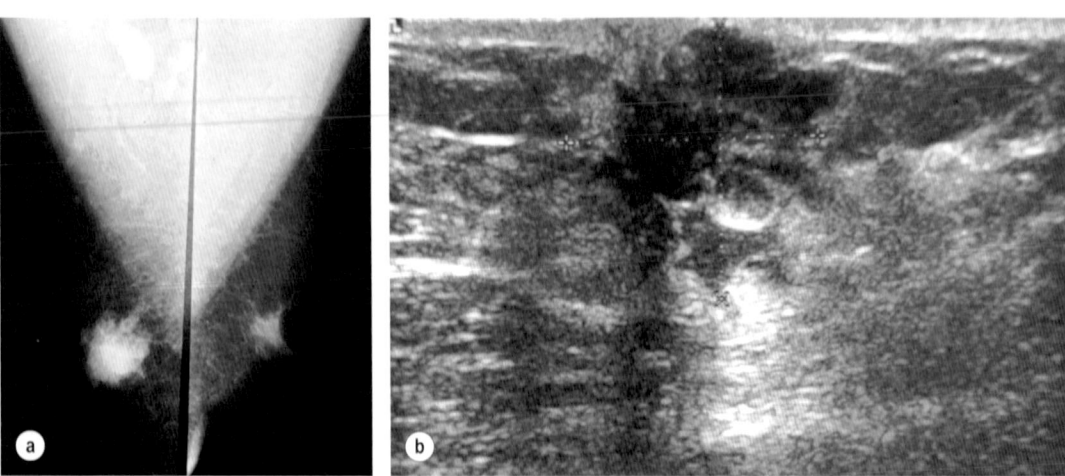

Figure 10.2 • (a) Mammogram of male breast cancer in right breast. **(b)** Ultrasound of male breast cancer in right breast.

HER-2/neu, p53, bcl-2, cyclin-D1 and epidermal growth factor receptor in MBC are limited, conflicting and inconclusive.

Clinical presentation

Though MBC can occur at any age, its incidence increases with age. The average age of diagnosis of breast cancer in men is approximately 10 years later than in women. Eighty-five per cent of MBCs present as a painless mass[32] and most MBCs are centrally located, with up to 50% demonstrating nipple retraction, discharge, pain or ulceration.[33] The time from the onset of symptoms to diagnosis is longer in men than in women – approximately 22 months. As a result, men often present at later stages.[34]

There are multiple risk factors for the development of MBC. Hormonal misbalance is one of these. Men with a history of undescended testes, congenital inguinal hernia, orchiectomy, orchitis, testicular injury, infertility, Klinefelter's syndrome, and obesity and cirrhosis (both of which induce a hyper-oestrogenic milieu) are at elevated risk.[35,36] In particular, Klinefelter's syndrome, which is characterised by a 47XXY karyotype, small testes and gynaecomastia, is associated with a 50-fold elevated risk.

Family history is another important risk factor. Between 15% and 20% of male patients with breast cancer have a family history of disease. The odds ratio for MBC increases with a positive family history and continues to increase as the number of affected first-degree relatives increases.[37,38] These factors probably reflect an increasing risk of *BRCA1* and *BRCA2* mutations, which predispose both men and women to breast cancer. Previous reports have focused on the association between MBC and *BRCA2* mutations. However, a recent report suggests that *BRCA1* and *BRCA2* carry equivalent elevations in risk.[39] Male *BRCA2* mutation carriers have a 6.3% cumulative risk of breast cancer.[37,38] In the United States, 4% of MBCs are in *BRCA2* mutation carriers; in Iceland, where a 'founder effect' is present, 40% of MBCs carry a mutation in *BRCA2*.[37]

As in women, radiation exposure is a risk factor for the development of breast cancer in men.[36] One evaluation of a national database of 324 799 men without breast cancer and 121 men with breast cancer found that a history of a bone fracture and obesity were associated with the development of MBC; relative risk ratios were 2.2 and 1.79 respectively.[40] Though gynaecomastia in and of itself was once thought to be a risk factor, it is no longer considered to be.[34,36] Indeed, it may be the case that obesity is associated with both gynaecomastia and MBC.

Diagnosis

The differential diagnosis of a breast mass in a man is somewhat limited: gynaecomastia is by far the most common cause, while abscess, sarcoma and metastasis are much less common. The work-up of a breast mass is similar in men and women, although imaging studies are less important in men. Physical examination characterises the size, shape and location of a mass, as well as the presence of nipple discharge or retraction, and skin changes. Examination of axillary, supraclavicular nodes and infraclavicular nodes should be performed. A diagnostic mammogram and focused ultrasound can be used to visualise and to characterise the lesion, but rarely obviates the need for histological diagnosis. Since mastectomy is the treatment of choice in the majority of MBCs, breast imaging is of limited utility unless a limited excision is planned. As in women, core-needle biopsy is the diagnostic technique of choice. Symptoms, laboratory values and clinical stage should guide the work-up for metastatic MBC.

Treatment

In a retrospective review, Scott-Conner et al. found significant differences in the treatment of matched men and women with breast cancer.[41] Given anatomical considerations, compared to women, men are less likely to undergo breast-conserving surgery. Also, compared to women, men who undergo breast-conserving surgery are less likely to receive adjuvant radiotherapy. Men are also less likely to receive adjuvant chemotherapy.

Local therapy

Surgery – specifically, mastectomy – is the primary therapy for MBC. Although breast-conserving surgery has been performed for MBC, the minimal amount of mammary tissue in most men and the central location of most tumours do not make this a particularly attractive option. If a tumour is in close proximity to or involves the pectoralis major, it may be necessary to resect a small portion of underlying muscle to ensure a negative margin; there is no longer a role for radical mastectomy. Locally advanced disease should be treated with neoadjuvant therapy followed by mastectomy.

Axillary staging guidelines are similar for men and for women. If axillary lymph nodes are clinically negative, SLNB should be performed. Sensitivity and specificity of SLNB in women and men are similar.[42] Clinically positive nodes should undergo core biopsy or FNA for histological confirmation, which will allow axillary dissection without an SLNB.

Adjuvant therapy

The same guidelines used to make recommendations for adjuvant therapy in women with breast cancer should be used in men. Two comprehensive reviews confirmed the benefits of adjuvant chemotherapy and hormonal treatment in MBC.[43,44] Although no trials have been conducted to determine indications for postmastectomy radiation for MBC, it has been reported to reduce rates of local recurrence, and guidelines for women are usually applied for men.[45]

Treatment of metastatic disease

For hormone receptor-positive metastatic MBC, endocrine therapy is the mainstay of treatment. In the past, ablative surgeries, including orchiectomy, were used. A variety of hormonal therapies have been used, including exogenous steroids, androgens, antiandrogens, oestrogens, progestins, aminoglutethimide and tamoxifen, and may improve survival.[46,47] Tamoxifen is the drug of choice. In men, the testes produce 20% and the periphery produces 80% of circulating oestrogens. Thus, aromatase inhibitors pose two potential problems in MBC, mitigating their efficacy. Firstly, they only partially block oestrogen production. Secondly, decreased levels of circulating oestrogens induce the hypothalamus to stimulate testicular hormone production. This may, in part, account for therapeutic resistance in aromatase inhibitors.[48] A 2010 consensus conference concluded that aromatase inhibitors should only be used in men in conjunction with surgical or medical orchiectomy.[49] A phase II trial examining the use of an aromatase inhibitor combined with goserelin acetate

for androgen suppression is ongoing. For hormone receptor-negative MBC, chemotherapy is the mainstay of therapy.[46]

Prognosis

Overall, despite delays in presentation, diagnosis and treatment, stage for stage, women and men with breast cancer have the same prognosis, which continues to improve as new diagnostic methods and treatments evolve.[50–52] The same factors predict outcome: node status, tumour size and grade, and hormone receptor status. As for women with breast cancer, axillary lymph node status – negative versus positive, and number of positive nodes – is the most important prognostic factor in men.[53] In a study of 335 cases of MBC, node-negative patients had a 5-year survival rate of 90%, whereas node-positive patients had a 5-year survival rate of 65%.[54] Also, 10-year survival for patients with one to three positive nodes was 44%; with four or more positive nodes, it was 14%.[53] Giordano et al. reported that, for MBC, rates of 5-year survival were 76% for grade 1 tumours, 66% for grade 2 tumours and 43% for grade 3 tumours.[31] Patients with oestrogen receptor- and progesterone receptor-positive tumours had significantly improved survival compared to those with oestrogen receptor- and progesterone receptor-negative tumours,[55] reflecting differences in both biology and treatment.

Paget's disease of the breast (Fig. 10.3)

In 1856, Alfred-Armand-Louis-Marie Velpeau, a French surgeon and anatomist, described a clinical condition in which patients suffered from bleeding and crusting ulcerations of the nipple and areola.[56] Velpeau believed that this condition was primarily dermatological in nature, failing to recognise that more than 95% of women with what we now know as Paget's disease of the breast have an underlying malignancy. Nearly two decades later, Sir James Paget, the British surgeon and pathologist, described this association.[57] He described 'an eczematous change in the skin of the nipple preceding an underlying mammary cancer'.

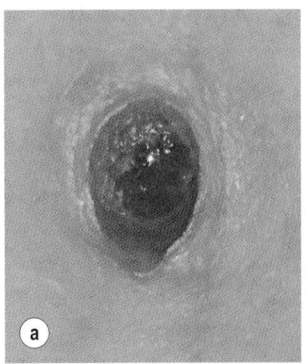 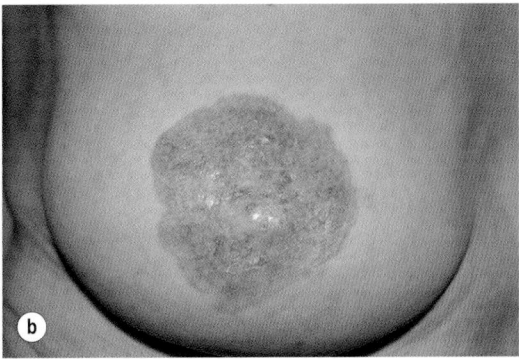

Figure 10.3 • (a) Early Paget's disease. **(b)** More extensive Paget's disease of the nipple.

Pathology

In Paget's disease of the breast, the epithelium of the nipple–areola complex displays two characteristic findings. First, Pagetoid cells are present – the *sine qua non* of Paget's disease of the breast. These are large, round or oval cells with enlarged pleomorphic and hyperchromatic nuclei, prominent nucleoli and abundant, clear, pale cytoplasm. Second, reactive changes in the epidermis and dermis, such as lymphocytic infiltration and angiogenesis, are also seen, giving rise to the hyperaemic, exudative appearance characteristic of Paget's disease of the breast.[58]

At present, there are two competing theories as to the pathogenesis of Paget's disease of the breast. One suggests that Pagetoid cells are keratinocytes that have undergone malignant transformation. According to this theory, Paget's disease of the breast represents an in situ carcinoma of the skin.[59,60] This theory is supported by the observation that, often, overlying skin changes and underlying malignancy are discontinuous. Another theory suggests that cells migrate along basement membranes and enter the epidermis and dermis of the nipple–areola complex.[61] Pagetoid cells and underlying carcinomas demonstrate similar immunohistochemical staining patterns, supporting this theory that it is cells from the cancer that migrate.[62]

Clinical presentation

Paget's disease of the breast occurs in both men and women. However, it is rare, accounting for 0.7–4.9% of breast malignancies.[59] Interestingly, age-adjusted rates of Paget's disease of the breast peaked in 1985 and have steadily decreased from 1.31 to 0.64 per 100 000.[63] The clear cause of this epidemiological phenomenon remains elusive, but it may be the case that as screening programmes are more widely available, clinically occult breast malignancies are detected prior to the development of dermatological nipple–areolar changes.

The first symptomatic manifestations are sensory – for example, lymphocytic infiltration and angiogenesis, which can produce burning or itching. Dermatological changes follow – crusty, erythematous flaking, and irregular, raised, scaly skin lesions may develop. Classically, these start within the nipple, spread to the areola and ultimately spread to the surrounding skin. This contrasts with eczema, which starts in the areola. As the disease progresses, bleeding, ulceration and destruction of the nipple–areola complex occur. Nipple discharge is rare and is usually a result of advanced local disease, rather than a consequence of Paget's disease. In approximately half of patients with Pagetoid changes of the nipple, an underlying malignancy is palpable.[64] Rarely, the underlying malignancy tethers the nipple–areola complex or adjacent skin, causing retractions and deformity of the natural contour of the breast.

In the absence of a palpable mass – in part because it is rare and has an innocuous appearance – misdiagnosis of Paget's disease as eczema and treatment with topical steroids is common.[60,65] Typically, the interval from the development of symptoms to definitive diagnosis and treatment is 10–12 months.[58]

Diagnosis

The diagnostic goals for suspected Paget's disease of the breast are twofold: confirmation that the cutaneous disease is Paget's and the detection of the underlying malignancy.

Eczematmous changes of the nipple–areola complex in the absence of a history suggestive of contact dermatitis should be biopsied. A punch biopsy can be performed and allows sampling of the epidermis, dermis and subdermis. If non-diagnostic, excisional biopsy is more invasive, but provides more tissue. Histology reveals Pagetoid cells. On immunohisto-chemistry, these cells stain for CK7, CAM-5.2, AE1/AE3 and S100; they do not stain for HMB-45 or keratins, differentiating them from melanoma.[66] Almost 90% of Paget's cells are HER-2 positive.

As with all breast cancers, bilateral mammography and ultrasound are the initial steps in the imaging work-up. If a lesion is seen, it is investigated in standard fashion. However, the sensitivity of mammography in this setting is limited; in one series, mammography detected only 32% of underlying carcinomas.[67] Breast MRI may be valuable in diagnosing clinically and mammographically occult underlying malignancies in patients with Paget's disease of the breast, with case reports and series demonstrating identification of carcinomas.[68,69] In a series of eight cases with a normal mammogram, MRI identified an underlying carcinoma in half.[67] Moreover, Morrogh et al. showed that MRI demonstrated the extent of occult disease in six of seven patients, thereby guiding surgical planning and the decision whether to pursue total mastectomy or breast conservation.[67,70]

Treatment (Table 10.1)

Surgery is the mainstay of treatment for Paget's disease of the breast – except for patients with significant comorbidities. For all patients, resection of the nipple–areola complex is necessary; small studies have demonstrated that preservation of the nipple–areola resulted in unacceptably high rates of local recurrence.[71] In patients with an identifiable primary tumour, the choice between total mastectomy and central lumpectomy is determined by the extent of disease. If disease is confined to the central breast, multiple small studies have demonstrated low rates of local recurrence after excision to negative margins and adjuvant radiotherapy. After a median follow-up of 6.4 years, one prospective study of 61 patients demonstrated a local recurrence rate of 5.2% after central lumpectomy to clear margins and 50 Gy of adjuvant radiotherapy.[72] When cancer is present at a distance from the nipple–areola complex, mastectomy is the treatment of choice. In the absence of an identifiable tumour within the breast, Paget's disease is considered to be ductal carcinoma in situ of the nipple–areolar region and can be treated with excision alone or excision and radiotherapy. In one small study of 48 patients, 40% of patients with Paget's disease of the breast treated with excision alone experienced a local recurrence after 4.6 years of median follow-up.[65]

Axillary staging with SLNB is performed when invasive cancer is present or if mastectomy is undertaken without a diagnosis of invasive cancer.

Guidelines for systemic therapy for women with and without Paget's disease of the breast are identical.

Prognosis

The underlying malignancy and the treatment thereof determine the prognosis of patients with Paget's disease of the breast.[73]

Table 10.1 • Conservative management of Paget's disease of the nipple

Reference	Year	n	Median follow-up (months)	Radiation	Recurrence (%)	No. of local recurrences	No. of distant recurrences	No. of deaths
Kawase et al.[74]	2005	12	84	Yes	8	1	0	0
Marshall et al.[75]	2003	36	113	Yes	11	4	0	0
Bijker et al.[72]	2001	61	77	Yes	5.2	4	2	1
Fu et al.[71]	2001	12	42	No	25	3	0	0
Kollmorgen et al.[76]	1998	10	71	No	20	0	2	2
Dixon et al.[65]	1991	10	56	No	40	4	0	0
Fourquet et al.[77]	1987	20	90	Yes	6.7	3	0	0

Other breast malignancies

Melanoma of the breast

Constituting 0.28% of all primary melanomas, primary melanoma of the breast is exceedingly infrequent.[78] Melanoma is more likely to present in the breast as a result of a metastasis from a non-mammary primary tumour.[79]

The investigation and treatment of melanoma of the breast is similar to the investigation and treatment of melanoma elsewhere. The history should focus on risk factors for its development – including cancer history, sun exposure and family history – and on changes in size or shape, ulceration or bleeding, and the presence of satellite, in-transit or distant lesions. Physical examination should include a comprehensive skin survey as well as examination of all nodal basins. Because it is a cutaneous lesion, mammography and ultrasound are generally not helpful in diagnosis or therapeutic planning. Rather, core-needle, punch or surgical biopsy of the thickest portion of the lesion should be performed, first to establish the diagnosis and second to determine the depth of invasion. Immunohistochemistry for HMB-45 and S100 may help differentiate melanoma from other cutaneous lesions. A thick lesion should prompt staging assessment, which may include measurement of serum lactate dehydrogenase (LDH) and imaging with CT, MRI or PET. Staging follows guidelines from the American Joint Committee on Cancer (AJCC) or International Union Against Cancer (UICC).

Surgical excision is the primary treatment for melanoma of the breast. In the past, mastectomy was considered the procedure of choice. Currently, it is recommended that patients undergo wide-local excision to margins determined by the depth of the lesion. SLNB is indicated for thin melanomas with poor prognostic features and for all intermediate and deep melanomas.[80] Clinically positive nodes and positive sentinel nodes should prompt axillary dissection.

Adjuvant treatment for primary melanoma of the breast follows current guidelines for adjuvant treatment of melanoma elsewhere.

Primary breast lymphoma (Fig. 10.4)

Primary breast lymphoma (PBL) constitutes 0.14% of all breast malignancies and 0.60–2.00% of all non-Hodgkin's lymphomas. It arises from

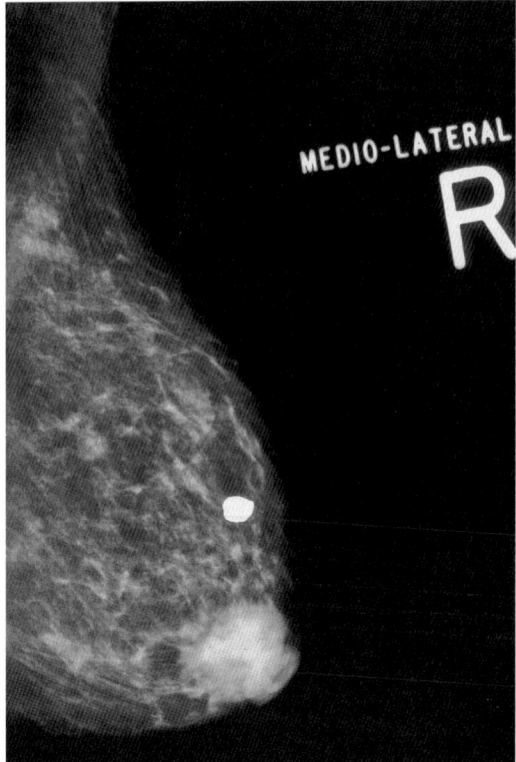

Figure 10.4 • Mammogram of a primary breast lymphoma in the subareolar space. The appearance is indistinguishable from that of a primary adenocarcinoma.

mammary lymphoid tissue and, by definition, is localised to the breast and its draining lymph node basins.[81,82] The most common subtype is diffuse large B-cell lymphoma.[81,82] PBLs are categorised using the Working Classification and the Ann Arbor Classification of lymphomas.

The mean age of patients with PBL is 65 years.[81,82] These lesions often present as a painless, enlarging and rubbery mass. Because mammographic and sonographic findings tend to be non-specific, PBL is usually not suspected (in the absence of constitutional symptoms) until a core-needle biopsy is obtained. Once the diagnosis is known, a complete history and physical examination should be obtained, focusing on constitutional symptoms and evaluation of lymph node basins. Additionally, CT of the chest, abdomen and pelvis, and bone marrow biopsy, are needed for adequate staging, though according to one pathological review, gene rearrangement analysis precluded the need for bone-marrow biopsy and histological evaluation in certain populations.[81]

In general, surgery is neither necessary nor recommended for PBL. According to single-institution reports, surgery either alone or in conjunction with radiation results in increased rates of local, regional or distant recurrence, and decreased rates of survival.[82,83] Surgery is no longer indicated for PBL except for situations in which the core-needle biopsy proves to be non-diagnostic. Chemotherapy directed to the histological type and targeted radiotherapy are the mainstays of treatment, and have proven to be modestly effective.[84–86] The role of rituximab continues to be evaluated.[87]

As with all lymphomas, the International Prognostic Index is helpful in predicting the aggressiveness of PBLs.[88] The 2-year overall survival of mammary lymphomas is 63%, which is consistent with the overall survival of extramammary lymphomas.[81] Immunohistochemical studies of PBLs have shown that tumours co-expressing bcl-6 and CD-10 have a better prognosis than those that do not.[83]

Angiosarcoma of the breast
(Fig. 10.5)

Angiosarcoma of the breast is rare, constituting 0.05% of all breast malignancies.[89] Primary angiosarcoma of the breast occurs sporadically; secondary angiosarcoma of the breast occurs in the setting of a history of radiotherapy and lymphoedema.[89] For an angiosarcoma of the breast to be considered radiotherapy induced, it must occur within the radiated field and

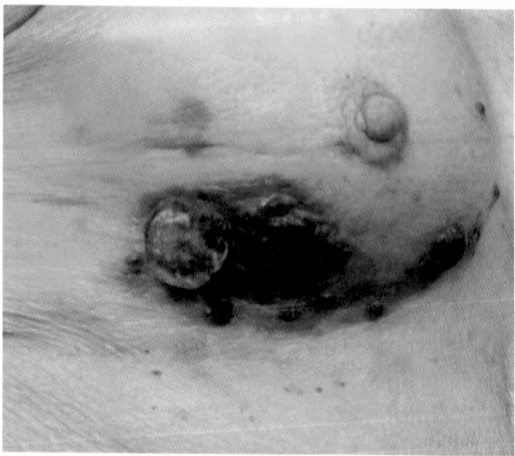

Figure 10.5 • Appearance of a radiation-induced angiosarcoma on the inferior-lateral aspect of a breast treated for invasive ductal carcinoma with lumpectomy and radiotherapy.

have a long latency. On average, the time interval from completion of radiotherapy to diagnosis of angiosarcoma of the breast is 75 months.[90] The first report of post-radiotherapy angiosarcoma of the breast was in 1981.[91] The incidence of angiosarcoma of the breast may be increasing – and may continue to increase – as more and more patients with breast cancer undergo breast-conserving therapy with irradiation.[92]

Primary angiosarcoma of the breast usually presents as a mass, while post-radiotherapy angiosarcoma of the breast usually presents as multifocal, painless, red, blue, purple or black skin nodules (Fig. 10.5).[93] The differential diagnosis of early skin lesions is fairly broad and includes benign radiation-associated skin changes, recurrent or de novo adenocarcinoma of the breast, and melanoma. Interestingly, the right breast is twice as likely to be affected as the left.[88]

Generally, mammography, ultrasound and MRI are not helpful.[94] Full-thickness punch, or incisional or excisional biopsy are diagnostic; FNA is not. Two molecular markers, factor VIII-related antigen and CD-34, are positive in most angiosarcomas, distinguishing angiosarcomas from other sarcomas.[92]

Staging of angiosarcomas of the breast mirrors staging of other sarcomas; it is based on tumour size, grade and depth. As in other sarcomas, grade is the most important determinant of prognosis. Whereas most primary angiosarcomas are low grade, most radiotherapy-induced angiosarcomas are high grade.[93]

Treatment consists of total mastectomy with wide resection of involved skin. The microscopic extent of disease is often greater than is clinically evident; every effort should be made to achieve widely negative skin margins. Axillary staging is not recommended since most sarcomas do not metastasise to regional lymph nodes. Adjuvant treatment follows recommendations for other sarcomas.[95] Recent case reports contend benefit for adjuvant radiotherapy, and in certain patients it may be considered.[89,95]

In one study of 58 patients, almost half were dead at an average follow-up period of 15 months.[90] In another study of 69 patients, the recurrence rate was 55% at a median follow-up of 40 months; the overall survival was 61% at 60 months.[95] In a third study of 49 patients, the local recurrence rate was 24% at 35 months, the distant recurrence rate was 58.5% at 34 months and the mortality was 44% at 29 months. These reports indicate that the prognosis is poor.

Metastasis to the breast

Metastasis to the breast is uncommon, accounting for 0.5–6.6% of breast malignancies.[96,97] The contralateral breast is the most common primary source.[92] Other primary sources include lymphoma, melanoma, rhabdomyosarcoma and small-cell lung cancer.[79]

Physical examination and imaging studies demonstrate masses indistinguishable from primary mammary carcinoma, although they are often circumscribed. In most cases, core-needle or excisional biopsy is preferred over FNA for pathological diagnosis since immunohistochemistry and the presence of an in situ component may play an important role in differentiating between primary and metastatic tumours.

Treatment is directed at the primary malignancy. Prognosis is poor: 80% of patients die within 1 year.[79]

Key points

Pregnancy-associated breast cancer

- A multidisciplinary approach and patient/family counselling are necessary.
- Mammography, sonography and image-guided biopsy are safe during pregnancy.
- Surgery can be performed during any trimester, though may be safest during the second. Radiotherapy is contraindicated. Chemotherapy can be given safely during the second and third trimesters.

Male breast cancer

- The investigation and treatment of male breast cancer mirror those of female breast cancer.
- Most male breast cancers are oestrogen receptor positive and the endocrine agent used most commonly is tamoxifen.
- The use of aromatase inhibitors in men is controversial.

Paget's disease of the breast

- Local treatment of Paget's disease of the breast includes either total mastectomy or central lumpectomy with adjuvant radiotherapy.
- SLNB is indicated when mastectomy is performed or in the presence of invasive carcinoma.
- Adjuvant treatment is determined by the receptor status of any underlying malignancy.

Other breast malignancies

- The investigation and treatment of other breast malignancies are determined by their pathological diagnosis.

References

1. Gemignani ML, Petrek JA, Borgen PI. Breast cancer and pregnancy. Surg Clin North Am 1999;79(5):1157–69.

2. Andersson TM, Johansson AL, Hsieh CC, et al. Increasing incidence of pregnancy-associated breast cancer in Sweden. Obstet Gynecol 2009;114(3):568–72.

3. Ishida T, Yokoe T, Kasumi F, et al. Clinicopathologic characteristics and prognosis of breast cancer patients associated with pregnancy and lactation: analysis of case–control study in Japan. Jpn J Cancer Res 1992;83(11):1143–9.

4. Guinee VF, Olsson H, Moller T, et al. Effect of pregnancy on prognosis for young women with breast cancer. Lancet 1994;343(8913):1587–9.

5. Barnes DM, Newman LA. Pregnancy-associated breast cancer: a literature review. Surg Clin North Am 2007;87:417–30.

6. Keleher AJ, Theriault RL, Gwyn KM, et al. Multidisciplinary management of breast cancer concurrent with pregnancy. J Am Coll Surg 2002;194(1):54–64.

7. Scott-Conner CE, Schorr SJ. The diagnosis and management of breast problems during pregnancy and lactation. Am J Surg 1995;170(4):401–5.

8. Woo JC, Yu T, Hurd TC. Breast cancer in pregnancy: a literature review. Arch Surg 2003;138(1):91–9.

9. Liberman L, Giess CS, Dershaw DD, et al. Imaging of pregnancy-associated breast cancer. Radiology 1994;191(1):245–8.

10. Schackmuth EM, Harlow CL, Norton LW. Milk fistula: a complication after core breast biopsy. Am J Roentgenol 1993;161(5):961–2.

11. Loibl S, von Minckwitz G, Gwyn K, et al. Breast carcinoma during pregnancy. International recommendations from an expert meeting. Cancer 2006;106(2):237–46.

12. Duncan PG, Pope WD, Cohen MM, et al. Fetal risk of anesthesia and surgery during pregnancy. Anesthesiology 1986;64(6):790–4.

13. Gentilini O, Cremonesi M, Toesca A, et al. Sentinel lymph node biopsy in pregnant patients with breast cancer. Eur J Nucl Med Mol Imaging 2010;37(1):78–83.

14. Ebert U, Loffler H, Kirch W. Cytotoxic therapy and pregnancy. Pharmacol Ther 1997;74(2):207–20.

15. Berry DL, Theriault RL, Holmes FA, et al. Management of breast cancer during pregnancy using a standardized protocol. J Clin Oncol 1999;17(3):855–61.

16. Hahn KM, Johnson PH, Gordon N, et al. Treatment of pregnant breast cancer patients and outcomes of children exposed to chemotherapy in utero. Cancer 2006;107(6):1219–26.

17. Mir O, Berveiller P, Ropert S, et al. Emerging therapeutic options for breast cancer chemotherapy during pregnancy. Ann Oncol 2008;19(4):607–13.

18. Isaacs RJ, Hunter W, Clark K. Tamoxifen as systemic treatment of advanced breast cancer during pregnancy – Case report and literature review. Gynecol Oncol 2001;80(3):405–8.

19. Kroman N, Jensen MB, Wohlfahrt J, et al. Pregnancy after treatment of breast cancer – a population-based study on behalf of Danish Breast Cancer Cooperative Group. Acta Oncol 2008;47(4):545–9.

20. Ives A, Saunders C, Bulsara M, et al. Pregnancy after breast cancer: population based study. Br Med J 2007;334(7586):194.

21. Beadle BM, Woodward WA, Middleton LP, et al. The impact of pregnancy on breast cancer outcomes in women ≤35 years. Cancer 2009;115(6):1174–84.

22. Love SM, Linsey K. Dr. Susan Love's breast book. 5th ed. Philadelphia: Da Capo Press; 2010.

23. Weir HK, Thun MJ, Hankey BF, et al. Annual report to the nation on the status of cancer, 1975–2000, featuring the uses of surveillance data for cancer prevention and control. J Natl Cancer Inst 2003;95(17):1276–99.

24. La Vecchia C, Levi F, Lucchini F. Descriptive epidemiology of male breast cancer in Europe. Int J Cancer 1992;51(1):62–6.

25. Stang A, Thomssen C. Decline in breast cancer incidence in the United States: what about male breast cancer? Breast Cancer Res Treat 2008;112(3):595–6.

26. Anderson WF, Devesa SS. In situ male breast carcinoma in the Surveillance, Epidemiology, and End Results database of the National Cancer Institute. Cancer 2005;104(8):1733–41.

27. Sasco AJ, Lowenfels AB, Pasker-de Jong P. Review article: epidemiology of male breast cancer. A meta-analysis of published case–control studies and discussion of selected aetiological factors. Int J Cancer 1993;53(4):538–49.

28. Stalsberg H, Thomas DB, Rosenblatt KA, et al. Histologic types and hormone receptors in breast cancer in men: a population-based study in 282 United States men. Cancer Causes Control 1993;4(2):143–51.

29. Giordano SH, Buzdar AU, Hortobagyi GN. Breast cancer in men. Ann Intern Med 2002;137(8):678–87.

30. Hittmair AP, Lininger RA, Tavassoli FA. Ductal carcinoma in situ (DCIS) in the male breast: a morphologic study of 84 cases of pure DCIS and 30 cases of DCIS associated with invasive carcinoma – a preliminary report. Cancer 1998;83(10):2139–49.

31. Giordano SH, Cohen DS, Buzdar AU, et al. Breast carcinoma in men: a population-based study. Cancer 2004;101(1):51–7.

32. Ribeiro G. Male breast carcinoma – a review of 301 cases from the Christie Hospital & Holt Radium Institute, Manchester. Br J Cancer 1985;51(1):115–9.

33. Goss PE, Reid C, Pintilie M, et al. Male breast carcinoma: a review of 229 patients who presented to the Princess Margaret Hospital during 40 years: 1955–1996. Cancer 1999;85(3):629–39.

34. Pant K, Dutta U. Understanding and management of male breast cancer: a critical review. Med Oncol 2008;25(3):294–8.

35. Lynch HT, Kaplan AR, Lynch JF. Klinefelter syndrome and cancer. A family study. JAMA 1974;229(7):809–11.

36. Thomas DB, Jimenez LM, McTiernan A, et al. Breast cancer in men: risk factors with hormonal implications. Am J Epidemiol 1992;135(7):734–48.

37. Thorlacius S, Olafsdottir G, Tryggvadottir L, et al. A single BRCA2 mutation in male and female breast cancer families from Iceland with varied cancer phenotypes. Nat Genet 1996;13(1):117–9.

38. Friedman LS, Gayther SA, Kurosaki T, et al. Mutation analysis of BRCA1 and BRCA2 in a male breast cancer population. Am J Hum Genet 1997;60(2):313–9.

39. Brose MS, Rebbeck TR, Calzone KA, et al. Cancer risk estimates for BRCA1 mutation carriers identified in a risk evaluation program. J Natl Cancer Inst 2002;94(18):1365–72.

40. Brinton LA, Richesson DA, Gierach GL, et al. Prospective evaluation of risk factors for male breast cancer. J Natl Cancer Inst 2008;100(20):1477–81.

41. Scott-Conner CE, Jochimsen PR, Menck HR, et al. An analysis of male and female breast cancer treatment and survival among demographically identical pairs of patients. Surgery 1999;126(4):775–81.

42. Port ER, Fey JV, Cody 3rd HS, et al. Sentinel lymph node biopsy in patients with male breast carcinoma. Cancer 2001;91(2):319–23.

43. Fentiman IS, Fourquet A, Hortobagyi GN. Male breast cancer. Lancet 2006;367(9510):595–604.

44. Agrawal A, Ayantunde AA, Rampaul R, et al. Male breast cancer: a review of clinical management. Breast Cancer Res Treat 2007;103(1):11–21.

45. Schuchardt U, Seegenschmiedt MH, Kirschner MJ, et al. Adjuvant radiotherapy for breast carcinoma in men: a 20-year clinical experience. Am J Clin Oncol 1996;19(4):330–6.

46. Jaiyesimi IA, Buzdar AU, Sahin AA, et al. Carcinoma of the male breast. Ann Intern Med 1992;117(9):771–7.

47. Ribeiro G, Swindell R. Adjuvant tamoxifen for male breast cancer (MBC). Br J Cancer 1992;65(2):252–4.

48. Doyen J, Italiano A, Largillier R, et al. Aromatase inhibition in male breast cancer patients: biological and clinical implications. Ann Oncol 2010;21(6):1243–5.

49. Korde LA, Zujewski JA, Kamin L, et al. Multidisciplinary meeting on male breast cancer: summary and research recommendations. J Clin Oncol 2010;28(12):2114–22.

50. Anderson WF, Jatoi I, Tse J, et al. Male breast cancer: a population-based comparison with female breast cancer. J Clin Oncol 2010;28(2):232–9.

51. Cutuli B, Le-Nir CC, Serin D, et al. Male breast cancer. Evolution of treatment and prognostic factors. Analysis of 489 cases. Crit Rev Oncol/Hematol 2010;73(3):246–54.

52. Miao H, Verkooijen HM, Chia KS, et al. Incidence and outcome of male breast cancer: an international population-based study. J Clin Oncol 2011;29(33):4381–6.

53. Cutuli B, Lacroze M, Dilhuydy JM, et al. Male breast cancer: results of the treatments and prognostic factors in 397 cases. Eur J Cancer 1995;31A(12):1960–4.

54. Guinee VF, Olsson H, Moller T, et al. The prognosis of breast cancer in males. A report of 335 cases. Cancer 1993;71(1):154–61.

55. Donegan WL, Redlich PN, Lang PJ, et al. Carcinoma of the breast in males: a multiinstitutional survey. Cancer 1998;83(3):498–509.

56. Velpeau A-A-L-M. A treatise on diseases of the breast and mammary region. London: Sydenham Society; 1856.

57. Paget J. On disease of the mammary areola preceding cancer of the mammary gland. St Bartholomews Hosp J 1874;10:87–9.

58. Sakorafas GH, Blanchard K, Sarr MG, et al. Paget's disease of the breast. Cancer Treat Rev 2001;27:9–18.

59. Lagios MD, Westdahl PR, Rose MR, et al. Paget's disease of the nipple. Alternative management in cases without or with minimal extent of underlying breast-carcinoma. Cancer 1984;54(3):545–51.

60. Kothari AS, Beechey-Newman N, Hamed H, et al. Paget disease of the nipple: a multifocal manifestation of higher-risk disease. Cancer 2002;95(1):1–7.

61. Jahn H, Osther PJ, Nielsen EH, et al. An electron microscopic study of clinical Paget's disease of the nipple. Acta Pathol Microbiol Immunol Scand 1995;103(9):628–34.

62. Fu W, Lobocki CA, Silberberg BK, et al. Molecular markers in Paget disease of the breast. J Surg Oncol 2001;77(3):171–8.

63. Chen CY, Sun LM, Anderson BO. Paget disease of the breast: changing patterns of incidence, clinical presentation, and treatment in the US. Cancer 2006;107(7):1448–58.

64. Kaelin C. Paget's disease. In: Harris JR, Lippman ME, Morrow M, et al., editors. Diseases of the breast. 2nd ed. Baltimore: Lippincott, Williams & Wilkins; 2000. p. 227–83.

65. Dixon AR, Galea MH, Ellis IO, et al. Paget's disease of the nipple. Br J Surg 1991;78(6):722–3.

66. Hitchcock A, Topham S, Bell J, et al. Routine diagnosis of mammary Paget's disease. A modern approach. Am J Surg Pathol 1992;16(1):58–61.

67. Morrogh M, Morris EA, Liberman L, et al. MRI identifies otherwise occult disease in select patients with Paget disease of the nipple. J Am Coll Surg 2008;206(2):316–21.

68. Echevarria JJ, Lopez-Ruiz JA, Martin D, et al. Usefulness of MRI in detecting occult breast cancer associated with Paget's disease of the nipple–areolar complex. Br J Radiol 2004;77(924):1036–9.

69. Frei KA, Bonel HM, Pelte M-F, et al. Paget disease of the breast: findings at magnetic resonance imaging and histopathologic correlation. Invest Radiol 2005;40(6):363–7.

70. Dominici LS, Lester S, Liao GS, et al. Current surgical approach to Paget's disease. Am J Surg 2012;204(1):18–22.

71. Fu W, Mittel VK, Young SC. Paget disease of the breast: analysis of 41 patients. Am J Clin Oncol 2001;24(4):397–400.

72. Bijker N, Rutgers EJ, Duchateau L, et al. Breast-conserving therapy for Paget disease of the nipple: a prospective European Organization for Research and Treatment of Cancer study of 61 patients. Cancer 2001;91(3):472–7.

73. Dalberg K, Hellborg H, Wärnberg F. Paget's disease of the nipple in a population based cohort. Breast Cancer Res Treat 2008;111(2):313–9.

74. Kawase K, Dimaio DJ, Tucker SL, et al. Paget's disease of the breast: there is a role for breast-conserving therapy. Ann Surg Oncol 2005;12(5):391–7.

75. Marshall JK, Griffith KA, Haffty BJ, et al. Conservative management of Paget disease of the breast with radiotherapy: 10- and 15-year results. Cancer 2003;97(9):2142–9.

76. Kollmorgen DR, Varanasi JS, Edge SB, et al. Paget's disease of the breast: a 33-year experience. J Am Coll Surg 1998;187(2):171–7.

77. Fourquet A, Campana F, Vielh P, et al. Paget's disease of the nipple without detectable breast tumor: conservative management with radiation therapy. Int J Radiat Oncol Biol Phys 1987;13(10):1463–5.

78. Ariel IM, Caron AS. Diagnosis and treatment of malignant melanoma arising from the skin of the female breast. Am J Surg 1972;124(3):384–90.

79. Bartella L, Kaye J, Perry NM, et al. Metastases to the breast revisited: radiological–histopathological correlation. Clin Radiol 2003;58(7):524–31.

80. Bedrosian I, Faries MB, Guerry DT, et al. Incidence of sentinel node metastasis in patients with thin primary melanoma (< or = 1 mm) with vertical growth phase. Ann Surg Oncol 2000;7(4):262–7.

81. Topalovski M, Crisan D, Mattson JC. Lymphoma of the breast. A clinicopathologic study of primary and secondary cases. Arch Pathol Lab Med 1999;123(12):1208–18.

82. Kuper-Hommel MJ, Snijder S, Janssen-Heijnen ML, et al. Treatment and survival of 38 female breast lymphomas: a population-based study with clinical and pathological reviews. Ann Hematol 2003; 82(7):397–404.

83. Fruchart C, Denoux Y, Chasle J, et al. High grade primary breast lymphoma: is it a different clinical entity? Breast Cancer Res Treat 2005;93(3):191–8.

84. Jeanneret-Sozzi W, Taghian A, Epelbaum R, et al. Primary breast lymphoma: patient profile, outcome and prognostic factors. A multicentre Rare Cancer Network study. BMC Cancer 2008;8:86.

85. Ryan G, Martinelli G, Kuper-Hommel M, et al. Primary diffuse large B-cell lymphoma of the breast: prognostic factors and outcomes of a study by the International Extranodal Lymphoma Study Group. Ann Oncol 2008;19(2):233–41.

86. Martinelli G, Ryan G, Seymour JF, et al. Primary follicular and marginal-zone lymphoma of the breast: clinical features, prognostic factors and outcome: a study by the International Extranodal Lymphoma Study Group. Ann Oncol 2009;20(12):1993–9.

87. Aviles A, Neri N, Nambo MJ. The role of genotype in 104 cases of diffuse large B-cell lymphoma primary of breast. Am J Clin Oncol 2012;35(2):126–9.

88. The International Non-Hodgkin's Lymphoma Prognostic Factors Project. A predictive model for aggressive non-Hodgkin's lymphoma. N Engl J Med 1993;329(14):987–94.

89. Nascimento AF, Raut CP, Fletcher CD. Primary angiosarcoma of the breast: clinicopathologic analysis of 49 cases, suggesting that grade is not prognostic. Am J Surg Pathol 2008;32(12):1896–904.

90. Rao J, DeKoven JG, Beatty JD, et al. Cutaneous angiosarcoma as a delayed complication of radiation therapy for carcinoma of the breast. J Am Acad Dermatol 2003;49(3):532–538.

91. Maddox JC, Evans HL. Angiosarcoma of skin and soft tissue: a study of forty-four cases. Cancer 1981;48(8):1907–21.

92. Monroe AT, Feigenberg SJ, Mendenhall NP. Angiosarcoma after breast-conserving therapy. Cancer 2003;97(8):1832–40.

93. Scow JS, Reynolds CA, Degnim AC, et al. Primary and secondary angiosarcoma of the breast: the Mayo Clinic experience. J Surg Oncol 2010;101(5):401–7.

94. Glazebrook KN, Magut MJ, Reynolds C. Angiosarcoma of the breast. Am J Roentgenol 2008;190(2):533–8.

95. Sher T, Hennessy BT, Valero V, et al. Primary angiosarcomas of the breast. Cancer 2007;110(1):173–8.

96. Paulus DD, Libshitz HI. Metastasis to the breast. Radiol Clin North Am 1982;20(3):561–8.

97. Amichetti M, Perani B, Boi S. Metastases to the breast from extramammary malignancies. Oncology 1990;47(3):257–60.

11

Treatment of ductal carcinoma in situ

Nicola L.P. Barnes
Nigel J. Bundred

Background

The introduction of screening mammography has resulted in a marked increase in the detection rates of ductal carcinoma in situ (DCIS) from 2% of newly diagnosed breast cancers before national screening to 20% of all screen-detected tumours.[1] DCIS is a preinvasive breast cancer; the proliferation of malignant ductal epithelial cells remains confined by an intact basement membrane, with no invasion into the surrounding stroma.[2] Over 90% of DCIS lesions currently diagnosed are impalpable, asymptomatic and detected by screening. These screening-detected cases are frequently small (<4 cm) and localised, and breast-conserving surgery is often possible. The remaining 10% present symptomatically, with a palpable breast lump, nipple discharge or Paget's disease of the nipple. If these symptoms are present, the underlying disease is often extensive and usually requires mastectomy.

Risk factors, natural history, pathology and receptors

Risk factors

Risk factors for the development of DCIS include a family history of breast cancer, older age at first childbirth and nulliparity.[3] Although breast epithelial proliferation is increased by the use of the oral contraceptive pill[4] and hormone replacement therapy (HRT), particularly combined oestrogen/progestogen HRT for over 5 years,[5] there is little evidence to date that either the oral contraceptive pill or HRT increases the risk of DCIS.[4] Two studies[6,7] have reported a relative risk of 1.4 for the development of DCIS following oestrogen-only HRT preparations and a relative risk of 1.7–2.3 with oestrogen- and progestogen-containing preparations.[8] In the Women's Health Initiative study there were 47 cases of DCIS in the HRT group compared with 37 cases in the control group (hazard ratio 1.18; weighted $P = 0.09$). Other studies have shown no increased risk following HRT use.[9,10]

Natural history

Although factors that pertain to an increased risk of developing DCIS have been identified, the natural history of this heterogeneous disease remains poorly understood. It is thought that developmental pathways for low- and intermediate-grade DCIS are distinct from the development of high-grade DCIS and can be explained partly by reference to biological markers. In the sequence of progression from normal breast to DCIS, there is a variable loss of chromosomal heterozygosity dependent on nuclear grade. Low- and intermediate-grade tumours show 16q loss, whereas there is 17q gain in high-grade lesions.[11] It is likely that low-grade lesions arise from oestrogen receptor-positive atypical ductal hyperplasia (ADH) or lobular intra-epithelial neoplasia carcinoma and progress to low-grade oestrogen receptor-positive DCIS. High-grade lesions have no obvious precursor, unless they arise from usual ductal hyperplasia or ADH that expresses 17q gain. The progression of well-differentiated/low-grade DCIS to poorly differentiated/high-grade DCIS or high-grade invasive cancer is an uncommon event.[12]

✔ A review of DCIS recurrences and their primary lesions from the EORTC 10853 trial[12,13] found concordant histology (similar grade) in 62% of cases, and identical marker expression (oestrogen receptor, progesterone receptor, p53 and c-erbB-2/HER-2/*neu*) in 63% of both invasive and non-invasive recurrences.[12] This high percentage of tumours with identical receptor profiles indicates that it is likely that residual disease after initial treatment recurs as detectable DCIS or progresses to invasive cancer.

Retrospective studies of low-grade DCIS misdiagnosed as benign conditions found that, 20 years after local excision, approximately 33% had developed an invasive cancer.[14] As not all cases of DCIS progress to invasive disease, detection by mammographic screening may lead to over-treatment of 'non-progressive DCIS', i.e. DCIS that would not progress to invasive disease if left untreated. It was hoped that breast screening programmes would, after a lag phase, result in a decreased incidence of invasive breast cancer, secondary to an increase in detection and treatment of DCIS. This has not been demonstrated, as there has been no corresponding decrease in invasive disease in a recent review of American screening data although there appears to be a reduction in grade 3 cancers in women of screening age over time.[15] There is therefore now concern that we may be over-treating DCIS and in particular 'low-risk' DCIS, and that such lesions may never pose a threat to a patient's life. Suggestions for alternative management strategies for these patients range from endocrine therapy alone (no surgery)[16] to, at the most extreme, 'watchful waiting'.[15] However, what constitutes 'low-risk' DCIS remains undefined.

The recent MAP.3 trial showed that exemestane reduces DCIS development in a prevention setting.[17] A study looking at ADH (which may be a precursor lesion of low-grade DCIS and has an approximately fivefold increase in risk of subsequent invasive cancer) showed that ADH (and by implication, low-grade DCIS) has become less common since women have stopped using as much HRT.[18] The low-grade lesions are the ones that are being potentially over-treated. They are nearly always oestrogen dependent. Removing the oestrogenic drive, either following menopause or with the use of aromatase inhibitors, may allow control of these low-grade cases so they progress to invasive cancer only rarely.

Stem cells

Recent evidence suggests that the breast has stem cells that can reconstitute the various cell types within the breast after trauma. Cancers (including DCIS) arise from accumulations of mutations within stem cells that disrupt their tightly controlled self-renewal and proliferation processes. Stem cells have recently been isolated from human DCIS. In this process, samples of human DCIS tissue have been separated into single cells and a subset of these cells (which are putative stem/progenitor cells) grows, in non-adherent culture conditions, to form three-dimensional branching structures (known as mammospheres). Mammosphere growth is dependent on growth simulation via the epidermal growth factor (EGF) and Notch receptor pathways.[19] The DCIS stem cell paradigm could explain the development of both multifocal DCIS and local recurrence. Stem cells could potentially survive after wide local excision with clear margins and regrow, which would also explain the 'identical' receptor expression seen in recurrent DCIS as well as early recurrences seen most often in high-grade DCIS, as there are more stem cells found in these high-grade lesions. Potentially, therefore, targeted inhibition of stem cells could reduce the rate of DCIS recurrence.

Pathology

Classification and features

DCIS has been classified into two major subtypes according to the presence or absence of comedo necrosis. DCIS is designated as comedo if atypical cells with abundant luminal necrosis fill at least one duct. In comedo, DCIS cells are large with pleomorphic nuclei and abnormal mitoses. The necrotic material often calcifies and this is what is visible on mammography.

Non-comedo DCIS encompasses all other subtypes and includes the following types:

- Solid – where tumour fills extended duct spaces.
- Micropapillary – where tufts of cells project into the duct lumen perpendicular to the basement membrane.
- Papillary – where the projecting tufts are larger than in the micropapillary type and contain a fibrovascular core.
- Cribriform – where the tumour takes on a fenestrated/sieve-like appearance.
- Clinging (flat) – where there are variable columnar cell alterations along the duct margins. (There remains controversy as to whether clinging DCIS is truly an in situ cancer or whether it should be considered as atypical hyperplasia rather than DCIS.)

Rarer subtypes also exist, including neuroendocrine, encysted papillary, apocrine and signet cell.

The UK- and EU-funded breast screening programmes classify DCIS as of low, intermediate and high nuclear grade. This definition is based on the characteristics of the lesion as seen with a high-power microscope lens (×40) and uses a comparison of tumour cell size with normal epithelial and red blood cell size:[20]

- Low nuclear grade DCIS has evenly spaced cells with centrally placed small nuclei and few mitoses and nucleoli that are not easily seen.
- High nuclear grade DCIS has pleomorphic irregularly spaced cells with large irregular nuclei (often three times the size of erythrocytes), prominent nucleoli and frequent mitoses. It is often solid with comedo necrosis and calcification.
- Intermediate-grade DCIS has features between those seen in low- and high-grade DCIS.

If a lesion contains areas of varying grade, it is awarded the highest grade present. A universally agreed classification system is yet to be established and will need to be observer independent and clinically relevant. The majority of DCIS lesions are high grade. Most cases of DCIS are unicentric.[21] Following extensive pathological sectioning of DCIS mastectomy specimens, only 1% show multicentric disease.[21] A **multicentric** tumour is defined as separate foci of tumour found in more than one breast quadrant, or more than 5 cm away from

the initial primary. A tumour is classified as **multifocal** if there are separate tumour foci in the same quadrant that are close to each other, although most such lesions have similar morphology and are linked.[22] The local spread of DCIS is along branching ducts that form the glandular breast. The ducts, which are ill defined, often extend beyond the borders of a quadrant. Most DCIS is continuous along the branching ductal network. Poorly differentiated high-grade lesions are reported to be more frequently multifocal.[23] Most DCIS recurrences are at or near the site of the initial tumour,[24] but some recurrences are remote from the initial lesion yet exhibit similar genotypical and phenotypical characteristics to the primary lesion.[12]

As well as documenting pathological type and grade on the histology report, the pathologist should detail the presence or absence of microinvasion. If microinvasion is detected histologically, a thorough examination of the entire specimen should be undertaken to exclude other previously unnoticed areas of invasive cancer. Lesions that can be mistaken for microinvasion include DCIS involving lobules, branching of ducts, distortion of ducts by acini or fibrosis, crush or cautery artefacts, and DCIS involving a benign sclerosing process (e.g. radial scar).[25-29]

Lobular intraepithelial neoplasia (LIN)

The current classification combines lobular carcinoma in situ (LCIS) and atypical lobular hyperplasia (ALH) into a single entity known as lobular intraepithelial neoplasia (LIN). Rather than a premalignant lesion, LIN is considered a marker of increased risk. It is often an incidental finding during breast biopsy and accounts for approximately 0.5% of symptomatic and 1% of screen-detected tumours. In situ ductal and lobular tumours show different pathological and clinical features. Compared with DCIS, patients developing LIN tend to be younger and premenopausal, and have bilateral and multicentric disease of lower grade and close to 100% oestrogen receptor expression (Table 11.1). There is an approximate eight- to ninefold increased risk of developing invasive carcinoma after a diagnosis of LCIS compared to the general population.[30] Sometimes it is difficult to distinguish histologically between LCIS and DCIS, and the

Table 11.1 • Comparative clinicopathological features of ductal carcinoma in situ (DCIS) and tabular carcinoma in situ (LCIS)

Clinicopatho-logical feature	DCIS	LCIS
Age at diagnosis (years)	54–58	44–47
Premenopausal	30%	70%
Absence of clinical signs	90%	99%
Mammographic findings	Microcalcifications	None
Multicentric disease	30%	90%
Bilateral disease	12–20%	90%
Histological grade	65% high grade	90% low grade
Oestrogen receptor status	65% positive	95% positive
Subsequent invasive disease	30–40%	25–30%
Ipsilateral–contralateral ratio	9:1	1:1

pathology report should state this. The clinical interpretation of the report should take into account the increased risks from both tumour subtypes.

If LIN is detected at core biopsy, the area of suspicion is usually excised to confirm the diagnosis and exclude an adjacent invasive focus. If LIN is diagnosed coincidentally following excision of a coexisting lesion, no further surgical treatment is necessary (even if the area of lobular neoplasia is not fully excised) and the patient should undergo regular review on a 'watch and wait' basis or be considered for a preventional strategy. The NSABP P-1 prevention trial showed a 56% reduction in the risk of developing subsequent invasive cancer in women with LCIS who received tamoxifen.[31] Further studies are ongoing with aromatase inhibitors in postmenopausal patients with LIN. Chemotherapy and radiotherapy have no place in the treatment of lobular neoplasia. A problem area is pleomorphic LCIS. The current perspective is that this should be treated like DCIS rather than lobular neoplasia but the scientific basis for this is minimal. Further studies and clarification of the behaviour and most appropriate treatment of pleomorphic LCIS is needed urgently.

Receptors and markers

To advance our understanding of the development and behaviour of DCIS, there has been interest in cell receptor expression and signalling pathways controlling growth. These studies have been mainly based on immunohistochemical assessment and show that poorly differentiated high-grade comedo DCIS has low oestrogen receptor expression, high rates of cell proliferation[32] (as expressed by Ki67, a nuclear antigen expressed in late G_1 S, G_2 and M phases of the cell cycle but not in the quiescent G_0),[33] high rates of apoptosis,[34] and over-expression of HER-2 and epidermal growth factor receptor (EGFR (HER-1)).[32] Low-grade lesions in contrast have high oestrogen receptor expression, with lower rates of cell proliferation[32] and apoptosis than high-grade lesions,[34] and they rarely overexpress HER-2.[32] Progesterone receptor expression correlates with oestrogen receptor expression in both low- and high-grade tumours.[32] In comparison, normal breast epithelium has low levels of expression of oestrogen receptor and progesterone receptor,[35] and a very low rate of apoptosis and HER-2 expression.

The increased rate of apoptosis seen in DCIS is lost on progression to invasive cancer, but the high proliferative rate is maintained.[36] Cyclin D1, an oncogene responsible for G_1 cell cycle proliferation/progression and induction of apoptosis, is overexpressed in approximately 90% of in situ and invasive ductal cancers.[37] It also appears to be associated with a loss of differentiation (measured by p27[Kip1]).[38] In oestrogen receptor-positive tumours, the driving force behind this increase in cell proliferation is the nuclear action of the activated oestrogen receptor, which increases growth-promoting gene transcription. In oestrogen receptor-negative DCIS, the driving pathway is thought to be predominantly via EGFR/HER-2/RAS/MAP kinase activation (**Fig. 11.1**). This leads to a subsequent increase in transcription of both proliferative and, via Akt, anti-apoptotic genes. Activation of this pathway also induces the expression of cyclo-oxygenase-2 (COX-2), which is an inducible enzyme that converts arachidonic acid to prostaglandins. It has been found to be overexpressed in up to 80% of DCIS.[39] COX-2-positive DCIS shows increased cell proliferation,

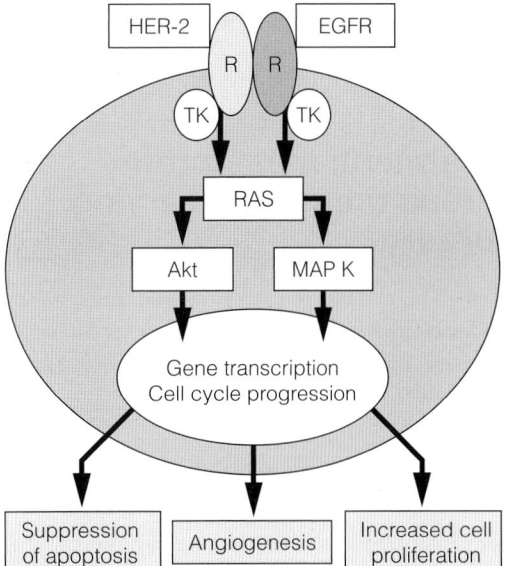

Figure 11.1 • The basic growth pathway in oestrogen receptor-negative breast tumour cells. The oestrogen receptor-positive signalling pathway is mediated via oestrogen attaching to its receptor, which then moves down its concentration gradient to the cell nucleus. The presence of oestrogen receptor in the cell nucleus subsequently increases gene transcription and expression of growth-promoting factors, leading to increased cell proliferation and tumour growth. In cells that do not express oestrogen receptors, the main signalling pathway for growth is via the epidermal growth factor (EGF)/c-erbB-2 receptor; this activates the RAS intracellular messenger, which increases cell proliferation and tumour growth via MAP kinase. RAS stimulation also leads to the suppression of the apoptosis cascade via Akt and BAD phosphorylation (an apoptotic protein). MAP K, MAP kinase; R, receptor; TK, tyrosine kinase.

and is related to increased tumour recurrence and decreased survival in invasive cancer.[40]

In addition to alterations in cell proliferation and apoptosis, the development of neovascularisation is necessary for the growth of solid tumours. It is driven in part by angiogenic factors expressed in hypoxic areas of the tumour. Hypoxic areas of DCIS show a less well differentiated, more malignant phenotype, with increased HIF-1α (a hypoxia-induced transcription factor), decreased oestrogen receptor expression and increased expression of cytokeratin-19 (a breast stem cell marker).[27] It is felt that hypoxia-induced dedifferentiation could be a factor promoting tumour progression.[41]

Presentation, investigation and diagnosis

Presentation

Over 90% of DCIS is detected by mammographic screening. Approximately 70% of these mammographically detected cases present as microcalcifications with no associated mass lesion. Calcifications may be heterogeneous, fine, linear, branching, malignant or of indeterminate appearance. Microcalcifications with an associated mass lesion are seen in approximately 30% of DCIS diagnosed by screening.[42] Circumscribed nodules, ill-defined masses, duct asymmetry and architectural distortion are sometimes seen in association with DCIS.[43] When diagnosed clinically, DCIS is often extensive or associated with a concurrent invasive tumour. It may present as a palpable mass, Paget's disease of the nipple or nipple discharge.[44]

Investigation and diagnosis

Thorough clinical examination is important to detect clinical signs of DCIS or coexisting pathology. In addition to clinical examination (often normal), ultrasound can be valuable to exclude an associated mass lesion. Diagnosis is confirmed by core biopsy, as cytology gives no information on stromal invasion. Image guidance is essential to ensure the accuracy of sampling. Mammographic magnification views are important in order to delineate accurately the extent of the microcalcifications.

Stereotactic core biopsy and vacuum-assisted biopsy

In the NHS Breast Screening Programme, the primary method of diagnosis was formerly by stereotactic core biopsy with a 14 G needle. If image-guided core biopsy was inconclusive then vacuum-assisted biopsy (VAB) using a device such as a Mammotome, which takes several contiguous biopsies of a wider calibre (11 G) during a single pass, can be used. A metal clip can be inserted during the procedure to aid future localisation. VAB has a higher sensitivity and specificity than core biopsy and is now the biopsy technique of choice for microcalcification,[45] but still underdiagnoses a coexisting invasive tumour in 10–20% of cases due to sampling error.[46] Other factors that have been shown to underestimate the presence of associated invasive disease include high-grade lesions, imaging size >2 cm, Breast Imaging and Reporting Data System (BI-RADS) score of 4 or 5, a visable mass at mammography (versus only calcification) and a palpable abnormality.[45] If the area of DCIS is extensive (>4 cm in size), two or more areas should be biopsied preoperatively to increase the chance of detecting any associated invasive component.

Localisation-guided biopsy

If a definitive histological diagnosis cannot be made with core biopsy or VAB, this due to failure to sample the calcification adequately, or doubt exists as to whether DCIS is present on histology, then open biopsy is necessary (see Chapter 1). The excised specimen should be sent for immediate radiography, after careful orientation with Liga-clips or metal markers, to confirm that all microcalcification of concern has been excised and is clear of margins. The guidelines of the Association of Breast Surgeons at BASO[47] recommends that 90% of diagnostic guided biopsies for screen-detected abnormalities should weigh less than 20 g. Due to improved preoperative diagnosis, wire-guided localisation procedures are usually therapeutic rather than diagnostic. However, DCIS is often pathologically larger than mammographically suggested; this is especially true if magnification views are not used, and up to 30% of cases need re-excision to clear margins adequately.[48] Accurate orientation of the specimen is essential to direct re-excision of the relevant margins and to minimise the volume of any re-excision.

Other diagnostic procedures
Ductoscopy

Ductoscopy (see Chapter 3) is an appealing option for DCIS. There has been interest in its use both in diagnosis and potential for treatment with direct instillation of chemotherapy into the ducts[49] (see Chapter 3).

Magnetic resonance imaging (MRI)

MRI can be used to image DCIS and is currently being investigated in a number of trials. DCIS may identify occult multifocal or contralateral disease, but there are concerns about the potential of MRI to overestimate the extent of disease, leading to wider than necessary excisions, and unnecessary mastectomy or identifying high numbers of contralateral lesions that turn out to be benign. There are also concerns that MRI might detect biologically insignificant disease that could increase 'over-treatment'. It therefore remains under investigation in trials and has no routine role in assessing DCIS.

Treatment: mastectomy versus breast-conserving surgery

Even though there is current debate over the potential over-treatment of some cases of DCIS, the accepted current standard of management is at present surgical.

Mastectomy

The long-term recurrence rate following mastectomy for DCIS is less than 1%.[50] As current evidence (see p. 181) points to DCIS being predominantly unicentric in origin, it is now recognised that mastectomy is over-treatment for the majority of patients.[50] In 1983 mastectomy was performed for 71% of cases of DCIS in the USA but this had dropped to 44% by 1992.[51] Mastectomy is now reserved for patients with larger areas of DCIS (arbitrarily considered as >4 cm), for multicentric disease and for patients where radiotherapy is contraindicated. Women should also be offered mastectomy if the excision margins are involved following breast-conserving surgery and the patient is not deemed suitable for re-excision. Rates of re-excision versus mastectomy vary widely in different units. Women with DCIS requiring mastectomy are excellent candidates for skin-sparing mastectomy and immediate breast reconstruction.

Breast-conserving surgery

Breast-conserving surgery is the treatment of choice for small localised areas of DCIS (generally those <4 cm in diameter). Larger areas of DCIS can be excised but often require a reshaping or an oncoplastic procedure combined with a contralateral breast reduction to achieve symmetry. Areas of DCIS usually need to be radiologically localised preoperatively, as they are predominantly impalpable (see p. 181). Multiple wires may assist the surgeon and thus increase the rates of complete excision. The lesion should be excised in one piece if possible and orientated with radio opaque markers. Before wound closure, the specimen should undergo radiography to ensure that all suspicious microcalcifications have been removed and are clear of the radial margins. Many surgeons use a four-quadrant cavity biopsy, with or without India ink, to assess the margins. The pathologist should assess the histological margin status and document this in the histology report. If the margins are close (<1 mm), the patient should undergo cavity re-excision, as margin status is a key prognostic factor for local recurrence.

The recommended treatment protocol for DCIS is shown in **Fig. 11.2**.

Axillary staging

The incidence of macroscopic lymph node metastasis in DCIS is less than 1% and should prompt thorough pathological examination for occult invasion. Formal axillary staging in women with DCIS should not be performed alongside breast-conserving surgery.[52] However, National Institute for Health and Clinical Excellence (NICE) guidelines recommend that a sentinel lymph node biopsy should be performed at the same time as mastectomy for DCIS[52] and women should be counselled as to the indications for this. The rationale for performing sentinel lymph node biopsy with mastectomy is the potential

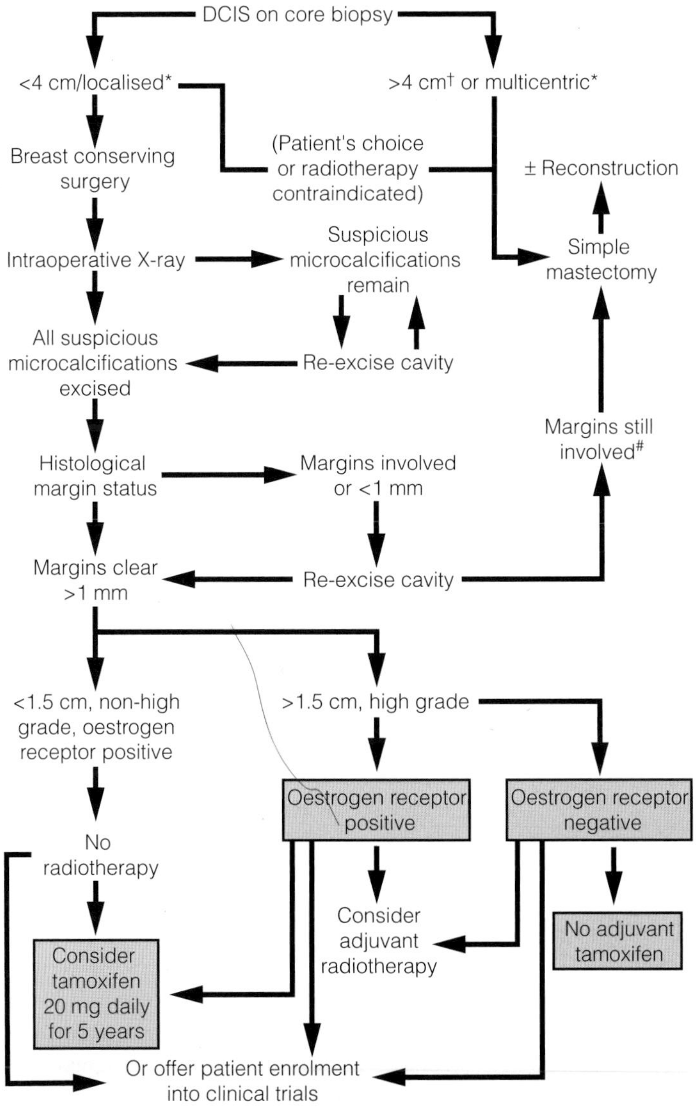

Figure 11.2 • Recommended treatment algorithm for ductal carcinoma in situ (DCIS). *Determined mammographically. Shaded boxes indicate those treatments suggested by the results of recent trials.[55,66] †Areas of DCIS >4 cm can be treated by breast conservation if unifocal and patient has large breasts, or is suitable for an oncoplastic procedure. #A further re-excision can be attempted providing the final cosmetic result is acceptable to the patient.

of occult invasive disease that may be identified histologically in a large area of DCIS. This would subsequently require axillary staging. A sentinel lymph node biopsy cannot easily be performed after a mastectomy. Patients found to have positive lymph nodes have occult invasive disease and should be managed accordingly. A study by Veronesi et al. of 508 patients with pure DCIS found that nine patients (1.8%) had epithelial cells found in the sentinel node (five of these nine cases were micrometastases alone). None of the cases showed further lymph node involvement at formal axillary dissection.[53] A further study that looked retrospectively at the NSABP B-17 and B-24 data, from patients who had undergone local excision of DCIS with clear margins (no axillary surgery at initial treatment), showed that the ipsilateral nodal recurrence rate was 0.83 per 1000 patient-years in the B-17 trial and 0.36 per 1000 patient-years in the B-24 trial. Meta-analysis of the published literature showed approximately 1.8% of DCIS (almost entirely G3 or high-grade disease) had involved sentinel nodes.[54]

Recurrence: rates and predictors

No trial has specifically evaluated breast-conserving surgery versus mastectomy in DCIS. The long-term recurrence rate following mastectomy is known to be very low at less than 1%.[50] The majority of these recurrences are invasive disease. This reflects the fact that after mastectomy no imaging is performed routinely of the ipsilateral side and further disease is only detected when it becomes clinically apparent – at which stage it is most likely to be invasive. The recurrence rate for breast-conserving surgery alone has been reported to be up to 25% at 8 years follow-up, with up to 50% of recurrences (i.e. 12.5% of all cases) being invasive disease.[13,48,55] The remaining 50% of recurrences are in situ tumours.[56] Reviews of clinical and pathological variables have demonstrated certain unfavourable tumour characteristics and these are outlined below. Recurrence rates have fallen significantly over time.

Assessment of excision margins

A fundamental risk factor for recurrence is inadequate excision following breast-conserving surgery.

This is judged as close (<1 mm) or involved margins[48] and/or failure to remove all suspicious microcalcifications.[57] Excision margin width has three times the power of tumour grade in predicting local recurrence.[58] The NSABP-B17, NSABP-B24 and EORTC clinical trials all revealed that the presence of clear margins after local excision significantly decreased tumour recurrence.[13,59-61] On multivariate analysis of the EORTC trial, non-specified, close or involved margins conferred a hazard ratio of 2.07 (95% confidence interval (CI) 1.35–3.16, P = 0.0008) compared with clear margins.[61] The NSABP-B24 trial found a covariate relative risk of 1.68 (95% CI 1.20–2.34) if the margins were involved.[59] No prospective trials have looked at the optimum excision width required for in situ or invasive cancer. When considering the extent of surgical excision there has to be balance between minimising recurrence and producing an acceptable cosmetic outcome. A retrospective study by Chan et al.[48] reported that women with clear margins (judged as greater than 1 mm) had an 8.1% recurrence at a median follow-up of 47 months compared with 37.9% recurrence where excision margins were close (1 mm). There was no improvement in recurrence rates in more widely excised lesions. The recent meta-analysis performed by Wang et al.[62] suggested a 10-mm margin was superior to lesser margins for local recurrence but this conflicts with an earlier meta-analysis, which suggested 2 mm.[63] Part of the problem of defining an optimum margin is that these analyses are affected by confounding factors. The 10- and 2-mm distances also rely on a small proportion of patients treated in very few centres. At present, as Morrow and Katz conclude, there is no compelling evidence that bigger is better for margins in DCIS.[64]

High-grade/comedo tumours

High-grade tumours and tumours showing comedo necrosis are independent risk factors for recurrence. In a review of the EORTC 10853 trial,[61] high nuclear grade had a hazard ratio of 2.23 (95% CI 1.41–3.51, P = 0.0011) for local recurrence, with 22% of high-grade tumours and 11% of intermediate-grade tumours developing either recurrent DCIS or invasive tumour. Comedo necrosis was also shown to be related to local recurrence, 18% of patients with DCIS having comedo necrosis developing recurrence (hazard ratio 1.80, 95% CI 1.08–3.00, P = 0.0183).

Histological type and tumour architecture

The degree of tumour differentiation is predictive of both local recurrence and metastatic disease. In the EORTC trial,[13,61] poorly differentiated tumours were at significantly higher risk of developing DCIS recurrence (hazard ratio 3.58, 95% CI 1.68–7.62, $P = 0.0001$) and metastasis (hazard ratio 6.65, 95% CI 1.46–30.22, $P = 0.00083$) compared with well-differentiated tumours. In this same trial, histological type was also strongly related to DCIS recurrence, though not to invasive recurrence. Both solid/comedo DCIS (hazard ratio 4.40, 95% CI 2.28–8.48, $P = 0.0001$) and cribriform DCIS (hazard ratio 3.74, 95% CI 1.91–7.30, $P = 0.0001$) were found to be much more likely to recur than clinging or micropapillary tumours. Within the well-differentiated group, no tumours with clinging DCIS recurred.[61] It has been suggested that this well-differentiated clinging DCIS should be reclassified separately as 'columnar alteration with prominent apical snouts and secretion',[65] with debate as to whether this subtype should be managed as atypical ductal hyperplasia or LCIS.

Age at diagnosis

A further risk factor for recurrence irrespective of tumour grade or type is young age (<40 years) at diagnosis. The EORTC 10853 trial[13,61] found that women less than 40 years at diagnosis were more likely to recur (hazard ratio 2.54, 95% CI 1.53–4.23, $P = 0.010$) than older women. The NSABP B-24 trial[59] found that the rate of ipsilateral breast tumours (in the placebo population) in women aged 49 years or less at diagnosis was 33.3 per 1000, compared with 13.0 for those aged 50 and above. In the UK/ANZ DCIS trial,[66,67] only a small proportion (9.5%) of women was less than 50 years old at diagnosis. The power of this study is thus limited, but of these younger women, 26% recurred after excision and tamoxifen compared with only 17% of women older than 50 years. Rodrigues et al.[68] studied women aged 42 years or less (mean age 38.5) or women aged 60 years or more (mean age 67.8) at diagnosis. They found that although there was no difference in tumour grade, comedo necrosis or overall histology (also found in the EORTC trial)

between the groups, compared with older patients HER-2 was more frequently overexpressed in the younger patient population. Approximately 65% of the younger age group were HER-2 positive compared with 38% of the older age group ($P = 0.06$). No significant difference was found between oestrogen receptor, progesterone receptor, p53, Ki67, cyclin D1 or bcl-2 expression.

Tumour size and palpability

None of the major trials have found any statistical significance between recurrence and size. The NSABP-B17 trial[55] found that the size of mammographically detected tumours was not significant in predicting ipsilateral recurrence. However, when researchers examined clustering of microcalcifications in women whose mammograms did not show a tumour mass, they found that clustered microcalcifications greater than 10 mm (relative risk 2.06, 95% CI 1.36–3.10) or scattered calcifications (relative risk 2.41, 95% CI 1.40–4.16) had a significantly higher ipsilateral recurrence than clustered calcifications of 10 mm or less. The problem is that there may be differences in histology between the groups, so counfounding the analysis of size. The EORTC 10853 trial[61] found no difference in recurrence rates between tumours less than 10 mm in size and those 10–20 mm or greater than 20 mm in size ($P = 0.2127$). However, tumours that were clinically apparent rather than mammographically detected were more likely to recur (covariate relative risk 2.17, 95% CI 1.53–3.08).[61]

Scoring systems

In order to bring together the most clinically relevant risk factors, Silverstein and Lagois[69] developed the Van Nuys Prognostic Index, with the aim of predicting which women would be at risk of recurrence following breast-conserving surgery. This numerical algorithm was derived from regression analysis of retrospective data pooled from patients with DCIS treated at two centres in the USA. Recurrence is clearly multifactorial but the problem with the Van Nuys Index is that the data derived were not randomised and used historical controls. The formula encompassed tumour size, margin width and pathological classification.

The index has since been modified as the University of Southern California/Van Nuys Prognostic Index (USC/VNPI) and now includes patient age.[69] Each criterion is weighted and scored 1, 2 or 3 and the individual scores combined to give an overall score from 4 to 12. Scores of 4–6, 7–9 and 10–12 are said to be at low, moderate and high risk of 5-year recurrence, respectively. It was designed to achieve a less than 20% recurrence rate at 12 years. The data are skewed by the fact that 80% of large tumours (>4 cm) recurred, whereas in the UK these women would have undergone mastectomy. These large tumours were also more likely high grade and incompletely excised. The value of the scoring system for a UK population, where the majority of cases of DCIS are small (<2 cm) and screen detected (patients usually over 50 years old), may be limited. For instance, Boland et al.[58] were unable to demonstrate that size was a marker of recurrence in screen-detected DCIS in the UK.

Markers of recurrence

✅ To improve the detection of specific patient groups at increased risk of recurrence, biological markers that might help determine recurrence potential in DCIS are being investigated. Provenzano et al.[70] found that oestrogen receptor, progesterone receptor and bcl-2 negativity and HER-2 and p21 positivity were associated with an increased risk of clinical recurrence. This was irrespective of tumour grade. Oestrogen receptor, progesterone receptor, bcl-2 and HER-2 were found to be interdependent of each other, whereas p21 was found to be independent of the above associations, and is thought to reflect the differing biological pathways of action between the markers.

There has also been interest in another member of the type 1 tyrosine kinase receptor family, HER-4. DCIS and invasive tumours that show co-expression of HER-2 and HER-4 have a better prognosis (reduced recurrence) than HER-2-positive, HER-4-negative tumours.[71–72] A summary of the risk factors for DCIS recurrence is shown in Table 11.2 (see Lari SA and Kuerer HM[73] review of DCIS biological prognostic markers).

The use of genomics looks as if it may have the potential to identify patients and high and low risk of recurrence. Oncotype DX marketed by Genomic Health is a scoring system for invasive cancer recurrence

Table 11.2 • Risk factors for recurrence of ductal carcinoma in situ

Excision margins	Margins <1 mm after breast-conserving surgery
Tumour grade	High grade (III)
Comedo necrosis	Present
Histological type	Poorly differentiated
Patient age	Younger age at diagnosis (<40 years)
Biological markers	
Negativity	Oestrogen receptor
	Progesterone receptor
	bcl-2
	HER-4
Positivity	HER-2
	p21
	p53
	Ki67 (high-percentage expression)
Patient presentation	Symptomatic
Tumour size	Not significant

Poor-prognosis tumours often possess multiple bad prognostic features, i.e. they tend to be poorly differentiated high-grade, comedo tumours that are oestrogen receptor negative and overexpress c-erbB-2.

based on a 21-gene assay. Researchers have recently shown that the use of a modified 12-gene DCIS assay (Oncotype DX DCIS) using data from the Eastern Cooperative Oncology Group study 5194 trial (see later) can identify 75% of women from this cohort with low- and intermediate-grade DCIS who have a low risk of recurrence after treatment for DCIS (and could therefore avoid radiotherapy).

Adjuvant therapy

Radiotherapy

Four main trials and a subsequent Cochrane review[74] have examined the value of radiotherapy following breast-conserving surgery for DCIS. The NSABP-B17,[55] EORTC 10853,[13] UK/ANZ DCIS[66,67] and SWEDCIS[75] trials each studied a radiation dose of 50 Gy in 25 fractions. All found a significant reduction in ipsilateral recurrence following radiotherapy. However, none of the trials have shown any impact on mortality (Table 11.3, **Fig. 11.3**).

The reduction in recurrence was similar for both in situ and invasive disease. In the EORTC trial,

Table 11.3 • Summary of major radiotherapy/tamoxifen clinical trials following breast-conserving therapy for ductal carcinoma in situ

	NSABP-17*		NSABP-24*		EORTC 10853[†]		UK/ANZ DCIS[‡]			
	BCS alone	BCS and XRT	BCS and XRT	BCS, XRT and tamoxifen	BCS alone	BCS and XRT	BCS alone	BCS and XRT	BCS and tamoxifen	BCS, XRT and tamoxifen
Number of patients	403	411	899	899	500	502	544	267	567	316
Number of local recurrences at median follow-up:										
43 months	64	28	–	–	–	–	–	–	–	–
48 months	–	–	–	–	83	53	–	–	–	–
53 months	–	–	–	–	–	–	119	22	101	21
74 months	–	–	130	84	–	–	–	–	–	–
90 months	140	47	–	–	–	–	–	–	–	–
126 months	–	–	–	–	132	75	–	–	–	–
152 months	–	–	–	–	–	–	174	35	135	32
Local recurrence rates:										
4-year all recurrences	–	–	–	–	16%	9%	–	–	–	–
4-year invasive	–	–	–	–	8%	4%	–	–	–	–
5-year all recurrences	–	–	13%	8.2%	–	–	15%	3%	12%	3%
5-year invasive	–	–	7%	4.1%	–	–	5%	1%	5%	2%
8-year all recurrences	27%	12%	–	–	–	–	–	–	–	–
8-year invasive	13%	4%	–	–	–	–	–	–	–	–
10-year all recurrences	–	–	–	–	26%	15%	–	–	–	–
10-year invasive	–	–	–	–	13%	8%	–	–	–	–
Annual recurrence rate	–	–	–	–	–	–	3.2%	1.2%	2.2%	0.9%
Number of distant metastases	6	9	7	3	20	23	–	–	–	–
Total number of contralateral breast events	19	20	36	18	28	39	29	7	11	9
Number of contralateral invasive breast cancers	16	12	23	15	19	28	20	5	7	7

(Continued)

Table 11.3 • (cont.) Summary of major radiotherapy/tamoxifen clinical trials following breast-conserving therapy for ductal carcinoma in situ

	NSABP-17*		NSABP-24*		EORTC 10853†		UK/ANZ DCIS‡			
	BCS alone	BCS and XRT	BCS and XRT	BCS, XRT and tamoxifen	BCS alone	BCS and XRT	BCS alone	BCS and XRT	BCS and tamoxifen	BCS, XRT and tamoxifen
Bilateral event-free survival at:										
4 years	–	–	–	–	82%	86%	–	–	–	–
5 years	74%	84%	83%	87%	–	–	85%	97%	88%	97%
8 years	60%	75%	–	–	–	–	–	–	–	–
10 years	–	–	–	–	74%	85%	–	–	–	–

BCS, breast-conserving surgery; XRT, radiotherapy.

*Fisher ER, Dignam J, Tan-Chiu E et al. Pathologic findings from the National Surgical Adjuvant Breast Project (NSABP) eight-year update of Protocol B-17: intraductal carcinoma. Cancer 1999; 86:429–38.

†Julien J, Bijker N, Fentimen I et al. Radiotherapy in breast-conserving treatment for ductal carcinoma in situ: first results of the EORTC randomized phase III trial 10853. EORTC Breast Cancer Cooperative Group and EORTC Radiotherapy group. Lancet 2000; 355:528–33. Bijker N, Meijnen P, Peterse JL et al. Breast-conserving treatment with or without radiotherapy in ductal carcinoma-in-situ: ten-year results of European Organisation for Research and Treatment of Cancer randomized phase III trial 10853 – a study by the EORTC Breast Cancer Cooperative Group and EORTC Radiotherapy Group. J Clin Oncol 2006; 24(21):3381–7.

‡UK Coordinating Committee on Cancer Research (UKCCCR). Ductal carcinoma in situ (DCIS) Working Party on behalf of DCIS trialists in the UK, Australia and New Zealand. Radiotherapy and tamoxifen in women with completely excised ductal carcinoma in situ of the breast in the UK, Australia and New Zealand: randomised controlled trial. Lancet 2003; 362:95–103. Cuzick J, Sestaka I, Pinder S, et al Effect of tamoxifen and radiotherapy in women with locally excised ductal carcinoma in situ: long-term results from the UK/ANZ DCIS trial. Lancet Oncol. 2010; 12(1): 21–9.

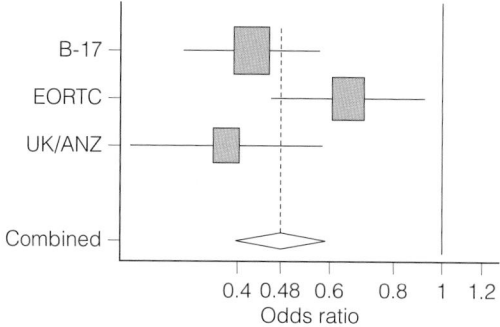

Figure 11.3 • Radiotherapy trials overview: ipsilateral ductal carcinoma in situ (DCIS) and invasive recurrences. This Forrest plot of the major randomised controlled trials of radiotherapy in DCIS (B17,[55] EORTC[13] and UK/ANZ[66]) shows a significant reduction in ipsilateral recurrence risk following radiotherapy for all trials, with a combined odds ratio for the reduction in recurrence of DCIS and invasive disease of 0.48 for all trials. Reproduced from Cuzick J. Treatment of DCIS – results from clinical trials. Surg Oncol 2003; 12:213–9. With permission from Elsevier.

radiotherapy reduced the risk of DCIS recurrence by 48% ($P = 0.0011$) and invasive local recurrence by 42% ($P = 0.0065$) at a median of 10.7 years' follow-up.[76] The UK DCIS trial found that after a median follow-up of 12.5 years there was a reduced incidence of ipsilateral invasive disease (0.32, 0.19–0.56; $P < 0.0001$) and ipsilateral DCIS (0.38, 0.22–0.63; $P < 0.0001$).[67] Both groups had similar low risks of metastases and death. No survival advantage following radiotherapy was found in any trial.

✅✅ Current NICE guidelines recommend that you should: 'Offer adjuvant radiotherapy to patients with DCIS following adequate breast-conserving surgery and discuss with them the potential benefits and risks.'[52]

The Cochrane review concluded that 'nine women require treatment with radiotherapy to prevent one ipsilateral recurrence'.[74]

Two studies have looked at avoiding radiotherapy in 'low-risk' cases of pure DCIS; one by Wong et al.[77] was stopped in line with the trial protocol because of high recurrence rates, although most recurrences were mammographically detected DCIS and the remainder node-negative invasive cancers and thus did not impact overall survival. They concluded that it remained unclear how to identify patients who had a low recurrence risk with excision alone, and that despite margins >1 cm (or having had re-excision) the local recurrence rate

was still high. The second, the Eastern Cooperative Oncology Group study 5194 (the study in which the Oncotype DX DCIS score was validated (see previously)),[78] included 558 cases of low- or intermediate-grade DCIS, which measured 2.5 cm or less, and 103 cases of high-grade DCIS of 1 cm or smaller which had been excised completely with 3-mm margins, none of which had radiation therapy but they may have had tamoxifen. The 5-year ipsilateral overall breast event rate for low/intermediate-grade DCIS was 6.1% (3% for invasive disease alone). For the high-grade lesions this was increased to 15.3% (7.5% for invasive disease). They concluded that a 6% 5-year ipsilateral breast event rate for low/intermediate-grade tumours may be acceptable to patients and physicians, but that the 15% high-grade event rate would not be. They suggested that specimens need to be rigorously evaluated to ensure they are actually 'low risk'. This study included patients with DCIS with a median size of 1 cm. Seventy-five per cent of the patients were classified by the Oncotype DX assay as low risk, 14% intermediate risk and 11% high risk. Low-risk patients had a 10-year event rate of 12% and a 5% rate of developing an invasive cancer with no radiotherapy. This event rate is higher than one currently sees in invasive cancer after breast conservation surgery and radiotherapy but many of these events will be further DCIS which can be treated effectively by further surgery +/− radiotherapy.

✅ The National Institutes for Health State-of-the-Science conference included a multiprofessional event of independent panels of health professionals and public representatives. This reviewed systematic literature on DCIS, with presentations by investigators working in wide-ranging areas of DCIS management (2009).[79] It concluded that for radiotherapy:

'Randomised clinical trials demonstrate that all subsets of patients benefit from radiotherapy in terms of decreased local recurrence. However, there may be a subgroup of women who have DCIS in which the risk of local recurrence is so low that radiotherapy may be of no benefit. In addition, there also may be a subset of women who can be monitored after biopsy in lieu of surgery or other therapies.'

Endocrine therapy

Although radiotherapy reduces tumour recurrence following breast-conserving surgery, there is still an overall recurrence rate of between 3% and 13%[13,55,66] at 5 years, and research into the use of additional adjuvant therapies for women with 'high-risk' DCIS remains important.

✅✅ The NSABP-B24 trial compared breast-conserving surgery and radiotherapy with or without adjuvant tamoxifen. The study found that tamoxifen following breast-conserving surgery and radiotherapy was of benefit in reducing recurrence. There were 43% fewer invasive breast cancer events and 31 % fewer non-invasive events in the tamoxifen-treated group.[59] The main advantage was in reducing invasive recurrence in the ipsilateral breast, although there was a significantly lower cumulative incidence of all breast cancer-related events in the tamoxifen group.

In this trial, 30% of women were younger than 50 years at diagnosis and the effect of tamoxifen was largely due to a 40% reduction in this younger age group, with only a 20% reduction in the age group greater than 50 years. On this basis adjuvant tamoxifen after wide local excision for DCIS could be discussed in this younger (under 50) age group; however, current NICE guidelines indicate that tamoxifen should not be used in DCIS.[52] A retrospective review of the NSABP-B24 results showed that tamoxifen was only beneficial in oestrogen receptor-positive cases, as one would expect. The relative risk of recurrence of any breast cancer in the oestrogen receptor-positive cohort was 0.41 (95% CI 0.25–0.65, $P = 0.0002$), whereas there was little benefit in the oestrogen receptor-negative cases (relative risk 0.80, $P = 0.51$).[80] The UK/ANZ DCIS trial found that adjuvant tamoxifen reduced overall DCIS recurrence (0.70, 0.51–0.86; $P = 0.03$) and contralateral tumours (0.44, 0.25–0.77; $P = 0.005$) but had no effect on ipsilateral invasive disease[67] (see Table 11.3). The UK/ANZ DCIS trial has not published a breakdown of tamoxifen response in relation to oestrogen receptor status, but tamoxifen was found to be more effective in low- and intermediate-grade compared with high-grade DCIS and this is likely a surrogate (though not completely accurate) reflection of oestrogen receptor status; low-grade DCIS tends to be nearly 100% oestrogen receptor positive, compared with only 60% of high-grade cases expressing oestrogen receptor.[81] The UK/ANZ DCIS trial authors suggested that the variation in findings, as to the benefit of tamoxifen in preventing ipsilateral invasive recurrence

between the two trials, may have been a product of the American B24 trial having approximately 34% of women aged under 50, whereas in the UK trial >90% of participants were older than 50.[67] No significant effects were seen on mortality with the use of tamoxifen in either trial.

In the randomised controlled trials, the rate of contralateral breast cancer after DCIS is 0.5% per year for 10 years. As tamoxifen can halve the risk of breast cancer in the contralateral breast, its effects in part are as a chemopreventive agent. This may possibly justify its use in some women with oestrogen receptor-positive disease. Approximately 60% of DCIS cases express HER-2. Oestrogen receptor-positive tumours that also express HER-2 are considered to be more often resistant to tamoxifen but do respond to aromatase inhibitors. The ERISAC trial showed that exemestane, at a dose of 25 mg/day, inhibits epithelial proliferation in DCIS by 39% (hazard ratio 0.61, 95% CI 0.41–0.91, $P = 0.016$) compared with placebo.[82] This suggests that aromatase inhibition of oestrogen receptor-positive DCIS could potentially be used to prevent local recurrence.

The use of aromatase inhibitors is currently being investigated in the IBIS II DCIS trial, which is a comparison of tamoxifen with anastrozole or placebo, after complete excision of oestrogen receptor-positive DCIS. The NSABPB35 trial is comparing anastrozole with tamoxifen for patients with DCIS after lumpectomy and radiation therapy. The NSABP P-1 chemoprevention trial[83] compared tamoxifen to placebo in patients at high risk of breast cancer. The study reported a 49% reduction in incidence of invasive cancer and a 50% reduction of DCIS in the tamoxifen-treated group. The reduction in contralateral breast cancer was only seen in oestrogen receptor-positive cases, with no benefit being seen for oestrogen receptor-negative patients.

The recent MAP.3 trial looked at exemestane in a prevention setting in postmenopausal women and showed a reduction in both new cases of DCIS and further breast events in women with a prior diagnosis of DCIS, though numbers were small.[17]

Follow-up and prognosis

Following confirmation that there has been complete excision of all suspicious microcalcifications with clear margins, patients should be given the opportunity to participate in clinical trials. One trial is investigating the role of boost radiotherapy in DCIS. Follow-up in outpatient clinics, after the initial postoperative reviews, should be by annual bilateral two-view mammography to detect recurrence. Most DCIS recurrence is impalpable and the only role for clinical examination may be in detecting invasive recurrences in premenopausal women. Breast cancer-specific mortality following breast-conserving surgery for DCIS is low at less than 2% at 10 years and is not influenced by adjuvant radiotherapy. This figure is similar to that following mastectomy for DCIS.

Management of recurrence

In situ recurrence

Patients with an in situ recurrence where the primary was treated initially with breast-conserving surgery alone can be offered re-excision (ensuring clear margins) followed by postoperative radiotherapy. Patients who have already received radiotherapy following their primary excision are usually advised to have completion mastectomy unless recurrence is many years later. A skin-sparing mastectomy with a myocutaneous flap breast reconstruction gives excellent results. Implant based reconstructions have an increased rate of complications if there has been prior radiotherapy.

Invasive recurrence

The management of invasive recurrence is dependent on the initial therapy for DCIS. If the patient did not receive radiotherapy after initial DCIS excision, then wide local excision and radiotherapy may be an option depending on the size and location of the invasive tumour. If wide local excision is not an option, then mastectomy and axillary staging is the treatment of choice, with adjuvant therapy dictated by standard protocols for primary invasive cancers. Studies following salvage treatment for both in situ and invasive recurrences of DCIS have shown overall cause-specific survival rates in excess of 90% at 8 years after recurrence.[57]

DCIS of the male breast

DCIS accounts for approximately 5% of breast cancers in men.[84] It usually presents clinically with symptoms of a retro-areola cystic-type mass or bloody nipple discharge. Clinical, rather than mammographic, detection possibly accounts for the different incidence of DCIS between men and women. The predominant histological subtypes of DCIS in men are papillary and cribriform. Standard treatment is total mastectomy with excision of the nipple–areola complex but wide excision and radiotherapy is being used more frequently.[85] Pure DCIS in men is usually of low or intermediate grade; less than 3% of cases are high grade. In a series of 114 patients, 84 with pure DCIS and 30 with DCIS and invasive cancer, there were no cases of high-grade comedo DCIS in men without an invasive tumour.[86] The percentage of men with DCIS that eventually develop an invasive cancer is not known.

The future

Ongoing trials

The IBIS II and NSABP B-35 trials (as discussed previously) are in active follow-up. The NSABP B-43 trial is currently recruiting patients to compare trastuzumab given during radiotherapy or radiotherapy alone in women with HER-2-positive DCIS treated with lumpectomy. The ICICLE trial is trying to identify genes that increase women's risk of developing DCIS, and also trying to identify which women with DCIS are at risk of developing an invasive recurrence if left untreated. A more novel treatment is being investigated in a phase I/II trial looking at vaccine therapy, where vaccines made from a patient's white blood cells mixed with peptides may help the body build an effective immune response to kill tumour cells. Neoadjuvant therapy with aromatase inhibitors in postmenopausal women with oestrogen receptor-positive cancers is showing promise as a short-term treatment to reduce tumour extent and as long-term treatment for some patients with low- and intermediate-grade DCIS.

UK National DCIS audit (Sloane Project)

The Sloane Project is a prospective audit that is collecting data on all screen-detected DCIS, LCIS, ADH and ALH in the UK. For each case the clinical, pathological, radiological and treatment characteristics are documented. It currently has over 10 000 cases submitted by participating UK breast screening units. The aim is to correlate initial characteristics with clinical outcomes – specifically recurrence and invasive cancer development. Data from this study to inform clinical management and restrict treatment to at-risk groups are awaited eagerly.

DCIS stem cell therapy

Breast cancers have been shown to consist of a mixture of stem cells and proliferating cells.[19] The stem cells appear to be more resistant to both chemotherapy and endocrine therapy than proliferating cells. Stem cells evade death and subsequently may re-grow and may be a source of breast recurrence. Farnie et al.[19] showed that primary cultures of DCIS using a mammosphere technique identified Notch and the epidermal growth factor receptor/HER-1 as key receptors that stem cells use to avoid death. Thus strategies aimed at inhibiting both stem cell self-renewal and proliferating progeny may increase the DCIS cure rate. HER-2-amplified DCIS has an increased stem cell population and this population is targeted by lapatinib, trastuzumab and other anti-HER-2 therapies but not by chemotherapy. In vitro lapatinib (an HER-1/2 inhibitor) has been shown to reduce stem cell renewal by 70% in HER-2-amplified DCIS.[87]

Therapies that target cancer stem cells may prevent recurrence of DCIS. There is concern that, in some patients with DCIS, there may be stem cells that are not identified by the standard methods of assessing margins. Treatment with anti-stem cell therapy given perioperatively or in combination with endocrine therapy should theoretically reduce the rate of recurrence. Additionally, new data utilising dual HER-2 inhibition with combinations of trastuzumab with either lapatinib or pertuzumab show complete response in up to 60% of oestrogen receptor-negative, HER-2-positive invasive cancers in association with chemotherapy and suggest that dual anti-HER-2 treatment might be effective in oestrogen receptor-negative, HER-2-positive DCIS at reducing disease burden and could avoid mastectomy in some women. This strategy is also an effective anti-stem cell strategy and so may have long-term benefits in reducing recurrence rates for women with HER-2-positive DCIS.

Optimising treatment

Controversies regarding the optimum management of this heterogeneous preinvasive lesion still reign. Surgeons should ensure complete pathological and radiological excision of DCIS and discuss the appropriateness of adjuvant therapy (radiotherapy or endocrine) with the patient in a multidisciplinary setting in order to minimise recurrence without over-treatment.

Key points

- DCIS is a preinvasive breast tumour; the proliferation of malignant epithelial cells is confined within an intact basement membrane. The developmental pathway for low- and intermediate-grade DCIS appears different from that for high-grade DCIS.
- DCIS accounts for approximately 20% of new screen-detected cancers.
- Small localised areas of DCIS (normally <4 cm) should be treated with breast-conserving surgery with or without radiotherapy. Larger lesions are usually treated by mastectomy and sentinel node biopsy unless they can be excised using oncoplastic techniques. Axillary surgery should be avoided after breast-conserving surgery.
- We are potentially over-treating a number of 'low-risk' cases of DCIS that may never progress to invasive disease.
- There are current controversies in management of DCIS with respect to over-treatment and in particular the widespread use of radiotherapy in this condition.
- Up to 13% of cases recur at 5 years following breast-conserving surgery and radiotherapy, 50% of which (i.e. up to 6.5% of all cases) are invasive disease.
- The key factor for decreasing tumour recurrence is to excise the lesion to clear margins at the time of surgery.

- Bad prognostic factors include younger age at diagnosis (<40 years), poorly differentiated high-grade tumours, the presence of comedo necrosis, HER-2 positivity and oestrogen receptor negativity.
- Tamoxifen is not indicated after mastectomy for DCIS but appears to have benefits and can be discussed with the patient in oestrogen receptor-positive lesions treated by breast-conserving surgery.
- Advances in genomics and proteomics may provide important information to select the most appropriate management for individual patients with DCIS.

References

1. NHS Cancer Screening Programmes. All breast cancer report. An analysis of all symptomatic and screen detected breast cancers diagnosed in 2006. NHS Breast Screening Programme; October 2009.

2. Lagios MD. Heterogeneity of ductal carcinoma in situ of the breast. J Cell Biochem Suppl 1993;17G:49–52.

3. Rakovitch E. Part 1 Epidemiology of ductal carcinoma in situ. Curr Probl Cancer 2000;24:100–11.

4. Williams G, Anderson E, Howell A, et al. Oral contraceptive (OCP) use increases proliferation and decreases oestrogen receptor content of epithelial cells in the normal human breast. Int J Cancer 1991;48:206–10.

5. Hofseth LJ, Raafat AM, Osuch JR, et al. Hormone replacement therapy with oestrogen or oestrogen plus medroxyprogesterone acetate is associated with increased epithelial proliferation in the normal post-menopausal breast. J Clin Endocrinol Metab 1999;84:4559–65.

6. Schairer C, Byrne C, Keyl PM, et al. Menopausal estrogen and estrogen–progestin replacement therapy and the risk of breast cancer (United States). Cancer Causes Control 1994;5:491–500.

7. Longnecker MP, Bernstein L, Paganini-Hill A, et al. Risk factors for in situ breast cancer. Cancer Epidemiol Biomarkers Prev 1996;5:961–5.

8. Chlebowski RT, Hendrix SL, Langer RD, WHI Investigators. Influence of estrogen plus progestin on breast cancer and mammography in healthy post-menopausal women: the Women's Health Initiative Randomized Trial. JAMA 2003;289(24):3243–53.

9. Henrick JB, Kornguth PJ, Viscoli CM, et al. Postmenopausal estrogen use and invasive versus in situ breast cancer risk. J Clin Epidemiol 1998;51:1277–83.

10. Gapstur SM, Morrow M, Sellars TA. Hormone replacement therapy and risk of breast cancer with a favourable histology: results of the Iowa Women's Health Study. JAMA 1999;281:2091–7.

11. Hwang ES, DeVries S, Chew KL, et al. Patterns of chromosomal alterations in breast ductal carcinoma in situ. Clin Cancer Res 2004;10(15):5160–7.

12. Bijker N, Peterse JL, Duchateau L, et al. Histological type and marker expression of the primary tumour compared with its local recurrence after breast-conserving therapy for ductal carcinoma in situ. Br J Cancer 2001;84:539–44.

13. Julien J, Bijker N, Fentimen I, et al. Radiotherapy in breast-conserving treatment for ductal carcinoma in situ: first results of the EORTC randomized phase III trial 10853. EORTC Breast Cancer Cooperative Group and EORTC Radiotherapy Group. Lancet 2000;355:528–33.

   The results of a multicentre, randomised, controlled trial of 1010 patients with DCIS treated with breast-conserving surgery, randomised to receive no further treatment or radiotherapy. The study found that radiotherapy reduced overall invasive (40% reduction, $P = 0.04$) and non-invasive (35% reduction, $P = 0.06$) ipsilateral recurrences (median follow-up 4.25 years).

14. Page DL, Dupont WD, Rogers LW, et al. Continued local recurrence of carcinoma 15–25 years after a diagnosis of low grade ductal carcinoma in situ of the breast treated only by biopsy. Cancer 1995;76:1197–200.

15. Ozanne EM, Shieh Y, Barnes J, et al. Characterizing the impact of 25 years of DCIS treatment. Breast Cancer Res Treat 2011;129(1):165–73.

16. Chen YY, DeVries S, Anderson J, et al. Pathologic and biologic response to preoperative endocrine therapy in patients with ER-positive ductal carcinoma in situ. BMC Cancer 2009;9:285.

17. Goss PE, Ingle JN, Alés-Martínez JE, et al. NCIC CTG MAP.3 Study Investigators. Exemestane for breast-cancer prevention in postmenopausal women. N Engl J Med 2011;364(25):2381–91.

18. Menes TS, Kerlikowske K, Jaffer S, et al. Rates of atypical ductal hyperplasia have declined with less use of postmenopausal hormone treatment: findings from the Breast Cancer Surveillance Consortium. Cancer Epidemiol Biomarkers Prev 2009;18(11):2822–8.

19. Farnie G, Clarke RB, Spence K, et al. Novel cell culture technique for primary ductal carcinoma in situ: role of Notch and epidermal growth factor receptor signaling pathways. J Natl Cancer Inst 2007;99:616–27.

20. NHS Breast Screening Programme. Pathology reporting of breast disease. Sheffield: National Pathology Co-ordinating Group; January 2005 Publication no. 58.

21. Holland R, Hendriks JH, Vebeek AL, et al. Extent, distribution, and mammographic/histological correlations of breast ductal carcinoma in situ. Lancet 1990;335:519–22.

22. Steering Committee on Clinical Practice Guidelines for the Care and Treatment of Breast Cancer. The management of ductal carcinoma in situ (DCIS). Can Med Assoc J 1998;158(Suppl):S27–34.

23. Faverley DRG, Burgers L, Bult P, et al. Three dimensional imaging of mammary ductal carcinoma in situ: clinical implications. Semin Diagn Pathol 1994;11:193–8.

24. Holland PA, Ghandi A, Knox WF, et al. The importance of complete excision in the prevention of local recurrence of ductal carcinoma in situ. Br J Cancer 1998;77:110–4.

25. Kerner H, Lichtig C. Lobular cancerisation: incidence and differential diagnosis with lobular carcinoma in situ of the breast. Histopathology 1986;10:621.

26. Fisher ER. Pathobiological considerations relating to the treatment of intraductal carcinoma (ductal carcinoma in situ) of the breast. CA Cancer J Clin 1997;47(1):52–64.

27. Eusebi V, Collina G, Bussolati G. Carcinoma in situ in sclerosing adenosis of the breast. An immunocytochemical study. Semin Diagn Pathol 1989;6:146.

28. Youngston BJ, Cranor M, Powell C, et al. Epithelial displacement in surgical breast specimens following needling procedures. Am J Surg Pathol 1994;18:896.

29. Akashi-Tanaka S, Fukotomi T, Nanasawa T, et al. Treatment of non-invasive carcinoma: fifteen-year results at the National Cancer Centre Hospital in Tokyo. Breast Cancer 2000;7:341–4.

30. O'Malley FP. Lobular neoplasia: morphology, biological potential and management in core biopsies. Mod Pathol 2010;23(Suppl. 2):S14–25.

31. Dunn BK, Ford LG. Breast cancer prevention: results of the National Surgical Adjuvant Breast and Bowel Project (NSABP) breast cancer prevention trial (NSABP P-1: BCPT). Eur J Cancer 2000;36(Suppl. 4):S49–S50.

32. Millis RR, Bobrow LG, Barnes DM. Immunohistochemical evaluation of biological markers in mammary carcinoma in situ: correlation with morphological features and recently proposed schemes for histological classification. Breast 1996;5:113–22.

33. Sullivan RP, Mortimer G, Muircheartaigh IO. Cell proliferation in breast tumours: analysis of histological parameters Ki67 and PCNA expression. Ir J Med Sci 1993;162:343–7.

34. Boland GP, Knox WF, Bundred NJ. Molecular markers and therapeutic targets in ductal carcinoma in situ. Microsc Res Tech 2002;59:3–11.

35. Shoker BS, Jarvis C, Clarke RB, et al. Estrogen receptor-positive proliferating cells in the normal and pre-cancerous breast. Am J Pathol 1999;155:1811–5.

36. Parton M, Dowsett M, Smith I. Studies of apoptosis in breast cancer. Br Med J 2001;322:1528–32.

37. Weinstat-Saslow D, Merino MJ, Manrow RE, et al. Overexpression of cyclin D mRNA distinguishes invasive and in situ breast carcinomas from non-malignant lesions. Nat Med 1995;1:1257–60.

38. Zhou Q, Hopp T, Fuqua SA, et al. Cyclin D1 in breast pre-malignancy and early breast cancer: implications for prevention and treatment. Cancer Lett 2001;162:3–17.

39. Soslow RA, Dannenberg AJ, Rush D, et al. COX-2 is expressed in human pulmonary, colonic and mammary tumours. Cancer 2000;89:2637–45.

40. Ristimaki A, Sivula A, Lundin J, et al. Prognostic significance of elevated COX-2 expression in breast cancer. Cancer Res 2002;62:632–5.

41. Helcynska K, Kronblad Å., Jögi A, et al. Hypoxia induces a dedifferentiated phenotype in ductal carcinoma in situ. Cancer Res 2003;63:1441–4.

42. Dershaw DD, Abramson MD, Kinne DW. Ductal carcinoma in situ: mammographic findings and clinical implications. Radiology 1989;170:411–5.

43. Ikeda DM, Andersson I. Ductal carcinoma in situ: atypical mammographic appearances. Radiology 1989;172:661–6.

44. Schuh ME, Nemoto T, Penetrante RB, et al. Intraductal carcinoma. Analysis of presentation, pathologic findings, and outcome of disease. Arch Surg 1986;121:1303–7.

45. Brennan ME, Turner RM, Ciatto S, et al. Ductal carcinoma in situ at core-needle biopsy: meta-analysis of underestimation and predictors of invasive breast cancer. Radiology 2011;260(1):119–28.

46. Lee CH, Carter D, Philpotts LE, et al. Ductal carcinoma in situ diagnosed with stereotactic core needle biopsy: can invasion be predicted? Radiology 2000;217:466–70.

47. Association of Breast Surgery at BASO. Surgical guidelines for the management of breast cancer. Eur J Surg Oncol 2009;35(Suppl. 1):1–22.

48. Chan KC, Knox WF, Sinha G, et al. Extent of excision margin width required in breast conserving surgery for ductal carcinoma in situ. Cancer 2001;91:9–16.

49. Tang S, Twelves D, Isacke C, et al. Mammary ductoscopy in the current management of breast disease. Surg Endosc 2010;25(6):1712–22.

50. Silverstein MJ, Barth A, Poller DN, et al. Ten year results comparing mastectomy to excision and radiation therapy for ductal carcinoma in situ of the breast. Eur J Cancer 1995;31A:1425–7.

51. Fonseca R, Hartmenn L, Petersen I, et al. Ductal carcinoma in situ of the breast. Ann Intern Med 1997;127:1013–22.

52. NICE clinical guideline 80. Early and locally advanced breast cancer: diagnosis and treatment. Developed by the National Collaborating Centre for Cancer, February 2009.

53. Veronesi P, Intra M, Vento AR, et al. Sentinel lymph node biopsy for localised ductal carcinoma in situ? Breast 2005;14(6):520–2.

54. Julian TB, Land SR, Fourchotte V, et al. Is sentinel node biopsy necessary in conservatively treated DCIS? Ann Surg Oncol 2007;14(8):2202–8.

55. Fisher ER, Dignam J, Tan-Chiu E, et al. Pathologic findings from the National Surgical Adjuvant Breast Project (NSABP) eight-year update of Protocol B-17: intraductal carcinoma. Cancer 1999;86:429–38.
    The 8-year update of 623 women in a randomised controlled trial of 814 women with DCIS treated with local excision who were randomised to receive radiotherapy or no additional treatment. The study found that women who received additional radiotherapy following breast-conserving surgery had a significant reduction in ipsilateral breast tumours (31% vs. 13% at 8 years, P = 0.0001). The authors also analysed a range of clinicopathological characteristics of the patients and the tumours to assess predictors of recurrence; findings suggested that the presence of comedo necrosis was an independent risk factor for recurrence.

56. Solin LJ, Fourquet A, Vincini FA, et al. Salvage treatment for local recurrence after breast-conserving surgery and radiation as initial treatment for mammographically detected carcinoma in situ of the breast. Cancer 2001;91:1090–7.

57. Sneige N, McNeese MD, Atkinson EN, et al. Ductal carcinoma in situ treated with lumpectomy and irradiation: histopathological analysis of 49 specimens with emphasis on risk factors and long term results. Hum Pathol 1995;26:642–9.

58. Boland GP, Chan KC, Knox WF, et al. Value of the Van Nuys Prognostic Index in prediction of recurrence of ductal carcinoma in situ after breast-conserving surgery. Br J Surg 2003;90:426–32.

59. Fisher B, Dignam J, Wolmark N, et al. Tamoxifen in the treatment of intraductal breast cancer: National Surgical Adjuvant Breast and Bowel Project B-24 randomised controlled trial. Lancet 1999;353:1993–2000.
    Double-blind, randomised, controlled trial of 1804 women with completely or incompletely excised DCIS at breast-conserving surgery who were randomised to receive radiotherapy plus or minus tamoxifen. The women receiving tamoxifen had fewer breast cancer events at 5 years compared with placebo (8.2 vs. 13.4, P = 0.0009), mainly due to a decrease in invasive cancer in the ipsilateral breast. A retrospective review of the results (Ref. 80) showed that this benefit was confined to oestrogen receptor-positive cases.

60. Fisher B, Constantino J, Redmond C, et al. Lumpectomy compared with lumpectomy and radiation therapy for the treatment of intraductal breast cancer. N Engl J Med 1993;328:1581–6.

61. Bijker N, Peterse JL, Duchateau L, et al. Risk factors for recurrence and metastasis after breast conserving therapy for ductal carcinoma in situ: analysis of EORTC trial. J Clin Oncol 2001;19:2263–71.
    A review of 843 women of the 1010 randomised cases from the EORTC 10853 trial (local excision of DCIS plus or minus radiotherapy) that examined the clinicopathological characteristics of the women. The authors found that clear margins were the most important factor in reducing local recurrence (hazard ratio 2.07, P = 0.0008). Patients with poorly differentiated DCIS were at higher risk of metastatic disease (hazard ratio 6.57, P = 0.01) and other poor prognostic factors included young age (<40 years) at diagnosis (hazard ratio 2.14, P = 0.02) and symptomatic detection (hazard ratio 1.8, P = 0.008).

62. Wang SY, Chu H, Shamliyan T, et al. Network meta-analysis of margin threshold for women with ductal carcinoma in situ. J Natl Cancer Inst 2012;104:507–16.

63. Dunne C, Burke JP, Morrow M, et al. Effect of margin status on local recurrence after breast conservation and radiation therapy for ductal carcinoma in situ. J Clin Oncol 2009;27(10):1615–20.

64. Morrow M, Katz SJ. Margins in ductal carcinoma in situ: is bigger really better? J Natl Cancer Inst 2012;104(7):494–5.

65. Fraser J, Raza S, Chorny K, et al. Columnar alteration with prominent apical snouts and secretions: a spectrum of changes frequently present in breast biopsies with microcalcifications. Am J Surg Pathol 1998;22:1521–7.

66. UK Coordinating Committee on Cancer Research (UKCCCR). Ductal Carcinoma In Situ (DCIS) Working Party on behalf of DCIS trialists in the UK, Australia and New Zealand. Radiotherapy and tamoxifen in women with completely excised ductal carcinoma in situ of the breast in the UK, Australia and New Zealand: randomised controlled trial. Lancet 2003;362:95–103.
    A 2 × 2 factorial design, randomised controlled trial of 1701 screen-detected patients with completely excised DCIS, randomised to receive tamoxifen, radiotherapy, both treatments or none. The authors found that radiotherapy reduced the incidence of both ipsilateral invasive recurrence (hazard ratio 0.45, P = 0.01) and DCIS recurrence (hazard ratio 0.36, P = 0.0004). Tamoxifen reduced overall DCIS recurrence (hazard ratio 0.68, P = 0.03) but not invasive disease. The trial has not yet published results with regard to oestrogen receptor status.

67. Cuzick J, Sestaka I, Pinder S, et al. Effect of tamoxifen and radiotherapy in women with locally excised ductal carcinoma in situ: long-term results from the UK/ANZ DCIS trial. Lancet Oncol 2010;12(1):21–9.

68. Rodrigues N, Dillon D, Parisot N, et al. Differences in the pathologic and molecular features of intraductal breast carcinoma between younger and older women. Cancer 2003;97:1393–403.

69. Silverstein MJ, Lagios MD. Choosing treatment for patients with DCIS: fine tuning the University of Southern California/Van-Nuys Prognostic Index. J Natl Cancer Inst Monogr 2010;41:193–6.

70. Provenzano E, Hopper JL, Giles GG, et al. Biological markers that predict clinical recurrence in ductal carcinoma in situ of the breast. Eur J Cancer 2003;39:622–30.

71. Witton CJ, Reeves JR, Going JJ, et al. Expression of the HER 1–4 family of receptor tyrosine kinases in breast cancer. J Pathol 2003;200:290–7.

72. Barnes NLP, Khavari S, Boland GP, et al. Absence of HER4 expression predicts recurrence of ductal carcinoma in situ of the breast. Clin Cancer Res 2005;11:2163–8.

73. Lari SA, Kuerer HM. Biological markers in DCIS and risk of Breast recurrence: A systematic review. J Cancer. 2011. May 1; 2; 232–61.

74. Goodwin A, Parker S, Ghersi D, et al. Post-operative radiotherapy for ductal carcinoma in situ of the breast. Cochrane Database Syst Rev 2009;(1)CD000563.

75. Emdin SO, Granstrand B, Ringberg A, et al. SweDCIS: radiotherapy after sector resection for ductal carcinoma in situ of the breast. Results of a randomised trial in a population offered mammography screening. Acta Oncol 2006;45(5):536–43.

76. Bijker N, Meijnen P, Peterse JL, et al. Breast-conserving treatment with or without radiotherapy in ductal carcinoma-in-situ: ten-year results of European Organisation for Research and Treatment of Cancer randomized phase III trial 10853 – a study by the EORTC Breast Cancer Cooperative Group and EORTC Radiotherapy Group. J Clin Oncol 2006;24(21):3381–7.

77. Wong J, Kaelin C, Troyan S, et al. Prospective study of wide local excision alone for ductal carcinoma in situ of the breast. J Clin Oncol 2006;24(7):1031–6.

78. Hughes L, Wang M, Page D, et al. Local excision alone without irradiation for ductal carcinoma in situ of the breast: a trial of the Eastern Cooperative Oncology Group. J Clin Oncol 2009;27(32):5319–24.

79. 2009 National Institutes for Health State-of-the-Science meeting on Ductal Carcinoma in Situ: Management and Diagnosis. J Natl Cancer Inst Monogr 2010;2010(41)111–222.

80. Allred DC, Anderson SJ, Paik S, et al. Adjuvant tamoxifen reduces subsequent breast cancer in women with estrogen receptor-positive ductal carcinoma in situ: a study based on NSABP Protocol B-24. J Clin Oncol 2012;30(12):1268–73.

81. Boland GP, McKeowan A, Chan KC, et al. Biological response to hormonal manipulation in oestrogen receptor positive ductal carcinoma in situ of the breast. Br J Cancer 2003;89:277–83.

82. Bundred NJ, Cramer A, Cheung KL, et al. ERISAC trial: evidence exemestane effects oestrogen receptor (ER) positive ductal carcinoma in situ (DCIS) proliferation. Breast Cancer Res Treat 2007;106(Suppl. 1):S5043.

83. Fisher B, Constantino JP, Wickerman DL, et al. Tamoxifen for prevention of breast cancer: report of the National Surgical Adjuvant Breast and Bowel Project P-1 Study. J Natl Cancer Inst 1998;90:1371–88.

84. Pappo I, Wasserman I, Halevy A. Ductal carcinoma in situ of the breast in men: a review. Clin Breast Cancer 2005;6(4):310–4.

85. Simmons RM. Male ductal carcinoma in situ presenting as bloody nipple discharge: a case report and literature review. Breast J 2002;8:112–4.

86. Hittmair AP, Liniger RA, Tavassoli FA. Ductal carcinoma in situ (DCIS) in the male breast. A morphological study of 84 cases of pure DCIS and 30 cases of DCIS associated with invasive carcinoma: a preliminary report. Cancer 1998;83:2139–49.

87. Li X, Lewis MT, Huang J, et al. Intrinsic resistance of tumorigenic breast cancer cells to chemotherapy. J Natl Cancer Inst 2008;100(9):672–9.

12

The role of adjuvant systemic therapy in patients with operable breast cancer

Rosalie Fisher
Ian Smith

Introduction

The mortality from breast cancer has fallen by over 15% in the UK over the last 15 years, despite a rising incidence. The improvement in survival coincides with the widespread uptake of adjuvant systemic therapy and increasing evidence of its survival benefit. The rationale for this treatment is that over half of women with operable breast cancer who receive local regional treatment alone will die from metastatic disease, indicating the presence of micrometastases at the time of initial clinical presentation. Traditionally, the major risk factors for recurrence have been the involvement of axillary nodes, poor histological grade, large tumour size and histological evidence of lymphovascular invasion around the tumour site. The absence of oestrogen and progestogen receptor and the over-expression of human epidermal growth factor receptor 2 (HER-2) also carry an adverse prognosis. The only way to improve survival for these women is to administer effective systemic medical treatment, using endocrine therapy, chemotherapy and targeted biological therapies, along with surgery and radiotherapy. It is now recognised that breast cancer comprises a number of subtypes, each with a distinct biological behaviour and prognosis, and increasingly molecular factors rather than classical histopathological features are being used to determine the degree of residual risk after breast cancer surgery, and all the judicious use of potentially toxic treatments.[1] Gene expression profiling has emerged as a new determinant of recurrence risk and a major current challenge is to assimilate this new technology into treatment planning.

Adjuvant endocrine therapy

Approximately 75% of invasive breast cancer patients present with hormone-receptor positive disease.[2] As the oestrogen receptor (ER) pathway is key to the growth of these cancers, modulation of ER activation is an essential component of treatment for these women. Since the observation by Beatson more than 100 years ago that oophorectomy could induce regression of advanced breast cancer,[3] endocrine treatment has proved one of the most valuables therapies in cancer medicine.

Tamoxifen

Until recently tamoxifen was the standard adjuvant endocrine therapy. The results of the most recent overview of tamoxifen trials involving around 21 000 women carried out by the Early Breast Cancer Trialists' Collaborative Group (EBCTCG) have shown that tamoxifen given for about 5 years reduces the risk of death by around one-third (relative risk (RR) = 0.71 ± 0.07).[4] The proportional reduction is not significantly affected by age, nodal status or use of chemotherapy; the absolute benefit of course relates to the absolute risk. The reduction in the risk of recurrence is seen both during the 5 years of treatment (RR = 0.53 ± 0.03) and extends into years 5–9 (RR = 0.70 ± 0.06), but there was no further reduction in risk beyond 10 years. The benefits were similar and highly significant in both ER-positive/progesterone receptor (PgR)-positive and ER-positive/PgR-negative disease. The reduction was greater in strongly positive ER disease (RR = 0.51 ± 0.07) than in marginally ER-positive disease (RR = 0.65 ± 0.07).

Tamoxifen is associated with a small but significantly increased risk of developing uterine carcinoma and of thromboembolism; when combined these two conditions result in a 10-year mortality of 0.2%.

Tamoxifen duration

The overview data indicate that 5 years of tamoxifen is more effective than shorter durations. Until very recently, there was no convincing evidence that more than 5 years of tamoxifen had a further advantage. Indeed, the largest published trial so far of tamoxifen for more than 5 years (National Surgical Adjuvant Breast and Bowel Project (NSABP) B14) showed that tamoxifen for more than 5 years had an unexpected adverse influence on disease-free survival (DFS) (78% vs. 82% with placebo, P = 0.03) and was also associated with higher rates of endometrial cancer, ischaemic heart disease and cerebral vascular disease.[5] Recently a much larger international trial involving 11 500 patients, the Adjuvant Tamoxifen Longer Against Shorter (ATLAS) trial, has addressed the question of long-term tamoxifen duration. Results have so far been presented only in abstract form, but showed a small but significant reduction in recurrence comparing 5 years with more than 5 years treatment (hazard ratio (HR) = 0.88).[6] Preliminary results from a similar UK trial (aTTom: adjuvant Tamoxifen – To offer more?) involving 8000 patients are reported to be consistent with those of ATLAS, but mature data are awaited.[7]

Aromatase inhibitors

First line

✓✓ The aromatase inhibitors anastrozole and letrozole have each been shown to improve DFS compared with tamoxifen when given as first-line adjuvant therapy for a planned 5 years in postmenopausal women with hormone receptor-positive early breast cancer[8,9] (**Fig. 12.1**).

In the ATAC (Arimidex, Tamoxifen, Alone or in Combination) trial involving over 9000 women, anastrozole was compared with tamoxifen and with a combination of the two drugs, and was shown to be superior to both in terms of DFS. With a median follow-up of 120 months, a 5-year DFS benefit of 4.3% (HR = 0.86) emerged in hormone receptor-positive patients.[10]

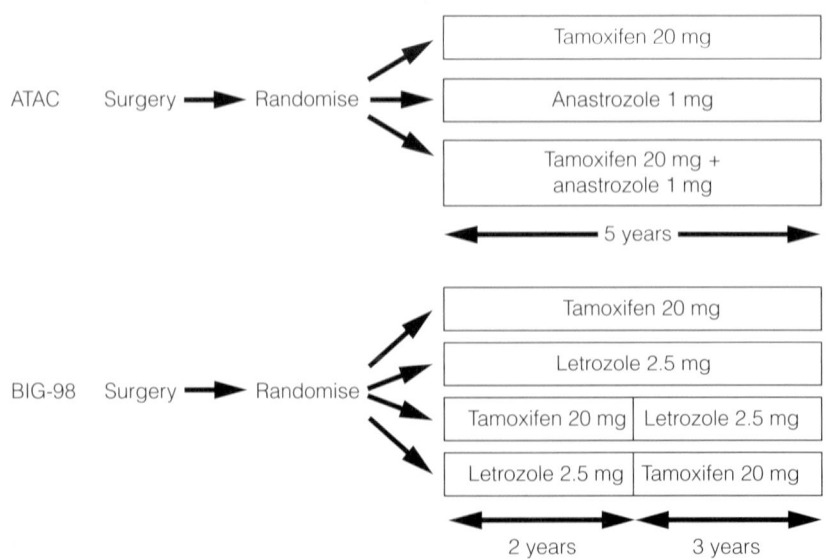

Figure 12.1 • The ATAC and BIG1-98 trial schemes.

In the BIG1-98 trial involving more than 8000 women, letrozole was compared with tamoxifen in a four-arm trial as follows: letrozole monotherapy; tamoxifen monotherapy; sequential tamoxifen then letrozole; sequential letrozole then tamoxifen; all for a total of 5 years. With a median follow-up period of 8.7 years, letrozole was significantly better than tamoxifen in terms of both DFS (HR = 0.82, 95% confidence interval (CI) 074–0.92) and overall survival (OS) (HR = 0.79, CI 0.69–0.90).[11] This is in contrast to the ATAC trial, where no overall survival benefit was seen for anastrozole over tamoxifen. The results of these two trials are summarised in Table 12.1.

First-line aromatase inhibitors: bad prognosis subgroups

ER-positive, PgR-negative breast cancers are recognised as having a poorer outcome.[12] In the EBCTCG analysis, patients with PgR poor tumours had a worse prognosis but nevertheless had a similar proportional benefit to adjuvant tamoxifen compared with control.[4]

The relative gain with anastrozole and letrozole respectively over tamoxifen is similar in both the ATAC and the BIG 1-98 trials,[13] but in both instances the absolute gain is greater in patients with PgR-negative cancers, because of the greater risk of recurrence.

HER-2-positive tumours have a worse prognosis than HER-2-negative cancers and in a neoadjuvant endocrine therapy trial comparing letrozole with tamoxifen, a large and highly significant benefit was seen for letrozole over tamoxifen in terms of clinical response in this small subgroup (88 vs. 21%, $P = 0.0004$).[14] In a similar neoadjuvant trial comparing anastrozole with tamoxifen, the IMmediate Preoperative Arimidex Compared with Tamoxifen (IMPACT) trial, a numerical although

non-significant difference was again seen in favour of the aromatase inhibitor for HER-2-positive tumours (58% vs. 22%, $P = 0.09$).[15]

These results were not, however, confirmed in the equivalent adjuvant trials. In the ATAC trial there was no evidence of a proportionately greater benefit for anastrozole over tamoxifen in HER-2-positive tumours compared with other subtypes.[13] A similar finding was true when letrozole was compared with tamoxifen in the BIG1-98 trial.[16] Invasive lobular cancers appear to benefit more from letrozole than tamoxifen.[17]

Comparative toxicities of front-line anastrozole/letrozole and tamoxifen

The ATAC and BIG1-98 trials have both shown that tamoxifen is associated with a small but significant increase in the incidence of hot flushes compared with anastrozole or letrozole (4.5–5% increase), vaginal bleeding (3.3–3.7% increase), vaginal discharge (8.6% increase), endometrial carcinoma (0.2–0.4% increase) and venous thromboembolism (1.4–2% increase). The ATAC trial has likewise shown a small but significant increase in ischaemic cerebral vascular disease (1.1% increase) with tamoxifen compared with anastrozole, but this has not been confirmed in the BIG1-98 trial with letrozole. In contrast, anastrozole and letrozole have been shown to be associated with a statistically significant increase in the incidence of musculoskeletal problems (6.5–8% increase) and fractures (1.7–2.2% increase).

Of note, tamoxifen is associated with a significant increase in gynaecological surgery compared with either of the aromatase inhibitors. In the ATAC trial 5.1% of women had hysterectomies compared with 1.3% on anastrozole.[18] In the BIG1-98 trial 288 women (9.1%) have required endometrial biopsies compared with 77 (2.3%) with letrozole.[9]

Sequential therapy with aromatase inhibitors after tamoxifen

Until recently, there was considerable interest in trials assessing the benefit of sequential adjuvant aromatase inhibitors given 2–3 years after tamoxifen. For example, in the Intergroup Exemestane Study (IES), 4274 patients who had already been on tamoxifen for around 2 years were randomised double-blind to continuing on tamoxifen or switching to exemestane to complete 5 years of treatment. Updated results with a median follow-up of 91 months have shown a significant reduction

Table 12.1 • Results from the ATAC and BIG1-98 trials

	ATAC*	BIG1-98*
No. of patients	6241	8010
Median follow-up (years)	10	8.7
DFS (hazard ratio)	0.91	0.82
5-year DFS difference (%)#	2.7	3.1
OS (hazard ratio)	0.97†	0.79

*Monotherapy groups only.
†Non-significant. #Absolute difference

in the risk of relapse and an improvement in OS (HR = 0.86, 95% CI 0.75–0.99) with the switch.[19] Three other sequential trials involving anastrozole have shown similar results.[20–22]

These results suggested possible superiority with sequential switching over the benefit achieved with first-line aromatase inhibitor therapy in ATAC and BIG1-98.

Two trials have addressed this issue directly, however, and recently reported results. Two of the arms in BIG1-98 compared tamoxifen for 2 years followed by a switch to letrozole with letrozole alone for 5 years and found no significant benefit of the switch compared with letrozole up front (8-year DFS 85.9% vs. 87.5%).[11] Likewise, in the TEAM (Tamoxifen Exemestane Adjuvant Multinational) trial, 9779 patients were randomised to tamoxifen for 2–3 years followed by exemestane to complete 5 years or to exemestane up front for 5 years. No significant difference was found in DFS (85% vs. 86%) with a median follow-up of 5.1 years.[23]

> ✅ Current evidence therefore suggests that it is easier and at least as effective to give aromatase inhibitors up front rather than after 2–3 years of tamoxifen.

Extended adjuvant therapy with aromatase inhibitors

The risk of recurrence of early breast cancer continues for at least 10 years after diagnosis and is greater in patients with hormone receptor-positive cancers.[24] In the EBCTCG overview analysis more than half of breast cancer recurrences occur after the 5-year mark.[4]

Against this background, the results of the MA17 trial evaluating the benefit of extended adjuvant therapy with letrozole in women still in remission after 5 years of tamoxifen were of great importance in that they demonstrated a significant DFS benefit in favour of letrozole.[25] This benefit has continued, and indeed increased with time, with an initial HR of 0.52 (95% CI 0.40–0.64) 12 months after randomisation, increasing to 0.19 (0.04–0.34) after 48 months. Recently a similar and perhaps even greater benefit has been reported for the subgroup of 889 younger women <50 and premenopausal at the time of diagnosis but who subsequently became postmenopausal during their 5 years of tamoxifen,

with an absolute gain in 4-year DFS of 10%.[26] This represents a risk reduction of 75% with extended adjuvant endocrine therapy compared with 33% in the much larger group who were postmenopausal from the outset.

In two similar but smaller trials, extended adjuvant anastrozole (ABCSG-6a) and extended adjuvant exemestane (NSABP-B33), both after 5 years of tamoxifen, showed that extended therapy with an aromatase inhibitor reduces the risk of recurrence significantly.[27,28]

The optimal duration of adjuvant aromatase inhibitor therapy has not yet been established. It is possible that for some women very lengthy or even lifelong treatment might be the most appropriate but this has to be balanced against the potential risks of very-long-term usage. Clinical trials are essential in this area. In this context, the MA17 trial is now running a second randomisation for women still in remission after 5 years of letrozole. Other trials are also addressing this key issue, including NSABP B-42 (5 vs. 10 years letrozole) and the ABCG-16 Secondary Adjuvant Long-term Study with Arimidex (SALSA) comparing a further 2 years versus a further 5 years of adjuvant treatment with anastrozole after an initial 5 years of adjuvant endocrine therapy.

Other aromatase inhibitor issues

Aromatase inhibitors are contraindicated in premenopausal women. Likewise, caution must be observed in their use in younger women following chemotherapy-induced amenorrhoea. In an audit carried out at the Royal Marsden Hospital 12 of 45 younger women (27%), median age 47, treated with an aromatase inhibitor following chemotherapy-induced amenorrhoea (27%) developed clinical or biochemical return of ovarian function (including up to the age of 53 years).[29] Aromatase inhibitors should therefore be used with great caution in this group of women and ideally serum oestradiol should be monitored using a high sensitivity assay.

Vaginal dryness, atrophy and dyspareunia are significant issues in women on aromatase inhibitors. In a small study, six of seven women given vaginal oestradiol (Vagifem®) while on an aromatase inhibitor developed a significant rise in serum oestradiol from less than 5 pmol/L to a mean of 72 pmo/L (maximum 219 pmol/L) at 2 weeks.[30]

✅ The majority of vaginal oestrogen preparations should not be used in women on aromatase inhibitors unless serum oestradiol levels can be monitored with a high sensitivity assay. Estring® releases very low levels of oestrogen continuously and appears to have very low levels of absorption when compared to oestrogen creams or pessaries. This may well be a better option, although confirmatory studies have not yet been done. The other option is to switch to tamoxifen, which is likely to be of similar efficacy except for high-risk cancers.

Endocrine therapy in premenopausal women

✅✅ The 2011 EBCTCG overview analysis shows no significant difference in the reduction in the risk of recurrence or mortality with tamoxifen in women less than 45 compared with older women (Table 12.2).[4]

A key question is whether ovarian suppression in addition to tamoxifen (and chemotherapy where appropriate) is superior to tamoxifen alone in the management of premenopausal breast cancer. In the INT-101 trial, the addition of goserelin and tamoxifen to standard adjuvant therapy with CAF (cyclophosphmide, adriamycin and fluorouracil) significantly improved DFS; 9-year DFS rates were 57% for CAF, 60% for CAF plus goserelin, and 68% for CAF plus goserelin and tamoxifen.[31] An unplanned retrospective analysis of these data suggested that the addition of goserelin to CAF was most beneficial in those women under the age of 40. A prospective trial, SOFT (Suppression of Ovarian

Function), is currently addressing this question and has recruited 3000 premenopausal women with hormone receptor-positive disease randomised to tamoxifen alone for 5 years or ovarian suppression with either tamoxifen or exemestane for 5 years in women post-chemotherapy who are still menstruating, or who have not received chemotherapy. It is currently in active follow-up. In a randomised trial involving 927 premenopausal women, no significant differences in risk reduction were seen after 12 years of follow-up between tamoxifen alone (27%) or a combination of tamoxifen with the luteinising hormone-releasing hormone (LHRH) analogue goserelin (24%).[32]

✅ Given the potential long-term morbidity of early treatment-induced menopause, the authors do not believe there is currently a strong evidence base for recommending ovarian suppression in addition to tamoxifen.

The SOFT trial also addresses the important question of whether an aromatase inhibitor is superior to tamoxifen in premenopausal patients who have undergone ovarian suppression. The only trial to present data on this so far is ABCSG-12 and the Austrian Group reported no significant difference in outcome for 1803 women randomised to tamoxifen or anastrozole, both given with goserelin, with a median 62 months follow-up.[33]

Obesity and adjuvant endocrine therapy

An increase in body mass index is associated with an increased risk of breast cancer recurrence[34,35] and this was recently confirmed in patients in the ATAC trial.[36] Moreover, the benefit of anastrozole over tamoxifen in terms of distant recurrence was lost in patients with a body mass index of 25 kg/m^2 or greater, and a similar trend was seen for all recurrences. The Austrian ABCSG-6 and -6a trials in which patients who had maintained a continued remission on tamoxifen for 5 years were randomised to a further 3 years of anastrozole or not have reported similar findings. Outcome was not influenced by body weight during tamoxifen therapy, but during extended adjuvant therapy an exploratory analysis found that women with normal body weight randomised to anastrozole had a significant gain in DFS

Table 12.2 • Outcomes for oestrogen receptor-positive patients with ~5 years tamoxifen, by age at trial entry

Age	<45 years	45–54 years	55–69 years
Risk reduction for recurrence	0.63	0.72	0.54
Risk reduction for breast cancer mortality	0.71	0.82	0.63

Table 12.3 • Summary of recommendations for adjuvant endocrine therapy

Menopausal status*	Recommendation
Premenopausal	Tamoxifen 5 years
Postmenopausal[†]	Anastrazole 5 years or Letrozole 5 years
Women who are menopausal after 5 years of tamoxifen	Consider: Anastrazole Letrozole Exemestane in high-risk patients
Women who have completed 5 years of aromatase inhibitor	Currently no data Consider option of continuing in high-risk patients

*Based on pre-chemotherapy menopausal status.
[†]Caution in women under the age of 50; return of ovarian function on aromatase inhibitor is possible.

(HR = 0.46, $P = 0.02$) and OS (HR = 0.37, $P = 0.02$), whereas no gain was seen in patients with a body mass index of greater than $25 \, kg/m^2$.[37] This raises the intriguing possibility that anastrozole, a relatively weak aromatase inhibitor, is unable to inhibit fully the excess aromatase associated with adiposity. In contrast, in the BIG 1-98 trial, the benefit of letrozole, a much more potent aromatase inhibitor than anastrozole, over tamoxifen was maintained whatever the body mass index.[38] Further data are required, but these results suggest that anastrozole may not be the optimal aromatase inhibitor in women with higher body mass indices.

See Table 12.3 for a summary of recommendations for adjuvant endocrine therapy.

Adjuvant chemotherapy

✓✓ Adjuvant chemotherapy is effective in the treatment of early breast cancer. The 2011 Oxford Overview meta-analysis[39] included outcome data from more than 100 polychemotherapy trials (including the oldest of 25 years) and for approximately 100 000 randomised women, and reported that combination chemotherapy reduces the annual risk of recurrence by almost 25% and reduces the risk of death by around 14%. Furthermore, greater reductions in breast cancer and overall mortality were shown in comparisons between trials of more modern and older chemotherapy regimens. Most of the effect of adjuvant chemotherapy on the risk of recurrence

is seen within the first 5 years after randomisation. Patient selection is critical to the effective and safe use of adjuvant chemotherapy; for some subgroups, the benefit is very much larger than the average and for others smaller. Adjuvant chemotherapy began in women with involved axillary lymph nodes for whom recurrence risk was highest. It is now clear that many women with node-negative disease also benefit; conversely it is likely that some with node-positive disease do not. The most recent Oxford meta-analysis suggests that the proportional risk reductions associated with taxane- or anthracycline-based chemotherapy regimens are not influenced by age, nodal status or tumour characteristics.[39] Currently, a great deal of research is focused on identifying with more precision than in the past which patients are likely to benefit from chemotherapy, and particularly those women with oestrogen receptor-positive cancers who benefit, as in these women adjuvant endocrine therapy also improves outcome. Indeed, a poll of international breast cancer specialists indicated that this was the top priority in breast cancer research.[40]

Age and chemotherapy

In general, the absolute gain from chemotherapy is higher for younger than older women.[39] It is likely, however, that this difference relates mainly to the biological characteristics of breast cancer being more favourable to chemotherapy response (ER negativity, for example) in younger women, rather than an intrinsic adverse interaction between age and chemotherapy efficacy.[41]

Elderly women with breast cancer have been under-represented in clinical trials to date, but this is changing. The Cancer and Leukaemia Group B (CALGB) 49907 trial demonstrated that standard adjuvant chemotherapy was superior to single-agent oral chemotherapy with capecitabine in women over the age of 65, and suggested that the benefit was more pronounced in women with hormone receptor-negative tumours.[42] However, it is also clear that older women experience significantly greater toxicity with adjuvant cytotoxic treatment,[43–46] and there are a number of trials under way that aim to define those elderly patients for whom chemotherapy is most appropriate.

Nodal status

Initially adjuvant chemotherapy tended to be reserved for patients with axillary node involvement on the basis of higher risk. It is now clear that the proportional reduction in the risk of recurrence is similar for those with node-negative as for node-positive disease.[39] Nevertheless, since the absolute risk is greater with nodal involvement, so is the absolute benefit. Although nodal involvement carries a worse prognosis, this does not necessarily imply chemotherapy benefit and we are now in an era when molecular markers are at least as important as nodal status in determining chemotherapy benefit (see below).

ER status

There has been considerable controversy over the years as to whether patients with ER-positive disease gain as much from adjuvant chemotherapy as those whose tumours are ER negative. The 2011 Oxford Overview data indicate that the proportional benefits are very similar, both in older and younger women.[39]

The Overview also indicates an additional benefit for combination chemotherapy over tamoxifen alone for ER-positive tumours, but again more so for younger than for older women. Recent evidence, however, suggests that the major chemotherapy benefit in ER-positive breast cancer is in selected subgroups and that for many patients with ER-positive cancers there is little or no benefit for chemotherapy (see below).

Anthracycline-based chemotherapy

Anthracyclines have been used widely for the last decade or more, and have largely replaced older CMF (cyclophosphamide/methotrexate/fluorouracil) regimens. The 2005 Overview data (including trials involving a total of around 40 000 women) established clearly the efficacy of anthracycline-based adjuvant regimens in early breast cancer, and indicated an additional proportional risk of recurrence of around 11% and a proportional reduction in mortality of around 16%.[47]

✓✓ Since this Overview, other studies have confirmed the greater benefits with anthracycline-based therapy,[48–50] including, in the UK, the National Epirubicin Adjuvant Trial (NEAT) trial.[51]

Dose of anthracyclines

The two main anthracyclines in current use are adriamycin (doxorubicin) and epirubicin. The Cancer and Leukaemia Group B (CALGB) 9344 trial randomised women with node-positive breast cancer to receive four courses of anthracycline chemotherapy to one of three different adriamycin dose levels (60, 75 or 90 mg/m^2), followed by four cycles of paclitaxel or not.[52] This important dose escalation trial showed no benefit for adriamycin doses above 60 mg/m^2 and this dose should now be considered standard.

The French Adjuvant Study Group (FASG)-05 trial randomised lymph node-positive women with poor prognosis and found a dose effect in favour of six cycles of FEC100 (epirubicin 100 mg/m^2) over six cycles of FEC50 (epirubicin 50 mg/m^2).[53] A significant improvement in the DFS (66.3 months vs. 54.8 months) and 5-year OS (77.4% vs. 65.3%) was seen in the FEC100 group but there were significantly more side-effects in the FEC100 group. These included neutropenia, anaemia, nausea and vomiting, stomatitis, alopecia and grade 3 infections. It is important to note that this trial does not determine that an epirubicin dose of 100 mg/m^2 is optimal. All that can be concluded is that 50 mg/m^2 is suboptimal and that a dose between the two is likely to achieve the best balance between efficacy and toxicity.

In the 2011 Oxford meta-analysis, four cycles of anthracycline chemotherapy appeared equivalent to six courses of standard CMF, but there was a clear improvement in recurrence and mortality when regimens with a cumulative anthracycline dosage of more than 240 mg/m^2 adriamycin or 360 mg/m^2 epirubicin (for example, fluorouracil/adriamycin/cyclophosphamide (FAC) or FEC) were compared with CMF (risk ratio 0.89 and 0.84 for recurrence and mortality respectively).[39]

Higher doses of anthracylines are related to long-term complications such as an increased incidence of acute myeloid leukaemia (AML)/myelodysplasia. In the EBC-1/MA.5 study by the NCIC CTG, which used the very high epirubicin dose of 120 mg/m^2, a disturbingly high incidence of AML/myelodysplasia was reported (2% at 10-year follow-up).[50] Likewise, in a study that analysed the toxicity of adjuvant chemotherapy treatment in elderly patients, there was a linear increase in the incidence of AML/myelodysplasia with advancing age ($P < 0.001$) with a reported incidence of 1.8% for the group of age >65 years.[43]

Cardiotoxicity is a further concern with the anthracyclines. Symptomatic congestive heart failure (CHF) is a rare but very serious complication in patients receiving an anthracycline-based chemotherapy regimen with an incidence that relates to the cumulative dose received.[54,55] As with secondary AML, there is an association between the risk of cardiotoxicity and increasing age. Recent long-term data on cardiac safety in more than 40 000 early breast cancer patients of an older age treated with adjuvant anthracycline regimens have shown an increased risk of cardiotoxicity compared with non-anthracycline chemotherapy treatment. This was statistically significant in the group of patients aged 66–70 with a 26% increased risk of developing CHF. This difference in rates of CHF continued to increase through more than 10 years of follow-up.[45]

For all these reasons, therefore, it is important to determine whether high doses of epirubicin (90 mg/m^2 and above) really are more effective than moderate doses of around 75 mg/m^2 to justify the additional toxicity, and trials addressing this issue are indicated.

Anthracyclines and HER-2-positive disease

The CALGB 8541 trial reported in 397 node-positive patients that high expression of HER-2 was associated with benefit from standard doses of doxorubicin (60 mg/m^2) but not from lower doses of anthracyclines.[56] In contrast, this dose–response effect was not seen in the majority whose tumours did not overexpress HER-2. An additional cohort of 595 patients showed an even stronger correlation between HER-2 overexpression and CAF dose efficacy with further follow-up.[57] No significant interaction was observed in the CALGB 9344 study between HER-2 status and the use of doses of doxorubicin >60 mg/m^2.[58]

In a retrospective study of 639 formalin-fixed paraffin-embedded specimens obtained from 710 premenopausal women with node-positive breast cancer who had received either cyclophosphamide, epirubicin and fluorouracil (CEF) or CMF, *HER2* amplification or overexpression was associated with a poor prognosis regardless of the type of treatment. In patients whose tumours showed amplification of *HER2*, CEF was superior to CMF in terms of recurrence-free survival (RFS) (HR = 0.52, 95% CI 0.34–0.80; P = 0.003) and OS (HR = 0.65,

95% CI 0.42–1.02; P = 0.06).[59] Similarly, a retrospective evaluation of patients in the Southwest Oncology Group study (SWOG) 8814 trial, which randomised postmenopausal patients with node-positive hormone receptor-positive tumours between tamoxifen and tamoxifen plus CAF chemotherapy, showed that CAF offered a substantial advantage for patients with HER-2-positive cancers but little, if any, advantage for those with HER-2-negative tumours.[60]

Recently, the Breast Cancer International Research Group (BCIRG)-006 trial published results of a non-anthracycline regimen combined with trastuzumab in patients with HER-2-positive early breast cancer.[61] This prospective study randomised 3222 women to one of three treatment arms: doxorubicin and cyclophosphamide followed by docetaxel (AC-T), the same regimen plus 52 weeks of trastuzumab (AC-TH), or docetaxel and carboplatin plus 52 weeks of trastuzumab (TCH). Predictably, both trastuzumab-containing regimens improved DFS and OS significantly compared to the AC arm, but there were no significant differences between AC-T and TCH in these outcome measures (DFS at 5 years 75%, 84% and 81% for AC, AC-T and TCH respectively, and OS 87%, 92% and 91% respectively). Anthracycline-based treatments resulted in significantly higher rates of cardiotoxicity and leukaemia, and TCH was better tolerated overall.

✓ BCIRG-006 was not designed as a non-inferiority trial, but it is reasonable to conclude that TCH is an acceptable standard of care in the adjuvant treatment of HER-2-positive early breast cancer, and should be considered for those patients who have a higher baseline risk for cardiac and other toxicities.

This trial raises the critical question of whether adjuvant chemotherapy regimens should always include an anthracycline. There has been much interest in defining the biological mechanism that underlies the anthracycline sensitivity of HER-2-positive breast cancers, and a number of studies have implicated alterations in topoisomerase II-α (*TOP2A*) in this process. The *TOP2A* gene regulates DNA replication and RNA transcription and is considered a target of anthracyclines. It is located on chromosome 17, in close proximity to the *HER2* gene, and the two are frequently co-amplified. However, despite a number of pre-clinical and clinical studies, (including a sub-study of the BCIRG-006 trial described above) suggesting a predictive role for *TOP2A* amplification and benefit from anthracyclines, other studies disagree, so at present there is no indication to look for *TOP2A* amplification when considering treatment selection.[62,63]

Taxanes

Paclitaxel (Taxol) and docetaxel (Taxotere) have emerged as two of the most active cytotoxic agents against breast cancer. In the metastatic setting, these compounds have been shown to be active in anthracyline-resistant breast cancers.[64] Several randomised trials have evaluated the benefit of taxanes combined with anthracyclines in the adjuvant treatment of early breast cancer,[52,65–69] but their exact role remains controversial. The majority have shown a DFS benefit, but some have failed to show a benefit in OS[65,70] and in endocrine receptor-positive tumours.[52,70] A meta-analysis of 13 randomised trials involving more than 22 000 patients assessing the addition of a taxane to an anthracycline-based regimen[71] showed an absolute improvement at 5 years of approximately 5% for recurrence and 3% for death. This benefit is present irrespective of the number of lymph nodes involved (N1–3 vs. N4+), ER status (ER positive vs. ER negative) or age/menopausal status (≤50 years/premenopausal vs. >50 years/postmenopausal). The most recent Oxford meta-analysis of polychemotherapy included data from 44 000 women in 33 taxane studies.[39] A significant reduction in breast cancer mortality (15–20%) was found when trials that added four separate cycles of a taxane to anthracycline chemotherapy (thereby prolonging adjuvant chemotherapy duration) were compared with anthracycline chemotherapy alone, but this benefit was much smaller (though still significant) when studies in which the number of anthracycline cycles was increased to balance treatment duration were analysed. The results of this meta-analysis suggest that the benefit from taxanes is independent of age, nodal status or hormone receptor status. It should also be noted, however, that results from the largest adjuvant taxane trial, the UK Taxotere as Adjuvant Chemotherapy Trial (TACT), involving 4162 patients, did not show a significant benefit for the addition of docetaxel to standard anthracycline chemotherapy.[70]

✅ Our interpretation of all these data is that the most convincing evidence of benefit for adjuvant taxanes is in patients with ER-negative and/or HER-2-positive disease. In a retrospective analysis of the CALGB 9344 trial, in which patients with node-positive breast cancer were randomised to receive paclitaxel (175 mg/m^2) or observation after four cycles of AC at doses of 60, 75 and 90 mg/m^2,[58] patients who gained from the addition of paclitaxel were those with HER-2-positive disease (including those with ER-positive and ER-negative disease) and those with HER-2-negative and ER-negative disease. In contrast, patients whose tumours were HER-2 negative and ER positive (by far the largest group) achieved no benefit from the addition of paclitaxel.

Adjuvant docetaxel has also been tested instead of an anthracycline in patients with early breast cancer. In a prospective US Oncology phase III trial, a total of 1106 patients were randomised to received either four cycles of standard AC (doxorubicin 60 mg/m^2 and cyclophosphamide 600 mg/m^2) or four cycles of TC (docetaxel 75 mg/m^2 and cyclophosphamide 600 mg/m^2) as adjuvant treatment for early breast cancer.[72] Treatment with TC achieved a significant improvement in 5-year DFS compared with AC (86% vs. 80% respectively, HR = 0.67; P = 0.015). With further follow-up a significant overall survival benefit has also emerged.[73] There was significantly more nausea and vomiting in patients receiving AC compared with TC, whereas patients receiving docetaxel experienced more oedema, myalgia, arthralgia and a higher rate of fever and neutropenia compared with AC (5% vs. 2.5%; P = 0.07).

Which taxane and which schedule?

The optimal schedule is determined by the type of taxane selected, as demonstrated by the pivotal ECOG 1199 trial.[74] Nearly 5000 women with node-positive or high-risk node-negative disease were enrolled and received standard AC chemotherapy for four cycles, followed by paclitaxel or docetaxel, either given every 3 weeks for four cycles or weekly for 12 cycles. Progression-free survival was superior in those treated with 3-weekly docetaxel (HR = 1.23), or weekly paclitaxel (HR = 1.27), when compared with the standard treatment of paclitaxel given 3-weekly. A survival gain was demonstrated in patients treated with weekly compared with 3-weekly paclitaxel (HR = 1.32). On the basis of these results, weekly paclitaxel or 3-weekly docetaxel are considered standards of care in adjuvant breast cancer treatment.

Duration of chemotherapy

The optimum duration of chemotherapy remains uncertain. The 1998 EBCTG meta-analysis assessed five CMF-based trials and found no survival benefit for more than 6 months treatment,[75] but the most recent data suggest that regimens utilising chemotherapy regimens longer than four cycles of AC (more cycles or higher cumulative dose) are more effective.[39] A French FASG-01 trial showed a significant benefit in DFS of six cycles of FEC50 over three cycles of FEC50 or 75, and improved OS with six cycles of FEC50 over three cycles.[76]

Preliminary results of the CALGB 40101 trial were presented recently in abstract form[77] and indicate that for women with early breast cancer and no or limited lymph node disease (0–3), four cycles of 3-weekly AC or weekly paclitaxel were equivalent in efficacy to six cycles of either. Further trials of chemotherapy duration are needed.

Dose density

Recently interest has developed in accelerated (also called dose-dense) chemotherapy in which treatment is given at 2-week rather than 3-week intervals with G-CSF (granulocyte colony-stimulating factor) support to overcome the risk of neutropenic sepsis. The CALGB 9741 trial has shown that accelerated 2-weekly AC × 4 followed by accelerated paclitaxel × 4 improved efficacy over the same eight courses given conventionally at 3-weekly intervals in women with node-positive breast cancer, with 4-year DFS of 82% and 75% respectively.[78] In addition, the accelerated arm was associated with less neutropenic sepsis. Likewise, an Italian trial, so far presented only in abstract form, has shown a similar increase in efficacy with reduced risk of neutropenic sepsis when six courses of FEC chemotherapy were given in accelerated fashion compared with the conventional approach.[79]

A recent systematic review and meta-analysis of dose-dense chemotherapy for early or locally advanced breast cancer reported improved outcomes with this approach, but included a number of trials with heterogeneous study designs and treatments, and for this reason did not provide meaningful conclusions.[80]

Which patients really benefit from adjuvant chemotherapy? The role of molecular markers

The EBCTCG Overview shows that, overall, the survival of patients with hormone receptor-positive disease is significantly improved by chemotherapy over and above tamoxifen, with an HR of 0.66.[39] The important question, however, is to identify those women for whom the gain is large enough to be of real clinical benefit when balanced against toxicity. Various guidelines for chemotherapy decision-making have been proposed; one of the best recognised is the St Gallen Consensus. In the most recent update, the 2011 St Gallen panel suggested that subtypes of breast cancer can be defined by gene array profiles, and that each subtype differs in its epidemiological risk factors, natural history, and response to systemic and local therapies.[1] Surrogate immunohistochemical markers of gene expression array information allow an approximate and simplified classification system of intrinsic subtypes (see Table 12.4). This latest consensus demonstrates a paradigm shift from the use of traditional clinico-pathological features to determine the risk of recurrence, towards an assessment of the underlying biology of the tumour. This is also evidenced by the fact that most of the panel supported further research into the role of molecular profiling techniques (discussed below) as prognostic and predictive tools in early breast cancer.

Table 12.4 • Intrinsic subtypes of breast cancer and approximation by immunohistochemistry (St Gallen 2011)

Intrinsic subtype	Clinico-pathological definition
Luminal A	ER positive HER-2 negative Ki67 low (<14%)*
Luminal B	ER positive HER-2 negative Ki67 high
HER-2 overexpression	HER-2 overexpressed ER absent
Basal-like	'Triple negative' ER, PgR absent HER-2 negative

*Definition of Ki67 low established by comparison with PAM50 intrinsic subtyping.[119]

Further insight into this issue comes from an analysis of the SWOG 8814 trial, in which post-menopausal women with node-positive hormone receptor-positive tumours were randomised to tamoxifen alone or tamoxifen with anthracycline-containing chemotherapy (cyclophosphamide, adriamycin and 5-fluorouracil).[81] Overall, there was a significant benefit in favour of those receiving chemotherapy concurrently with tamoxifen but in a retrospective subset analysis, patients with a high ER score (Allred score 7 or 8) showed no benefit from the addition of chemotherapy even in the presence of involved nodes. Likewise, women whose tumours were HER-2 negative showed no benefit from the addition of chemotherapy unless they had four or more nodes involved. This analysis should be considered by hypothesis generation rather than being definitive, but emphasises the need to identify molecular markers to predict which patients really benefit from chemotherapy.

Multiple gene expression assays including Oncotype DX

DNA micro array analysis has classified breast cancers according to gene expression signatures, to quantify more accurately the likelihood of breast cancer recurrence and predict the magnitude of chemotherapy benefit. Currently, the most widely used of these is a 21-gene assay now offered as a commercial reference laboratory test (Oncotype DX Genomic Health Inc.). This is based on formalin-fixed material from which the level of gene expression is used to determine a recurrence score predicting the likelihood of distant recurrence.[82] The Oncotype DX assay has been applied to a subset of patients in the NSABP B-20 trial, randomising women with node-negative disease to tamoxifen and chemotherapy (CMF or MF) versus tamoxifen alone. It was found that women with a low recurrence score had no significant benefit from chemotherapy, whereas those with a high recurrence score had a major and significant benefit with an absolute decrease in the 10-year rate of distant recurrence of 28% (88% vs. 60% free of distant recurrence).[83] Patients with an intermediate recurrence score had a relatively small benefit and such patients are now being included in a trial randomising women with cancers with

intermediate scores to chemotherapy or not in addition to endocrine therapy (TAILORx). Oncotype DX has also been validated in ER-positive patients in the ATAC trial[84] and in node-positive patients in SWOG 8814;[85] the key message from these data is that many patients, even those with node-positive disease, may not benefit from chemotherapy. The question with regard to Oncotype DX is its additional benefit over standard immunohistochemistry. This was addressed in a study where proliferation as measured by Ki67, were combined with ER, PgR and HER-2 to form the IHC4 score.[86] The score appeared to further risk-stratify those patients deemed intermediate risk by the Adjuvant Online and Nottingham Prognostic Index (NPI) and correlated closely with Oncotype DX. The main issue with the IHC4 is quality control; measuring Ki67 in a reproducible manner continues to be a problem in many laboratories.[87] Similarly, a 70-gene signature has also shown strong correlation with outcome[88,89] and identifies a good and a poor prognosis group. A second trial, MINDACT, is assessing the value of this signature, in predicting which patients with hormone receptor-positive tumours might also benefit from chemotherapy.

Bisphosphonates

Two of three early trials indicated a benefit for the use of oral clodronate compared with placebo in the adjuvant setting in early breast cancer.[90–93] Both positive trials observed a reduction in bone metastases and improvement in overall survival. The NSABP B-34 study is the largest trial to compare clodronate with placebo in addition to adjuvant chemo- or hormone therapy and results were presented recently. The trial's primary end-point of superior disease-free survival was not met, but there appeared to be distinct benefits of clodronate for women over the age of 50, including a trend toward improved overall survival.[94]

The results of two large trials of a much more potent bisphosphonate, zoledronic acid, have been published recently. The Austrian Breast and Colorectal Cancer Study Group trial-12 (ABSCG-12) randomised premenopausal women with hormone receptor-positive early breast cancer to anastrazole or tamoxifen, with or without zoledronic acid.[33] All patients received goserelin for ovarian suppression.

The investigators reported that disease-free survival was improved with the addition of zoledronic acid (HR = 0.68), although zoledronic acid did not significantly affect overall survival. More recently, the AZURE trial randomising pre- and postmenopausal women to receive standard adjuvant systemic therapy with or without zoledronic acid produced complex results.[95] Overall, no difference in disease-free survival was observed between these two groups, but in a pre-planned analysis of AZURE, postmenopausal patients (similar to the premenopausal population of ABSCG-12 who were rendered 'postmenopausal' with goserelin) had a small but significant disease-free survival advantage, which was apparent early after diagnosis. The results of ABSCG-12 and AZURE suggest that there may be an interaction between menopausal status and effect of bisphosphonates. This hypothesis was supported by the results of two further studies of adjuvant bisphosphonates presented in late 2011. In an unplanned analysis of the ZO-FAST study, disease-free survival and overall survival were improved by the addition of zoledronic acid to adjuvant endocrine therapy in women who were established to be postmenopausal,[96] while the GAIN (German Adjuvant Intergroup Node-Positive) study,[97] although negative overall, suggested a beneficial effect of bisphosphonates in older women.

The weight of evidence increasingly favours a benefit for adjuvant zoledronic acid in women whose ovarian function has ceased or been suppressed, but further confirmatory data are required.

Trastuzumab (Herceptin)

Trastuzumab is a recombinant humanised monoclonal antibody specific to the human HER-2 receptor. HER-2 is amplified in 15–20% of breast cancers. It plays a critical role in tumour development, and is an independent marker of survival, with amplification/ overexpression carrying an adverse prognosis.[98,99] Trastuzumab was developed as targeted therapy against HER-2[100] and has established efficacy, including a significantly improved survival benefit in metastatic breast cancer.[101,102]

Four large, multicentre randomised adjuvant trials involving more than 12 000 women have assessed whether trastuzumab given concurrently with a taxane after anthracycline chemotherapy (adriamycin/cyclophosphamide, AC) (NSABP B-31;

Intergroup N9831; BCIRG 006)[61,103] or concurrently with a non-anthracycline regimen of taxotere and carboplatin (BCIRG 006),[61] or sequentially after any standard chemotherapy schedule (Herceptin in Adjuvant Breast Cancer (HERA) trial),[104] or sequentially after AC and a taxane (Intergroup N9831)[105] can improve disease-free survival and overall survival (Table 12.4). In all these trials trastuzumab was given for 1 year; in the HERA trial a third arm is also evaluating treatment for 2 years (**Fig. 12.2**).

✅✅ The most recent results from these trials confirm that, with longer follow-up, there is a consistent disease-free and overall survival benefit from the addition of trastuzumab to adjuvant chemotherapy, establishing adjuvant trastuzumab as improving survival in women with HER-2-positive breast cancer.[61,103,104] The hazard ratios for disease-free survival range from 0.52 to 0.76, and for overall survival range from 0.61 to 0.77, in these large trials. A much smaller trial, FinHer, randomised 232 HER-2-positive patients to adjuvant docetaxel or vinorelbine with or without trastuzumab for three cycles, followed by FEC in both groups for three cycles.[106] The initial results of this trial also indicated a significant disease-free survival benefit in favour of trastuzumab. There was no difference in outcome for 2 years vs 1 year trastuzumab in the HERA trial.[107]

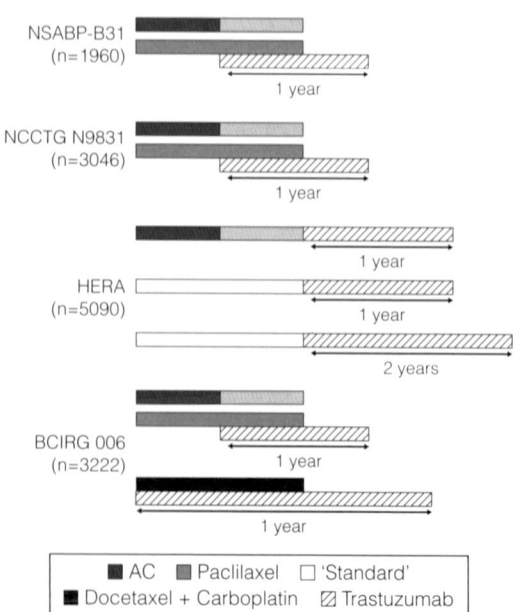

Figure 12.2 • Schematic of the main trials testing trastuzumab in the adjuvant setting.

Table 12.5 • Adjuvant trastuzumab trials: concurrent and sequential

Trial	Treatment	Number	HR for DFS	HR for OS	Median follow-up (years)
Concurrent					
Combined US (NSABP B-31 and N9831)	NSABP: AC-T vs. AC-TH N9831: AC-T vs. AC-T-H vs. AC-TH	3968	0.52	0.61	4
BCIRG-006	AC-T	2147	0.64	0.63	4
	TCH	2148	0.75	0.77	4
FinHER	TH-FEC vs. T-FEC	232	0.65 (NS)	0.42 (NS)	5
Sequential					
HERA	Standard adjuvant chemotherapy then trastuzumab	3501	0.76	0.85 (NS)	4
PACS 004	FEC100-T Epirubicin/docetaxel-T	540	0.86 (NS)	1.27	3

DFS, disease-free survival; HR, hazard ratio; NS, not significant; OS, overall survival.

Chemotherapy and trastuzumab: concurrent or sequential?

Indirect comparisons of these trials suggest improved benefit when trastuzumab is given concurrently with chemotherapy (NSABP B-31; Intergroup N9831; BCIRG 006; FinHer) rather than when it is administered sequentially (HERA) (Table 12.5). Likewise, a much smaller French PACS 004 trial involving 540 women also assessed trastuzumab given sequentially after chemotherapy and so far this is the only negative trial.[108] The inferior results of the PACS trial raises the important issue of whether trastuzumab given sequentially after chemotherapy may be inferior to concurrent administration. The definitive answer to this question comes from the N9831 trial, in which patients were randomised to control (AC followed by weekly paclitaxel, arm A), versus AC followed by weekly paclitaxel and thereafter trastuzumab sequentially (arm B), versus AC followed by weekly paclitaxel with concurrent trastuzumab (arm C).

✔ After 6 years of follow-up, comparison of arms B and C revealed that trastuzumab given concurrently with chemotherapy resulted in a significant improvement in disease-free survival, compared to sequential chemotherapy and trastuzumab (HR = 0.77).[105]

Duration of trastuzumab

The optimal duration of adjuvant trastuzumab therapy is unknown. Results of the 2-year treatment arm from the HERA trial showed no benefit over 1 year. The preliminary results of the FinHer randomised study suggested similar results with only 9 weeks of trastuzumab treatment combined with nonanthracycline chemotherapy,[107] with an increase in 3-year RFS compared with those receiving chemotherapy alone (89% vs. 78%, HR = 0.32; P = 0.02).[78] This effect lost statistical significance with longer follow-up, but results may have been influenced by crossover in the control arm once the first results were announced.[109] A confirmatory trial, the Synergism or Long Duration (SOLD) study, is currently randomising 3000 patients with HER-2-positive early breast cancer to 9 or 52 weeks of adjuvant trastuzumab in an attempt to clarify this issue.

Small HER-2-positive breast cancers

It is becoming clear that small (less than 10 mm) HER-2-positive cancers have a worse prognosis than similarly small HER-2-negative tumours.[110-112] The adjuvant trials of trastuzumab largely excluded patients with tumours of this size, but in the HERA trial patients with small (1.1–2 cm) node-negative breast cancers had a very similar benefit to those with larger tumours from the addition of trastuzumab (HR = 0.53),[113] and it is reasonable to expect that this group would derive a similar reduction in risk from adjuvant chemotherapy and trastuzumab. The issue of whether to give a modified, shorter chemotherapy regimen with trastuzumab in this situation remains controversial: a US group has recently carried out a non-randomised phase II study of single agent paclitaxel with trastuzumab in 400 patients with small HER-2-positive breast cancer and results are awaited (clinical trials NCT 00542451).

Cardiotoxicity with trastuzumab

The only significant toxicity associated with trastuzumab (and one that was quite unexpected from preliminary experimental studies) is cardiotoxicity, particularly when given concurrently with or after anthracyclines. Updated cardiac safety data from three of the adjuvant trastuzumab trials were presented in 2010. Independent retrospective review of the NSAPB B-31 and N9831 trials reported that the risk of symptomatic CHF from trastuzumab was low, but that it increased from 0.45% for patients treated with chemotherapy alone to 2% when trastuzumab was added to chemotherapy.[114] The majority of patients (86.1%) experienced complete or partial recovery. A second, similar analysis of the HERA trial confirmed a low incidence of cardiac end-points; severe CHF occurred in 0.8% versus 0% and significant decreases in left ventricular ejection fraction (LVEF) occurred in 3.6% versus 0.6% in the trastuzumab and control arms respectively.[115] Approximately 80% of patients who suffered a cardiac event achieved 'acute recovery', defined as two or more sequential LVEF measurements of 50% or more, after the initial low ejection fraction.

> ✔ In summary, therefore, the risk of significant and/or long-term cardiotoxicity is low with trastuzumab. There is accumulating evidence that older patients with borderline LVEF function and hypertension might be at increased risk of cardiotoxicity, and for this population it is appropriate to consider a non-anthracycline-based chemotherapy regimen in combination with trastuzumab.

Triple-negative breast cancer

Triple-negative breast cancers are defined as lacking expression of the ER, PgR, and HER-2 receptors.[116] They are usually associated with a high histological grade[117] and are recognised to have a more aggressive natural history than other breast cancer subtypes. Although considered as one group, they consist of basal cancers, metaplastic cancers and a heterogeneous mixture of other true tumour types. Some triple negatives have low levels of expression of ER rather than being true ER zero. Standard adjuvant anthracycline chemotherapy results in poorer outcomes for triple-negative patients,[118] and retrospective data from CALGB 9344 suggest that triple-negative breast cancers specifically benefit from adjuvant taxanes.[58] New therapies for this subtype, including the angiogenesis inhibitor bevacizumab, are also being investigated. The value of bevacizumab in breast cancer is, however, far from clear and its use outside clinical trials cannot be justified.

Conclusion

Adjuvant medical therapy after surgery represents the most important advance in the treatment of breast cancer over the last four decades and is largely responsible for the very significant improvement in mortality.

Adjuvant endocrine therapy is indicated for all but the very best prognosis hormone receptor-positive tumours. Tamoxifen remains the standard treatment for premenopausal women with ER-positive cancers, and current evidence suggests that there may be some, if limited, additional benefit with concomitant ovarian suppression. Aromatase inhibitors are marginally better than tamoxifen as first-line or sequential treatment in postmenopausal women, and in particular those at higher risk. Extended adjuvant therapy with an aromatase inhibitor beyond 5 years of tamoxifen is also an important new development for women at prolonged risk.

Adjuvant chemotherapy is likewise of major importance, particularly for women with hormone receptor-negative disease. Many patients with hormone receptor-positive disease undoubtedly also benefit, but the challenge is to define these more accurately using modern molecular marker technology to determine exactly who will benefit from chemotherapy.

Adjuvant trastuzumab has been a major breakthrough for patients whose tumours amplify or overexpress HER-2, and the likelihood is that evidence will continue to accumulate in the near future to support the use of adjuvant bisphosphonates.

Key points

- Adjuvant treatment for breast carcinoma after surgery is responsible for significant improvements in outcome.
- Tamoxifen remains the standard for premenopausal patients with oestrogen receptor-positive early breast cancer and an aromatase inhibitor for postmenopausal patients, with tamoxifen still a reasonable alternative if tolerability is poor.
- Adjuvant chemotherapy reduces the risk of recurrence and death from breast cancer, particularly for oestrogen receptor-negative and/or HER-2-positive disease. A key current challenge is to identify which patients with oestrogen receptor-positive disease also benefit from chemotherapy.
- Adjuvant trastuzumab in addition to adjuvant chemotherapy confers a very significant further benefit in patients with HER-2-positive disease.
- The weight of evidence increasingly favours a benefit for adjuvant zoledronic acid in women whose ovarian function has ceased or been suppressed, but this has not yet been approved as standard treatment.

References

1. Goldhirsch A, Wood WC, Coates AS, et al. Strategies for subtypes – dealing with the diversity of breast cancer: highlights of the St. Gallen International Expert Consensus on the Primary Therapy of Early Breast Cancer 2011. Ann Oncol 2011;22(8):1736–47.

2. Li CI, Daling JR, Malone KE. Incidence of invasive breast cancer by hormone receptor status from 1992 to 1998. J Clin Oncol 2003;21(1):28–34.

3. Beatson G. On the treatment of inoperable cases of carcinoma of the mamma: suggestions for a new method of treatment, with illustrative cases. Lancet 1896;ii:104–7.

4. Davies C, Godwin J, Gray R, et al. Relevance of breast cancer hormone receptors and other factors to the efficacy of adjuvant tamoxifen: patient-level meta-analysis of randomised trials. Lancet 2011;378(9793):771–84.
   The updated meta-analysis of adjuvant tamoxifen confirms that 5 years of adjuvant tamoxifen confers a mortality benefit to women with hormone receptor-positive breast cancer, regardless of age, nodal status and use of adjuvant chemotherapy.

5. Fisher B, Jeong JH, Bryant J, et al. Treatment of lymph-node-negative, oestrogen-receptor-positive breast cancer: long-term findings from National Surgical Adjuvant Breast and Bowel Project randomised clinical trials. Lancet 2004;364(9437):858–68.

6. Peto R, Davies C, on Behalf of the ATLAS Collaboration, ATLAS (Adjuvant Tamoxifen, Longer Against Shorter). International randomized trial of 10 versus 5 years of adjuvant tamoxifen among 11 500 women: preliminary results. on Behalf of the Breast Cancer Res Treat 2007;106(Suppl. 1):48:abstract.

7. Gray RG, et al. aTTom (adjuvant Tamoxifen – To offer more?): randomized trial of 10 versus 5 years of adjuvant tamoxifen among 6,934 women with estrogen receptor-positive (ER+) or ER untested breast cancer – preliminary results. J Clin Oncol 2008;26(May 2 – Suppl; abstract 513).

8. Baum M, Budzar AU, Cuzick J, et al. Anastrozole alone or in combination with tamoxifen versus tamoxifen alone for adjuvant treatment of post-menopausal women with early breast cancer: first results of the ATAC randomised trial. Lancet 2002;359(9324):2131–9.

9. Thurlimann B, Keshaviah A, Coates AS, et al. A comparison of letrozole and tamoxifen in post-menopausal women with early breast cancer. N Engl J Med 2005;353(26):2747–57.

10. Cuzick J, Sestak I, Baum M, et al. Effect of anastrozole and tamoxifen as adjuvant treatment for early-stage breast cancer: 10-year analysis of the ATAC trial. Lancet Oncol 2010;11(12):1135–41.

11. Regan MM, Neven P, Giobbie-Harder A, et al. Assessment of letrozole and tamoxifen alone and in sequence for postmenopausal women with steroid hormone receptor-positive breast cancer: the BIG 1-98 randomised clinical trial at 8.1 years median follow-up. Lancet Oncol 2011;12(12):1101–8.

The ATAC and BIG1-98 trials (Refs 8–11) established upfront aromatase inhibitors as superior treatment over tamoxifen for postmenopausal women with hormone receptor-positive breast cancer.

12. Arpino G, Weiss HL, Clark GM, et al. Hormone receptor status of a contralateral breast cancer is independent of the receptor status of the first primary in patients not receiving adjuvant tamoxifen. J Clin Oncol 2005;23(21):4687–94.

13. Dowsett M, Allred C, and on Behalf of the TransATAC Investigators. Relationship between quantitative ER and PgR expression and HER2 status with recurrence in the ATAC trial. and on Behalf of the San Antonio Breast Cancer Symp 2006;48, abstract.

14. Ellis MJ, Coop A, Singh B, et al. Letrozole is more effective neoadjuvant endocrine therapy than tamoxifen for ErbB-1- and/or ErbB-2-positive, estrogen receptor-positive primary breast cancer: evidence from a phase III randomized trial. J Clin Oncol 2001;19(18):3808–16.

15. Smith IE, Dowsett M, Yap YS, et al. Neoadjuvant treatment of postmenopausal breast cancer with anastrozole, tamoxifen, or both in combination: the Immediate Preoperative Anastrozole, Tamoxifen, or Combined with Tamoxifen (IMPACT) multicenter double-blind randomized trial. J Clin Oncol 2005;23(22):5108–16.

16. Viale G, Regan M, Dell'Orto P, et al. Central review of ER, PgR and HER-2 in BIG 1-98 evaluating letrozole vs. tamoxifen as adjuvant endocrine therapy for postmenopausal women with receptor-positive breast cancer. San Antonio Breast Cancer Symp 2005;44:abstract.

17. Metzger O, Giobbie-Hurder A, Mallon E, et al. Relative effectiveness of letrozole compared with tamoxifen for patients with lobular carcinoma in the BIG 1-98 trial. Cancer Res 2012;72(24 suppl):S1-1.

18. Duffy S, Jackson TL, Lansdown M, et al. The ATAC ('Arimidex', Tamoxifen, Alone or in Combination) adjuvant breast cancer trial: first results of the endometrial sub-protocol following 2 years of treatment. Hum Reprod 2006;21(2):545–53.

19. Bliss JM, Kilburn LS, Coleman RE, et al. Disease-related outcomes with long-term follow-up: an updated analysis of the intergroup exemestane study. J Clin Oncol 2012;30(7):709–17.

20. Jonat W, Gnant M, Boccardo F, et al. Effectiveness of switching from adjuvant tamoxifen to anastrozole in postmenopausal women with hormone-sensitive early-stage breast cancer: a meta-analysis. Lancet Oncol 2006;7(12):991–6.

21. Boccardo F, Rubagotti A, Puntoni M, et al. Switching to anastrozole versus continued tamoxifen treatment of early breast cancer: preliminary results of the Italian Tamoxifen Anastrozole Trial. J Clin Oncol 2005;23(22):5138–47.

22. Jakesz R, Jonat W, Gnant M, et al. Switching of postmenopausal women with endocrine-responsive early breast cancer to anastrozole after 2 years' adjuvant tamoxifen: combined results of ABCSG trial 8 and ARNO 95 trial. Lancet 2005;366(9484):455–62.

23. van de Velde CJ, Rea D, Seynaeve C, et al. Adjuvant tamoxifen and exemestane in early breast cancer (TEAM): a randomised phase 3 trial. Lancet 2011;377(9762):321–31.

24. Saphner T, Tormey DC, Gray R. Annual hazard rates of recurrence for breast cancer after primary therapy. J Clin Oncol 1996;14(10):2738–46.

25. Goss PE, Ingle JN, Martino S, et al. A randomized trial of letrozole in postmenopausal women after five years of tamoxifen therapy for early-stage breast cancer. N Engl J Med 2003;349(19):1793–802.

26. Goss P, et al. Outcomes of women who were premenopausal at diagnosis of early stage breast cancer in the NCIC CTG MA17 trial. Cancer Res 2009;69(Suppl. 3; 24).

27. Jakesz R, et al. Extended adjuvant treatment with anastrozole: results from the Austrian Breast and Colorectal Cancer Study Group Trial 6a (ABCSG-6a). Proc Am Soc Clin Oncol 2005;527, abstract.

28. Mamounas EP, Jeong JH, Wickerham DL, et al. Benefit from exemestane as extended adjuvant therapy after 5 years of adjuvant tamoxifen: intention-to-treat analysis of the National Surgical Adjuvant Breast And Bowel Project B-33 trial. J Clin Oncol 2008;26(12):1965–71.

29. Smith IE, Dowsett M, Yap YS, et al. Adjuvant aromatase inhibitors for early breast cancer after chemotherapy-induced amenorrhoea: caution and suggested guidelines. J Clin Oncol 2006;24(16):2444–7.

30. Kendall A, Dowsett M, Folkerd E, et al. Caution: Vaginal estradiol appears to be contraindicated in postmenopausal women on adjuvant aromatase inhibitors. Ann Oncol 2006;17(4):584–7.

31. Davidson NE, O'Neill AM, Vukov AM, et al. Chemoendocrine therapy for premenopausal women with axillary lymph node-positive, steroid hormone receptor-positive breast cancer: results from INT 0101 (E5188). J Clin Oncol 2005;23(25):5973–82.

32. Sverrisdottir A, Johansson H, Johansson U, et al. Interaction between goserelin and tamoxifen in a prospective randomised clinical trial of adjuvant endocrine therapy in premenopausal breast cancer. Breast Cancer Res Treat 2011;128(3):755–63.

33. Gnant M, Mlineritsch B, Stoeger H, et al. Adjuvant endocrine therapy plus zoledronic acid in premenopausal women with early-stage breast cancer: 62-month follow-up from the ABCSG-12 randomised trial. Lancet Oncol 2011;12(7):631–41.

34. Reeves GK, Pirie K, Beral V, et al. Cancer incidence and mortality in relation to body mass index in the Million Women Study: cohort study. Br Med J 2007;335(7630):1134.

35. Loi S, Milne RL, Friedlander ML, et al. Obesity and outcomes in premenopausal and postmenopausal breast cancer. Cancer Epidemiol Biomarkers Prev 2005;14(7):1686–91.

36. Sestak I, Distler W, Forbes JF, et al. Effect of body mass index on recurrences in tamoxifen and anastrozole treated women: an exploratory analysis from the ATAC trial. J Clin Oncol 2010;28(21):3411–5.

37. Pfeiler G, et al. Impact of body mass index (BMI) on the efficacy of endocrine therapy in postmenopausal breast cancer patients – an analysis of the ABCSC 6 and 6a trial. Cancer Res 2010;70(24):Suppl 2, abstract PD09-05.

38. Ewertz M, Gray KP, Regan MM, et al. Obesity and risk of recurrence or death after adjuvant endocrine therapy with letrozole or tamoxifen in the breast international group 1-98 trial. J Cin Oncol 2012;30(32):3967–75.

39. Early Breast Cancer Trialists' Collaborative Group. Comparisons between different polychemotherapy regimens for early breast cancer: meta-analyses of long-term outcome among 100,000 women in 123 randomised trials. Lancet 2012;379(9814):432–44. The 2011 Oxford Overview demonstrates that adjuvant chemotherapy produces a proportional reduction in recurrence and mortality, independently of age, nodal status and hormone receptor status. It also confirms that modern chemotherapy regimens are more effective than older ones.

40. Dowsett M, Goldhirsch A, Hayes DF, et al. International Web-based consultation on priorities for translational breast cancer research. Breast Cancer Res 2007;9(6):R81.

41. van der Hage JA, Mieog JS, van de Vijver MJ, et al. Efficacy of adjuvant chemotherapy according to hormone receptor status in young patients with breast cancer: a pooled analysis. Breast Cancer Res 2007;9(5):R70.

42. Muss HB, Berry DA, Cirrincione CT, et al. Adjuvant chemotherapy in older women with early-stage breast cancer. N Engl J Med 2009;360(20):2055–65.

43. Muss HB, Berry DA, Cirrincione CT, et al. Toxicity of older and younger patients treated with adjuvant chemotherapy for node-positive breast cancer: the Cancer and Leukemia Group B Experience. J Clin Oncol 2007;25(24):3699–704.

44. Muss HB, Woolf S, Berry D, et al. Adjuvant chemotherapy in older and younger women with lymph node-positive breast cancer. JAMA 2005;293(9):1073–81.

45. Pinder MC, Duan Z, Goodwin JS, et al. Congestive heart failure in older women treated with adjuvant anthracycline chemotherapy for breast cancer. J Clin Oncol 2007;25(25):3808–15.

46. Patt DA, Duan Z, Fang S, et al. Acute myeloid leukemia after adjuvant breast cancer therapy in older women: understanding risk. J Clin Oncol 2007;25(25):3871–6.

47. Early Breast Cancer Trialists' Collaborative Group. Effects of chemotherapy and hormonal therapy for early breast cancer on recurrence and 15-year survival: an overview of the randomised trials. Lancet 2005;365(9472):1687–717.

48. Bergh J, Wiklund T, Erikstein B, et al. Tailored fluorouracil, epirubicin, and cyclophosphamide compared with marrow-supported high-dose chemotherapy as adjuvant treatment for high-risk breast cancer: a randomised trial. Scandinavian Breast Group 9401 study. Lancet 2000;356(9239):1384–91.

49. Hutchins LF, Green SJ, Ravdin PM, et al. Randomized, controlled trial of cyclophosphamide, methotrexate, and fluorouracil versus cyclophosphamide, doxorubicin, and fluorouracil with and without tamoxifen for high-risk, node-negative breast cancer: treatment results of Intergroup Protocol INT-0102. J Clin Oncol 2005;23(33):8313–21.

50. Levine MN, Bramwell VH, Pritchard KI, et al. Randomized trial of intensive cyclophosphamide, epirubicin, and fluorouracil chemotherapy compared with cyclophosphamide, methotrexate, and fluorouracil in premenopausal women with node-positive breast cancer. National Cancer Institute of Canada Clinical Trials Group. J Clin Oncol 1998;16(8):2651–8.

51. Poole CJ, Earl HM, Hiller L, et al. Epirubicin and cyclophosphamide, methotrexate, and fluorouracil as adjuvant therapy for early breast cancer. N Engl J Med 2006;355(18):1851–62. A number of trials, including the United Kingdom's NEAT trial, confirm the greater efficacy of adjuvant anthracycline-based chemotherapy regimens in early breast cancer.

52. Henderson IC, Berry DA, Demetri GD, et al. Improved outcomes from adding sequential Paclitaxel but not from escalating Doxorubicin dose in an adjuvant chemotherapy regimen for patients with node-positive primary breast cancer. J Clin Oncol 2003;21(6):976–83.

53. French Adjuvant Study Group. Benefit of a high-dose epirubicin regimen in adjuvant chemotherapy for node-positive breast cancer patients with poor prognostic factors: 5-year follow-up results of French Adjuvant Study Group 05 randomized trial. J Clin Oncol 2001;19(3):602–11.

54. Perez EA, Suman VJ, Davidson NE, et al. Effect of doxorubicin plus cyclophosphamide on left ventricular ejection fraction in patients with breast cancer in the North Central Cancer Treatment Group N9831 Intergroup Adjuvant Trial. J Clin Oncol 2004;22(18):3700–4.

55. Swain SM, Whaley FS, Ewer MS. Congestive heart failure in patients treated with doxorubicin: a retrospective analysis of three trials. Cancer 2003;97(11):2869–79.

56. Wood WC, Budman DR, Korzun AH, et al. Dose and dose intensity of adjuvant chemotherapy for stage II, node-positive breast carcinoma. N Engl J Med 1994;330(18):1253–9.

57. Thor AD, Berry DA, Budman DR, et al. erbB-2, p53, and efficacy of adjuvant therapy in lymph node-positive breast cancer. J Natl Cancer Inst 1998;90(18):1346–60.

58. Hayes DF, Thor AD, Dressler LG, et al. HER2 and response to paclitaxel in node-positive breast cancer. N Engl J Med 2007;357(15):1496–506.

59. Pritchard KI, Shepherd LE, O'Malley FP, et al. HER2 and responsiveness of breast cancer to adjuvant chemotherapy. N Engl J Med 2006;354(20):2103–11.

60. Ravdin PM, Green S, Albain KS, et al. Initial report of the SWOG biological correlative study of c-erbB-2 expression as a predictor of outcome in a trial comparing adjuvant CAF T with tamoxifen alone. Proc Am Soc Clin Oncol 1998;17(97):abstract.

61. Slamon D, Eiermann W, Robert N, et al. Adjuvant trastuzumab in HER2-positive breast cancer. N Engl J Med 2011;365(14):1273–83.

62. Press MF, Sauter G, Buyse M, et al. Alteration of topoisomerase II-alpha gene in human breast cancer: association with responsiveness to anthracycline-based chemotherapy. J Clin Oncol 2011;29(7):859–67.

63. Gianni L, Norton L, Wolmark N, et al. Role of anthracyclines in the treatment of early breast cancer. J Clin Oncol 2009;27(28):4798–808.

64. Ghersi D, Wilcken N, Simes RJ. A systematic review of taxane-containing regimens for metastatic breast cancer. Br J Cancer 2005;93(3):293–301.

65. Mamounas EP, Bryant J, Lembersky B, et al. Paclitaxel after doxorubicin plus cyclophosphamide as adjuvant chemotherapy for node-positive breast cancer: results from NSABP B-28. J Clin Oncol 2005;23(16):3686–96.

66. Fountzilas G, Skarlos D, Dafni U, et al. Postoperative dose-dense sequential chemotherapy with epirubicin, followed by CMF with or without paclitaxel, in patients with high-risk operable breast cancer: a randomized phase III study conducted by the Hellenic Cooperative Oncology Group. Ann Oncol 2005;16(11):1762–71.

67. Martin M, Pienkowski T, Mackey J, et al. Adjuvant docetaxel for node-positive breast cancer. N Engl J Med 2005;352(22):2302–13.

68. Evans TR, Yellowlees A, Foster E, et al. Phase III randomized trial of doxorubicin and docetaxel versus doxorubicin and cyclophosphamide as primary medical therapy in women with breast cancer: an Anglo-Celtic cooperative oncology group study. J Clin Oncol 2005;23(13):2988–95.

69. Roche H, Fumoleau P, Spielmann M, et al. Sequential adjuvant epirubicin-based and docetaxel chemotherapy for node-positive breast cancer patients: the FNCLCC PACS 01 Trial. J Clin Oncol 2006;24(36):5664–71.

70. Ellis P, Barrett-Lee P, Johnson L, et al. Sequential docetaxel as adjuvant chemotherapy for early breast cancer (TACT): an open-label, phase III, randomised controlled trial. Lancet 2009;373(9676):1681–92.

71. De Laurentiis M, Cancello G, D'Agostino D, et al. Taxane-based combinations as adjuvant chemotherapy of early breast cancer: a meta-analysis of randomized trials. J Clin Oncol 2008;26(1):44–53.

72. Jones SE, Savin MA, Holmes FA, et al. Phase III trial comparing doxorubicin plus cyclophosphamide with docetaxel plus cyclophosphamide as adjuvant therapy for operable breast cancer. J Clin Oncol 2006;24(34):5381–7.

73. Jones SE, Holmes F, O'Shaughnessy J, et al. Extended follow-up and analysis by age of the US Oncology Adjuvant trial 9735: docetaxel/cyclophosphamide is associated with an overall survival benefit compared to doxorubicin/cyclophosphamide and is well-tolerated in women 65 or older. San Antonio Breast Cancer Symp 2007;12, abstract.

74. Sparano JA, Wang M, Martino S, et al. Weekly paclitaxel in the adjuvant treatment of breast cancer. N Engl J Med 2008;358(16):1663–71.

75. Early Breast Cancer Trialists' Collaborative Group. Polychemotherapy for early breast cancer: an overview of the randomised trials. Lancet 1998;352(9132):930–42.

76. Fumoleau P, Kerbrat P, Romestaing P, et al. Randomized trial comparing six versus three cycles of epirubicin-based adjuvant chemotherapy in premenopausal, node-positive breast cancer patients: 10-year follow-up results of the French Adjuvant Study Group 01 trial. J Clin Oncol 2003;21(2):298–305.

77. Shulman LN, et al. Four vs 6 cycles of doxorubicin and cyclophosphamide or paclitaxel as adjuvant therapy for breast cancer in women with 0–3 positive axillary nodes: CALGB 40101 – a 2 × 2 factorail phase III trial: first results comparing 4 vs 6 cycles of therapy. Cancer Res 2010;70(24):Suppl 2, abstract S6-3.

78. Citron ML, Berry DA, Cirrincione C, et al. Randomized trial of dose-dense versus conventionally scheduled and sequential versus concurrent combination chemotherapy as postoperative adjuvant treatment of node-positive primary breast cancer: first report of Intergroup Trial C9741/Cancer and Leukemia Group B Trial 9741. J Clin Oncol 2003;21(8):1431–9.

79. Venturini M, Del Mastro L, Aitini E, et al. Dose-dense adjuvant chemotherapy in early breast cancer patients: results from a randomized trial. J Natl Cancer Inst 2005;97(23):1724–33.

80. Bonilla L, Ben-Aharon I, Vidal L, et al. Dose-dense chemotherapy in nonmetastatic breast cancer: a systematic review and meta-analysis of randomized controlled trials. J Natl Cancer Inst 2010;102(24):1845–54.

81. Albain KS, Barlow WE, Ravdin PM, et al. Adjuvant chemotherapy and timing of tamoxifen in postmenopausal patients with endocrine-responsive, node-positive breast cancer: a phase 3, open-label, randomised controlled trial. Lancet 2009;374(9707):2055–63.

82. Paik S, Shak S, Tang G, et al. A multigene assay to predict recurrence of tamoxifen-treated, node-negative breast cancer. N Engl J Med 2004;351(27):2817–26.

83. Paik S, Tang G, Shak S, et al. Gene expression and benefit of chemotherapy in women with node-negative, estrogen receptor-positive breast cancer. J Clin Oncol 2006;24(23):3726–34.

84. Dowsett M, Cuzick J, Wale C, et al. Prediction of risk of distant recurrence using the 21-gene recurrence score in node-negative and node-positive postmenopausal patients with breast cancer treated with anastrozole or tamoxifen: a TransATAC study. J Clin Oncol 2010;28(11):1829–34.

85. Albain KS, Barlow WE, Shak S, et al. Prognostic and predictive value of the 21-gene recurrence score assay in postmenopausal women with node-positive, oestrogen-receptor-positive breast cancer on chemotherapy: a retrospective analysis of a randomised trial. Lancet Oncol 2010;11(1):55–65.

86. Barton S, Zabaglo L, A'Hern R, et al. Assessment of the contribution of the IHC4+C score to decision making in clinical practice in early breast cancer. Br J Cancer 2012;106(11):1760–5.

87. Dowsett M, Nielsen TO, A'Hern R, et al. Assessment of Ki67 in breast cancer: recommendations from the International Ki67 in Breast Cancer Working Group. J Natl Cancer Inst 2011;103(22):1656–64.

88. van de Vijver MJ, He YD, van't Veer LJ, et al. A gene-expression signature as a predictor of survival in breast cancer. N Engl J Med 2002;347(25):1999–2009.

89. van't Veer LJ, Dai H, van de Vijver MJ, et al. Gene expression profiling predicts clinical outcome of breast cancer. Nature 2002;415(6871):530–6.

90. Diel IJ, Jaschke A, Solomayer EF, et al. Adjuvant oral clodronate improves the overall survival of primary breast cancer patients with micrometastases to the bone marrow: a long-term follow-up. Ann Oncol 2008;19(12):2007–11.

91. Diel IJ, Solomayer EF, Costa SD, et al. Reduction in new metastases in breast cancer with adjuvant clodronate treatment. N Engl J Med 1998;339(6):357–63.

92. Powles T, Paterson S, Kanis JA, et al. Randomized, placebo-controlled trial of clodronate in patients with primary operable breast cancer. J Clin Oncol 2002;20(15):3219–24.

93. Saarto T, Blomqvist C, Virkkunen P, et al. Adjuvant clodronate treatment does not reduce the frequency of skeletal metastases in node-positive breast cancer patients: 5-year results of a randomized controlled trial. J Clin Oncol 2001;19(1):10–7.

94. Paterson AHG, et al. NSABP protocol B-34: a clinical trial comparing adjuvant clodronate vs placebo in early stage breast cancer patients receiving systemic chemotherapy and/or tamoxifen or no therapy – final analysis. Cancer Res 2011;71(24):Suppl, abstract S2-3.

95. Coleman RE, Marshall H, Cameron D, et al. Breast-cancer adjuvant therapy with zoledronic acid. N Engl J Med 2011;365(15):1396–405.

96. de Boer R, et al. Long-term survival outcomes among postmenopausal women with hormone receptor-positive early breast cancer receiving adjuvant letrozole and zoledronic acid: 5-year follow-up of ZO-FAST. Cancer Res 2011;71(24):Suppl, abstract S1-3.

97. Mobus V, et al. GAIN (German Adjuvant Intergroup Node Positive) study: a phase III multicenter trial to compare dose dense, dose intense ETC vs EC-TX and ibandronate vs observation in patients with node-positive primary breast cancer – first interim efficacy analysis. Cancer Res 2011;71(24):Suppl, abstract S2-4.

98. Slamon DJ, Clark GM, Wong SG, et al. Human breast cancer: correlation of relapse and survival with amplification of the HER-2/neu oncogene. Science 1987;235(4785):177–82.

99. Slamon DJ, Godolphin W, Jones LA, et al. Studies of the HER-2/neu proto-oncogene in human breast and ovarian cancer. Science 1989;244(4905):707–12.

100. Finn RS, Slamon DJ. Monoclonal antibody therapy for breast cancer: herceptin. Cancer Chemother Biol Response Modif 2003;21:223–33.

101. Slamon DJ, Leyland-Jones B, Shak S, et al. Use of chemotherapy plus a monoclonal antibody against HER2 for metastatic breast cancer that overexpresses HER2. N Engl J Med 2001;344(11):783–92.

102. Marty M, Cognetti F, Maraninchi D, et al. Randomized phase II trial of the efficacy and safety of trastuzumab combined with docetaxel in patients with human epidermal growth factor receptor 2-positive metastatic breast cancer administered as first-line treatment: the M77001 study group. J Clin Oncol 2005;23(19):4265–74.

103. Perez EA, Romond EH, Suman VJ, et al. Four-year follow-up of trastuzumab plus adjuvant chemotherapy for operable human epidermal growth factor receptor 2-positive breast cancer: joint analysis of data from NCCTG N9831 and NSABP B-31. J Clin Oncol 2011;29(25):3366–73.

104. Gianni L, Dafni U, Gelber RD, et al. Treatment with trastuzumab for 1 year after adjuvant chemotherapy in patients with HER2-positive early breast cancer: a 4-year follow-up of a randomised controlled trial. Lancet Oncol 2011;12(3):236–44.

105. Perez EA, Suman VJ, Davidson NE, et al. Sequential versus concurrent trastuzumab in adjuvant chemotherapy for breast cancer. J Clin Oncol 2011;29(34):4491–7.

These three randomised trials (along with Ref. 60) of adjuvant concurrent trastuzumab with chemotherapy demonstrate a reduction in recurrence and death in women with HER-2-positive breast cancer. All trials published updated results in 2011, confirming that these benefits are maintained with longer follow-up.

106. Joensuu H, Kellokumpu-Lehtinen PL, Bono P, et al. Adjuvant docetaxel or vinorelbine with or without trastuzumab for breast cancer. N Engl J Med 2006;354(8):809–20.

107. Goldhirsch A, Piccart-Gebhart M.J, Procter M, et al. HERA Trial: 2 years versus 1 year of trastuzumab after adjuvant chemotherapy in women with HER2-positive early breast cancer at 8 years of median follow up. Cancer Res 2012;72(24 suppl):S5-2.

108. Spielmann M, Roché H, Delozier T, et al. Trastuzumab for patients with axillary-node-positive breast cancer: results of the FNCLCC-PACS 04 trial. J Clin Oncol 2009;27(36):6129–34.

109. Joensuu H, et al. FinXX final 5-year analysis: results of the randomised, open-label, phase III trial in medium-to-high risk early breast cancer. Cancer Res 2010;70(24):Suppl 2, abstract S4-1.

110. Curigliano G, Viale G, Bagnardi V, et al. Clinical relevance of HER2 overexpression/amplification in patients with small tumor size and node-negative breast cancer. J Clin Oncol 2009;27(34):5693–9.

111. Park YH, Kim ST, Cho EY, et al. A risk stratification by hormonal receptors (ER, PgR) and HER-2 status in small (< or = 1 cm) invasive breast cancer: who might be possible candidates for adjuvant treatment? Breast Cancer Res Treat 2009;119(3):653–61.

112. Chavez-MacGregor M, Gonzalez-Angulo AM. HER2-neu positivity in patients with small and node-negative breast cancer (pT1a,b,N0,M0): a high risk group? Clin Adv Hematol Oncol 2009;7(9):591–8.

113. Untch M, Gelber RD, Jackisch C, et al. Estimating the magnitude of trastuzumab effects within patient subgroups in the HERA trial. Ann Oncol 2008;19(6):1090–6.

114. Russell SD, Blackwell KL, Lawrence J, et al. Independent adjudication of symptomatic heart failure with the use of doxorubicin and cyclophosphamide followed by trastuzumab adjuvant therapy: a combined review of cardiac data from the National Surgical Adjuvant breast and Bowel Project B-31 and the North Central Cancer Treatment Group N9831 clinical trials. J Clin Oncol 2010;28(21):3416–21.

115. Procter M, Suter TM, de Azambuja E, et al. Longer-term assessment of trastuzumab-related cardiac adverse events in the Herceptin Adjuvant (HERA) trial. J Clin Oncol 2010;28(21):3422–8.

116. Foulkes WD, Smith IE, Reis-Filho JS. Triple-negative breast cancer. N Engl J Med 2010; 363(20):1938–48.

117. Reis-Filho JS, Tutt AN. Triple negative tumours: a critical review. Histopathology 2008;52(1): 108–18.

118. Tan DS, Marchió C, Jones RL, et al. Triple negative breast cancer: molecular profiling and prognostic impact in adjuvant anthracycline-treated patients. Breast Cancer Res Treat 2008;111(1):27–44.

119. Cheang MC, Chia SK, Voduc D, et al. Ki67 index, HER2 status, and prognosis of patients with luminal B breast cancer. J Natl Cancer Inst 2009;101(10):736–50.

Locally advanced breast cancer

Douglas J.A. Adamson
Alastair M. Thompson

Introduction

Locally advanced breast cancer (**Fig. 13.1**) includes primary breast tumours with diameters of greater than 5 cm, breast cancers with frank skin or chest wall involvement, and any size of tumour with certain degrees of nodal involvement, but excludes cancers that have spread further than local, supra/infraclavicular and internal mammary chain nodes.[1] Locally advanced breast cancer includes all cancers of 'TNM' stage III, but also a subset of stage II cancers (Table 13.1). The definition of locally advanced breast cancer includes inflammatory breast cancer (**Fig. 13.2**), which is characterised by involvement of the dermal lymphatic vessels by cancer cells that produces an inflamed, erythematous appearance to the whole breast. The management of locally advanced breast cancer should be multidisciplinary in nature, and based on the extent of the disease, as assessed with computed tomography (CT) scanning of chest, abdomen and pelvis, and, if required, isotope bone scanning, magnetic resonance imaging (MRI) or positron emission tomography (PET) to detect or confirm metastatic disease (Chapter 1). Histological confirmation of the tumour type along with appropriate immunohistochemistry for oestrogen receptor and human epidermal growth factor (HER-2) receptor (supplemented by fluorescence in situ hybridisation (FISH) analysis of HER-2 status) is required before embarking on therapy (Chapter 2). Multimodal therapy is generally needed and the timing and nature of treatments will vary depending on whether the disease is confined to operable areas, whether there is involvement of internal mammary or supraclavicular lymph nodes, and above all the general fitness of the patient.

The general principles of the oncological management of locally advanced breast cancer are similar to those for less advanced disease and draw on appropriate use of surgery, including plastic and reconstructive techniques, radiotherapy, chemotherapy, endocrine treatments, and therapy with biological agents targeting specific cellular proteins. The management of recurrent breast cancer in the breast, chest wall and regional nodes is also guided by these same principles.

Surgical management

Breast surgery

Pathological confirmation of the clinical diagnosis of locally advanced breast cancer should be made by core biopsy to distinguish invasive breast cancer from ductal carcinoma in situ (DCIS) or metastatic disease to the breast from another primary site. If the patient is likely to be a candidate for neoadjuvant therapy, placement of a radiological marker in the tumour immediately following the core biopsy is required to facilitate accurate surgical resection or to localise the site of the cancer for the pathologist if mastectomy is subsequently performed.[2] However, on occasion, excision of a skin nodule under local anaesthetic may be useful to confirm the diagnosis

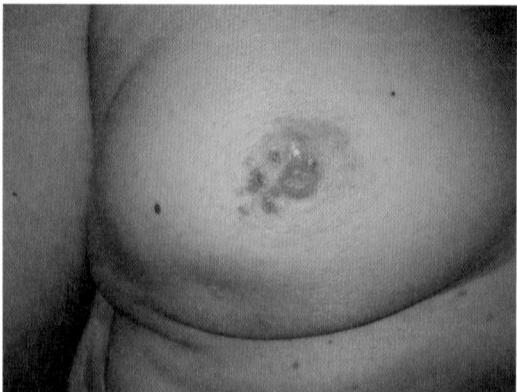

Figure 13.1 • Locally advanced breast cancer: still operable by mastectomy.

Table 13.1 • Locally advanced breast cancer stage and TNM

Stage	TNM		
IIB	T3	N0	M0
IIIA	T any	N2	M0
IIIA	T3	N1–2	M0
IIIB	T4a, b, c, d	N0–2	M0
IIIC	T any	N3	M0

and get tissue for receptor analysis. Resectional surgery aims to secure clear surgical margins around the cancer. There is a balance between the completeness of excision (margin involvement is linked to recurrence) versus poorer cosmetic results from more extensive surgery. If the cancer is not excisable by conventional means then neoadjuvant therapy or radiotherapy are the only treatment options. Radical mastectomy (including excision of pectoralis major and level III axillary clearance) does not improve survival over total mastectomy (odds ratio of death 0.98 over 10 years[3]) and is rarely, if ever, indicated even in locally advanced breast cancer. Since survival following breast conservation is not significantly different from that following mastectomy, this has led most centres to use neoadjuvant therapy for locally advanced breast cancer as initial treatment followed by surgery, including the option of breast conservation where appropriate. Where neoadjuvant therapy has produced an excellent clinical and radiological response, effective surgery is possible only if a surgical marker was inserted prior to commencing neoadjuvant treatment, as the tumour may not be visible radiologically. As for all

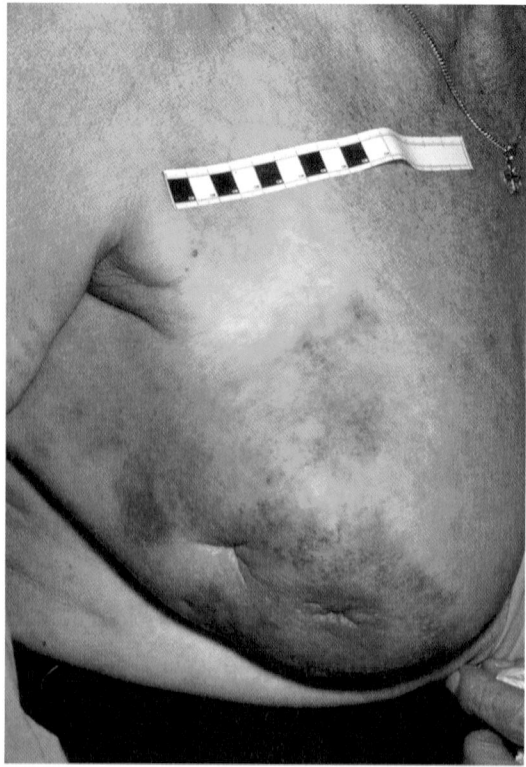

Figure 13.2 • Inflammatory breast cancer demonstrating skin erythema (with indrawn nipple and skin tethering) and a visible axillary nodal mass.

breast conservation surgery (Chapter 4), complete surgical excision with clear margins of at least 1 mm on pathology review is required to reduce disease recurrence. The term 'toilet mastectomy' has historically been applied to mastectomy performed to excise locally advanced breast cancer. Surgery alone rarely controls such cancers and combination with radiotherapy and/or systemic therapy is now standard. Excision of bulky disease in the breast previously led to difficulties in skin closure with the need for split-skin grafting or application of an omental flap to the chest wall but the widespread use of skin-bearing autologous flaps, particularly the latissimus dorsi flap, has made primary closure possible in all but a few patients.

Axillary surgery

Previously, level III axillary node clearance was the axillary surgery of choice in patients with locally advanced breast cancer due to the high probability of axillary lymph node involvement. Given the significant morbidity associated with level III axillary clearance, for patients undergoing neoadjuvant therapy who were node negative at diagnosis or have a good clinical response this is being challenged. Sentinel lymph node biopsy of the post-treatment axilla is now being used to guide therapy and is of similar efficacy to that in patients who have not received neoadjuvant therapy[4] (see Chapter 7). Although some advocate sentinel node biopsy prior to neoadjuvant therapy this is illogical and denies those whose nodes are cleared by this treatment the option of sentinel node biopsy after completion of their systemic therapy. It is useful, however, to consider sentinel node biopsy prior to a definitive surgical procedure in patients who are having mastectomy and undergoing breast reconstruction, in order to guide the extent of the axillary node dissection. Axillary nodes are converted to node negative in approximately 35% of patients by neoadjuvant chemotherapy. The rate of conversion from positive to negative relates to tumour type. Between 25% and 50% of involved nodes in triple negative cancers, 40–60% in HER-2-positive patients who receive trastuzumab but less than 10% of nodes in patients with oestrogen receptor-positive breast cancers are converted from positive to negative.

✅✅ Sentinel lymph node biopsy after neoadjuvant chemotherapy in patients with a good response should be considered in place of axillary node clearance.[4]

Breast reconstruction in locally advanced breast cancer

For those patients undergoing mastectomy either as primary treatment or following neoadjuvant therapy, there remains controversy regarding immediate breast reconstruction (Chapter 9). Although there may be concerns that delayed wound healing (on the chest wall or at donor sites for autologous reconstruction) may delay the delivery of postoperative adjuvant chemotherapy or postoperative radiotherapy[5] and the need to avoid radiotherapy following reconstruction with prostheses, few patients experience significant delays. Some surgeons do not offer immediate reconstruction to patients with locally advanced disease because of the likelihood postoperative radiotherapy will be required. Over the past 15 years, US practice has swung from

immediate reconstruction for patients with locally advanced breast cancer to a more conservative approach of delayed breast reconstruction. There is the option for patients wishing reconstruction of a skin-sparing mastectomy and placement of a tissue expander that is deflated during radiotherapy and reflated shortly after completion of radiation. Thereafter, an autologous reconstruction with a myocutaneous flap utilises the preserved skin. Autologous abdominal flap reconstruction at the time of mastectomy has been reported by some to produce unsatisfactory long-term outcomes following radiotherapy, and with modern postoperative radiotherapy techniques in the UK it does not appear to prejudice the cosmetic outcome nor the oncological management.[6]

Radiotherapy

Radiotherapy is thought to work mainly by causing damage to the DNA of tumour cells, which is repaired more slowly than the damage caused in the adjacent normal tissue. Tumour tissue is therefore preferentially destroyed compared with the normal tissue over a course of radiotherapy treatment. In general, the chance of tumour control increases with increasing total dose of radiotherapy given, but so does the chance of permanent radiotherapy-related side-effects, some of which have been implicated in treatment-related mortality[7] (Box 13.1).

Certain tissues (termed 'late-responding tissues') such as nerves and, to some extent, lung can withstand a higher total dose of radiotherapy without giving rise to symptomatic damage if the dose of each separate radiotherapy treatment (or 'fraction') is kept low. Traditionally, a course of radiotherapy

---

Box 13.1 • Side-effects of breast cancer radiotherapy

Acute skin toxicity: erythema, dry desquamation, moist desquamation

Late skin toxicity: pigmentation, telangiectasia, fibrosis

Shoulder stiffness (if axilla treated)

Arm oedema (if lymphatics treated)

Pneumonitis (increasing likelihood with increasing lung volume in treatment field)

Oesophagitis (uncommon, self-limiting)

Bone radionecrosis (rare with modern treatments)

Brachial plexopathy

that was thought to give the best chance of long-term tumour control comprised a relatively large total dose given over several weeks by using small daily fractions. Whilst shorter palliative courses of treatment may be considered for less fit patients, the total dose has to be reduced to minimise the toxicity of the treatment, because the fraction size for such short courses is by necessity large.[8] The reduction in the total radiotherapy dose for such short courses often means that any benefit obtained from radiotherapy is short-lived and may not be worth the inconvenience to the patient of the treatment, and so many oncologists advocate longer courses over several weeks for advanced breast cancer. This view is being challenged, partly because of the results of large randomised radiotherapy studies such as the START trial,[9] which has demonstrated that shorter, 'hypofractionated' regimens using a lower total dose than has been traditional produce good outcome results with a trend towards fewer side-effects. It remains to be seen whether further research into much shorter hypofractionated courses yields similar results.

Before considering radiotherapy, the patient with locally advanced breast cancer should be assessed to ensure she can comply with the treatment. Radiotherapy is generally given with the patient lying flat: patients with severe orthopnoea, for example (whether due to breast cancer metastasis or cardiorespiratory comorbidities), may not be able to cope with this position. During radiotherapy, the patient will be left on her own in the planning and treatment room, and will be raised off the concrete floor by several feet. If there is any chance she may fall off the treatment couch, for example if she has dementia, then the treatment cannot be given safely. In additon, if the locally advanced disease prevents abduction of the ipsilateral arm to less than 90°, then it is difficult to give conventional radiotherapy treatment to breast and axilla.

Adjuvant (postoperative) radiotherapy

When treating locally advanced breast cancer, whatever surgery is performed on the breast, postoperative radiotherapy significantly reduces locoregional recurrence and improves overall survival for both premenopausal[10] and postmenopausal[11] women, and modern techniques do not have the cardiac morbidity of older treatments.[12] Postoperative radiotherapy (which may be given after adjuvant chemotherapy) reduces local recurrence from 35% without radiotherapy to 8% with radiotherapy and improves disease-free survival at 10 years from 24% to 36%.

✔✔ Postoperative radiotherapy following surgery for advanced breast cancer reduces locoregional recurrence and improves survival.[10,11]

Radiotherapy following the surgical treatment of locally advanced breast cancer is given in the same way as treatments for early breast cancer, the aim being to reduce local relapse by about two-thirds and improve survival.[13] Locally advanced breast cancer, by definition, has many features that predict for local relapse (large tumour size, lymph node involvement, close or positive margins despite adequate surgery). Thus, postoperative radiotherapy is usually given,[14] even if there has been a good response to neoadjuvant treatment, as the risk of local relapse in larger tumours is higher than for less advanced cancers.[15] The chest wall or residual conserved breast is treated and the peripheral lymphatics are irradiated as appropriate[16] (see Chapter 15). It is unusual to irradiate the internal mammary chain nodes, as evidence for the efficacy of this treatment is lacking, although much of the data relates to trials that are decades old.[17]

Primary radical radiotherapy

If the patient is not fit for or declines surgery, and is fit for radiotherapy, then radiotherapy may be used as the principal local treatment. It is unusual to 'cure' a locally advanced breast cancer without surgery, but sometimes excellent local control can be obtained (**Figs 13.3** and **13.4**) and unpleasant symptoms of the tumour, such as pain, discharge, bleeding and odour, can be partially or completely removed following radiotherapy treatment.

While there is little evidence to support the use of routine radiotherapy prior to definitive surgery, radiotherapy has been used as an alternative to surgery following neoadjuvant chemotherapy. In women with stage III disease given neoadjuvant chemotherapy, disease control, median survival (39 months) and relapse rates appear similar in studies that randomised patients to radiotherapy or

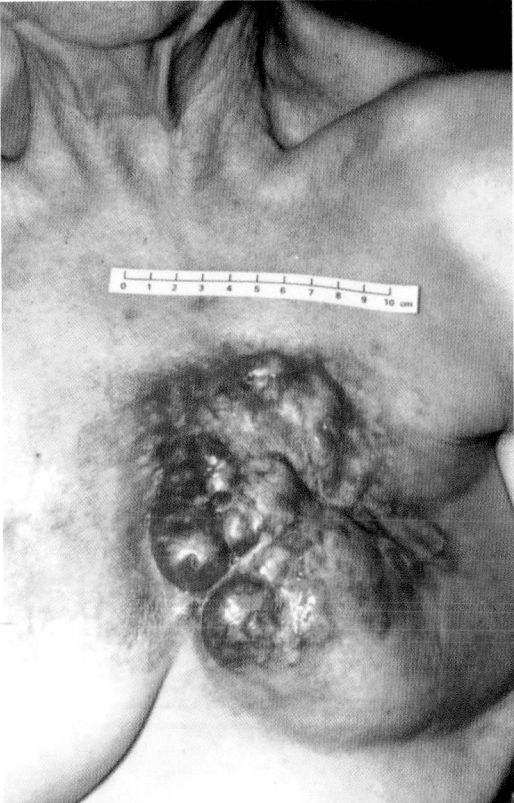

Figure 13.3 • Inoperable locally advanced breast cancer prior to radiotherapy.

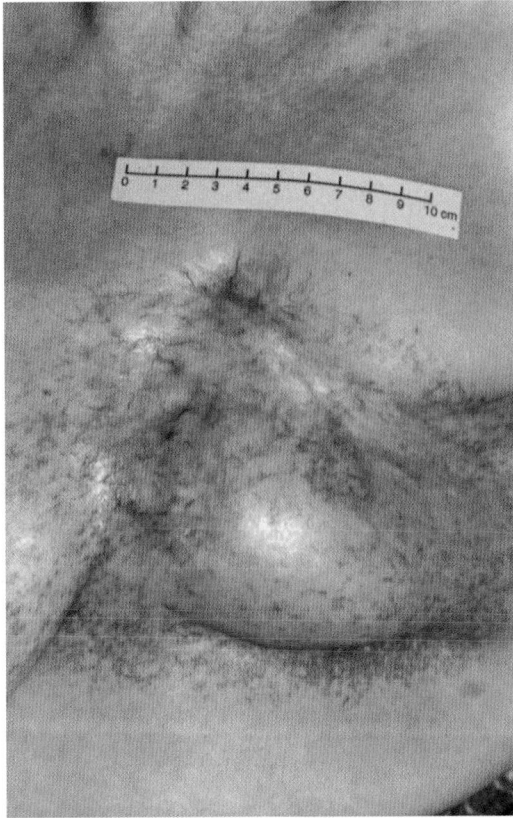

Figure 13.4 • Locally advanced breast cancer as in Fig. 13.3 following radiotherapy.

surgery.[18,19] For patients with disease suitable for breast-conserving surgery, the combination of excision and radiotherapy improves local control compared to radiotherapy alone.

Systemic treatment

If the patient has locally advanced disease and is fit for treatment, then systemic therapy is usually considered, as the risk of relapse in locally advanced breast cancer is high. In addition, neoadjuvant treatment is often needed to 'downstage' some patients with locally advanced breast cancer to allow surgery to be completed successfully and sometimes thereafter breast conservation can be achieved. Although cancer that has spread to the ipsilateral supraclavicular lymph nodes was formerly considered 'metastatic' disease, patients with isolated supraclavicular disease as the only site of distant disease do just as well in terms of survival as those patients with lesser stages of locally advanced breast cancer.[20]

Neoadjuvant treatment

Treatment options include neoadjuvant chemotherapy ± trastuzumab (for HER-2-positive breast cancer) and neoadjuvant endocrine therapy (for oestrogen receptor-positive breast cancer).

> ✓✓ Neoadjuvant chemotherapy is as effective as adjuvant chemotherapy in terms of survival benefit for locally advanced breast cancer.[21]

Neoadjuvant chemotherapy

Neoadjuvant chemotherapy is as effective as adjuvant chemotherapy in terms of survival in locally advanced breast cancer. Randomised trials have shown a possible long-term advantage for neoadjuvant chemotherapy, particularly in young women (**Fig. 13.5a,b**). Neoadjuvant chemotherapy is associated with a 31% reduction in overall infective episodes compared to adjuvant chemotherapy.[22] The choice of agents for locally advanced breast cancer is determined by emerging trial data and by local preferences, but is often similar

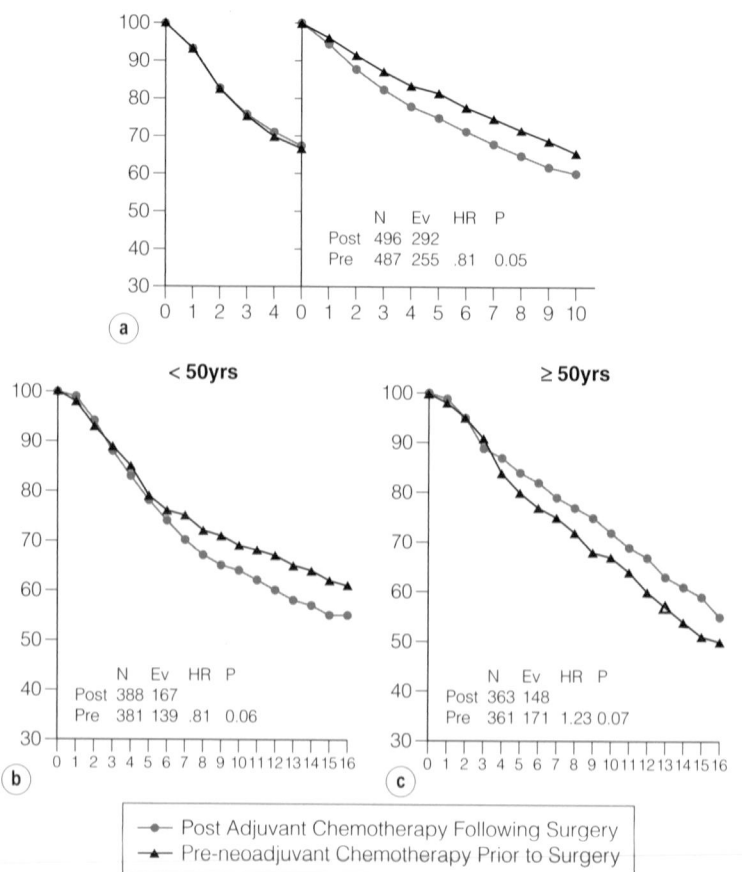

Figure 13.5 • Disease-free survival in National Surgical Adjuvant Breast and Bowel Project (NSABP) B18 from 0–5 and 5–15 years **(a)** and overall survival split into age groups **(b)** <50 and ≥50 **(c)** years of age. N = number of events; Ev = Events; HR = hazard ratio. Overall, disease free survival is increased. This reaches significance beyond 5 years in patients treated with neoadjuvant rather than adjuvant chemotherapy. However, the benefit may be confined to premenopausal women.

or the same as the chemotherapy regimens given for adjuvant therapy. There are no compelling data on the optimum number of cycles of chemotherapy but there may be some advantage in delivering the whole chemotherapy course at once rather than in a perioperative fashion, as splitting it may give the worst of both worlds, by exposing the patient to side-effects both before and after their surgery with no evidence of marked clinical advantage. It has been shown that HER-2-positive tumours are more likely (by about three times) to show a complete pathological response after treatment with conventional neoadjuvant chemotherapy compared to HER-2-negative cancers, although the overall outlook for such tumours is not as good as for those that are HER-2 negative.[23] Neoadjuvant trastuzumab has been used in conjunction with chemotherapy and has shown improved rates of complete pathological response compared to chemotherapy alone, even in groups of patients that

include a significant proportion of more advanced disease.[24] Trials are underway, and showing promising results, from other inhibitors of this signalling pathway, using the agents lapatinib, pertuzumab and T-DM1 in different combinations with trastuzumab. A combination of chemotherapy and trastuzumab together with either lapatanib or pertuzumab appears superior to chemotherapy or trastuzumab alone.

The primary tumour should be assessed prior to treatment, with documentation of its position in the breast, accurate measurements of dimensions of the mass both clinically and on imaging, and a description of the appearance of the lump and any changes associated with it (Figs 13.1 and 13.2). A clinical photograph often helps with future assessments if there is a visible mass or abnormality and helps assess response to treatment. Any palpable local lymph nodes that are thought to be involved should be measured carefully in the same way. Imaging,[25] including ultrasonography, mammography,

MRI or PET/CT scanning, is required to obtain an accurate assessment of the extent of disease before treatment and assessment of response after chemotherapy has been given if baseline images are obtained. Marker placement can complement imaging by locating the original position of the tumour, and facilitates tumour site localisation following successful neoadjuvant therapy. Some are now placing tumour markers in involved lymph nodes to confirm that in patients with a negative sentinel node biopsy after an excellent response to neoadjuvant therapy the node known to be involved prior to therapy has been removed. There are some data suggesting that MRI scanning after one cycle may yield information about likely response to chemotherapy.[26] There are also data to indicate that MRI is accurate in most patients at assessing response, but in a significant number can overestimate or underestimate the extent of residual disease following neoadjuvant chemotherapy.[27] Assessment is usually performed after two or three cycles of treatment and if the tumour responds, then chemotherapy should continue for up to eight cycles[28] and the patient then proceeds to definitive curative surgery.

When using adjuvant treatment, the clinician has no idea whether the chemotherapy produces an effect on micrometastatic disease. This is not the case for neoadjuvant chemotherapy. If the tumour fails to respond, then the chemotherapy agents should be changed and the assessment process repeated, unless the tumour is deemed operable at that time, in which case it may be better to stop neoadjuvant chemotherapy and proceed directly to surgery. Lack of response to the first-line neoadjuvant chemotherapy is a poor prognostic sign.

Despite much research into markers to predict prognosis after neoadjuvant chemotherapy (Chapter 2), the degree of involvement of axillary nodes following neoadjuvant chemotherapy remains the best predictor of subsequent relapse.[29] Pathological complete response is associated with improved overall survival[22] and is more likely to be seen in younger women with higher grade invasive ductal carcinoma that is oestrogen receptor/progesterone receptor negative and HER-2 positive.[30] It is important to remember that both tumour grade and receptor immunohistochemistry can change following treatment[31] when pre- and post-chemotherapy pathological specimens are examined after neoadjuvant chemotherapy for advanced breast cancer.

Neoadjuvant/therapeutic endocrine therapy

If the tumour is positive for oestrogen or progesterone receptor immunohistochemistry, then the patient may be treated with neoadjuvant oestrogen blockade instead of with chemotherapy. The side-effects are less with endocrine therapy than with chemotherapy, although time to response is generally slower and complete pathological response less likely. The majority of patients treated with neoadjuvant hormone therapy have been postmenopausal. The pathological changes seen following neoadjuvant treatment with an aromatase inhibitor such as letrozole appear to be different from those seen with neodjuvant chemotherapy, with more 'central scarring' using this type of oestrogen blockade, compared with more cancers showing diffuse changes and a complete pathological response rate with chemotherapy.[32] Neoadjuvant therapy with oestrogen blockade can potentially increase anxiety in patients (and clinicians) and could potentially lead to delay in switching to an effective treatment should the first agent used be ineffective, as about 3 months of anti-oestrogen treatment are needed before a true impression of response can be obtained. Progression during treatment is rare with endocrine therapy and occurs in less than 5% of patients. The relative lack of side-effects, and the potential for excellent tumour response,[33] make neoadjuvant endocrine treatment an attractive prospect. Primary endocrine blockade also acts as a chemotherapy-sparing treatment strategy, allowing more options in the future as the patient is chemotherapy naive. Some work has been done comparing neoadjuvant oestrogen blockade with neoadjuvant chemotherapy in older women with hormone-sensitive breast cancers; the results of the two treatments, in one small study, appeared to be equivalent for outcomes such as response rate and time to response,[34] with a suggestion of a greater rate of conversion from planned mastectomy to breast-conserving surgery with endocrine therapy. The optimal duration for endocrine therapy is a matter for debate, but it is clear that treatments of around 9 months or more are clinically acceptable and appear to produce better results than treatments of shorter duration.[35]

For many years, it has been clear that postmenopausal women with advanced disease, including metastatic disease, respond to an aromatase inhibitor at least as well[36] or better[37] than to tamoxifen. In the treatment of locally advanced and metastatic breast cancer in postmenopausal women, treatment failure rate is lower with anastrozole (79%) compared with tamoxifen (84%), with a median time to progression of 11.1 months for anastrozole and 5.6 months for tamoxifen.[38] Letrozole is superior to tamoxifen in terms of objective response rate (30% vs. 20%) and treatment failure (85% vs. 75%).[39]

✓✓ Aromatase inhibitors appear more effective than tamoxifen in the neoadjuvant treatment of locally advanced breast cancer.[39]

The difference could be related to a genuine difference between different classes of oestrogen blocking drugs. In addition, it is known that tamoxifen metabolism by the cytochrome P450 system varies in different individuals according to genotype, adherence to taking the medication and potential interaction with other drugs, but the influence of individual variation in the metabolism of tamoxifen (and indeed aromatase inhibitors) and their subsequent efficacy is unclear.[40] The pure oestrogen antagonist, fulvestrant, is as effective as anastrozole in postmenopausal women with advanced breast cancer progressing after prior endocrine treatment,[41] but the place of this drug, which must be given parenterally, in the treatment of locally advanced breast cancer is still under evaluation.

Adjuvant systemic treatment

Adjuvant systemic treatment for advanced breast cancer that has been treated successfully by surgery is very similar to that given for early-stage breast cancer. Locally advanced breast cancer has a higher risk of relapse than early-stage breast cancer, and so it is likely that following surgery the patient will be offered adjuvant oestrogen blockade, local radiotherapy and therapies targeting specific signalling pathways such as the HER-2/neu transmembrane receptor, assuming that the tumour is found to be of the correct biological type for the patient to potentially benefit from such targeted agents (Chapter 2). Certainly, adding chemotherapy or endocrine therapy or both with radiotherapy for stage IIIB disease reduces locoregional recurrence from 60% to 50% but may not secure a long-term survival advantage.

Problems of locally recurrent disease after previous treatment

Local recurrence of advanced breast cancer may occur in isolation or in conjunction with overt metastatic disease. Since histological confirmation of disease recurrence is required and the oestrogen, progesterone or HER-2 receptor status may change between the primary and the recurrent disease for one in six patients,[42] biopsy of the locally recurrent cancer should be performed. It is essential to know what treatment a patient has received in the past to be able to advise them on future treatment for a recurrent cancer. For example, if the patient has only had a sentinel node biopsy or axillary sampling procedure, and further breast surgery is required to treat recurrent disease, then an axillary clearance should be considered.

The patient who has already been treated with radiotherapy and who develops disease recurrence in the treated area poses a problem. For the reasons given above, there is a limit to how much radiotherapy can be delivered to one area of the body. Accurate written information on previous radiotherapy prescriptions is therefore vital before further treatment can be administered safely. Previous permanent skin marks tattooed during radiotherapy planning may help accurately delineate which areas may be irradiated in the event of recurrence, but not if further local surgery or reconstruction has been performed following the tattoo, repositioning the markings.

A recent study has shown chemotherapy prolongs survival for isolated or regional recurrence of breast cancer.[43] The use of systemic treatment for advanced, recurrent disease will depend on what was given as adjuvant therapy at the time of the original diagnosis. In general, different chemotherapy agents are used to treat the recurrent disease, on the basis that the ones used originally did not sterilise the tumour completely, and also because some, notably the anthracyclines, have cumulative cardiac toxicity that can be serious. Likewise, there may be some gain from rotating oestrogen-blocking agents to palliate locally advanced cancers when there are no other treatment options. Tamoxifen may work when aromatase inhibitors start to fail and vice versa. Sometimes older agents such as megestrol acetate or newer agents such as fulvestrant are effective when other agents fail to control the cancer.

The use of biological agents continues to evolve. Trastuzumab in locally advanced disease typically mimics the efficacy in metastatic disease (for inoperable locally advanced cancers) or as adjuvant treatment (in those advanced cancers amenable to more radical treatment). However, trastuzumab is seldom used as a single agent, as the response rates in combination with chemotherapy are much better,[44] although ongoing work on the use of other agents such as lapatinib in combination with trastuzumab, pertuzumab, T-DM1, chemotherapy and other biologicals may provide new advances in the care of these patients.

There remains considerable uncertainty around the optimum management of locally advanced breast cancer. The accuracy of detecting systemic disease, the value of data that are 20–30 years old, and the relevance of agents and regimens in old trials to the use of newer therapies and current radiotherapy fractionation are unclear, and for operable locally advanced breast cancer surgery remains a good treatment option.

Key points

- Locally advanced breast cancer should be treated by a multidisciplinary team.
- Surgery is an option for operable locally advanced breast cancer but most patients are best treated initially by systemic therapy.
- The surgeon removing the primary tumour as primary therapy or after neoadjuvant therapy should aim for clear resection margins.
- Sentinel node biopsy is appropriate after successful neoadjuvant therapy.
- Immediate breast reconstruction can and should be considered following mastectomy for locally advanced breast cancer.
- Postoperative radiotherapy significantly reduces local recurrence and improves survival in locally advanced breast cancer.
- Neoadjuvant chemotherapy is as effective as adjuvant chemotherapy in prolonging survival for patients with locally advanced breast cancer.
- After neoadjuvant chemotherapy, radical radiotherapy or surgery have similar efficacy.
- Neoadjuvant endocrine therapy with aromatase inhibitors is more effective than tamoxifen.

References

1. Giordano S. Update on locally advanced breast cancer. Oncologist 2003;8:521–30.

2. Coles CE, Wilson CB, Cumming J, et al. Titanium clip placement to allow accurate tumour bed localisation following breast conserving surgery: audit on behalf of the IMPORT Trial Management Group. Eur J Surg Oncol 2009;35:578–82.

3. Early Breast Cancer Trialists' Collaborative Group. Effects of radiotherapy and surgery in early breast cancer: an overview of the randomised trials. N Engl J Med 1995;333:1444–55.

4. Xing Y, Foy M, Cox DD, et al. Meta-analysis of sentinel lymph node biopsy after preoperative chemotherapy in patients with breast cancer. Br J Surg 2006;93(5):539–46.
   Sentinel lymph node biopsy of the post-treatment axilla may be used to guide therapy.

5. Motwani SB, Strom EA, Schechter NR, et al. The impact of immediate breast reconstruction on the technical delivery of postmastectomy radiotherapy. Int J Radiat Oncol Biol Phys 2006;66(1):76–82.

6. Chatterjee JS, Lee A, Anderson A, et al. The effects of post-operative radiotherapy on autologous Deep Inferior Epigastric Perforator (DIEP) flap volume in immediate postmastectomy breast reconstruction. Br J Surg 2009;96:1135–40.

7. Early Breast Cancer Trialists' Collaborative Group. Radiotherapy for early breast cancer (Cochrane Review). In: The Cochrane Library, Issue 2. Oxford: Update Software; 2002.

8. Adamson DJA. The radiobiological basis of radiation side effects. In: Faithfull S, Wells M, editors. Supportive care in radiotherapy. Edinburgh: Churchill Livingstone; 2003. p. 71–96.

9. The START Trialists' Group. The UK Standardisation of Breast Radiotherapy (START) Trial A of radiotherapy hypofractionation for treatment of early breast cancer: a randomised trial. Lancet Oncol 2008;9(4):331–41.

10. Overgaard M, Hansen PS, Overgaard J, et al. Postoperative radiotherapy in high-risk premenopausal women with breast cancer who receive adjuvant radiotherapy. N Engl J Med 1997;337:949–55.

11. Overgaard M, Jensen MB, Overgaard J, et al. Postoperative radiotherapy in high-risk postmenopausal women with breast cancer given adjuvant tamoxifen: Danish Breast Cancer Cooperative Group DBCG 82c randomised trial. Lancet 1999;353:1641–8.
    The above two papers show that postoperative radiotherapy reduces locoregional recurrence and improves survival.

12. Hojris I, Overgaard M, Christensen JJ, et al. Morbidity and mortality of ischaemic heart disease in high-risk breast-cancer patients after adjuvant postmastectomy systemic treatment with or without radiotherapy: analysis of DBCG 82b and 82c randomised trials. Radiotherapy Committee of the Danish Breast Cancer Cooperative Group. Lancet 1999;354(9188):1425–30.

13. Whelan TJ, Julian J, Wright J, et al. Does loco-regional radiation therapy improve survival in breast cancer? A meta-analysis. J Clin Oncol 2000;18(6):1220–9.

14. Chua B, Olivotto IA, Weir L, et al. Increased use of adjuvant regional radiotherapy for node-positive breast cancer in British Columbia. Breast J 2004;10(1):38–44.

15. Rouzier R, Extra J-M, Carton M, et al. Primary chemotherapy for operable breast cancer: incidence and prognostic significance of ipsilateral breast tumour recurrence after breast-conserving surgery. J Clin Oncol 2001;19(18):3828–35.

16. Recht A, Edge SB, Solin LJ, et al. Postmastectomy radiotherapy: clinical practice guidelines of the American Society of Clinical Oncology. J Clin Oncol 2001;19(5):1539–69.

17. SIGN Clinical Guideline Number 84. Management of breast cancer in women. Edinburgh: Scottish Intercollegiate Guidelines Network; 2005.

18. Perloff M, Lesnick GJ, Korzun A, et al. Combination chemotherapy with mastectomy or radiotherapy for stage III breast carcinoma: a Cancer and Leukaemia Group B Study. J Clin Oncol 1988;6:261–9.

19. De Lena M, Varini M, Zucali R, et al. Multimodality treatment for locally advanced breast cancer. Results of chemotherapy–radiotherapy versus chemotherapy–surgery. Cancer Clin Trials 1981;4:229–36.
    After neoadjuvant chemotherapy, radical radiotherapy may have equivalent relapse and survival to surgical resection.

20. Wolff AC. Systemic therapy. Curr Opin Oncol 2001;13:436–49.

21. Deo SV, Bhutani M, Shukla NK, et al. Randomized trial comparing neo-adjuvant versus adjuvant chemotherapy in operable locally advanced breast cancer (T4b N0–2 M0). J Surg Oncol 2003;84(4):192–7.
    Paper showing equivalence of neoadjuvant chemotherapy compared with adjuvant in terms of survival.

22. Mieog JSD, van der Hage JA, van de Velde CJH. Neoadjuvant chemotherapy for operable breast cancer. Br J Surg 2007;94:1198–200.

23. Penault-Llorca F, Abrial C, Mouret-Reynier M-A, et al. Achieving higher pathological complete response rates in HER-2-positive patients with induction chemotherapy without trastuzumab in operable breast cancer. Oncologist 2007;12:390–6.

24. Limentani SA, Brufsky AM, Erban JK, et al. Phase II study of neoadjuvant docetexel, vinorelbine, and trastuzumab followed by surgery and adjuvant doxorubicin plus cyclophosphamide in women with human epidermal growth factor receptor 2-overexpressing locally advanced breast cancer. J Clin Oncol 2007;25(10):1232–8.

25. Hsiang DJ, Yamamoto M, Mehta RS, et al. Predicting nodal status using dynamic contrast-enhanced magnetic resonance imaging in patients with locally advanced breast cancer undergoing neoadjuvant chemotherapy with and without sequential trastuzumab. Arch Surg 2007;142(9):855–61.

26. Melsamy S, Bolan PJ, Baker EH, et al. Neoadjuvant chemotherapy of locally advanced breast cancer: predicting response with in vivo 1H MR spectroscopy – a pilot study at 4 T. Radiology 2004;233:424–31.

27. Kwong MS, Chung GC, Horvath LJ, et al. Postchemotherapy MRI overestimates residual disease compared with histopathology in responders to neoadjuvant therapy for locally advanced breast cancer. Cancer J 2006;12(3):212–21.

28. Rastogi P, Anderson SJ, Bear HD, et al. Preoperative chemotherapy: updates of National Surgical Adjuvant Breast and Bowel Project Protocols B-18 and B-27. J Clin Oncol 2008;26(5):778–85.

29. Escobare PF, Patrick RJ, Rybicki LA, et al. Prognostic significance of residual breast disease and axillary node involvement for patients who had primary induction chemotherapy for advanced breast cancer. Ann Surg Oncol 2006;13(6):783–7.

30. Huober J, von Minckwitz G, Denkert C, et al. Effect of neoadjuvant anthracycline–taxane-based chemotherapy in different biological breast cancer phenotypes: overall results from the GeparTrio study. Breast Cancer Res Treat 2010;124:133–40.

31. Shet T, Agrawal A, Chinoy R, et al. Changes in the tumor grade and biological markers in locally advanced breast cancer after chemotherapy – implications for a pathologist. Breast J 2007;13(5):457–64.

32. Thomas JSJ, Julian HS, Green RV, et al. Histopathology of breast carcinoma following neoadjuvant systemic therapy: a common association between letrozole therapy and central scarring. Histopathology 2007;51:219–26.

33. Dixon JM, Love CDB, Bellamy COC, et al. Letrozole as primary medical therapy for locally advanced and large operable breast cancer. Breast Cancer Res Treat 2001;66(3):191–9.

34. Semiglazov VF, Semiglazov VV, Dashyan GA, et al., Phase 2 randomized trial of primary endocrine therapy versus chemotherapy in postmenopausal patients with oestrogen receptor-positive breast cancer. Cancer 2007;110(2):244–54.

35. Llombart-Cussac A, Guerrero A, Galan A, et al. Phase II trial with letrozole to maximum response as primary systemic therapy in postmenopausal patients with ER/PgR[+] operable breast cancer. Clin Transl Oncol 2012;14(2):125–31.

36. Bonneterre J, Thürlimann B, Robertson JFR, et al. Anastrozole versus tamoxifen as first-line therapy

for advanced breast cancer in 668 postmenopausal women: results of the tamoxifen or arimidex randomized group efficacy and tolerability study. J Clin Oncol 2000;18(22):3748–57.

37. Macaskill EJ, Renshaw L, Dixon JM. Neoadjuvant use of hormonal therapy in elderly patients with early or locally advanced hormone receptor-positive breast cancer. Oncologist 2006;11:1081–8.

38. Nabholtz JM, Buzdar A, Pollak M, et al. Anastrozole is superior to tamoxifen as first-line therapy for advanced breast cancer in postmenopausal women: results of a North American multicenter randomized trial. J Clin Oncol 2000;18(22):3758–67.

39. Mouridsen H, Gershanovich M, Sun Y, et al. Superior efficacy of letrozole (Femara) versus tamoxifen as first-line therapy for postmenopausal women with advanced breast cancer: results of a phase III study of the International Breast Cancer Group. J Clin Oncol 2001;19(10):2596–606.

Aromatase inhibitors may be more effective than tamoxifen in the neoadjuvant treatment of locally advanced breast cancer.

40. Thompson AM, Johnson A, Quinlan P, et al. Comprehensive CYP2D6 genotype and adherence affect outcome in breast cancer patients treated with tamoxifen monotherapy. Breast Cancer Res Treat 2010;125:279–87.

41. Osborne CK, Pippen J, Jones SE, et al. Double-blind, randomized trial comparing the efficacy and tolerability of fulvestrant versus anastrozole in postmenopausal women with advanced breast cancer progressing on prior endocrine therapy: results of a North American trial. J Clin Oncol 2002;20(16):3386–95.

42. Thompson AM, Jordan JB, Quinlan P, et al- The Breast Recurrence in Tissues Study Group. Prospective comparison of switches in biomarker status between primary and recurrent breast cancer: the Breast Recurrence in Tissues Study (BRITS). Breast Cancer Res 2010;12:R92.

43. Aebi S, Gelber S, Lang I, et al. Chemotherapy prolongs survival for isolated or regional recurrence of breast cancer: The CALOR trial (Chemotherapy as Adjuvant for Locally Recurrent breast cancer; IBCSG 27-02, NSABP B-37, BIG 1-02). Cancer Res 2012;72(24):96s.

44. Lewis R, Bagnall A-M, Forbes C, et al. The clinical effectiveness of trastuzumab for breast cancer: a systematic review. Health Technol Assess 2002;6(13):1–71.

14

Metastatic disease and palliative care

John A. Dewar
Pamela Levack

Introduction

Metastatic spread is defined as spread of breast cancer beyond the breast and ipsilateral axillary and/or internal mammary lymph nodes. With current therapies, metastatic disease is incurable and treatment is, by definition, palliative. Such patients may, however, benefit considerably from treatment. The principles and practice of treatment include a combination of active disease management, active symptom management, and appropriate support for patient and family. A more detailed review of the evidence is provided in the National Institute of Health and Clinical Excellence (NICE) guideline.[1]

Historically, palliative care and terminal care were one and the same. However, modern palliative care includes symptom and supportive care for patients 'upstream' in their illness. As cancer advances, patients' symptom burden increases, and they need the best of symptom control as well as the best of cancer treatment. All surgeons should be able to provide high-quality basic palliative care for their patients, and specialist palliative care staff should be available to support staff to manage the most complex and persisting problems.

A frequent dilemma is how much and how intensively to both treat and provide care aimed at comfort. The issues faced by staff working at this interface between intensive palliative surgical (or medical) treatment and intensive symptom control are demanding and complex.

Presentation and prognosis

A minority of breast cancer patients (<10%) present initially with metastatic disease.[2] Most metastatic patients, however, present months or years after their primary treatment (surgery and appropriate adjuvant therapy). The natural history of breast cancer can be very long – patients still die from breast cancer 20 years and more after their initial treatment.[3]

Most patients present with symptoms of metastatic disease between follow-up visits;[4] screening asymptomatic patients is not worthwhile.[5,6] The common sites of metastatic spread are listed in Table 14.1; among other sites is the peritoneum, to which infiltrating lobular carcinoma, in particular, can spread and cause non-specific abdominal symptoms and/or obstruction.

Staging

All patients presenting with locally advanced, inoperable or locally recurrent breast cancer should undergo a series of investigations to stage their disease adequately. In addition, patients presenting with metastatic disease at one site (e.g. bone) should have investigations to assess the extent of spread to other organs. The principal sites of spread are the thorax, bone and liver. Thus, tests to assess the extent of spread and organ function include a full blood count, clinical chemistry (urea and electrolytes, bone

Table 14.1 • Symptoms commonly associated with metastatic spread to different organs

Site	Common symptoms
Pleura	Dyspnoea (due to effusion)
Bone	Pain
	Pathological fracture
	Nausea and thirst (due to associated hypercalcaemia)
Lung	Dyspnoea
	Cough (dry cough is often seen with lymphangitis carcinomatosa)
Liver	Fatigue
	Nausea
	Anorexia
	Pain over liver
Brain	Headache (often worse first thing in the morning)
	Unilateral weakness
	Unsteady gait

chemistry and liver function tests), tumour markers (carcinoembryonic antigen and carbohydrate antigen 15-3, which can be useful to assess response[7]), bone scintigram and computed tomography (CT) scan of thorax abdomen and pelvis. Alternatives are a liver ultrasound or magnetic resonance imaging (MRI). Increased long bone activity identified on bone scintigraphy should be further assessed by plain X-ray, supplemented by MRI if necessary, to assess degree of destruction and risk of pathological fracture. The brain should be assessed (CT or MRI) if the patient has symptoms suggestive of intracranial metastases. Urgent MRI of the whole spine is required if the patient has symptoms of spinal cord compression.

Clinicians need to understand the limitations of these investigations. Although bone scintigraphy is more sensitive than plain X-ray, it will not detect all bone metastases. If a patient has persistent bony symptoms and a negative bone scan (or negative in the symptomatic area) then an MRI should be requested, since it is more sensitive than bone scintigraphy. Discrete liver metastases are well visualised by most techniques, but diffuse infiltration may not be apparent on liver ultrasound. Positron emission tomography (PET)-CT cam be useful[8] in resolving whether lymph nodes or isolated lesions seen in the lung or liver are indeed metastases (albeit infected or inflammatory conditions can also be positive on fluorodeoxyglucose PET).

Treatment

Management is palliative and the aim of treatment is to give the patient the best quality of life with the minimum of side-effects. Successful management of symptoms will tend to prolong survival, but the emphasis of treatment is on the quality of the life lived rather than its length. Patients need to understand from their clinician the nature of their illness and the aims of treatment before discussing treatment options, likely side-effects and potential benefits.

Broadly speaking, systemic therapies control breast cancer and specific therapies control specific symptoms. The two are not mutually exclusive and most patients will need both.

Systemic therapy

In general, a durable response to systemic therapy offers the best quality of life (see guidance in **Fig. 14.1**).

> ✔ Most patients with oestrogen receptor (ER)-positive tumours will be initially treated with hormone therapy: it is generally less toxic than chemotherapy, responses are of longer duration and there is no evidence that patients with ER-positive metastatic disease do better with chemotherapy first.[9]

Exceptions are patients with lymphangitis carcinomatosa or extensive liver metastases – hormone-induced response rates at both these sites are low, and one may not be able to wait 6–8 weeks for a response, hence chemotherapy is indicated. Endocrine therapy is ineffective in ER-negative breast cancer. If patients respond well to either endocrine or chemotherapy, then they may respond to second-line agents on relapse.

Endocrine therapy

Premenopausal women

In 1896, Beatson[10] demonstrated the endocrine sensitivity of breast cancer for the first time, by undertaking surgical oophorectomy for advanced breast cancer. Current therapy (Table 14.2) aims to either decrease levels of circulating oestrogen (ovarian ablation) or block its effect on the oestrogen receptor (anti-oestrogens). Ovarian ablation can be performed either by surgical removal (usually laparoscopically), by a short course of radiotherapy to the pelvis (infrequent – because of gastrointestinal side-effects),

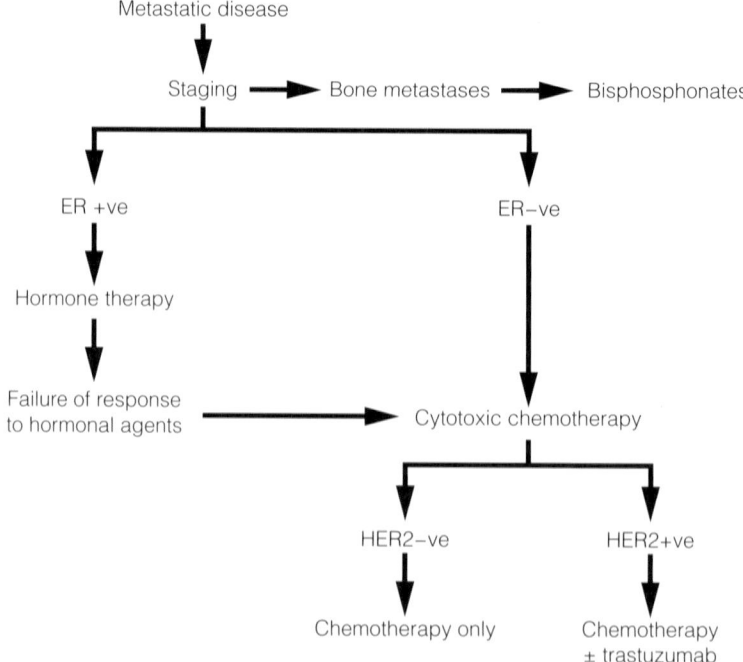

Figure 14.1 • Outline of systemic therapy. Oestrogen receptor positive (ER +ve) includes all ER-positive and/or progesterone receptor-positive patients. ER-positive patients with lymphangitis carcinomatosa or liver metastases would normally be considered for chemotherapy in preference to hormone therapy.

Table 14.2 • Endocrine agents used in breast cancer

Class of agent	Examples	Main side-effects
Ovarian ablation	Surgical oophorectomy Radiation menopause LH-RH agonists	Menopausal symptoms
Anti-oestrogens	Tamoxifen Fulvestrant	Menopausal symptoms Thrombo-embolism
Aromatase inhibitors	Anastrozole Letrozole Exemestane	Menopausal symptoms Arthralgia Osteoporosis
Progestagens	Megesterol acetate	Weight gain Increased appetite Thrombo-embolism Glucocorticoid suppression

or the use of a luteinising hormone-releasing hormone (LH-RH) agonist, e.g. goserelin. The latter is given by monthly injection into the anterior abdominal wall and is reversible; thus, if there is no tumour response, the patient's periods can be restored and menopausal symptoms abolished. Tamoxifen is a partial oestrogen agonist but its effects on breast cancer cells are to antagonise oestrogen. It is effective in both pre- and postmenopausal women.

> ✔ Response to ovarian ablation is improved if tamoxifen is added.[11]

Aromatase inhibitors (AIs; see next section) work in postmenopausal but not in premenopausal women. Particular caution should be taken with women who have chemotherapy-induced amenorrhoea, as they may still have some ovarian function, making AIs ineffective.[12] In premenopausal women, a combination of LH-RH agonist plus AI has shown responses.[13]

Progestagens (e.g. megesterol acetate, medroxyprogesterone) at high dose have been used for many years, for their anti-oestrogenic action. Their main side-effects are significant weight gain and increased risk of thromboembolic disease. Suppression of glucocorticoid production has been reported,[14] so patients may need hydrocortisone to cover physiological stress (e.g. pinning of pathological fractures, infections, etc.).

Thus, first-line therapy would be tamoxifen ± ovarian ablation, with an AI/LH-RH agonist as second line and progestagens as third line. Choice will, however,

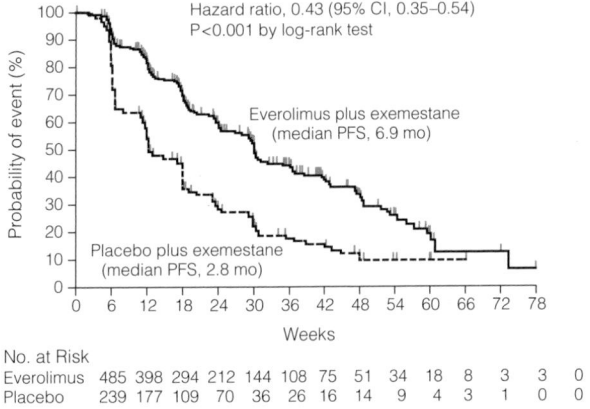

Figure 14.2 • Progression-free survival on the basis of local assessment of radiographic studies. Reproduced from N Engl J Med 2012; 366(6): 520–9.

be influenced by prior adjuvant therapy, though if it is >1 year since the last endocrine therapy (e.g. tamoxifen), it may be worth retrying it.

Postmenopausal patients

Ovarian ablation has no role. Oestrogen in postmenopausal women is produced by conversion of androstenedione to oestrone by aromatase,[15] mostly in peripheral fat but also in liver, normal breast tissue and some breast cancers. Aromatase inhibitors (Table 14.2) reduce circulating oestrogen to nearly immeasurable levels.

There are two types of AI: non-steroidal (anastrozole and letrozole) and steroidal (exemestane). Their side-effects are, however, similar (Table 14.2), implying that these are due to their reduction of circulating oestrogen.

> ✓✓ AIs are more effective[16] than tamoxifen (appropriate second-line agent) and progestagens (third line).

Fulvestrant is a pure oestrogen antagonist, as unlike tamoxifen it has no agonist action. It binds to, blocks and degrades the oestrogen receptor. Clinical trials in postmenopausal women have shown it to be as active as anastrozole.[17] It is given monthly by intramuscular injection – a potential advantage where oral compliance is a problem. Studies with higher doses, 500 mg instead of the standard 250 mg dose, have shown that these higher doses appear effective.

Adding biological agents such as mTOR (mammalian target of rapamycin) inhibitors to endocrine agents such as tamoxifen or aromatase inhibitors appears to increase response rate, duration of response and even overall survival (**Fig. 14.2**). Studies

with these agents are continuing, although as yet they are not used outside clinical trials.

Chemotherapy

Chemotherapy is used to treat ER-negative breast cancer, ER-positive breast cancer that is no longer sensitive to endocrine agents, and advanced ER-positive visceral disease. The main classes of drugs and their side-effects are listed in Table 14.3. These drugs are toxic and should only be prescribed by clinicians (usually oncologists) experienced in their use.

Table 14.3 • Main cytotoxic chemotherapy drugs used in breast cancer

Group of drugs	Examples	Main side-effects*
Anthracyclines	Doxorubicin Epirubicin	Mouth ulcers Cardiomyopathy
Alkylating agents	Cyclophosphamide	
Antimetabolites	5-Fluorouracil (capcitabine) Methotrexate	Coronary spasm Hand–foot symdrome
Taxanes	Docetaxel Paclitaxel	Peripheral and autonomic neuropathy Mouth ulcers
Vinca alkaloids	Vinorelbine	Peripheral neuropathy
	Gemcitabine	
Platinum	Carboplatinum Cis-platinum	Neuropathy Renal failure

*Nearly all these drugs can cause fatigue, nausea, vomiting, myelosuppression, cessation of periods (premenopausal women) and alopecia, so they are not listed individually.

> ✔✔ Drug combinations appear more effective than single agents partly because combinations of drugs with different modes of action increase efficacy and reduce the risk of drug resistance but are associated with more toxicity.[18] Nonetheless, it is not uncommon in clinical practice to use sequential single agents.

The drug groups with the highest activity are the anthracyclines and the taxanes. The major limitation to anthracycline use is cardiomyopathy – the risk increasing as cumulative dose increases. A course of anthracyclines cannot, therefore, usually be repeated. Taxanes are active and more effective than some other regimens.[19] Capecitabine is an oral prodrug of 5-fluorouracil. It is metabolised into the active component in the liver and possibly in the tumour itself.

As more agents are used in the adjuvant (or neo-adjuvant) setting, the use of other active drugs such as vinorelbine, gemcitabine and platinum agents in metastatic disease is likely to increase. Platinum salts may have particular activity in the treatment of patients with basal-type tumours[20] and are currently being studied in clinical trials.

The choice of chemotherapy agents is influenced by prior therapy, the general health of the patient, and what agent is most likely to produce useful palliation with minimal side-effects.

Trastuzumab

A growth factor receptor gene, human epidermal growth factor (HER-2), is amplified in about 14% of breast cancers and is associated with a poorer prognosis.[21] Trastuzumab is a humanised monoclonal antibody that targets the HER-2 receptor in patients whose tumours overexpress HER-2 as assessed by immunohistochemistry and/or fluorescence in situ hybridisation (FISH) testing.

> ✔✔ Whilst it has some activity as a single agent (response rates of 20–50% partly depending on previous treatments), it increases the response rate and survival of patients when added to taxane chemotherapy.[22]

Trastuzumab is generally well tolerated except for cardiac toxicity, so is not usually given concurrently with anthracyclines. It should be used with caution in patients with prior anthracycline exposure or significant cardiac disease; patients require cardiac monitoring by multiple-gated acquisition (MUGA) scan or echocardiogram.

With these provisos, trastuzumab can be used in HER-2-positive patients. It is generally given with a course of taxane chemotherapy and continued as a single agent whilst response is maintained. Response may last months and even years. Trastuzumab is a large molecule and does not pass the blood–brain barrier, so patients who respond may develop brain metastases as the sole site of active disease. The brain metastases should be treated actively (see later), trastuzumab continued and the patient may regain remission. Other drugs targeting HER-2-positive breast cancers including pertuzumab and T-DM1 are in clinical trials. Combination of pertuzumab and trastuzumab looks particularly promising in patients with metastatic breast cancer (**Fig. 14.3**).

Lapatinib inhibits the tyrosine kinases of HER-2 and has been shown to be active in combination with capecitabine in patients who have relapsed on trastuzumab.[23]

Assessment of response

The most important method of assessing benefit is whether the patient's symptoms have improved. Nevertheless, symptoms can improve independently of systemic therapy (e.g. analgesics for pain). Thus, it is also important to assess response to systemic therapy objectively. Locally recurrent disease can be assessed by regular photography and compared with previous clinical photographs. Similarly, monitoring measurable lesions on CT provides objective evidence of response. Assessment of bony metastases can be difficult. Plain

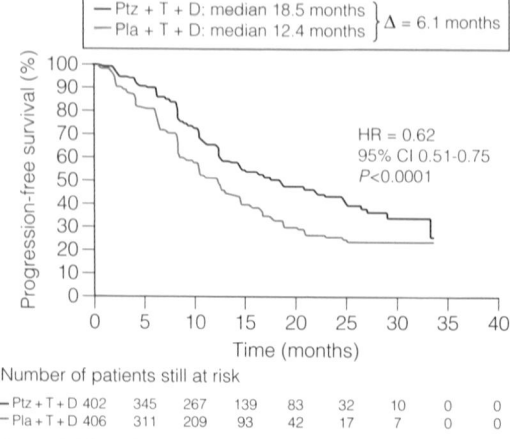

Figure 14.3 • Progression free survival in the CLEOPATRA Trial of Docetaxel + Trastuzumab +/– Pertuzumab. Ptz = pertuzumab; T = trastuzumab; D = docetaxel; Pla = placebo. Reproduced from N Engl J Med 2012; 366(2): 109–19.

X-ray changes are slow to develop with response, and responding sclerotic lesions will show little change. Bone scintigraphy can be misleading; 3 months after starting therapy, there may be increased uptake at sites of disease ('flare') indicating response and this can be indistinguishable from progression. Changes in the levels of tumour markers at 3 months can predict response[24] or individual lesions can be monitored by MRI.[1]

Surgery

For patients presenting with metastatic disease it was formerly the case that surgery to the primary site was contraindicated because it will not help symptoms nor influence prognosis. This has now been questioned by a series of studies that have shown improved outcome in patients who have had surgery. Whether this improved outcome is due to selection bias or is genuine is not clear.[25] Ongoing randomised trials will provide the answers. In those patients who are responding and have stable metastatic disease, surgery to control local disease in the breast and on the chest wall and in regional nodes should be considered.

Control of symptoms

> ✔ Patients with advanced malignancy can have a high burden of distressing symptoms, frequently under-reported by patients and underestimated and undertreated by clinicians.[26]

Despite the absence of evidence, staff, patients and families are often concerned that intensive symptom management prevents further palliative treatment of underlying cancer and that it inevitably causes sedation and may even hasten death. Uncontrolled symptoms affect quality of life and the ability of the patient to make considered treatment decisions, hence meticulous symptom control should be available as part of comprehensive cancer management.

Pain

Sixty-five per cent of patients with advanced cancer suffer pain.[27] One-third of those with pain have one pain, another third have two different types of pain and the remaining third have three or more types of pain. Cancer-related nerve pain is common; 70–90% of pain responds to potent opioids if properly prescribed[28] and the key to managing pain is careful assessment using a simple structured tool such as 'NOPQRST' (Box 14.1).

Box 14.1 • NOPQRST tool for effective pain history taking

N: Number of pains
O: Origin of pain
P: Palliate and potentiate
Q: Quality, e.g. is it neuropathic
R: Radiation
S: Severity *or* Suffering – 7–10 is a serious problem, >10 overwhelming
   Suffering is the impact pain has on the patient
T: Timing, including incident pain, for example moving or dressing changes

Analgesic requirements are likely to increase as illness advances.

> ✔ Morphine is the strong opioid of choice for cancer pain management.[29]

Other strong opioids are used when the transdermal route is preferred or the patient has unacceptable side-effects with morphine.

Non-oral routes (e.g. by a subcutaneous syringe driver) are preferable when nausea and vomiting are present and do *not* mean that the patient is dying, merely that an alternative route to deliver medication is needed – for example, a patient with pain who is vomiting due to hypercalcaemia and constipation. Morphine (10 mg given by intermittent intravenous boluses) may lead to erratic pain control and sleepiness, which can be avoided by using lower doses by subcutaneous infusion, until the situation has resolved and oral medications are appropriate.

Common concerns over opioid analgesics

Whilst morphine is the drug of first choice, side-effects or inadequate pain relief may limit benefit in 10–30% of patients. Switching opioids may reduce side-effects (Box 14.2) but if the pain is not opioid sensitive and toxicity is not a problem, switching from one to the other alone will not solve uncontrolled pain.[30]

Pain flares

Transient flares of severe pain are common and may be due to end of dose failure, a spontaneous worsening of pain or incident pain. The first two usually respond to an increased 24-hour dose of opioid.

✔ Incident pain occurs in two-thirds of patients with pain[31] and is common in patients with bone metastases. It is the result of an intervention such as weight bearing, coughing or moving.

Analgesia sufficient to manage an incident pain peak may cause toxicity in relation to background pain; therefore, a fast, short-acting rescue analgesic such as transmucosal or intranasal fentanyl may be more effective than breakthrough oral morphine.

Liver capsule pain from liver metastases usually responds to dexamethasone 4–12 mg p.o. daily or, for speed and if pain is associated with nausea or vomiting, 12 mg over 24 hours by subcutaneous syringe driver for a few days until symptoms have resolved. The dose should then be reduced to the smallest effective oral maintenance dose.

Neuropathic pain

Patients often find it difficult to describe accurately nerve pain that typically has burning, shooting, stabbing, knife-like or tingling character and patients frequently accompany their description by rubbing the dermatome where the pain is felt. It has a distressing quality, which may not be adequately reflected in a simple 0–10 scale; hence a simple neuropathic pain screening tool has been recently developed.[32] It is critical to recognise neuropathic pain, and to diagnose the underlying pathology, as it usually represents new and potentially treatable metastatic disease.

Neuropathic pain responds to opioids in approximately one-third of patients, but the remaining two-thirds may be difficult to manage. Nerve root involvement is most likely to result from brachial plexus involvement or epidural disease as a result of vertebral metastases and subsequent bony collapse. Drugs used primarily for reasons other than analgesia may help,[33,34] such as low doses of antidepressants (amitriptyline or nortriptyline[35]), anticonvulsants (gabapentin, pregabalin[36]) or specific N-methyl-D-aspartate antagonists (ketamine[37]). Methadone (specialist use only) is helpful when pain consists of a mixture of neuropathic and non-neuropathic pain, but there is insufficient published evidence on its use in cancer-induced pain.[38] Finally, interventional procedures – cordotomy (unilateral nerve root pain) or epidural followed by an intrathecal implant – may be considered following consultation with the local pain or anaesthetic service.

Spinal cord compression

Patients with severe increasing back pain plus neuropathic pain referred around the chest wall, abdomen or down one or both legs should be assessed for the risk of spinal cord compression.

✔ Waiting until the patient has neurological signs of compression (loss of power and/or a sensory level) will almost certainly be too late to institute effective treatment.[39]

If spinal cord compression is suspected, then an urgent MRI scan of the whole spine should be organised. If the diagnosis is confirmed, radiotherapy or surgical intervention is indicated.[40,41]

Bony metastases

This is the commonest site of metastatic disease and can cause significant pain and morbidity.

✔ Specific treatment guidelines have been published.[24]

Bisphosphonates

Bisphosphonates inhibit osteoclast activity, leading to decreased bone absorption.

✔✔ There is good evidence[42,43] that regular treatment with bisphosphonates for 6 months or longer reduces 'skeletal morbidity', namely reduction in pathological fractures, need for palliative radiotherapy and hypercalcaemia.

The drugs used are most commonly the third-generation drugs zoledronate and ibandronate. Zoledronate is given intravenously every 4 weeks (or 3-weekly with chemotherapy); ibandronate can be given orally (on an empty stomach 1 hour before food). They are usually reasonably well tolerated but can cause flu-like symptoms, gastrointestinal disturbance and rarely osteonecrosis of the jaw.[44] They should be given with caution in patients with renal impairment. Intravenous bisphosphonates can also reduce pain in patients with widespread bony metastases.[45] A monoclonal antibody against rank ligand, denosumab, looks promising and is at least as effective as zoledronate and can be administered by subcutaneous injection.

Bone pain

Non-steroidal analgesics are helpful and are opioid sparing. The most common drug used by palliative medicine physicians is diclofenac (75 mg, slow release twice daily). A slow-release preparation reduces early morning pain due to overnight immobility. When pain is severe and distressing, immediate relief may need a non-oral prescription, e.g. 48-hour syringe driver with, for example, an opioid and a non-steroidal such as ketorolac, before returning to oral medication.

✓✓ Palliative radiotherapy to painful bony metastases can be very helpful in reducing pain and single fractions are as effective as multiple fractions.[46]

Fractures

Pathological fractures cause severe bony pain. Orthopaedic interventions can stabilise fractures of long bones (commonly femur or humerus). The results of orthopaedic interventions are usually better if done prophylactically rather than as an emergency. In either case, surgery will normally be followed by palliative radiotherapy. Most vertebral fractures are managed by palliative radiotherapy but selected cases may benefit from surgical stabilisation and/or decompression, especially where there is a risk of spinal cord compression.[41]

Effusions

Pleural spread is common, especially on the ipsilateral side. The patient usually presents with dyspnoea, and drainage with pleurodesis (using talc[47]) gives good symptomatic relief. Ascites is less common than pleural spread and is managed by repeated percutaneous drainage.

Cerebral metastases

This is typically a relatively late site of metastases. Occasionally, it may be the sole site of metastases. Presentation is usually with headache (characteristically worst in the morning if the patient has raised intracranial pressure), weakness and/or altered sensation, difficulty walking or severe persisting nausea. Diagnosis is confirmed by CT or MRI. A short course (five fractions) of palliative radiotherapy to the whole brain may provide useful palliation for patients whose clinical condition is reasonably well preserved. A patient who is in good general condition and has a single cerebral metastasis may get a more prolonged remission from neurosurgical removal followed by radiotherapy.

Nausea, vomiting and retching

These are common, distressing symptoms and are reported in 50–60% of patients suffering from advanced cancer. Numerous neurotransmitters and receptor types are involved; thus, antiemetics are mainly neurotransmitter blockers (Table 14.4).[48]

Constipation

Constipation is present in half of all patients with advanced cancer. It causes pain, distension, anorexia, nausea, malaise and embarrassment, and diagnostic confusion if it results in 'overflow' diarrhoea. Contributory factors include opioid use, reduced fluid and fibre intake, and reduced mobility. A recent Cochrane systematic review[49] concluded that all laxatives assessed were ineffective for a significant proportion of patients, and some patients required multiple 'rescue' laxatives. Patients on opiates should be routinely prescribed a stimulant and a softener. Methylnaltrexone is a novel treatment for opioid-induced constipation.[50]

Overall care of the patient approaching death

On approaching the terminal phase, patient and clinicians need to recognise that active treatment becomes less appropriate, although active symptom palliation remains paramount. The primary care team and the hospital specialists involved in the care of the patient will often have known the patient for some considerable time and have some knowledge of the family circumstances. But if the patient does not understand the reality of their situation,

Table 14.4 • Management of nausea/vomiting due to cancer or its treatment

	Anti-emetic
Metabolic, e.g. hypercalcaemia	Haloperidol 1.5 mg nocte/b.d.
Drug/toxin induced, e.g. opioid	Levomepromazine 6 mg tab nocte
	Haloperidol 1.5 mg nocte/b.d.
	Levomepromazine 6 mg nocte
Chemotherapy	Ondansetron
	Dexamethasone
Radiotherapy	Ondansetron
Raised intracranial pressure (cerebral metastases, brain stem or meningeal disease)	Cyclizine 50 mg t.d.s. or 150 mg/24 h s.c.
	Dexamethasone 4–16 mg in morning
Bowel obstruction	Cyclizine 50 mg p.o. t.d.s./150 mg/24 h s.c.
(if surgery inappropriate)	Hyoscine butyl bromide 40–100 mg/24 h s.c.
	Octreotide 300–1000 mg/24 h s.c.
	Ondansetron 8–24 mg/24 h p.o., i.v., s.c.
Gastric stasis/outlet obstruction	Metochlopramide or domperidone 10–20 mg q.d.s. or
	Metochlopramide 30–100 mg/24 s.c.
Vestibular disease (base skull tumour)	Cyclizine 50 mg p.o. t.d.s.
	Levomepromazine 6 mg p.o.
	Haloperidol 1.5 mg b.d.
	Trial dexamethasone

then important issues may not have been discussed. For example, the young single mother will need to address the future care of her children, an older woman the care of a frail elderly spouse.

Patients may have survived many relapses over the years, and they and their families may believe that they will recover from the current episode. Clinical staff need to recognise a patient's likely prognosis – is she ill with very advanced metastatic breast cancer and is she perhaps dying?

What does the patient understand? Although clinical prediction of survival is a useful independent predictor for survival, it tends to be over-optimistic and for many patients it will be inaccurate. Broadly speaking, when deterioration in health is noted over months, survival is likely to be months, when it has been over weeks, survival is likely weeks and when it has been over days, survival is likely to be days.

In advanced malignancy, symptoms rather than test results may be more useful in predicting survival. Patients with low performance status (Palliative or Karnofsky Performance Scales) have a poorer survival, although higher performance status does not necessarily predict for longer survival. Certain symptoms such as nausea, breathlessness and weakness have independent value as prognostic factors. Combining clinical prediction with other factors to produce a prognostic score (Table 14.5) gives simple and clinically more accurate useful bedside prognostic information.[51]

Table 14.5 • Palliative Prognostic Index (PPI; palliative. info/teaching material/Prognosis.pdf)

		Maximum possible	
Palliative	10–20	4	4
Performance	30–50	2.5	
Scale	≥60	0	
Oral intake	Severely reduced	2.5	2.5
	(≤ mouthfuls)	1	
	Moderately reduced	0	
	(> mouthfuls)		
	Normal		
Oedema	Present	1	1
	Absent	0	
Dyspnoea at	Present	3.5	3.5
rest	Absent	0	
Delirium	Present	4	4
	Absent	0	
	Total		15

If PPI >6, survival is less than 3 weeks.

Recognition and communication that the patient may be dying

'Is this a patient who could die during this admission?'

Making and communicating a diagnosis that 'this patient may be dying' is the key to good end-of-life care, but it is a difficult skill. It is not exclusively a nursing responsibility – the doctor's role in diagnosis and prognostication is vital. If there is no gap between aggressive or interventional palliative treatments and terminal care, the patient and family will be unprepared – a change from 'doing everything' to 'doing nothing'.

'The physician does and does not want to pronounce a death sentence and the patient does and does not want to hear it'

The patient and family value communication of information and support that will come from a variety of sources (e.g. doctors, specialist and general nurses, palliative care staff) at different times and stages.

Patients, families and professionals need to understand that death is a possibility before they can discuss management options. Several consultations may need to take place over a few days as people psychologically edit what they are told.

Communication in difficult situations is difficult, and easy for professionals to avoid. Some patients prefer not to discuss these matters, as do some professionals. Both patients and professionals may collude to limit such discussions.[52]

There is usually more agreement about the most appropriate approach when a patient is actively dying, i.e. the last few days or hours, and the use of care pathways[53] may be helpful in ensuring that all pre-emptive medications for distress, pain, etc. are prescribed and that the goals of care are clear to the patient, family and staff. Requests for transfer to hospice are common during this time, even when the patient is comfortable and their needs are being met. Other patients may wish to be at home and many specialist palliative care services can help with a swift, supported discharge.

Key points

- Metatastic breast cancer can be treated actively and many patients will survive with a good quality of life for months and often years.
- Most of this time patients will be in the community and care will be shared between primary and secondary care. Good communication between the two is vital.
- The patient will need considerable support from a multidisciplinary team during management of metastatic breast cancer and will need help from many different members of the team that will vary over time.
- Care will be a combination of active oncological management and meticulous symptom control.
- Metastatic breast cancer is ultimately a fatal condition and it is the duty of the staff looking after the patient to optimise survival but also to recognise that the final phase of life needs to be actively and sympathetically managed in line with the wishes of the patient and her family.

References

1. National Institute of Health and Clinical Excellence (NICE). Advanced breast cancer: diagnosis and treatment. Full Guideline, www.nice.org.uk; 2009.

2. Scottish Breast Cancer Focus Group and Scottish Cancer Therapy Network. Scottish Breast Cancer Audit 1987 and 1993: Report to the Chief Scientist and CRAG. Edinburgh: SCTN, ISD; 1996.

3. Brinkley D, Haybittle JL. The curability of breast cancer. Lancet 1975;ii:95–7.

4. Dewar JA, Kerr GR. Value of routine follow up of women treated for early carcinoma of the breast. Br Med J 1985;291:1464–7.

5. Givio Investigators. Impact of follow-up testing on survival and health-related quality of life in breast cancer patients: a multicentre randomized controlled trial. JAMA 1994;271:1567–92.

6. Rosselli Del Turci M, Palli D, Cariddi A, et al. Intensive diagnostic follow-up after treatment of primary breast cancer: a randomized trial. National Research Council Project on Breast Cancer follow-up. JAMA 1994;271:1593–7.

7. Harris L, Fritsche H, Mennel R, et al. American Society of Clinical Oncology 2007 update of recommendations for the use of tumour markers in breast cancer. J Clin Oncol 2007;25(33):5287–312.

8. Brunetti JC. PET and PET-CT imaging of breast cancer. Appl Radiol 2009;38:9–16.

9. Wilcken N, Hornbuckle J, Ghersi D. Chemotherapy alone versus endocrine therapy alone for metastatic breast cancer. Cochrane Database Syst Rev 2003;2:CD002747.

10. Beatson GT. On the treatment of inoperable cases of carcinoma of the mamma: suggestions for a new method of treatment, with illustrative cases. Lancet 1896;ii:104–7,162–5.

11. Robertson JF, Blamey R. The use of gonadotrophin-releasing hormone (GnRH) agonists in early and advanced breast cancer in pre- and perimenopausal women. Eur J Cancer 2003;7:861–9.

12. Smith IE, Dowsett M, Yap YS, et al. Adjuvant aromatase inhibitors for early breast cancer after chemotherapy induced amenorrhoea: caution and suggested guidelines. J Clin Oncol 2006;24:2444–7.

13. Forward DP, Cheung KL, Jackson L, et al. Clinical and endocrine data for goserelin plus anastrozole as second-line endocrine therapy for premenopausal advanced breast cancer. Br J Cancer 2005;92:416–7.

14. Naing KK, Dewar JA, Leese GP. Megesterol acetate (Megace) therapy and secondary adrenal suppression. Cancer 1999;86(6):1044–9.

15. Miller WR. Aromatase inhibitors:mechanism of action and role in the treatment of breast cancer. Semin Oncol 2003;30(4, Suppl. 14):3–11.

16. Gibson LJ, Dawson CK, Lawrence DH, et al. Aromatase inhibitors for the treatment of advanced breast cancer in postmenopausal women. Cochrane Database Syst Rev 2007;1: CD003370.
This meta-analysis of all the trials comparing AIs with other endocrine therapies confirms the advantages of AIs.

17. Howell A, Pippen J, Elledge RM, et al. Fulvestrant versus anastrozole for the treatment of advanced breast cancer: a prospectively planned combined analysis of two multicentre trials. Cancer 2005;104:236–9.

18. Carrick S, Parker S, Thornton CE, et al. Single agent versus combination chemotherapy for metastatic breast cancer. Cochrane Database Syst Rev 2009;2: CD003372.
A systematic review of 43 trials and, although the results are summarised in the text, there is heterogeneity between the trials reflecting differences in efficacy of the drugs used.

19. Ghersi D, Wilcken N, Simes J, et al. Taxane containing regimes for metastatic breast cancer. Cochrane Database Syst Rev 2005;2:CD003366.

20. Brody LC. Treating cancer by targeting a weakness. N Engl J Med 2005;353:949–50.

21. Purdie CA, Baker L, Ashfield A, et al. Increased mortality in HER2 positive, oestrogen receptor positive invasive breast cancer: a population based study. Br J Cancer 2010;102(4):719–26.

22. Slamon DJ, Leyland-Jones B, Shak S, et al. Use of chemotherapy plus a monoclonal antibody against HER2 for metastatic breast cancer that overexpresses HER2. N Engl J Med 2001;344:783–92.
The first randomised trial to demonstrate the activity of a monoclonal antibody in human breast cancer.

23. Geyer CE, Forster J, Lindquist D, et al. Lapatinib plus capecitabine for HER2-positive advanced breast cancer. N Engl J Med 2006;355:2733–43.

24. Breast Speciality Group of the British Association of Surgical Oncology. Guidelines for the Management of Metastatic Bone Disease in Breast Cancer in the United Kingdom. Eur J Surg Oncol 1999;25:3–23.

25. Rapiti E, Verkooijen HM, Vlastos G, et al. Complete excision of primary breast tumor improves survival of patients with metastatic breast cancer at diagnosis. J Clin Oncol 2006;24:2743–9.

26. Grossman SA, Sheidler VR, Swedeen K, et al. Correlation of patient and caregiver ratings of cancer pain. J Pain Symptom Manage 1991;6:53–7.

27. Van den Beuken, van Everdingen MHJ, de Rijke JM, et al. Prevalence of pain in patients with cancer: a systematic review of the past 40 years. Ann Oncol 2007;18:1437–49.

28. David MP, Glare P, Quigley C, et al. Opioids in cancer pain. 2nd ed. Oxford: Oxford University Press; 2009.

29. King S, Forbes K, Hanks GW, et al. A systematic review of the use of opioid medication for those with moderate to severe cancer pain and renal impairment: a European Palliative Care Research Collaborative opioid guidelines project. Palliat Med 2011;25:525–52.

30. Fine PG, Portnoy RK. Ad hoc expert panel on evidence review and guidelines for opioid rotation. J Pain Symptom Manage 2009;38(3):418–25.

31. Dale O, Moksnes K, Kaasa S. European Palliative Care Research Collaborative pain guidelines: opioid switching to improve analgesia or reduce side effects. A systematic review. Palliat Med 2011;25:494–503.

32. Portenoy R. Development and testing of a neuropathic pain screening questionnaire: ID Pain. Curr Med Res Opin 2006;22(8):1555–65.

33. Attal N, Cruccu G, Baron R, et al. EFNS guidelines on the pharmacological treatment of neuropathic pain: 2010 revision. Eur J Neurol 2010;17:1113–23.

34. Bennett MI. Effectiveness of antiepileptic and anti-depressant drugs when added to opioids for cancer pain: systematic review. Palliat Med 2011;25:553–9.

35. Saarto T, Wiffin PJ. Antidepressants for neuropathic pain. Cochrane Database Syst Rev 2005;3:CD005454. Updated 2007.

36. Wiffen PJ, McQuay HJ, Edwards JE, et al. Gabapentin for acute and chronic pain. Cochrane Database Syst Rev 2005;3:CD005452.

37. Bell RF, Ecclestone C, Kalso E. Ketamine as an adjuvant to opioids for cancer pain. Cochrane Database Syst Rev 2003;1:CD003351. Updated 2009.

38. Nicholson AB. Methadone for cancer pain. Cochrane Database Syst Rev 2004;2:CD003971. Reviewed 2007.

39. Levack P, Graham J, Collie D, et al. Don't wait for a sensory level – listen to the symptoms: a prospective audit of the delays in the diagnosis of malignant spinal cord compression. Clin Oncol 2002;14:472–80.

40. Loblaw DA, Perry J, Chambers A, et al. Systematic review of the diagnosis and management of malignant cord compression: the Cancer Care Ontario Practice Guidelines Initiative's Neuro-Oncology Disease Site Group. J Clin Oncol 2005;23(9):2028–37.

41. Metastatic spinal cord compression: diagnosis and management of adults at risk of and with metastatic spinal cord compression. NICE; 2008.

42. Pavlakis N, Schmidt R, Stockler M. Bisphosphonates for breast cancer. Cochrane Database Syst Rev 2005;3:CD003474.

43. Ross JR, Saunders Y, Edmonds PM, et al. Systematic review of role of bisphosphonates on skeletal morbidity in metastatic cancer. Br Med J 2003;327:469–72.
    Both of these reviews (Refs 42 and 43) confirm from large randomised studies in women with advanced breast cancer that bisphosphonates when given in addition to systemic endocrine or chemotherapy reduce the risk of skeletal morbidity.

44. Marx RE, Sawatari Y, Fortin M, et al. Bisphosphonate-induced exposed bone (osteonecrosis/osteopetrosis) of the jaws: risk factors, recognition, prevention and treatment. J Oral Maxillofac Surg 2005;63:1567–75.

45. Wong R, Wiffen PJ. Bisphosphonates for the relief of pain secondary to bone metastases (Cochrane review). The Cochrane Library, Issue 2. Chichester, UK: John Wiley; 2004.

46. Chow E, Harris K, Fan G, et al. Palliative radiotherapy trials for bone metastases: a systematic review. J Clin Oncol 2007;25(11):1423–36.
    A systematic review of 16 trials comparing single fractions vs. multiple fractions confirms that both are as effective in relieving pain, but patients who had a single fraction are more likely to be retreated.

47. Tan C, Sedrakyan A, Browne J, et al. The evidence on the effectiveness of management for malignant pleural effusion: a systematic review. Eur J Cardiothorac Surg 2006;29:829–38.

48. Hallenbeck JL. Palliative care perspectives. Oxford University Press; 2003.

49. Miles CL, Fellowes D, Goodman ML, et al. Laxatives for the management of constipation in palliative care patients. Cochrane Database Syst Rev 2006;4:CD003448.

50. Candy B, Jones L, Goodman ML, et al. Laxatives or methylnaltrexone for the management of constipation in palliative care patients. Cochrane Database Syst Rev 2011;CD003448.

51. Lau F, Cloutier-Fischer D, Kuziemsky C, et al. A systematic review of prognostic tools for estimating survival time in palliative care. J Palliat Care 2007;23(2):93–112.

52. The A-M, Hak T, Koeter G, et al. Collusion in doctor–patient communication about imminent death: an ethnographic study. Br Med J 2000;321:1376–81.

53. National Care of the Dying – Audit of Hospitals (England). http://www.mcpcil.org.uk/files/hospital_pathway.pdf; December 2011.

15

The role of adjuvant radiotherapy in the management of breast cancer

Ian Kunkler

Introduction

Adjuvant radiotherapy (RT) remains, with surgery and systemic therapy, a core component of the adjuvant treatment of breast cancer. There have been innovations in breast radiation planning and delivery, the role of adjuvant radiotherapy after breast-conserving surgery (BCS) and mastectomy, partial breast irradiation and altered fractionation.

Advances in radiotherapy planning and delivery

Major improvements in radiation planning and delivery include the wider dissemination and use of three-dimensional computed tomography (CT) planning and intensity-modulated radiotherapy (IMRT). These developments may contribute to improved locoregional control and survival while reducing acute and late radiation-induced morbidity.

Three-dimensional CT planning has improved dose homogeneity both within the breast and/or to regional nodal areas while reducing dosage to critical normal tissues, particularly the lungs, heart and brachial plexus. In addition, breathing-adapted gating techniques have reduced cardiac irradiation.[1]

Achieving a homogeneous dose distribution is challenging in the breast because its contour changes in both cranio-caudal and sagittal planes. Homogeneity is poorer in the upper and lower regions of the breast, resulting in 'hot spots' in areas of the breast distant from the central axis.[2] Tangential beam plans can be optimised to ensure that the volumes of the breast exceeding 105% of the prescribed dose are minimised. With IMRT the X-ray beam is dynamically collimated to modify its fluence, allowing a therapeutic dose to be 'painted' to the breast/chest wall and peripheral lymphatics while minimising dosage to critical adjacent structures. The 'field-in-field' technique (the addition of supplementary photon fields) reduces 'hot spots' such as the inframammary fold and the thin breast tissue close to the nipple–areola complex.[2,3]

✔✔ A randomised trial comparing IMRT to standard three-dimensional planning postoperative radiotherapy after BCS showed that IMRT reduced acute breast toxicity (breast pain and moist desquamation) and improved quality of life.[4]

✔ Patients with larger breasts where homogeneous dose distribution is difficult to achieve should be considered for IMRT. Longer term follow-up will be needed to see if local control is improved and late radiation changes such as breast fibrosis are reduced by IMRT.

The role of adjuvant radiotherapy in ductal carcinoma in situ (DCIS)

In principle, DCIS should be as sensitive as invasive breast cancer (IBC) to irradiation. However, its role in the conservative management of DCIS is less firmly established than for IBC and use of adjuvant RT varies across the UK with no clear standard of care.[5]

✅✅ There are four randomised trials that have investigated the value of the addition of whole-breast irradiation and/or tamoxifen to BCS.[6–12]
All show that postoperative radiotherapy reduces the risk of in ipsilateral recurrence of DCIS and development of invasive breast cancer.

All these trials used a dose fractionation schedule of 50 Gy in 25 fractions over 5 weeks. The EORTC trial[6] randomised 1010 women with clinically or mammographically detected DCIS ≤5 cm in size to wide local excision alone or wide local excision plus whole breast irradiation (50 Gy in 25 fractions over 5 weeks). The 10-year local relapse-free rate was 85% with RT compared to 74% with surgery alone (hazard ratio (HR) 0.53, $P < 0.001$). In situ local recurrence rates were 7% and 13% respectively and invasive rates were also 7% and 13%. In the NSABP B-17 trial[7] 818 patients were randomised to +/– whole-breast radiotherapy (WBRT) after lumpectomy. RT reduced the local relapse rate from 16.8% to 7.7% (relative risk (RR) 0.38, 95% confidence interval (CI) 0.25–0.59; $P < 0.00001$). In a recent update of the trial with 10-year follow-up, invasive recurrence within the ipsilateral breast was associated with a slightly higher risk of death. In contrast, recurrence of DCIS was not.[8] The UK/ANZ trial[9] recruited 1701 patients treated by BCS. Patients were randomised into four treatment groups (BCS alone, BCS + RT, BCS + tamoxifen and BCS + RT + tamoxifen). Approximately 90% of patients were ≥50 years and screen detected. Median follow-up was 53 months. Local recurrence rates were 22%, 8%, 18% and 6% respectively. Adjuvant RT was associated with a significant reduction for both DCIS and IBC ipsilateral recurrence (HR 0.38, $P < 0.0001$). Radiotherapy reduced the risk of recurrence by 64% for DCIS ($P = 0.0004$) and by 55% for invasive year cancer ($P = 0.01$). The Swedish DCIS trial (SweDCIS)[10] randomised 1067 patients after wide excision for DCIS to WBRT or no WBRT. There was a risk reduction of 16% in ipsilateral events (in situ or invasive carcinoma) at 10 years from RT (95% CI 10.3–21.6%) and a relative risk of 0.40 (95% CI, 0.30–0.54%). The effect of RT in women was lower in women younger than 50, but there was a substantial benefit in women >60 years. Results of the four trials

were pooled in a Cochrane review[11] and showed that the risk of ipsilateral invasive recurrence was halved by radiotherapy at 10 years (HR 0.50, 95% CI 0.32–0.76) with about 50% of the ipsilateral breast tumour recurrence (IBTR) being invasive and 50% DCIS. In a subgroup analysis according to age (</>50 years, presence or absence of comedo necrosis and tumour size >/<10 mm) all subgroups derived benefit from RT. Women >50 years appeared to experience a greater reduction in recurrence than compared to younger women (HR 0.35 (>50) vs. 0.67 (<50)). What limits interpretation, as others have pointed out,[5] is that none of the trials were designed prospectively for subgroup analyses. In addition, there have been criticisms of the quality of the DCIS trials, summarised in a review,[13] and problems with these trials include deficiencies in radiological–pathological correlation, measurement of tumour size,[14] routine imaging of pathology specimens, postoperative imaging, definition and classification of lesions,[7] definition of tumour-free margins,[15] consistency in inclusion/exclusion criteria, randomisation procedures and insufficient statistical power to detect small differences in survival.[12] Attempts have been made to define a subset of patients from whom postoperative radiotherapy might be omitted. In the E5194 non-randomised study of wide local excision alone in 711 patients with low- or intermediate-grade DCIS ≤2.5 cm or high-grade ≤1 cm with margins ≥3 mm with median follow-up of 6.7 years, the 5-year ipsilateral recurrence rate was 6.1%.[16] A continued increase in the rate of IBTR beyond 5 years is of concern and long-term follow-up will be needed to determine if omission of radiotherapy is safe.

The absolute benefits of radiotherapy on local control are greater in high-grade compared to low-grade DCIS. The thresholds for recommending radiotherapy vary widely internationally. In some centres radiotherapy is confined to patients with high-grade DCIS, whereas other women with all grades of DCIS are treated following BCS on the basis[17] that there is no group that does not benefit. One of the arguments for a more conservative approach to selection is that these patients are subject to the same risks of radiation-induced morbidity (including cardiac damage, rib fractures and pneumonitis) as patients with invasive breast cancer. In some groups of women with DCIS mortality rates are <1% and so this encourages a more cautious approach in recommending adjuvant breast irradiation. That said, the risks, for example, of cardiopulmonary morbidity have been substantially reduced by the use of three-dimensional CT planning.

✅ At present it can be argued that since all subgroups of patients with DCIS benefit from RT after BCS, all should receive it.

In clinical practice, radiotherapy is used selectively based on patient age, the size of the DCIS, grade of DCIS, adequacy of excision, the patient's general health and their wishes.

Is there a role for a boost dose after whole-breast irradiation for DCIS?

✅ Whether giving a boost dose to the site of excision of DCIS after whole-breast irradiation confers similar benefit to that seen in invasive breast cancer is unclear. Retrospective pooled data[18] suggest there may be a benefit.

A multi-institution retrospective study comparing wide local excision alone, wide local excision and whole-breast radiotherapy among 373 patients ≤45 years showed a reduced risk of relapse at 10 years in patients treated with a boost dose (86%) compared to no boost (72%).[18] However, this study was potentially subject to selection bias, with the possibility that higher risk patients were more likely to have received a boost.[19] The role of the boost and of hypofractionation is currently under investigation in the international BIG 3-07 trial. Patients with non-low-risk DCIS are randomised after whole-breast irradiation to a boost of 16 Gy in eight fractions or no boost. An external beam dose fractionation regimen (the standard of 50 Gy in 25 fractions over 5 weeks) or a hypofractionated regimen of 42.5 Gy in 16 daily fractions are options that are included in the randomisation or can be selected in the trial. The primary end-point is time to local recurrence.

✅ There is a limited evidence base for hypofractionation in DCIS. In a retrospective study from Toronto of patients with DCIS treated with conventional (50 Gy in 25 fractions) or hypofractionated (42.4 Gy in 16 fractions or 40 Gy/16 + 12.5 Gy boost) WBRT after breast-conserving surgery for DCIS (median follow-up 3.76 years), there was no difference in local control or toxicity.[20]

Role of adjuvant radiotherapy in invasive breast cancer

The Oxford overview

The overall impact of radiotherapy on local recurrence and survival is best appreciated from the 5-yearly updates of the Oxford overview of randomised trials of radiation after both breast-conserving surgery and mastectomy. The conclusions have changed dramatically since the first overview in 1978, which showed an adverse effect of RT on survival after mastectomy,[21] largely due to the adverse effects of excessive cardiac irradiation from now obsolete orthovoltage techniques.

✅✅ In the 2000 overview of radiotherapy trials, a 2% benefit in 20-year survival was counterbalanced by an excess of non-breast cancer mortality, predominantly vascular, again a residual effect of older trials.[22] This provides a strong rationale for radiotherapy techniques that reduce cardiac dose.

However, in 2005, the first evidence emerged of the beneficial effect of a reduction in local recurrence from RT on the overall survival[23] of 42 000 women in 78 randomised trials.

✅✅ A key observation from the Oxford overview of radiotherapy trials was that for every four local recurrences prevented, one breast cancer death was avoided, now known as the '4:1 ratio'.[23]

This ratio was confirmed in a more recent meta-analysis confined to over 10 000 women of trials of breast-conserving surgery with or without adjuvant whole breast irradiation.[24] It should be noted that the primary end-point in the latter overview has been changed from previous radiotherapy overviews to include any first recurrence, whether this is locoregional or metastatic. The overall impact of adjuvant radiotherapy is an impressive 50% reduction in the risk of any first recurrence. However, the absolute benefits of radiotherapy are less in older lower-risk patients (**Fig. 15.1**). The 10-year risk of any recurrence was reduced by radiotherapy by 15.7% (35% to 19.3%; 95% CI 13.7–17.7, $2P < 0.00001$) and the 15-year mortality fell from 25.2% to 21.4% (an absolute reduction of 3.8%; 95% CI 1.6–6.0, $2P = 0.00005$). In 7287 pN0 patients, the equivalent risk was reduced from 31% to 15.6%, which is a 15.4% absolute reduction (95%

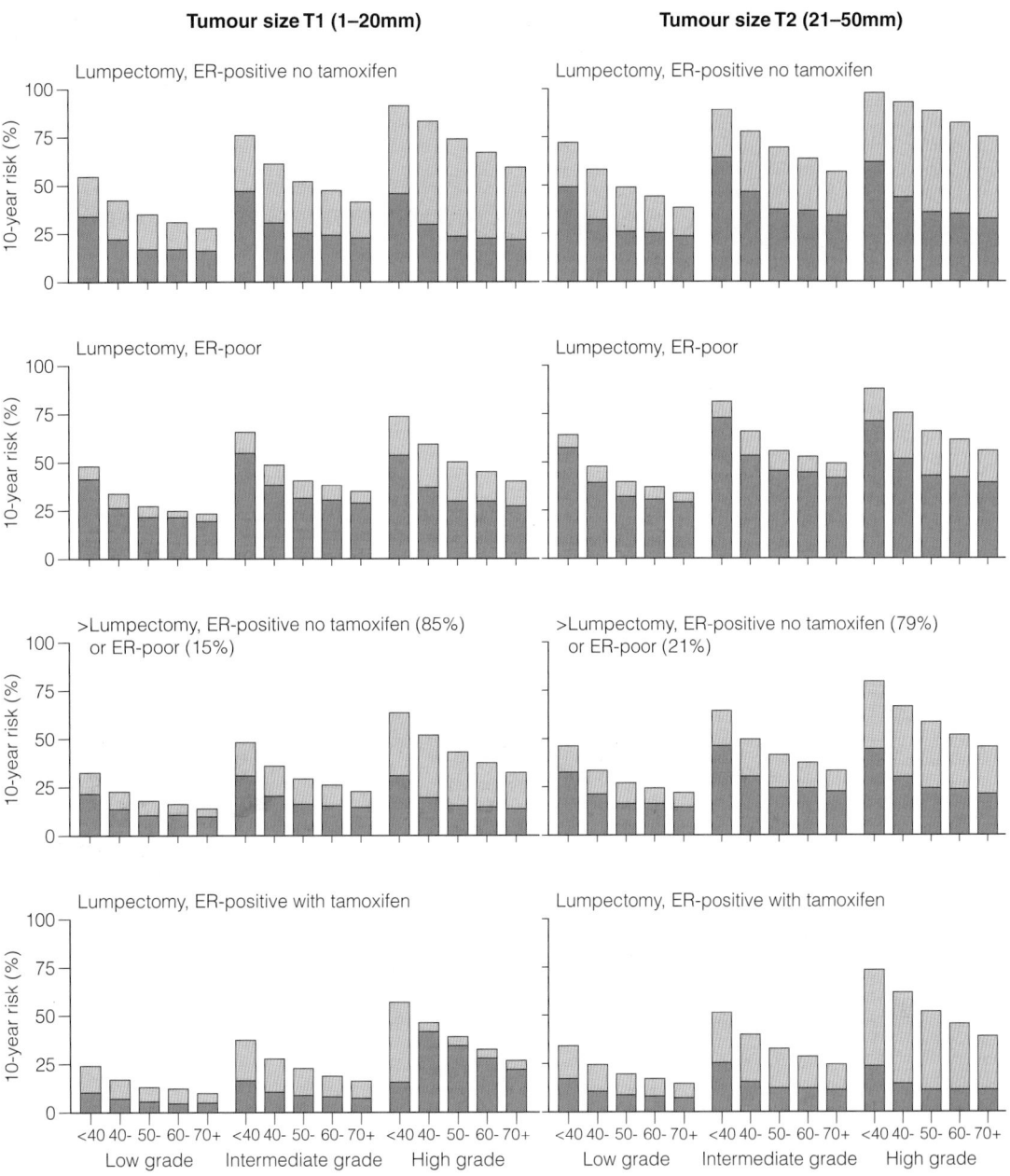

Figure 15.1 • Absolute 10-year risks (%) of any (locoregional or distant) first recurrence with and without radiotherapy (RT) following breast-conserving surgery (BCS) in pathologically node-negative women by patient and trial characteristics, as estimated by regression modelling of data for 7287 women. Bars show 10-year risks in women allocated to BCS only. Dark sections show 10-year risks in women allocated to BCS plus RT, light sections show absolute reduction with RT. ER, oestrogen receptor. Reprinted from The Lancet. Early Breast Cancer Trialists' Collaborative (EBCTCG). Effect of radiotherapy after breast-conserving surgery on 10-year recurrence and 15-year breast cancer death: meta-analysis of individual patient data for 10 801 women in 17 randomised trials. Lancet 2011; 378 (9804):1707–16. With permission from Elsevier.

CI 13.2–17.6, 2P < 0.00001) with a 3.3% absolute reduction in mortality from 20.5% to 17.2%. In pN1 (1050 patients) the 10-year reduction in risk of recurrence was greater (21.2%; 95% CI 14.5–27.9, 2P < 0.00001) from 63.7% to 42.5% with an 8.5% reduction in 15-year breast cancer mortality (95% CI 1.8–15.2, 2P = 0.01) from 51.3% death to 42.8%. The risk of any first recurrence at 10 years was influenced by tumour size, age, grade, use of tamoxifen, oestrogen receptor (ER) status and extent of local breast surgery (**Fig. 15.2**). The proportional reduction in first recurrence is similar irrespective of age. However, the absolute reduction in risk is much less for women >70 years. Most recurrences (75%) were locoregional and were higher in the no RT groups (25%) compared to 8% in the RT

arms. The dominant effect on locoregional recurrence from RT was in the first year but there was a lesser but still substantial impact up to 9 years.

Is there a subgroup of patients from whom postoperative radiotherapy can be omitted?

✔ It remains controversial as to whether there is any subgroup of patients from whom postoperative radiotherapy can be omitted.

This would be attractive, particularly in older patients who may find attendance for several weeks of radiotherapy burdensome. The current consensus is that no group has as yet been identified. Whole-breast radiotherapy reduces the risk of IBTR in all subgroups, although the absolute benefit in low risk, small (<2 cm), well differentiated, hormone receptor-positive, node-negative tumours is small.

✔✔ The only randomised trial to address the issue of the omission of postoperative radiotherapy in 'low-risk' women after breast-conserving surgery is the US Cancer and Leukemia Group B (CALGB) trial.[25,26]

Six hundred and thirty-six women, 70 years or older with T1, N0, M0 breast tumours, were randomised after breast-conserving surgery and tamoxifen to whole-breast irradiation or no further treatment. The difference in local recurrence was 3% at 5 years (4% vs. 1%) in favour of adjuvant irradiation.[25]

Breast oedema, skin fibrosis and pain were all more frequent in the irradiated group. In an accompanying editorial[27] the value of radiotherapy was questioned given the small difference in local recurrence. However, no axillary surgical staging procedure was included in this study so it is possible that the some higher risk, node-positive patients were enrolled. In addition, as the authors acknowledge, the trial was underpowered. It is well recognised that there is a persistent pattern of local recurrence of up to 1% per year at least up to 10 years.[28] This concern is validated by the update of the CALGB trial showing that at a median follow-up of 10.5 years, the difference in local recurrence has increased to 7% (9% vs. 2%).[26] Of the 43% of patients who had died only 7% of deaths were due to breast cancer, reflecting the competing risks of death from non-breast cancer causes, predominantly vascular, in older patients with breast cancer.

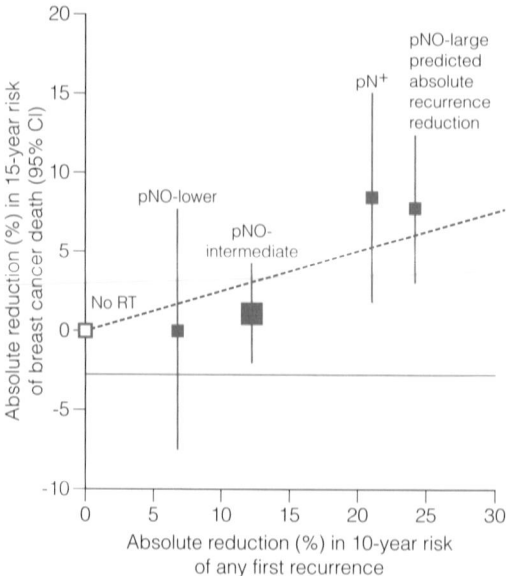

Figure 15.2 • Absolute reduction in 15-year risk of breast cancer death with radiotherapy (RT) after breast-conserving surgery versus absolute reduction in 10-year risk of any (locoregional or distant) recurrence. Women with pN0 disease are subdivided by the predicted absolute reduction in 10-year risk of any recurrence suggested by regression modelling (pN0 large ≥ 20%, pN0 intermediate 10–19%, pN0 lower<10%). Vertical lines are 95% CIs. Sizes of dark boxes are proportional to amount of information. Dashed line: one death from breast cancer avoided for every four recurrences avoided. pN0, pathologically node negative; pN+, pathologically node positive. Reprinted from The Lancet. Effect of radiotherapy after breast-conserving surgery on 10-year recurrence and 15-year breast cancer death: meta-analysis of individual patient data for 10 801 women in 17 randomised trials. Lancet 2011; 378(9804):1707–16. With permission from Elsevier.

Two additional trials shed light on the possibility of the omission of RT in some patients. The Italian 55-75 trial[29] randomised 749 women with T (<2.5 cm) N0/1, M0 breast cancer to whole-breast irradiation (50 Gy in 2-Gy fractions) after quadrantectomy and systemic therapy. For N0 patients, sentinel lymph node biopsy (SLNB) was undertaken. SLNB-positive patients were additionally treated by axillary clearance. This trial is not directly comparable to the CALGB trial since it was not exclusive to older patients and higher risk patients with one to three involved nodes were included as well as hormone receptor-positive and -negative tumours. At a median follow-up of 53 months, the cumulative incidence of IBTR was 2.5% in the surgery-alone arm and 0.7% in the surgery plus radiotherapy arm. The smaller difference in IBTR (1.8%) in the Italian 55-75 trial compared to the CALGB trial largely reflects the greater volume of breast tissue resected by quadrantectomy compared to lumpectomy. The PRIME II trial,[30] currently in the follow-up phase, included over 1300 patients ≥65 years with T<3 cm pathologically axillary node-negative breast cancer after breast-conserving surgery (minimum 1 mm clear margin) and adjuvant endocrine therapy who were randomised to whole-breast irradiation (40–50 Gy) or no whole-breast radiotherapy. Other randomised trials of breast-conserving surgery with or without postoperative radiotherapy that have included but were not limited to older patients do not provide an answer to the question of the omission of postoperative radiotherapy after breast-conserving surgery. In a Canadian trial,[31] age was an independent risk factor with a higher locoregional recurrence rate (LRR) in women over the age of 50. However, a low-risk group with an LRR <10% could not be identified. In the Milan III trial, women over the age of 55 years had a lower risk of recurrence (3.8% vs. 8.8% for the whole population).[32] In the Scottish conservation trial,[33] there was a trend to a lower recurrence rate with age, particularly between 60 and 70 years. No difference in local recurrence was observed in the NSABP B-06 trial for women older or younger than 50 years.[34] The upper age of the trial, however, is not stated.

> ✓✓ At present international consensus is that postoperative radiotherapy after breast-conserving surgery should be the standard of care for all fit patients irrespective of age.[35]

It should be noted, however, that 5-year local recurrence rates in more recently published studies of breast conservation are falling to around 3%.[36] In part this is due to better imaging, screening, surgery and systemic therapy, particularly the introduction of aromatase inhibitors. So the absolute benefits in local control from whole-breast irradiation for older patients are likely to diminish. There is a need to identify better markers of women who are genuinely at low risk of local recurrence to better define clinical 'low-risk' categories and then provide level I evidence to underpin this approach.

Breast boost after breast-conserving surgery for invasive breast cancer

There is level I evidence that a boost of irradiation to the site of excision after breast-conserving surgery improves local control in older as well as young patients. The EORTC boost trial randomised over 5000 T1/2, N0, NIM0 patients after breast-conserving surgery with clear margins and whole-breast irradiation (50 Gy) to a boost of 16 Gy in eight fractions or no boost. The original analysis[37] at 5 years of follow-up showed that the benefit in local control was only statistically significant in women under the age of 50. However, at 10 years of follow-up,[38] all age groups were shown to benefit, although the reduction in local recurrence (7.3% vs. 3.8%) was only 3.5% in the over 60 years of age group.

> ✓✓ On this basis[37,38] all patients, including patients over the age of 60, should be considered for a breast boost and whole-breast irradiation.

Impact of adjuvant whole-breast radiotherapy on quality of life

It might be assumed that the quality of life of older patients treated with postoperative radiotherapy would be worse than for patients treated by breast-conserving surgery and adjuvant endocrine therapy alone due to the burden of attending for several weeks of radiotherapy. However, there is good evidence that adjuvant radiotherapy is well tolerated by the majority of older patients.[39,40] The only trial to address this issue is the PRIME I trial.

It randomised 255 T1/2, N0, M0 patients treated by breast-conserving surgery and endocrine therapy to whole-breast radiotherapy (40–50 Gy) or no further therapy. There was no overall difference in global quality of life measured by the EORTC breast QoL measures[41] at 5 years.

> ✓✓ This implies that, while quality of life is in general a relevant issue in selecting patients for treatment, it should not be a major factor in determining whether or not older patients are recommended to receive postoperative radiotherapy.[41]

Hypofractionated dose fractionation regimens

Shorter radiation regimens than the internationally recognised standard of whole-breast irradiation of 50 Gy in 25 fractions over 5 weeks would be particularly attractive to older patients to reduce the burden of lengthy periods of outpatient attendance and associated fatigue.

> ✓✓ While there is no randomised trial testing hypofractionation in older patients, the results of two UK trials[42,43] and one Canadian trial[44] are likely to be practice changing for patients of all ages. Both trials show that breast cancer is sensitive to fraction size and that fewer larger fractions provide equivalent local control with similar or reduced breast toxicity.

In the UK START A trial, two postoperative hypofractionated dose fractionation regimens, 39 Gy in 13 fractions of 3.2 Gy and 41.6 Gy in 13 fractions of 3 Gy, were compared with 50 Gy in 25 fractions in 2236 women treated by mastectomy or breast-conserving surgery. All regimens were given over 5 weeks. The 5-year LRR was 3.6%, 3.5% and 5.2% for 50 Gy, 41.6 Gy and 39 Gy respectively.[42] In the START B trial, 40 Gy in 15 fractions over 3 weeks was compared to 50 Gy in 25 fractions over 5 weeks in 2215 women after primary surgery. The 5-year locoregional recurrence rates were 2.2% and 3.3% for 40-Gy and 50-Gy regimens respectively. Breast cosmesis was superior in the 40-Gy arm. In both trials the shorter regimens provided similar locoregional control to the standard 50 Gy. The National Institute for Clinical Excellence (NICE) has adopted a 40 Gy in 15 fractions dose fractionation regimen as the new UK standard for adjuvant postoperative

radiotherapy.[45] In the Canadian trial,[44] 1234 patients with T1/2 axillary node-negative breast cancer were randomised after breast-conserving surgery with clear margins to a hypofractionated regimen (42.5 Gy in 16 fractions over 3.5 weeks) of whole-breast irradiation or to 50 Gy in 25 fractions over 5 weeks. No boost was given to the site of excision. At 10 years the local recurrence rate was 6.7% in the standard arm and 6.2% in the test arm. Breast cosmesis was similar in both arms of the trial. There has been little consensus on the generalisability of the findings of the START and Canadian hypofractionation trials. The recent ASTRO Consensus statement recommends that hypofractionated whole-breast irradiation (HF-WBI) is confined to women 50 years or older with T1/2 N0 disease not receiving chemotherapy or nodal irradiation.[46] There is uncertainty about the long-term effects of hypofractionated radiotherapy on the heart. The ASTRO consensus statement therefore advises that HF-WBI should only be used where the heart is excluded from the radiation fields. In contrast, 40 Gy in 15 fractions has been endorsed by the guidelines of the National Institute for Clinical Excellence for postconservation and postmastectomy irradiation,[45] a much broader application of shortened fractionation.

The results of other hypofractionated dose fractionation regimens have been reported in nonrandomised studies. Kirova et al.,[47] in a series of 317 patients aged 70 years or over treated with 32.5 Gy in five fractions once weekly of 6.5 Gy, found similar all-cause-free, local recurrence-free and metastasis-free survival to conventionally fractionated radiotherapy of 50 Gy in 25 daily fractions over 5 weeks. Acute skin toxicity with the HF-WBI regimen was acceptable and no different from the conventionally fractionated patients of similar age. Cosmesis was also similar. However, late complications measured on the LENT-SOMA (late effects normal tissue – subjective, objective management, analytic) showed a higher incidence of grade 1–2 fibrosis (33%) with HF-WBI compared with conventionally fractionated therapy (15%). Similar rates of late effects were seen using the same hypofractionated regimen.[48]

Partial breast irradiation

Partial breast irradiation (PBI) in which adjuvant irradiation is delivered exclusively or in higher dosage to the primary site than the rest of the breast is being investigated in a number of randomised trials. The rationale for this approach is that local recurrences occur predominantly at or close to the site of excision.[34,49] A number of techniques are being studied in clinical trials, including external beam import low,[50] intraoperative kilovoltage (TARGIT)[51] (**Fig. 15.3**)/electron therapy (ELIOT)[52] and intraoperative or postoperative brachytherapy.[53] The rationale and indications for these techniques have recently been reviewed.[54] Of particular interest to older patients are single fraction intraoperative techniques, which avoid the inconvenience of attendance for several weeks of daily outpatient radiotherapy. The only published randomised trial of PBI is the TARGIT A trial,[51] which randomised predominantly low-risk postmenopausal patients randomised to intraoperative radiotherapy (IORT) with the Intrabeam device (Fig. 15.3) using 50 kV X-rays (20 Gy to the surface of the applicator) or to whole-breast irradiation. The local recurrence rate was very low in both arms of the trial but the follow-up was relatively short (4 years). The Kaplan–Meier estimate of ipsilateral breast tumour recurrence at 4 years was 1.20% (95% CI 0.53–2.71) in the targeted intraoperative radiotherapy group (Fig. 15.3) and 0.95% (95% CI 0.39–2.31) in the external beam radiotherapy group. The results, however, are confounded by the option of investigators to supplement IORT with external beam if the investigator considered that there were additional risk factors for recurrence on the excision specimen.[55,56]

The main drawback of the technique is that irradiation is delivered before the margins of excision are assessed on the operative specimen. Intraoperative electrons (3–12 MeV) using a mobile linear accelerator delivering 21 Gy to the 90% isodose are being studied by the Milan group, shielding the chest wall with lead if required.[52]

Postoperative brachytherapy after lumpectomy using low-dose-rate implants over 4–5 days or high dose rate typically twice daily for 5 days has yielded low local recurrence rates.[57,58] Largely in response to the adoption of PBI outside of clinical trials predominantly in the USA and some parts of Europe, consensus guidelines for the use of PBI have been published by ASTRO and GEC, ESTRO.[46,53] While these guidelines may be a pragmatic approach to PBI, they are not based on level I evidence.

> ✅ In the absence of level I evidence, it is important that older patients are not recommended to have PBI outside the confines of clinical trials. Patients should be made aware, as the ASTRO guidelines endorse,[46] that whole-breast irradiation has a much longer track record of safety and efficacy. Until more level I evidence is published, PBI should remain investigational.

Postmastectomy irradiation

It has long been established that postmastectomy radiation therapy (PMRT) reduces the relative risk of locoregional recurrence by about two-thirds in

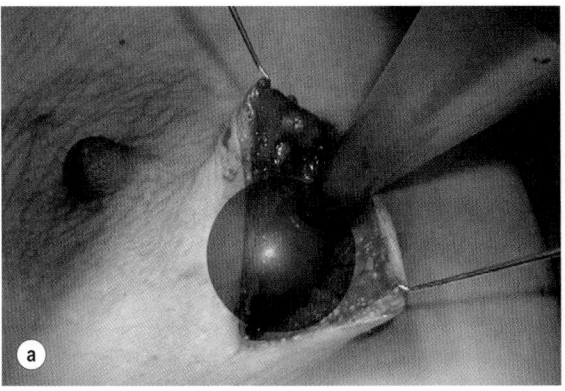
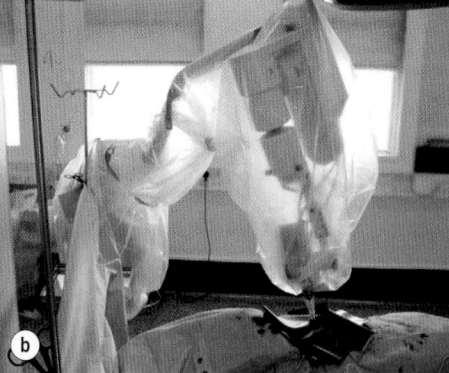

Figure 15.3 • Targeted intraoperative radiotherapy techniques with the Intrabeam system. **(a)** The applicator being placed in the tumour bed. **(b)** The X-ray source is delivered to the tumour bed by use of a surgical support stand. The sterile applicator is joined with a sterile drape that is used to cover the stand during treatment delivery. Reprinted from The Lancet. Vaidya JS, Joseph DJ, Tobias JS et al. Targeted intraoperative radiotherapy versus whole breast radiotherapy for breast cancer (TARGIT-A trial): an international, prospective, randomised, non-inferiority phase 3 trial. Lancet 2010; 376(9735):91–102. With permission from Elsevier.

randomised trials.[59-62] However, the impact on overall survival has been controversial.[22,63,64]

✅✅ A key watershed in the delivery of locoregional radiotherapy of patients after mastectomy was the publication in 1997 of the Danish and Canadian randomised trials that demonstrated a 10-year 9% survival benefit from the addition of comprehensive locoregional radiotherapy after mastectomy to systemic therapy in high-risk premenopausal[59,61] and postmenopausal women.[60]

An explanation for this survival benefit is that tumour cells in local recurrence may have a greater proclivity to metastasise than the original primary tumour.[65] Support is lent to this idea by the fact that patients with local recurrence have a higher breast cancer mortality than patients with a new primary breast tumour.[66,67] As Chung and Harris[65] point out, there is a reduction in local failure rate from chemotherapy alone (50% in ER-positive disease at 5 years and one-third irrespective of ER status), although where the combination of chemotherapy and radiation achieves more impact on local control than either treatment alone.[68,69]

Role of postmastectomy radiotherapy in intermediate risk breast cancer

The role of PMRT in the intermediate-risk group (i.e. women with a 10–19% 10-year risk of locoregional recurrence) with one to three involved axillary nodes or axillary node negative but with other risk factors, e.g. grade 3 histology and/or lymphovascular invasion remains controversial with proponents and sceptics of routine PMRT in this setting.[70,71] What is unclear is the generalisability of the Danish and British Columbia trials to contemporary practice. The locoregional failure rate in the Danish and Canadian trials was greater than in many contemporary non-randomised American series. This might in part be explained by suboptimal axillary surgery with a median of only seven nodes removed in the Danish trials and 11 in the British Columbia trial. An additional criticism was the intensity of chemotherapy.[72] Furthermore, the duration of cyclophosphamide, methotrexate and 5-fluorouracil (CMF) changed over the course of the Danish premenopausal trial. Early in the trial CMF was given for 12 months but this was subsequently shortened to 6 months. In addition only 1 year of adjuvant tamoxifen was given in the Danish 82b trial in contrast to the current standard of 5 years. The risk of local relapse in intermediate-risk patients was of the order of 5–15%[73] and better quality surgery and anthracycline-based adjuvant chemotherapy will reduce this so that further reductions in risk by PMRT might be too low to justify giving irradiation to all such women.

In response to concerns about the adequacy of axillary surgery in the Danish trials, a subgroup analysis of 1000 patients from the DBCG 82b and 82c trials was undertaken. It showed a survival advantage in women with one to three involved nodes as well as those with four or more nodes. The authors and others[74] interpreted this analysis as implying that all node-positive patients should receive postmastectomy irradiation. Others have argued that the somewhat historic Danish trial data are not translatable to contemporary practice[71] since patients with similar levels of risk are now treated with anthracycline-based chemotherapy rather than the CMF-based regimens used in the Danish and Canadian high-risk premenopausal studies.[59,61]

The role of PMRT in 'intermediate-risk' breast cancer is currently being investigated in the MRC/ EORTC BIG 2-04 SUPREMO trial.[75] This includes a biological substudy TRANS-SUPREMO designed to analyse molecular markers associated with risk of relapse. Biological factors may be important in selecting patients for PMRT. Of note, an unplanned subgroup analysis of more than 1000 patients in the Danish 82b and 82c trials by ER, progesterone receptor and human epidermal growth factor receptor (HER-2) status showed that the survival benefit of PMRT was confined to hormone receptor-positive patients and that hormone receptor-negative or triple negative or HER-2-positive patients did not derive a survival advantage.[76] A possible explanation is that these high-risk patients already have disseminated disease on which PMRT is likely to have little impact.

Adjuvant radiotherapy in older patients

Local control in breast cancer is as important for older patients as it is for their younger counterparts, whether after mastectomy or after breast-conserving surgery. Radiotherapy, in conjunction with surgery, continues to play a key role in achieving this. The Oxford overview of randomised trials of adjuvant radiotherapy demonstrates that good local control contributes to reducing breast cancer mortality.[77] There is, however, little level I evidence for the role of adjuvant radiotherapy in breast cancer in older patients largely due to the historical exclusion of patients over the age of 70 from clinical trials. Extrapolation of the results of trials of adjuvant radiotherapy in younger patients to older patients may not be appropriate given the different biology of breast cancer in older patients and the competing risks of non-breast cancer death in this age group. In general older patients tend to have more favourable biological prognostic factors than younger patients with a higher proportion of hormone receptor-positive tumours. This advantage is counterbalanced by exclusion of older patients from national breast screening programmes. As a result, presentation with locally advanced disease with associated poor prognosis is still seen in older women.

For older patients with breast cancer, postoperative whole-breast irradiation after breast-conserving surgery remains the standard of care. Postmastectomy radiotherapy is advised for 'high-risk' older patients. In 'intermediate-risk' breast cancer, its role is controversial. Tolerance of radiotherapy in general is good in older patients and does not impair quality of life. Multimodality therapy should not be withheld from older patients.

Axillary irradiation

With the rapid replacement of routine axillary clearance by sentinel node biopsy as a less morbid method of staging the axilla, the optimal management of patients with micro- or macrometastases in the axillary nodes and the role of axillary irradiation is a focus of ongoing current debate. Central to this discussion is the interpretation of the American College of Surgeons Oncology Group Z0011 phase III trial,[78] which randomised patients with T1–T2 sentinel node biopsy-positive invasive breast cancer treated by breast-conserving surgery to no further surgery or to axillary lymph node dissection (ALND). Patients with micro- or macrometastases in one or two sentinel nodes were included. The whole breast was irradiated by tangential fields and systemic therapy given as appropriate. This was a non-inferiority trial with an intended target accrual of 1900 patients, although less than half were actually accrued. At a median follow-up of 6.3 years there was no difference found in 5-year rates of locoregional recurrence (1.6% for SLNB alone compared

to 3.1% in the ALND arm) or in overall survival (92.5% vs. 91.8% respectively). The hazard ratio for overall survival was 0.79 (90% CI 0.56–1.11) When adjusted for age and systemic therapy, the HR rose to 0.87 (90% CI 0.62–1.23). Both these figures were interpreted by the authors as demonstrating non-inferiority of the SLNB-alone arm and endorsing a policy of observation only in SLNB patients without the need for axillary irradiation. However, there are major issues with this trial. Firstly, the trial was closed prematurely after the accrual of 900 patients, less than half of the planned target accrual of 1900 patients. The trial was therefore potentially underpowered to detect the primary end-point of overall survival (500 deaths were needed to have 90% power to confirm non-inferiority of SLNB compared to axillary node dissection) although it did reach its statistical end-point. Secondly, there was no quality assurance of the radiotherapy of the trial to confirm that there was no difference in field placements between the two arms of the trial. In the SLNB arm, radiation oncologists might have been tempted to raise the upper border of tangential fields in order to cover more of the axillary nodes. This is currently being investigated. If there was genuinely no difference then this would be reassuring that there was no bias in RT technique. A number of possible explanations for the low event rates in the axilla have been postulated,[79] including the low-risk population studied, the impact of systemic therapy and immune surveillance mechanisms suppressing axillary disease. Certainly event rates in contemporary trials of therapy in early breast cancer have been falling. However, the impact of immune surveillance mechanisms in dealing with axillary disease is poorly understood and remains speculative. To address concerns about leaving residual axillary disease untreated after SLNB, a number of algorithms have been developed to predict the probability of non-sentinel lymph node involvement. These algorithms have been tested retrospectively, generally in small cohorts of a few hundred patients with positive sentinel nodes. In the recent study, for example, on a cohort of 159 patients from China,[80] the Cambridge and Mou models outperformed the Mayo, Tenon, MD Anderson, Memorial Sloan Kettering, Turkish, Llubjana, SNUH and Louisville models. However, there remain limitations to these models in predicting residual axillary disease. There is at present limited data to inform best practice, and such data may not be an argument to convince all surgeons that observation only is an option for selected patients with involved nodes following SLNB. An option to complete axillary dissection is axillary irradiation, as it is proven therapy to control axillary disease, although there is limited level I evidence. The Edinburgh randomised trial included patients treated by BCS and mastectomy and compared ALND to axillary RT in axillary lymph node sample-positive patients.[81] It showed no difference in regional control at 5 years or in overall survival. The trial provided excellent data on axillary morbidity showing a low incidence of lymphoedema in the axillary RT arm but some long-term limitation of shoulder mobility. Higher levels of persistent lymphoedema complicated ANLD. The ongoing AMAROS trial[82] is comparing ANLD and axillary irradiation in patients with sentinel node metastases. Identifying more reliably the subset of patients with sentinel node macrometastases who need axillary irradiation requires more level I evidence. In the absence of such evidence, a pragmatic approach to selecting higher risk patients on the basis of number of positive sentinel nodes, tumour size,

ER status and presence or absence of lymphovascular invasion proposed by Haffty et al.[79] (Table 15.1) is a reasonable pragmatic approach.

Minimising radiation-induced cardiac morbidity

Older radiotherapy techniques that led to excess radiation-induced cardiac toxicity and mortality have been replaced by three-dimensional planning[84] and breath holding techniques[1] to minimise cardiac irradiation in left-sided tumours. In successive cohorts of patients treated in the USA, radiation-induced cardiac mortality has fallen.[85] This almost certainly reflects the introduction of three-dimensional planning for breast cancer. Ischaemic heart disease is commoner in older patients. While the cardiac sequelae of adjuvant breast irradiation may take 10 years to manifest themselves, this latency may be within the life expectancy of older patients with early breast cancer. At least the same priority should be given to minimising cardiac irradiation in older as in younger patients.

Table 15.1 • Suggested approach for radiation field design in patients with positive sentinel node biopsy without axillary lymph node dissection

Clinical and pathological parameters	No. of positive sentinel nodes	Total no. of sentinel nodes sampled	Probability of additional nodes* (%)	Probability of additional nodes† (%)	Probability of four or more nodes involved‡ (%)	Field design
IDC, 1.0 cm, LVI negative, ER positive	1 (IHC only)	3	3	8	<1	Tangents only
IDC, 1.8 cm, G3, LVI negative, ER positive, unifocal	1 (macro)	2	27	24	2	High tangents
IDC, 2.0 cm, ER negative, LVI positive	2 (macro)	2	63	55	30	High tangents/ consider full nodal irradiation
ILC, 4.0 cm, ER positive, multifocal, LVI negative	2 (macro)	2	77	64	40	High tangents/ consider full nodal irradiation
IDC, 3.0 cm, ER negative, LVI positive, multifocal	3 (macro with ENE)	3	78	95	80	Full nodal irradiation

Abbreviations: ENE, extranodal extension; ER, oestrogen receptor; G, grade; IDC, infiltrating ductal carcinoma; IHC, immunohistochemistry; ILC, infiltrating lobular carcinoma; LVI, lymphovascular invasion; Macro, macroscopic.
*On the basis of the Memorial-Sloan Kettering Cancer Center nomogram.
†On the basis of the MD Anderson Center nomogram.
‡Katz et al.[83]
Modified from Haffty BG, Hunt KK, Harris JR et al. Positive sentinel nodes without axillary dissection: implications for the radiation oncologist. J Clin Oncol 2011; 29:4479–81.

Key points

- All patients with DCIS after breast-conserving surgery potentially benefit from postoperative radiotherapy, although the absolute benefits in small, low-grade lesions are small.
- There is no subgroup of patients from whom postoperative whole breast radiotherapy can be omitted after breast-conserving surgery for invasive breast cancer.
- Hypofractionated dose fractionation schedules are suitable for most patients requiring adjuvant radiotherapy after breast-conserving surgery or mastectomy.
- More research is needed to identify a subgroup of sentinel node-positive patients from whom axillary irradiation can be omitted in the absence of axillary node dissection.
- A breast boost after breast-conserving surgery and whole-breast irradiation benefits all age groups, although the absolute gain in patients >60 years is small.
- The role of partial breast irradiation remains investigational.
- Adjuvant local/locoregional irradiation after mastectomy is recommended in T3, T4 tumours and those patients with four or more involved axillary nodes.
- The role of postmastectomy irradiation in the one to three node-positive group is controversial.

References

1. Korreman SS, Pedersen AN, Nottrup TJ, et al. Breathing adapted radiotherapy for breast cancer: comparison of free breathing gating with breath-hold technique. Radiother Oncol 2005;76:311–8.

2. Haffty BG, Buchholz TA, McCormick B, et al. Should intensity-modulated radiation therapy be the standard of care in the conservatively managed breast cancer patient? J Clin Oncol 2008;26:2072–4.

3. Hoover S, Bloom E, Patel S. Review of breast conservation therapy: then and now. ISRN Oncol 2011;2011:617593.

4. Pignol JP, Olivotto I, Rakovitch E, et al. A multi-center randomized trial of breast intensity-modulated radiation therapy to reduce acute radiation dermatitis. J Clin Oncol 2008;26:2085–92.
   In this trial, 358 patients with early breast cancer were randomised to standard radiotherapy (RT) with wedged fields or to intensity-modulated radiotherapy (IMRT); 331 patients were analysed. IMRT significantly improved the dose distribution compared with standard radiation. Fewer patients treated with IMRT (31.2%) experienced moist desquamation during or up to 6 weeks after RT compared to 47.8% with standard treatment ($P = 0.002$). On multivariate analysis breast IMRT ($P = 0.003$) and smaller breast size ($P < 0.001$) were significantly associated with a lower risk of moist desquamation. The application of IMRT did not correlate with pain and quality of life, but moist desquamation did significantly correlate with pain ($P = 0.002$) and impaired quality of life ($P = 0.003$).

5. Barnes NL, Ooi JL, Yarnold JR, et al. Ductal carcinoma in situ of the breast. Br Med J 2012;344:e797.

6. EORTC Breast Cancer Cooperative Group, EORTC Radiotherapy Group, Bijker N, Meijnen P, Peterse JL, et al. Breast-conserving treatment with or without radiotherapy in ductal carcinoma-in-situ: ten-year results of European Organisation for Research and Treatment of Cancer randomized phase III trial 10853 – a study by the EORTC Breast Cancer Cooperative Group and EORTC Radiotherapy Group. J Clin Oncol 2006;24:3381–7.
   This randomised trial provides evidence of the effectiveness of postoperative radiotherapy in reducing ipsilateral DCIS and invasive recurrence (level I evidence).

7. Fisher B, Land S, Mamounas E, et al. Prevention of invasive breast cancer in women with ductal carcinoma in situ: an update of the National Surgical Adjuvant Breast and Bowel Project experience. Semin Oncol 2001;28:400–18.

8. Wapnir IL, Dignam JJ, Fisher B, et al. Long-term outcomes of invasive ipsilateral breast tumor recurrences after lumpectomy in NSABP B-17 and B-24 randomized clinical trials for DCIS. J Natl Cancer Inst 2011;103:478–88.
   This paper provides the longest follow-up data among randomised trials of postoperative radiotherapy (RT) for DCIS (207 months for the B-17 trial and 163 months for the B-24 trial). RT reduced IBTR by 52% in the lumpectomy+RT arm compared with lumpectomy alone (B-17, HR of risk of IBTR=0.48, 95% CI=0.33–0.69, $P<0.001$). Lumpectomy+RT+tamoxifen reduced IBTR by 32% compared with lumpectomy+RT+placebo (B-24, HR of risk of IBTR=0.68, 95% CI=0.49–0.95, $P=0.025$). The 15-year cumulative incidence of IBTR was 19.4% for lumpectomy alone, 8.9% for lumpectomy+RT (B-17), 10.0% for lumpectomy+RT+placebo (B-24), and 8.5% for lumpectomy+RT+tamoxifen (level I evidence).

9. Houghton J, George WD, Cuzick J, et al., UK Coordinating Committee on Cancer Research, Ductal Carcinoma In Situ Working Party, DCIS trialists in the UK, Australia, and New Zealand. Radiotherapy and tamoxifen in women with completely excised ductal carcinoma in situ of the breast in the UK, Australia, and New Zealand: randomised controlled trial. Lancet 2003;362:95–102.
This was a randomised controlled trial with a 2 × 2 factorial design in which investigators could elect to give radiotherapy and randomise to +/– tamoxifen or elect tamoxifen and randomise to +/– radiotherapy. Radiotherapy reduces ipsilateral DCIS and invasive recurrence (level I evidence).

10. Holmberg L, Garmo H, Granstrand B, et al. Absolute risk reductions for local recurrence after postoperative radiotherapy after sector resection for ductal carcinoma in situ of the breast. J Clin Oncol 2008;26:1247–52.
This randomised trial showed a particular benefit of adjuvant postoperative in older patients and less impact in women under the age of 50. There was no confounding effect on age by focality, lesion size, completeness of excision or method of detection. There was no subgroup that had a low risk without radiotherapy (level I evidence).

11. Goodwin A, Parker S, Ghersi D, et al. Post-operative radiotherapy for ductal carcinoma in situ of the breast. Cochrane Database Syst Rev 2009;4: CD000563.
This is a meta-analysis of the four randomised trials assessing the role of adjuvant radiotherapy after wide local excision of DCIS (level I evidence).

12. Julien JP, Bijker N, Fentiman IS, et al. Radiotherapy in breast-conserving treatment for ductal carcinoma in situ: first results of the EORTC randomised phase III trial 10853. EORTC Breast Cancer Cooperative Group and EORTC Radiotherapy Group. Lancet 2000;355:528–33.
This is the first publication of the EORTC DCIS trial assessing the role of adjuvant irradiation at a median follow-up of 4.25 years. The 4-year local relapse-free rate was 84% with local excision alone compared to 91% with wide local excision + radiotherapy (log rank P = 0.005; hazard ratio 0.62). There were similar reductions in the risk of invasive (40%, P = 0.04) and non-invasive (35%, P = 0.06) local recurrence (level I evidence).

13. Patani N, Cutuli B, Mokbel K. Current management of DCIS: a review. Breast Cancer Res Treat 2008;111:1–10.

14. Bijker N, Peterse JL, Duchateau L, et al. Risk factors for recurrence and metastasis after breast-conserving therapy for ductal carcinoma-in-situ: analysis of European Organization for Research and Treatment of Cancer Trial 10853. J Clin Oncol 2001;19:2263–71.

15. Page DL, Lagios MD. Pathologic analysis of the National Surgical Adjuvant Breast Project (NSABP) B-17 trial. Unanswered questions remaining unanswered considering current concepts of ductal carcinoma in situ. Cancer 1995;75:1219–22.

16. Hughes LL, Wang M, Page DL, et al. Local excision alone without irradiation for ductal carcinoma in situ of the breast: a trial of the Eastern Cooperative Oncology Group. J Clin Oncol 2009;27:5319–24.

17. Fisher ER, Dignam J, Tan-Chiu E, et al. Pathologic findings from the National Surgical Adjuvant Breast Project (NSABP) eight-year update of Protocol B-17: intraductal carcinoma. Cancer 1999;86:429–38.

18. Omlin A, Amichetti M, Azria D, et al. Boost radiotherapy in young women with ductal carcinoma in situ: a multicentre, retrospective study of the Rare Cancer Network. Lancet Oncol 2006;7:652–6.

19. Stillie A, Kunkler I, Kerr G, et al. Is a radiotherapy boost truly beneficial? Lancet Oncol 2006;7:795–6.

20. Williamson D, Dinniwell R, Fung S, et al. Local control with conventional and hypofractionated adjuvant radiotherapy after breast-conserving surgery for ductal carcinoma in-situ. Radiother Oncol 2010;95:317–20.

21. Cuzick J, Stewart H, Peto R, et al. Overview of randomized trials comparing radical mastectomy without radiotherapy against simple mastectomy with radiotherapy in breast cancer. Cancer Treat Rep 1987;71:7–14.

22. Early Breast Cancer Trialists' Collaborative Group. Favourable and unfavourable effects on long-term survival of radiotherapy for early breast cancer: an overview of the randomised trials. Lancet 2000;355:1757–70.

23. Early Breast Cancer Trialists' Collaborative Group (EBCTG). Effects of chemotherapy and hormonal therapy for early breast cancer on recurrence and 15-year survival: an overview of the randomised trial. Lancet 2005;365:1687–717.
This was the first Oxford overview of radiotherapy trials that identified a link between locoregional control by radiotherapy and survival.

24. Early Breast Cancer Trialists' Collaborative Group. Effects of radiotherapy on 10-year recurrence and 15-year breast cancer death: meta-analysis of individual patient data for 10,801 women in 17 randomised trials. Lancet 2011;378:1707–16.
This, the latest overview of randomised trials of radiotherapy after breast-conserving surgery, uses first recurrence of any type (locoregional or metastatic) in contrast to first locoregional recurrence in previous overviews of breast radiotherapy. It provides longer term data that the '4:1 ratio' (for every four local recurrences avoided, one breast cancer death is avoided) still holds.

25. Hughes KS, Schnaper LA, Berry D, et al. Lumpectomy plus tamoxifen with or without irradiation in women 70 years of age or older with early breast cancer. N Engl J Med 2004;351:971–7.
This is the only randomised trial addressing the need for radiotherapy in low-risk hormone receptor breast cancer in older patients after breast-conserving surgery receiving adjuvant tamoxifen.

75. Kunkler IH, Canney P, van Tienhoven G, et al., MRC/EORTC (BIG 2-04) SUPREMO Trial Management Group. Elucidating the role of chest wall irradiation in 'intermediate-risk' breast cancer: the MRC/EORTC SUPREMO trial. Clin Oncol 2008;20:31–4.

76. Kyndi M, Sørensen FB, Knudsen H, et al., Danish Breast Cancer Cooperative Group. Estrogen receptor, progesterone receptor, HER-2, and response to postmastectomy radiotherapy in high-risk breast cancer: the Danish Breast Cancer Cooperative Group. J Clin Oncol 2008;26:1419–26.

77. Clarke M, Collins R, Darby S, et al. Effects of radiotherapy and of differences in the extent of surgery for early breast cancer on local recurrence and 15-year survival: an overview of the randomised trials. Lancet 2005;366:2087–106.

78. Giuliano AE, Hunt KK, Ballman KV, et al. Axillary dissection vs no axillary dissection in women with invasive breast cancer and sentinel node metastasis: a randomized clinical trial. JAMA 2011;305:569–75.

79. Haffty BG, Hunt KK, Harris JR, et al. Positive sentinel nodes without axillary dissection: implications for the radiation oncologist. J Clin Oncol 2011;29:4479–81.

80. Chen K, Zhu L, Jia W, et al. Validation and comparison of models to predict non-sentinel lymph node metastasis in breast cancer. Cancer Sci 2012;103:274–81.

81. Chetty U, Jack W, Prescott RJ, et al. Management of the axilla in operable breast cancer treated by breast conservation: a randomized clinical trial. Edinburgh Breast Unit. Br J Surg 2000;87:163–9.

82. Hurkmans CW, Borger JH, Rutgers EJ, et al., EORTC Breast Cancer Cooperative Group, Radiotherapy Cooperative Group. Quality assurance of axillary radiotherapy in the EORTC AMAROS trial 10981/22023: the dummy run. Radiother Oncol 2003;68:233–40.

83. Katz A, Smith BL, Golshan M, et al. Nomogram for the prediction of having four or more involved nodes for sentinel lymph node-positive breast cancer. J Clin Oncol 2008;26:2093–8.

84. Das IJ, Cheng EC, Freedman G, et al. Lung and heart dose volume analyses with CT simulator in radiation treatment of breast cancer. Int J Radiat Oncol Biol Phys 1998;42:11–9.

85. Giordano SH, Kuo YF, Freeman JL, et al. Risk of cardiac death after adjuvant radiotherapy for breast cancer. J Natl Cancer Inst 2005;97:419–24.

16

Psychosocial issues in breast cancer

Lesley Fallowfield
Valerie Jenkins

Introduction

The diagnosis of breast cancer, for women at any age and stage, brings with it a myriad of emotions, provoked by the decisions needed and concerns about the surgery, systemic treatments and likely prognosis. Conveying options to anxious patients is not easy. The increasingly complex nature of the disease, in terms of its molecular profile and appropriate novel targeted therapies, necessitates ever more advanced communication skills if patients are to make informed choices.

This chapter deals with many of the psychosocial issues associated with treatments for breast cancer, but is not exhaustive. It reflects some of the most topical questions of the day, which include delay in presentation, quality of life associated with adjuvant and targeted therapies, and dilemmas associated with ductal carcinoma in situ. We also discuss the efficacy of interventions aimed at preventing or ameliorating some of the problems associated with diagnosis and treatment.

Delay in presentation

Despite efforts to increase awareness, many women in the UK present late with their breast cancer; this delay can be due to patient or provider factors. Patient delay refers to the interval between first detection of symptoms and first medical consultation. The period that most authors accept as prolonged delay is 12 weeks or more,[1] although others regard patient delay as 4 weeks or more.[2] Provider or system delay is usually taken to be the interval between first presentation to the GP and initial treatment, and is not easy to define. Some of the reasons for patient delay can be ignorance of the symptoms, or fears about breast cancer and its associated treatments.

Unfortunately, delay of greater than 3 months is associated with worse outcomes. In the UK it has been shown to contribute to the difference in survival between rich and poor[3] and ethnic groups, especially Black African women.[4] Also, older women who have lower levels of knowledge about the signs and symptoms of breast cancer are more likely than younger women to present late. In a survey of 712 older (67–73 years) British women, 50% believed their lifetime risk of developing breast cancer was 1 in 100 and 75% were not aware that age was a risk factor.[5] In an attempt to improve breast awareness, Linsell et al. conducted a randomised controlled trial (RCT) with 867 women attending for their final routine appointment on the UK NHS Breast Screening Programme.[6] Women were randomised to receive a scripted 10-minute interaction with a radiographer plus a booklet that conveyed key breast awareness messages, the booklet alone or usual care. The primary outcome was the proportion of women achieving breast cancer awareness at 1 month. Results from this RCT did show an increased awareness in the intervention group compared with usual care at 1 month (32.8% vs. 4.1%), and the booklet versus usual care (12.7% vs. 4.1%), which was largely maintained at 12 months. Whether knowledge translates into a change in behaviour is yet to be determined. A systematic review of the efficacy of interventions to promote cancer awareness and early presentation reveals some evidence that interventions delivered at an individual level can promote cancer awareness in the short term, but insufficient evidence that these promote early presentation with cancer symptoms.[7] Individuals' behaviours are not governed by a single set of attitudes and can change over time, therefore predicting which factors determine change is involved and complex.

Psychosocial issues with breast cancer surgery

Decision-making

Although surgeons perform breast-conserving surgery (BCS) wherever possible, this does not always translate into measurable reductions in psychological morbidity. Some have suggested that psychological morbidity could be prevented if only women were allowed to choose their preferred surgical treatments. Although the proponents of more consumerist approaches strongly assert the putative benefits of active participation in treatment decision-making, these benefits are not well supported by firm data. In one study, the decision-making preferences of 150 women with newly diagnosed breast cancer were established and compared with those of 200 women with benign breast disease. The majority of women with breast cancer preferred a more passive role, whereas the majority of the benign disease group wished for a more collaborative role.[8]

Data from the USA examined decision-making in 1884 women with ductal carcinoma in situ (DCIS) and invasive breast cancer. Results showed that although only 11.5% had clinical contraindications to BCS, 30% had mastectomy as their initial surgical treatment. The majority of the women (41%) reported that they had been the primary decision-maker, 37% felt that the decision was shared with the surgeon and 22% felt that the decision had been made by their surgeon.[9] Intriguingly, the greater the patient involvement in decision-making the more likely that mastectomy was the preferred surgery. After adjusting for clinical and demographic variables, significant correlations were found. Only 5.8% of women whose surgeon made the decision had a mastectomy compared with 16.8% of the women who shared decision-making and 27% of those who made the decision themselves ($P = 0.003$). The primary reason for a mastectomy preference was fear about recurrence. Although 80% of women expressed a high degree of confidence about their decisions, fewer than 50% were able to answer correctly a true/false question about the lack of a survival difference between mastectomy and BCS.

Effects of type of surgery

Many have asserted that the type of surgery makes a difference to patients' quality of life (QoL). However, except for differences in perception of body image, the literature comparing the other psychosocial sequelae of BCS with mastectomy is ambiguous and shows a lack of substantial benefits.[10-12] Few have examined QoL prospectively beyond a 2-year period, yet approximately 80% of women with breast cancer survive ≥ 5 years.[13] Engle et al.[14] measured long-term QoL in women ($n = 990$) treated with BCS or mastectomy at regular intervals over 5 years. The cross-sectional data showed that mastectomy patients had significantly ($P<0.01$) lower satisfaction with body image, role and sexual functioning scores, and their lives were more disrupted than BCS patients. Another study showed that at 5 years women who had BCS had a significant increase in overall QoL compared with those who had a mastectomy.[15] Surprising differences were found by Collins et al. examining QoL in women ($n = 549$) who had BCS, mastectomy or mastectomy plus reconstruction.[16] The researchers adjusted the analysis to take account of the severity of surgical side-effects by type of operation. In the model without surgical side-effect severity, women who underwent mastectomy plus reconstruction reported poorer body image than those who had BCS at all time points except the last (T4: 2 years post op). When they adjusted for surgical side-effect severity, body image scores did not differ significantly from patients with BCS. Also, women who had mastectomy alone had a better body image at T2 (6 months) than those who had reconstruction ($P = 0.011$). The authors explained that dissatisfaction with body image can be explained in part by patients' experience of surgical side-effects, including wound infections. However, the severity of the side-effects did not substantially weaken the effects of an elevated depressed mood on patients' body image problems.

Impact of axillary surgery on quality of life

Sentinel lymph node biopsy (SLNB) is now established as an accurate, minimally invasive means of providing regional staging for primary breast cancer, and the standard of care for patients with clinically node-negative breast cancer.[17] In the UK ALMANAC (Axillary Lymphatic Mapping Against Nodal Axillary Clearance) trial of 1031 patients, data showed that women who received standard axillary treatment recovered more slowly than those in the SLNB group (P<0.01).[18] The ALMANAC trial showed that the benefits of sentinel node biopsy are not only reduction of unnecessary resection of the axilla, but also a marked reduction in unwanted sequelae such as arm morbidity, thus permitting a better quality of life, without sacrificing any staging accuracy. However, 25% of the SLNB group required further axillary surgery or radiotherapy to the axilla because of spread of disease. Additional surgery is normally conducted 2 weeks later and this two-stage procedure has advantages and disadvantages. The latter include the psychological and physical stress associated with a second operation; conversely, the delay could be viewed as a benefit by some, giving time to adjust to the knowledge that their breast cancer has spread. Recently some units are able to offer intraoperative SLNB analysis, which allows immediate progression to axillary clearance in patients found to have positive nodes. However, there is still debate amongst clinicians on the accuracy of intraoperative analysis,[19,20] but findings from women who had and had not experienced this diagnostic technique revealed a positive inclination towards the one-step axillary surgery. The advantages included: knowing the result straight away, less anaesthesia, fewer days in hospital and consequently more cost-effectiveness for the NHS.[21]

Ductal carcinoma in situ

Women given the diagnosis of ductal carcinoma in situ (DCIS), be it low, moderate or high grade, can be left wondering whether or not they have breast cancer. Some describe it as 'a very early form of breast cancer'[22] or pre-cancerous condition. Most often it is found through mammographic screening and the incidence is increasing. Although mortality risk is low, treatments are similar to that demanded of invasive breast cancer (surgery, radiotherapy, endocrine therapy) and women are left confused. The psychological and QoL impacts of having a label of DCIS and how it affected women's lives have been subject to review.[23] Studies show that although those with low/intermediate-grade DCIS have an excellent prognosis and normal life expectancy, many women experience substantial psychological distress. Cross-sectional studies have compared psychosocial outcomes of women with DCIS with those with early invasive breast cancer (EBC).[24,25] Findings suggest DCIS patients have better physical health, sex life and social functioning than women with invasive breast cancer. However, despite the relatively good prognosis, DCIS patients held perceptions about the risk of recurrence and dying comparable to women with EBC. Other research showed that women had inaccurate perceptions about their risk of invasive disease and spread of DCIS to other parts of their body that changed little across an 18-month period; these perceptions were strongly related to distress.[26]

Lauszier et al. reported similar levels of psychological distress in women with DCIS and those with invasive disease who had a worse prognosis.[27] So although women with DCIS reported significantly better physical health, it did not offset the psychological distress felt of having a cancer diagnosis. This finding is supported from results of a UK-based study with 50 women with DCIS, whose QoL, psychological functioning and body image were measured at three time points (baseline, 6 and 9 months). The results provide a valuable insight of emotional distress during the first year post-diagnosis, with some women experiencing significant levels of distress both in the short and long term.[28] Previous DCIS research has proposed that some of the influencing factors for this distress are confusion about the diagnosis and prognosis, together with inaccurate risk perceptions.

There remains considerable controversy about the natural history of low-grade DCIS and it is now commonly diagnosed by routine breast cancer screening. The diagnosis and treatment of a condition that may not cause problems during the patient's lifetime is considered by some to be both overdiagnosis and overtreatment.[29] There are few conclusive data demonstrating that low-grade DCIS commonly develops into invasive cancer, prompting some to question the use of the word carcinoma in the diagnosis. Conducting randomised trials to determine whether or not active surveillance or giving endocrine therapy is as safe an option as immediate surgery is important but fraught with difficulty. Outcomes of both the safety and psychosocial sequelae of hormone therapy (IBIS II) are awaited. Clinical trials comparing surgery with active monitoring or hormone therapy for low-grade DCIS are urgently required.

Hormone therapy

RCTs have demonstrated the efficacy of selective oestrogen receptor modulators (SERMs) such as tamoxifen in preventing recurrence in oestrogen receptor (ER)-positive early breast cancer, and in other studies the superiority of the aromatase inhibitors (AIs). Recommendations worldwide mean that most women will have to endure at least 5 years of therapy. Unfortunately there is still uncertainty as to which women really benefit from these drugs. ER positivity is not a sensitive enough marker. A substantial number of women at low risk of recurrence with small tumours, who have had complete local excision and radiotherapy, derive no extra benefit from this therapy but experience considerable iatrogenic harm. Many of these side-effects go under-reported, unrecognised and untreated.

Studies comparing clinician-reported (via case report forms in trials) and patient-reported (via validated questionnaires and interviews) quality of life rather than life-threatening side effects show little concordance.[30–33] Apart from this inaccurate reporting, severe and/or untreated side-effects can lead to discontinuation of therapy or non-adherence in between 25% and 55% of patients.[34,35] Ameliorative interventions are consequently an important and neglected area of research. In the section below we present an overview of some of the evidence for various interventions aimed at the primary side-effects: vasomotor complaints, gynaecological/sexual issues and musculoskeletal problems, especially arthralgia.

Vasomotor problems

Hot flushes and drenching night sweats are some of the most commonly reported problems (30–45%) associated with all hormone treatments.[34,35] Not only are they extremely unpleasant but they interfere with sleep and impact on numerous other activities of daily living and quality of life. Mechanisms are complex but are probably oestrogen withdrawal rather than related to absolute levels of circulating oestrogen. Hormone replacement therapy (HRT) is of course a useful treatment for menopausal hot flushes but HRT is not appropriate for breast cancer, as shown in the HABITS trial.[36] Other ameliorative interventions are shown in Table 16.1.

The evidence for efficacy for most of the dietary changes, herbal remedies and practical interventions is very thin, and there have been reports that some of the unregulated herbal supplements may be dangerous and potentiate the adverse events of orthodox anticancer treatments. Other interventions are worthy of more examination.

Acupuncture

A systematic review of acupuncture in breast cancer showed that of the three RCTs employing sham acupuncture control arms, only one was favourable in reducing hot flush frequency; however, a meta-analysis has suggested a benefit overall ($P = 0.05$), although there was marked heterogeneity in the data.[37] One study of acupuncture compared with HRT favoured HRT, another two comparing acupuncture versus venlafaxine or relaxation therapy found a small benefit for acupuncture but no differences between groups. All these studies suffer from small numbers. A more comprehensive study enrolled women who had experienced more than seven hot flushes per day for 7 consecutive days.[38] Patients were randomised to acupuncture or control. Primary outcome was hot flush frequency with

Table 16.1 • Ameliorative interventions for side-effects

Complementary therapies	Acupuncture, relaxation, paced breathing, yoga, t'ai chi, mindfulness, hypnosis
Dietary changes	Avoidance of alcohol, caffeine and spicy foods
Supplements and herbal remedies	Dong quai, primrose oil, red clover, Black Cohosh, Mexican yam
Practical advice	Dressing in layers, menopausal pyjamas and chillows, air-conditioning, fans and drinking cold water
SSRIs and SNRIs	e.g. venlafaxine, paroxetine

a wide variety of other secondary end-points. Both frequency and intensity of hot flushes were significantly reduced in the acupuncture arm ($P<0.001$). There were also reductions in sleep disturbance and other somatic symptoms as measured with the Women's Health Questionnaire (WHQ).[39]

Relaxation, mindfulness, yoga, hypnosis

Stress and anxiety are common features associated with the diagnosis and treatment of breast cancer and appear to contribute to the frequency and intensity of symptoms.[40,41] It seems a reasonable hypothesis therefore that any behavioural technique that reduces stress may help vasomotor complaints. As with acupuncture these studies often lack good controls and include only small numbers but there does appear to be some beneficial evidence in support of hypnosis,[42] relaxation/paced breathing,[43,44] yoga[45] and group cognitive behavioural therapy.[46] From a clinical point of view all these interventions have the advantages of being inexpensive, very acceptable and attractive to women, and importantly have no adverse events.

Selective serotonin reuptake inhibitors (SSRIs) and selective norepinephrine reuptake inhibitors (SNRIs)

Clinicians who are sceptical about the previously mentioned interventions are often more comfortable recommending drug therapies such as the selective serotonin or norepinephrine uptake inhibitors. Venlafaxine has been tested in numerous studies. An important double-blind placebo-controlled RCT of different doses revealed a significant reduction in hot flush scores ($P<0.001$) but some side-effects, including a dry mouth, appetite loss and constipation.[47] A double-blind crossover study with paroxetine showed a significant reduction in hot flushes ($P<0.001$); furthermore, patients were less likely to discontinue a 10-mg dose compared with 20 mg, as the latter dose resulted in greater toxicity.[48] In a double-blind crossover RCT of fluoxetine there was a 24% improvement in hot flush reduction favouring fluoxetine ($P = 0.02$).[49] Likewise, another randomised double-blind crossover study favoured sertraline.[50] This project also examined preference and demonstrated that 48% of patients preferred sertraline, 11% placebo and 41% had no preference. Anxieties still exist about the potential effects

of CYP 2D6 inhibition for some patients taking tamoxifen and SSRIs, although most recent research has failed to offer compelling cause for concern. The benefits of SSRIs and SNRIs in hot flush reduction are clear, but the side-effects sometimes outweigh these and may lead to discontinuation. Research on efficacy and safety with newer antidepressants such as mirtazapine or citalopram is ongoing, and also with the anticonvulsant gabapentin, to see if they have fewer side-effects. Gabapentin produces a 35–66% reduction in hot flash score but patients prefer venlafaxine 2:1 over gabapentin. Likewise, there are several comparative trials being conducted of different treatments using reductions of vasomotor problems and patient preference as outcomes.[51] Most recent research has suggested that escitalopram (Cipralex) conveys benefits without too many side-effects.[52]

Gynaecological/sexual problems

The AIs and SERMs create numerous gynaecological and sexual problems for patients. Discharge (5–17%) is probably higher in tamoxifen than in the AIs but vaginal dryness affects between approximately 16% and 40% of women taking anastrozole, exemestane or letrozole.[33] As a consequence, previously sexually active women may experience dyspareunia (15–18%) and a loss of libido (16–45%). In extreme cases patients may develop very unpleasant and painful vulvo-vaginal atrophy. The most appropriate ameliorative intervention for dryness and dyspareunia is regular use of moisturisers such as Replens®. Lubricants alone are insufficient. For vulvo-vaginal atrophy there are suggestions from early phase trials that progesterone and testosterone creams may help.[53] For clinicians worried about oestrogen in breast cancer, studies have shown that Estring® has a low systemic uptake of oestrogen.[54]

Musculoskeletal problems and arthralgia

Adjuvant trials of anastrozole,[55] letrozole[56] and exemestane[57] show reports of joint pains and stiffness or arthralgia to be common (20–30%). A survey of UK clinicians reported that AI-induced arthralgia is a distinct clinical problem, with limited data on its aetiology and management.[58] Arthralgic pain and stiffness can be an important reason for discontinuation of AI therapy. Unfortunately, these do not always respond to analgesia, they negatively impact on QoL and can lead to non-adherence. The mechanism remains uncertain and is certainly different from the normal aches and pains of ageing. Oestrogen deprivation, together with the release of pro-inflammatory cytokines (interleukin-1β, tumour necrosis factor-α), is the most likely cause.[59]

Crew et al. conducted a small crossover study of full-body and auricular acupuncture, 30 min, twice weekly for 6 weeks on 27 women who had been taking an AI for at least 6 months and who were experiencing arthralgia.[60] Using numerous validated patient-reported outcome measures (PROs), the authors reported significant improvements in worst pain ($P = 0.01$), pain severity ($P = 0.02$), functional interference ($P = 0.02$), functional ability ($P = 0.02$) and overall physical well-being ($P = 0.04$).

SSRIs and SNRIs

Duloxetine is an SNRI used for multiple chronic pain. Henry et al. reported a small pilot study for postmenopausal women on AIs with new or worsening pain.[61] Duloxetine 30 mg daily was administered for 7 days, then increasing to 60 mg daily. The study employed many patient-reported outcome (PRO) measures, looking at quality-of-life symptoms, sleep quality, menopause and hot flushes, but the primary end-point was a 30% decrease in pain. Results showed that 21 of 29 evaluable patients reported ≥30% decreased pain. The authors also reported other significant improvements including the amount of interference caused by pain and improvement in hot flushes, depression and sleep. Although 78% of patients continued on treatment, it did cause fatigue, xerostomia and headache. This was a very small study but the drug seems worthy of examination in a larger RCT. In an observational study vitamin D deficiency was suggested as the cause of musculoskeletal pain[62] and a double-blind placebo-controlled RCT of high-dose vitamin D seemed to improve pain reports.[63]

Hormone therapy undoubtedly benefits many women with breast cancer but quality-of-life-threatening toxicities may be much more of a problem than commonly acknowledged. We require systematic assessment of the impact of treatment using validated PROs so that evidence-based interventions can be offered in a timely manner. It is also clear that we need to conduct much more high-quality research into ameliorative interventions with sensible numbers of patients and using robust outcome measures.

Exercise

In the past, cancer patients were usually advised to rest and avoid physical effort. However, it is now well established that excessive rest and lack of physical activity may result in severe deconditioning and reduced physical functioning. Women undergoing chemotherapy or radiation therapy as adjuvant treatment for breast cancer commonly experience debilitating side-effects including nausea,[64] fatigue,[65] weight gain[66] and mood disturbances.[67] These side-effects can interfere with daily activities such as self-care or return to work and exercise for patients with cancer is strongly supported by national cancer charities. A report by Macmillan suggested that patients who are receiving cancer treatments engage in two and a half hours of exercise a week.[68] This advice is in line with the Department of Health guidelines that recommend two and a half hours of moderate to vigourous intensity exercise for adults each week, moderate exercise defined as swimming or a brisk walk.[69] Adherence to exercise programmes is, however, a problem and the mean dropout rate from supervised exercise programmes has remained at 50% over the decades.[70] However, being diagnosed with a serious illness can prompt an individual to change their lifestyle and there are media reports of individuals running half-marathons even whilst undergoing treatments for breast cancer.[71]

Whilst these are uplifting accounts, running a half-marathon will not appeal to the majority of women undergoing treatments for breast cancer. However, there are reports that less intensive exercise can be of benefit, both during and following treatment. Courneya and colleagues have been involved in this area of research for many years, examining via RCTs which exercise programmes engage patients and also the barriers and predictors of exercise behaviour. In one study they randomised 242 women initiating chemotherapy treatment to resistance training, aerobic exercise or usual care for the duration of their chemotherapy regimens (mean of 17 weeks).[72] Although neither aerobic nor resistance exercise significantly improved QoL in breast cancer patients receiving chemotherapy, the programmes improved self-esteem, physical fitness, body composition and chemotherapy completion rate without causing lymphoedema or significant adverse events. At 6-month follow-up, the women were sent a questionnaire that assessed QoL, self-esteem, fatigue, anxiety, depression and exercise behaviours.[73] Eighty-three per cent (201/242) responded; compared to usual care, those who participated in the resistance training maintained an increase in self-esteem. There was a reduction in anxiety in the aerobic group that had not been observed during chemotherapy. The authors also measured which factors, personal and clinical, predicted exercise training responses.[74] They found patients who had a preference for resistance training had improved QoL when they were assigned to receive it, compared with usual care (P = 0.008). Patients who had no preference had improved QoL when they were assigned to receive either programme (P = 0.014). The barriers to supervised exercise varied but over half were directly attributed to the disease and side-effects of treatments.[75] Exercise behaviour 6 months after the trial was predicted by a wide range of demographic, medical, behavioural, fitness, psychosocial and motivational variables, which highlights the difficulties with promoting and maintaining fitness.[76] A Cochrane review of exercise in women receiving adjuvant therapy for breast cancer that included nine controlled trials involving 452 patients concluded that physical exercise can improve physical function even during cancer treatment. This review also considered that there was still not enough evidence about the effect of exercise on outcomes such as fatigue, mood disturbances, immune function and weight gain.[77]

There are other forms of 'exercise' that may appear more attractive to patients with breast cancer, including yoga and Pilates. An evidence-based review of yoga as a complementary therapy for patients with cancer, including six RCTs, concluded that yoga helped improve mood, QoL and decrease anxiety.[78] More research is warranted on whether yoga can improve specific physical damage, for example arm morbidity following axillary surgery.

Conclusion

There are a large number of studies showing that the adjuvant systemic therapies that form part of

the management pre- and post-breast cancer surgery impact on the quality of patients' lives. In a recent report of 653 women with breast cancer, substantial numbers sought help with symptoms: hot flushes (41%), night sweats (36%), loss of interest in sex (30%), difficulty sleeping (25%), fatigue (22%) and extreme vaginal dryness (19%).[79] Chemotherapy-induced ovarian failure was reported by 29% of the breast cancer patients seen. A wide range of management approaches were offered, with 55% of the women prescribed non-hormonal pharmacological therapies for vasomotor symptoms, including vitamin E 400 IU twice daily (21%), venlaflaxine 75 mg CR once daily (13%), clonidine 50 μg twice daily (11%), or gabapentin 300 mg three times daily (4%). As found in other studies, vasomotor symptoms, sexual dysfunction and sleep disturbance are the most distressing menopausal symptoms requiring attention. Menopausal symptom management after breast cancer is complex and demands a multidisciplinary approach with interventions appropriately tested and monitored.

Summary

The treatments available to women with breast cancer continue to improve, offering many the prospect of cure or lengthier lives. Despite these advances and improvements in the delivery of care and provision of support services, the diagnosis of breast cancer still causes considerable distress. Women cope in many different ways with the knowledge that they have a potentially life-threatening disease requiring unpleasant treatments. For some it is a major emotional and social catastrophe, whereas others approach it with a degree of equanimity and/or stoicism. It is sometimes difficult to predict how women will react, adapt and adjust to what lies ahead. Greater awareness of some of the psychosocial, sexual and cognitive dysfunction associated with different treatments should enable us to design interventions to prevent or ameliorate their problems. The importance of provision of good clear information delivered in a supportive, honest and empathic manner should not be overlooked. The communication skills of a surgeon can exert a surprisingly useful psychotherapeutic impact on a woman and her ability to cope with the disease and its treatment.

Key points

- Despite efforts to increase awareness, many women in the UK present late with their breast cancer; there is some evidence that interventions delivered at an individual level can promote cancer awareness in the short term, but insufficient evidence that these promote early presentation of cancer symptoms.
- There is considerable controversy as to whether or not screening results in overdiagnosis and overtreatment, especially for patients with low-grade DCIS.
- Despite the vast improvement in the last decade in diagnostic procedures, surgical techniques and other systemic therapy offering the prospect of cure or longer life, many patients still experience significant anxiety/depression and sexual dysfunction.
- The adjuvant systemic therapies that accompany surgery significantly reduce recurrence but have many quality-of-life-threatening side-effects that demand more attention and research into ameliorative interventions.

References

1. Ramirez AJ, Westcombe AM, Burgess CC, et al. Factors predicting delayed presentation of symptomatic breast cancer: a systematic review. Lancet 1999;353(9159):1127–31.

2. Nosarti C, Crayford T, Roberts J, et al. Delay in diagnosis in breast cancer. Lancet 1999;353(9170):2154.

3. Downing A, Prakash K, Gilthorpe MS, et al. Socioeconomic background in relation to stage at diagnosis, treatment and survival in women with breast cancer. Br J Cancer 2007;96(5):836–40.

4. Jack RH, Davies EA, Meller H. Breast cancer incidence, stage, treatment and survival in ethnic groups in South East England. Br J Cancer 2009;100:545–50.

5. Linsell L, Burgess CC, Ramirez AJ. Breast cancer awareness among older women. Br J Cancer 2008;99:1221–5.

6. Linsell L, Forbes LJL, Kapari M, et al. A randomised controlled trial of an intervention to promote early presentation of breast cancer in older women: effect on breast cancer awareness. Br J Cancer 2009;101:S40–S48.

7. Austoker J, Bankhead C, Forbes LJL, et al. Interventions to promote cancer awareness and early presentation: a systematic review. Br J Cancer 2009;101(S2):S31–9.

8. Beaver K, Luker KA, Owens RG, et al. Treatment decision making in women newly diagnosed with breast cancer. Cancer Nurs 1996;19(1):8–19.

9. Katz SJ, Lantz PM, Janz NK, et al. Patient involvement in surgery treatment decisions for breast cancer. J Clin Oncol 2005;23(24):5526–33.

10. Fallowfield L. Offering choice of surgical treatment to women with breast cancer. Patient Educ Couns 1997;30:209–14.

11. Ganz PA, Schag CAC, Lee JJ, et al. Breast conservation versus mastectomy: Is there a difference in psychological adjustment or quality of life in the year after surgery? Cancer 1992;69(7):1729–38.

12. De Haes JCJM, Curran D, Aaronson NK, et al. Quality of life in breast cancer patients aged over 70 years, participating in the EORTC 10850 randomised clinical trial. Eur J Cancer 2003;39(7):945–51.

13. Survival statistics for the most common cancers: http://info.cancerresearchuk.org/cancerstats/survival/latestrates/; [accessed 19.11.11].

14. Engle J, Kerr J, Schlesinger-Raab A, et al. Quality of life following breast conserving therapy or mastectomy: results of a 5 year prospective study. Breast 2004;10(3):223–31.

15. Arndt V, Stegmaier C, Ziegler H, et al. Quality of life over 5 years in women with breast cancer after breast conserving therapy versus mastectomy: a population based study. J Cancer Res Clin Oncol 2008;134(12):1311–8.

16. Collins KK, Liu Y, Schootman M, et al. Effects of breast cancer surgery and surgical side effects on body image over time. Breast Cancer Res Treat 2011;126:167–76.

17. Layfield DM, Agrawal A, Roche H, et al. Intraoperative assessment of sentinel lymph nodes in breast cancer. Br J Surg 2011;98(1):4–17.

18. Fleissig A, Fallowfield LJ, Langridge CI, et al. Postoperative arm morbidity and quality of life. Results of the ALMANAC randomised trial comparing sentinel node biopsy with standard axillary treatment in the management of patients with early breast cancer. Breast Cancer Res Treat 2006;95(3):279–93.

19. Tamaki Y, Akiyama F, Iwase T, et al. Molecular detection of lymph node metastases in breast cancer patients: results of a multicenter trial using the one-step nucleic acid amplification assay. Clin Cancer Res 2009;15(8):2879–84.

20. Khaddage A, Berremila S-A, Forest F, et al. Implementation of molecular intra-operative assessment of sentinel lymph node in breast cancer. Anticancer Res 2011;31(2):585–90.

21. Jenkins V, Harder H, Babar M, et al. A pilot study to examine the experiences and attitudes of women with breast cancer towards one versus two-step axillary surgery. Breast 2012;21(1):72–6.

22. DCIS: http://cancerhelp/type/breast cancer/about/types/dcis-ductal carcinoma in situ; [accessed 03/12/2011].

23. Ganz P. Quality of life issues in patients with ductal carcinoma in situ. J Natl Cancer Inst Monogr 2010;41:218–22.

24. Rakovitch E, Franssen E, Kim J, et al. A comparison of risk perception and psychological morbidity in women with ductal carcinoma in situ and early invasive breast cancer. Breast Cancer Res Treat 2003;77(3):285–93.

25. van Gestel YR, Voogd AC, Vingerhoets AJ, et al. A comparison of quality of life, disease impact and risk perception in women with invasive breast cancer and ductal carcinoma in situ. Eur J Cancer 2007;43(3):549–56.

26. Partridge A, Adloff K, Blood E, et al. Risk perceptions and psychosocial outcomes of women with ductal carcinoma in situ: longitudinal results from a cohort study. J Natl Cancer Inst 2008;100(4):243–51.

27. Lauszier S, Maunsell E, Levesque P, et al. Psychological distress and physical health in the year after diagnosis of DCIS or invasive breast cancer. Breast Cancer Res Treat 2010;120:685–91.

28. Kennedy F, Harcourt D, Rumsey N, et al. The psychosocial impact of ductal carcinoma in situ (DCIS): A longitudinal prospective study. Breast 2010;19(5):382–7.

29. Raftery J, Chorozoglou M. Possible net harms of breast cancer screening: updated modelling of Forrest report. Br Med J 2011;343:d7627.

30. Fallowfield L, Cella D, Cuzick J, et al. Quality of life of postmenopausal women in the Arimidex, Tamoxifen, Alone or in Combination (ATAC) Adjuvant Breast Cancer Trial. J Clin Oncol 2004;22(21):4261–71.

31. Ruhstaller T, Von Moos R, Rufibach K, et al. Breast cancer patients on endocrine therapy reveal more symptoms when self-reporting than in pivotal trials: an outcome research study. Oncology 2009;76(2):142–8.

32. Oberguggenberger A, Hubalek M, Sztankay M, et al. Is the toxicity of adjuvant aromatase inhibitor therapy underestimated? Complementary information from patient-reported outcomes (PROs). Breast Cancer Res Treat 2011;128(2):553–61.

33. Cella D, Fallowfield LJ. Recognition and management of treatment-related side effects for breast cancer patients receiving adjuvant endocrine therapy. Breast Cancer Res Treat 2008;107(2):167–80.

34. Fallowfield L, Cella D, Cuzick J, et al. Quality of life of postmenopausal women in the Arimidex, Tamoxifen, Alone or in Combination (ATAC) Adjuvant Breast Cancer Trial. J Clin Oncol 2004;22(21):4261–71.

35. Fallowfield LJ, Bliss JM, Porter LS, et al. Quality of life in the intergroup exemestane study: a randomized trial of exemestane versus continued tamoxifen after 2 to 3 years of tamoxifen in postmenopausal women with primary breast cancer. J Clin Oncol 2006;24(6):910–7.

36. Holmberg L, Anderson H. HABITS (hormonal replacement therapy after breast cancer – is it safe?): a randomized comparison: trial stopped. Lancet 2004;363(9407):453–5.

37. Lee MS, Kim KH, Choi SM, et al. Acupuncture for treating hot flashes in breast cancer patients: a systematic review. Breast Cancer Res Treat 2009;115(3):497–503.

38. Borud EK, Alraek T, White A. The Acupuncture on hot flushes among menopausal women (ACUFLASH) study: a randomized controlled trial. Menopause 2009;16(3):484–93.

39. Hunter MS. The Women's Health Questionnaire (WHQ): the development, standardisation and application of a measure of mid-aged women's emotional and physical health. Qual Life Res 2000;9:733–8.

40. Freeman EW, Sammel MD, Lin H, et al. The role of anxiety and hormonal changes in menopausal hot flashes. Menopause 2005;12(3):258–66.

41. Gold EB, Colvin A, Avis N, et al. Longitudinal analysis of the association between vasomotor symptoms and race/ethnicity across the menopausal transition: study of women's health across the nation. Am J Public Health 2006;96(7):1226–35.

42. Elkins G, Marcus J, Stearns V, et al. Randomized trial of a hypnosis intervention for treatment of hot flashes among breast cancer survivors. J Clin Oncol 2008;26(31):5022–6.

43. Nedstrand E, Wijma K, Wyon Y, et al. Vasomotor symptoms decrease in women with breast cancer randomized to treatment with applied relaxation or electro-acupuncture: a preliminary study. Climacteric 2005;8(3):243–50.

44. Nedstrand E, Wyon Y, Hammar M, et al. Psychological well-being improves in women with breast cancer after treatment with applied relaxation or electro-acupuncture for vasomotor symptom. J Psychosom Obstet Gynaecol 2006;27(4):193–9.

45. Booth-LaForce C, Thurston RC, Taylor MR. A pilot study of a Hatha yoga treatment for menopausal symptoms. Maturitas 2007;57(3):286–95.

46. Hunter MS, Coventry S, Hamed H, et al. Evaluation of a group cognitive behavioural intervention for women suffering from menopausal symptoms following breast cancer treatment. Psychooncology 2009;18(5):560–3.

47. Loprinzi CL, Kugler JW, Sloan JA, et al. Venlafaxine in management of hot flashes in survivors of breast cancer: a randomised controlled trial. Lancet 2000;356(9247):2059–63.

48. Stearns V, Slack R, Greep N, et al. Paroxetine is an effective treatment for hot flashes: results from a prospective randomized clinical trial. J Clin Oncol 2005;23(28):6919–30.

49. Loprinzi CL, Sloan JA, Perez EA, et al. Phase III evaluation of fluoxetine for treatment of hot flashes. J Clin Oncol 2002;20(6):1578–83.

50. Kimmick GG, Lovato J, McQuellon R, et al. Randomized, double-blind, placebo-controlled, cross-over study of sertraline (Zoloft) for the treatment of hot flashes in women with early stage breast cancer taking tamoxifen. Breast J 2006;12(2):114–22.

51. Bordeleau L, Pritchard K, Goodwin P, et al. Therapeutic options for the management of hot flashes in breast cancer survivors: an evidence-based review. Clin Ther 2007;29(2):230–41.

52. Freedman RR, Kruger ML, Tancer ME. Escitalopram treatment of menopausal hot flashes. Menopause 2011;18(8):893–6.

53. Chin SN, Trinkaus M, Simmons C, et al. Prevalence and severity of urogenital symptoms in postmenopausal women receiving endocrine therapy for breast cancer. Clin Breast Cancer 2009;9(2):108–17.

54. Pfeiler G, Glatz C, Königsberg R, et al. Vaginal estriol to overcome side-effects of aromatase inhibitors in breast cancer patients. Climacteric 2011;14(3):339–44.

55. Baum M, Buzdar AU, Cuzick J, et al. Anastrozole alone or in combination with tamoxifen versus tamoxifen alone for adjuvant treatment of postmenopausal women with early breast cancer: first results of the ATAC randomised trial. Lancet 2002;359(9324):2131–9.

56. Goss PE, Ingle JN, Jose MD, et al. Exemestane for breast cancer prevention in post menopausal women. N Engl J Med 2011;364:2381–91.

57. Coombes RC, Hall E, Gibson LJ. A randomized trial of exemestane after two to three years of tamoxifen therapy in postmenopausal women with primary breast cancer. N Engl J Med 2004;350(11):1081–92.

58. Din OS, Dodwell D, Winter MC, et al. Current opinion of aromatase inhibitor-induced arthralgia in breast cancer in the UK. Clin Oncol 2011;23(10):674–80.

59. Henry NL, Giles JT, Stearns V. Aromatase inhibitor-associated musculoskeletal symptoms: etiology and strategies for management. Oncology 2008;22(12):1401–8.

60. Crew KD, Capodice JL, Greenlee H, et al. Randomized, blinded, sham-controlled trial of acupuncture for the management of aromatase inhibitor-associated joint symptoms in women with early-stage breast cancer. J Clin Oncol 2010;28(7):1154–60.

61. Henry D, Robertson J, O'Connell D. A systematic review of the skeletal effects of estrogen therapy in postmenopausal women. I. An assessment of the quality of randomized trials published between 1977 and 1995. Climacteric 1998;1(2):92–111.

62. Waltman NL, Ott CD, Twiss JJ, et al. Vitamin D insufficiency and musculoskeletal symptoms in breast cancer survivors on aromatase inhibitor therapy. Cancer Nurs 2009;32(2):143–50.

63. Rastelli AL, Taylor ME, Gao F, et al. Vitamin D and aromatase inhibitor-induced musculoskeletal symptoms (AIMSS): a phase II, double-blind, placebo-controlled, randomized trial. Breast Cancer Res Treat 2011;129(1):107–16.

64. Ganz PA, Kwan L, Stanton AL, et al. Physical and psychosocial recovery in the year after primary treatment of breast cancer. J Clin Oncol 2011;29(9):1101–9.

65. Bower JE, Ganz PA, Desmond KA, et al. Fatigue in breast cancer survivors: occurrence, correlates, and impact on quality of life. J Clin Oncol 2000;18(4):743–53.

66. Irwin ML, McTiernan A, Baumgartner RN, et al. Changes in body fat and weight after a breast cancer diagnosis: influence of demographic, prognostic, and lifestyle factors. J Clin Oncol 2005;23(4):774–82.

67. Montel S. Mood and anxiety disorders in breast cancer: an update. Curr Psychiat Rev 2010;6(1):56–63.

68. www.macmillan.org.uk/movemore; [accessed 8.08.11].

69. Department of Health UK Physical Activity Guidelines. http://www.dh.gov.uk/health/2011/07/physical-activity-guidelines/; [accessed 11.07.11].

70. Morgan WP, Dishman RK. Adherence to exercise and physical activity. Quest 2001;53:277–8.

71. http://www.thisisbristol.co.uk/Fundraising-couple-race-line/story-11284208-detail/story.html, http://runningtimes.com/Print.aspx?articleID=12936; [accessed 29.06.12].

72. Courneya KS, Segal RJ, Mackey JR, et al. Effects of aerobic and resistance exercise in breast cancer patients receiving adjuvant chemotherapy: a multicenter randomised controlled trial. J Clin Oncol 2007;25:4396–404.

73. Courneya KS, Segal RJ, Gelmon K, et al. Six month follow up of patient rated outcomes in a randomised controlled trial of exercise training during breast cancer chemotherapy. Cancer Epidemiol Biomarkers Prev 2007;16:2572–8.

74. Courneya KS, Segal RJ, Gelmon K, et al. Barriers to supervised exercise training in a randomised controlled trial of breast cancer patients receiving chemotherapy. Ann Behav Med 2008;35:116–22.

75. Courneya KS, Friedenreich CM, Reid R, et al. Predictors of follow-up exercise behavior 6 months after a randomised trial of exercise training during breast cancer chemotherapy. Breast Cancer Res Treat 2009;114:179–87.

76. Courneya KS, Karvinen KH, McNeely ML, et al. Predictors of adherence to supervised and unsupervised exercise in the Alberta physical activity and breast cancer prevention trial. J Phys Act Health 2011;Sept 13. Epub ahead of print.

77. Markes M, Brockow T, Resch K-L. Exercise for women receiving adjuvant therapy for breast cancer. Cochrane Database Syst Rev 2006;4:CD005001. http://dx.doi.org/10.1002/14651858.CD005001.pub281.

78. Smith K, Pukall C. An evidence-based review of yoga as a complementary intervention for patients with cancer. Psychooncology 2009;18(5):465–75.

79. Hickey M, Emery LI, Gregson J, et al. The multidisciplinary management of menopausal symptoms after breast cancer: a unique model of care. Menopause 2010;17(4):727–33.

17

Benign breast disease

Steven Thrush
J. Michael Dixon

Introduction

Over 90% of patients presenting to a breast clinic have normal breasts or benign breast disease.[1] An understanding of the aetiology, symptoms and management will ensure correct treatment and patient satisfaction. The expectation that the breast surgeon's role is simply to diagnose or exclude breast cancer has long disappeared. Benign breast disease causes considerable morbidity and anxiety, and with increasing patient awareness and expectations, the number of such patients attending clinics is increasing. Effective treatment includes accurate diagnosis followed by adequate explanation of the condition, provision of relevant information related to the diagnosis and how it is best managed. This is a rewarding part of a breast specialist's workload.

Benign breast disease can be divided into congenital abnormalities, aberrations of normal breast development and involution (ANDI) and conditions secondary to some extrinsic precipitatory factors (non-ANDI).

Congenital abnormalities

Although not diseases as such, developmental abnormalities of the breast can cause considerable concern and are not uncommon reasons for referral to a breast clinic.

Supernumerary nipples and accessory breast tissue

Accessory breast tissue is usually found in the axilla and supernumerary or *accessory* nipples are usually seen below the breast and above the umbilicus. Accessory nipples vary and are usually just rudimentary but can include glandular tissue (accessory breast). Accessory nipples in the bra line can be excised if they cause irritation.

Accessory breast tissue tends to become more prominent or obvious during pregnancy (**Fig. 17.1**). Reassurance and an explanation of the cause of the 'lump' are usually all that is required. Surgical excision should be reserved for those truly symptomatic, as they are difficult to excise cosmetically and surgery is associated with significant morbidity.[2] Liposuction during excision helps define the planes between the accessory breast and the fascia of the axilla. As with normal breast tissue, both benign and malignant conditions can develop within accessory breast tissue.[3]

Breast hypoplasia

This is failure of one or both (rarely) breasts to develop fully and can be congenital or acquired. Genetic causes include Poland's syndrome and ulnar–mammary syndrome. Poland's syndrome is a group of conditions

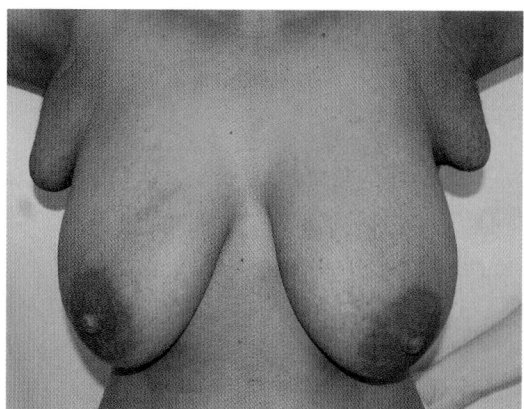

Figure 17.1 • Bilateral accessory breasts in axilla.

associated with the absence of hypoplasia of the pectoralis major muscle, the chest wall and varying degrees of syndactyly.[4] It is rare and usually only partial in nature. It is more common in men than in women. Acquired abnormalities in breast development can be caused by iatrogenic trauma or radiotherapy.

Treatment of hypoplasia and Poland's syndrome depends on the degree of deformity. Mild asymmetry is a common problem and usually only reassurance is needed. If the asymmetry is marked, augmentation of the smaller breast with or without tissue expansion and/or reduction or augmentation of the opposite breast may be required (**Fig. 17.2**). Tissue expansion is often required as there are differing amounts of skin on the two breasts. A pedicled or free myocutaneous flap, with or without an implant, can be used to reconstruct any muscle defect and produce symmetry in cases of severe hypoplasia or aplasia. Fat transfer (lipofilling) has also been described as a technique to correct or aid correction of breast hypoplasia either alone or combined with a breast implant.[5,6]

Hypoplasia can also be associated with tubular or tuberous breasts. This deformity can affect one or both breasts and the breast shape is caused by a constricting ring at the base of the breast, limiting vertical and horizontal growth. The surgical management of this group of conditions is challenging and often unsatisfactory. Tissue expansion combined with radial incisions on the deep aspect of the breast to divide the constricting ring usually improves contour. The large nipple–areola complex may need to be reduced in size. Lipofilling is being used increasingly in such patients.[6]

Macromastia is the excessive development of the breasts. This tends to occur during puberty (juvenile hypertrophy) or with onset of lactation (gestational). Prepubertal breast enlargement may occur very rarely in conjunction with a hormone-secreting tumour. Juvenile hypertrophy results from excessive proliferation of ducts and stromal tissue but no lobule formation. Significant psychological and physical problems can be caused by macromastia and patients with significant breast enlargement benefit from breast reduction. This procedure is not

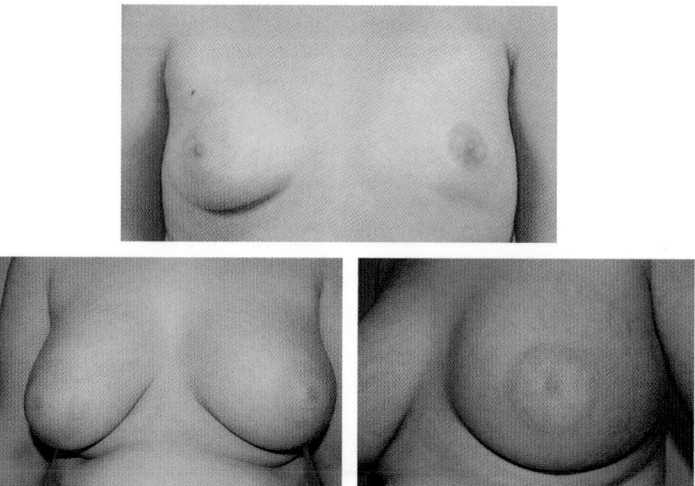

Figure 17.2 • Hypoplasia pre- and post-surgery with expansion followed by implant.

without complications and should be performed by an appropriately trained surgeon.[7]

Aberrations of normal breast development and involution

Defining what represents breast disease and what is normal is not a new problem. The ANDI classification[8] was developed to provide a framework to help understanding of the pathogenesis and subsequent management of benign breast disease. Most benign diseases arise from normal physiological processes and range from normality to mild abnormality (aberration) to severe abnormality (disease). The breast passes through phases related to the levels of circulating hormones and their effects on the ducts, lobule and stroma. The phases are breast development, cyclical change and involution (Table 17.1).

Fibroadenomas

A fibroadenoma is classified as an aberration of normal breast development and is made up of a combination of connective tissue and proliferatory epithelium (**Fig. 17.3**).[9] It is not a neoplasm or benign tumour as it does not arise from a single cell. Fibroadenomas arise from the hormone-dependent terminal duct lobular unit and are influenced by hormones, e.g. increasing in size during pregnancy. The stromal element of these tumours defines their classification and behaviour. A 'simple' fibroadenoma contains stroma of low cellularity and

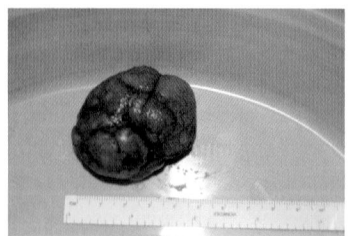

Figure 17.3 • Fibroadenoma.

regular cytology. Phyllodes tumours may or may not arise from fibroadenomas but contain stroma with much more marked cellularity and atypia. Although phyllodes tumours cannot always be differentiated on core biopsy with 100% certainty from fibroadenomas, it is usually possible to tell whether phyllodes is likely and when the lesion is a simple fibroadenoma. All discrete masses over the age of 23 should have a core biopsy – multiple passes with three samples of the lesion. Although ultrasound can usually differentiate fibroadenomas from cancers and guidelines indicate ultrasound is safe under 25, experience from medicolegal practice indicates the cut-off should be younger at 24 or below.

Simple fibroadenomas

These are benign, extremely mobile, discrete, rubbery masses that present symptomatically in young women or are an incidental finding during breast imaging. They are a 'frequent' condition and are seen most commonly at the time of greatest lobular development in the late teens and early twenties. They are usually solitary findings but some women develop multiple lesions in one or both breasts. The aetiology is unknown but has been linked to the oral contraceptive and Epstein–Barr virus following immunosuppression. They are highly mobile due to encapsulation and pliability of the breast tissue. This can make them appear to be much more superficial on examination than their true position, important to appreciate when embarking on removal under local anaesthetic.

> ✔ Fibroadenomas were observed for 2 years in women under 40 years of age: the majority did not change in size (55%), some got smaller or resolved (37%) and only a small number increased in size (8%), the majority of which were in women under the age of 20.[10]

Table 17.1 • Aberrations of normal breast development and involution

Age (years)	Normal process	Aberration
<25	Breast development	
	Stromal	Juvenile hypertrophy
	Lobular	Fibroadenoma
25–40	Cyclical activity	Cyclical mastalgia
		Cyclical nodularity (diffuse or focal)
35–55	Involution	
	Lobular	Macrocysts
	Stromal	Sclerosing lesions
	Ductal	Duct ectasia

In older women (>23 years of age) it is clearly essential to differentiate a fibroadenoma from breast cancer by triple assessment including core biopsy. Rapid growth of a fibroadenoma is rare but can occur in either adolescence (juvenile fibroadenoma) or in the perimenopausal age group (**Fig. 17.4**). Tumours over 5 cm are termed 'giant fibroadenoma' and are seen more commonly in African countries.[11] On macroscopic appearance fibroadenomas are discrete, bosselated, whitish tumours that appear to bulge when cut through. Only rarely does cancer develop within a fibroadenoma but when it does it tends to be non-invasive and lobular in nature.[12]

Management

The management of fibroadenomas depends on the patients' age and preference as well as the results of triple assessment. Core biopsy (multiple cores) is now preferred to cytology to confirm the diagnosis of a fibroadenoma. In patients with lesions under 4 cm, where histology confirms the diagnosis, the patient can then be reassured and discharged. In women presenting with multiple clinical and radiological fibroadenomata, core biopsy should be undertaken of the largest lesions – either one from both breasts or two from the same breast.

Excision is rarely indicated unless the fibroadenoma is obviously symptomatic, it increases significantly in size or causes significant distortion of the breast profile. Lesions measuring over 4 cm in size are usually removed, as should those with histological concern about stromal activity. Large fibroadenomas can be observed providing they have been adequately sampled. Although it is important to take account of the wishes of the patient when considering surgery, these are influenced by the manner in which the facts are presented. All patients should be given written information, which is available online from Breast Cancer Care.

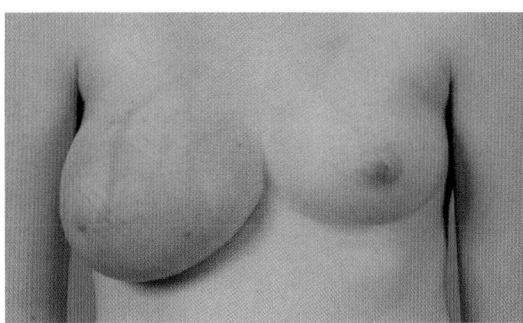

Figure 17.4 • Juvenile fibroadenoma right breast.

Excision should be performed through a cosmetically placed incision, which includes a submammary, axillary and circumareolar incision. Another option is to remove fibroadenomas with a mammotome.[13] With larger lesions (>5 cm where histology has shown no suggestion that it could be a phyllodes tumour), it is safe to section the tumour in situ and remove it through a small incision below the breast to improve cosmetic outcome. Large lesions are best be removed cosmetically through an inframammary incision. Removal of excess skin is rarely required in young women, particularly when removing a large juvenile fibroadenoma (Fig. 17.4). In some very large lesions later revisional surgery is required but it is important to leave this for up to a year after the initial excision as skin retracts and the breast reshapes itself over this period. Recurrence of a fibroadenoma can occasionally occur but is rare and it may be due to undiagnosed adjacent lesions rather than incomplete excision.

Tubular and lactating adenomas

A fibroadenoma consists of fibroconnective stroma containing glandular structures. The glandular element is lined by a single or multiple layers of epithelial cells. When the entire lesion consists of glands with very little intervening stroma, this is termed a tubular adenoma. Lactating adenomas are similar to tubular adenomas, but occur in the pregnant or lactating breast and are often multiple. Tubular adenomas in non-pregnant women are clinically similar to fibroadenomas and are managed identically. Mammographically punctuate microcalcification within the acini may be visible. Lactating adenomas can be managed conservatively once a diagnosis has been established through breastfeeding unless there is clinical concern. They tend to regress following cessation of breastfeeding.

Hamartoma

Hamartomas are common benign breast lesions and are composed of variable amounts of adipose, glandular and fibrous tissues. They are usually asymptomatic but may be palpable and feel like soft fibroadenomas. Most occur in women over 35. Mammographically they usually have a classical appearance (circumscribed area consisting of both soft tissue and lipomatous elements, surrounded by a thin radiolucent zone). They also differ subtly on ultrasound and are often misdiagnosed as fibroadenomas. Management is similar to that of fibroadenomas. It is important when performing a core biopsy of a possible hamartoma to inform the pathologist that the lesion may be a hamartoma as otherwise they are often reported as normal breast tissue on core biopsy.

Phyllodes tumour and sarcoma

The aetiology of phyllodes (leaf-like) tumours is unknown. They are less common than fibroadenomas (ratio of presentation 1:40[14]) and constitute about 2.5% of all fibroepithelial tumours. The age of onset is 15–20 years later than fibroadenomas. They can grow rapidly, sometimes producing marked distortion and cutaneous venous engorgement, which occasionally can lead to ulceration. The majority are benign in nature and feel like large fibroadenomas, and are diagnosed only following core biopsy. They are rarely fixed to skin or muscle. When cut during removal they are more brownish in colour than fibroadenomas and can have areas of necrosis within. Most diagnoses of phyllodes tumour are made before operation, on core biopsy, and the aim of surgery should be to remove the lesion with a clear macroscopic margin.

Differentiating benign from malignant phyllodes can be difficult and involves assessment of the size, ratio of stroma and epithelium, the border of the lesion, stromal cellularity and the number of stromal mitoses, and the presence or absence of necrosis. Current classification identifies benign, borderline and malignant phyllodes tumours.

Overall, phyllodes tumours recur locally in approximately 20% of patients. Most locally recurrent tumours are histologically similar to the original lesions but occasionally benign phyllodes recur as borderline lesions. Malignant phyllodes tumours recur earlier on average than benign lesions. For benign lesions, total excision with clear margins (≥1 mm) is sufficient.[15] For borderline and malignant lesions a wider margin is recommended and this may necessitate mastectomy with or without a myocutaneous flap for skin cover or breast reconstruction in large lesions. Regional lymph node metastases are seen rarely in malignant phyllodes tumours, with nodes being affected in approximately 5%. Metastatic spread, when it occurs, is similar in pattern to that of sarcomas. Fewer than 5% of all phyllodes tumours metastasise and approximately 25% of those classified as malignant metastasise,

depending on the exact criteria used for classification. Treatment of metastatic disease is discouraging, with no sustained remissions reported from radiation, hormonal treatment or chemotherapy.

Nipple discharge

Nipple discharge accounts for 5% of referrals to a breast clinic,[16] with up to 20% of these caused by in situ or malignant disease.[17] The important features to assess are whether the discharge is from a single or multiple ducts, is coloured or bloodstained, is induced or spontaneous, and is affecting one or both breasts. The frequency, colour and consistency of the discharge should be noted. Blood-coloured discharge or discharge that contains significant amounts of blood on testing has been reported by some but not all authors to be more likely to arise from a cancer than coloured discharge that contains no blood on testing.[18] The sensitivity and specificity of blood in the discharge is, however, not high. Persistent discharge (≥2 per week) is also more likely to be associated with a significant causative lesion (such as a papilloma or cancer). The aim is to differentiate between physiological causes and ductal pathology (**Fig. 17.5**). Discharge can be elicited by squeezing around the nipple in 20% of women[19] and is often noted following mammography. If discharge is associated with a lump, then management is directed to the diagnosis of the lump.

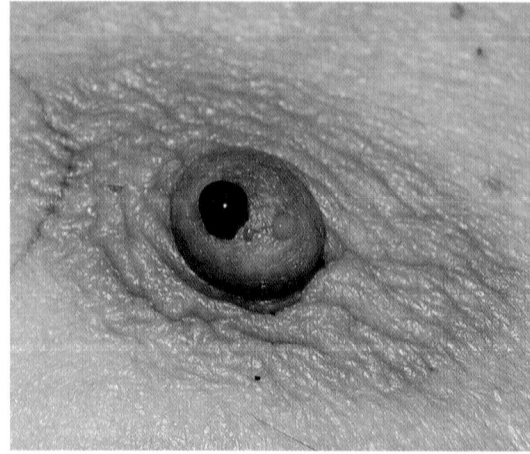

Figure 17.5 • Multiduct physiological discharge. Note the range of colours characteristic of physiological discharge.

Galactorrhoea should only be diagnosed if the discharge is bilateral, copious, pale milky in colour and from multiple ducts. Some women continue to produce milk for many months after they have stopped breastfeeding but galactorrhoea usually develops long after cessation of breastfeeding. Prolactin levels should be checked and, if raised (>1000 mIU/L), the cause can be secondary to medication or a pituitary tumour. If the serum prolactin is normal, then reassurance and a full explanation of the aetiology are often all that is required. If there are persistent symptoms, the ducts underneath the nipple can be ligated.

Coloured opalescent discharge, from multiple ducts, is common. It is usually physiological discharge. In older women thick yellow discharge can result from duct ectasia. Serosanguineous and/or bloody discharge from a single duct is more likely to be associated with papillomas, epithelial hyperplasia, ductal carcinoma in situ (DCIS) or an invasive carcinoma.

Investigation

Assessment includes a careful breast examination to identify the presence or absence of a breast mass. Firm pressure applied around the areola can help to identify the site of any dilated duct (pressure over a dilated duct will produce the discharge); this is helpful in defining where an incision should be made for any subsequent surgery. The nipple is squeezed with firm digital pressure and if fluid is expressed, the site and character of the discharge are recorded. Testing of the discharge for haemoglobin determines whether blood is present but this is of limited value, although bloodstained discharge is more likely to be associated with malignancy. Fewer than 20% of patients who have a bloodstained discharge or who have a discharge containing moderate or large amounts of blood have an underlying malignancy. Age is said to be an important predictor of malignancy; in one series, 3% of patients younger than 40, 10% of patients between ages 40 and 60, and 32% of patients older than 60 years who presented with nipple discharge as their only symptom were found to have cancers.[20] The absence of blood in nipple discharge is not an absolute indication that the discharge is unrelated to an underlying malignancy, as demonstrated in a series of 108 patients where the sensitivity of haemoccult testing was only 50%. Nipple discharge cytology is of little use due to its poor sensitivity.[21,22]

A number of techniques have evolved to determine the aetiology and avoid unnecessary surgery. Ductoscopy, using a microendoscope passed into the offending duct, allows direct visualisation. There are encouraging reports of its use (see Chapter 3), especially in directing duct excision at surgery[23] and detecting deeper lesions that may be missed by blind central excision.[24] Ductal lavage is a technique in which the duct is cannulated, irrigated with saline and the subsequent discharge examined cytologically. This technique increases cell yield by 100 times that of simple discharge cytology.[25] Ductography (imaging of the ductal system) can identify intraductal lesions. Although this investigation has only a 60% sensitivity for malignancy, a filling defect or duct cut-off has a high positive predictive value for the presence of either a papilloma or a carcinoma.[26,27] Ductography, however, is a painful procedure and is not widely practised.

At present, the major role of ductoscopy is as an adjunct to surgery; by using simple transillumination of the skin overlying the lesion during ductoscopy, limited duct excision is possible. The role of ductal lavage has been questioned due to large variations in its sensitivity and specificity.[28,29] During ductoscopy, visualised lesions can be biopsied and in one report 38 of 46 women with biopsy-proven papillomas were observed for 2 years with no reported missed cancers.[24] The role of ductoscopy in the assessment of nipple discharge is set to increase as the quality of equipment improves and it becomes more widely available. A benefit of both ductography and ductoscopy is that they allow identification of the site of any lesion in younger women, allowing localisation and excision of the causative lesion while retaining the ability to lactate (**Fig. 17.6**). A mammogram should be performed as part of the assessment of patients over 35 years of age with a discharge. The sensitivity in this group of patients is low, at 57%.[21] Digital mammography has been shown to have a greater pick-up rate than film mammography in women under 50 or with dense breasts.[30] Ultrasound can sometimes identify papillomas and malignant lesions in the ducts close to the nipple.[31] Papillomas visualised on ultrasound can then be biopsied or removed using a vacuum-assisted core biopsy device.[32]

If no abnormality is found on clinical or mammographic examination, patients are managed according to whether the discharge is from a single duct or multiple ducts (Fig. 17.6). Any patient with

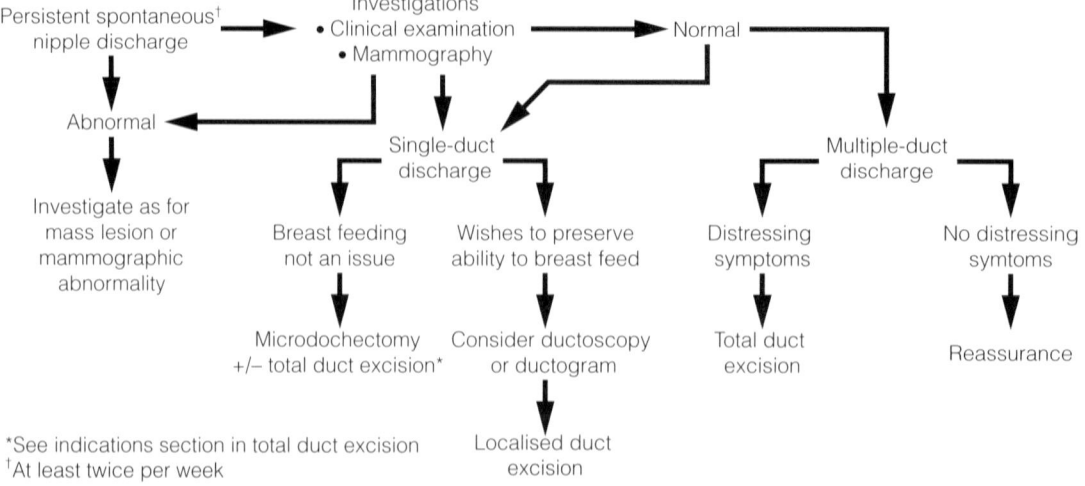

Figure 17.6 • Investigation of nipple discharge.

spontaneous single-duct discharge should undergo surgery to determine the cause of the discharge if it is:

- bloodstained or contains moderate to large amounts of blood on testing;
- persistent (at least twice per week);
- associated with a mass;
- a new serosanguineous discharge in a postmenopausal woman.

Aetiology

Duct ectasia

This is benign dilatation and shortening of the terminal ducts within 3 cm of the nipple. It is a common condition and increases in incidence with age. It should not be confused with periductal mastitis, which occurs in younger women and is secondary to cigarette smoking. Duct ectasia can present as nipple discharge, nipple retraction (giving a slit-like appearance) or a palpable mass. It is usually asymptomatic. The discharge is usually creamy and cheesy in nature. Bilateral multiduct green discharge is physiological and not related to duct ectasia.

Ductal papillomas

There are three main forms: a solitary-duct discrete papilloma, multiple papillomas or juvenile papillomatosis (Swiss cheese disease). Papillomas are characterised by formation of epithelial fronds that have both the luminal epithelial and the outer myoepithelial cell layers, supported by a fibrovascular stroma. The epithelial component can be subject to a spectrum of morphological changes ranging from metaplasia to hyperplasia, atypical hyperplasia and in situ carcinoma. A solitary intraductal papilloma, which occurs in a large duct (within 5 cm of the nipple), is the commonest form and is the most common aetiology of a bloody nipple discharge. They are most frequently seen in the 30–50 age group and can be palpated in one-third of patients. As papillomas have a thin stalk, they have the potential to tort and necrose. Half of women with papillomas have bloody discharge while the other half have a serous discharge.[33]

Women with multiple intraductal papilloma syndrome have many peripheral duct papillomas. There has to be a minimum of five clearly separate papillomas within a localised segment of breast tissue, usually in a peripheral location. These tend not to present as nipple discharge but as a palpable lump and usually occur at a younger age than single papillomas. They are only associated with an increased risk of malignancy if they contain areas of atypical hyperplasia. Repeated excision of papillomas in patients with multiple intraductal papillomas can result in significant breast asymmetry. One option in such patients is to excise such lesions with a vacuum-assisted core biopsy device. This provides sufficient material for the pathologist to assess that all excised lesions are benign. Surgery to excise the affected duct system with an oncoplastic procedure to reshape the breast is preferential to mastectomy if biopsies show atypia.

Juvenile papillomatosis is a very rare condition defined as severe ductal papillomatosis occurring in young women <30 years old and usually presents as a painless, mobile mass (similar to fibroadenoma).

Treatment is by complete excision. Patients with this condition (and their close family) may be at some increased risk of subsequent breast cancer, especially if the lesion is bilateral and there is significant family history. Close clinical surveillance is indicated.

Ductal carcinoma in situ

Bloody nipple discharge with or without the presence of Paget's disease constitutes one-third of all symptomatic in situ patients.[34] Only rarely does an invasive cancer cause nipple discharge in the absence of a clinical mass. In most series, ductal carcinoma in situ (DCIS) is responsible for less than 20% of unilateral single-duct nipple discharge.[19] The diagnosis is often made only following surgical excision of the affected duct.

Bloody nipple discharge in pregnancy

Bilateral bloody nipple discharge detected either visibly or on testing during pregnancy or lactation is common. In 20% of women who develop nipple discharge during pregnancy, blood is evident on testing. The likely cause is hypervascularity of developing breast tissue; provided that the discharge is multiductal and/or bilateral it is benign, resolves spontaneously and requires no specific treatment.[35]

Nipple adenoma

Nipple adenomas present as a non-discrete, palpable growth of the papilla of the nipple (see **Fig. 17.7**). There may be nipple discoloration and contour change noted. Nipple adenomas tend to cause erosion of the nipple tip and commonly present as a bloody discharge from the surface of the nipple. They are benign in nature and definitive treatment is complete excision. It is caused by ductal hyperplasia of the lactiferous ducts and is seen most commonly in women of between 40 and 50 years of age.

Surgery
Microdochectomy

A single duct can be removed by microdochectomy. This is performed through either a radial incision or preferably a circumareolar incision. Expression of the discharge should not be performed until the patient is in theatre and fully draped in order to provide the best chance of identifying the offending duct. The discharging duct is cannulated and either a lacrimal probe placed or methylene blue injected and an incision made. The probe aids identification of the relevant duct and dissection of this from surrounding ducts/breast tissue. A length of at least 2–3 cm should be removed. The excised duct should be opened to

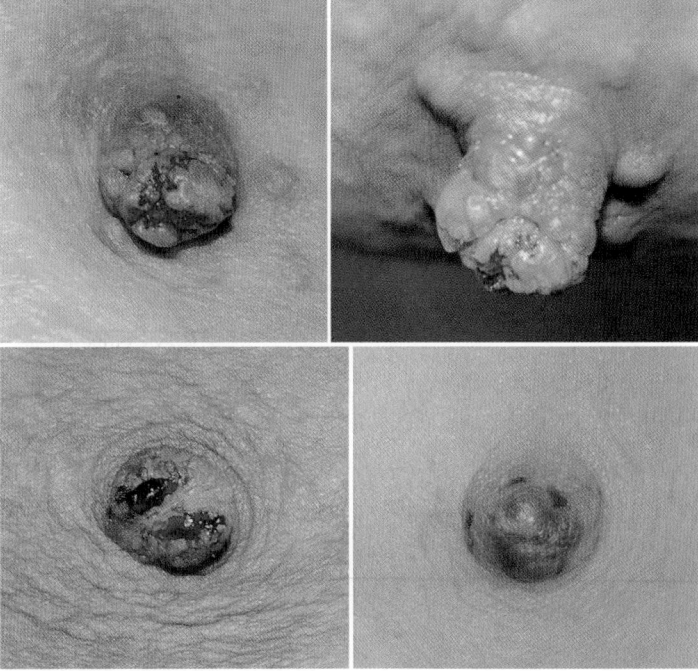

Figure 17.7 • Nipple adenomas.

ensure a cause for the discharge is present and the distal remnant inspected to ensure that the entire dilated duct has been excised. If the residual duct is dilated, then it should be split, opened and inspected. Microdochectomy should not damage surrounding normal ducts and allows subsequent breastfeeding. If performing a duct excision directed by ductoscopy, then having identified an abnormality in the duct, the light is used to direct the surgical excision. Once the excision has been performed, the nipple should be squeezed gently to ensure that the discharging duct has been excised.

Total duct excision or division

In women of non-childbearing age, total duct excision is an option for a single-duct discharge. Current evidence suggests that total duct excision is more likely to result in a specific diagnosis and less likely to miss underlying malignancy than microdochectomy.[36] Total duct excision can also be used for multiple-duct discharge if the discharge is copious and affecting quality of life, and is often performed for periductal mastitis. The operation involves dividing all the ducts from the underside of the nipple and removing surrounding breast tissue to a depth of 2 cm behind the nipple–areola complex.[37] A circum-areolar incision is used. Patients should be warned that there is a small risk of nipple tip necrosis (<1%), reduced sensation (40%) and nipple inversion associated with this operation. Patients undergoing surgery for periductal mastitis require total removal of all ducts from behind the nipple; leaving even small remnants of ducts predisposes to recurrence. Because the lesions of periductal mastitis usually contain organisms, patients should receive appropriate systemic antibiotic treatment during the operation and for 5 days after surgery. Options for antibiotic therapy include amoxicillin–clavulanate or a combination of erythromycin and metronidazole.

For patients having cosmetic nipple eversion, the procedure can be performed through a limited incision and the ducts divided, ensuring that the nipple everts naturally without the need for sutures.

Mastalgia

Most women at some point during their lives will suffer from breast pain. The aim for clinicians is to differentiate between true mastalgia (pain originating within the breast) and referred pain. Women with referred pain describe the pain as unilateral, associated with activity and reproduced by pressure on the chest wall. Non-steroidal anti-inflammatory drugs, either taken orally or applied topically, can relieve such symptoms. True mastalgia is associated with swelling and nodularity of the breasts. It resolves spontaneously in 20–40% of women but can recur.

Due to the hormonal aetiology, true breast pain is often worse before and relieved after menstruation. Exacerbating factors include the perimenopausal state (where hormone levels fluctuate) and the use of exogenous hormones (hormone replacement therapy or the oral contraceptive pill). The cause of cyclical mastalgia is unknown but studies have implicated excess production of prolactin,[38] excess oestrogen,[39] insufficient progesterone,[40] or increased receptor sensitivity in breast tissue caused by a raised ratio of saturated fatty acids to essential fatty acids.[41]

Assessment

A full history and examination should be performed. The patient should be rolled and the underlying chest wall – often the site of the pain – palpated. In women over 40 years of age, mammography should be performed to exclude an occult malignancy (approximately 5% of women with breast cancer complain of pain,[14] while 2.7% of women presenting with pain as their main symptom are diagnosed with breast cancer[42]). If a dominant lump or lumpiness is palpable, then this will dictate further management. Most breast pain, and this includes many women with cyclical breast pain, arises in the chest wall. Analgesia, a firm bra worn 24 hours a day and gentle stretching exercises such as swimming are effective treatments.

Treatment

Reassurance that the symptoms are not related to an underlying malignancy is the most effective treatment for mastalgia.[43] Following this, the majority will require no further treatment.

Evening primrose oil (EPO) is not effective, as two double-blind, randomised, crossover trials comparing EPO versus placebo showed no benefit for EPO.[44,45] The original work that advocated its use has never been published other than in abstract form.[46] Other agents that have been shown to have some benefit include phyto-oestrogens (e.g. soya milk)[47] and Agnus castus (a fruit extract).[48]

Reducing fat intake to less than 15% of dietary calories has been shown to improve symptoms in cyclical mastalgia.[49] The patients who responded showed changes in their serum lipid profiles but the study was not blinded so placebo effects cannot be excluded and the diet is not easy to adhere to in the long term.

In severe pain, medication can be used but complications of these treatments need to be outlined to the patient. Treatment should be either tamoxifen 10 mg daily or danazol. Tamoxifen 20 mg daily was superior to placebo in a double-blind, randomised, controlled trial and pain relief was maintained in 72% of women 1 year after use.[50] Tamoxifen restricted to the luteal phase of the menstrual cycle abolished pain in 85% of women. Recurrent pain at 1 year was seen in 25% and the rate of adverse effects was 21%.[51] Tamoxifen 10 mg daily has fewer side-effects and is as effective as 20 mg when compared with danazol 200 mg daily.[52]

✓✓ Tamoxifen is superior to danazol, with fewer adverse effects: 53% of patients receiving tamoxifen were pain free at 1 year compared with 37% of patients receiving danazol. Tamoxifen 10 mg daily or danazol can be given only during the luteal phase of the menstrual cycle and results in similar improvements in symptoms, but with a marked reduction in adverse effects.[51,53]

Tamoxifen is not licensed for use in mastalgia. Toremifene, another selective oestrogen receptor modulator, has also recently demonstrated its effectiveness in treating mastalgia. In a randomised, double-blind trial of 195 women with persistent (lasting longer than 6 months) mastalgia, they assigned patients to toremifene 30 mg daily or a matched placebo for three menstrual cycles. This demonstrated a significant benefit for toremifene but with no significant difference in adverse events between the two groups.[54]

A phase II trial using afimoxifene (4-hydroxytamoxifen) delivered locally to the breast as a transdermal hydroalcoholic gel daily over four cycles has shown statistically significant improvements in signs and symptoms of cyclical mastalgia across patient- and physician-rated scales, with excellent tolerability and safety. There is strong evidence that this tamoxifen metabolite is absorbed into the breast tissue but does not have the systemic effects associated with tamoxifen.[55] It is not used in the UK.

Bromocriptine should not be used, due to its high rate of adverse effects (80%).[56] Selective serotonin reuptake inhibitors have been reported as being of some benefit in mastalgia as part of premenstrual syndrome;[57] they also have effects on fatty acid profiles.

Breast cysts

Palpable breast cysts are a common presentation to a breast clinic and affect 7% of all women.[14] Small cysts have no significance except their potential to grow. Larger cysts present typically in the fifth decade and are usually multiple in nature. Cysts can be divided into apocrine and non-apocrine, depending on the consistency of the fluid found within the cyst. The only relevance of this classification is that apocrine cysts have a higher tendency to recur.[58]

Imaging

Mammographically, breast cysts have characteristic haloes but ultrasound is essential to the management of cystic disease. Not only does ultrasound distinguish between solid and cystic lesions, it also provides information on the cyst wall and fluid consistency. It is also an adjunct in ensuring accurate differentiation of simple from complex cysts, as well as allowing complete aspiration. A simple cyst has a smooth outline with no internal echoes and posterior enhancement. Complex (or complicated or atypical) cysts are characterised by internal echoes or thin septations, thickened and/or irregular wall, and absent posterior enhancement. Complex cysts are rarely malignant and require aspiration or review with a follow-up scan several months later. If the cyst wall shows any projections into the centre of the cyst, this may indicate the presence of an intracystic papilloma or carcinoma and core biopsy of the projected area is indicated.

Management

Asymptomatic cysts should be left alone. Large, symptomatic or painful cysts should be aspirated to dryness. If the fluid is bloodstained it should be sent for cytology; otherwise it should be discarded. If a palpable mass is still present after aspiration, further imaging and biopsy are indicated. If the cyst recurs, then repeat aspiration can be performed. There is a slightly increased relative risk of developing breast cancer in women with cysts but this is not significant enough to warrant surveillance.

Sclerotic/fibrotic lesions

Stromal involution can produce areas of fibrosis within the breast supporting tissues. Three different groups of such lesions are described: sclerosing adenosis, radial scars and complex sclerosing lesions (CSLs). Sclerosing adenosis can present with a palpable mass and breast pain. Mammographically, it can be associated with microcalcificaton. It differs histologically from radial scars and CSLs in the degree of excessive myoepithelial proliferation seen together with the fibrosis. Radial scars and CSLs are considered to be part of the same process but are differentiated on size (radial scar, ≤1 cm; CSL, >1 cm). Radial scars and CSLs are usually asymptomatic and discovered as part of mammographic screening but can rarely present as a palpable mass. Both lesions may serve as a background for the development of atypical epithelial proliferations, including atypical hyperplasia and carcinoma in situ. Even in the absence of atypia there is some suggestion that the presence of such lesions increases the individual's risk of malignancy.[59] All these lesions, though benign in nature, are difficult to distinguish from malignancy mammographically, macroscopically and histologically. Percutaneous biopsy of these lesions with a large-gauge vacuum-assisted core needle is reliable, providing there is no associated atypia, at least 12 cores are performed and there is concordance with radiological findings.[60] Malignancy cannot be excluded reliably when there is limited sampling, the presence of atypia or discordance with the radiological appearance of the lesion. Then open excision is recommended.

Pseudoangiomatous stromal hyperplasia of the breast (PASH)

PASH is a benign myofibroblastic proliferation of non-specialised mammary stroma. It is frequently a microscopic incidental finding in breast biopsies performed for benign or malignant disease. It has been reported to form breast masses and some of these have been reported to be sizeable. Whether PASH is the cause of these masses or an epiphenomenon, for instance extensive PASH is seen commonly within a juvenile fibroadenoma, is not clear. The aetiology is not known and assuming that PASH explains the cause of any localised mass is unwise. The histological appearance has caused confusion with mammary angiosarcoma, so immunohistochemical vascular markers may be required to distinguish these two conditions.

Fibromatosis

Fibromatosis or *desmoid tumour* of the breast is an extremely rare entity. Fibromatosis is an infiltrative fibroblastic and myofibroblastic proliferation with significant risk for local recurrence, but no metastatic potential. Fibromatosis is uncommon in the mammary gland and accounts for less than 0.2% of all primary breast lesions. It probably arises from the fascia of the underlying chest wall muscles rather than on the breast tissue itself. It may be indistinguishable from malignancy on ultrasound, mammography, physical examination and on gross evaluation. Fibromatosis is a spectrum of conditions from extremely indolent areas principally of fibrosis to a more proliferative infiltrative lesion. Establishing the diagnosis can be difficult on core biopsy and larger vacuum-assisted needle biopsies provide more tissue for the pathologist to assess. Open biopsy may be necessary if a diagnosis is not evident on needle biopsy. Once it is established that the diagnosis is fibromatosis (this may involve sending the biopsy for an expert opinion), then the initial treatment is observation only. If the lesion increases in size and becomes symptomatic, particularly if it infiltrates the chest wall and encases the intercostal nerves, when it can cause marked discomfort and pain, then surgical excision should be considered. If the lesion recurs and becomes symptomatic or the initial excision involves removal of portions of the chest wall, then surgery should aim to remove all the disease with a 1-cm clear margin. There is little evidence of a benefit of chemotherapy or radiotherapy in recurrent or incompletely excised disease. Tamoxifen has been reported to be of benefit but these lesions are oestrogen receptor (ER) alpha negative, although reports suggest they are ER beta rich. Symptomatic recurrence is an issue only for a small percentage of patients with fibromatosis following excision and is often evident because of nerve entrapment, which results in local pain.

Non-ANDI conditions

Breast infections

Infection is a common problem affecting the breast,[61] and can be divided into lactational, non-lactational and postsurgical. The skin overlying the breast can also become infected either primarily or secondarily because of infection developing in an existing lesion such as an epidermoid cyst or as a consequence of a generalised skin condition such as hidradenitis suppurativa.

Lactational infections

Mastitis secondary to breastfeeding occurs in approximately 5% of puerperal women and is most common during the first month or during weaning as the baby's teeth develop. *Staphylococcus aureus* is the usual organism and it enters the duct system through the nipple. There is usually a history of a cracked nipple and/or problems with milk flow. Patients initially present with pain, localised erythema and swelling. If this progresses, the inflammation can affect large areas of the breast and the patient can become toxic. Promoting milk flow by continuing to breastfeed and the early use of appropriate antibiotics markedly reduces the rate of subsequent abscess formation. Infections developing within the first few weeks may result from organisms transmitted in hospital and may be resistant to commonly used antibiotics. Over half of organisms that cause breast infection produce penicillinase.[62] Co-amoxiclav or flucloxacillin and erythromycin are the antibiotics of preference. Tetracycline, ciprofloxacin and chloramphenicol should not be used to treat infection in breastfeeding women because these drugs enter breast milk and may harm the child.

Non-lactational infections

Non-lactational infections are grouped into peripheral or periareolar. Those infections in the periareolar area are seen in young women and are often secondary to periductal mastitis (associated with heavy cigarette smoking).[63] Substances in cigarette smoke may directly or indirectly damage the wall of subareolar ducts. Accumulation of toxic metabolites, such as lipid peroxidase, epoxides, nicotine and cotinine in the breast ducts has been demonstrated to occur in smokers within 15 minutes of a woman starting to breastfeed.[64] Smoking has also

been shown to inhibit growth of Gram-positive bacteria, leading to an overgrowth of Gram-negative bacteria.[65] This may affect the normal bacterial flora and allow overgrowth of pathogenic aerobic and anaerobic Gram-negative bacteria, and would explain the presence of these organisms in the lesions of periductal mastitis. Microvascular changes have also been recorded and it could be that cigarettes cause some local ischaemia. The view is that the combination of damage due to toxins, microvascular damage by lipid peroxidases, and altered bacterial flora produces the clinical manifestations of periductal mastitis.

Patients present with periareolar inflammation often associated with a mass or abscess. The organisms causing this infection are usually mixed and include anaerobes. Periareolar sepsis has a high rate of recurrence.

Peripheral non-lactational breast abscesses are three times more common in premenopausal women than in menopausal or postmenopausal women. The aetiology of these infections is unclear but although it was reported that these are commonly associated with diabetes, rheumatoid arthritis, steroid treatment and trauma, this is untrue.[66] The usual organism responsible is *S. aureus*. Very rarely, an infection is related to underlying comedo necrosis in DCIS. For this reason a mammogram should be performed in women over 35 years of age after resolution of the inflammation.

Postsurgical infection

Infections can present in the acute postsurgical period or after the wound has healed. There was formerly conflicting evidence of the benefit of prophylactic antibiotics during clean breast surgery, although studies have now shown a small but consistent benefit from a single perioperative dose of a broad-spectrum antibiotic such as co-amoxiclav.[67] The most common organisms causing early infection include normal skin flora, *S. aureus* or organisms derived from the terminal ducts.[68] Most surgeons give antibiotics routinely to patients having implants inserted. Patients having surgery for periductal mastitis are at increased risk of postoperative infection and all these patients should have intraoperative and postoperative antibiotics that cover the range of organisms isolated from this condition. 'Seromas' are frequent and can become infected following aspiration or as a result of reduced resistance to infection during chemotherapy. Radiotherapy interferes with both the blood and lymphatic flow to the breast, and its effect is to increase rates of infection in the treated area; when infection occurs, prolonged and high-dose antibiotic therapy may be required in such pateints. Redness and oedema of the breast following breast-conserving surgery are not uncommon (especially after radiotherapy). This usually occurs between 3 and 12 months following surgery. This is unresponsive to antibiotics and has an incidence of 3–5% in patients following radiotherapy for breast-conserving surgery.[69] It appears to be related to obstructed lymphatic flow and responds to manual lymphatic drainage.

If an implant becomes infected, intensive antibiotic therapy is occasionally effective but usually the prosthesis has to be removed. Replacing an infected implant following thorough lavage has been reported to be effective but is rarely performed.[70] It is not uncommon for implants to become infected after a minor surgical intervention (such as dental work) or during chemotherapy given as adjuvant therapy or as treatment for metastatic disease. Prophylactic antibiotics should be considered for patients with implants undergoing major dental work.

Treatment

The basis of treatment for all breast infections is use of a broad-spectrum antibiotic and draining any collections of pus.

✅ Due to the difficulty of predicting the presence of pus within an inflamed breast, ultrasound with or without aspiration should be performed.[71] The need for open drainage in breast abscesses has been superseded by the use of aspiration.[72–74]

This has allowed management of breast infection to become outpatient based. Protocols validated within the Edinburgh Breast Unit have demonstrated that few if any breast abscesses require incision and drainage under general anaesthesia.[75] All abscesses should be assessed by ultrasound and if pus is present the surgeon or radiologist aspirates this, usually under ultrasound guidance (**Figs 17.8** and **17.9**). Patients are reviewed every 2–3 days and any further collections aspirated until no further pus forms. Drainage of pus by making a small stab incision in the skin under local anaesthesia is performed in patients where the overlying skin is thinned or necrotic (**Fig. 17.10**). The incision to drain any breast abscess should be just large enough to allow the pus to drain (1 cm or less), which minimises later scarring. Ultrasound provides a simple method for differentiating an abscess from cellulitis, allows assessment of any loculation, which is rare, and permits complete aspiration of all pus. Experience in the Edinburgh Breast Unit of using ultrasound to assist aspiration of breast abscesses is that it is quick and simple to learn and use. Local anaesthetic (1% lignocaine with 1:200 000 adrenaline) is injected into non-inflamed skin away from the abscess and along the needle track and is then irrigated into the abscess cavity. Aspiration is then relatively painless and the local anaesthetic helps if the pus is thick by diluting the pus to allow aspiration. Periareolar non-lactational abscesses can be treated and cured by repeated aspiration. Due to the recurrent nature of periareolar infection, recurrent abscess formation is common and in such patients when all signs of acute infection have settled, which takes at least 6 weeks, careful surgical excision of any residual abscess and affected ducts is often required. A mammary duct fistula (a connection between the infected and damaged duct and the skin, usually at the edge of the areola) develops

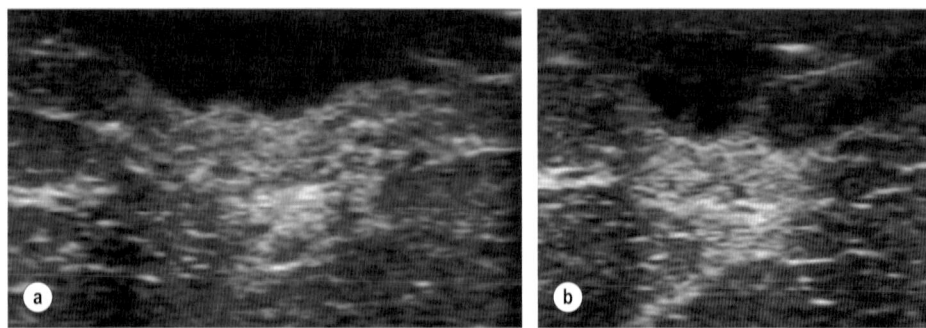

Figure 17.8 • Aspiration of abscesses under ultrasound guidance. **(a)** Ultrasound view of a breast abscess. **(b)** The needle can be seen entering the abscess on the right, allowing aspiration to be performed.

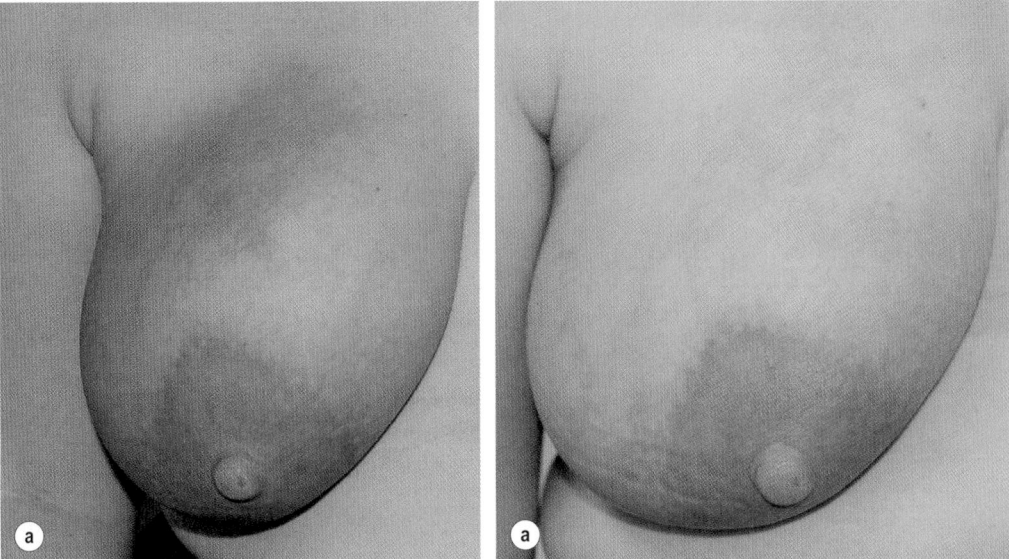

Figure 17.9 • (a) Lactating abscess: skin red but normal at presentation. **(b)** Lactating abscess following aspiration.

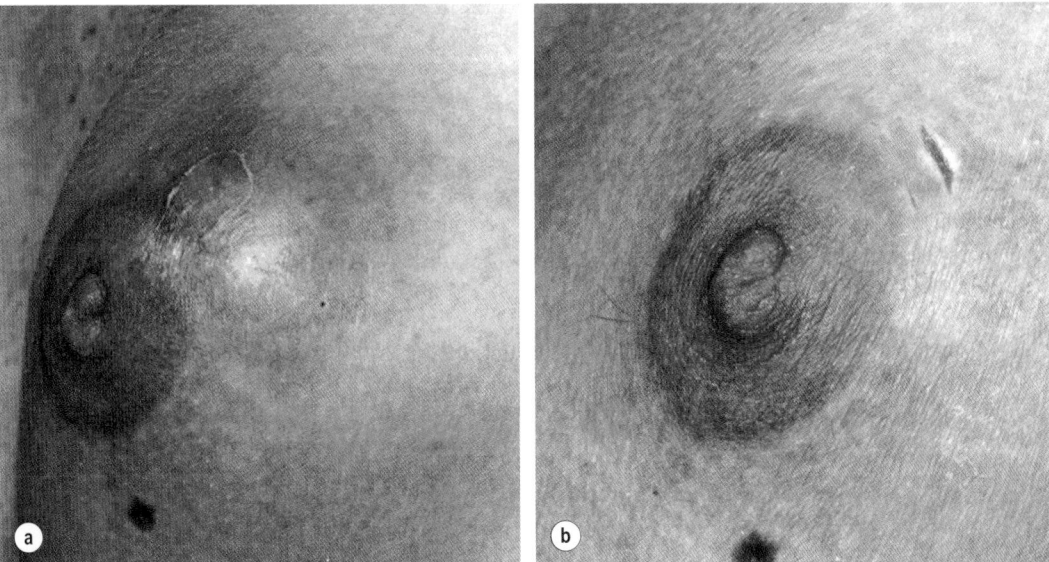

Figure 17.10 • Abscess of the left breast with thinned overlying skin: **(a)** before incision; **(b)** after incision and drainage through a small stab incision.

in up to one-third of patients after incision and drainage of a periareolar abscess.[76] Fistulas require definitive surgical management. Options include fistulotomy, cutting down on a probe into the fistula and allowing healing by secondary intention, which is painful after surgery and produces an ugly scar, and fistula excision and primary closure. Excising a fistula is easier through a radial scar, but circumareolar incision produces the best cosmetic outcome. Complete excision of the granulation tissue lined tract (plus the affected ducts under the nipple) and primary closure requires antibiotic cover (**Fig. 17.11**). There is a high risk of recurrence in the presence of postoperative wound infection.[77]

An important aspect of the management of puerperal breast infections is the continued expression of

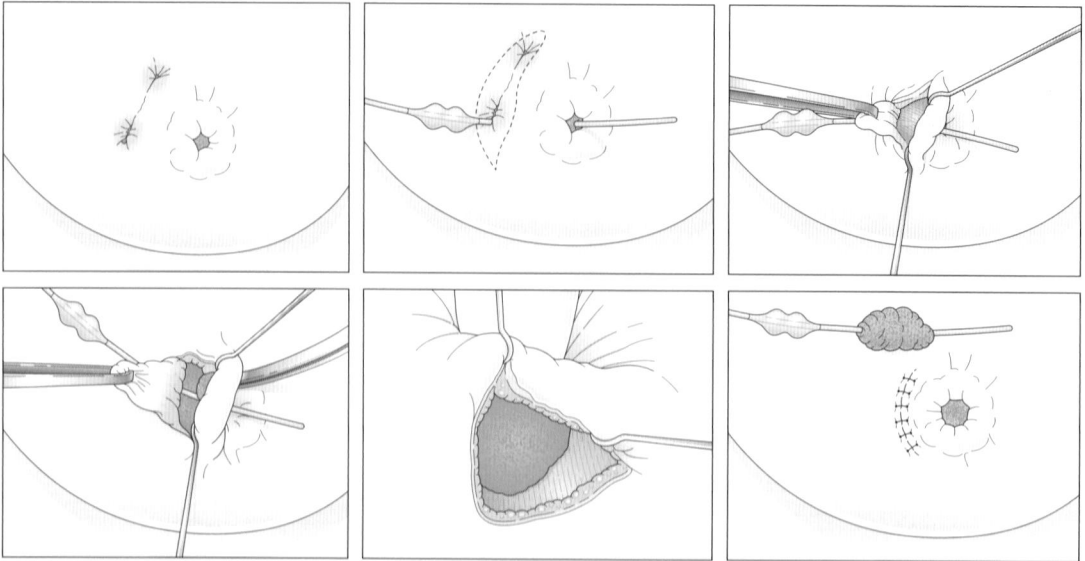

Figure 17.11 • Diagrammatic illustration of the steps involved in excision of a mammary duct fistula performed through a circumareolar incision with primary wound closure under antibiotic cover.

milk, with the most efficient breast pump being the baby's mouth. Emptying the breast increases the rate of a good outcome in infective mastitis[78] and although bacteria and the antibiotic are present in the milk, this does not appear to harm the child.[79] It is rarely necessary to suppress lactation but in severe unremitting or repeated infections, the prolactin antagonist cabergoline is effective at stopping milk flow.

It is essential to remember that inflammatory carcinoma can be difficult to differentiate from breast infection. If the inflammatory mass does not settle on appropriate management, then core biopsy of any abnormal area should be considered.

Other infections

Granulomatous mastitis

This is a rare condition, characterised by non-caseating granulomas and microabcesses confined to a breast lobule.[80] Patients present with a firm irregular mass (which is often indistinguishable from a carcinoma) or multiple or recurrent abscesses (**Fig. 17.12**). The mass can be extremely tender. Young parous women are most frequently affected and there is no association with smoking. The role of organisms in the aetiology of this condition is unclear but one study did isolate corynebacteria from nine of 12 women with granulomatous lobular mastitis.[81]

The most common species isolated was the newly described *Corynebacterium kroppenstedtii*, followed by *Corynebacterium amycolatum* and *Corynebacterium tuberculostearicum*. These organisms are, however, sensitive to penicillin and tetracycline, and treatment with these antibiotics does not produce resolution of granulomatous lobular mastitis so it is unlikely that these organisms have a major role. In patients diagnosed as having granulomatous lobular mastitis on core biopsy, excision of the mass should be avoided, as it is often followed by persistent wound discharge and failure of the wound to heal. Steroids and other immunosuppressive agents have been used with varying reports of their efficacy.[82] There is no convincing evidence that steroids alter the course of this condition. They do improve symptoms during administration of high doses but the condition then worsens when the dose is reduced. Reports of the benefit of injecting depot steroid are emerging. We no longer use steroids in this condition. It resolves spontaneously over a period of 6–18 months. Treatment is supportive and is aimed at treating associated infection and abscesses.

Hidradenitis suppurativa

Hidradenitis is a condition affecting the apocrine glands of the skin, including the axillae, perineum and/ or breast areas. It is much commoner in smokers and the organisms responsible are similar to those present

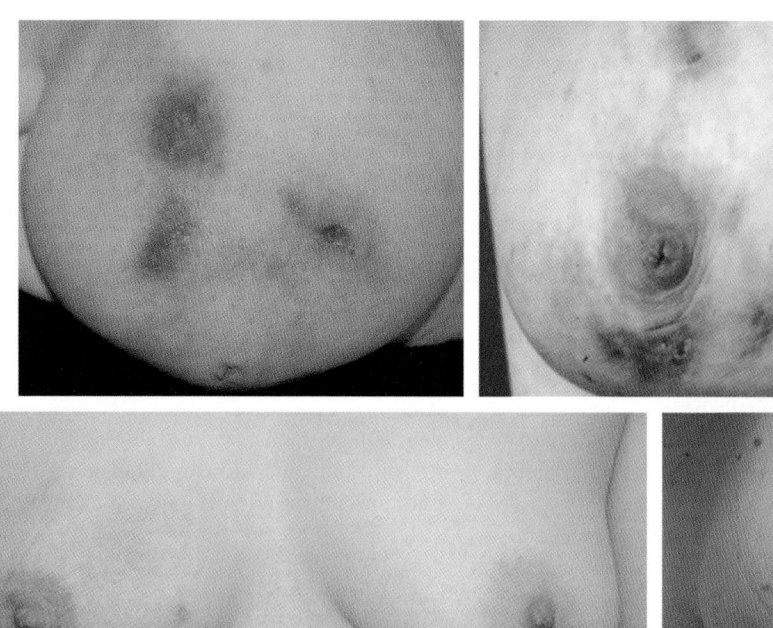

Figure 17.12 • Granulomatous lobular mastitis in its various presentations with skin changes, a mass and abscesses.

in periareolar sepsis. Treatment in the acute phase comprises management of any infection/abscesses by appropriate antibiotics and aspiration or drainage of any abscess. Excision of the affected area with skin grafting has been reported to be effective in approximately 50% of patients and may be the only long-term option for some patients. Smoking cessation is also beneficial.

Miscellaneous benign lesions

Montgomery's gland problems

Throughout the areola are blind-ending glands that produce fluid to lubricate the areola during breast-feeding. These glands can become blocked, forming hard nodules on the periphery of the areola. Occasionally these can become infected. Unless symptomatic, the management of these prominent Montgomery's glands is reassurance.

Fat necrosis

Following trauma to the breast, fat necrosis can occur. Fat necrosis can produce either a mass that can feel similar on palpation and appear similar on imaging to a breast carcinoma or a cystic oily collection. Patients usually give a history of direct trauma (or surgery) to the affected breast and examination may reveal bruising. It is important to assess such patients with imaging and not dismiss dimpling and bruising as fat necrosis. Histologically, fat necrosis is characterised by anucleate fat cells, surrounded by histiocytic giant cells and foamy macrophages. Severe fat necrosis can follow seat-belt damage and such patients often have a significant defect in the breast with significant distortion at the site where the seat-belt has disrupted a significant area of breast fat.

Lipomas

Due to the fatty nature of the breast it is not surprising that lipomas are common. They tend to present in the fifth decade[14] and have to be distinguished from any sinister cause. Imaging shows a radiolucent lobulated mass. Fine-needle aspiration is often reported as inadequate (C1) due to fat only being aspirated and is not recommended. A pseudolipoma is a mass that clinically appears to be a simple lipoma but is actually caused by a small cancer that produces compressed fat lobules as the suspensory ligaments of the breast shorten. Liposarcomas occur only very rarely in the breast.[83] Larger or symptomatic lipomas can be excised. Some of the larger lipomas develop deep in the fascia overlying the chest wall muscles.

Granular cell tumours

This is an uncommon, usually benign neoplasm that originates from Schwann cells of peripheral nerves in the breast. About 6% of all granular cell tumours involve the breast. The mean age at diagnosis is 40 years. Clinically and on imaging they are difficult to differentiate from a breast carcinoma due to their fibrous consistency, fixation to the pectoral fascia and skin retraction. Granular cell tumours are usually benign but there have been reports of malignant cases. Treatment is by local excision, ensuring a narrow clear margin to prevent recurrence.

Diabetic mastopathy

This is a form of sclerosis occurring in premenopausal women, and occasionally men, with long-standing type I diabetes, often associated with other diabetic complications, particularly retinopathy. It can result clinically in one or more hard masses within the breast that have features making it indistinguishable clinically from malignancy, but on histology the findings are of sclerosing lymphocytic lobulitis or 'diabetic mastopathy'. The disease probably represents an immune reaction to the abnormal accumulation of altered extracellular matrix in the breast, which is a manifestation of the effects of hyperglycaemia on connective tissue. It does not seem to predispose to breast carcinoma or lymphoma and in patients without diabetes it is not clear why some get it and others do not.[84]

Haematomas

These most commonly follow trauma such as a road traffic incident, but can occur after core biopsy, fine-needle aspiration or open biopsy. In extremely unusual circumstances a breast carcinoma may present with a spontaneous haematoma. Breast haematoma can also occur spontaneously in patients on anticoagulant therapy.

Para areola cysts

These cysts are rare and occur in pubertal and post-pubertal teenagers (11–16 years), presenting as discrete superficial cystic masses at the areola margin; occasionally they become infected. They can be interpreted as solid on ultrasonography because of numerous internal echoes. Diagnosis and treatment can be by aspiration, although if they cause no symptoms and ultrasonography shows a cystic lesion, no intervention is required as they disappear with time.

Mondor's disease

Mondor's disease is spontaneous superficial thrombophlebitis of a breast vein. It is often initially painful and often there may be a history of trauma or surgery to the breast. Clinically, there may be a thickened palpable cord with associated erythema. Its aetiology in the absence of surgery, trauma or infection is unknown. It is a self-limiting condition that normally resolves within a couple of weeks but can be very painful. Non-steroidal anti-inflammatory agents massaged over the area of tenderness improve the pain. Mondor's disease most commonly involves one or more of three venous channels: the thoracoepigastric vein, the lateral thoracic vein and the superior epigastric vein. The upper, inner portion of the breast is never involved.

Gynaecomastia

True gynaecomastia is caused by hyperplasia of the stromal and ductal tissue of the male breast. It is responsible for considerable embarrassment and worry and is the commonest condition affecting the male breast (**Fig. 17.13**). Pseudogynaecomastia gives a similar appearance but is due to excess adipose tissue with no increase in stromal or ductal tissue. Both types can present together.[85] Gynaecomastia associated with Klinefelter syndrome is associated with actual lobule formation and a risk of breast cancer approaching that of the female population.

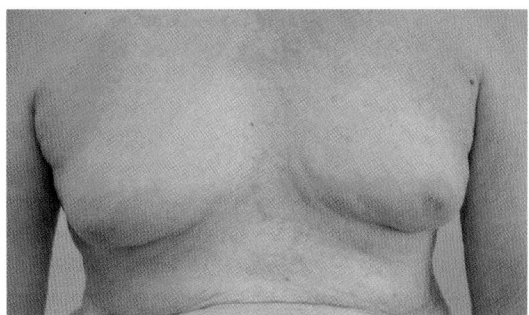

Figure 17.13 • Bilateral senescent gynaecomastia.

Gynaecomastia can occur from any age and presents as a concentric painful swelling. It is a common condition, occurring in at least 35% of men at some time in their life. It is benign and usually reversible. An important differential diagnosis is a primary breast cancer but breast cancers present with eccentric masses that are usually painless.

The aetiology of gynaecomastia is due to a relative hyperoestrogenism.[86] This is caused by decreased androgen production, increased oestrogen production or an increase in peripheral aromatisation. In patients where no endocrine abnormality or drug is found, the cause may be a reduction in androgen receptors and/or a local increase in aromatase activity.[87] Causes can be divided into physiological, pathological, drug induced (medicinal and recreational) and idiopathic. Excess intake of beer or lager can result in gynaecomastia as a consequence of the phyto-oestrogens present in these drinks. A combination of regular cannabis use and drinking large volumes of lager is particularly potent at causing gynaecomastia.

1. Physiological, or primary, gynaecomastia shows a trimodal pattern, with peaks in the neonatal period, puberty and senescence. It is often self-limiting but will occasionally require treatment.
2. Pathological causes are listed in Box 17.1.
3. Common drugs that produce gynaecomastia include: spironolactone (antiandrogen); histamine H$_2$ antagonists, antipsychotics and methyldopa (gonadotrophin disturbance); digoxin, cannabis and griseofulvin (oestrogen receptor competitors); and anabolic steroids (Box 17.2). HIV treatment with highly active anti-retrovirals is also commonly associated.

The degree of gynaecomastia is classified using appearance (Table 17.2). A thorough history will

Box 17.1 • Pathological causes of gynaecomastia

Decreased androgens

Reduced production
- Chromosomal abnormalities, e.g. Klinefelter's syndrome
- Bilateral cryptorchidism
- Hyperprolactinaemia
- Bilateral torsion
- Viral orchitis
- Renal failure

Androgen resistance
- Testicular feminisation

Increased oestrogens

Increased secretion
- Testicular tumours
- Carcinoma of the lung

Increased peripheral aromatisation
- Liver disease
- Adrenal disease
- Thyrotoxicosis

usually elicit the underlying cause. Examination of breast, axilla, testes and abdomen should be performed.

Investigations of gynaecomastia are directed to excluding a primary breast carcinoma or a secondary pathological cause. Biochemical assessment (liver and renal function tests, γ-glutamyltransferase, prolactin, α-fetoprotein, β-human chorionic gonadotrophin and total testosterone) is only required in rapidly growing gynaecomastia. Imaging (with mammography and/or ultrasound) plus biopsy (fine-needle aspiration cytology and/or core biopsy) can be performed if the cause of the gynaecomastia is indeterminate, or if surgery is being considered or cancer is suspected.

Treatment

Reassurance of the transient and benign nature is often all that is required in the management of potential gynaecomastia. More than 80% resolve within 2 years without any treatment. In drug-related gynaecomastia, withdrawal of the drug or change to an alternative should be considered. For pathological gynaecomastia, the underlying cause needs to be addressed.

For those cases requiring treatment there are two options: medical treatment and surgical excision.

Medical management benefits from a high success rate and avoidance of an operation.

> ✅ The evidence for the three commonly prescribed drugs (danazol,[88] tamoxifen[89] and clomifene[90]) is based on small non-randomised trials and does not include recurrence rates, optimum dose, length of treatment or associated long-term risks. Tamoxifen at a dose of 10 mg is the agent of choice.

In the UK, danazol is the only drug licensed for the treatment of gynaecomastia. A short 6-week course is recommended, with 100 mg b.d. for the

Box 17.2 • Drugs associated with gynaecomastia

Hormones
- Anabolic steroids (bodybuilders)
- Oestrogenic agonists
- Antiandrogens (treatment of prostate cancer), e.g. cyproterone acetate, goserelin

Recreational drugs
- Alcohol
- Cannabis
- Heroin

Cardiovascular drugs
- Digoxin
- Spironolactone
- Captopril
- Enalapril
- Amiodarone
- Nefedipine
- Verapamil

Antiulcer drugs
- Cimetidine
- Ranitidine
- Omeprazole

Antibiotics
- Ketoconazole
- Metronidazole
- Minocycline

Psychoactive agents
- Tricylic antidepressants
- Diazepam
- Phenothiazines

Others
- Domperidone
- Metoclopramide
- Penicillamine
- Phenytoin
- Theophylline

Table 17.2 • Classification of gynaecomastia

Grade	Clinical appearance
I	Small but visible breast development with little redundant skin
IIa	Moderate breast development with no redundant skin
IIb	Moderate breast development with redundant skin
III	Marked breast development with much redundant skin

From Simon BE, Hoffman S, Kahn S. Classification and surgical correction of gynecomastia. Plast Reconstr Surg 1973; 51:48–52.[105] With permission from Lippincott, Williams & Wilkins. © American Society of Plastic Surgeons.

first week followed by 100 mg t.d.s. for the second to sixth weeks, response being assessed at the eighth week. Imaging and clinical photography can be used to evaluate success of treatment. Repeat courses may be required. Tamoxifen at a daily dose of 10 mg produces excellent response rates and is the drug we use in the limited number of patients we treat with medication.

Due to the high risk of poor cosmesis associated with gynaecomastia surgery and subsequent risk of litigation, operation should only be considered after medical failure or where the gynaecomastia is large (class IIa/III). Marking the extent of the gynaecomastia prior to surgery is essential. Patients with limited gynaecomastia can have excision performed through a periareolar incision to reduce scarring. The use of lighted retractors and diathermy aids surgery. A disc of breast tissue should be left behind the nipple combined with an intact pectoral fascia and overlying fat to prevent retraction and fixation to the muscle (saucer deformity). Skin flaps are kept thick to prevent deformity and skin necrosis. Patients should be warned about nipple necrosis, sensory changes and recurrence, as well as cosmetic problems. In larger cases excess skin is removed, requiring repositioning of the nipple and even free nipple grafts.[91] In young patients, excess skin often corrects itself without need for excision. The use of liposuction alone or combined with limited surgery or mammotomy improves cosmetic outcomes. Ultrasound-assisted liposuction allows

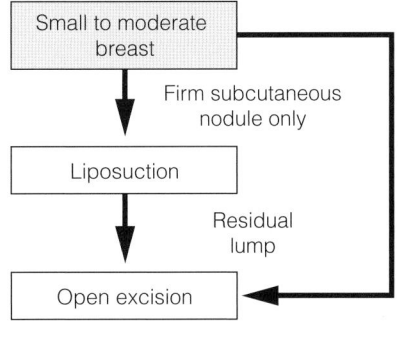

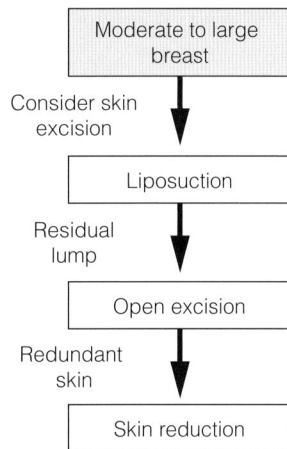

Figure 17.14 • Algorithm for management of gynaecomastia.

treatment of more fibrous areas and increases the number of patients suitable for this technique.[92] An approach to management including liposuction is outlined in **Fig. 17.14**.[93] In those for whom surgery has produced an unsatisfactory cosmetic result, further liposuction and lipofilling can be effective in achieving a satisfactory final result.

Common complications of cosmetic breast surgery

Cosmetic surgical procedures to the breast are increasing in popularity. The frequency of patients presenting with symptoms either as a consequence of previous operations or with an unrelated problem in a patient who has undergone cosmetic surgery means an understanding of such procedures and their complications can allow rapid diagnosis and that the treatment is appropriate. It is *highly* recommended that if there are complications from recent surgery the operating surgeon assesses their own patient runs better. However, it is not uncommon for these patients to be referred to a breast clinic.

Assessment involves a detailed history of the original procedure as well as standard triple assessment. In the augmented patient it is useful to know the type of implant used (particularly with the recent knowledge that some implants have a high rate of leakage and rupture) as well as the size, shape, composition and its position (subpectoral or submammary). The time since surgery and any postoperative surgical complications (e.g. haematoma)

should also be recorded. Examination will show if any breast reductions or mastopexy (breast lift) have been performed. In the patient who has undergone a reduction mammaplasty it is useful to know the approximate volume reduction and whether there were wound healing problems.

Imaging of breasts post-cosmetic surgery can pose technical challenges. Scarring and calcification from fat necrosis is commonly seen after breast reduction and can make mammographic interpretation difficult. Assessment of the augmented breast should include mammography (using the Ekland technique) and ultrasound. Magnetic resonance imaging (MRI) is useful in assessing disease extent and is the technique of choice if implant rupture is suspected. Due to the obvious risk of implant damage, any needle biopsy of an augmented breast should be performed under image guidance.

Breast augmentation complications

Capsular contraction

Any foreign tissue placed within a body will produce a reaction or scar. The scarring around an implant produces a capsule, which contracts over time. Due to the relative inertness of silicone and the textured surface of modern implants, capsular contracture causing symptoms or significant distortion is less common than it used to be. It can be exacerbated by postoperative complications such as haematoma or a subclinical infection. Capsular contraction tends to produce pain, change in shape and hardness of the breast. A grading for capsular contraction is shown in Box 17.3. Treatment depends on severity of symptoms and patient wishes. Removal plus capsulotomy or capsulectomy for rupture is the standard treatment with or without re-augmentation.

Rippling/palpable implant edge

Due to the pressure effect of the implant on the breast tissue, some degree of glandular atrophy can occur. This can make the underlying implant more palpable, especially in the thin woman. Round, non-cohesive implants, due to their softness and fluid nature, can have a palpable 'rippling'. This is commonly felt superiorly when placed submammary in a slim patient or if there is marked ptosis. Rippling and sometimes the implant edge can be felt on the medial or lateral edges if there is a large implant or paucity of glandular cover. Treatment is reassurance and explanation, lipofilling the area above the rippling or revisional surgery to place the implant in the submuscular plane.

Implant rupture

Rupture is most commonly due to implant failure over time but may be caused by trauma or iatrogenic injury. Modern silicone breast implants tend to contain cohesive gel, which tends not to have the same frequency of rupture seen with liquid silicone implants.

Women with rupture present with pain, change in breast shape or a lump. Once identified, treatment is removal of implant plus capsule. Residual silicone can leak into the breast and chest wall and cause a reaction producing hard lumps

(silicone granulomas). Silicone can also migrate to axillary nodes, which can become quite large. They have a snowstorm appearance on ultrasound, which is quite typical. Care should be taken in removing such nodes. They are the sentinel nodes of the breast and aggressive removal of nodes containing silicone can cause both breast and arm oedema. Therefore, these nodes should only be removed if there is definite evidence they are causing symptoms.

Breast reduction problems

Fat necrosis

Scarring and fat necrosis can result from devascularisation of fatty breast tissue or following wound healing problems. This may not be noticed until some time has passed postsurgery. Triple assessment will rule out any malignancy and allow for reassurance. Large areas that are symptomatic can be treated by a combination of liposuction and lipofilling.

Inclusion cyst

An inclusion cyst occurs due to implantation of keratinising squamous epithelium within the dermis if an area of incomplete de-epithelialised skin (usually the pedicle for the nipple) has been buried during a breast reduction operation. A discrete lump may be palpable or an impalpable lesion may be discovered on subsequent mammographic screening.

Assessment of patients with benign breast disease

The current issues include:

- Is a one-stop clinic the best method of diagnosing breast disease?
- Fine-needle aspiration cytology, core biopsy or both?
- Should benign breast disease become the remit of nurse specialists?

One-stop clinics

The aim of the one-stop clinic is to provide the patient with all the relevant investigations and to establish a diagnosis at the initial visit. This requires

---

Box 17.3 • Classification of capsular contraction

Grade I (absent)

The breast is soft with no palpable capsule and looks natural.

Grade II (minimal)

The breast is slightly firm, with a palpable capsule but looks normal.

Grade III (moderate)

The breast is firm with an easily palpable capsule and looks abnormal.

Grade IV (severe)

The breast is hard, cold, painful and distorted.

the availability of a breast radiologist to provide immediate interpretation of the examination and investigations. Even with all these available, a definitive diagnosis is not always possible.[94] There are benefits in reducing anxiety in such a service (*especially in the majority with normal breasts or benign disease*) but this benefit is only in the short term.[95] Patients like these clinics and they reduce the number of clinic visits and letters, improving administration efficiency. Although there have been concerns that immediate reporting may affect accuracy and that there may be a possible detrimental psychological aspect for those with cancer,[96] these are more than offset by the benefits. It is well recognised that at the time when a patient is given bad news, little other information provided in the consultation is remembered. By concentrating on establishing and delivering a diagnosis at the first visit, it is then possible to have a more useful and constructive second visit to consider management of any cancer detected.

Fine-needle aspiration cytology, core biopsy or both?

Fine-needle aspiration cytology was the mainstay of diagnosis of symptomatic breast lumps for more than 30 years. Its introduction allowed preoperative diagnosis and avoided a large number of open excision biopsies. It has the benefit of being easy to perform, but can cause patient discomfort and has a high sensitivity and specificity (in experienced hands[97]). The result can be interpreted quickly, allowing rapid diagnosis. Its major disadvantage is that it does not provide architectural information on the area examined and therefore cannot differentiate in situ and invasive disease. It has been reported that it is possible to grade tumours on cytology[98] and although it can provide oestrogen receptor status,[99] full profiling is not possible from cytology.

✅ Core biopsy has taken over as the preoperative technique of choice for diagnosing palpable breast lumps and areas of nodularity.[100] The improved sensitivity and specificity and greater information available (architecture, oestrogen receptor and human epidermal growth factor receptor 2 (HER-2) status, grade, presence of vascular invasion or calcification) with core biopsy is the reason for this change.

There is little if any benefit from combining fine-needle aspiration (FNA) and core biopsy as FNA disrupts the cancer, makes it more difficult to visualise and this may adversely affect subsequent core biopsy accuracy. The only continuing role of FNA in patients with breast cancer is in assessment of suspicious lymph nodes. If recurrence is suspected core biopsy should be performed of the recurrence because knowledge of the current ER and HER-2 status of the cancer is essential and these can differ from the initial primary tumour.

There is increasing evidence that symptomatic lumps should be biopsied under ultrasound guidance.[101] This ensures that the abnormality is visualised with the biopsy needle within it, improving sensitivity. Suitably trained surgeons or breast physicians, as well as radiologists, can undertake these biopsies safely.[102]

Future management of benign breast disease

The last few years have seen the expansion of breast physicians, nurse specialists and the formation of nurse consultants. Their roles have expanded to help with the increasing breast workload and the lack of breast specialists. There is evidence that such professionals can play an important part in symptomatic clinics, perform follow-up clinics and run symptom-specific clinics (e.g. mastalgia clinics) as long as there is specialist back-up.[103,104] The future roles of these individuals are likely to expand. One note of caution: in a clinic of 30 symptomatic patients run by three or four individuals, there will be an average three cancers – that is, one per individual in the clinic. If a nurse specialist does one new patient clinic once a week, they may only see 40–45 cases of breast cancer per year. Some breast abnormalities and cancer types are rare. What is not clear is what is adequate training for such individuals. If any individual is to give a 'consultant' opinion in such clinics, then ideally they should have seen hundreds of breast cancers and the whole range of common and rare presentations before they make final decisions on whether patients can be discharged. This is also true for trainees who cover for consultant surgeons in such clinics. The breast surgeons of the future may be less involved in diagnosis and more active surgically.

Key points

- The majority of patients seen in a breast clinic have normal breasts or benign disease.
- Many conditions occur so commonly against the background of breast development, cyclical activity and involution that they are best considered aberrations of this process.
- Following a diagnosis of benign disease, reassurance alone is insufficient. An explanation of the cause, possible risks and treatment options is required.
- Spontaneous, single-duct persistent (>2 per week) or bloodstained nipple discharge requires a definitive diagnosis that may only be obtained by duct excision.
- Breast pain is common and the majority originates in the underlying chest wall, not the breast itself.
- For true cyclical breast pain, tamoxifen is effective.
- Breast cysts diagnosed on ultrasound require aspiration only if symptomatic or complex on scan.
- Breast infection requires early antibiotic therapy and rapid referral to hospital if it does not settle rapidly on antibiotics.
- Breast abscesses should be assessed by ultrasound and treated by repeated aspiration or mini-incision and drainage.
- Gynaecomastia is an increasing problem. The cause should be ascertained and surgery only performed after other options have been exhausted.

References

1. Thrush S, Sayer G, Scott-Coombes D, et al. Is the grading of referrals to a specialist breast unit appropriate or effective? Br Med J 2002;324:1279.

2. Down S, Barr L, Baildam AD, et al. Management of accessory breast tissue in the axilla. Br J Surg 2003;90:1213–4.

3. Aydogan F, Baghaki S, Celik V, et al. Surgical treatment of axillary accessory breasts. Am Surg 2010;76(3):270–2.

4. Nerakha GJ. In: Gallager HS, Leis HP, Synderman RK, et al., editors. The breast. St Louis, MO: Mosby; 1978. p. 442–51.

5. Pinsolle V, Chichery A, Grolleau JL, et al. Autologous fat injection in Poland's syndrome. J Plast Reconstr Aesthet Surg 2008;61(7):784–91.

6. Delay E, Garson S, Tousson G, et al. Fat injection to the breasts: technique, results and indications based on 880 procedures over 10 years. Aesthet Surg J 2009;29:360–76.

7. Hall-Findlay EJ. Vertical breast reduction using the superomedial pedicle. In: Speark SL, editor. Surgery of the breast, principles and art. Philadelphia: Lippincott Williams & Wilkins; 2006. p. 1072–92.

8. Hughes LE, Mansel RE, Webster DJ. Aberrations of normal development and involution (ANDI): a new perspective on pathogenesis and nomenclature of benign breast disorders. Lancet 1987;ii:1316–9.

9. World Health Organisation. Histological typing of breast tumours. 2nd ed. Geneva: WHO; 1981.

10. Dixon JM, Dobie V, Lamb J, et al. Assessment of the acceptability of conservative management

of fibroadenoma of the breast. Br J Surg 1996;83:264–5.

11. Hughes LE, Mansel RE, Webster DJT. Benign disorders of the breast. London: Bailliére Tindall; 2001.

12. Ozzello L, Gump FE. The management of patients with carcinomas in fibroadenomatous tumors of the breast. Surg Gynecol Obstet 1985;160:99–104.

13. Sperber F, Blank A, Metser U, et al. Diagnosis and treatment of breast fibroadenomas by ultrasound guided vacuum-assisted biopsy. Arch Surg 2003;138:796–800.

14. Haagenson CD. Diseases of the breast. 3rd ed. Philadelphia: WB Saunders; 1986.

15. Guillot E, Couturaud B, Reyal F, et al. Management of phyllodes breast tumors. Breast J 2011;17(2):129–37.

16. Dixon JM, Mansel RE. ABC of breast diseases: symptoms, assessment and guidelines for referral. Br Med J 1994;309:722–6.

17. King EB, Chew KC, Petrakis NL, et al. Nipple aspiration cytology for the study of pre-cancer precursors. J Natl Cancer Inst 1983;71:1115–21.

18. Chen L, Zhou WB, Zhao Y, et al. Bloody nipple discharge is a predictor of breast cancer risk: a meta-analysis. Breast Cancer Res Treat 2012;132(1):9–14.

19. Ambrogetti D, Berni D, Catarzi S, et al. The role of ductal galactography in the differential diagnosis of breast carcinoma. Radiol Med (Torino) 1996;91:198–201.

20. Selzer MH, Perloff LJ, Kelley RI, et al. Significance of age in patients with nipple discharge. Surg Gynecol Obstet 1970;131:519.

21. Simmons R, Adamovich T, Brennan M, et al. Nonsurgical evaluation of pathologic nipple discharge. Ann Surg Oncol 2003;10:113–6.

22. Groves AM, Carr M, Wadhera V, et al. An audit of cytology in the evaluation of nipple discharge: a retrospective study of 10 years' experience. Breast 1996;5:96.

23. Dooley WS. Routine operative breast endoscopy for bloody nipple discharge. Ann Surg Oncol 2002;9:920–3.

24. Matsunaga T, Ohta D, Misaka T, et al. A utility of ductography and fibreoptic ductoscopy for patients with nipple discharge. Breast Cancer Res Treat 2001;70:103–8.

25. Shen KW, Wu J, Lu JS, et al. Fiberoptic ductoscopy for breast cancer patients with nipple discharge. Surg Endosc 2001;15:1340–5.

26. King BL, Love SM, Rochman S, et al. The Fourth International Symposium on the Intraductal Approach to Breast Cancer, Santa Barbara, California, 10–13 March 2005. Breast Cancer Res 2005;7(5):198–204.

27. Ambrogetti D, Berni D, Catarzi S, et al. The role of ductal galactography in the differential diagnosis of breast carcinoma. Radiol Med (Torino) 1996;91:198–201.

28. Khan SA, Baird C, Staradub VL, et al. Ductal lavage and ductoscopy: the opportunities and the limitations. Clin Breast Cancer 2002;3:185–95.

29. Van Zee KJ, Ortega Perez G, Minnard E, et al. Preoperative galactography increases the diagnostic yield of major duct excision for nipple discharge. Cancer 1998;82:1874.

30. Pisano ED, Gatsonis C, Hendrick E, et al., The Digital Mammographic Imaging Screening Trial (DMIST) Investigators Group. Diagnostic performance of digital versus film mammography for breast-cancer. N Engl J Med 2005;353(17):1773–83.

31. Cabioglu N, Hunt KK, Singletary SE, et al. Surgical decision making and factors determining a diagnosis of breast cancer in women presenting with nipple discharge. J Am Coll Surg 2003;196:354–64.

32. Helbich TH, Matzek W, Fuchsjager MH. Stereotactic and ultrasound-guided breast biopsy. Eur Radiol 2004;14:383–93.

33. Van Zee KJ, Ortega Perez G, Minnard E, et al. Preoperative galactography increases the diagnostic yield of major duct excision for nipple discharge. Cancer 1998;82:1874–80.

34. Rosen PP, Cantrell B, Mullen DL, et al. Juvenile papillomatosis (Swiss cheese disease) of the breast. Am J Surg Pathol 1980;4:3–12.

35. Lafreniere R. Bloody nipple discharge during pregnancy: a rationale for conservative treatment. J Surg Oncol 1990;43:228–30.

36. Sharma R, Dietz J, Wright H, et al. Comparative analysis of minimally invasive microductectomy versus major duct excision in patients with pathologic nipple discharge. Surgery 2005;138(4):591–7.

37. Dixon JM, Kohlhardt SR, Dillon P. Total duct excision. Breast 1998;7:216–9.

38. Peters F, Pickardt CR, Zimmerman G, et al. TSH and thyroid hormones in benign breast disease. Klin Wochenschr 1981;59:403–7.

39. England PC, Skinner LG, Cotterell KM, et al. Serum oestradiol-17β in women with benign and malignant breast disease. Br J Cancer 1974;30:571–6.

40. Sitruk-Ware R, Sterkers N, Mauvais-Jarvis P. Benign breast disease. 1. Hormonal investigation. Obstet Gynecol 1979;53:457–60.

41. Gateley CA, Maddox PR, Pritchard GA, et al. Plasma fatty acid profiles in benign breast disorders. Br J Surg 1992;79:407–9.

42. Mansel RE. ABC of breast diseases: breast pain. Br Med J 1994;309:866–8.

43. Barros AC, Mottola J, Ruiz CA, et al. Reassurance in the treatment of mastalgia. Breast J 1999;5:162–5.

44. Khoo SK, Munro C, Battistutta D. Evening primrose oil and treatment of premenstrual syndrome. Med J Aust 1990;153:189–92.

45. Blommers J, de Lange-De Klerk ES, Kuik DJ, et al. Evening primrose oil and fish oil for severe chronic mastalgia: a randomised, double blind controlled trial. Am J Obstet Gynecol 2002;187:1389–94.

46. Pashby NH, Mansel RE, Hughes LE, et al. A clinical trial of evening primrose oil in mastalgia. Br J Surg 1981;68:801–24.

47. McFayden IJ, Chetty U, Setchell KDR, et al. A randomized double blind crossover trial of soya protein for the treatment of cyclical breast pain. Breast 2000;9:271–6.

48. Halaska M, Raus K, Beles P, et al. Treatment of cyclical mastodynia using an extract of *Vitex agnus castus*: results of a double blind comparison with a placebo. Cesk Gynekol 1998;63:388–92.

49. Boyd NF, McGuire V, Shannon P, et al. Effect of a low-fat high-carbohydrate diet on symptoms of clinical mastopathy. Lancet 1988;ii:128–32.

50. Fentiman IS, Caleffi M, Brame K, et al. Double blind controlled trial of tamoxifen therapy for mastalgia. Lancet 1986;i:287–8.

51. GEMB Group Argentine. Tamoxifen therapy for cyclical mastalgia: dose randomised trial. Breast 1997;5:212–3.

52. Kontostolis E, Stefanidis K, Navrozoglou I, et al. Comparison of tamoxifen with danazol for treatment of cyclical mastalgia. Gynecol Endocrinol 1997;11:393–7.

53. O'Brien PM, Abukhalil IE. Randomised controlled trial of the management of premenstrual syndrome and premenstrual mastalgia using luteal phase-only danazol. Am J Obstet Gynecol 1999;180:18–23.

54. Mansel R, Goyal A, Le Nestour E, et al., Afimoxifene (4-OHT) Breast Pain Research Group A phase II trial of Afimoxifene (4-hydroxytamoxifen gel) for cyclical

mastalgia in premenopausal women. Breast Cancer Res Treat 2007;106(3):389–97.

55. Gong C, Song E, Jia W, et al. A double-blind randomized controlled trial of toremifen therapy for mastalgia. Arch Surg 2006;141(1):43–7.

56. Blichert-Toft M, Anderson AN, Henrikson D, et al. Treatment of mastalgia with bromocriptine: a double blind crossover study. Br Med J 1979;1:273.

57. Eriksson E. Serotonin reuptake inhibitors for the treatment of premenstrual dysphoria. Int Clin Psychopharmacol 1999;14(Suppl. 2):S27–33.

58. Dixon JM, McDonald C, Elton RA, et al. Risk of breast cancer in women with palpable breast cysts. Lancet 1999;353:1742–5.

59. Jacobs TW, Byrne C, Colditz G, et al. Radial scars in benign breast-biopsy specimens and the risk of breast cancer. N Engl J Med 1999;340(6):430–6.

60. Brenner RJ, Jackman RJ, Parker SH, et al. Percutaneous core needle biopsy of radial scars of the breast: when is excision necessary? AJR Am J Roentgenol 2002;179(5):1179–84.

61. Thrush S, Banergee S, Sayer G, et al. Breast sepsis: a unit's experience. Br J Surg 2002;89(Suppl. 1):75–6.

62. Goodman MA, Benson EA. An evaluation of the current trends in the management of breast abscesses. Med J Aust 1970;1:1034–9.

63. Schafer P, Furrer C, Merillod B. An association between smoking with recurrent subareolar breast abscess. Int J Epidemiol 1988;17:810–3.

64. Petrakis NL, Maack CA, Lee RE, et al. Mutagenic activity of nipple aspirates of breast fluid. Cancer Res 1980;40:188–9.

65. Ertel A, Eng R, Smith SM. The differential effect of cigarette smoke on the growth of bacteria found in humans. Chest 1991;100:628–30.

66. Rogers K. Breast abscess and problems with lactation. In: Smallwood JA, Talor I, editors. Benign breast disease. London: Edward Arnold; 1990. p. 96.

67. Gupta R, Sinnett D, Carpenter R, et al. Antibiotic prophylaxis for post-operative wound infection in elective breast surgery. Eur J Surg Oncol 2000;26:363–6.

68. Collis N, Mirza S, Stanley PR, et al. Reduction of potential contamination of breast implants by the use of 'nipple shields'. Br J Plast Surg 1999;52:445–7.

69. Zippel D, Siegelmann-Danieli N, Ayalon S, et al. Delayed breast cellulitis following breast conservation operations. Eur J Surg Oncol 2003;29:327–30.

70. Nahabedian MY, Tsangaris T, Momen B, et al. Infectious complications following breast reconstruction with expanders and implants. Plast Reconstr Surg 2003;112:467–76.

71. Hayes R, Mitchell M, Nunnerley HB. Acute inflammation of the breast: the role of breast ultrasound in diagnosis and management. Clin Radiol 1991;44:253–6.

72. Dixon JM. Repeated aspiration of breast abscesses in lactating women. Br Med J 1988;297:1517–8.

73. O'Hara RJ, Dexter SPL, Fox JN. Conservative management of infective mastitis and breast abscesses after ultrasonographic assessment. Br J Surg 1996;83:1413–4.

74. Dixon JM. Outpatient treatment of non-lactational breast abscesses. Br J Surg 1992;79:56–7.

75. Dixon JM, editor. ABC of breast. London: BMJ Publications; 2000.

76. Bundred NJ, Dixon JM, Chetty U, et al. Mammary fistula. Br J Surg 1991;78:1185.

77. Hanavadi S, Pereira G, Mansel RE. How mammillary fistulas should be managed. Breast J 2005;11(4):254–6.

78. Thomsen AC, Espersen T, Maigaard S. Course and treatment of milk stasis, non-infectious inflammation of the breast and infectious mastitis in nursing women. Am J Obstet Gynecol 1984;149:492–5.

79. Anonymous, Single dose cabergoline versus bromocriptine in inhibition of puerperal lactation: randomised, double blind, multicentre study. European Multicentre Study Group for Cabergoline in Lactation Inhibition. Br Med J 1991;302:1367–71.

80. Howell JD, Barker F, Gazet J-C. Granulomatous lobular mastitis: report of further two cases and comprehensive literature review. Breast 1994;3:119–23.

81. Paviour S, Musaad S, Roberts S, et al. *Corynebacterium* species isolated from patients with mastitis. Clin Infect Dis 2002;35:1434–40.

82. Taylor GB, Paviour SD, Musaad S, et al. A clinicopathological review of 34 cases of inflammatory breast disease showing an association between corynebacteria infection and granulomatous mastitis. Pathology 2003;35:109–19.

83. Blanchard DK, Reynolds CA, Grant CS, et al. Primary nonphylloides breast sarcomas. Am J Surg 2003;186:359–61.

84. Kudva YC, Reynolds CA, O'Brien T, et al. Mastopathy and diabetes. Curr Diab Rep 2003;3:56–9.

85. Daniels IR, Layer GT. How should gynaecomastia be managed? Aust N Z J Surg 2003;73:213–6.

86. Carlson HE. Gynecomastia. N Engl J Med 1980;303:795–9.

87. Ismail AA, Barth JH. Endocrinology of gynaecomastia. Ann Clin Biochem 2001;38:596–607.

88. Jones DJ, Holt SD, Surtees P, et al. A comparison of danazol and placebo in the treatment of adult idiopathic gynaecomastia: results of a prospective study in 55 patients. Ann R Coll Surg Engl 1990;72:296–8.

89. Khan HN, Blamey RW. Endocrine treatment of physiological gynaecomastia. Br Med J 2003;327:301–2.

90. Plourde PV, Kulin HE, Santner SJ. Clomiphene in the treatment of adolescent gynecomastia. Clinical and endocrine studies. Am J Dis Child 1983;137:1080–2.

91. Wray Jr RC, Hoopes JE, Davis GM. Correction of extreme gynaecomastia. Br J Plast Surg 1974;27:39–41.

92. Samdal F, Kleppe G, Amland PF, et al. Surgical treatment of gynaecomastia. Five years' experience with liposuction. Scand J Plast Reconstr Surg Hand Surg 1994;28:123–30.

93. Fruhstorfer BH, Malata CM. A systematic approach to the surgical treatment of gynaecomastia. Br J Plast Surg 2003;56:237–46.

94. Eltahir A, Jibril JA, Squair J, et al. The accuracy of 'one stop' diagnosis for 1110 patients presenting to a symptomatic breast clinic. J R Coll Surg Edinb 1999;44:226–30.

95. Dey P, Bundred N, Gibbs A, et al. Costs and benefits of a one stop clinic compared with a dedicated breast clinic: randomised controlled trial. Br Med J 2002;324:507–10.

96. Harcourt D, Ambler N, Rumsey N, et al. Evaluation of a one-stop breast clinic: a randomised controlled trial. Breast 1998;7:314–9.

97. Dixon JM, Lamb J, Anderson TJ. Fine needle aspiration of the breast: importance of the operator. Lancet 1983;ii:564.

98. Robinson IA, McKee G, Nicholson A, et al. Prognostic value of cytological grading of fine-needle aspirates from breast carcinomas. Lancet 1994;343:947–9.

99. Zoppi JA, Rotundo AV, Sundblad AS. Correlation of immunocytochemical and immunohistochemical determination of estrogen and progesterone receptors in breast cancer. Acta Cytol 2002;46:337–40.

100. Britton PD. Fine needle aspiration or core biopsy? Breast 1999;8:1–4.

101. Hatada T, Ishii H, Ichii S, et al. Diagnostic value of ultrasound-guided fine needle aspiration biopsy, core needle biopsy, and evaluation of combined use in the diagnosis of breast lumps. J Am Coll Surg 2000;190:299–303.

102. Whitehouse PA, Baber Y, Brown G, et al. The use of ultrasound by breast surgeons in outpatients: an accurate extension of clinical diagnosis. Eur J Surg Oncol 2001;27:611–6.

103. Garvican L, Grimsey E, Littlejohns P, et al. Satisfaction with clinical nurse specialists in a breast care clinic: questionnaire survey. Br Med J 1998;316:976–7.

104. Earnshaw JJ, Stephenson Y. First two years of a follow-up breast clinic led by a nurse practitioner. J R Soc Med 1997;90:258–9.

105. Simon BE, Hoffman S, Kahn S. Classification and surgical correction of gynaecomastia. Plast Reconstr Surg 1973;51:48–52.

18

Litigation in breast surgery

Tim Davidson
Tom Bates

Introduction

Litigation for clinical negligence has accelerated at an alarming rate. In 2009/10 the NHS paid out £787 m (including £164 m for defence and claimant legal costs).[1] In the USA, the value of malpractice claims for delay in the diagnosis of breast cancer 15 years ago was second only to that for neurological damage to neonates[2,3] and today this situation remains unchanged.[4] Poor cosmetic outcome is also a frequent cause for litigation and heightened public awareness has increased patients' expectations of recompense for real or perceived injury following both cosmetic and reconstructive breast surgery.

Basic principles

The legal process differs between countries and although this chapter is based on civil law in England and Wales, the general principles in use elsewhere are similar.[5] For a claimant to succeed in law, she must satisfy the court (in the UK a judge, or in some countries a jury) that there was a failure or breach of duty of care (*liability*) and that as a foreseeable result she suffered an injury (*causation*). For the case to succeed, the court must find in favour of the claimant with regard both to liability and to causation. Clinical negligence cases are heard in civil court and the judge determines *on the balance of probabilities* whether the

defendant is liable. This is entirely different from a criminal court determining guilt or innocence where the level of proof is *beyond all reasonable doubt* (which many equate to a degree of confidence >95%). If the court finds in favour of the claimant, the court awards financial recompense to redress, as far as money is able, the injury that she has suffered.

Breach of duty

Duty of care

Any doctor – GP, radiologist, surgeon or pathologist – owes each individual patient a duty of care. This is rarely an issue. In the NHS the doctor acts as an employee of the hospital or health board, which is covered by the NHS Litigation Authority, which administers a scheme that acts as a mutual insurer for participating trusts (Clinical Negligence Scheme for Trusts).[6] When acting in a private capacity, the doctor is covered by a professional defence organisation of his or her choice.

The Bolam test

A doctor is not negligent if he or she acts in accordance with a practice accepted at the time as proper by a responsible body of medical opinion. The Bolam test arises from the case of a patient who received electroconvulsive therapy and sustained fractures.[7] Negligence was alleged because the patient was not given muscle relaxants and was inadequately restrained. Some doctors would have used muscle relaxants and restraints, others not. The doctor was not found negligent because he acted in accordance with a practice accepted at the time, even though other doctors may have advocated a different practice.

The Bolitho modification of Bolam adds the requirement that for the practice or opinion formed to be acceptable, it must be based on logical argument; an irrational practice cannot be argued as reasonable in court simply because a body of medical opinion agrees with its use.[8]

The Bolam test requires a higher degree of skill from a specialist in his or her own field than from a GP. If a patient is referred to a breast surgeon and the standard of care falls below that which the patient could reasonably have expected from a breast specialist, there has been a breach of the duty of care. The standard of care needs to be determined by an appropriate peer group, so a GP expert would be asked by the court to advise on breach of duty on the part of a GP whereas a specialist expert would be asked to give an opinion on the standard of care delivered by a breast surgeon.

Guidelines

National and local guidelines of good clinical practice are now in use throughout the NHS with guidelines covering patient referral, diagnosis, treatment and organisational arrangements within breast units.[9,10] Breaches of guidelines are not indicative of, or equivalent to, negligent practice and guidelines are constantly being amended in the light of scientific knowledge, healthcare resources, government targets, etc. Consideration must always be given to the time at which the alleged breach of duty took place and for a guideline to be relevant it must have been in the public domain at the time.

Clinical practice that complies with guidelines is inevitably much easier to defend against allegations of negligence. A diagnostic excision biopsy exceeding 20 g, as set out in NHS Breast Screening Programme guidelines, does not equate to negligent practice; however, a patient claiming excessive deformity after such a procedure is unlikely to succeed in litigation if her biopsy specimen weighed under 20 g. There is ongoing debate regarding the medicolegal implications of surgical guidelines.[11] Carrick et al.[12] reported that whereas 41% of surgeons surveyed believed that guidelines would protect them against litigation, 37% believed that they would increase their exposure to claims.

Consent

Doctors have been made increasingly aware of the need to warn patients of the risks involved with any diagnostic or therapeutic procedure, to involve patients in decision-making and to seek fully informed consent. Patient information leaflets, involvement of breast-care nurses and more detailed consent forms signed by the operating surgeon are now standard practice but have done little to stem the tide of litigation as expectations continue to rise. Consent obtained by a junior doctor without the knowledge and skill to undertake the intended procedure or to discuss the possible complications is no longer considered acceptable. The degree of disclosure is primarily a matter of clinical judgment, but major complications (such as loss of a flap in breast reconstruction) must be included even if their occurrence is rare.[5,13] Where a procedure (such as breast reduction) is being undertaken primarily for cosmetic reasons, the surgeon is advised to include even minor potential consequences in the documentation of informed consent.

Causation

The second hurdle to be overcome by the claimant is to prove that the negligent act caused an injury that was forseeable. Causation may be obvious (from clinical examination or photographic records) where there is a poor cosmetic outcome from breast reduction, but may be difficult to prove where there has been a delay in the diagnosis of breast cancer.

The award of damages

The sole remedy available to the successful claimant is an award of damages – a sum of money intended to restore the claimant to the position she would have been in but for the negligent act. Explanation and apology to the claimant or her family, desirable though they may be, are not within the power of civil law, nor are recommendations for retraining, suspension or deregistration of doctors who find themselves as defendants. Patients seeking to hold their doctor to account are, however, increasingly turning to the fitness to practice procedures of the

General Medical Council (GMC), with such enquiries rising 30% between 2004 and 2009.[14] An unhappy patient may both embark on litigation and report the doctor to the GMC, with the practitioner facing so-called double jeopardy.

The award comprises two components, general and special damages. General damages compensate for pain, suffering and loss of amenity, and are based upon judicial guidelines that are upgraded regularly to allow for inflation. Special damages are specific to the individual claimant and include past losses, which can be identified with some accuracy, and estimated future losses. It is the future loss of earnings and the costs of providing care for the claimant or dependants that generate very high claims. A young woman with children and a high income will attract a high value award if she (or her surviving family) can demonstrate that her premature death resulted from substandard care.

In English law the perceived culpability or magnitude of the negligent act has no bearing on the sum awarded. This contrasts with the position in the USA, where cases that proceed to trial (the minority) rely on jury decisions that often incorporate an element of punitive or exemplary damages, a sum the jury considers warranted by the wrongfulness of the defendant's act. The extent to which this affects the size of the award can be seen by comparing the average value of claims concluded by settlement ($282 000) with that secured by jury verdict ($870 000).[3]

The Woolf report

In a review of the UK civil justice system, Lord Woolf singled out clinical negligence cases[15] because the difficulty in proving both liability and causation accounts for much of the excessive cost and the high proportion of cases that fail. The root of the problem, however, lies less in the complexity of the law than in the climate of defensiveness. The patient's disappointment when treatment goes wrong is heightened by what she perceives to be a refusal to acknowledge fault and an attempt to cover up.

The general rule is that 'costs follow the event' – so the unsuccessful party is responsible for the costs of both sides. Privately financed claimants or lawyers acting on a no-win, no-fee basis are therefore reluctant to pursue actions where the chances of success are small. However, if the claimant is supported by legal aid and loses the case, costs are not recoverable by the defendant. Most claims in the UK are legally aided because of the high costs of litigation; often the defendant is an NHS Trust, hence expenses incurred by both the claimant and defendant are funded from the public purse. In cases valued at less than £12 500, the median figure for the costs of litigation was 137% of the value of the claim. This explains the pressure to settle low-value claims even if defensible and a reluctance to appeal a doubtful judgment.

The recommendations of the Woolf report are intended to improve the resolution of disputes between patients and doctors, and reduce delay and costs while treating both parties fairly:

- Pre-litigation protocol where claimants should notify defendants with a written intention to sue 3 months before action. If liability is disputed, defendants should provide a reasoned answer.
- Lists on the Queen's Bench to include a list of judges familiar with clinical negligence cases and training of trial judges in medical issues.
- Fast-track options for claims under £10 000 so that these can be litigated on a modest budget with a single expert acceptable to both parties appointed by the court.
- The medical expert is now required to address his report to the court and not to the instructing party,[16] with an overriding duty 'to provide objective unbiased opinion to the court on matters within his expertise, never assuming the role of an advocate'.

The burden (level) of proof

In civil litigation the court determines the facts, which means that the judge makes a decision *on the balance of probabilities*. This means that the successful claimant will normally recover damages in full, although in one case where the claimant was held to have lost an 80% chance of cure, a deputy high court judge directed that damages should be calculated accordingly.[17]

The all-or-none nature in awarding damages is arguably the most troubling aspect for experts involved in clinical negligence.[18] For example, if the court finds that as a result of negligence a woman has suffered a reduction in her chance of survival from 60% to 40%, she will be awarded the full amount to compensate her (or her family) as though the loss had already occurred, on the basis that on balance she is now more likely to die. If the court finds, however, that her chance of survival has reduced from 90% to 60%, it may award her nothing on the basis that on balance her chance of survival remains unchanged.

In the case of *Hotson* v. *East Berkshire Area Health Authority* (1987), the House of Lords formulated the current UK position on causation. The defendant was in breach of duty in failing to diagnose a fracture of a femoral epiphysis following a fall. The child developed avascular necrosis with significant disability. The evidence was that the child had a 75% risk of developing this complication due to the accident and the trial judge and the Court of Appeal held that he was entitled to 25% of his damages for the 25% loss of a chance that prompt treatment might have prevented the complication. However, the House of Lords overturned the decision and held that on balance he was going to develop it even in the absence of negligence or, put another way, he had failed to establish that he was within the 25% who would not develop it.

The position on causation was again recognised in the appeal case of *Gregg* v. *Scott* (2002), a claim for failure to diagnose an axillary lump as non-Hodgkin's lymphoma. The Court of Appeal held that the delay had reduced his chance of survival, although this had always been less than 50%, from 42% to 25% survival at 10 years. The case was appealed to the House of Lords who dismissed the claimant's appeal for loss of a chance and upheld the traditional approach. So the burden of proof in deciding causation, for the time being at least, remains unchanged.

Delay in the diagnosis of breast cancer

Delay in diagnosis may occur as a result of failure to refer the patient from primary care or, once referral has taken place, for example with false-negative mammography, failure to perform triple assessment, misinterpretation of equivocal results or the misfiling of a positive test result.[19]

Litigation arising from delay in diagnosis concerns two main areas:

- Did the delay necessitate more extensive treatment?
  Where the patient has had a mastectomy on the basis of tumour size, it is often claimed that earlier diagnosis would have made breast conservative surgery an option. For multifocal tumours, it can be argued that mastectomy would have been needed from the outset. With the advent of sentinel node biopsy, a claimant who has undergone axillary clearance for involved nodes may contest that earlier diagnosis at a time when her nodes were clear would have allowed less radical axillary surgery. When the patient has received chemotherapy it might be argued that this would not have been necessary if the diagnosis had been made sooner when, for example, the axillary nodes would on balance have been negative.

- Did the delay in diagnosis reduce the chance of cure?
  This is a controversial area since there is public expectation, promoted over the years by health campaigners, that earlier diagnosis offers better chance of a cure. Where expert opinion is divided, the court often prefers the evidence in favour of the delay having caused a reduced survival time. A review of claims for diagnostic delay in breast cancer in Sweden over a 10-year period concluded that delays had an impact on treatment in 23% of cases and adversely affected prognosis in 11% of those patients for whom the delay was longer than 12 months.[20]

Delay in primary care

The GP who sees many cases with benign breast symptoms each year but only one or two breast cancers is in a difficult position and GPs are increasingly facing litigation for delays in referral. The main area of contention is where long-standing or recurrent breast nodularity coexists with an (initially) undetected lump. Relying on a negative mammogram without an expert clinical examination, ultrasound or needle biopsy may increase the risk of false reassurance.[19]

GPs today are therefore faced with referring most women with breast symptoms for a specialist opinion and referral guidelines have been in use in the UK since 1995.[21-23]

Delay after specialist referral

Breast units throughout the UK submit audit data on compliance with 2-week *target* referrals for suspected cancers.[24] The prioritisation of referral letters can be counter-productive if non-urgent cases have to wait longer, but current NHS guidelines stipulate all symptomatic breast referrals are now seen within 2 weeks. NHS '31/62' cancer targets (allowing 31 days from urgent referral to diagnosis and 62 days to commencing treatment) will identify units in breach of national guidelines.

The role of triple assessment, and the circumstances in which it fails, are critical. The specialist centre is also faced with the problem that women under 35 form the majority of the diagnostic workload (66%) but the fewest number of breast cancers (3%).[21]

The North American experience

Two studies commissioned by the Physician Insurers Association of America (PIAA)[2,3] showed delay in the diagnosis of breast cancer to be the commonest cause of clinical litigation, and a striking feature of both studies was young age: women under 50 accounted for 69% of claimants and received 84% of the damages paid, whereas only 25% of cancers occur in women under 50.

The most common reasons cited for the delay were (in descending order):

- physical findings failed to impress;
- failure to follow up the patient;
- negative mammogram report or misreading of the mammogram;
- failure to perform a biopsy.

In 487 cases where liability was admitted, the mean delay was 14 months. The mean payout was $301 000, with higher damages for longer delays and to younger patients.[3]

Diagnosis of breast cancer

Triple assessment is the foundation upon which clinicians diagnose breast lumps. However, the extent to which the accuracy of these tests is reduced in younger women is not well appreciated (**Fig. 18.1**). It has been suggested that perfection of diagnosis will require removal of every solid mass,[25] but this would represent a retrograde step. The practice of defensive medicine, in place of conventional wisdom, may well be encouraged by a litigious public and diagnostic tests where the sensitivity falls below 95%.

Physical examination

About 70% of all breast cancers are palpable, but with tumours of 0.6–1 cm diameter this figure falls

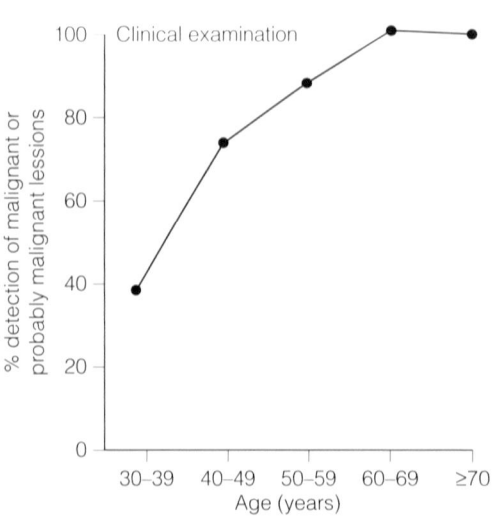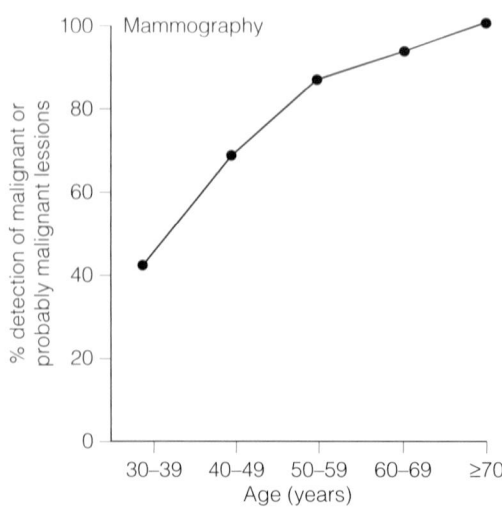

Figure 18.1 • Sensitivity of clinical and mammographic examination by age. Reproduced from Dixon JM, Mansel RE. Symptoms, assessment and guidelines for referral. In: Dixon JM (ed.) ABC of breast diseases, 2nd edn. London: BMJ Books, 2000; p. 6. With permission from Wiley Publishing Ltd.

to 50%.[26] The larger the breast and the greater the density of breast tissue, the more difficult physical examination becomes. Cyclical changes in breast parenchyma may require repeat examination at different phases of the menstrual cycle. Coexisting benign lumps, scars and distortion from previous surgery, the ridge of tissue above the inframammary fold, changes during pregnancy and lactation, and the underlying ribs all add to the uncertainty of clinical examination. Other difficulties include: inflammatory cancers masquerading as infection; the presence of implants with an associated fibrous capsule; and the effect of hormone replacement therapy, which increases the density of breast parenchyma both clinically and radiologically.

The sensitivity of clinical examination in women aged 30–39 can be as low as 25%.[26] A sensitivity over 90% can only be expected in older women, when the atrophic nature of the breast parenchyma and the low incidence of benign disease combine to make clinical diagnosis a relatively simple task. The low sensitivity of clinical examination, coupled with the low incidence of breast cancer and the considerable numbers of young women attending breast clinics, must largely explain why failure of physical findings to impress the clinician was one of the most common reasons for delay in diagnosis in the PIAA study.[3]

Mammography

False-negative mammography is one of the principal reasons for delay in diagnosis,[3,27] since it gives the clinician and patient false reassurance. Age is an important factor in false-negative reporting (Fig. 18.1), with the number of cancers missed inversely proportional to age: 36% of cancers in women aged 40 compared with just 9% in those aged 75. The net result of medicolegal pressure on breast radiologists has been an increase in recall and biopsy rates.[28,29]

Ultrasound

The use of ultrasound is now an integral part of breast imaging in a patient of any age with a lump (see Chapter 1), especially when an abnormality is not detectable on clinical or mammographic examination. Ultrasound-guided core biopsy has replaced fine-needle aspiration cytology (FNAC) in screen-detected tumours, although both techniques are currently acceptable in the symptomatic clinic. The expertise required for ultrasound examination and guided core biopsy has placed breast imaging outside the competency of the general radiologist. The breast surgeon using ultrasound in the clinic may be similarly compromised unless training in the technique can be verified.

Cytology

For many years FNAC has allowed rapid and cost-effective tissue diagnosis of a palpable lump. How reliable is FNAC? Dixon et al.[26] reported that the sensitivity of FNAC could be increased from 66% to 99% by restricting the biopsy to one aspirator. In comparison, the sensitivity of FNAC in women under 36 was as low as 78%,[25] though Dixon et al.[26] found that accuracy was not related to age if inadequate samples were excluded from the calculations.

In a review of 112 reports of FNAC of breast masses by Layfield et al.[30] the overall accuracy was over 95% but delays in diagnosis of greater than 50 days still occurred, and 85% of such delays were in women under 55[31] and with smaller tumours.[32] In small tumours, a sampling error is probably more common than misinterpretation of the cytology and ultrasound-guided core biopsy is advisable.

Efficacy of triple assessment

If it is assumed that breast cancer detection by clinical examination, imaging and FNAC are independent of each other, it is possible to calculate the theoretical rate at which all three tests will give a false-negative result. The false-negative rates of the three investigations have been multiplied and expressed as a percentage in **Table 18.1**. It is probable that the sensitivities of these tests are not totally independent of each other, and therefore the predicted rate that all three tests will be false negative for an individual is a conservative estimate. For a woman under 35 with breast cancer, there may be a 12% chance that all three tests will give a false-negative result. Using optimal sensitivities, the chance that all three tests will produce a false-negative result falls to approximately 1 in 1000 patients with these data skewed towards the older age groups; the likely overall rate of false-negative triple assessment in the clinic is between 1.4% and 4%.[32,33]

Table 18.1 • False-negative rates of triple assessment for women under 35 compared with the generally quoted results[19,31]

	False-negative rate	
	Women <35 years	Optimal
Clinical examination	0.75	0.12
Mammography	0.75	0.12
Fine-needle cytology	0.22	0.05
All three false negative	12.3%	0.072%

Tumour doubling time

The usual threshold diameter for detection of a breast cancer by physical examination is 1 cm; such a tumour consists of 10^9 cells and is the result of 30 doublings. It is possible for mammography to detect tumours as small as 2 mm, which equates to a tumour of 10^7 cells and about 23 doublings.

Assuming a constant doubling time, early detection of breast cancer is a misnomer, since at least two-thirds of the biological life of the tumour will have been completed by the time of detection.[34] In medicolegal terms, if the alleged delay in diagnosis was 14 months for a cancer with a doubling time of 90 days, such a delay would equate to the number of cells increasing by one order of magnitude (i.e. from 10^9 to 10^{10} cells). This represents a major increase in tumour load but is a very short period in the lifespan of the tumour and it is difficult to be sure that this period of delay would have a significant effect. In civil law, however, the court wants to know whether such an effect is more likely than not to alter the patient's prognosis or treatment.

Lymph node status remains the most important prognostic indicator at the time of primary treatment. Tubiana and Koscielny[35] suggested that breast cancer represents a continuum from slow-growing tumours with late axillary involvement and distant dissemination to the most aggressive, rapidly growing and early metastasising subtype. Assuming the growth rate of the nodal metastasis approximates to that of the primary tumour, it is possible to estimate the theoretical time at which the tumour must have

metastasised, and not infrequently this would have occurred before the threshold size for detection of the primary tumour.[34]

It is generally accepted that breast cancer begins as a single cell or a small group of cells that exhibit an exponential growth pattern. The time taken for a tumour to double in *volume* is known as the doubling time. Doubling times for breast cancers have been estimated by measuring the size of mastectomy scar recurrences[36] and by serial mammographic evaluation.[37]

Pearlman[36] categorised patients as having fast- (<25 days), intermediate- (26–75 days) and slow-growing (>76 days) tumours based on measurement of tumour doubling time; 5-year survival rates were 5%, 62% and 100% respectively. Peer et al.[38] estimated mean doubling time in women under 50 to be 80 days (confidence limits 44–147 days) and in women over 50 to be 157 days (confidence limits 121–204 days). Although lymph node metastases are more commonly found in fast-growing tumours, it would be wrong to assume that the survival of patients was entirely a consequence of tumour doubling time. Galante et al.[37] emphasised the importance of the metastatic potential of the tumour, suggesting that within fast-, intermediate- and slow-growing tumours there may be subsets with high and low metastasising potential.

The premise that early detection of a tumour will lead to cure depends on the concept that at the time of earlier treatment the tumour has not metastasised. The period of time between the earliest possible detection of the cancer and the time at which the tumour metastasises has been described as the cancer control window.[39] If the tumour has already metastasised by the time it reaches the threshold size for detection, there is no window and only effective systemic therapy might cure the patient. It is often argued by the claimant and her legal team that delay in treatment is the cause of metastasis rather than the inherent biology of the tumour itself.

Vignettes on breach of duty

The following vignettes illustrate areas of breach of duty that have arisen in medicolegal breast cases and the comments following each vignette raise issues that might be discussed in conference with counsel.

Vignette 1: False-positive cytology, lymphoedema and alteration of records

A 60-year-old patient was referred to a breast clinic with a clinically suspicious breast lump. Mammography was suspicious (M4) and FNAC was malignant (C5). The patient underwent wide local excision and axillary clearance for what subsequently proved to be a histologically benign condition. She complained of a poor cosmetic outcome and a painful swollen arm, which she had not been warned about. The nursing records stated 'patient was warned of the risk of lymphoedema'.

Comments

- A false-positive cytology result is a rare but potentially devastating event. From a medicolegal standpoint, an expert review of the cytology should be the first step. If experts are agreed that the cytologist acted reasonably in reporting the slides as malignant, attention will then focus on the surgeon.
- The surgeon has to be aware that a false-positive cytology can occur and for this reason most surgeons will not carry out mastectomy without histological confirmation from a core biopsy. Histology is mandatory in the absence of a fully concordant malignant triple assessment and should have been obtained in this case. Axillary clearance for a benign condition is a potentially significant injury and it is unfortunate that this patient developed lymphoedema.
- The tense of the warning suggested to the judge that this was a retrospective note. Judges place most reliance on contemporaneous records and alterations to the notes are often quite obvious. Any addition to the notes must be clearly identified as such by signing and dating the record and any temptation to alter the record after the event must be firmly resisted.

Vignette 2: Failure of preoperative assessment and postoperative management

A 69-year-old woman presented with a small but obvious carcinoma in the tail of the breast. The surgeon performed FNAC, which showed malignant cells (C5), and he carried out wide local excision of the tumour without preliminary breast imaging and without performing axillary staging. The tumour was grade 2 but the resection margins were not reported. The patient was started on tamoxifen but was not referred for consideration of radiotherapy.

Comments

- The management of this patient falls short of an acceptable standard in a number of respects (breach of duty), but until such time as she develops evidence of recurrence, which may never occur, any resultant harm (causation) remains potential.
- A preoperative mammogram might have shown widespread microcalcification or multifocal tumour and in this situation conservative surgery would not have been appropriate. There might also have been an undetected cancer in the contralateral breast.
- To fail to report the margin status and managing a patient with conservative surgery without consideration of radiotherapy is unacceptable.
- It is clear that this case was not discussed at a multidisciplinary meeting.
- Axillary node status should have been assessed and has been recommended in UK guidelines since 1995.[9]

Vignette 3: False-negative cytology, trainees in the clinic and lobular carcinoma

A 38-year-old patient was referred to a breast clinic with a breast lump. Mammography was negative and a specialist registrar found an indefinite lump of which he was not suspicious. He carried out FNAC but failed to achieve an adequate specimen (C1). At follow-up 6 weeks later a repeat FNAC showed an adequate benign sample (C2). She was discharged from the clinic but re-presented 6 months later with an invasive lobular carcinoma at the same site.

Comments

- Trainees must be adequately supervised and only permitted to see patients by themselves when their trainer is satisfied that they are competent and understand local protocols.[10]

- There is a learning curve in achieving adequate samples with FNAC. The rate of inadequate FNAC samples should be monitored for each clinician.
- Clinicians should be aware that lobular cancers are prone to false-negative mammography. There is also an increased difficulty with false-negative cytology interpretation.
- The diagnosis of breast cancer in young women is difficult and in the situation where a patient complains of a lump but on clinical examination or mammography nothing is obvious, ultrasound is advisable, with guided biopsy if a lesion is seen.

Vignette 4: Pneumothorax following FNAC

A dental nurse aged 32 presented with a lump in the tail of the breast. An experienced clinical assistant in the breast clinic carried out FNAC. Unfortunately, he pierced the pleura and caused a pneumothorax that required hospitalisation and pleural drainage. The patient was not warned of the risk and complained of persistent chest pain over a period of many months.

Comments

- Did the clinician fail in his duty of care by advancing the needle too far or by failing to warn the patient? The literature suggests a risk of around 1 in 10 000.[40–42] It is not rare to strike a rib with the needle at FNAC. Piercing the pleura may be more common because a trivial pneumothorax may go undetected.
- In several cases the court has found pneumothorax to be a rare but recognised complication that can occur without breach of duty, although one case ruled this injury to be negligent, which was an unexpected judgment.[42] There is often a reluctance on the part of trusts to defend or appeal low-value cases under £10 000 (as would be the case for damages here).
- In defending a claim of negligence, it is important to be able to show that the clinician was experienced in the technique. Were this to be a trainee, it would be necessary to establish that he or she had been properly supervised.

- Pneumothorax has been reported following needle localisation by a radiologist and following aspiration of axillary seroma, performing FNAC and core biopsy. Using image guidance should theoretically reduce the risk.

Delay in diagnosis: causation issues

In a case of delay in diagnosis, it is often relatively straightforward to establish whether there has been a breach of duty of care. The next hurdle to be overcome by the claimant is to satisfy the court, on the balance of probabilities, that this delay caused her harm. Expert opinion is often divided and if the experts cannot agree then the court makes a judgment. The public and the judiciary have the expectation that early diagnosis carries a better outlook. It is not surprising therefore that counter-arguments of lead-time bias and innate tumour biology tend to fall on deaf ears.

Having established breach of duty, the issue of causation may include the allegation that less treatment would have been required. It may also be argued that psychological damage has ensued. However, the main issue centres around whether the claimant has suffered a reduced expectation of life or, if she has died by the time the matter comes to court, whether she would have lived longer. Richards et al.,[43] after a systematic review, concluded that there is an average reduction in 5-year survival of 7% with a delay of 3–6 months and 12% with a delay of more than 6 months. Dische et al.[44] extrapolated a 1.8% decrease in survival from Richards et al.'s data for each 1-month delay up to 6 months. In the same issue of the *Lancet*, Sainsbury et al.[45] reported no such effect but produced the apparently contradictory finding that patients with the shortest delay had the worst prognosis, a finding previously reported by Afzelius et al.[46]

The survival in patients with the best-prognosis tumours (small, special type, grade 1, node negative) approaches that of the normal population, and clearly a formula attributing a reduction in survival for each month of delay would be inappropriate in such tumours. However, if one accepts this, then for some tumours with a worse prognosis there must be a greater loss of survival.[44] It would nevertheless seem intuitive that the most aggressive tumours with rapid metastatic potential are likely to be incurable from early in their natural history, suggesting diagnostic delays in such cancers are less likely to have an impact on survival.

Vignettes on causation

The following vignettes illustrate some of the causation issues that have arisen once liability has been established. Delay in diagnosis remains an area of considerable uncertainty and the comments reflect our experience of differing arguments presented to the court.

Vignette 5: 12-month delay in diagnosis of node-positive carcinoma

A 32-year-old woman was referred to a breast clinic with a lump in the breast. Ultrasound showed an indeterminate opacity 1 cm in diameter consistent with a fibroadenoma but no sample was taken by FNAC or core biopsy. She was discharged from the clinic but returned a year later with a clinical carcinoma at the same site. This measured 2.1 cm on both ultrasound and histology and was grade 3; one of four nodes was positive. Liability for delay in diagnosis was admitted in failing to carry out a biopsy at the first visit.

Comments

- The Nottingham Prognostic Index (NPI)[47–49] and Adjuvant!Online[50] are often used to determine the difference in outcome over the period of delay.
- Both NPI and Adjuvant!Online rely on the following assumptions about the individual case:
  Assumption 1: the tumour grade remains constant – this is usually agreed by both sides.
  Assumption 2: earlier tumour size. In this particular case a record of tumour size at the first visit was available, but if no clinical measurement was recorded and there was no imaging, an approximate tumour size has to be derived by working back from the tumour volume at diagnosis using tumour doubling times. This calculation assumes (i) that tumour growth is exponential, (ii) that in calculating tumour diameter the tumour approximates a sphere or an ellipsoid, and (iii) that the doubling time chosen is appropriate. Tumour size itself is a weak determinant of prognosis but the derived earlier tumour size is further used to calculate the likely nodal status.
  Assumption 3: the nodal status at the time of the breach of duty is usually unknown and often disputed by the experts. Axillary node status is invariably presumed to have been negative by the claimant, and this claim is supported by tables for tumour grade and tumour size that show the probability of positive nodes.[51] Only in grade 2 and 3 tumours greater than 2.5 cm does the probability of positive nodes rise above 50%. Therefore, *on balance* it may often be argued that the nodes would have been negative at the earlier time when the tumour was smaller.

Vignette 6: 2-year delay in diagnosis of node-negative grade 1 carcinoma

A 40-year-old woman presented with a lump in the breast and a triple assessment was carried out. The tumour measured 1.5 cm on ultrasound and mammography, and FNAC was reported as benign (C2). She was discharged but 2 years later returned with a carcinoma 3 cm in diameter on histology. The patient was treated by breast conservation and post-operative radiotherapy.

The tumour was grade 1 and four nodes sampled were clear. Review of the original cytology indicated that this had been under-reported and an expert opinion graded the slides unequivocally malignant (C5). Breach of duty was admitted.

Comments

- The standard of care must be judged against the standard reasonably to be expected of a cytologist working at the same level and not that of a world expert in the field.
- Although the tumour doubled in diameter over the 2-year period of delay, it remained within the good prognosis group. The treatment would have been the same with an earlier diagnosis and therefore the case did not succeed on causation.

Vignette 7: 3-year delay in diagnosis of a carcinoma missed on screening

A woman of 50 responded to an invitation for screening and was recalled for a localised area of microcalcification. There was a soft-tissue opacity and the appearance was judged benign on further magnification views and ultrasound. She was returned to routine screening but 3 years later the screening films showed an obvious carcinoma at the same site. This was a 2-cm grade 2 infiltrating carcinoma with an extensive in situ component; four of 10 nodes were positive. An expert opinion from a breast-screening radiologist rated the original films as suspicious for ductal carcinoma in situ (DCIS; M4) and stated that the microcalcification should have been biopsied by any competent breast radiologist.

Comments

- Delay due to radiological misinterpretation tends to be a matter of years rather than months. Screening by 3-yearly mammography probably reduces breast cancer deaths by up to 25%, and it is likely that a delay in diagnosis of 3 years will affect survival in a proportion of cases.
- The potential loss of survival in this case would be considerable since the original lesion would, on the balance of probabilities, have been an area of high-grade DCIS with a near-normal expectation of life if adequately treated at age 50. At age 53 the patient now has a relatively poor prognosis but on balance is still more likely to survive 10 years (Table 18.2).

Table 18.2 • Nottingham Prognostic Index groups

Group	NPI value	10-year survival (%)
Excellent (EPG)	2.0–2.4	96
Good (GPG)	2.41–3.4	93
Moderate I (MPGI)	3.41–4.4	82
Moderate II (MPGII)	4.41–5.4	75
Poor (PPG)	5.41–6.4	53
Very poor (VPG)	≥6.41	39

From the Nottingham Primary Breast Cancer Series. Data relate to patients with primary operable breast cancer, treated from 1990 to 1996.[47]

Vignette 8: 14-month delay in the breast clinic and failure to recommend chemotherapy

A 30-year-old woman was referred with a lump in the breast and was seen by a succession of specialist registrars. An initial ultrasound showed a 1-cm opacity consistent with a fibroadenoma but the FNAC was reported as mildly atypical (C3) and the pathologist advised 'consider biopsy to confirm' but no action was taken. A series of 6-month follow-up appointments were given. Finally the GP referred the patient again to the consultant, who immediately diagnosed breast cancer. The tumour was 4 cm, grade 3 and heavily node positive. The patient was treated by wide local excision, axillary clearance and radiotherapy. She was not given chemotherapy or hormone treatment until she developed bone secondaries 16 months later. Breach of duty was admitted for the delay in diagnosis and the failure to give chemotherapy at the time of diagnosis.

Comments

- Discussion of the discordant triple assessment at the breast multidisciplinary meeting (MDM) did not take place.
- Arranging a 6-month follow-up for a breast lump that is presumed benign is illogical.
- The judge took evidence from five expert witnesses. It was agreed that when first seen the tumour would have been grade 3, 1 cm in diameter and node negative. The tumour had increased in size to 4 cm in the 14 months of delay and opinion was divided as to whether this was ever potentially curable. The experts for the claimant were far more optimistic than those for the defence but in the event the judge preferred the latter.[52]
- The judge considered that, on balance, the breach of duty 'caused her to die 18 months before, sadly, she would have died anyway'.
- Unfortunately, the damages amounted to less than the defence had already paid into court. Civil litigation rules resulted in the family winning the case but receiving none of the settlement.

Vignette 9: 8-month delay in diagnosis in primary care

A 46-year-old woman attended her GP with a new lump that the GP assessed as a 1.5-cm smooth benign lump; in view of the past history of benign breast nodularity, the GP recommended a conservative approach and it was only when she saw a different GP 8 months later that referral to the clinic and a diagnosis of breast cancer was made. She underwent mastectomy and axillary clearance for a 42-mm grade 2 carcinoma with seven of 20 nodes involved, followed by chemotherapy, radiotherapy, trastuzumab and endocrine therapy. She had suffered persistent shoulder discomfort since the time of axillary surgery.

Comments

- Following an opinion from a GP expert, breach of duty on the part of the GP was admitted and the claim for causation was both for more extensive treatment and loss of chance of survival.
- The claimant's breast expert maintained that she would had undergone wide excision and sentinel node biopsy at the earlier time and that her expected survival had been reduced from 93% to 53%.
- At a pre-trial meeting of experts, they agreed jointly that the nodes would still have been involved at the earlier time and that the axillary surgery would have been unchanged, and agreed that she was, on balance, still more likely to survive than die from the breast cancer.
- The experts agreed that she had lost the chance of breast conservation as a result of the delay and following their joint report the case was settled for £50 000 on the basis that she had undergone mastectomy and would require future breast reconstruction.
- Less than 5% of clinical negligence cases are contested in court with over 95% of cases either dropped or settled before the trial date.
- Since the discussion of discordant triple assessments in breast MDMs has become widespread good practice, claims for delay in diagnosis against breast specialists have reduced and are now mainly against GPs who fail to refer cases to the breast clinic.

Poor cosmetic outcome

The mastectomy rate in the UK remains close to 40%, and where mastectomy is required the increasing demand for reconstruction has been addressed in national guidelines[53] and detailed audit.[54] Litigation has risen in line with patients' expectations,[55] although the typical size of claim for an unsatisfactory cosmetic outcome is considerably less than for delay in diagnosis.

Clinical notes should record evidence of discussions with the patient regarding either immediate or later breast reconstruction and should document that alternative treatment options and potential complications of surgery have been discussed. The presence of the breast-care nurse to augment and further document the surgeon's counselling is advisable and her written record, usually kept separately from the clinical notes, can make all the difference when allegations of inadequate preoperative information are part of a claim for breach of duty on the part of the reconstructive surgeon.

Preoperative markings should be made on the ward by the operating surgeon, explained to and agreed with the patient without pressure of time, and a record kept of this operative planning. Hasty skin marking in the anaesthetic room or on a patient already anaesthetised are not compatible with a reasonable standard of care.

A request for immediate reconstruction can present difficulties in offering the most appropriate reconstruction and yet not breach guidelines for commencing treatment. This tension has presented medicolegally with a patient offered a more basic form of reconstruction with a subpectoral implant in order to expedite mastectomy who, once the cancer had been dealt with, felt that the advice fell below a reasonable standard. The breast surgeon must make available to the patient the appropriate range of reconstructive options, including those that might require the involvement of a plastic surgical colleague.

Should a patient pursue litigation for her cosmetic outcome, the Bolam principle[7] would apply in determining breach of duty, i.e. the practice would be compared with that held to be reasonable by a similar body of professionals, in this case breast surgeons trained to undertake breast reconstruction. An audit of the surgeon's operative results is not currently expected by the court, nor are there prescribed minimum numbers of procedures to comply with good practice. At present there is no certificate of competency in training in breast reconstruction within the UK, but current reconstructive guidelines[53] outline the requirements for good practice.

When a poor cosmetic outcome is due to a recognised complication rather than poor judgment and provided the patient has been warned of the risk, she does not have a case against the surgeon.

Reduction mammoplasty, breast augmentation and surgery for gynaecomastia remain high-risk areas for patient dissatisfaction and should never be undertaken on an occasional basis. Breast operations represent the biggest group of plastic surgical procedures giving rise to claims.[56] It is vital that evidence of appropriate discussions about potential problems is adequately recorded in the notes and the correspondence, together with the use of appropriate information leaflets and clinical photographs to explain the proposed procedure. Consent forms should record the signed informed consent as well as documenting that the literature has been received and understood. Operation notes, where relevant, should include details of implant type, serial and lot number, and manufacturer, for possible future reference.[57]

Vignette 10: Poor cosmetic outcome after immediate breast reconstruction

A 52-year old patient with multifocal cancer was advised to have a mastectomy by a breast surgeon and after discussion with the breast-care nurse she requested immediate reconstruction. He offered her a tissue expander, which was inserted at the time of mastectomy, but it was not possible to achieve symmetry with the large contralateral breast. Contralateral breast reduction was carried out, with a poor cosmetic outcome. She was subsequently referred to a plastic surgeon for revision surgery and then sued her first surgeon.

Comments

- With cosmetic and reconstructive surgery, the damage is self-evident, i.e. causation is less of an issue than breach of duty. With delay in diagnosis the converse is often the case.

- Patient expectation of a good cosmetic outcome is arguably less demanding for postmastectomy reconstruction than for purely cosmetic surgery of the breast. Nevertheless, there is growing demand for a wider choice and more sophisticated reconstruction techniques.

- The first question that must be addressed is the adequacy of training in reconstructive surgery. If the level of training was appropriate, the second question is whether the standard of advice and operative skill met that which the patient could reasonably have expected. Unless the answer to both questions is in the affirmative, the surgeon is liable.

- Most breast surgeons undertaking reconstruction in the UK have attended training courses on the use of subpectoral and latissimus dorsi techniques. Some breast surgeons undertake pedicled transverse rectus abdominis muscle reconstruction, but free tissue transfer is beyond the training and theatre time constraints of most breast surgeons.

Risk management

Failure of communication and poor rapport often prompt patients into taking legal action. A woman who feels that her complaints have been taken seriously and investigated thoroughly is less likely to sue. In cases where the doctor–patient relationship breaks down, referral to another specialist may be the best course of action.

A rapid and timely diagnosis will best be achieved by establishing and adhering to a multidisciplinary approach in the care of breast patients, and for the breast clinician this is arguably the most robust safeguard of good practice in both diagnostic and treatment aspects of breast surgery.

Key points

- Missed diagnosis of breast cancer is the commonest cause of litigation, and the settlements highest, in premenopausal women.
- False reassurance from a negative mammogram is a common factor: always obtain a tissue diagnosis in a palpable mass with a negative mammogram.

- Triple assessment should be reviewed in the breast multidisciplinary meeting.
- Discordant triple assessment always need further consideration.
- Clinical practice that complies with guidelines is easier to defend.
- For reconstructive surgery, provide and document written information about the risks and benefits of the procedure.
- Ensure the patient's expectations about reconstruction are realistic and that her consent is fully informed.

References

1. Lawyers' fees and NHS savings. Br Med J 2011;343:d4035–6.

2. Physician Insurers Association of America. Breast cancer study. Rockville, MD: PIAA; 1990.

3. Physician Insurers Association of America. Breast cancer study. Rockville, MD: PIAA; 1995. p. 1–27.

4. Physician Insurers Association of America. Claim trend analysis. 2011 ed. Rockville, MD: PIAA; 2011.

5. Branthwaite M. Law for doctors: principles and practicalities. London: Royal Society of Medicine Press; 2000.

6. NHS Litigation Authority. Available at http://www.justice.gov.uk/courts/procedure-rules/civil/rules/part35; [accessed 30.06.12].

7. Bolam v. Friern Hospital Management Committee [1957] 2 All ER 118; [1957] 1 WLR 582.

8. Bolitho v. City & Hackney Health Authority [1997] 4 All ER 771; [1997] 3 WLR 1151.

9. Breast Surgeons Group of the British Association of Surgical Oncology. Guidelines for surgeons in the management of symptomatic breast disease in the United Kingdom. Eur J Surg Oncol 1995;21(Suppl. A):1–13.

10. The Association of Breast Surgery at BASO. Guidelines for the management of symptomatic breast disease. Eur J Surg Oncol 2005;31:1–21.

11. Hurwitz B. Clinical guidelines and the law. Br Med J 1995;311:1517–8.

12. Carrick SE, Bonevski B, Redman S, et al. Surgeons' opinions about the NMRC clinical practice guidelines for the management of early breast cancer. Med J Aust 1998;169:300–5.

13. Chester v. Afshar [2004] UKHL 41.

14. GMC 2009 annual statistics: fitness to practise. Available at http://www.gmc-uk.org; Annual.statistics.pdf.33097340.pdf; [accessed 30.06.12].

15. Woolf HK. Medical negligence. In: Access to justice: final report to the Lord Chancellor on the civil justice system in England and Wales. London: HMSO; 1996. p. 169–96.

16. Civil Procedure Rules. Available at www.justice.gov.uk/courts/procedure-rules/civil/rules/part35.

17. Brahams D. Loss of chance of survival. Lancet 1996;348:1604.

18. Davidson T. The medico-legal issue of causation – current status. Association of Breast Surgery at BASO Yearbook; 2006. Available at http://www.associationofbreastsurgery.org.uk[accessed 30.06.12].

19. Salih A, Webb MW, Bates T. Does open-access mammography and ultrasound delay the diagnosis of breast cancer? Breast 1999;8:129–32.

20. Hafstrom L, Johansson H, Ahlberg J. Diagnostic delay of breast cancer – an analysis of claims to Swedish Board of Malpractice. Breast 2011;20:539–42.

21. Andrews BT, Bates T. Delay in the diagnosis of breast cancer: medico-legal implications. Breast 2000;9:223–7.

22. Davidson T. Delay in diagnosing breast cancer: medicolegal implications. Trends Urol Gynaecol Sexual Health 1998;3:11–2.

23. Austoker J, Mansel R, Baum M, et al. Guidelines for referral of patients with breast problems. Sheffield: NHS Breast Screening Programme; 1995.

24. Dr Foster guide to hospitals and consultants. Available at http://www.drfosterhealth.co.uk.

25. Yelland A, Graham MD, Trott PA, et al. Diagnosing breast carcinoma in young women. Br Med J 1991;302:618–20.

26. Dixon JM, Anderson TJ, Lamb J, et al. Fine needle aspiration cytology, in relationship to clinical examination and mammography in the diagnosis of a solid breast mass. Br J Surg 1984;71:593–6.

27. Joensuu H, Asola R, Holli K, et al. Delayed diagnosis and large size of breast cancer after a false negative mammogram. Eur J Cancer 1994;30A:1299–302.

28. Elmore JG, Taplin SH, Barlow WE, et al. Does litigation influence medical practice? The influence of community radiologists' medical malpractice perceptions and experience on screening mammography. Radiology 2005;236(1):37–46.

29. Halpin SF. Medico-legal claims against English radiologists: 1995–2006. Br J Radiol 2009;82(984):982–8.

30. Layfield LJ, Glasgow BJ, Cramer H. Fine needle aspiration in the management of breast masses. Pathol Annu 1989;24:23–62.

31. Bates AT, Bates T, Hastrich DJ, et al. Delay in the diagnosis of breast cancer: the effect of the introduction of fine needle aspiration cytology to a breast clinic. Eur J Surg Oncol 1992;18:433–7.

32. Jenner DC, Middleton A, Webb WM, et al. Inhospital delay in the diagnosis of breast cancer. Br J Surg 2000;87:914–9.

33. Barber MD, Jack W, Dixon JM. Diagnostic delay in breast cancer. Br J Surg 2004;91(1):49–53.

34. Plotkin D, Blankenberg F. Breast cancer: biology and malpractice. Am J Clin Oncol 1991;14:254–66.

35. Tubiana M, Koscielny S. Cell kinetics, growth rate and the natural history of breast cancer. The Heuson Memorial Lecture. Eur J Clin Oncol 1988;24:9–14.

36. Pearlman AW. Breast cancer: influence of growth rate on prognosis and treatment evaluation. A study based on mastectomy scar recurrences. Cancer 1976;38:1826–33.

37. Galante E, Gallus G, Guzzon A, et al. Growth rate of primary breast cancer and prognosis: observations on a 3- to 7-year follow up in 180 breast cancers. Br J Cancer 1986;54:833–6.

38. Peer PG, van Dijk JA, Hedriks JH, et al. Age-dependent growth rate of breast cancer. Cancer 1993;71:3547–51.

39. Spratt JS, Spratt SW. Medical and legal implications of screening and follow-up procedures for breast cancer. Cancer 1990;66:1351–62.

40. Christie R, Bates T. The risk of pneumothorax as a complication of diagnostic fine needle aspiration or therapeutic needling of the breast: should the patient be warned? Breast 1999;8:98–9.

41. Gately CA, Maddox PR, Mansel RE. Pneumothorax: a complication of fine needle aspiration of the breast. Br Med J 1991;303:627–8.

42. Bates T, Davidson T, Mansel R. Litigation for pneumothorax as a complication of fine-needle aspiration of the breast. Br J Surg 2002;89:134–7.

43. Richards MA, Westcombe AM, Love SB, et al. Influence of delay on survival in patients with breast cancer: a systematic review. Lancet 1999;353:1119–26.

44. Dische S, Bentzen G, Bond S. The influence of delay in diagnosis of breast cancer upon outlook. Clin Risk 2000;6:4–6.

45. Sainsbury R, Johnston C, Haward B. Effect on survival of delays in referral of patients with breast-cancer symptoms: a retrospective analysis. Lancet 1999;353:1132–5.

46. Afzelius P, Zedeler K, Sommer H, et al. Patients' and doctors' delay in primary breast cancer. Acta Oncol 1994;33:345–51.

47. Thompson AM, Pinder SE. Prognostic factors. In: Dixon JM, editor. The ABC of breast diseases. 3rd ed. Oxford: Blackwell Publishing; 2006. p. 77–80.

48. Blamey RW, Ellis IO, Pinder SE, et al. Survival of invasive breast cancer according to the Nottingham Prognostic Index in cases diagnosed in 1990–1999. Eur J Cancer 2007;43(10):1548–55.

49. Blamey RW, Pinder SE, Ball GR, et al. Reading the prognosis of the individual with breast cancer. Eur J Cancer 2007;43(10):1545–7.

50. Adjuvant!Online. Available at hppt//:www.adjuvantonline.com; [accessed 30.06.12].

51. Yiangou C, Shousha S, Sinnett HD. Primary tumour characteristics and axillary lymph node status in breast cancer. Br J Cancer 1999;80:1974–8.

52. Taylor v. West Kent Health Authority [1997] 8 Med LR 251–7.

53. Association of Breast Surgery at BASO; Association of Breast Surgery at BAPRAS; Training Interface Group in Breast Surgery. Baildam A, Bishop, H, Boland, G. Oncoplastic breast surgery – A guide to good practice. Eur J Surg Oncol 2007;33:S1–23.

54. National Mastectomy and Breast Reconstruction Audit (Fouth Annual Report); Available at www.ic.nhs.uk/mbrreports; 2011[accessed 30.06.12].

55. Richards E, Vijh R. Analysis of malpractice claims in breast care for poor cosmetic outcome. Breast 2011;20:225–8.

56. Claims analysis. MDU J 2011;27(2):19–21.

57. O'Dowd A. UK launches rapid inquiry into the safety of PIP breast implants. Br Med J 2012;344:e11.

Index

NB: Page numbers followed by *f* indicate figures, *t* indicate tables and *b* indicate boxes.

A

Index

Index

M

S

City ... 03 7... - Fas ...
.uk ...

SPORT
PSYCHOLOGY
Interventions

Shane M. Murphy, PhD

Editor

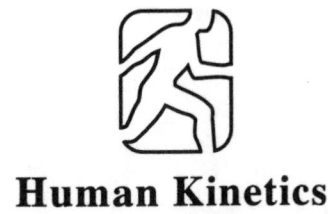

Human Kinetics

Library of Congress Cataloging-in-Publication Data

Sport psychology interventions / [edited by] Shane M. Murphy.
    p.   cm.
   Includes index.
   ISBN 0-87322-659-3
    1. Athletes--Mental health.   2. Athletes--Mental health services.
   3. Athletes--Counseling of.   4. Sports--Psychological aspects.
   I. Murphy, Shane M., 1957-
   RC451.4.A83S66   1995
   616.89'008'8796--dc20   94-10390
                                          CIP

ISBN: 0-87322-659-3

Developmental Editor: Mary E. Fowler; **Assistant Editors:** Sally Bayless, Hank Woolsey, Karen Bojda, Erik Dafforn, and Jacqueline Blakley; **Copyeditor:** Tom Plummer; **Proofreader:** Pam Johnson; **Indexer:** Joan K. Griffitts; **Production Manager:** Kris Ding; **Typesetter:** Sandra Meier; **Text Designer:** Keith Blomberg; **Layout Artist:** Tara Welsch; **Photo Editor:** Karen Maier; **Cover Designer:** Jack Davis; **Illustrator:** Craig Ronto; **Printer:** Braun-Brumfield

Printed in the United States of America   10 9 8 7 6 5 4

Human Kinetics
Web site: www.HumanKinetics.com

United States: Human Kinetics, P.O. Box 5076, Champaign, IL 61825-5076
800-747-4457
e-mail: humank@hkusa.com

Canada: Human Kinetics, 475 Devonshire Road, Unit 100, Windsor, ON N8Y 2L5
800-465-7301 (in Canada only)
e-mail: orders@hkcanada.com

Europe: Human Kinetics, 107 Bradford Road, Stanningley
Leeds LS28 6AT, United Kingdom
+44 (0) 113 255 5665
e-mail: hk@hkeurope.com

Australia: Human Kinetics, 57A Price Avenue, Lower Mitcham, South Australia 5062
08 8277 1555
e-mail: liaw@hkaustralia.com

New Zealand: Human Kinetics, Division of Sports Distributors NZ Ltd.
P.O. Box 300 226 Albany, North Shore City, Auckland
0064 9 448 1207
e-mail: info@humankinetics.co.nz

CONTENTS

Chapter 4   Competitive Recreational Athletes: A Multisystemic Model   71
James P. Whelan, PhD, Andrew W. Meyers, PhD, and Charlene Donovan, MA

Chapter 5   Invisible Players: A Family Systems Model   117
Jon C. Hellstedt, PhD

**Chapter 6   The Coach and the Team Psychologist:
An Integrated Organizational Model   147**
Frank Gardner, PhD

**Chapter 7   Providing Psychological Services to Student Athletes:
A Developmental Psychology Model   177**
Michael Greenspan, PhD, and Mark B. Andersen, PhD

PREFACE

Sport in the United States is in serious trouble. Front page stories in the sports section of any metropolitan newspaper describe a pattern of turmoil and discontent.

- At a Little League baseball game a father argues angrily with the umpire over an *out* call on his son. After the game another argument breaks out, and the umpire is stabbed and seriously wounded.
- A feature story describes the experiences of a former professional female tennis player who burned out and retired from the sport at age 17.
- Another story presents the startling statistic that 40% of children leave competitive sport every year. The story includes interviews with parents and teachers describing the pressure of competitive sport and what can be done about it.
- Three starters on a Division I football team are arrested and charged with the gang rape of a college student.
- An aging professional comes back from retirement twice in one season and is arrested on a charge of cocaine distribution. He explains that his gambling debts were so large that he "couldn't see any other way out."
- A promising young Olympic athlete is arrested after the car she was driving crashes, killing a passenger. The Olympian's blood alcohol level was .12, and she later pleaded guilty to manslaughter.

Such stories tempt the jaded observer to question whether sport itself produces these problems. The answer is probably that such problems are a reflection of society as a whole but that the intense scrutiny that accompanies high-level sports competition in our society produces greater publicity when athletes are involved. *Sport* is still synonymous with *play* and is meant to be fun. But in professional and elite sport environments, there is often little fun.

This book is about ways of helping athletes cope with the special circumstances of committed sports involvement. The focus is on psychological interventions—ways to produce change in the individual athlete. Several other texts have been written that discuss psychological interventions aimed at increasing athletic performance. Performance is not the focus of this text. Instead, the underlying philosophy here is that athletes who can learn to manage their lives successfully, who can grow and develop as individuals, and who can experience sport as a positive learning process will enjoy their participation more and perform better.

Sport Psychology Interventions is written for all helping professionals who are working with or interested in helping athletes. It addresses the practical concerns that are typically encountered by physicians, athletic trainers, psychologists, counselors, and health care professionals working with athletes. Because understanding the psychology of sport, competition, and training is critical to the effectiveness of any intervention with athletes, this book is a necessity for all helping professionals who work in sport, but it also will interest anyone—athlete, coach, parent, or fan—who wants to understand sports participation and how to gain the maximum positive benefit from being an athlete.

In editing this book, I turned to the top professionals in the field of sport psychology. Knowledge in an applied area grows in proportion to the number of professionals working in that area, and the application of the science of psychology to athletics was still in its infancy a decade ago. Fortunately many professionals throughout the United States now are working with athletes and sport organizations to help improve the athletic experience for participants, and it is that group with whom I began this venture. Thus this book is written by authors familiar with the struggles of athletes.

Part I presents a variety of models of intervention in sport, encompassing systemic, educational, cognitive-behavioral, and marital therapy, with each model examined in the context of application to a specific sport group. In this way the issues specific to a variety of athlete populations are addressed for the first time in the sport psychology literature. Intervention issues in working with elite athletes are described along with issues specific to helping female, competitive, recreational, student, and child athletes.

In Part II, experts address issues commonly encountered by helping professionals in the sport setting. Injury, alcohol and drug use, eating disorders, career transitions, and overtraining are discussed, and interventions are described.

Each chapter in this book contains extensive case-study material, allowing the authors to use real-life illustrations of the issues they address. The case studies help focus the book on applied issues and prevent the discussions from becoming too theoretical. You will find that the case studies bring the chapters to life in an exciting and enriching manner.

Sport Psychology Interventions presents a new philosophy of helping athletes, recognizing that athletes face special challenges and sometimes unique problems. As editor, I am pleased to present the stimulating and thoughtful ideas of some of the nation's leading sport psychologists on how to tackle these issues. I believe that the ideas we discuss can profoundly change the sporting experience in this society. I hope this book will serve all of us who care about sport and about athletes.

Shane Murphy

ACKNOWLEDGMENTS

Many people assisted in the development of this book, and I would like to publicly thank them.

First, all the chapter authors, who met their deadlines and suffered my continual questions with gentle patience. Their expertise is highly valued.

The sport psychology staff at the United States Olympic Committee, who helped me continually refine my ideas, especially Sean McCann, Chris Carr, Bob Swoap, Frank Perna, Megan Neyer, Suzie Tuffey, Kirsten Peterson, Shirley Durtschi, Mike Greenspan, Doug Jowdy, Vance Tammen, Michael Lesser, and Alan Budney.

My ever-patient and always smiling secretary, Sally Bowman.

My developmental editor at Human Kinetics, Mary Fowler, for all her patient help. And many, many thanks to Rainer Martens, whose personal vision for sport psychology inspired this book.

The staff of the United States Olympic Committee, whose dedication to helping athletes reach their potential serves as a wonderful model for the sporting community, and in particular Harvey Schiller, Charles Davis, Jim Page, Jay T. Kearney, Tom Crawford, Steve Fleck, Sarah Smith, Leonard Jansen, Sheryl McSherry, and Peter Van Handel, who all have taught me so much.

Rob Woolfolk, who supported my interest in sport psychology from the very beginning.

All the athletes I have known over the years—those many wonderful people I have learned so much from.

Jerry May, who has been a wise and valued mentor.

My wife, Annemarie, and my children, Bryan and Theresa, for their support and patience through the missing weekends and long nights.

And lastly, my father, Tom, and mother, Nola, who taught me everything I know about being a good sport, the thrill of participating, and the love of the game. With that training, is it any wonder I became a sport psychologist?

CHAPTER 1

INTRODUCTION TO SPORT PSYCHOLOGY INTERVENTIONS

Shane M. Murphy, PhD
United States Olympic Committee

The effect sport has on our lives and how individuals adjust to sport are topics that have been too long ignored in the psychological community. Using psychological interventions to help athletes manage the stresses of intensive sport involvement is a relatively new enterprise. It differs from the more traditional *sport psychology* that mainly seeks to understand and optimize athletic performance.

You might wonder if the subject of psychological interventions with athletes deserves an entire book. I argue that it is important to explore how people can develop healthier, more productive athletic lifestyles. Professional sport is a pervasive feature of American society. For good or bad many Americans, young and old, identify strongly with sports figures. Recreational athletic activity has never been more actively promoted, as an aging population grapples with its lifestyle choices, preventive medicine, the costs of health care, and the quality of life. Sport and exercise are integral to our lives and deserve no less serious attention by health care professionals than our work and relationships.

Psychological interventions are required with sports issues such as treating the emo-

tional effects of athletic injury, preventing overtraining and burnout, helping athletes with eating disorders, attacking drug and alcohol abuse in sport, heightening awareness of gender issues in sport, and assisting athletes who are making the transition out of competitive sport into the business world. We discuss these issues in *Sport Psychology Interventions*. Before describing these sport psychology interventions, however, we must first review the broader history of sport psychology.

WHAT IS SPORT PSYCHOLOGY?

The term *sport psychology* has developed two separate, entirely different meanings, resulting in a great deal of confusion and even stress in sport psychology organizations. One meaning relates to the practice of psychology by professionals who specialize primarily in working with athletes in a variety of sport settings. After World War II, the practice of psychology flourished (see Napali, 1981 and Pryzwansky & Wendt, 1987, for a history),

1

and subspecialties began to appear, such as clinical psychology, school psychology, industrial-organizational psychology, and rehabilitation psychology. These subspecialties were defined primarily by setting and type of clients: Thus school psychologists work in school settings with students, and industrial-organizational psychologists work with employers and employees in companies and organizations. Similarly, as some psychologists began to specialize by working with athletes in sport organizations they called themselves sport psychologists.

Most psychologists who practice in the area of sport have received little formal education in a content area called sport psychology. There is a clear reason for this situation: Few psychology training programs offer formal course work in the sport area. The study of the psychological issues confronted by athletes is almost nonexistent in graduate psychology programs. This situation has characterized other specialty areas: in the early years of school psychology, its practitioners received their training in other specialties, such as clinical or counseling psychology. As the demand for psychologists grew in school settings, training programs were developed to prepare psychology students for working in schools. It remains to be seen whether a similar growth will occur in sport psychology. (I will return to this issue later.)

But a second, very different view of sport psychology emerges if we examine the development of the academic discipline known as sport psychology, usually found in university departments of sport science, human movement, or physical education. Here the study of sport psychology is "concerned with both the psychological factors that influence participation in sport and exercise and the psychological effects derived from that participation" (Williams & Straub, 1986, p. 1).

Many universities in the United States offer courses and programs in sport psychology, and many of the faculty in these programs call themselves sport psychologists. Yet the training and interests of this group of sport psychologists differ greatly from the first group's. It is tempting to say that a major difference between the groups is that the first works in the applied area—the practice of psychology in sport settings—whereas the second group is academically based, working with research issues, theory development, and education. Although this might have been true in the past, it no longer is. In the last decade interest has grown in applying the knowledge gained from academic sport psychology in the sporting arena. Books like *Applied Sport Psychology* (Williams, 1986) and *Psyching for Sport* (Orlick, 1986) demonstrate this growing interest. Simple generalizations do not work in the complex, rapidly evolving area of sport psychology. We need to take a closer look at the historical development of both strands to understand the rope known as sport psychology.

TRACING THE HISTORY

The history of psychologists working with athletes is more difficult to trace than the development of academic sport psychology, because practicing psychologists usually experience less pressure to publish than their academic colleagues. I have traced the development of practice with athletes through presentations, professional publications, and occasional books. The development of the academic discipline of sport psychology, described as "the youngest of the sport sciences" (Williams & Straub, 1986, p. 11), was traced more directly through the publication of foundational works in the field.

Psychologists in Sport Settings

It seems that before the 1960s few psychologists specialized in working with athletes.

City (03 7 - Fas   I/
.uk

SPORT
PSYCHOLOGY
Interventions

Shane M. Murphy, PhD

Editor

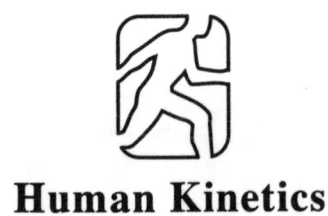

Human Kinetics

SPORT
PSYCHOLOGY
Interventions

Shane M. Murphy, PhD

Editor

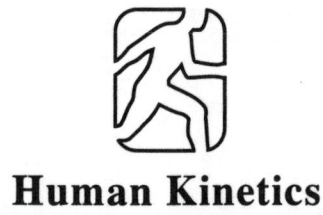

Human Kinetics

Library of Congress Cataloging-in-Publication Data

Sport psychology interventions / [edited by] Shane M. Murphy.
     p.   cm.
   Includes index.
   ISBN 0-87322-659-3
     1. Athletes--Mental health.   2. Athletes--Mental health services.
   3. Athletes--Counseling of.   4. Sports--Psychological aspects.
   I. Murphy, Shane M., 1957-
   RC451.4.A83S66   1995
   616.89'008'8796--dc20   94-10390
                                      CIP

ISBN: 0-87322-659-3

Developmental Editor: Mary E. Fowler; **Assistant Editors:** Sally Bayless, Hank Woolsey, Karen Bojda, Erik Dafforn, and Jacqueline Blakley; **Copyeditor:** Tom Plummer; **Proofreader:** Pam Johnson; **Indexer:** Joan K. Griffitts; **Production Manager:** Kris Ding; **Typesetter:** Sandra Meier; **Text Designer:** Keith Blomberg; **Layout Artist:** Tara Welsch; **Photo Editor:** Karen Maier; **Cover Designer:** Jack Davis; **Illustrator:** Craig Ronto; **Printer:** Braun-Brumfield

Printed in the United States of America   10 9 8 7 6 5 4

Human Kinetics
Web site: www.HumanKinetics.com

United States: Human Kinetics, P.O. Box 5076, Champaign, IL 61825-5076
800-747-4457
e-mail: humank@hkusa.com

Canada: Human Kinetics, 475 Devonshire Road, Unit 100, Windsor, ON N8Y 2L5
800-465-7301 (in Canada only)
e-mail: orders@hkcanada.com

Europe: Human Kinetics, 107 Bradford Road, Stanningley
Leeds LS28 6AT, United Kingdom
+44 (0) 113 255 5665
e-mail: hk@hkeurope.com

Australia: Human Kinetics, 57A Price Avenue, Lower Mitcham, South Australia 5062
08 8277 1555
e-mail: liaw@hkaustralia.com

New Zealand: Human Kinetics, Division of Sports Distributors NZ Ltd.
P.O. Box 300 226 Albany, North Shore City, Auckland
0064 9 448 1207
e-mail: info@humankinetics.co.nz

CONTENTS

Chapter 4   Competitive Recreational Athletes: A Multisystemic Model   71
James P. Whelan, PhD, Andrew W. Meyers, PhD, and Charlene Donovan, MA

Chapter 5   Invisible Players: A Family Systems Model   117
Jon C. Hellstedt, PhD

**Chapter 6   The Coach and the Team Psychologist:
An Integrated Organizational Model   147**
Frank Gardner, PhD

**Chapter 7   Providing Psychological Services to Student Athletes:
A Developmental Psychology Model   177**
Michael Greenspan, PhD, and Mark B. Andersen, PhD

PREFACE

Sport in the United States is in serious trouble. Front page stories in the sports section of any metropolitan newspaper describe a pattern of turmoil and discontent.

- At a Little League baseball game a father argues angrily with the umpire over an *out* call on his son. After the game another argument breaks out, and the umpire is stabbed and seriously wounded.
- A feature story describes the experiences of a former professional female tennis player who burned out and retired from the sport at age 17.
- Another story presents the startling statistic that 40% of children leave competitive sport every year. The story includes interviews with parents and teachers describing the pressure of competitive sport and what can be done about it.
- Three starters on a Division I football team are arrested and charged with the gang rape of a college student.
- An aging professional comes back from retirement twice in one season and is arrested on a charge of cocaine distribution. He explains that his gambling debts were so large that he "couldn't see any other way out."
- A promising young Olympic athlete is arrested after the car she was driving crashes, killing a passenger. The Olympian's blood alcohol level was .12, and she later pleaded guilty to manslaughter.

Such stories tempt the jaded observer to question whether sport itself produces these problems. The answer is probably that such problems are a reflection of society as a whole but that the intense scrutiny that accompanies high-level sports competition in our society produces greater publicity when athletes are involved. *Sport* is still synonymous with *play* and is meant to be fun. But in professional and elite sport environments, there is often little fun.

This book is about ways of helping athletes cope with the special circumstances of committed sports involvement. The focus is on psychological interventions—ways to produce change in the individual athlete. Several other texts have been written that discuss psychological interventions aimed at increasing athletic performance. Performance is not the focus of this text. Instead, the underlying philosophy here is that athletes who can learn to manage their lives successfully, who can grow and develop as individuals, and who can experience sport as a positive learning process will enjoy their participation more and perform better.

Sport Psychology Interventions is written for all helping professionals who are working with or interested in helping athletes. It addresses the practical concerns that are typically encountered by physicians, athletic trainers, psychologists, counselors, and health care professionals working with athletes. Because understanding the psychology of sport, competition, and training is critical to the effectiveness of any intervention with athletes, this book is a necessity for all helping professionals who work in sport, but it also will interest anyone—athlete, coach, parent, or fan—who wants to understand sports participation and how to gain the maximum positive benefit from being an athlete.

In editing this book, I turned to the top professionals in the field of sport psychology. Knowledge in an applied area grows in proportion to the number of professionals working in that area, and the application of the science of psychology to athletics was still in its infancy a decade ago. Fortunately many professionals throughout the United States now are working with athletes and sport organizations to help improve the athletic experience for participants, and it is that group with whom I began this venture. Thus this book is written by authors familiar with the struggles of athletes.

Part I presents a variety of models of intervention in sport, encompassing systemic, educational, cognitive-behavioral, and marital therapy, with each model examined in the context of application to a specific sport group. In this way the issues specific to a variety of athlete populations are addressed for the first time in the sport psychology literature. Intervention issues in working with elite athletes are described along with issues specific to helping female, competitive, recreational, student, and child athletes.

In Part II, experts address issues commonly encountered by helping professionals in the sport setting. Injury, alcohol and drug use, eating disorders, career transitions, and overtraining are discussed, and interventions are described.

Each chapter in this book contains extensive case-study material, allowing the authors to use real-life illustrations of the issues they address. The case studies help focus the book on applied issues and prevent the discussions from becoming too theoretical. You will find that the case studies bring the chapters to life in an exciting and enriching manner.

Sport Psychology Interventions presents a new philosophy of helping athletes, recognizing that athletes face special challenges and sometimes unique problems. As editor, I am pleased to present the stimulating and thoughtful ideas of some of the nation's leading sport psychologists on how to tackle these issues. I believe that the ideas we discuss can profoundly change the sporting experience in this society. I hope this book will serve all of us who care about sport and about athletes.

Shane Murphy

ACKNOWLEDGMENTS

Many people assisted in the development of this book, and I would like to publicly thank them.

First, all the chapter authors, who met their deadlines and suffered my continual questions with gentle patience. Their expertise is highly valued.

The sport psychology staff at the United States Olympic Committee, who helped me continually refine my ideas, especially Sean McCann, Chris Carr, Bob Swoap, Frank Perna, Megan Neyer, Suzie Tuffey, Kirsten Peterson, Shirley Durtschi, Mike Greenspan, Doug Jowdy, Vance Tammen, Michael Lesser, and Alan Budney.

My ever-patient and always smiling secretary, Sally Bowman.

My developmental editor at Human Kinetics, Mary Fowler, for all her patient help. And many, many thanks to Rainer Martens, whose personal vision for sport psychology inspired this book.

The staff of the United States Olympic Committee, whose dedication to helping athletes reach their potential serves as a wonderful model for the sporting community, and in particular Harvey Schiller, Charles Davis, Jim Page, Jay T. Kearney, Tom Crawford, Steve Fleck, Sarah Smith, Leonard Jansen, Sheryl McSherry, and Peter Van Handel, who all have taught me so much.

Rob Woolfolk, who supported my interest in sport psychology from the very beginning.

All the athletes I have known over the years—those many wonderful people I have learned so much from.

Jerry May, who has been a wise and valued mentor.

My wife, Annemarie, and my children, Bryan and Theresa, for their support and patience through the missing weekends and long nights.

And lastly, my father, Tom, and mother, Nola, who taught me everything I know about being a good sport, the thrill of participating, and the love of the game. With that training, is it any wonder I became a sport psychologist?

CHAPTER 1

INTRODUCTION TO SPORT PSYCHOLOGY INTERVENTIONS

Shane M. Murphy, PhD
United States Olympic Committee

The effect sport has on our lives and how individuals adjust to sport are topics that have been too long ignored in the psychological community. Using psychological interventions to help athletes manage the stresses of intensive sport involvement is a relatively new enterprise. It differs from the more traditional *sport psychology* that mainly seeks to understand and optimize athletic performance.

You might wonder if the subject of psychological interventions with athletes deserves an entire book. I argue that it is important to explore how people can develop healthier, more productive athletic lifestyles. Professional sport is a pervasive feature of American society. For good or bad many Americans, young and old, identify strongly with sports figures. Recreational athletic activity has never been more actively promoted, as an aging population grapples with its lifestyle choices, preventive medicine, the costs of health care, and the quality of life. Sport and exercise are integral to our lives and deserve no less serious attention by health care professionals than our work and relationships.

Psychological interventions are required with sports issues such as treating the emo-

tional effects of athletic injury, preventing overtraining and burnout, helping athletes with eating disorders, attacking drug and alcohol abuse in sport, heightening awareness of gender issues in sport, and assisting athletes who are making the transition out of competitive sport into the business world. We discuss these issues in *Sport Psychology Interventions*. Before describing these sport psychology interventions, however, we must first review the broader history of sport psychology.

WHAT IS SPORT PSYCHOLOGY?

The term *sport psychology* has developed two separate, entirely different meanings, resulting in a great deal of confusion and even stress in sport psychology organizations. One meaning relates to the practice of psychology by professionals who specialize primarily in working with athletes in a variety of sport settings. After World War II, the practice of psychology flourished (see Napali, 1981 and Pryzwansky & Wendt, 1987, for a history), and subspecialties began to appear, such as clinical psychology, school psychology, industrial-organizational psychology, and rehabilitation psychology. These subspecialties were defined primarily by setting and type of clients: Thus school psychologists work in school settings with students, and industrial-organizational psychologists work with employers and employees in companies and organizations. Similarly, as some psychologists began to specialize by working with athletes in sport organizations they called themselves sport psychologists.

Most psychologists who practice in the area of sport have received little formal education in a content area called sport psychology. There is a clear reason for this situation: Few psychology training programs offer formal course work in the sport area. The study of the psychological issues confronted by athletes is almost nonexistent in graduate psychology programs. This situation has characterized other specialty areas: in the early years of school psychology, its practitioners received their training in other specialties, such as clinical or counseling psychology. As the demand for psychologists grew in school settings, training programs were developed to prepare psychology students for working in schools. It remains to be seen whether a similar growth will occur in sport psychology. (I will return to this issue later.)

But a second, very different view of sport psychology emerges if we examine the development of the academic discipline known as sport psychology, usually found in university departments of sport science, human movement, or physical education. Here the study of sport psychology is "concerned with both the psychological factors that influence participation in sport and exercise and the psychological effects derived from that participation" (Williams & Straub, 1986, p. 1).

Many universities in the United States offer courses and programs in sport psychology, and many of the faculty in these programs call themselves sport psychologists. Yet the training and interests of this group of sport psychologists differ greatly from the first group's. It is tempting to say that a major difference between the groups is that the first works in the applied area—the practice of psychology in sport settings—whereas the second group is academically based, working with research issues, theory development, and education. Although this might have been true in the past, it no longer is. In the last decade interest has grown in applying the knowledge gained from academic sport psychology in the sporting arena. Books like *Applied Sport Psychology* (Williams, 1986) and *Psyching for Sport* (Orlick, 1986) demonstrate this growing interest. Simple generalizations do not work in the complex, rapidly evolving area of sport psychology. We need to take a closer look at the historical development of both strands to understand the rope known as sport psychology.

TRACING THE HISTORY

The history of psychologists working with athletes is more difficult to trace than the development of academic sport psychology, because practicing psychologists usually experience less pressure to publish than their academic colleagues. I have traced the development of practice with athletes through presentations, professional publications, and occasional books. The development of the academic discipline of sport psychology, described as "the youngest of the sport sciences" (Williams & Straub, 1986, p. 11), was traced more directly through the publication of foundational works in the field.

Psychologists in Sport Settings

It seems that before the 1960s few psychologists specialized in working with athletes.

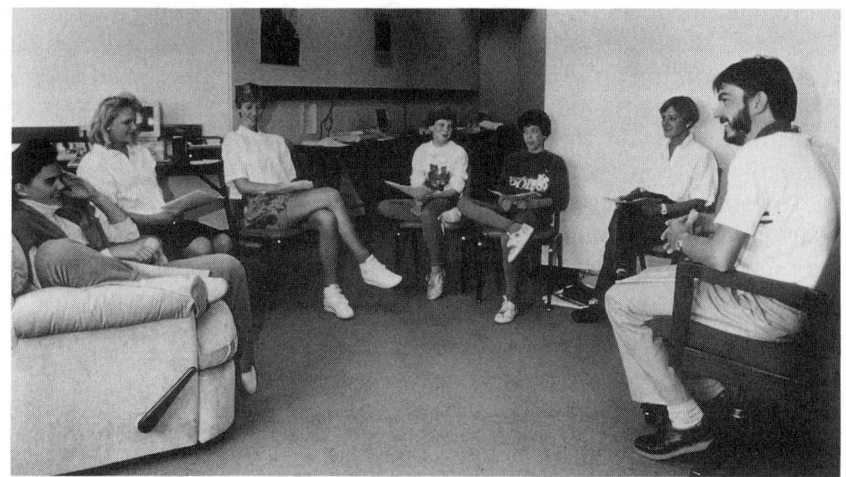

Courtesy USOC

Those who did seemed to be "isolated individuals without any recognizable training who applied techniques such as hypnosis to sport without any special rationale" (Nideffer, 1987, p. 2). In the 1960s and 1970s, however, a small group of psychologists became interested in the practice of psychology as it relates to athletes. The publication of such books as *Problem Athletes and How to Handle Them* (Ogilvie & Tutko, 1966) and *The Madness in Sport* (Beisser, 1977) and such articles as "The Psychologist's Contribution to Sport Organizations and the Athlete" (Butt, 1979) indicate that the psychological concerns of athletes were seriously addressed during this period.

A major factor in the increasing involvement of psychologists with sport organizations has been the increasing professionalism of sport itself. The advent of two factors in the 1960s and 1970s transformed the face of sport in America: sports television and sports sponsorship. Money was the common element. As networks paid organizations to air their competitions and as companies paid them for the right to associate products with star athletes, the profitability of sport organizations grew. Athletes in turn began to receive substantial sums for their sports participation. This trend was evident across all areas

of major sport: professional, collegiate, and Olympic. Although many lament the demise of "playing for the love of the game," the influx of money into the sporting arena was inevitable. Sport organizations began to view athletes as valuable assets. Without great athletes, success was out of reach—success that bred bigger television contracts and bigger sponsorship deals. An organization that had spent years developing a scouting and coaching system to create successful athletes was averse to losing them, especially to factors perceived as psychological problems. Thus psychologists were hired as consultants to work with athletes, in a sense protecting the investment of the organization. Although some might decry this analysis as overly economic, ample evidence suggests it is a viable model that explains the development of sport over the past 20 years (in particular see the analysis of the development of the Olympic movement in *The Lords of the Rings* by Simson and Jennings, 1992).

The result for psychologists has been increased opportunities to work in sport settings, a blessing for those who love sport and who enjoy helping athletes. Individual psychologists have been hired to work with professional sport organizations and national

Olympic sport organizations and by college counseling centers to work primarily with college athletes. Many of the contributors to this book work in such settings. Overall, however, the opportunities remain few. Compared to other areas of professional specialization in psychology, sport psychology is too small to warrant subspecialty status. The future of the field remains a mystery.

One indication that an interest area is becoming a subspecialty is the development of professional organizations to address the needs of professionals in that area. As more psychologists worked with athletes over the long term, a move began in the national organization of psychologists in the United States, the American Psychological Association (APA), to develop a separate area for psychologists interested in sport and exercise. In the early 1980s, APA instituted a freeze on the development of new subareas, called divisions of APA, so psychologists interested in sport formed a special interest group. Thanks largely to the tireless efforts of leaders such as Steve Heyman and William Morgan, APA approved a new Division of Sport and Exercise (Division 47) in 1985; it is one of the fastest-growing divisions in APA. Division 47 has addressed many professional concerns in the field and has published a small pamphlet for students interested in careers in sport and exercise psychology, describing the opportunities available and the training required for different career tracks.

Academic Sport Psychology

The beginnings of the academic discipline of sport psychology were *Psychology of Coaching* (1926) and *Psychology of Athletics* (1928) by Griffith. The publication record shows a long gap until the appearance of another *Psychology of Coaching* in 1951, by Lawther, but by the 1960s a variety of research was published in journals such as *Research Quarterly for Sport*. In 1967 a group of teachers and researchers formed the North American Society for the Psychology of Sport and Physical Activity (NASPSPA), the first sport psychology organization in the United States. It took another decade for the first separate sport psychology journal, the *Journal of Sport Psychology*, to appear, but the 1980s witnessed an explosion of interest in the area. Wiggins (1984) has written an excellent history of the development of academic sport psychology.

Sport psychology grew in the 1980s as a result of increasing interest in its applied aspects. Although it is difficult to infer a causal relationship in such matters, the publication of an important article by Rainer Martens in 1979 seemed to signal the growth of interest in applied issues. "About Smocks and Jocks" criticized much of contemporary sport psychology research for being conducted in artificial laboratory settings and contained a call to arms for researchers to emphasize field research, which is directly relevant to athletes and coaches. The article also emphasized that new multivariate theories that would not assume unidirectional causality would need to be developed in sport psychology. The increase in methodologically sound field research in the following decade seemed to answer Martens's call for action.

It thus became logical to study the impact of educating athletes and coaches about this body of knowledge. For example, if research indicates that certain factors might promote team cohesion, a logical follow-up line of inquiry is to determine if structuring the team to promote those factors increases cohesion. As researchers began working with sport groups, interest grew among coaches and athletes in understanding the psychological factors involved in their sporting vocation. As consumer demand for information grew, it was filled by educators formally trained in the academic discipline of sport psychology. What distinguished them from the psychologists just described is that few were graduates of psychology training programs or were licensed psychologists. Thus an entirely separate group of professionals interested in applying the principles of psychology to sport came to be identified as "sport psychologists" in the eyes of the public. Given the age-old instinct of territoriality, it was inevitable that clashes between the two groups would occur.

The transformation of academic sport psychology to include application as a major focus can be seen in the advent of books, journals, and organizations centering on the topic. The journal *The Sport Psychologist* began publication in 1987 and was followed by the appearance of the *Journal of Applied Sport Psychology* in 1989. Perhaps most significantly, an organization devoted entirely to applied issues, the Association for the Advancement of Applied Sport Psychology (AAASP), held its first conference in 1986 at Jekyll Island, Georgia. AAASP was the first in the new field to attract a representative mixture of professionals from both university psychology departments and the sport sciences. Almost from the first, however, members intensely debated whether the proper focus of sport psychology was primarily educational, focusing on performance issues, or psychological, focusing on personal development of athletes. As would be expected, individual training was often the decisive factor in determining on which side of the issue members stood.

THE CURRENT STATUS OF SPORT PSYCHOLOGY

As you might expect from this history, considerable confusion exists in the field of sport psychology concerning its nature, goals, and priorities, primarily because two groups of professionals regard themselves as sport psychologists. However, because of their different educational experiences and training,

these groups see many issues from different perspectives, and hostility can arise when one group perceives the other as imposing its worldview on an issue.

The sport psychology literature is filled with debate over basic questions: Who is a sport psychologist? What are the boundaries of sport psychology? How should sport psychologists be trained? What services should sport psychologists supply? (Brown, 1982; Clarke, 1983; Danish & Hale, 1981, 1982; Dishman, 1983; Gardner, 1991; Harrison & Feltz, 1979; Heyman, 1982; LaRose, 1988; McAuley, 1987; Monahan, 1987; Newburg, 1992; Nideffer, DuFresne, Nesvig, & Selder, 1980; Nideffer, Feltz, & Salmela, 1982; Rejeski & Brawley, 1988; Silva, 1989). As the debate has evolved, some basic concerns have been addressed repeatedly. For sport psychology to develop as a profession, at least the following issues must be resolved.

- *Competency.* A specialized area of practice assumes that the professionals working in it are competent to practice. There are several ways to address competency of practitioners, including requirements for minimal educational qualifications and competency-based exams or practice reviews.
- *Knowledge base.* Practitioners should agree on the general knowledge base that guides their practice. This might be based on research, be based on a set of codes or rules, relate to a body of experiential knowledge, or represent a combination of these.
- *Training.* Those wishing to enter the profession must participate in a recognized training experience that adequately prepares them for practice. Such training usually involves both academic study at a university and a structured practical experience under the guidance of recognized professionals.
- *Ethics.* All professions have their own set of ethical guidelines that guide proper

and appropriate practice. Each of the previously mentioned issues might involve various ethical questions. For example, an ethical guideline on competency could be that professionals practice only in areas within their competency. Professions have varying procedures for ensuring adherence to ethical guidelines.

These issues have been debated again and again in the literature but have not yet been resolved. Some, for example, argue that sport psychology services should not be provided because not enough is known about the psychological factors that affect sport and exercise participation; others feel that sport psychology should be a separate profession with its own structure and specialized training. I will deal with these issues again when I examine the future of sport psychology. But at this point I will examine the nature of the issues and concerns that professionals typically encounter when working in the area of applied sport psychology, however it is defined.

ISSUES IN THE PRACTICE OF SPORT PSYCHOLOGY

It does not matter whether one's professional training is in the sport sciences or in psychology; the concerns of athletes are the same in either case. Most issues or problems that lead athletes to seek assistance from a sport psychology consultant are related to the environmental stressors that committed athletes inevitably face in a modern sport context. At the Olympic Training Center in Colorado Springs we have kept records for 6 years on more than 1,000 athletes seeking consultation with our sport psychology staff, and more than 60% of the identified issues leading to consultation involve performance concerns. Typical concerns include anxiety at competitions, concentration during performance,

lack of motivation in the face of grueling training schedules, worry over whether success will be gained and efforts rewarded, and problems communicating with a coach or fellow athlete.

Discussion of interventions for such issues is infrequent in the applied sport psychology literature. In reading the major books in the applied sport psychology area, one is struck by their uniformity of approach. Typically these books take a mental-skills-training approach to working with athletes, an approach that has grown out of the cognitive-behavioral model in psychology. The mental-skills approach assumes that sport performance is managed largely by athletes' thought processes and emotional states. Athletes are taught these "effective" ways of cognitively managing their performance in the expectation that these methods will lead to better performance. Much of this literature assumes that athletes have few problems and that their primary concern is simply better performance. Williams and Straub, for example, state that "some data suggest that over 90% of all athletes are very stable psychologically" (1986, p. 9). This assumption can be dangerous, as it leads practitioners toward a complacent attitude that few athletes have serious problems. Given the extent of the problems facing sport, as any casual reading of a newspaper sports section will indicate, this view is naive. The reality is that athletes operate in a stressful world with challenges that few of us can imagine. Athletes encounter a variety of problems in their sports participation, and the interventions described in this book have grown out of a need to help athletes with these problems.

Also strikingly uniform in the applied sport psychology literature is the common focus on techniques. Every applied sport psychology book has chapters on techniques such as visualization or imagery, relaxation, concentration, and goal setting. Little attention is paid to the wide variety of concerns athletes in different performance settings encounter. Consider, for example, the different needs and concerns of athletes in the following situations:

- Youth sport athletes
- Recreational adult athletes
- Collegiate female athletes
- Masters athletes
- Minority athletes in high school sports
- Professional athletes
- Olympic hopefuls
- Collegiate athletes in revenue-producing sports

This sample list indicates how much the concerns and issues of athletic participants can vary. Some issues are common to all athletes, but even the meaning of a common problem, say injury, will be different for a first-year pro than for an active 60-year-old masters participant. In this book, the issues faced by different levels of sports participants are addressed for the first time.

THE FUTURE OF SPORT PSYCHOLOGY

It is perilous to look into the crystal ball for revelations about a professional area as young as sport psychology. Yet the brief historical overview of the field presented earlier includes many issues that remain unresolved and demand further discussion. Resolution of these issues will require much debate among those working in this field, but it is possible to predict some resolutions based on current trends. This final section of this introduction deals with possible developments in the sport psychology areas discussed previously.

Academic Sport Psychology

In some ways the future of the sport science subdiscipline known as sport psychology looks bright. There exists a great and still growing interest in the psychological processes related to athletic performance and the effects of sports participation on individual athletes. Research in this area will continue to grow, and it is natural to expect it to be conducted in sport science or physical education departments. These faculty have the keenest interest in athletes and sport, and the results of their research directly impacts their teaching. Funding for such research may expand as society commits some of its resources to tackling some of the problems associated with sports involvement: on-the-ice and off-the-field violence, cheating, blood doping and drug abuse, sex-related problems, and academic–sport conflicts. On a more positive note, the benefits of athletic participation and exercise will also have a higher research priority as society strives to find ways to encourage everyone to be fit and to adopt healthy lifestyles. As the baby boom generation ages and a greater percentage of the U.S. population reaches the senior years, a focus on the benefits of a preventive approach to containing health care costs will be critical.

Yet there might be storm clouds on the horizon of this optimistic outlook, and indeed the first signs of a coming tempest might have appeared. As interest in applied sport psychology has grown, more and more students have enrolled in sport psychology programs at both the undergraduate and graduate levels. This could cause problems if students graduating from these programs wish to enter careers in applied sport psychology and find few job possibilities. This career issue was addressed at length in a recent AAASP presidential address by Michael Sachs (1992). Problems can arise for students if (a) few job openings that fit their training are available when they graduate and (b) if the available job openings are more likely to be filled by graduates of other types of training programs.

The first situation apparently already exists. Typically, the most appropriate type of position for sport psychology graduates is a teaching and research appointment at a college or university. As has occurred in most university areas, the number of teaching positions in sport psychology has steadily decreased over recent years; at the same time student enrollment in sport psychology graduate programs has increased. Combine this situation with the apparent preference of many current graduate students to enter primarily applied careers and it is clear that a discrepancy exists between student expectations and job possibilities.

The second situation is a potential problem because many jobs that require direct intervention with athletes are likely to be described as "psychologist" positions, because they require applicants to have a state license to practice psychology. This is true of positions such as counselor or clinician for a sport organization or university counselor, and certainly anyone working in private practice as a "sport psychologist" must be licensed. Graduate student frustration can result if job positions are perceived as going to graduates with less training in sport psychology.

The immediate implications of this development for graduate training programs in sport psychology are twofold. First, students must be clearly educated about potential careers in sport psychology when they enter a program. Second, administrators of graduate programs must reexamine their priorities and determine if changes need to be made in areas such as the number of positions available for incoming graduates, the curricula offered, and the types of training experiences made available to students. The content of appropriate training programs for students interested in applied sport psychology careers is examined on page 10.

The academic discipline of sport psychology is in a turbulent period. Even as new opportunities emerge, several prominent physical education programs have been merged with other departments or closed down entirely. As several leaders of the field have noted (Bunker & McQuire, 1985; Silva, 1989), the discipline might have to undergo dramatic structural changes to keep pace with the changing demands of sport, students, and society.

Psychologists in Sport Settings

As this book makes clear, many psychological issues and problems encountered in the athletic domain are unique to sport. Psychologists practicing in this area without an adequate understanding of these issues are likely to experience many problems. Yet the current sport psychology literature does not often address these practice issues, and until this book's publication the practicing psychologist had no place to seek information on issues such as injury concerns among professional athletes, challenges to confidentiality in sport settings, approaches to drug education in sport, ethical issues encountered in working with a sport organization, and so on.

It is interesting to speculate on reasons for this apparent lack of interest on the part of the psychological community toward the problems of athletes and exercise participants. That a possible negative bias exists toward the serious study of sport in psychology is indicated by a comment made by the head of a clinical psychology program in response to a survey by LeUnes and Hayward: "The idea that one should devote one's life to 'bringing out the best' in sports performance is repulsive to me . . . it's a sign that we have a lot of misordered values in our society" (1990, p. 18). A personal anecdote also gives some measure of the extent of the problem. When I was in graduate school I chose a sport psychology topic for my dissertation research, only to have a senior faculty member take me aside and caution that I was "wasting my time" in sport psychology because "there are no careers" in this area.

The basic problem with the study of sport in psychology departments seems to be that because sport is a form of play, it is widely viewed as frivolous or trivial. Yet Freud himself said that life is made up of three essential elements, "love, work and play." Although courses on the study of love and relationships and on work and business can be found in all psychology departments, LeUnes and Hayward (1990) found that just 10 psychology programs of 102 respondents offered any type of graduate course work in the psychology of sport. Further, 92% of respondents indicated they had no plans to create such a course in the future. Although some of the paucity of courses on the psychology of sport might be explained by the existence of such courses in physical education departments, it is clear that there is little drive toward establishing the study of the athletic domain as a serious specialty for future psychologists.

The growth of sport as an area of serious study in psychology looks much less promising than it does in physical education. Without student interest, course offerings, and career possibilities, there is simply no impetus to establish applied sport psychology training in existing psychology programs. Instead, the study of the types of issues described in this book might become a postdoctoral specialization for psychologists who are interested in expanding their practice to include working with athletes. Evidence for such a trend is given by the popularity of continuing education courses in sport psychology that I have offered at the last several meetings of the APA. According to the APA continuing education staff, the sport psychology workshops are always among the first to be filled, and many more people apply than the 40 who are accepted each year. It is likely that the two major applied sport psychology organizations, AAASP and Division 47 of APA, will begin in the near future to offer more

extensive and coordinated continuing education courses in sport psychology to conference attendees.

The future of psychologists in sport settings is uncertain. It remains to be seen whether enough psychologists will continue to practice in the sport world to warrant serious attention to issues concerning the profession and its practice. It is the hope of all the contributors to the present volume that our work is of enough concern to stimulate much more research.

Training Programs in Applied Sport Psychology

Some leaders in the sport psychology community have argued that to accommodate the interests of students in applied issues graduate programs should change to incorporate more applied training experiences. Silva, for example, recommends that "the training of future sport psychologists who wish to practice or apply their specialization should be differentiated from that of research specialists by the formal establishment of intervention observation, supervised experiences with interventions, and structured internships" (1989, p. 269). Likewise, Feltz argues that the future of graduate education in sport psychology will be tied to more integration with mainstream psychology departments, but she argues strongly that the courses and faculty in sport psychology should stay in human movement or sport science programs (1987).

The issue of what constitutes proper training for a consultant in sport psychology has been tackled head-on by the AAASP. In 1990 it finally published, after several years of deliberation, a set of certification criteria by which applicants would be judged qualified for the designation *Certified Consultant, AAASP*. In publishing these criteria, AAASP noted that several benefits are to be gained by establishing a certification program, including increased accountability, more recognition for individuals and the field, enhanced credibility, increased public awareness, and further definition of appropriate professional preparation. With respect to the last point, the AAASP certification materials note that the process ". . . will provide colleges and universities with guidelines for programs, courses, and practicum experiences in the field of sport psychology."

Because they represent the culmination of intense debate among many leaders in the field of sport psychology, the AAASP certified consultant criteria are important and are worth examining closely. The criteria follow:

1. A doctoral degree
2. Knowledge of scientific and professional ethics and standards
3. Three courses in sport psychology
4. Courses in biomechanics or exercise physiology
5. Courses in the historical, philosophical, social, or motor behavior bases of sport
6. Course work in psychopathology and its assessment
7. Training in counseling (e.g., course work, supervised practica)
8. Supervised experience with a qualified person in sport psychology
9. Knowledge of skills and techniques in sport or exercise
10. Courses in research design, statistics, and psychological assessment

(At least two of the following four criteria must be met through educational experiences that focus on general psychological experiences rather than sport-specific ones.)

11. Knowledge of the biological bases of behavior
12. Knowledge of the cognitive-affective bases of behavior

13. Knowledge of the social bases of behavior
14. Knowledge of individual behavior

Several points concerning these criteria should be noted. First, in order to meet all criteria, a graduate student currently in training would probably have to take courses in at least two, perhaps more, different departments in the university. Few graduate training programs could currently offer all the necessary courses and practica to a student to ensure certification. Second, the criteria heavily emphasize training in two areas: psychology and sport. Except for Criteria 3 and 4, the guidelines do not emphasize a sport science background. Third, there remains some ambiguity in the criteria. For example, exactly what constitutes a qualified person in sport psychology?

It remains to be seen whether the AAASP criteria will be widely accepted by the sport psychology community, by universities and colleges, and by the general public. If the existing criteria (or some modified version) can be agreed on by other groups, such as Division 47 of APA and NASPSPA, then the chances of long-term success for the endeavor to establish criteria are probably greater. The criteria have not existed long enough to accurately judge whether they will have the hoped-for impact on the types of curricula offered by sport psychology training programs.

Potential Opportunities in Applied Sport Psychology

Having been a full-time sport psychologist in the most applied sense of the word for the last 7 years, I would like to conclude this introductory chapter with my own thoughts on resolution of the issues I have raised in this chapter. I would like to thank the many colleagues whose discussions have stimulated the thoughts expressed here, but I take sole responsibility for the opinions expressed.

It might be possible to resolve an issue that is currently receiving a lot of attention, namely, whether those interested in the application of sport psychology principles should abandon the term *sport psychology* entirely and adopt a new title, for example, *performance enhancement consultant* or *life skills specialist*. I believe the opposite, however—that the term sport psychologist is more relevant today than ever. This is true because (a) the term accurately describes the nature of the profession and (b) it is recognized as meaningful by the public.

Some of those who recommend that the term *sport psychologist* be abandoned argue that those who intervene with athletes and performance issues draw from many disciplines: ". . . the consultant reaches into an ever-expanding tool kit. In this tool kit are ideas from the world of psychology, as well as many other tools, such as philosophy, coaching strategies, interpersonal skills" (Newburg, 1992, p. 23). The argument has also been put forward that sport psychology is fundamentally different from other areas of psychology. "In most cases psychologists are helping unhappy, dysfunctional people to be normal. That is not what we're trying to accomplish at all" (Rotella, cited in Newburg, 1992, p. 16). Yet when a separate field of *performance enhancement* is promoted, the descriptions of this field end up being descriptions of psychological interventions:

> "What I do is teach people to think good thoughts, to think effectively. We spend a great deal of time talking about having a free will." (Rotella, cited in Newburg, 1992, p. 16)

> "We usually are working on human potential in an athletic setting. This work includes dealing with the athlete's attitudes, thoughts, and beliefs. . . . We help

them learn life skills that match their situation. Maybe the best way to say it is we teach self-management." (Halliwell, cited in Newburg, 1992, pp. 17-18)

> "When it comes to performance, they need a myriad of tools to succeed, to even take the first step. They need the right thoughts, mechanics, execution, attitude, commitment, intentions. And then throw in their feelings, affect. They need connection, immersion." (Ravizza, cited in Newburg, 1992, p. 17)

Psychologists and educators will recognize each of these approaches as variants of various psychological theories drawn from the work of such theorists as Ellis, Beck, Frankl, Perls, and Meichenbaum. It seems unwise to deny the historical and theoretical roots of such approaches. The danger of "reinventing the wheel" is apparent. As this book illustrates, there is much more to be gained from recognizing the intellectual roots of the field and drawing on them in fresh and creative ways. The variety of intervention models described in this book are a testament to the vibrancy of the field of psychology and to the opportunities for incorporating a variety of approaches into the applied practice of sport psychology.

As well, it is not necessary or advisable to change the meaning of sport psychology or to come up with a new descriptor of the field, because the present term already has a well-accepted meaning in the eyes of the public. This was brought home to me forcefully at a recent sport psychology conference when a young college athlete was asked to comment on whether his coach could also be his sport psychologist. The athlete pondered this question carefully and researched his answer. He concluded that it would be acceptable for his coach to teach him visualization techniques, to set goals with him, and to teach him how

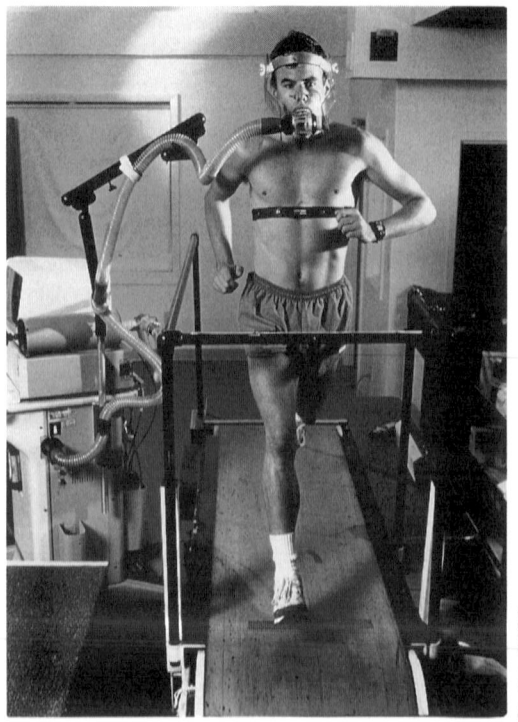

Courtesy USOC

an applied profession? My own belief is that the education of future sport psychologists is the critical issue facing the field. The important issue is not where students receive their training, but the nature of the training they receive, the skills they develop, and the impact they can have on the fields of sport, exercise, and recreation. As the AAASP certification criteria suggest, current education programs in sport psychology are inadequate and do not properly prepare students to be practitioners in this field. Yet there is a tremendous interest on the part of students in applying the principles of sport psychology in the real world of sports.

A potential solution to this problem is to restructure graduate training programs in sport psychology, much along the lines suggested by the AAASP certification criteria. Such programs would give students a strong background in both sport and psychology. Such programs should continue to be housed in academic departments of sport science, physical education, and human movement. The reason is simple. As explained previously, it is only in these departments that sport is taken seriously as an area of study. Psychology departments are unlikely to ever devote the resources necessary to investigate the myriad of psychological dimensions of sport. However, sport science programs will have to develop strong relationships with companion departments of counseling or clinical psychology. Training in counseling, psychotherapy, and abnormal psychology together with supervised training in practicum settings will require a far larger psychological component to graduate education programs in sport psychology than has ever existed. The rewards should be great, producing well-trained people who are adept at applying psychological interventions in a variety of sports and athletic settings.

Should these sport psychologists of the future be licensable as psychologists? A strong

to relax under pressure. But in one area the athlete believed that the roles of coach and sport psychologist were incompatible: "If I had a problem in performance, I couldn't go to my coach to talk about it. I couldn't say 'I'm having a problem at the free throw line in the last five minutes of a game.' The coach would yank me from the game at the end. I would have to go to a sport psychologist to get help for a problem like that" (Walker & Griess, 1992). This athlete clearly delineated the important role that athletes expect a sport psychologist to play in the athletic setting.

So the term *sport psychologist* is an accurate descriptor for applied practitioners of sport psychology, and the term has a clear meaning to athletes, coaches, and the public. Yet the field itself is in a state of confusion, beset by questions of competency, identity, education, and practice. How can the field meet these challenges and continue to move forward as case could be made for arguing the affirmative. As licensed psychologists, these people would have a greater variety of career paths open to them, a bonus in the present workplace environment. Additionally, they could legally use the term *sport psychologist* in offering their skills on a fee-for-service basis. To gain the types of experience that would prepare them to use most of the intervention models described in this book, students would meet most training criteria required of licensed psychologists. It would not, therefore, be an onerous extra requirement to meet the criteria for licensing. Such an attitude on the part of programs of sport psychology would require some psychology departments to relinquish some control and cooperate with programs preparing psychologists outside psychology departments. This battle has been won before, for example, by school psychology and educational psychology programs. This attitude also would require some sport psychology programs to adopt a new role, that of preparing professional practitioners rather than academic educators and researchers. Such changes will probably require enormous effort on the part of individual leaders in the field of sport psychology.

CONCLUSION

The field of sport psychology is in a controversial period in its history. Yet it is also an enormously exciting period. New areas of investigation are constantly being explored and new knowledge in the applied area is constantly being acquired. Many of the chapters in this book break new ground in the areas they tackle and the intervention models they present. We hope that the research and ideas presented in this book help many professionals assist athletes in enjoying and benefiting from their sports experience. Sports involvement can be a positive experience for all participants, but only if the experience is properly structured with the physical and psychological needs of the participants in mind.

REFERENCES

Beisser, A. (1977). *The madness in sport*. Bowie, MD: Charles Press.

Brown, J.M. (1982). Are sport psychologists really psychologists? *Journal of Sport Psychology*, **4**, 13-18.

Bunker, L.K., & McQuire, R.T. (1985). Give sport psychology to sport. In L.K. Bunker, R. Rotella, & A. Reilly (Eds.), *Sport psychology: Psychological considerations in maximizing sport performance* (pp. 3-15). Ann Arbor, MI: McNaughton & Gunn.

Butt, D.S. (1979). the psychologist's contribution to sport organizations and the athlete: An example. In P. Klavora & J.V. Daniel (Eds.), *Coach, athlete, and sport psychologist* (pp. 74-81). Champaign, IL: Human Kinetics.

Clarke, K. (1983). US Olympic Committee establishes guidelines for sport psychology services. *Journal of Sport Psychology*, **5**, 4-7.

Danish, S.J., & Hale, B.J. (1981). Toward an understanding of the practice of sport psychology. *Journal of Sport and Exercise Psychology*, **3**, 90-99.

Danish, S.J., & Hale, B.J. (1982). Let the discussions continue: Further considerations on the practice of sport psychology. *Journal of Sport Psychology*, **4**, 10-12.

Dishman, R.K. (1983). Identity crises in North American sport psychology: Academics in professional issues. *Journal of Sport and Exercise Psychology*, **5**, 123-134.

Feltz, D.L. (1987). The future of graduate education in sport and exercise science: A sport psychology perspective. *Quest*, **39**, 217-223.

Gardner, F.L. (1991). Professionalization of sport psychology: A reply to Silva. *Sport Psychologist*, **5**, 55-60.

Griffith, C.R. (1926). *The psychology of coaching*. New York: Scribner's.

Griffith, C.R. (1928). *The psychology of athletics*. New York: Scribner's.

Harrison, R.P., & Feltz, D.L. (1979). The professionalization of sport psychology: Legal considerations. *Journal of Sport and Exercise Psychology*, **1**, 182-190.

Heyman, S.R. (1982). A reaction to Danish and Hale: A minority report. *Journal of Sport Psychology*, **4**, 7-9.

LaRose, B. (1988). What can the sport psychology consultant learn from the educational consultant? *Sport Psychologist*, **2**, 141-153.

Lawther, J.D. (1951). *Psychology of coaching*. Englewood Cliffs, NJ: Prentice Hall.

LeUnes, A., & Hayward, S.A. (1990). Sport psychology as viewed by chairpersons of APA-approved clinical psychology programs. *Sport Psychologist*, **4**, 18-24.

Martens, R. (1979). About smocks and jocks. *Journal of Sport Psychology*, **1**, 94-99.

McAuley, E. (1987). Sport psychology in the eighties: Some current developments. *Medicine and Science in Sports and Exercise*, **19**, 95-97.

Monahan, T. (1987). Sport psychology: A crisis of identity? *Physician and Sportsmedicine*, **15**, 203-212.

Napali, D.S. (1981). *Architects of adjustment: The history of the psychological profession in the United States*. Port Washington, NY: Kennikat Press.

Newburg, D. (1992). Performance enhancement: Toward a working definition. *Contemporary Thought on Performance Enhancement*, **1**, 10-25.

Nideffer, R.M. (1987). Applied sport psychology. In J.R. May & M.J. Asken (Eds.), *Sport psychology: The psychological health of the athlete* (pp. 1-18). New York: PMA.

Nideffer, R.M., DuFresne, P., Nesvig, D., & Selder, D. (1980). The future of applied sport psychology. *Journal of Sport Psychology*, **2**, 170-174.

Nideffer, R., Feltz, D., & Salmela, J. (1982). A rebuttal to Danish and Hale: A committee report. *Journal of Sport Psychology*, **4**, 3-6.

Ogilvie, B., & Tutko, T.A. (1966). *Problem athletes and how to handle them*. London: Pelham Books.

Orlick, T. (1986). *Psyching for sport: Mental training for athletes*. Champaign, IL: Human Kinetics.

Pryzwansky, W.B., & Wendt, R.N. (1987). *Psychology as a profession: Foundations of practice*. Elmsford, NY: Pergamon Press.

Rejeski, W.J., & Brawley, L.R. (1988). Defining the boundaries of sport psychology. *Sport Psychologist*, **2**, 231-242.

Sachs, M. (1992, October). *AAASP Presidential Address*. Paper presented at the annual meeting of the Association for the Advancement of Applied Sport Psychology, Colorado Springs, CO.

Silva, J.M. III. (1989). Toward the professionalization of sport psychology. *Sport Psychologist*, **3**, 265-273.

Simson, V., & Jennings, A. (1992). *The lords of the rings: Power, money and drugs in the modern Olympics*. London: Simon & Schuster.

Walker, A., & Griess, A. (1992, October). Dual roles: The coach/sport psychologist—conflict or compatibility? Symposium conducted at the annual meeting of the Association for the Advancement of Applied Sport Psychology, J.M. Silva, Chair, Colorado Springs, CO.

Wiggins, D.K. (1984). The history of sport psychology in North America. In J. Silva & R. Weinberg (Eds.), *Psychological foundations of sport* (pp. 9-22). Champaign, IL: Human Kinetics.

Williams, J. (Ed.) (1986). *Applied sport psychology*. Palo Alto, CA: Mayfield.

Williams, J.M., & Straub, W.F. (1986). Sport psychology: Past, present, future. In J. Williams (Ed.), *Applied sport psychology* (pp. 1-13). Palo Alto, CA: Mayfield.

PART I

MODELS OF INTERVENTION

CHAPTER 2

PSYCHOLOGICAL INTERVENTIONS: A LIFE DEVELOPMENT MODEL

Steven J. Danish, PhD
Virginia Commonwealth University

Al Petitpas, EdD
Springfield College

Bruce D. Hale, PhD
Staffordshire University, United Kingdom

This chapter describes Life Development Intervention (LDI), a framework for the practice of sport psychology based on a psychoeducational-developmental perspective. Following an explanation of the concept of critical life events (the concept that serves as a structure for understanding the life course of an athlete), we will present a number of LDI strategies and techniques. We define a *technique* as a specific procedure or method and a *strategy* as a detailed plan to reach a goal. Within a strategy several techniques might be used (Danish & D'Augelli, 1983). A number of techniques will be mentioned but will not be described in detail, due to space constraints. Throughout the chapter we use a specific case study to provide examples of how the life-event perspective applies to sport psychology and how LDI is used.

We will also delineate the training and roles necessary for an LDI specialist to practice sport psychology. At the outset it is important to clarify that the LDI framework, although multidisciplinary, borrows heavily from psychology. Whereas most sport psychologists seem to equate the term *psychologically trained* with clinical psychology (LeUnes & Haywood, 1990), a number of "psychologically trained" sport psychologists are actually trained in counseling psychology. The differences between clinical and counseling psychology can be considerable, depending on an individual's training. Perhaps Super (1977) delineated the differences most succinctly:

> It is the difference between developmental and remedial help, between education and medicine, between pathology and hygieology. Clinical psychologists tend to look for what is wrong and how to treat it, while counseling psychologists tend to look for what is right and how to help use it.

Though the distinctions between counseling and clinical psychologists might not be as great as they once were, the contrast between a focus on proactive versus remedial interventions still exists. Proponents of LDI design and implement both proactive and remedial interventions, although the proactive predominates.

■ THE CASE OF CHUCK ■

Chuck was a highly recruited middleweight wrestler in high school. He earned all-state honors his last 3 years and was state champion twice. Chuck's father, a national-caliber coach, pushed him to excel, and his younger brother, just 2 years his junior, also was an excellent wrestler who had won all-state honors. Chuck accepted a scholarship to a top-ranked collegiate wrestling program with a goal of becoming an NCAA champion.

Even though Chuck had been a *B*-student in high school, school was not particularly important to him. His dreams and goals revolved around wrestling. He knew he would have to work harder in college to succeed academically, but his energy and concerns had little to do with school. He would do what he had to in the classroom to please his mother and his counselor. However, his main focus was on what happened in the wrestling room, not the classroom.

Early in his first year Chuck began to experience disappointments. It became evident almost immediately that he was not the best wrestler on the squad; he was uncertain whether he was even the best freshman. He was continually being decked by upper-class middleweights. No one had ever taken him down so easily. He began to lose confidence and doubt his abilities. His schoolwork suffered, and his girlfriend from home broke off their 2-year relationship. He competed intercollegiately just twice his first year, winning once.

During his second year Chuck had to deal with the first of two potentially debilitating injuries that were turning points in his development. A chronic shoulder weakness would not allow him to wrestle, and surgery was required. He spent a "redshirt" year rehabilitating his shoulder and trying to redevelop his psychological strengths. As it turned out, this injury was a catalyst for his future development as a wrestler and student. During his rehabilitation Chuck enrolled in a sport psychology class, where he learned many mental skills that improve sport performance, including goal setting, stress reduction, imagery, and positive self-talk. He also learned how to apply these same skills in non-sport-related areas, such as school, work, home, interpersonal relationships, and even coping with injuries.

As a result of his sport psychology class Chuck came to realize how important his early training with his father and brother had been and how what he had learned during these formative years had contributed to his success as a wrestler. Chuck also recognized how he had failed to understand the role some of these mental skills played in his success. It seemed as if he thought he could win in college by strength and quickness, yet in his previous successes his ability to concentrate, plan, and be positive had been critical to his success. He began to refocus on using and strengthening these and other mental skills he learned, and he began to apply these skills in school. The psychological skills Chuck learned during this period helped him to earn a starting position, and during his third and fourth years he earned All-America honors.

In Chuck's fifth year, when he was a senior, an acute bout of mononucleosis a month before the NCAA championships seriously jeopardized his final attempt to attain his goal of being a national champion. Chuck began to panic. He temporarily forgot how to apply some of the psychological coping skills he had learned in the sport psychology class and in subsequent consultations with the LDI specialist. Chuck felt weak and quickly became fatigued when he tried to maintain his fitness level for the championships. He was frustrated, angry, and on the verge of quitting on his goal of becoming national champion. The LDI specialist reminded him to apply the goal-setting model to his short but critical daily workouts. It was important to view an increase of a minute longer on the stationary bicycle as improvement and a successful step toward his ultimate training goal. Focusing on his end result and his inability to train at the desired level would have been counterproductive. But with small, progressive training steps Chuck was able to regain his fitness level by the tournament date. His confidence level was revived, because he could focus on his successes no matter how small they were. As a result of his refocused efforts, he won his weight class in the regional tournament and attained All-America status for the third time.

Another critical life event occurred when Chuck was about to graduate. While on work-site practicum, he realized that he had probably made the wrong career choice and did not want to become an investment counselor. First, he wanted to try out for the Pan-American Games team (he ended up not qualifying for the team, as he had a reoccurrence of mononucleosis). Chuck also needed to choose an alternative career. Initially he was somewhat confused and unsure about the next step, but by applying the life skills he had learned, he used the decision-making process and decided to pursue his interest in sport and communication. Chuck obtained an interview and ultimately a job in the advertising office at a major television network (where he recently received a promotion).

LIFE-SPAN DEVELOPMENT: A FRAMEWORK FOR INTERVENTION

The LDI model described in this chapter is based on the perspective of human develop-

ment. The major assumption of this framework is its emphasis on continuous growth and change. To understand both we must examine several disciplines, namely, the biological, social, and psychological. Thus the study of behavior, development, and change is multidisciplinary and should be considered against the backdrop of prevailing norms and present environment. Furthermore, because change is sequential it is necessary to consider any stage of life in the context of both past and future events. Finally, although changes in one's life might result in problems or crises, these are to be viewed not as pathological but rather as critical life events (Baltes, Reese, & Lipsett, 1980).

In the case study of Chuck we can see the changes he encounters and the effects they have on many of his life domains. The problems he faced when he first entered college were difficult for him, and it could be said that he was "in crisis." Despite how we commonly interpret the word *crisis*, it is not synonymous with being mentally ill and in need of psychotherapy. The word is derived from the Greek word meaning *decision*. The Random House *Dictionary of the English Language* defines crisis as "a stage in a sequence of events at which the trend of all future events, especially for better or for worse, is determined; turning point."

Most of us do not like change in our lives, because change disrupts our routines and relationships with others and can result in stress. We like continuity without having to confront life decisions and change. Systems, like families, teams, and work units, resist change for the same reasons (Watzlawick, Weakland, & Fisch, 1974). For this reason a change resulting from life situations has been called a critical life event. We experience many such events throughout life. In the year he applied to colleges, Chuck had to decide to attend a certain college, to leave the security of his home to go away to school, to change the nature of his relationship with his girlfriend (who still had a year of high school left), and to commit himself to work harder in school. Yet despite his willingness to make these decisions, several other decisions (crises) were thrust upon him. Perhaps the most important was the result of his failure to immediately live up to his own expectations as a wrestler. This sense of personal failure was the event that gave Chuck the most difficulty during his transition and first year in college.

Sometimes an individual anticipates a change but it does not take place. These non-events can also result in considerable stress (Schlossberg, 1984). An example of a non-event for Chuck in the sport domain was his realization that he would not make the starting team during his first season.

Although we often regard *events* as occurring in a discrete moment of time, critical life events are really processes that begin before and continue well after ''events.'' Critical life events, then, have histories—from the time we anticipate them, through their occurrence, and until their aftermath has been determined and assessed.

Coping With Critical Life Events

As noted earlier and as discussed in detail by Danish and D'Augelli (1983), Falek and Britton (1974), Haerle (1975), and Mayer and Andrews (1981), among others, critical life events are not the same as crises. As depicted in Figure 2.1, critical life events can result

in debilitation or decreased functioning; they might result in little change in one's life; or they might result in increased opportunities for growth.

Which result occurs is dependent on a person's resources before the event, level of preparation for the event (preoccurrence priming), and past history in dealing with similar events. For example, Chuck was able to overcome his mononucleosis, despite some difficult times, because he had experienced similar events (his shoulder injury) and had developed resources through the mental skills learned in the sport psychology course he took and because he worked individually with the LDI specialist to cope with the difficult situation.

All critical life events are similar to each other. If an athlete has handled past critical life events successfully and knows how it was done, being able to cope with a present event will be easier due to feelings of confidence and anticipation of success. In Chuck's case, because he had not been pampered in high school and college by his teachers, coaches, and parents and because he had been expected to make his own decisions, he was better able to cope with new events as they arose and to benefit from his ability to have successfully encountered past events.

THE STRATEGIES AND TECHNIQUES OF LDI

The central strategy of the LDI approach is the teaching of goal setting as a means of

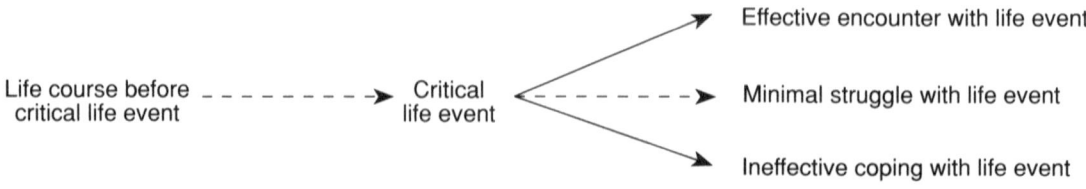

Figure 2.1 People have three basic ways to cope with critical life events.
Note. From *Life Development Skills* (p. 3) by S.J. Danish and A.R. D'Augelli, 1983, New York: Human Sciences Press. Copyright 1983 by Human Sciences Press, Inc. Adapted by permission.

empowerment. In this section we will begin with a discussion of goal setting. Other strategies and techniques that enable a person to learn skills to successfully encounter critical life events will be considered as well.

Setting Goals

Proponents of a life-span development framework assume that individual behavior is intentional. Thus people shape rather than respond to their environments. Goals are the source of energy that motivates people to action. A person without goals is like a computer without a program. The key to developing *personal competence*—defined as the ability to do life planning, be self reliant, and seek the resources of others (Danish, D'Augelli, & Ginsberg, 1984)—is to be able to identify, set, and attain goals. When people can set and attain goals they are able to gain control over their lives, because they feel able to direct their future. As a result, they feel empowered (Rappaport, 1981) and have a greater sense of self-efficacy (Bandura, 1977). Once people are able to accomplish this step they can then acquire the necessary interpersonal and intrapersonal skills. *Interpersonal* skills are those used to communicate with others in a variety of situations. *Intrapersonal* skills include both physical and mental skills; however, in LDI this term usually refers to what Vealey (1988) has called psychological skills. Interpersonal and intrapersonal skills are useful in the athletic domain but are not strictly athletic related. They are life skills.

By *goals* we mean actions undertaken to reach some desired end, not the end itself. Goals are different from results: Goals are actions over which the participant has control. For example, when Chuck chose to reconsider his career objective and focus on identifying the skills he had learned in sport that are transferable to the workplace, he was working on attaining a goal. If Chuck had

chosen as a "goal" to secure a non-athletic-related job, he would actually have chosen a result. Similarly, when Chuck was in rehabilitation following his shoulder injury or mononucleosis, developing a rehabilitation plan was a goal; wanting full recovery and the ability to wrestle was a result. People have control over their goals and only partial control over the results they want.

Three other elements are crucial for effective goal setting:

- Setting goals that the goal setter is motivated to attain
- Making sure the goal is stated in positive terms
- Having a specifically defined goal

Having people set goals for themselves is critical. If a goal is more important to others it is unlikely to be achieved. Unimportant goals rarely are. Goal statements that include words like *should* or *ought to* inspire lower levels of commitment than goal statements including words like *want*. Therefore, to increase the energy level invested in attaining a goal it is important to help a person ascertain whether goals are *should* or *want*, to change *should* goals to *want* goals, or to identify *want* goals.

When goals are not positively stated, the focus is on the negative and considerable energy is wasted trying not to do something. Setting a negative goal almost always produces a negative result. Goal statements that include words like *not*, *avoid*, *less than*, and *limit* should be changed to positive statements so the image of the goal is something to be achieved and worked toward. Having a positive goal means being able to identify the actions that must be done to reach the goal.

The goal should also be behaviorally stated and defined clearly. Goals that include vague terms such as *do better* or *improve* do not allow the goal setter the satisfaction of truly knowing whether or not the goal has been attained.

When the lack of clear feedback about goal attainment occurs, frustration and loss of motivation usually result and often lead to quitting. A rule of thumb when developing behaviorally stated goals is to answer this question: How many times, when, and under what conditions will the action occur?

Being willing to take an active role in setting a goal is one thing; being able to reach or attain the goal is another. There are roadblocks to reaching goals, whether athletic goals (improving concentration when attempting takedowns), career goals (making a decision about what to do following graduation), or personal goals (learning to be a better public speaker). The four major roadblocks are a lack of skill, a lack of knowledge, the lack of ability or courage to take appropriate risks, and the lack of adequate social support. In the case study, Chuck had many roadblocks throughout his career. He lacked knowledge of the therapy regimen he could undergo to strengthen his shoulder; he lacked the skill of talking positively to himself when he first came to college and experienced some setbacks; and when he became disaffected with his major he had to risk failure to find an alternative career.

Intervention requires that roadblocks be removed to enable people to work toward their goals. Removing roadblocks can become a goal in itself. Much of what the LDI specialist does is to teach or coach others, individually or in groups, to set goals, identify and overcome roadblocks, and reach their goals—by developing new skills, acquiring new knowledge, learning to take risks, and developing effective social support systems.

Attaining the goal involves developing a specific plan, a *goal ladder*, to reach the goal. Developing a goal ladder involves breaking the goal down into achievable, small steps. Too often people try to reach the goal all at once. If the goal can be broken down into 8 to 10 steps, the likelihood of achieving it increases tremendously. For example, Chuck's goal ladder for reaching his goal of rehabilitating his shoulder is depicted in Table 2.1.

Goals are identified and plans developed to help people encounter critical life events successfully. The fact that athletes are accustomed to goal setting is both a help and a hindrance. The familiarity with goals allows athletes to feel comfortable during the intervention process. However, because athletes are often taught or encouraged to set outcomes (results) as opposed to goals, some relearning might be necessary.

Developing LDI Strategies

As noted in our discussion of the life-span development framework, development is continuous. Critical life events produce a state of imbalance that precedes change and growth and might actually make growth possible. Consequently, the major focus of LDI becomes optimizing rather than remediating performance so that change is viewed as a challenge rather than a threat. Critical life events, whether sport- or non-sport-related, will occur; helping enhance or enrich a person's ability to encounter the event constructively through goal setting and other strategies is an empowering act (Danish & Hale, 1981; Danish, Petitpas, & Hale, 1990). In other words, the LDI specialist must help the person prepare to encounter the event, contend with the event during its occurrence, and cope with it following its occurrence (Danish, Smyer, & Nowak, 1980). Thus it is essential to consider the timing of the intervention in determining what strategies are to be used.

For the LDI specialist, the emphasis is on growth. Life events are considered processes that include anticipation, actual occurrence, and aftermath. Interventions occurring before an event are considered *enhancement* strategies; those occurring during an event are *supportive* strategies; once an event has

Table 2.1   Goal Ladder

End result

   To rehabilitate my shoulder by the end of spring semester so that strength and flexibility measures equal or surpass what they were last fall before my injury

Goal

   (Performance goals): Be able to military-press 175 lb; be able to clench my hand behind my back by reaching over my shoulder

Process-oriented

   Physical skills: New exercises for strength and flexibility

   Mental skills: Goal-setting plan for rehabilitation, exercises, and kinesthetic imagery for shoulder moves on takedown

   Knowledge: Ask the trainer about progressive resistance exercises and flexibility program

   Risk taking: None

   Social support: Talk with trainer and coach about feedback

Steps	Progress	Problems or roadblocks
Ask trainer for information about rehabilitation exercises for my shoulder	January 15	
Develop daily rehabilitation training program with trainer for the semester and begin a journal	January 20	
Record training sessions and have trainer evaluate once a week	January 21-April 21	Spring break means I will be at home for 1 week
Attend practice at least 3 times a week to watch demonstrations and coach freshmen	January 15-March 15	
Spend 15 min 5 times a week imagining takedowns, escapes, defenses	January 15-April 15	Will I get frustrated and lose my motivation?
Learn new mental images for coping with injury, work with trainer and LDI specialist to become confident that my shoulder can handle the stress	April 1	
Begin regular strength training with Nautilus and free weights 5 days a week	April 1	Might be too sore
Be able to military-press 160 lb	April 30	
Meet with coach to assess strengths and weaknesses and plan summer workouts	May 1	
Test my performance goals with trainer	May 15	

occurred, interventions are considered *counseling* strategies (see Figure 2.2).

Enhancement Strategies

Enhancement interventions are designed to prepare people for future events by

- helping them anticipate normative events,
- assisting them in recognizing how skills they have acquired in one domain apply to other life areas, and
- teaching skills that enhance their abilities to cope with future events.

Helping Anticipate Life Events. Understanding the nature of the future events that are likely to occur and having confidence in these strategies to cope with the future event increases self-efficacy. With this increased self-efficacy comes a sense of predictability

and control that translates into lower levels of stress (Meichenbaum, 1985).

When life events are examined to determine their effect on a person, three characteristics are usually considered: the timing of the event, the duration of the event, and the contextual purity of the event. The *timing* of the event refers to the congruence of the event with either the personal or societal expectations of when the event should occur (Neugarten, 1968). For example, Chuck's failure to make the Pan-American Games team following graduation and his subsequent retirement from competitive wrestling is an instance of an off-time event.

When we experience events that are on time we usually have the support of informal and formal networks to help us through the transition. When the event is one that is experienced by most or all people there also exists an opportunity for *preoccurrence priming* (Schlossberg, 1984). This form of anticipation

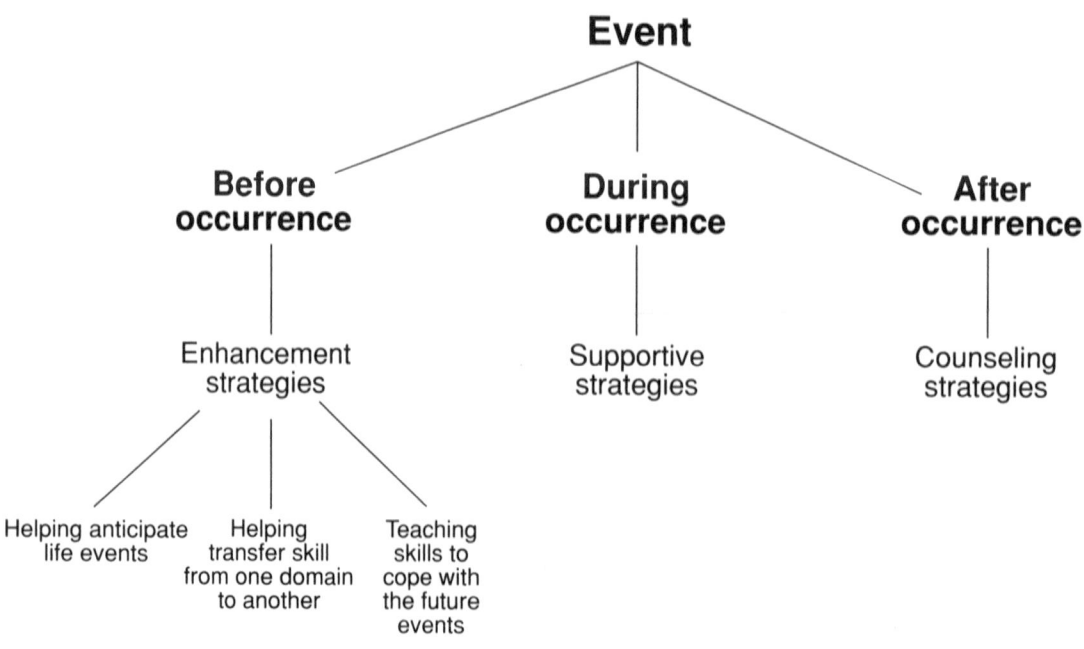

Figure 2.2 The type of intervention used must be related to the timing of the intervention.

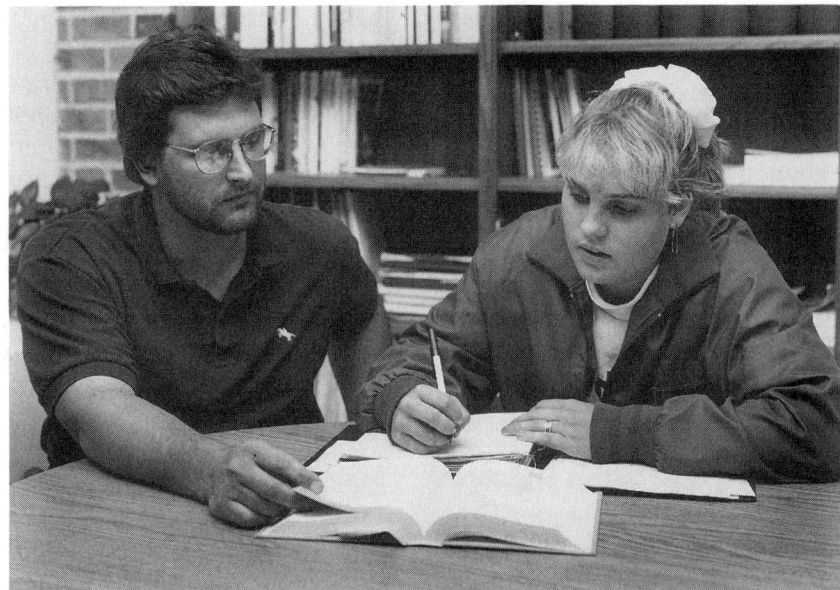

Courtesy University of Illinois Sports Information

provides a rehearsal period (an opportunity to try out different responses to the event). However, when the event is off time, such as athletic retirement in one's 20s (Baillie & Danish, 1992), coping becomes more difficult. A greatly off-time event, such as a sport injury that forces retirement before most athletes are ready, does not allow any preparation time for adaptation and teammates and coaches tend not to offer the social support that is essential in coping (Pearson & Petitpas, 1990). Moreover, when athletes retire as a result of injury they tend to feel unfulfilled, making the retirement process more problematic (Kleiber, Greendorfer, Blinde, & Samdahl, 1987).

Retirement from sport is not the only event athletes experience that can involve timing problems. The adulation, the time demands of practice, the loss of a normal childhood, and the expectations of success thrust upon young national-level elite athletes are all off-time events for adolescent athletes.

The *duration* of an event relates to its perceived length. Life events can be perceived as temporary, permanent, or uncertain and evaluated as positive, negative, or mixed (Schlossberg, 1984). A person's interpretation of a life event affects the type and severity of emotional and behavioral responses. For example, during Chuck's rehabilitation from injury and recuperation from illness he was often confused and anxious. However, as with other athletes in similar situations (McDonald & Hardy, 1990), once he believed that his condition was temporary and that he was making progress toward recovery, he became more goal directed and his emotions returned to normal. Had his injury been permanent, he probably would have experienced a more severe and protracted grief reaction (Rotella & Heyman, 1986). There is evidence that managing life events with uncertain durations produces the most stress (Chodoff, 1976). It should also be noted that perception of duration is often colored by the value one places on an event. As a sophomore Chuck knew he was redshirting, and he was able to design a more long-term recovery plan for his shoulder; his reaction to mononucleosis was panic, and his recuperation was probably slowed by his failure to manage the anxiety and to adhere to a carefully designed recovery program.

Contextual purity refers to the number of events being experienced simultaneously. Events usually don't occur in isolation. The more events being experienced simultaneously, the more difficult the adjustment. Events can be divided into a number of domains, such as familial, occupational, biological, or psychosocial. For example, as Chuck was learning that other middlewight, higher-class wrestlers were stronger and more experienced (biological domain), he experienced a loss of confidence and self-esteem (psychosocial domain), his grades suffered (career domain), and he and his girlfriend broke up (family and interpersonal domain). Although the latter event might not have been related to the others, it occurred at the same time and made coping more difficult. Thus even with a single event other issues intercede. Therefore, successful coping involves dealing with the perceived primary event as well as other events.

Athletes face many critical events in their careers. Injury, the annual team selection process, and forced retirement are but three of the events that can rob athletes of their prime sources of identity. These events typically occur much earlier in life for an athlete than they would in the career of a businessperson or medical professional. Assisting athletes in anticipating these events is but one of the goals of intervention programs like the United States Olympic Committee's (USOC) Career Assistance Program for Athletes (CAPA) (Petitpas, Danish, McKelvain, & Murphy, 1992) or the Ladies Professional Golf Associations' (LPGA) Preparing for Future Careers Program (Petitpas & Elliott, 1987).

The LPGA program was designed to assist members of the tour to prepare for their transition off the tour. The main goals of the program were to (a) provide athletes with a supportive environment where they could share their concerns; (b) help identify their values, needs, interests, and skills; (c) assist them in understanding and implementing a life-work plan; (d) enhance their self-confidence to assure successful career transition; and (e) establish peer and tour-alumni support groups.

Helping Transfer Skill From One Domain to Another. A second enhancement strategy is helping athletes recognize and use skills in other life areas that they have acquired through sport. The NCAA and other sport governing bodies have widely promoted the belief that sport is good preparation for life. This notion is true only if skills acquired through sport generalize to other life domains. Research on generalizability of skills indicates that skills acquired in one domain do not automatically transfer to other domains (Auerbach, 1986; Meichenbaum & Turk, 1987). For skills to generalize, many factors must be present:

- A belief that the acquired skills and qualities are valued in other settings.
- Awareness of current skills, both physical and psychological.
- Knowledge of how and in what context skills were learned.
- Confidence in the ability to apply skills in different settings.
- A willingness to explore nonsport roles.
- The desire and ability to seek out sources of social support.
- The ability to adjust to initial failures or setbacks. (Danish, Petitpas, & Hale, 1992)

Athletes must believe that they have skills and qualities valued in other settings. Many athletes do not recognize that many skills they have acquired to excel in sport are transferable to other life areas. For example, during one of the LPGA's Preparing for Future Careers programs, a tour veteran was teaching a group of 150 children and adults the basics of the golf swing using towels to demonstrate the proper mechanics and tempo. Her audience consisted of a large number of English-, French-, and Spanish-speaking people. She instructed and told stories in all three languages. The group was alive with laughter and enthusiasm. After this 90-min lesson, this same golfer was asked about her career plans. She immediately responded by stating, "I have no skills, the only thing I know how to do is hit a golf ball." Yet it seemed that the athlete had a number of skills and qualities that have considerable value in nonsport environments. Unfortunately, because she did not recognize that these qualities have value they will not transfer.

Athletes must learn that they possess both physical and psychological skills. There is a lot more to sport than just throwing a ball or running fast. Athletes plan, set goals, make decisions, seek out instruction, and manage arousal levels as a routine part of their athletic participation. Without mental skills it is unlikely that a person can qualify for elite levels of participation. When Chuck recognized that the mental skills he possessed had been a key to his success as a high-school wrestler and then committed himself to applying these skills in college, he became a much-improved wrestler. However, if athletes do not recognize that they possess mental skills it is unlikely that they will be able to use these skills in other nonsport domains.

For athletes, it is not enough to know that they possess physical and mental skills. They must also know how and in what context these skills were learned. Both types of skills are learned in the same fashion. For example, skills can be acquired through formal instruction. A skill is named and described and a rationale for its use is given. Then, the skill is demonstrated so the athlete can observe correct and incorrect use. Lastly, the athlete is given numerous opportunities to practice the skill

under supervision to insure continuous feedback.

Skills can also be learned by trial and error. People practice skills they observe in the playground or on television. They attempt to imitate these skills on their own, and with continual trial and error they acquire their own version.

It is helpful for athletes to understand why they wanted to learn the skill and whether they have tried to use the skill in different contexts or settings. If they have tried to use the skill in other settings, it is helpful to explore levels of success. In Chuck's case, he had learned how to set goals in his sport psychology class. When he later needed to apply this skill for his injury rehabilitation he was confident he knew how. If athletes have not attempted to use the skill in other settings, it might be helpful to explore what has held them back.

Athletes can lack confidence in their abilities to apply skills in different settings. They might fear failure or "looking bad." For example, when Chuck came to college his father chose Chuck's initial major. His father chose a "safe" major because Chuck was unwilling to examine his career interests and skills at the time. If athletes lack understanding of a new setting, this fear of the unknown can add to their hesitancy in attempting a skill. The LDI specialist can help by providing information about the new domain and coach the athlete through the process of preparing for and implementing the skill. By providing domain-specific information the LDI specialist can help to reduce the unknown and lessen the anxiety that can block an athlete from using a skill.

Some athletes have so much of their personal identity tied up in sport that they have little motivation to explore nonsport roles. They view themselves as successful athletes, not successful people. This mind-set can rob them of their confidence and prevent them from exploring nonsport roles. If they do not think they can be successful in other settings they might choose not to explore other options.

In addition, many athletes have internalized the belief that to succeed they must "give 110%" to their sport. This view can block athletes from investing time and energy in nonsport pursuits. It can also promote a narrowness of self-esteem and a lack of confidence in the ability to function effectively in other domains.

An LDI specialist can assist athletes by helping them understand that they possess valuable, transferable skills. The specialist can also promote the notion that having alternative activities can help generate a freshness and enthusiasm for sport that can protect against staleness and burnout and improve quality and concentration.

If a fear of failure blocks an athlete from trying the skill in another setting, the athlete and the LDI specialist should examine the perceived costs and benefits of the action. If the perceived benefits of the action outweigh potential costs, it is likely the athlete will risk the new behavior. If the perceived costs outweigh the benefits, the costs must be minimized and the benefits raised for the athlete to feel safe enough to take the risk. LDI specialists can teach risk-taking behavior using the process outlined by Danish and D'Augelli (1983).

Athletes might have difficulty seeking out sources of social support necessary to help them transfer their skills. Some athletes view seeking assistance as a sign of weakness. They might avoid opportunities to test out their skills in new settings, preferring to concentrate on their sport. Other athletes might not know the types of support they need or the best resource to supply the support. For example, Chuck did not realize that the LDI specialist could help him deal with the psychological reactions he experienced as a result of his mononucleosis and help him develop a rehabilitation goal. Too often coaches are viewed as the primary source of many types of support for athletes. Unfortunately, coaches are not always good sources of emotional support, and many coaches are not supportive of activities that, in their opinion, might detract emphasis from sport.

LDI specialists can assist athletes by teaching them how to identify types and sources of support. They can also help athletes understand the importance of support in the overall framework of personal competence so that they view seeking support as a sign of strength, not weakness. Two models of teaching how to identify the types and sources of support and how to seek out such support are outlined by Danish and D'Augelli (1983) and Pearson (1990).

Athletes can have difficulty adjusting to initial failures or setbacks in attempts to transfer skills to different settings, even though these skills are valuable in many nonsport settings. Such initial failures might be due to the lack of information and experience necessary to quickly adapt these skills into larger strategies required in new settings. This domain-specific knowledge might take some time to acquire and athletes who are used to elite levels of performance might become frustrated with their progress in new settings. In addition, plateaus and setbacks in skill attainment are common, and athletes might view these events as failures and begin to doubt their abilities. The slow pace of Chuck's recovery from mononucleosis was difficult for him, as he was used to more rapid success in other endeavors.

LDI specialists can assist athletes by preparing them for the pace of skill transfer by initiating a goal-setting procedure that may insure some initial success experiences. Using the goal-ladder process described earlier, the LDI specialist can help athletes plan out realistic time tables for skill transfer and plan strategies for overcoming any roadblocks to skill attainment that emerge. In addition, LDI specialists can use a relapse-prevention model to assist athletes in coping with any plateaus or setbacks that develop (Meichenbaum, 1985). The LDI specialist should also help athletes recall the time and processes involved in becoming elite athletes. Too often, athletes have short memories of the efforts they have expended in reaching elite-athlete status.

Teaching Skills to Cope With Future Events. Another type of enhancement strategy is teaching life skills that augment a person's ability to cope with future events. We have referred to these skills as life skills (interpersonal and intrapersonal skills); Vealey (1988) calls them psychological skills. Among the skills Vealey includes are arousal management, attention control, decision making, goal setting, positive self-talk, stress management, and time management, among others. These skills can be used in a number of life areas such as life-work planning, self-exploration and self-appraisal, and preparation for competition.

ATHLETES' VALUABLE LIFE SKILLS

To perform under pressure
To be organized
To meet challenges
To handle both success and failure
To accept others' values and beliefs
To be flexible to succeed
To be patient
To take risks
To make a commitment and stick to it
To know how to win and how to lose
To work with people you don't necessarily like
To respect others
To have self-control
To push yourself to the limit
To recognize your limitations
To compete without hatred

To accept responsibility for your behavior
To be dedicated
To accept criticism and feedback as a part of learning
To evaluate yourself
To be flexible
To make good decisions
To set and attain goals
To communicate with others
To be able to learn
To work within a system
To be self-motivated

Psychological skills can be taught through a series of interactive steps (Danish & Hale, 1981). The skill is described in behavioral terms, and a rationale is given for its use. This step is critical in assuring that people not only understand what the skill looks like but also have some faith that it can improve their performance. If athletes question the utility of a particular skill, it is doubtful that they will invest sufficient time and energy to acquire it. Once athletes understand how and why a particular skill can improve performance, the skill should be demonstrated. Many people must see both successful and unsuccessful attempts at using the skill to learn to differentiate the two and refine their mental picture of what is necessary for successful execution. From this point athletes are ready to attempt the skill, and with continual feedback based on their progress they can establish reasonable levels of mastery. Homework assignments and in vivo practice with continual supervision from the LDI specialist further enhance skill mastery.

Once athletes have reached adequate levels of skill attainment, LDI specialists can provide information on how individual skills fit into larger intervention strategies. For example, mastery of dribbling will not insure excellence as a basketball player. Acquisition of domain-specific strategies requires knowledge and understanding of the norms, processes, and structures of the new environment (Martin, 1990). LDI specialists assist people in acquiring this knowledge by providing information and experiences in the new domain as they provide support and feedback.

Supportive Strategies

Interventions that occur during an event or transition are called support. Some people require types of social support that cannot be provided by their natural system of family and friends. For example, the USOC has developed CAPA (referred to earlier), a service for present and transitional national-sport-team athletes. The goal of this program is to enhance participants' abilities to engage in the career-development process. Feedback from many CAPA participants indicates that one of the most significant elements of their experience was the ability to share feelings and concerns with other athletes "who really knew what we are going through" (Petitpas et al., 1992). The support groups that developed out of the CAPA workshops validated feelings, brainstormed job-hunting strategies, and supported both self-exploration and career exploration.

Chuck also commented that the life-skills course he took in his first year of college was critical for "helping me get back on track" during that year as well as for his future development. Although he believed that some of the skills he had learned were valuable, he commented that knowing other athletes experience some of the same feelings and worries about the future put him at ease. Until then, he worried that what he was experiencing was not normal.

Support can range from regular team meetings to group sessions for injured athletes. An LDI specialist can provide considerable personal support for transitional athletes through active listening and other aspects of rapport building. Other types of support would include

- organizing support groups for normative and paranormative transitional events such as injury or retirement;
- assisting in the development of personal support networks by assessing support needs and organizing resources;
- identifying potential mentors and role models;
- linking people to appropriate organizational resources;
- educating people about their own support-person roles; and
- advocacy.

In providing these services the LDI specialist becomes an important part of a person's support network.

An example of a support-based intervention now being conducted is the Going for the Goal program for the U.S. Diving Federation. This program involves having high-school–aged divers who have qualified for Junior Nationals teach a life-skills program for younger, less-experienced divers. It is expected that in addition to teaching skills, the older divers will serve as positive role models and mentors to the younger athletes.

Counseling Strategies

Another type of intervention, counseling strategies, takes place after a life event has occurred. These strategies help people to cope with difficulties confronting the impact or aftermath of a life event. The goal of counseling is to enable people to grow through a life event.

Unfortunately, many people experience emotional difficulties as a result of life events (Ogilvie & Howe, 1986). Often this occurs because a person's strategies for coping with the difficulty have now become the problem. For example, an athlete who was having difficulty managing his emotions due to a career-threatening injury was given pain medication to help manage the physical discomfort. The athlete soon realized that increased doses of the pain killer would also deaden the emotional pain. Quickly the athlete adopted a self-defeating pattern of self-medication that gave him short-term pain relief, but at the cost of commitment to his rehabilitation. In addition, his increased dependence on various types of medication superseded his need for family and friends. The end result of the athlete's attempts at managing his emotional pain was a substance-abuse problem.

Counseling interventions in an LDI framework attempt to assist people in identifying and developing resources to more effectively cope with significant life events. The approach is more educational than remedial. The first goal of counseling is to understand the problem from a person's perspective. This includes identifying the original intent of any maladaptive self-cure strategies. The second goal is to assess the coping resources, sources of support, and domain-specific variables. The third goal is to mobilize existing resources and teach new skills. The fourth goal is to give opportunities to practice the new skills in vivo with continual feedback, support, and follow-up. The fifth and last goal is to plan for future events and terminate the counseling relationship. A more inclusive example of the LDI counseling perspective as it relates to injury rehabilitation is presented in chapter 11.

In sum, LDI is designed to enhance personal competence in dealing with a number of life domains, both sport- and non-sport-related.

THE ROLE OF THE LDI SPECIALIST

As noted in the previous section, the strategies employed relate to the timing of an intervention vis-à-vis the occurrence of a critical life event. The education, training, and skills needed by LDI specialists are dependent on what strategies (enhancement, supportive, or counseling) are used. In this section we provide a general perspective on the requisite knowledge and skills needed by LDI specialists depending on the interventions and strategies they wish to implement.

Listening and Understanding

LDI specialists, regardless of what strategies they intend to implement, must be good listeners and be able to develop an understanding of the person or persons receiving the intervention. Understanding the critical life event from another's perspective is a difficult but necessary prerequisite. Too often we assume that we understand others and their problems and then rapidly begin the problem-solving attempt. When we initiate a problem-solving approach prematurely, we impede development of rapport, curtail self-exploration, and run a high risk of failure.

Attempting to solve a problem before it is fully understood can happen if the LDI specialist lacks training in sport sciences and misses or ignores important data about the athletes' experience (e.g., the centrality of sport in the athlete's life); has extensive experience in sport and assumes that this experience is identical to the athlete's; or uses the same methods in all situations due to the lack of a range of intervention skills or strategies.

Listening to and understanding others is the first essential phase of the helping process. LDI specialists must have such training. There are many effective listening-skills programs. These programs include *Helping Skills: A Basic Training Program* (Danish, D'Augelli, & Hauer, 1980), *The Skilled Helper* (Egan, 1986), and *Intentional Interviewing and Counseling* (Ivey, 1983).

Effective helpers, however, must not only understand the individual skills involved in listening, such as reflection of feelings and paraphrasing, but must understand the larger strategies of building rapport and gaining a commitment to action. Ineffective helpers come with a few skills and tend to force them on their clients. They do not understand the sport and intervention domains and assume that the few skills they have will work with everyone. LDI specialists must possess specific knowledge about both sport and the helping process to enable them to understand the unique dynamics presented.

The Training of the LDI Specialist

Although developing rapport with an athlete or group of athletes is a necessary first step, it is not sufficient if the goal is to enhance athletes' life development or athletic development. LDI specialists must have training to work with athletes experiencing a variety of critical life events. The training will differ depending on whether the intervention is implemented prior to, during, or after the event

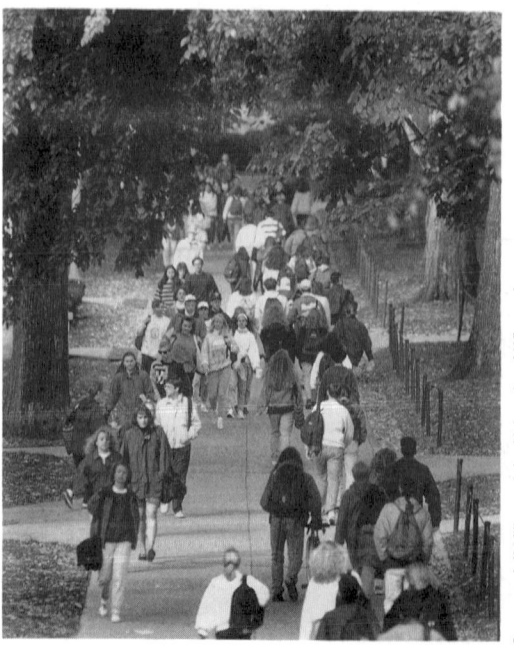

Courtesy Jeff Miller and the University of Wisconsin

and whether the target of the intervention is an individual or group. Whereas other chapters in this book cover some of these topics in greater detail, we discuss several training issues here only briefly. As a preface for this discussion it is important to note that other sport psychologists, especially those trained as psychologists, might disagree with this perspective.

Organizations such as the USOC and the Association for the Advancement of Applied Sport Psychology (AAASP) have developed guidelines for identifying the training needed for sport psychologists. The USOC has developed the Registry for the Psychology of Sport; AAASP has developed a certification system. One of the major distinctions underlying both credentialing systems is the discipline in which the sport psychologist is trained. Sport psychologists trained in physical education are viewed as educators; those trained in psychology are viewed as clinicians. What seems most important to us is whether a person has the requisite skills and knowledge to implement the intervention (strategy or technique) chosen; has the understanding of potential consequences, both intended and unintended, of the intervention; and has an understanding of human behavior (individual development, personality theory, abnormal behavior) so as to put both person and personal reactions into social context. Other necessary requisite knowledge and skills pertain to the area of sport. These include a knowledge of sport psychology subdisciplines, biomechanics, history and sociology of sport, physiology of exercise, motor learning, coaching strategies, and training and supervised practice working with athletes to enhance athletic performance. Additionally, people preparing to work in this field need experience in working with the coach–athlete relationship as well as with athletes who are training and participating in competitive sports.

From the LDI perspective, when the intervention occurs prior to the event, the major task of the LDI specialist is to teach life skills. To be an effective life-skills teacher requires a knowledge of how skills are taught and how learning takes place. Additionally, knowledge of the cognitive-affective and social bases of behavior as well as an understanding of human behavior (as detailed previously) are necessary. Regardless of what kind of intervention is being conducted, such knowledge is essential. This knowledge can be gained from a variety of sport- and psychology-related courses. The intervention agent must also have training and supervised practice in how to teach skills. We have described such a process earlier in this chapter as well as in other works (Danish & Hale, 1983; 1981). Gould (1983) has also delineated this process in considerable detail.

When the intervention occurs during an event, the focus of the intervention becomes threefold: to provide support; to help the person or group deal with the potential negative emotions and reactions being experienced as a result of the event; and to teach the new skills to encounter and, if possible, to grow from the event. The knowledge and skills required of an intervener providing support are diverse. In addition to the knowledge delineated above, knowledge of the social support and crisis intervention processes is critical. A *crisis* as we are referring to it here is something different than the denotative meaning of a turning point; it is the connotative meaning and is synonymous with emergency. Crises occur when an event has a sudden onset, is of great intensity, and represents a threat to important life goals (Danish & D'Augelli, 1983). When an event is being experienced, the LDI specialist must be prepared to contend with a crisis and its accompanying disorientation, confusion, and distraught emotion, even though these do not always occur.

Lastly, when the intervention occurs after the event, counseling becomes the intervention of choice. Although as we noted earlier an LDI perspective is different than a remedially oriented approach, the intervener must be knowledgeable about life-skills development as well as psychopathology. To understand normal development, one must have a knowledge of abnormal development and functioning. Training in counseling, both on a one-to-one basis and in groups, should be gained. The intervener should have supervised practica with an appropriate client population. For the intervener to be fully prepared to function in this context, training as a psychologist will most likely be needed. Such training, specified by the American Psychological Association, requires a doctoral degree in either clinical or counseling psychology. The application of psychological principles to sport is also essential.

In this section we have only touched on the issue of professional training. The topic is fraught with emotion, and we hope that these comments stimulate a reasoned discussion of the educational needs of a specific kind of sport psychologist, one who has training in two disciplines—physical education and psychology—and practices as an LDI specialist.

CONCLUSION

In this chapter we have described an educational-developmental model for the practice of sport psychology. We believe that the model provides a framework in which individuals trained in both psychology and physical education can design, implement, and evaluate a wide range of interventions with a variety of athletic populations. These athletes might be young or old, active or retired, able or disabled, or recreational or professional athletes; because of the emphasis on life-span development and the critical life events encountered throughout life, athletes at all levels can be considered. The primary focus of LDI is enhancement and social support, yet in some cases postevent adjustments might necessitate more clinically oriented strategies.

More importantly, an LDI perspective emphasizing optimization and the acquisition of life skills provides a framework for the practitioner to evaluate why, how, and for what purpose interventions are attempted. The LDI model recognizes that development is multidimensional. Change occurs in a variety of domains and affects not only the person but the system in which the person exists. By understanding the biopsychosocial context in which the person functions, the LDI specialist is less likely to rely on interventions targeting individuals when system-level problems exist. Additionally, having an LDI focus allows the specialist to be better able to identify the conditions that build character and enhance personal competence.

We recognize that other models for the practice of sport psychology exist. They must be shared so that appropriate roles and functions can be delineated. Following an examination of the various models, sport psychology will be able to begin the process of establishing itself as a unique discipline and profession.

REFERENCES

Auerbach, S. (1986). Assumptions of crisis theory and a temporal model of crisis intervention. In S.M. Auerbach & A.L. Stolberg (Eds.), *Crisis intervention with children and families* (pp. 3-37). Washington, DC: Hemisphere/Harper & Row.

Baillie, P.H.F., & Danish, S.J. (1992). Understanding the career transition of athletes. *Sport Psychologist*, **6**, 77-98.

Baltes, P., Reese, H., & Lipsett, L.P. (1980). Life-span developmental psychology. *Annual Review of Psychology*, **31**, 65-110.

Bandura, A. (1977). Self-efficacy: Toward a unifying theory of behavioral change. *Psychological Review*, **84**, 191-215.

Chodoff, P. (1976). The German concentration camp as a psychological stress. In R. Moos (Ed.), *Human adaptation: Coping with life stress*. Lexington, MA: Heath.

Danish, S.J. (1991). *Assessing the impact of a mentoring program to teach life skills*. Proposal submitted to the United States Olympic Committee, Sports Medicine and Science Committee.

Danish, S., & D'Augelli, A.R. (1983). *Helping skills II: Life development intervention*. New York: Human Sciences.

Danish, S., D'Augelli, A.R., & Ginsberg, M. (1984). Life development intervention: Promotion of mental health through the development of competence. In S. Brown & R. Lent (Eds.), *Handbook of counseling psychology* (pp. 520-544). New York: Wiley.

Danish, S.J., D'Augelli, A.R., & Hauer, A.L. (1980). *Helping skills: A basic training program* (2nd ed.). New York: Human Sciences Press.

Danish, S.J., & Hale, B.D. (1981). Toward an understanding of the practice of sport psychology. *Journal of Sport Psychology*, **3**, 90-99.

Danish, S.J., & Hale, B.D. (1983). Teaching psychological skills to athletes and coaches. *Journal of Physical Education, Recreation, and Dance, 57*, 11-12, 80-81.

Danish, S.J., Petitpas, A.J., & Hale, B.D. (1990). Sport as a context for developing competence. In T. Gullotta, G. Adams, and R. Monteymar (Eds.), *Developing social competency in adolescence: Vol. 3* (pp. 169-194). Newbury Park, CA: Sage.

Danish, S., Petitpas, A., & Hale, B. (1992). A developmental-educational intervention model of sport psychology. *Sport Psychologist, 6*, 403-415.

Danish, S., Smyer, M.A., & Nowak, C.A. (1980). Developmental intervention: Enhancing life-event processes. In P.B. Baltes & O.G. Brim, Jr. (Eds.), *Life-span development and behavior: Vol. 3* (pp. 339-366). New York: Academic Press.

Egan, G. (1986). *The skilled helper: A systematic approach to effective helping* (3rd ed.). Monterey, CA: Brooks/Cole.

Falek, A., & Britton, S. (1974). Phases in coping: The hypothesis and its implications. *Social Biology, 21*, 1-7.

Gould, D. (1983). Developing psychological skills in young athletes. In N. Wood (Ed.), *Coaching science update* (pp. 4-10). Ottawa, ON: Coaching Association of Canada.

Haerle, R. (1975). Career patterns and career contingencies of professional baseball players: An occupational analysis. In D.W. Ball & J.W. Loy (Eds.), *Sport and social order* (pp. 461-519). Reading, MA: Addison-Wesley.

Ivey, A.E. (1983). *Intentional interviewing and counseling*. Monterey, CA: Brooks/Cole.

Kleiber, D.A., Greendorfer, S.L., Blinde, E., & Samdahl, D. (1987). Quality of exit from university sports and subsequent life satisfaction. *Journal of Sport Sociology, 4*, 28-36.

LeUnes, A., & Haywood, S.A. (1990). Sport psychology as viewed by chairpersons of American Psychological Association—Approved clinical psychology programs. *Sport Psychologist, 4*, 18-24.

Martin, J. (1990). Confusions in psychological skills training. *Journal of Counseling and Development, 68*, 402-407.

Mayer, T., & Andrews, H.B. (1981). Changes in self-concept following a spinal cord injury. *Journal of Applied Rehabilitation Counseling, 12*, 135-137.

McDonald, S.A., & Hardy, C.J. (1990). Affective response patterns of the injured athlete: An exploratory analysis. *Sport Psychologist, 4*, 261-274.

Meichenbaum, D. (1985). *Stress inoculation training*. Elmford, NY: Pergamon Press.

Meichenbaum, D., & Turk, D.C. (1987). *Facilitating treatment adherence: A practitioner's guide*. New York: Plenum Press.

Neugarten, B. (1968). *Middle-age and aging*. Chicago: University of Chicago Press.

Ogilvie, B., & Howe, M. (1986). Trauma of termination from athletics. In J.M. Williams (Ed.), *Applied sport psychology: Personal growth to peak performance*. Palo Alto, CA: Mayfield.

Pearson, R. (1990). *Counseling and social support: Perspectives and practice*. Newbury Park, CA: Sage.

Pearson, R., & Petitpas, A. (1990). Transitions of athletes: Developmental and prevention perspectives. *Journal of Counseling and Development, 69*, 7-10.

Petitpas, A., Danish, S., McKelvain, R., & Murphy, S. (1992). A career assistance program for elite athletes. *Journal of Counseling and Development, 70*, 383-386.

Petitpas, A., & Elliott, W. (1987, November). *Preparing for future careers*. Presentation at the Annual Sponsor's Meeting of the Ladies Professional Golf Association, Pine Isle, GA.

Rappaport, J. (1981). In praise of paradox: A social policy of empowerment over prevention. *American Journal of Community Psychology, 9*, 1-25.

Rotella, S.A., & Heyman, S.J. (1986). Stress, injury, and the psychological rehabilitation of athletes. In J.M. Williams (Ed.),

Applied sport psychology: Personal growth to peak experience (pp. 343-364). Palo Alto, CA: Mayfield.

Schlossberg, N.K. (1984). *Counseling adults in transition: Linking practice with theory.* New York: Springer.

Super, D.E. (1977). The identity crisis of counseling psychologists. *Counseling Psychologist,* **7,** 13-15.

Vealey, R.S. (1988). Future directions in psychological skills training. *Sport Psychologist,* **2,** 318-336.

Watzlawick, P., Weakland, J., & Fisch, R. (1974). *Change: Principles of problem formation and problem resolution.* New York: Norton.

The authors appreciate the comments and suggestions of Patrick Baillie, Britt Brewer, Jennifer English, and Douglas Jowdy.

CHAPTER 3

CHILDREN IN SPORT: AN EDUCATIONAL MODEL

Maureen R. Weiss, PhD
University of Oregon

From 1930 until the early 1950s, the "experts" governing children's school and community athletic programs in the United States strongly urged the discontinuance of competitive sport for children of elementary and junior high school age (Wiggins, 1987). In particular, physical educators, health directors, and school administrators concluded that interscholastic and agency-sponsored competition among children and young adolescents was harmful for their developing bodies and minds. The experts instead recommended that these youngsters be involved in physical education and intramural programs, so as to maximize the positive physical and psychological benefits of participation in physical activity.

These recommendations had a strong impact on the prevalence of competitive sport programs in the elementary schools but had little effect on the community- or agency-sponsored programs governed outside the schools. Picking up the slack where elementary schools left off, agency-sponsored sport organizations at the national, regional, and local levels flourished. Organizations such as the YMCA, Catholic Youth Organization (CYO), and Boys and Girls Clubs stepped up the pace that they started earlier in the century. Little League Baseball was founded

in 1939, and the number of nonschool programs continued with Biddy Basketball, American Youth Soccer Association, USOC developmental programs, and millions of local organizations in every sport imaginable. In the end, the real experts prevailed—the youngsters themselves, their parents, and their coaches, who in many cases were also parents. In short, the overriding belief that sport contributes positively to children's physical, psychological, and social development has resulted in the participation of nearly 25 million children in nonschool-agency–sponsored competitive sport programs (Martens, 1986).

Despite the popularity and success of youth sport programs today, the debate continues regarding the potential benefits and costs of organized competitive sport for children. The key word in all these discussions is *potential*. The potential benefits of sport include physical development, such as skill learning and fitness, development of psychological characteristics, such as positive self-esteem and the ability to cope with stress, and development of social qualities, such as empathy for others and the development of lifetime friendships. However, these benefits are not automatically transmitted through mere participation in games and matches.

Rather, both positive or negative attitudes and behaviors are potentially taught in the sport setting by significant adults and peers and are learned by young athletes over time. If the physical, psychological, and social benefits available through sport are to occur, they must be purposely planned, structured, and taught as well as positively reinforced. This does not always happen.

This chapter provides knowledge about the development of children's self-perceptions, enjoyment, and motivation through sport experiences. Knowledge comes from theory, research, and personal experiences, and all are targeted at helping the practitioner maximize the probability of positive experiences and minimize the negative ones in the youth-sport competitive setting. Special attention is given to developmental or age-related differences in children's perceptions of their competence, of their coaches' and parents' feedback, and of their own performance outcomes. The objective is to determine how to structure the sport setting so that it develops youngsters physically, psychologically, and socially. If children sustain their activity involvement, then the value of sport in terms of self-confidence, enjoyment, and friendships will be optimally realized.

The chapter is organized into several sections. First I introduce three young athletes who serve as case studies to make developmental concepts and particular sport experiences more vivid as they are discussed. Next I describe a philosophy for understanding children's development through sport, with particular emphasis on an integrated sport science approach. Third, I review the literature on children's psychosocial development, emphasizing motivational theories and research and the salient characteristics influencing motivated behavior in children and adolescents. In the fourth section I focus on methods for enhancing psychological skills in children using a skill development model that describes the relationships among competence, self-confidence, and motivation. These constructs are further addressed using a psychological methods model that emphasizes the essential links among observation of behavior, instructional responses, and personal reflection of behavioral changes. I conclude the chapter with a return to the case studies and explore the intervention possibilities suggested by the information in the chapter.

■ THE CASE OF LAURA ■

At 14 Laura was an outstanding rhythmic gymnast who excelled in all of her events as well as at ballet. She had competed since she was 8 years old, and her coach's high expectations of her future in the sport were justified by scores in competitive meets and her improvement each season. Just after the start of one season Laura's coach contacted me, a sport psychology consultant, and expressed concern over Laura's decline in self-confidence, strength, and endurance during tricks and routines, and her subsequent overall performance decrements. Moreover, Laura was now self-conscious and constricted in her body movements and artistic expression, as exemplified by her wearing oversized T-shirts during practice. Laura's mother told me that Laura had grown several inches over the previous year and had gone through numerous physical changes in height, weight, and sexual development. Talking to Laura confirmed the observations of her coach and her mother. In particular, she expressed self-doubts and anxiety about upcoming meets and questioned her commitment to her sport in light of preparations for high school. New opportunities, such as academic courses, more time with friends, and specializing in ballet and theater, were becoming more and more attractive. Her parents and brother were extremely supportive in whatever route she decided to take. Despite Laura's attempts to understand that the reasons for her performance decrements were due to normal maturity changes, she decided to withdraw from rhythmic gymnastics and pursue other interests.

■ THE CASE OF RAUL ■

Raul's love for sports was unmatched among his 9-year-old peers. He loved all sports—basketball, track and field, baseball, swimming, and wrestling. In spite of his undying love for sports, he wished he could be as good an athlete as Roberto, his older brother. Roberto was one of the best football and baseball players in his high school. But Raul was small for his age, especially for football. And he wasn't as good in baseball as his brother, who was already being approached by college recruiters. Although Raul tried not to lose enthusiasm, it was clear that sibling comparison weighed heavily on his mind, and he wondered whether his parents, coaches, and friends would continually compare him to Roberto. Then one year at a summer sports program, the wrestling instructor observed Raul's enthusiasm and motivation as well as definite performance potential for the sport of wrestling. His size did not matter—he could be matched with similar-sized boys for practicing moves and competing in simulated matches. His instructor encouraged Raul to join a local USA Wrestling club, which he did, and he continued his involvement in wrestling at the middle school level. By the time Raul entered high school, he was still small for his age, but he was an accomplished wrestler with lots of room for improvement. He continued to improve steadily throughout his high school years, culminating in a district championship in the 136-lb (62-kg) class his senior year. During the summers of high school years, Raul often returned to the sports program to help teach children in the wrestling room, where he served as an excellent role model for youngsters much like him.

■ THE CASE OF JULIA ■

Julia, an 11-year-old, had competed for a gymnastics club since she was 6 years old. Her father drove her 45 mi (72 km) to practice each day so she could benefit from the best instruction in the state. For some time Julia had been distressed because her coach was *encouraging* her to practice harder, try more difficult moves, and generally "go for it" even when she did not feel confident that she could execute a trick. Competition against teammates, rather than participation with them, escalated when the coach started to encourage intrateam rivalries and to offer or withhold affection and attention based on the outcomes. What made matters worse for Julia was an ankle injury that did not seem to be healing; this affected her performance and self-confidence. Julia used to enjoy gymnastics because it gave her a sense of being good at something and allowed her to be with her friends, but lately the sport had turned from play to work. Thoughts of quitting gnawed at her, but she often heard her coaches and teammates call former gymnasts "quitters" and "losers." Moreover, she knew how proud her parents were and how they loved to show off about her talent, and she did not want to let them down. What should she do? She did not want to continue going to gymnastics, but she didn't want to quit either. On the long drive each day, she repeatedly rehearsed telling her father about her desire to quit, but she could not seem to get the words out. The anxiety of practice and the unrealistic demands of her coach were stressful, but so was the thought of telling her father she wanted to quit. Haunted by the anxiety of indecision, Julia finally made a choice. At practice one day, she purposely overshot a trick and twisted her knee on landing. Her self-imposed injury put her out for the season: she could avoid the stigma of being called a loser because she could claim that she had been "forced to discontinue gymnastics participation."

A PHILOSOPHY FOR UNDERSTANDING CHILDREN'S PSYCHOLOGICAL DEVELOPMENT THROUGH SPORT

My philosophy of working with children and understanding their development in sport settings revolves around three major themes. Personal development and a healthy lifestyle through positive sport experiences are the primary focus, with performance enhancement a secondary goal. More specifically, positive self-perceptions, intrinsic motivation, enjoyment, positive attitude toward the value of physical activity, ability to cope with stress, and sportspersonlike attitudes form the core of characteristics that provide the justification for children's competitive sport (Wiggins, 1987). However, little substantive evidence supports this claim. Instead, many parents and coaches come to expect that these personal qualities and skills will emerge as a result of mere participation and exposure to the rigors of competitive play. But if we are to claim that sport builds character then we must purposefully target these areas in our consulting with parents and coaches and especially help them structure sporting experiences to maximize the probability that these positive outcomes will occur.

Another theme of my philosophical approach with children in sport is the notion of a theory-to-practice and practice-to-theory perspective. That is, both the developmental and sport-psychology literatures provide tremendous insights about the nature of children's self-esteem, motivational orientations, and cognitive abilities as they relate to motor skills and behaviors. The solid knowledge base about children's cognitions and perceptions can help us in understanding and explaining their sport participation and performance. However, just as important are children's expressions of their own experiences, which can provide unique information not found in books and journals. Together, the empirical and experiential knowledge about children and adolescents provides a rich source of information for helping practitioners understand children's perceptions of sport experiences and the selection of appropriate intervention strategies for influencing positive changes.

Lastly, I have found it useful to adopt an integrated sport science approach to understanding children's attitudes and behaviors in sport settings. An integrated approach combines scientific knowledge from such areas as sport psychology, sport sociology, motor behavior (development, learning, control), exercise physiology, and biomechanics to describe, explain, and predict participation behavior and performance. It thus describes the interaction among biological, psychological, social, and physical differences in the social context of the developing child in sport. Such an approach should help to explain more of the variance in sport participation behaviors as well as provide practitioners with information that they can use to solve sport-specific problems, such as attrition from sport programs, effects of game and rule modifications, and readiness for sports competition.

The logic and rationale of such a multidisciplinary perspective can be seen with our three case-study athletes, Laura, Raul, and Julia. Before Laura entered an intense growth spurt at age 12, she was by far the best performer in her club. Her routines were exceptional in the rope, ball, hoop, ribbon, and clubs events. As a result of biological and physical changes associated with her maturation, mechanical and neuromuscular constraints influenced her ability to execute well-learned tricks and techniques. Having to adjust to her new body parameters to execute routines affected her psychologically, especially in terms of self-confidence, anxiety, and enjoyment. In addition, expectations of her coach and the elite structure of rhythmic gymnastics elevated feelings of anxiety and doubt about further performance. The combination of biological, psychological, and physical factors along with important social influences by family and coach influenced her eventual decision to quit gymnastics.

Raul's small size as a result of being a late-maturing youngster was a barrier to pursuing football as his brother had done, and his skills in baseball were not as good as Roberto's. But his extreme enthusiasm and motivation for sports kept him involved and determined to achieve in his own way. Strong encouragement from his instructors and coaches, a desire to excel in a unique area of achievement, and his physical size combined to make him a perfect match for wrestling. His successful experiences and positive feedback from peers and adults motivated his

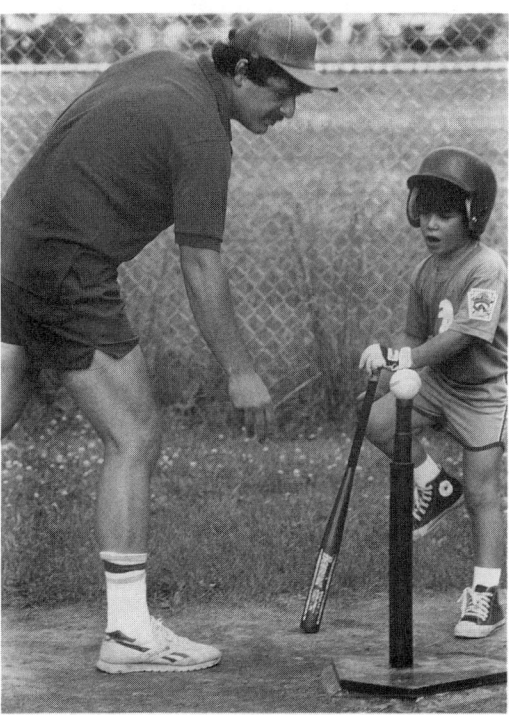

desire to excel in the sport, resulting in superior achievements at the high school level. Thus we again see that physical, biological, psychological, and social environmental factors influenced participation behaviors and performance in sport.

Lastly, we have the negative experiences and outcome for Julia. When Julia began her gymnastics participation, it was fun for her because of all the opportunities to learn new skills and to be with friends. As she got older and more talented in the sport, her own self-imposed demands as well as those of her parents and coach resulted in less enjoyment and the propensity for injury. The injuries had both physical and psychological consequences, which in turn affected the quality of her performance. The potential stigma of being called a quitter by significant adults and peers only made matters worse. She neither enjoyed her participation nor found a way to discontinue the sport without significant harm to her self-esteem. Her only way out was to incur an injury that gave her no choice but to withdraw from competition. The influence by significant others and the structure of sport in combination with individual differences along physical, social, and psychological lines contributes to our understanding of Julia's final decision.

An integrated perspective provides a holistic way of explaining children's participation and performance in sport. By considering the range of biological, physical, psychological, and social individual difference factors influencing the child as well as environmental factors, such as significant adults and peers, the particular level or structure of sport, and one's ascribed attributes, such as gender, race, and culture, researchers and practitioners alike can maximize their understanding of children's experiences in sport. Moreover, pinpointing the various influences in a child's life in sport can help practitioners decide on what psychological skills and methods should be chosen.

The focus on an integrated sport-science approach to understanding children's participation and performance in sport lends itself well to a focus on personal development and lifestyle skills. *Personal development* refers to the psychological skills or qualities to be attained through experiences in sport and physical activity, whereas *psychological methods* refer to the techniques or strategies for ensuring that these skills are developed (Vealey, 1988). Psychological skills can infer either those characteristics needed to facilitate optimal performance or those needed to maintain a positive attitude toward and enjoyment of physical activity. The psychological skills that I emphasize in my work with children along with strategies for developing them appear in Table 3.1.

The focus of my presentation on developing psychological skills in young athletes is on self-perceptions, affect, and motivation.

In order to understand antecedents, correlates, and consequences of these characteristics in children's lives, I will review the social, developmental, and sport psychology literatures on motivation theories and research. Following this presentation, I will derive from this literature intervention strategies or psychological methods for influencing positive self-perceptions, affect, and motivation.

PSYCHOSOCIAL DEVELOPMENT IN CHILDREN: REVIEWING THE LITERATURE

The research on participation motivation and attrition, although largely descriptive in nature, has provided a wealth of data on why children and adolescents participate in sport

Table 3.1   Psychological Skills and Methods in Working With Children in Sport

Psychological skills	Psychological methods
Positive self-perceptions	Environmental strategies
Intrinsic motivation	Skill development methods
Interpersonal skills	Structure of practice and competitions
Positive attitude toward value of	Game and rule modifications
physical activity	Motivational climate
Coping with competitive stress	Parent and coach education
Moral development and sportspersonship	Communication styles
Positive affect	Social reinforcement principles
	Leadership effectiveness
	Expectancy effects
	Modeling techniques
	Individual control strategies
	Imagery
	Goal setting
	Relaxation
	Self-talk

(Gould & Petlichkoff, 1988; Weiss & Chaumeton, 1992; Weiss & Petlichkoff, 1989). Several common themes for participation reasons have emerged based on the number of studies conducted. These include

- competence (learning and improving skills),
- affiliation (being with and making friends),
- team identification (being part of a group, team spirit),
- health and fitness (getting and staying in shape),
- competition (excitement, demonstrating skills), and
- fun.

The reasons cited are primarily intrinsic, rather than extrinsic, in their orientation. Less consensus exists about reasons for discontinuing involvement. Early research efforts identified lack of playing time, reduction in fun, dislike for the coach, and an overemphasis on competition as predominant reasons for discontinuing involvement. Subsequent studies reported reasons such as "conflicts of interest," time demands, and "other things to do" (Weiss & Chaumeton, 1992). An encouraging finding of the few studies that were specifically designed to follow up on athletes who withdrew from a sport was that the large majority are not permanent dropouts but rather that they often transfer to another sport or to the same sport at a lower intensity (Weiss & Petlichkoff, 1989). Nevertheless, a common theme of these findings is that reasons for leaving a sport are often linked to issues related to perceptions of competence, dissatisfaction with the social environment (e.g., coach, competitive emphasis), or no longer enjoying participation.

Although the research on participation motivation primarily tells us what reasons predominate for athletes' participation in sport, the underlying processes explaining *why* these reasons exist and how they are developed in the young athlete are not as clear. To understand the underlying social and cognitive mechanisms that might explain why athletes participate or discontinue sport involvement, I will review the developmental and social psychology literatures. Most of these theories have been supported primarily in the academic domain, but recent research in sport psychology strongly suggests that they are also valid when applied to physical achievement situations.

Children's Motivation According to Harter

Harter's competence-motivation theory (1978, 1981) emphasizes an understanding of children's psychological development as they strive to demonstrate competence in a particular achievement domain. According to competence-motivation theory, children are motivated to become competent in their social environments and do so by engaging in mastery attempts. When these efforts are successful in the child's eyes, perceptions of competence and internal locus of control increase, resulting in heightened positive affect and the maintenance of competence motivation. Thus the person continues to be motivated toward seeking challenges that will result in competent performance accomplishments.

Harter identifies other salient components that contribute to the development of these self-perceptions, affect, and motivation. In particular, the child's socialization history in the form of modeling, feedback, and reinforcement from significant adults and peers in response to performance plays a large role in psychosocial development. Moreover, adoption of a reward system and standard of goals are shaped through the quality of communication received from these significant others. Children who are reinforced for independent mastery attempts and encouraged to try harder, to persist in the face of skill barriers, and to use self-referenced information to judge competence (e.g., skill improvement, enjoyment of sport) will likely develop an intrinsic motivational orientation in which a self-reward system and mastery goals are embraced. In contrast, the child who is encouraged to view competence primarily in relation to the performance of others will most likely adopt an extrinsic motivational orientation, where a dependence on external rewards and the adoption of outcome goals predominate.

Relation of Perceived Competence to Affect and Motivation

The relationships among several of the salient components in Harter's model have been strongly supported by research in both the academic and sport domains (Weiss & Chaumeton, 1992). For example, Klint and Weiss (1987) found a strong relationship between perceived competence and motives for participating in competitive youth gymnastics. Specifically, athletes high in perceived physical competence indicated that skill development reasons were most important for their participation, whereas those athletes who registered higher perceived peer-acceptance scores identified affiliation and team aspects as most salient for their participation. Thus children were motivated by reasons related to opportunities for demonstrating their competence in the competitive sport setting and, in turn, perceptions of competence contributed to continued motivation.

Several studies have substantiated consistent relationships among perceptions of competence and control, affect in the form of enjoyment and anxiety, and intrinsic motivation. For example, Weiss and Horn (1990)

were interested in children's accuracy of perceived competence and its relation to achievement characteristics. They found that children who underestimated their abilities (i.e., their perceived competence scores were considerably lower than teachers' ratings of their actual competence) indicated higher trait anxiety, an external locus of control, and lower challenge-seeking behaviors in comparison to their accurate- and over-estimating peers. Weiss, McAuley, Ebbeck, and Wiese (1990) found a strong relationship between self-perceptions and causal attributions for performance in the physical domain. Specifically, children who were higher in perceived competence made causal attributions for perceived success that were more internal, stable, and personally controllable than did those lower in competence perceptions. Lastly, Weiss, Bredemeier, and Shewchuk (1986) investigated the relationships among perceived competence, perceived control, intrinsic motivation, and physical achievement in children participating in a variety of sports. Results revealed that children higher in perceived competence demonstrated higher achievement scores and a more intrinsic motivational orientation than children low in perceived competence.

Taken together, the results of these three studies (Weiss et al., 1986; Weiss et al., 1990; Weiss & Horn, 1990) suggest that children with high levels of physical competence perceptions follow a pattern of functional achievement behaviors, reflected by success perceptions, appropriate causal attributions for success and failure, an intrinsic motivational orientation, and positive affective outcomes. Conversely, children who evidence low (or inaccurate) perceptions of competence are characterized by psychological characteristics describing a more extrinsically oriented individual: low in challenge-seeking behavior and high on negative affect such as anxiety, inappropriate attributions for performance outcomes, and low future performance expectations.

Sources of Competence Information

A particularly interesting and insightful line of research testing Harter's predictions has been the investigation of developmental differences in the sources of information children use to judge their competence in the physical domain. Horn and her colleagues (Horn, 1991; Horn & Hasbrook, 1986, 1987; Horn & Weiss, 1991) have conducted several studies to investigate the developmental nature of preferences for sources of information. This research indicates that younger children (ages 8 and 9) prefer the use of adult feedback and evaluation; as children get older (ages 10 to 14) preference for adult feedback declines and reliance on peer comparison and evaluation becomes dominant. The later adolescent years are characterized by a tendency toward the use of multiple sources of criteria to judge competence, particularly a decline in the use of peer comparison and evaluation, and an increase in the use of internal criteria, such as goal achievement, self-improvement, speed, ease in learning new skills, and enjoyment of the activity.

Research has also found a relationship between sources of competence information and patterns of self-perceptions in children and adolescents. Specifically, Horn and Hasbrook (1987) found that children who were low in perceived competence and high in external perceptions of performance control indicated a preference for external sources of information, such as parental feedback and evaluation. Conversely, children high in perceived competence and internal locus of control were more likely to prefer internal sources of criteria to judge their physical competence, such as degree of skill improvement, ease in learning skills, and effort. These relationships were found in children 10 to 14 years of age, but a nonsignificant relationship between information sources and self-perceptions was found for the 8- to 9-year-old group, indicating that a certain developmental level of cognitive sophistication,

socialization history, or both must be in place for these relationships to unfold.

Dimensions of Self-Esteem

Another developmental finding in Harter's framework concerns the differentiation and salience of dimensions of self-esteem in early childhood through adolescence. Factor analyses have determined how self-esteem dimensions are integrated or differentiated with increases in maturity. More specifically, children younger than 8 years old do not distinguish between cognitive and physical competence, which load together on one factor, nor between social acceptance and behavioral conduct, which load on a second factor. Children in middle childhood (ages 8 to 12 years), however, clearly differentiate among five salient domains: scholastic competence, athletic competence, physical appearance, peer acceptance, and behavioral conduct. With adolescence, four unique dimensions emerge: close friendships, romantic relationships, job competence, and morality. Thus, with cognitive and physical maturity changes come concomitant changes in the importance of various competence or behavioral domains.

Accuracy of Children's Perceived Physical Competence

The accuracy of children's estimates of competence also exhibit a developmental shift. With increasing age, children show both a decline in levels of perceived competence and an increase in the accuracy of these judgments. Both Harter (1978, 1981) and Nicholls (1984) contend that accuracy of perceived competence increases as a function of two developmental phenomena: (a) children's cognitive ability to analyze the causes of performance outcomes in terms of ability, effort, and task difficulty, and (b) a shift in the sources of information used by children to judge performance capabilities. This phenomenon was demonstrated in an investigation by Horn and Weiss (1991). They found that perceived competence declined and accuracy increased over the age range of 8 to 13 years based on correlations between ratings of perceived competence and teachers' ratings of actual competence. The greatest differences in accuracy were between children 8 and 9 years of age with those 10 to 13 years old. These accuracy differences in age were associated with changes in the criteria children used to judge competence. Older children indicated a reliance on peer comparison and evaluation as preferred sources of information, whereas younger children were more dependent on parental feedback and evaluation.

In addition to accuracy judgments as a function of age, Horn and Weiss (1991) were interested in the relationship between accuracy of perceived competence and sources of information preferred by children. Children were divided into groups representing underestimators, accurate estimators, and overestimators, based on discrepancy scores between perceived and actual competence ratings. Results revealed that differences in accuracy estimates of physical ability were strongly related to preferences for competence-information sources. Underestimators and accurate estimators indicated primary reliance on peer comparison and evaluation, whereas overestimators scored highest on self-comparison sources such as skill improvement and effort exerted.

These findings are of great interest in light of their possible implications for consultants and practitioners. Although it is reasonable to understand that accurate estimators were influenced by peer-comparison and peer-evaluation sources of information, this same source was found for the children who seriously underestimated their physical competencies. What could be going on here? One interpretation is that a different standard of reference in peer comparison was used for the underestimators compared to the accurate estimators. It is possible that those who were low and inaccurate were comparing their abilities to a more select and talented group of peers, such as the star fourth graders or the best athletes in the class, whereas the accurate estimators were using a more similar group of peers (i.e., teammates in the program or age-mate peers of similar ability and experience).

Coaching Behavior Influences

Given the important role of the coach in youth sport, it is surprising that just a handful of studies have examined coaching behaviors on psychological development. Two studies were specifically designed within Harter's framework to examine coaches' influence on self-perceptions, affect, and motivation in young athletes. Horn (1985) was particularly interested in whether observed coaching behaviors would contribute to self-perceptions above and beyond improvement in skill level, using a sample of female junior-high-school softball players ages 13 to 15. Results revealed that skill improvements accounted for the most variance in self-perceptions of ability, but certain coaching behaviors also significantly contributed to these changes. Specifically, players who received more frequent positive reinforcement scored lower in perceived physical competence, and players who received higher frequencies of criticism were found to be higher in competence perceptions.

At first glance, these results directly contradict predictions based on Harter's competence-motivation theory. However, Horn (1985) observed that positive reinforcement statements frequently were given to lower ability players, often unconditional to their skill behaviors. That is, praise was frequently given in the form of "good job" or "way to go" without specific reference to the desirable skill technique or strategy displayed or combined with informational feedback on how to improve. Therefore these athletes might have inferred low performance expectations conveyed by the coach and this influenced perceptions of competence. In contrast, the criticism given for skill errors usually was directed at the high-ability players and contained skill-relevant information on how to improve on the next attempt (e.g., "Use two hands when you are trying to catch a pop fly!"). These results are important in demonstrating that the quantity of reinforcement and the mere use of positive statements is not sufficient to effect changes in ability perceptions and motivation. Rather, the quality of coaches' communication, specifically the contingency to behavior and the appropriateness of the information provided, are crucial for influencing children's perceptions about skill capabilities.

A recent study conducted by Black and Weiss (1992), using athletes' perceptions of coaching behaviors, also found that coaches' contingent feedback and reinforcement responses affected self-perceptions, affect, and motivation in youth swimmers. For children 12 to 18 years of age, perceptions of coaches' use of praise plus corrective information following performance successes were associated with higher perceptions of success and competence, higher enjoyment levels, and higher intrinsic motivation in the form of optimal challenge seeking. Similarly, athletes' ratings of their coaches' frequent use of encouragement plus corrective feedback in response to unsuccessful performances were also associated with more positive self-perceptions and intrinsic motivation.

In sum, Harter's (1978, 1981) theory of competence motivation provides a useful framework for understanding the development of children's self-perceptions and motivation in achievement domains. The findings reported here strongly suggest that there are consistent and strong relationships among self-perceptions of competence and control, affect, and motivation. Children who are high in perceived physical competence show functional achievement behaviors in the form of an internal locus of control and appropriate causal attributions for performance, greater enjoyment toward their participation, and higher intrinsic motivation in the form of challenge-seeking and mastery attempts. Second, sources of information for judging physical competence vary developmentally, from early childhood through adolescence, and this shift in information sources helps explain the decline in perceived competence or increase in accuracy with age. Lastly, significant others such as coaches (as well as parents and peers) can directly influence perceived physical competence, affect, and motivation, primarily through the quality of feedback and reinforcement they provide for performance outcomes.

Children's Motivation According to Nicholls and Dweck

An alternative approach to Harter's competence-motivation theory is the view from achievement-goal theorists such as Nicholls (1984, 1989) and Dweck (1986; Dweck & Elliott, 1983; Elliott & Dweck, 1988). These theories focus on children's motivation as a function of the types of goals adopted toward achievement and the way in which ability is construed as a result of this goal orientation. Like Harter, these achievement theorists strongly believe that the demonstration of competence is the central issue for understanding and explaining children's motivation and self-perceptions in achievement domains. Although the terminology used by these theorists is different from Harter's, I strongly believe that their theories and approaches are more similar than different. Therefore, after discussing these theories, I

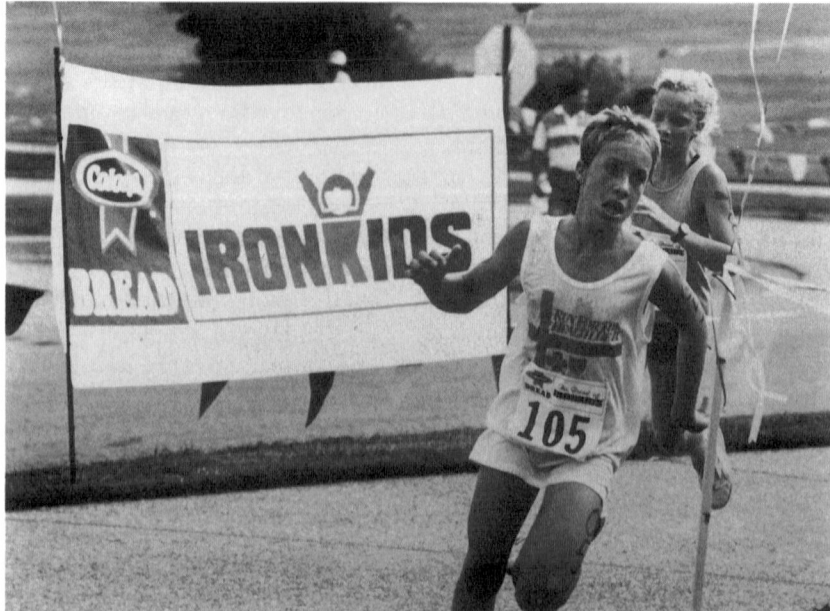

Courtesy Colonial Bread

will summarize their commonalities to identify interventions that would comply with both approaches.

According to both Nicholls and Dweck, children interpret their performances based on two goal perspectives. The first is a task, or learning-goal, perspective in which people rely primarily on self-referenced information to judge their level of competence. In this perspective, mastery of personally challenging goals is the focus, and sources such as effort, positive affect, learning, and improvement are used to judge level of ability. With a task, or learning-goal, perspective, individuals who are high or low in perceived competence are hypothesized to choose moderately difficult challenges, exert effort and persistence to attain these challenges, show task interest and enjoyment, and use effort attributions to maintain progress toward meeting goals as well as to respond to unsuccessful performances. When these mastery-oriented people encounter failure, they view it as a temporary setback and a cue to increase effort

or to determine what factors they can modify to maximize the probability of future success.

In contrast to the task, or learning-goal, perspective, Nicholls and Dweck describe the ego- or performance-goal-oriented person as one who seeks to maximize the display of high ability and minimize the display of low ability. These people define competence in relation to the performance of others and thus primarily depend on social comparison and evaluation to judge their abilities. According to Nicholls and Dweck, the ego- or performance-goal-oriented person who is high in perceived competence should evidence the same types of achievement behaviors as the task- or learning-goal-oriented person: selection of optimal challenges, intrinsic interest, effort, persistence, and enjoyment. However, the ego- or performance-goal-oriented person who is low in competence perceptions avoids moderate challenges so as not to risk demonstrating low ability. Such people (labeled as helpless-oriented by Dweck) choose very easy or very difficult tasks to protect evaluation of their ability: Easy tasks guarantee success and the demonstration of ability, whereas failure at difficult tasks would not necessarily signify low ability. In addition, the ego–low-confidence person is expected to exert little effort and persistence, thereby increasing the probability of low performance attainments. The helpless-oriented person experiences little enjoyment and low levels of intrinsic motivation and attributes negative outcomes to low ability, which is viewed as predictive of future failures.

Achievement-goal theorists also state that goal perspectives vary as a function of situational and individual difference factors. Situations that emphasize interpersonal competition, public evaluation, and normative feedback are likely to invoke an ego or performance-goal orientation, whereas situations characterized by a focus on learning, participation, skill mastery, and problem solving increase the probability of invoking a task, or learning-goal, orientation. Goal perspectives also vary as a function of individual differences, such as disposition, gender, culture, and age. Dispositional goal orientations, as well as those that are gender and culture related, are largely the function of childhood socialization experiences (Duda, 1987, 1992). Specifically, studies by Duda (1985, 1986) have shown that white males tend to be more ego involved in their sport-related achievement goals than black, Hispanic, and Navajo athletic participants. Similarly, males are more likely to emphasize ego-involved goals in the form of competitive outcomes and social comparison than females, who show a preference for skill mastery and self-comparison sources of information.

Developmental Trends in Goal Perspectives

The adoption of task and ego-goal perspectives also follows a cognitive-developmental pattern (Duda, 1987; Nicholls & Miller, 1983). Developmental differences revolve around children's ability to differentiate the concepts of ability, effort, and task difficulty in analyzing performance outcomes. Up until about age 9, children hold an undifferentiated view of the concept of ability, where effort is viewed as equal to ability in explaining successful performance. That is, children believe that a person who tried hard and succeeded has displayed high ability. At about age 9 through 11, children's cognitive ability to analyze the causes of performance becomes partially differentiated. That is, children come to understand that athletes must be highly skilled to be successful in a challenging competition, regardless of the level of effort exerted. But children do not employ this reasoning systematically. Lastly, at the completely differentiated view of ability, which is attained at about ages 11 to 12, children view ability as a capacity, where additional effort on a task might have limited impact on performance outcome, depending on the level of ability a person possesses.

According to Nicholls and Dweck, once children attain the cognitive maturity to view ability as a capacity that limits the effect of effort on performance, they can adopt either the undifferentiated or differentiated conception of ability. The undifferentiated view is consistent with the notion of a task, or learning-goal, orientation, with its focus on effort to attain personal mastery and use of self-referenced criteria to judge competence. The differentiated view is consistent with an ego, or performance-goal, orientation, with its emphasis on maximizing the demonstration of ability in comparison to others and use of normative criteria for self-ability judgments. These developmental findings in relation to achievement-goal perspectives have implications for the types of feedback and goals used with children in the competitive sport setting. For example, Horn (1987) cautions that using effort attributions in response to skill errors with a young child might result in a perception of low ability, whereas with an older child or adolescent, who can differentiate ability from effort as causes for performance outcomes, effort attributions should imply that with greater effort, attention, and strategy selection the child might be successful.

Nicholls's and Dweck's theories of achievement motivation have been widely supported in the academic domain (Elliott & Dweck, 1988; Nicholls, 1989), and the concepts and relationships these theories provide are intuitively appealing for application to the sport domain. However, testing of the relationships posited by achievement-goal theories among attributions for success and failure outcomes, goal perspectives, task choice, effort and persistence, and affect is scarce in the developmental sport psychology literature. The few published research studies have been primarily conducted with adult populations (Duda, 1992). However, given the support of achievement-goal theories in the academic domain and the competitive sport setting to date, I believe interventions that logically derive from such theoretical predictions definitely are important.

Consolidating Knowledge

Although Harter's competence-motivation theory and Nicholls's and Dweck's achievement-motivation theories take slightly different approaches to the understanding of children's development of self-perceptions and motivation, their similarities far outweigh their differences. For this reason, I propose an integrated model of motivation that takes into consideration the common constructs and relationships found in these theories (see Figure 3.1). This consolidation will provide the framework for identifying intervention strategies that can be used with children in

the context of the competitive sport setting (Weiss & Chaumeton, 1992).

Each of the theories distinguishes the child who is mastery- as opposed to performance-outcome-oriented in his or her motivational perspective. Both types of motivated children seek to demonstrate competence (e.g., learning and improving skills, attaining goals) and this is the central construct for explaining reasons for participating in sport. When demonstration of competence takes the form of mastery attempts followed by successful or unsuccessful outcomes, reinforcement by significant adults and peers helps to establish a standard of goals and a reward system. If independent mastery attempts and the skill learning process are encouraged and rewarded, the child tends to use internal or self-references criteria (e.g., skill improvement, effort) to judge ability and adopts a self-reward system and task or learning goals as a standard. If performance outcome (e.g., winning, performing better than others) is emphasized and rewarded by significant others, the child is expected to become dependent on external or normative criteria (e.g., peer comparison and evaluation) and adopt an extrinsic reward system and ego or performance goals as their preferred motivational orientation.

These motivational orientations, in turn, influence perceptions of competence and performance control, affect, and motivated behavior. The mastery-oriented child will derive positive perceptions of competence and an internal locus of control (or adaptive attributions for success and failure) and enjoyment and pleasure, and will choose optimally challenging skills and display maximal effort and persistence. Ultimately, high levels of personal performance achievement will be attained. The performance-outcome-motivated youngster, in contrast, will be susceptible to negative perceptions of competence and an external locus of control (and maladaptive attributions) and negative affect

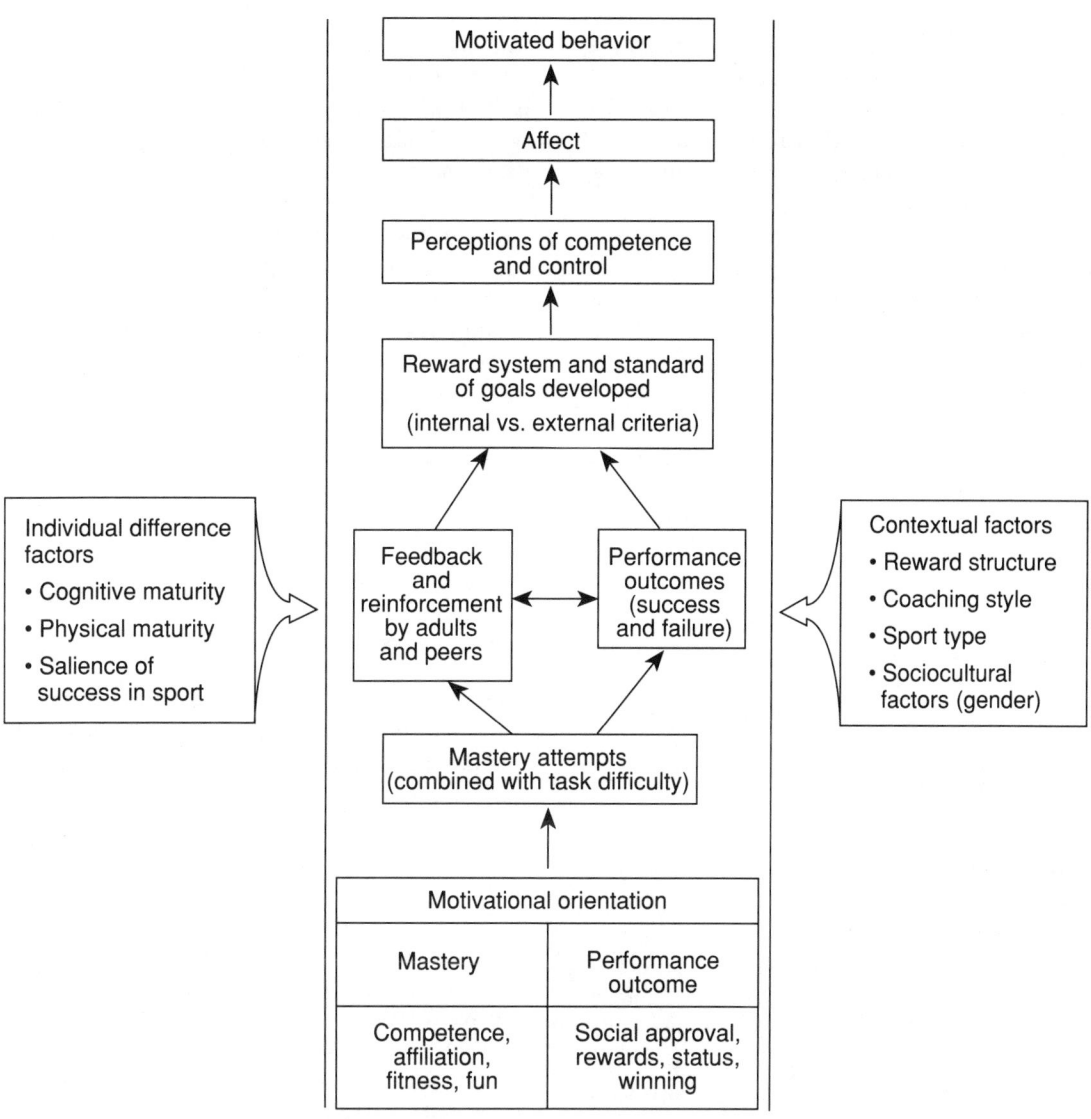

Figure 3.1 A proposed integrated model of sport motivation.

Note. From "Motivational Orientations in Sport" by M.R. Weiss and N. Chaumeton. In *Advances in Sport Psychology* (p. 90) by T.S. Horn (Ed.), 1992, Champaign, IL: Human Kinetics. Copyright 1992 by Human Kinetics. Reprinted by permission.

in the form of anxiety and embarrassment, and will choose easy or difficult tasks and display little effort and low-persistence behaviors. This orientation should result in less-than-optimal personal performance.

In addition to the major relationships among motivation and self-perception constructs, each of the theories suggests that developmental differences exist in children's perceptions of competence, their preference for internal and external sources of criteria to judge their ability, and their ability to analyze the causes of performance outcomes. Research indicates that children's perceptions of competence steadily decline, on average, but become more accurate with age. Thus younger children are more likely to be higher and less accurate in their judgments of competency than older children. These differences were associated with age-related differences in preferences for sources of competence information: younger children preferred parental feedback as criteria for judging their abilities, older children primarily relied on peer comparison and evaluation, and adolescents used internal standards (self-set goals, effort, improvement) more frequently.

Children also vary in their cognitive abilities to distinguish ability, effort, and task difficulty in their attempts to analyze performance outcomes. Specifically, Nicholls's theorizing contended that younger children (up to about age 11 or 12) cannot fully differentiate the concepts of ability and effort. However, a child capable of a differentiated conception of ability can separate the contributions of effort and skill in relation to the challenge of mastering a task. Thus younger children might deem themselves successful based on effort and simple task mastery, whereas older children are more likely to perceive success when their ability compares favorably with similar peers. After becoming capable of taking a differentiated view of ability (at about age 11 or 12), a child might choose to adopt a task or ego motivational orientation. The orientation choice has implications for subsequent motivated behavior and psychosocial development.

The information gleaned from motivational theory and research provides a number of recommendations concerning intervention techniques for enhancing intrinsic motivation, self-perceptions, and performance in the youth-sport setting. Each theory suggests that environmental factors (e.g., significant others, competitive emphasis) as well as individual difference factors (e.g., age, intrinsic vs. extrinsic orientations) influence motivation and performance in social achievement settings such as competitive sport. The next section focuses on psychological methods that consultants and practitioners can incorporate to maximize the probability of developing psychological skills in children, primarily via strategies for nurturing in sport the intrinsically oriented child (i.e., a child who displays positive self-perceptions, affect, and motivated behaviors).

ENHANCING PSYCHOLOGICAL SKILLS IN CHILDREN

The emphasis on a developmental approach to positive achievement behaviors in youth leads naturally to the selection of particular psychological skills or personal qualities to be gained from participation in sport. These skills represent those needed for optimal enjoyment and performance in competitive sport settings. Specifically, I focus on the psychological skills of self-perceptions of competence and control, positive affect, and intrinsic motivation. The psychological methods I advocate include strategies categorized as environmental, or social, influences and individual control, or self-regulated, learning strategies.

Environmental Influences

Based on motivational theories and research, coaches and parents significantly influence children's formation of favorable or unfavorable self-perceptions and subsequent motivated behavior. Their verbal and nonverbal behaviors in the form of modeling, feedback and reinforcement, and emphasis on mastery or performance-outcome goals strongly impact children's motivational orientation toward sport participation. The objective of our work with children is the development of mastery-oriented youngsters who are characterized by positive perceptions of competence and an internal locus of control, enjoyment, and pleasure with sport participation, and behavior in the form of optimal challenge-seeking, maximal effort, and persistence in the face of skill obstacles.

A key practical implication for consultants in the area of environmental strategies is providing educational workshops to coaches and parents about the importance of demonstrating appropriate attitudes and effective behaviors in response to children's performance in sport settings. To provide a systematic way of effecting changes in children's self-perceptions and motivation through mediating coach and parent behaviors, two models are presented. One model (see Figure 3.2) is a schematic representing the relationships among competence in meeting skill challenges, self-confidence (perceived competence and control), and motivation as suggested by theory and research (Bressan & Weiss, 1982). Thus self-confidence is seen as both a consequence of successful

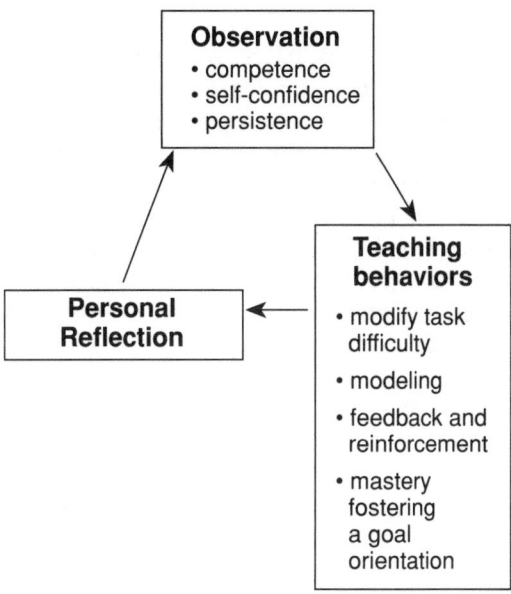

Figure 3.3   The psychological methods model describes the interrelationships among observation, teacher behavior, and personal reflection.

mastery attempts as well as a mediator of task choice, effort, and persistence. The diagram reveals that increases in skill competence with optimal challenges result in heightened self-confidence that, in turn, positively influences intrinsic interest and task persistence. Sustained effort or persistence increases the probability of further performance gains and the demonstration of competence in meeting skill challenges. I call this the skill development model.

The skill development model highlights the specific skill components for which instructional guidelines should be established. The consultant, through coach and parent education workshops, can systematically provide information on methods for positively influencing competence, self-confidence, and intrinsic motivation in the youth-sport setting. Another schematic, which I will call the psychological methods model (see Figure 3.3), identifies the essential

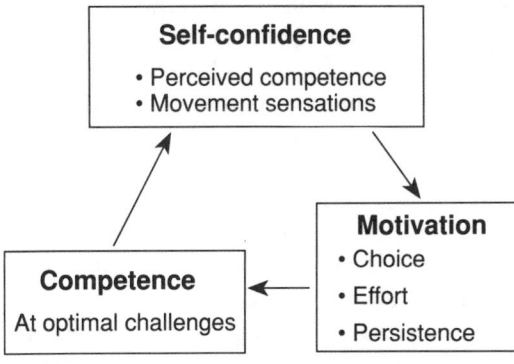

Figure 3.2   The skill development model describes the interrelationships among competence, self-confidence, and motivation.

skills of observation, teacher (instructional) behavior, and personal reflection for effecting changes in skill competence and psychological development of youth (Barrett, 1977). This model describes the process by which coaches and parents can effectively promote the development of an intrinsically motivated child in sport, primarily through the use of specific strategies designed to focus the child's efforts on mastery attempts for moderately difficult tasks and enhance perceptions of competence and performance control. For intervention strategies to be successful, coaches and parents must be made aware of or observe for competence, self-confidence, and persistence, respond with appropriate instructional behaviors, and personally reflect or evaluate whether the method chosen to implement change achieved its purpose.

Observation Skills

Careful observation of what is going on in the learning environment is the critical first step to initiating behavioral change in the youth-sport setting. Coaches and parents must realize that they need to purposefully and systematically search for verbal and non-verbal behaviors that convey information about children's levels of competence, self-confidence, and persistence behaviors. Competence pertains to both the child's actual skill capabilities in meeting certain task demands of a sport and the child's knowledge base related to declarative (facts), procedural (rules), and conditional (when to apply facts and rules) features of successful sport execution. The actual demands or challenges of the sport situation are also important in being able to accurately assess actual competence levels. Assessment methods that outline accurate sport techniques and strategies can be used to determine children's demonstration of competence.

Self-confidence refers to perceptions of competence and performance control manifested by the performer in relation to task demands. Parents and coaches can infer high levels of confidence when children verbalize a positive attitude toward participation, convey optimism about learning a sport skill, approach opportunities for trying challenging skills, demonstrate effort and persistence while struggling to approximate proper skill technique, and make personally controllable attributions, such as effort or incorrect strategy for unsuccessful performances. In contrast, children with low levels of self-confidence typically manifest avoidance behaviors, give up easily when trying to learn new skills, set unrealistic performance standards (too low or too high), and adopt strategies to avoid the demonstration of low ability (e.g., make excuses).

Self-confidence in executing sport skills might also be considered in relation to anticipated positive or negative sensations that might be experienced. These movement sensations include effects such as the physical contact in taking a charge in basketball, the disorienting vertigo when performing a flip on the trampoline, and the tension of entering a cold swimming pool. Behavioral manifestations of expected sensory effects can provide coaches and parents with indices of self-confidence in youngsters. For example, the eagerness of trying new physical skills and strategies, seeking out repetitive practice opportunities, and positive affect in the form of excitement and curiosity might indicate positive sensory anticipation and high self-confidence. In contrast, hesitation or avoidance of skill patterns, inappropriate fixation or attention to single elements in the performance environment (e.g., the trampoline bed), extraneous or protective movements, and facial expressions of uncertainty and fear might exemplify negative sensory perceptions and low self-confidence.

Observation of persistence behaviors is also critical for determining children's levels of self-confidence and motivation and thus the appropriate selection of intervention methods. The element of persistence is one of the prime indices of mastery or performance-outcome motivational orientations. Thus accurate determination of this psychological characteristic in children will convey important information about underlying cognitions and perceptions. Siedentop (cited in Bressan & Weiss, 1982) suggested that high levels of persistence can be inferred when children maintain their efforts on learning and performing skills under the following conditions: (a) instruction comes from indirect sources (e.g., videotape, workout sheet) rather than directly from the coach; (b) the athlete is not under direct coach supervision (e.g., coach is working one-on-one with another athlete); (c) athletes are willing to work toward deferred rather than immediate rewards (e.g., refining a technique or strategy rather than reverting to an old habit that usually results in successful outcomes); and (d) athletes continue to work toward skill mastery despite the frustrations and setbacks incurred from unsuccessful performance.

Coaches, parents, and consultants must be able to identify by observation behavioral indicators of competence, self-confidence, and persistence as outlined in this section. These observations provide a baseline from which the practitioner can establish levels of positive or negative physical skills (e.g., sport ability) and psychological skills (e.g., perceptions of competence, locus of control) in children. Once competence, confidence, and motivation levels can be ascertained, recommendations for implementing psychological methods for enhancing these skills can be made. These recommendations target instructional behaviors on the part of coaches and parents that are consistent with theoretical notions of developing intrinsic motivation.

Instructional Behaviors

The skill development model can be set into motion by first targeting changes in physical competence to meet skill challenges. According to developmental motivation theories and research, performance accomplishments based on mastery attempts are critical to forming positive self-perceptions and subsequent motivation. Harter, Nicholls, and Dweck concur that successful performance at moderately difficult or "optimal" challenges has the greatest chance of heightening perceptions of competence, perceptions of performance control, and intrinsic motivation. Consequently, consultants should facilitate coaches and parents in modifying the task difficulty for the purpose of challenging young learners at a level that is difficult but attainable. I like to view this concept of optimal challenges and modifying task difficulty as fitting the activity to the child, not the child to the activity.

Modifying Task Difficulty. To optimally challenge child athletes one must be able to carefully analyze what physical skill elements are necessary for successful performance. For example, coaches need to outline developmental progressions for each sport skill, so that the most simple tasks precede and transfer to more difficult executions. Learning to perform a dive from the side of the pool, for example, requires a progression of teaching steps to maximize the probability of performance success, enhanced self-confidence, and continued efforts to attain the skill. USA Wrestling developed the "Seven Basic Skills" (proper execution of body position, mobility, changing levels, penetration, lifting, back step, and back arch), where each skill depends on proficiently learning the skill preceding it. Other strategies for modifying task difficulty include providing physical guidance under conditions where athletes will not attempt the skill (e.g., a new trick in gymnastics), physical prompts (e.g., spotting belt), and physical aids (e.g., sliding pads for baseball; volleyball spike-it). It is important that use of these external aids is gradually eliminated so that athletes are performing the skill on their own and can attribute performance success to their own ability and effort.

The modifications of equipment, facilities, and rules to match the developmental capabilities of athletes also comprise ways of modifying task difficulty. For example, an 8-ft (2.4-m) rather than 10-ft (3.0-m) basketball goal, a Size 4 soccer ball, an "incredi-ball" rather than a hardball, and narrower and shorter fields increase opportunities for children to practice specific skills, receive informational feedback, and be reinforced for positive performances. Modifying task difficulty combined with ample practice opportunities in a positive social climate will enhance children's chances of increasing their competence in meeting skill challenges and thus positively influence self-perceptions and motivation.

Instructional behaviors can also directly target the area on the skill development model depicting self-confidence, which includes such characteristics as perceived competence, perceived control, and attributions for performance. Educational support strategies refer to those behaviors that can modify the performer's perceptions of the challenge inherent in the movement situation or their feelings of confidence about their chances for success (Bressan & Weiss, 1982). According to motivational theory and research, variables that directly or indirectly influence perceptions of competence and self-determination in the sport setting include modeling; feedback and reinforcement by adults and peers; and the nature of the climate (mastery or performance outcome). Each of these influential variables infer prescriptions for intervention methods in the youth competitive environment.

Modeling. *Modeling* refers to the cognitive, affective, and behavioral changes that occur as a result of observing adults and peers, whereas *models* are persons whose behaviors, verbalizations, and nonverbal expressions serve as cues for subsequent modeling (Schunk, 1989). Thus modeling can serve both an informational and a motivational function, and these functions have been strongly supported in the sport psychology and motor behavior literatures (McCullagh, Weiss, & Ross, 1989; Weiss, Ebbeck, & Wiese-Bjornstal, 1993). Adults can affect children's self-perceptions of ability through verbal (e.g., positive self-talk) and nonverbal (e.g., behaving calmly in a tight situation) behaviors that denote confidence and individual control in the sport setting. More importantly, peer modeling strategies have been found to be highly successful in affecting self-confidence and motivation in observers (Schunk & Hanson, 1985; Schunk, Hanson, & Cox, 1987). For example, same-age, or same-gender, or same-age-and-gender peers represent similarity between the model and observer, thus maximizing attention and motivation of learners. Similar models are likely to invoke the perception that "if she (he) can do it, so can I," and encourage mastery attempts. Coping models initially verbalize and demonstrate the same fears and hesitations of observers but gradually overcome uncertainties and perform the skill successfully. Coping models can influence self-confidence and motivation through both an informational function, conveying strategies for overcoming fears and performing successfully, and a motivational function, by invoking perceived similarity and bonding between observer and model. Thus coaches can be taught how to be aware of their own modeling behaviors as well as how to use teammates as effective models for children low in self-confidence for learning certain athletic skills.

Feedback and Reinforcement. Feedback and reinforcement by adults and peers provide salient sources of information to children and adolescents about their abilities. Younger children (under age 10) primarily rely on adult feedback and evaluation, while preference for peer comparison and evaluation becomes predominant from ages 10 to 14. Lastly, use of social comparison sources decline and preference for self-referenced criteria emerge among 14- to 18-year-old adolescents. Although preferred sources of information show developmental trends, it is important to remember that individual differences in age level also exist. This was seen in the study by Horn and Weiss (1991) where children between ages 8 and 13 who were low and inaccurate in their estimations of ability indicated preference for the use of peer comparison and evaluation. It is also important to remember that although one or more sources might be preferred by youngsters of particular age levels, many other sources are also available and used to some extent by children and adolescents. Based on these findings, then, consultants need to educate coaches and parents about the importance of using contingent and appropriate feedback in response to children's performance successes and errors as well as the need to de-emphasize the frequent use of peer comparison during the middle childhood years. That is, because children are prone to stacking up their skills against those of similar age or gender, it can be easy for them to fall into a rut of only defining success in peer-comparison terms. Adults can facilitate positive self-perceptions and motivation in youngsters by emphasizing improvement in personal performance capabilities rather than outcome-related goals.

Horn (1987) recommends three major guiding principles for developing positive self-perceptions in young athletes through coach and parental communication. These are (a) contingency and quality of praise and criticism; (b) frequency and contingency of skill-relevant feedback; and (c) appropriate attributional feedback for performance outcomes. These principles are strongly supported by intervention and correlational research in both the academic and sport psychology literatures (see Horn, 1987; Horn & Lox, 1993; Schunk, 1989). More specifically, contingent praise provides children with information about their competence, the performance standard they are expected to reach, and the criteria (i.e., winning or skill mastery) by which their competence will be evaluated (Horn, 1987). Appropriate use of praise means providing reinforcement in proportion to the difficulty of the skill attained. If children succeed at a simple task or demonstrate only mediocre performance, excessive praise for these behaviors might convey negative information and expectations. It is not the quantity of positive reinforcement that makes a difference, but rather the quality of the content in terms of contingency and appropriateness.

Another principle, providing appropriate skill-relevant feedback, is a crucial one for influencing perceptions of competence and performance control in children. In the area of competitive sport, the opportunities for committing skill errors are numerous and have the potential for being negatively evaluated by young athletes as indicants of low ability. However, research in the academic domain consistently shows that when unsuccessful performances are viewed as temporary setbacks or a natural part of the learning process by teachers and students, then perceptions of performance control are increased and competence perceptions are not negatively affected. More specifically, when coaches and parents respond to children's skill errors with encouragement and corrective instruction, self-perceptions of ability and control are enhanced, and effort and persistence increases.

Lastly, attributional feedback plays a large role in the formation of self-perceptions and motivation. Effort attributions made for performance errors in the sport setting are likely to enhance perceptions of control and motivation, because effort is usually a temporary quality and one that is under the young athlete's control. However, it is important to note that children must perceive that they have the requisite skills to eventually achieve success; otherwise, greater effort will not be perceived as effective. To do this, coaches and parents can make effort attributions for unsuccessful performance and combine them with instruction on how to modify the skill technique on the next attempt. Age differences in the capacity to distinguish ability and effort as causes of performance outcomes must also be considered. Young children who hold an undifferentiated view of the concept of ability might best benefit from effort attributions for success, whereas ability attributions for success might likely be more credible and effective for older children and adolescents.

Fostering a Mastery-Goal Orientation. Fostering a mastery-goal orientation is another educational support strategy that can be employed to positively influence psychological development. According to achievement-goal theories, children are more likely to develop self-confidence, positive affect, effort attributions for performance failures, intrinsic task interest, and persistence when they adopt a mastery- or learning-goal orientation to participation rather than a performance-outcome goal orientation. The central focus of a mastery-goal orientation is on learning and developing skills, and information about competence is primarily self-referenced. The child asks questions such as, How can I get better than I was before? and What strategies will help me improve from my unsuccessful performance? The performance-outcome goal orientation is

concerned with social comparison criteria as the main indicant of achievement (Did I win? Was my performance better than the rest of the class?). In the setting of competitive sport, it is difficult to avoid at least some orientation toward performance goals, with emphases on competing against others and striving toward the goal of winning. But Ames (1986; 1992; Ames & Archer, 1988) suggests that coaches and parents can learn to stem the tide of a highly competitive emphasis and foster a mastery-goal orientation in their young athletes.

One strategy for fostering a mastery-goal orientation is an emphasis on individualistic, rather than competitive, reward structures. Ames (1986) defines a competitive-goal structure as one in which athletes work against each other for a reward or recognition (e.g., coach's praise, starter role), whereas an individualistic-goal structure is one where athletes work toward independent goals (e.g., personal skill improvement, attainment of a technique). Ames contends that goal structures provide performance information and influence attributions, cognitive strategies, and affective outcomes. More specifically, a competitive-goal structure invokes the use of social-comparison criteria to evaluate ability and encourages an emphasis on the achievement outcome (e.g., winning). Attributions for failure revolve around inadequate ability, resulting in negative affect and a decline in motivation. An individualistic-goal structure is likely to invoke the use of self-referenced information for judging ability (e.g., effort, improvement) and encourages an emphasis on the process of learning skills. Effort attributions for unsuccessful performances predominate, resulting in perceptions of control and motivation to persist on the part of the athlete.

Despite the obvious benefits for employing individualistic-goal structures to influence psychosocial development, competitive sport by its nature maximizes the likelihood of invoking a competitive-goal structure, where winning and being number one are highly valued. However, competitive-goal structures give added salience to the natural use of peer comparison cues while decreasing the salience of self-referenced cues. If praise and criticism for children's performance are given primarily for the outcome of an event or competition, young athletes are likely to adopt peer comparison and evaluation as a primary source of judging ability. But if adults also praise the quality of performance success, provide corrective instruction in response to performance failures, and encourage the use of effort attributions, then children also learn to use internal sources such as self-improvement, degree of effort, and quality of skill technique to judge their competence.

Ames and Archer (1987) found that mothers' beliefs about the role of school learning could be classified as mastery- or performance-oriented, and these orientations were related to children's beliefs about the role of ability and effort in academic competence. Thus significant adults in the sport setting can help balance the child's motivational or goal perspective by emphasizing individualistic-goal structures in the context of competitive youth sport.

Similar to the notion of goal structures is the nature of the motivational or psychological climate of the classroom (Ames, 1992; Ames & Archer, 1988). Athletic "classrooms" are the gymnasiums, natatoriums, and the fields where daily practices and competitive events are held—where learning takes place and performance is demonstrated. According to Ames, there should be a positive relationship between a mastery climate and positive motivational characteristics (e.g., attributions, intrinsic task interest, persistence). Ames and Archer (1988) tested this notion by examining children's perceptions of classroom climate in relation to a number of motivational indicators. They defined a mastery-goal climate as one in which success is defined as improvement or progress (versus high grades and high normative performance): Value was placed on effort and learning; the teacher was oriented toward how students were learning (versus performing); errors were viewed as part of the learning process; and evaluation criteria were focused on absolute standards or individual progress (versus normative standards). Results revealed that students who perceived mastery goals as salient in their classroom preferred challenging tasks, had a more positive attitude toward the class, and had a stronger belief that success follows from one's effort. Students who perceived performance-goal orientations in their classroom focused on their normative ability, evaluated their ability negatively, and attributed failure to lack of ability. Thus adoption of a motivational climate that focuses on learning, improvement, and individual goal attainment is more likely to result in adaptive motivational patterns on the part of athletes than would emphasis on normative criteria for determining one's level of sport ability.

Personal Reflection

The selection of particular instructional strategies to influence changes in competence, self-confidence, and motivation included task modification, modeling, contingent feedback and reinforcement, effort attributions for failure, and emphasizing a mastery motivational climate. These methods require that consultants, coaches, and parents subsequently engage in personal reflection. Personal reflection entails the judgment and monitoring of the effectiveness of one's teaching or intervention methods (Barrett, 1977). That is, it requires that change agents actively compare what is happening in the learning environment with what was intended by the particular psychological method of intervention. Did the use of contingent feedback and reinforcement result in higher competence perceptions and continued motivation? Did a coping model effectively reduce anxiety induced from anticipated negative sensory experiences and motivate the learner to attempt the skill? Did an emphasis on self-referenced criteria to judge competence influence perceptions of performance control? In sum, personal reflection completes the psychological-methods-model cycle by comparing whether interventions used in response to observations about competence, self-perceptions, and motivation resulted in positive changes.

Individual Control Strategies

Consistent with a focus on developing mastery-oriented young athletes, the emphasis of this section is on identifying strategies that will help children and adolescents in competitive sport become self-regulated learners (see Zimmerman & Schunk, 1989). According to Schunk (1989), self-regulated learning occurs from children's self-generated behaviors that are systematically designed to maximize attainment of their goals. Thus children are active agents in their choice, control, and achievement of specific goals. Children who are effective in using self-regulation strategies to guide motivated behavior are characterized by favorable self-perceptions, high perceived performance control, accurate estimation of their abilities, steady progression toward self-set goals, and a tendency to thrive under a cooperative leadership style (McCombs, 1989; Schunk, 1989). The combined knowledge from motivational theory and the empirical research on self-regulated learning lends itself nicely to the view that consultants can work directly with young athletes on developing self-regulation skills.

Self-regulated learning is comprised of three subprocesses: self-observation, self-judgment, and self-reaction (Bandura, 1986), which are highlighted in Table 3.2. Self-observation entails monitoring one's behaviors regularly and proximally through some means of self-recording. Self-observation serves both an information function by showing progression toward goals and a motivational function by encouraging behavior change as a function of increased awareness through behavioral recording. Self-judgment is a process where learners compare present

Table 3.2   Components of Self-Regulated Learning

Component	Description	Acquisition strategy (for all 3 components)
Self-observation	• Monitors behaviors • Shows progress toward goals and encourages behavior change through increased awareness	Modeling Attributional feedback Social comparison
Self-judgment	• Compares present performance level with desired level	Reward contingencies Goal setting
Self-reaction	• Positive or negative evaluations of progress toward goals	Self-monitoring progress Strategy training Self-instructional talk Attribution retraining Anxiety management

performance level with desired goals. This process can be influenced by the types of goals adopted (e.g., mastery versus performance outcome); specificity, task difficulty, and proximity of goals; the importance of goal attainment; and attributions made for one's performance outcomes. Lastly, self-reaction refers to positive or negative evaluations concerning progress toward goal attainment. Positive evaluations of acceptable progress raise self-perceptions and motivation, whereas negative evaluations need not deter motivation if people believe themselves capable of improving in the future. Self-reaction can include evaluations from sources of information provided by self-reinforcement or external rewards and feedback.

Schunk (1989) provides a comprehensive literature review on the development and acquisition of these self-regulatory skills. Interventions include social influences such as modeling (e.g., peer models, coping models), attributional feedback, social comparison information from similar others, and reward contingencies. These methods were discussed previously in conjunction with educating coaches and parents on the content and quality of their communication with young athletes. Consultants working in the competitive youth sport system can employ these strategies one-on-one with athletes to help develop self-regulatory skills and subsequently enhance self-perceptions and motivation. (Because these topics were discussed on pages 57-62, they will not be repeated here.)

Other intervention techniques for developing self-observation, self-judgment, and self-reaction skills include athlete-centered or control strategies such as self-monitoring progress, goal setting, and strategy training. Strategy training can include such areas as self-instructional talk, attribution retraining, and anxiety-management skills. Goal-setting skills have been discussed extensively in the academic, industrial, and sport psychology literatures (Gould, 1986; Locke & Latham, 1990) and emphasize the importance of setting specific and measurable, moderately challenging, mastery rather than performance, and short- and long-term goals. Developmental considerations in the use of goal setting center on children's accuracy in making self-ability judgments and thus their ability to determine if progress is being made. As seen in developmental research, younger children tend to be higher in perceived competence and less accurate than older children and adolescents. Thus it becomes imperative for consultants and coaches to provide accurate feedback concerning children's progress toward skill-learning goals.

Self-instructional talk and attribution retraining go hand in hand because of their emphasis on modifying cognitions and thus influencing performance and motivation. Self-instructional talk has been primarily examined through the use of strategy verbalizations by children in attempting to achieve goals. These strategy verbalizations often take the initial form of overt self-talk, then proceed to faded and finally covert self-instruction. Considerable research by Schunk (1989) has shown that strategy verbalization skills enhance self-efficacy, performance, and ability attributions for success. Attribution retraining is a strategy recommended and used by Dweck (1986; Dweck & Elliott, 1983) to encourage children with maladaptive behavior patterns to view performance failures in a different light. Specifically, this technique involves training children to make effort—rather than ability—attributions for failure, and thus come to see future performance as changeable and under their personal control. Dweck has found that attribution retraining has positively influenced children's persistence on challenging tasks, in comparison merely to guaranteeing success experiences and not providing opportunities for dealing with failure.

Lastly, young athletes can be taught to monitor cognitive appraisals and physiological arousal before competition and to employ anxiety-management skills. These skills include progressive and cognitive relaxation techniques, mental imagery, task- or strategy-oriented rather than worry-oriented self-talk, mastery rather than outcome goals for competitive events, and general coping skills, such as planned alternative strategies in the case of a sudden change of events (e.g., weather, injuries). Again, developmental characteristics that might differentiate younger and older children and adolescents should be taken into account. For example, Ballinger and Heine (1991) recommend that relaxation scripts for children be modified to be interesting, meaningful, and conveyed in understandable language.

INTERVENTION POSSIBILITIES FOR LAURA, RAUL, AND JULIA

A review of the developmental psychology literature reveals that numerous factors directly or indirectly influence self-perceptions and motivation in the young athlete. These factors include cognitive-developmental level, perceptions of success, feedback and reinforcement from significant adults and peers, adoption of a mastery- or performance-outcome-goal orientation, and preference for internal or external criteria for judging competence levels. As a reminder, self-perceptions include the athlete's self-confidence, perceptions of competence, and perceptions of performance control, whereas motivation reflects choice, effort, and persistence behaviors exhibited in the pursuit of competitive sport goals. Taking a closer look at the developmental process of self-perceptions and motivation in each of our case studies will help us understand what

dynamics were taking place and decide which intervention strategies were or could have been successfully employed.

Laura

Laura's 6-year participation in rhythmic gymnastics indicates a high level of commitment to the sport. Several developmental and social factors, however, had a bearing on Laura's changed attitude and her eventual decision to withdraw from elite competition. Besides the obvious biological and physical changes affecting her performance of well-learned gymnastic tricks, Laura's cognitive maturity was reflected by changes in the salience of certain dimensions of self-esteem. In particular, physical appearance and close friendships intensify in importance during the adolescent years. For Laura, body changes caused by sexual development, and affective outcomes based on hormonal changes strongly influenced her perceptions of her physical appearance. These perceptions dramatically declined at this point in her life, which led to behaviors such as protecting evaluation of her body through the use of oversized T-shirts and constrained movements during athletic performance.

Anticipation of high-school academic demands and the potential distancing of close friendships due to excessive time demands of gymnastics practice were also influential factors in Laura's negative self-image. These changes in self-perceptions of ability, in combination with the competitive reward structure and the performance-goal climate of the gym contributed to low perceptions of performance control for Laura. Positive social support from her parents and brother as well as her school friends provided the impetus for finally deciding to call it quits after 6 years of committed participation. Although Laura ended up dropping out of highly competitive rhythmic gymnastics, she continued to be physically active, pursued ballet more seriously, and took advantage of every opportunity to cheer her former teammates on during subsequent competitions.

Possible intervention strategies that could have been used to sustain Laura's level of commitment and enjoyment of the sport would include both Laura and her coach. Laura would have benefited by learning about the interacting influence of biological, physical, and psychological factors on performance. Her physical growth and development took her by surprise, and she was never quite sure what was going on with her body, her emotions, and her perceptions of others' evaluations of her physical appearance. Additionally, Laura probably would have been a successful student of self-regulatory skills, especially in the modification of her goals based on her growth and development, anxiety-management skills, and attribution retraining. Retraining her attributions of low ability for unsuccessful performances to personally controllable reasons, such as inadequate practice time or poor strategy selection, would have helped her adapt more realistically to the newly defined internal demands being made on her.

The coach would have benefited by learning from a sport psychology consultant about the multidisciplinary nature of performance changes. This would have helped in the coach's handling of younger girls who would eventually go through the same process as Laura. The coach also needed to learn to become more aware of her reinforcement patterns and to focus on rewarding effort and technique in defining more of a mastery orientation, rather than criticizing lapses in performance and emphasizing skill errors as failures attributable to low ability. Lastly, the coach could have modified the climate of the gym so that athletes felt more comfortable in performing to the best of their ability through maximal effort and persistence, thereby contributing to the development of athletes' mastery motivation.

Raul

Raul was a lucky boy—social and individual control factors positively influenced his motivational orientation, self-perceptions, and sport-achievement levels. First, Raul's social support network, including peers, parents, and coach, provided contingent and appropriate praise for his performances, encouraged his efforts to try wrestling, and employed effective modeling techniques to influence Raul's perceptions of himself as a wrestler. Raul was a late-maturing boy, which accounted for his small size, but his coach had educational training and recognized this individual difference factor and so advised Raul accordingly. Wrestling provided the perfect optimal challenge for Raul—he could be matched in size with other athletes of similar ability and experience. Raul was also fortunate to have participated in athletic environments that encouraged an individualistic-reward structure and a mastery motivational climate. All his coaches at the elementary, middle-school, and high-school levels encouraged the use of self-referenced criteria to judge competence, focused on learning and effort goals, and viewed unsuccessful performances as cues for incorporating new strategies rather than as failures. Lastly, these positive social influences plus a focus on a mastery orientation helped Raul develop into a self-regulated learner, which maximized his self-perceptions of competence and performance control and his motivation to continue participating at moderately challenging levels. Raul's high level of intrinsic motivation guided him to influence others as he had been when he was a youngster; and I hope that his modeling behaviors, positive attitude, and mastery-goal orientation will have the same positive effect on other youngsters.

Julia

The case of Julia is troubling. Neither her social environment nor her own individual skills provided her with opportunities for positively affecting self-perceptions, motivation, and participation in gymnastics. The competitive-reward structure and performance-goal climate of the gym were not conducive to feelings of confidence, control, or intrinsic motivation. The coaches emphasized normative criteria for judging competence, which together with the salience of peer comparison and evaluation common to her age group caused undue levels of anxiety.

The coaches' use of a negative approach to skill learning included constant criticism for skill errors, nonreinforcement for improvements in technique, and frequent disapproval for any off-task behavior in the gym (e.g., talking with friends). As her skill levels improved, the environment did not offer Julia as much fun and enjoyment as it once had. Peer modeling of the labels *quitter* and *loser* had a strong impact on Julia, and this influence from her peers as well as the fact that her teammates were her closest friends made it especially difficult for her to decide to quit. Making matters worse was Julia's perception that she would be letting her parents down if she no longer continued.

All of these factors, combined with her recent injury, negatively affected her perceptions of control, affect, and competence. All were in the negative direction. Julia might be considered what Dweck called helplessoriented: being performance-goal-oriented, using ability attributions for performance errors, avoiding optimal challenges, and lacking persistence at difficult skills. Her conscious and deliberate attempt to injure herself

so that she could leave gymnastics without being called a loser was an extreme action that would have been unnecessary had appropriate intervention occurred.

A sport psychology consultant asked to intervene in this situation would need to proceed on many levels. Julia's support system needed attention and training. Her coaches and parents were, directly and indirectly, negatively influencing her self-perceptions and motivation. They needed to be taught how to nurture a mastery-goal orientation and an emphasis on self-referenced criteria for judging competence levels. Her coaches especially needed intense training on reward contingencies, attributional feedback, and methods of keeping practices fun and enjoyable for young children. Julia could benefit from self-regulatory skills to positively influence the development of self-perceptions and a learning-goal orientation. These would include attribution retraining, realistic goal setting, anxiety management techniques, and strategy verbalizations. Julia was in need of constructive strategies for controlling her own behaviors and performance as well as major changes in her social environment. When children no longer feel they can honestly participate at a level they are capable of because of anticipated disapproval, punishment, negative sensory anticipation, and emphasis on normative criteria, they have no choice but to withdraw. Julia had long ago withdrawn psychologically . . . it was withdrawing herself physically from her sport that she found difficult. She eventually figured out how to do it.

CONCLUSION

Children and adolescents participate in sport for reasons related to developing competence, affirming friendships, enhancing physical fitness, and experiencing fun. I have described a developmental framework of psychosocial growth in children and youth that includes development of positive affect, perceptions of physical competence and peer acceptance, perceptions of performance control, and intrinsic motivation. Empirical research demonstrates that cognitive-developmental differences exist in self-perceptions, that significant adults and peers strongly impact the psychological development of youngsters, and that qualitative differences in motivated behavior are evident based upon the adoption of a mastery- or performance-outcome-goal orientation. With an understanding of the processes involved in developing intrinsically motivated children in sport, I considered many environmental- and individual-control strategies for effecting positive changes in psychological skills. These psychological methods, when made available to coaches, parents, and young athletes, have the potential for developing self-regulated learners who feel in control of their performance outcomes, convey favorable perceptions of their ability, display a positive attitude toward participation in sport, seek optimal challenges in striving for mastery-oriented goals, and show persistence in their pursuit of learning skills and demonstrating competence.

REFERENCES

Ames, C. (1986). Conceptions of motivation within competitive and noncompetitive goal structures. In R. Schwarzer (Ed.), *Self-related cognitions in anxiety and motivation* (pp. 229-245). Hillsdale, NJ: Erlbaum.

Ames, C. (1992). The relationship of achievement goals to motivation in classroom settings. In G.C. Roberts (Ed.), *Motivation in sport and exercise* (pp. 161-176). Champaign, IL: Human Kinetics.

Ames, C., & Archer, J. (1987). Mothers' beliefs about the role of ability and effort in school learning. *Journal of Educational Psychology*, **79**, 409-414.

Ames, C., & Archer, J. (1988). Achievement goals in the classroom: Students' learning strategies and motivation process. *Journal of Educational Psychology*, **80**, 260-267.

Ballinger, D.A., & Heine, P.L. (1991). Relaxation training for children: A script. *Journal of Physical Education, Recreation, and Dance*, **62**(2), 67-69.

Bandura, A. (1986). *Social foundations of thought and action: A social cognitive theory*. Englewood Cliffs, NJ: Prentice Hall.

Barrett, K. (1977). Studying teaching: A means for becoming a more effective teacher. In B. Logsdon, K. Barrett, H. Ammons, M. Broer, L. Halvorson, R. McGee, & M. Roberton (Eds.), *Physical education for children* (pp. 249-287). Philadelphia: Lea & Febiger.

Black, S.J., & Weiss, M.R. (1992). The relationship among perceived coaching behaviors, perceptions of ability, and motivation in competitive age-group swimmers. *Journal of Sport and Exercise Psychology*, **14**, 309-325.

Bressan, E.S., & Weiss, M.R. (1982). A theory of instruction for developing competence, self-confidence and persistence in physical education. *Journal of Teaching Physical Education*, **2**, 38-47.

Duda, J.L. (1985). Goals and achievement orientations of Anglo- and Mexican-American adolescents in sport and the classroom. *International Journal of Intercultural Relations*, **9**, 131-155.

Duda, J.L. (1986). Perceptions of sport success and failure among white, black, and Hispanic adolescents. In J. Watkins, T. Reilly, & L. Burwitz (Eds.), *Sport science* (pp. 214-222). London: E. & F.N. Spon.

Duda, J.L. (1987). Toward a developmental theory of motivation in sport. *Journal of Sport Psychology*, **9**, 130-145.

Duda, J.L. (1992). Motivation in sport settings: A goal perspective approach. In G. Roberts (Ed.), *Motivation in sport and exercise* (pp. 57-91). Champaign, IL: Human Kinetics.

Dweck, C.S. (1986). Motivational processes affecting learning. *American Psychologist,* **41**, 1040-1048.

Dweck, C.S., & Elliott, E.S. (1983). Achievement motivation. In E.M. Hetherington (Ed.), *Socialization, personality, and social development* (pp. 643-691). New York: Wiley.

Elliott, E.S., & Dweck, C.S. (1988). Goals: An approach to motivation and achievement. *Journal of Personality and Social Psychology,* **54**, 5-12.

Gould, D. (1986). Goal setting for peak performance. In J.M. Williams (Ed.), *Applied sport psychology: Personal growth to peak performance* (pp. 133-148). Palo Alto, CA: Mayfield.

Gould, D., & Petlichkoff, L.M. (1988). Participation motivation and attrition in young athletes. In F. Smoll, R. Magill, & M. Ash (Eds.), *Children in sport* (3rd ed.) (pp. 161-178). Champaign, IL: Human Kinetics.

Harter, S. (1978). Effectance motivation reconsidered. *Human Development,* **21**, 34-64.

Harter, S. (1981). A model of intrinsic mastery motivation in children: Individual differences and developmental change. In W.A. Collins (Ed.), *Minnesota Symposium on Child Psychology: Vol. 14* (pp. 215-255). Hillsdale, NJ: Erlbaum.

Horn, T.S. (1985). Coaches' feedback and changes in children's perceptions of their physical competence. *Journal of Educational Psychology,* **77**, 174-186.

Horn, T.S. (1987). The influence of teacher-coach behavior on the psychological development of children. In D. Gould & M.R. Weiss (Eds.), *Advances in pediatric sport sciences: Vol. 2. Behavioral issues* (pp. 121-142). Champaign, IL: Human Kinetics.

Horn, T.S. (1991, October). *Sources of information underlying personal competence judgments in high school athletes.* Paper presented at the AAASP Annual Conference, Savannah, GA.

Horn, T.S., & Hasbrook, C.A. (1986). Information components influencing children's perceptions of their physical competence. In M.R. Weiss & D. Gould (Eds.), *Sport for children and youths* (pp. 81-88). Champaign, IL: Human Kinetics.

Horn, T.S., & Hasbrook, C.A. (1987). Psychological characteristics and the criteria children use for self-evaluation. *Journal of Sport Psychology,* **9**, 208-221.

Horn, T.S., & Lox, C. (1993). The self-fulfilling prophecy theory: When coaches' expectations become reality. In J.M. Williams (Ed.), *Applied sport psychology: Personal growth to peak performance* (2nd ed.) (pp. 68-81). Palo Alto, CA: Mayfield.

Horn, T.S., & Weiss, M.R. (1991). A developmental analysis of children's self-ability judgments in the physical domain. *Pediatric Exercise Science,* **3**, 310-326.

Klint, K.A., & Weiss, M.R. (1987). Perceived competence and motives for participating in youth sports: A test of Harter's competence motivation theory. *Journal of Sport Psychology,* **9**, 55-65.

Locke, E.A., & Latham, G. (1990). *A theory of goal setting and task performance.* Englewood Cliffs, NJ: Prentice Hall.

Martens, R. (1986). Youth sports in the USA. In M.R. Weiss & D. Gould (Eds.), *Sport for children and youths* (pp. 27-33). Champaign, IL: Human Kinetics.

McCombs, B.L. (1989). Self-regulated learning and academic achievement: A phenomenological view. In B.J. Zimmerman & D.H. Schunk (Eds.), *Self-regulated learning and academic achievement* (pp. 51-82). New York: Springer-Verlag.

McCullagh, P., Weiss, M.R., & Ross, D. (1989). Modeling considerations in motor skill acquisition and performance: An integrated approach. In K.B. Pandolf (Ed.), *Exercise and sport sciences reviews: Vol. 17* (pp. 475-513). Baltimore: Williams & Wilkins.

Nicholls, J.G. (1984). Achievement motivation: Conceptions of ability, subjective experience, task choice, and performance. *Psychological Review*, **91**, 328-346.

Nicholls, J.G. (1989). *The competitive ethos and democratic education*. Cambridge, MA: Harvard University Press.

Nicholls, J.G., & Miller, A. (1983). The differentiation of the concepts of difficulty and ability. *Child Development*, **54**, 951-959.

Schunk, D.H. (1989). Social cognitive theory and self-regulated learning. In B.J. Zimmerman & D.H. Schunk (Eds.), *Self-regulated learning and academic achievement* (pp. 83-110). New York: Springer-Verlag.

Schunk, D.H., & Hanson, A.R. (1985). Peer models: Influence on children's self-efficacy and achievement. *Journal of Educational Psychology*, **77**, 313-322.

Schunk, D.H., Hanson, A.R., & Cox, P.D. (1987). Peer model attributes and children's achievement behaviors. *Journal of Educational Psychology*, **79**, 54-61.

Vealey, R.S. (1988). Future directions in psychological skills training. *Sport Psychologist*, **2**, 318-336.

Weiss, M.R., Bredemeier, B.J., & Shewchuk, R.M. (1986). The dynamics of perceived competence, perceived control, and motivational orientation in youth sports. In M.R. Weiss & D. Gould (Eds.), *Sport for children and youths* (pp. 89-101). Champaign, IL: Human Kinetics.

Weiss, M.R., & Chaumeton, N. (1992). Motivational orientations in sport. In T.S. Horn (Ed.), *Advances in sport psychology* (pp. 61-99). Champaign, IL: Human Kinetics.

Weiss, M.R., Ebbeck, V., & Wiese-Bjornstal, D.M. (1993). Developmental and psychological factors related to children's observational learning of sport skills. *Pediatric Exercise Science*, **5**, 301-317.

Weiss, M.R., & Horn, T.S. (1990). The relation between children's accuracy estimates of their physical competence and achievement-related characteristics. *Research Quarterly for Exercise and Sport*, **61**, 250-258.

Weiss, M.R., McAuley, E., Ebbeck, V., & Wiese, D.M. (1990). Self-esteem and causal attributions for children's physical and social competence in sport. *Journal of Sport and Exercise Psychology*, **12**, 21-36.

Weiss, M.R., & Petlichkoff, L.M. (1989). Children's motivation for participation in and withdrawal from sport: Identifying the missing links. *Pediatric Exercise Science*, **1**, 195-211.

Wiggins, D.K. (1987). A history of organized play and highly competitive sport for American children. In D. Gould & M.R. Weiss (Eds.), *Advances in pediatric sport sciences: Vol. 2. Behavioral issues* (pp. 1-24). Champaign, IL: Human Kinetics.

Zimmerman, B.J., & Schunk, D.H. (1989). *Self-regulated learning and academic achievement*. New York: Springer-Verlag.

CHAPTER 4

COMPETITIVE RECREATIONAL ATHLETES: A MULTISYSTEMIC MODEL

James P. Whelan, PhD

Andrew W. Meyers, PhD

Charlene Donovan, MA

The University of Memphis

Some people might consider the term *competitive recreational athlete* an oxymoron. Although *competition* connotes intensity and seriousness, *recreation* suggests play, amusement, and relaxation. Such an apparent contradiction might be unsettling. Some people who might be labeled competitive recreational athletes are quite serious about their sports and might have great difficulty thinking about them as play. These people get up early every morning, rain or shine, to run or swim. They are willing to forgo sleep Saturday mornings to travel several hours to a race, a match, a meet, or a game. These are the sort of people who are conversant with air-cushion soles, carbon fiber, Lycra, a sweet spot, or metal woods. Most of these people do not consider themselves duffers or joggers; they do not refer to their sport as play. They think of themselves as athletes— serious, competitive athletes. They value the health benefits of regular exercise, but they love the competitive goals and experience, even though they might be competing primarily against themselves.

However, we would not argue that the term *competitive recreational athlete* should be abandoned. In fact, the original meaning of the word *competition*, from the latin *com petere*, is to seek or search together. The origin of the word *recreation* is the latin word *recreare*, meaning to restore or refresh. This suggests that recreational competition is a process of self-challenge or self-discovery directed toward restoration. The term also serves a valuable descriptive function. Competitive recreational athletes are different from other athletes considered in these chapters. Their sport involvement is what they choose to do with their free time. Although achievement and excellence in their sports might be valued objectives, training and racing must fit into the rest of their lives. These people typically have spouses, and often children, to whom they have responsibilities. They have jobs with supervisors, customers, deadlines, and obligations. Their self-identity is not solely dependent on their status as athletes.

This group also presents heterogeneous backgrounds, with a variety of athletic achievements and aspirations. Some approach their sports with a long history of athletic involvement; others, with little or no involvement. These competitors possess varying degrees of physical talent, and they have varying amounts of time to devote to training. Unlike elite junior national athletes, collegiate athletes, national team members, and professional competitors, these people compete for reasons other than the ability to perform.

Competitive recreational athletes also offer heterogeneous reasons for sport involvement, such as to establish a social support network, manage stress, moderate mood, control body weight, improve physical function, or combat the aging process. Consequently, competitive recreational athletes face a complex balancing task. Free to select among a variety of activities, they choose to train and compete. This decision must be balanced against the demands of family and work, the limitations of their physical skills, and the feasibility of their athletic and personal goals.

It is important to note that this group of athletes is probably the largest classification of athletes in the United States, and nearly every sport boasts a share of loyal participants. The United States Tennis Association (1990) has about 150,000 people currently playing in its adult recreational leagues, and a survey by the National Sporting Goods Association (1990) found that more than 3 million men and women over age 18 consider themselves to be "very frequent" tennis players (playing more than 30 days a year). According to the National Bowling Council (1990), there are 6 million adult men and women league bowlers in the United States, and the National Golf Foundation (1991) reports that about 10% of adult males and 2% of adult females in the United States play golf. The Athletic Congress, the governing body of track and field in the United States,

estimated that over 4 million people participate in sanctioned road-running races each year (Honikman & Honikman, 1991). United States Masters Swimming (1991) records indicate that 25,000 people participated in masters swim meets in 1990. The United States Cycling Federation (1990) licensed over 30,000 competitive cyclists in 1990.

Despite the distinctions between these athletes and other classifications of athletes and between these athletes and nonathletes, the differences within the population of competitive recreational athletes appear greater than the differences between this population and others. We are cautious, therefore, not to propose that psychological intervention for competitive recreational athletes must be unique. Knowledge and awareness of sport, athletes, and sport science is necessary to work with any athlete. But the process of creating change does not appear to be population specific. The available meta-analysis reviews of psychotherapy support the notion that the science of behavior change has not evolved to the point that we can identify particular change mechanisms for particular problems (for a review see Lambert, Shapiro, & Bergin, 1986).

Therefore, in this chapter we adopt a holistic personal enhancement model, similar in nature to psychotherapy, to address the complaints of competitive recreational athletes. We would not argue that therapy can be generically applied without consideration of individual uniqueness. We argue instead that sport participation is only one aspect in the lives of athletes. Directing efforts to resolve athletes' problems based on a snapshot of the athletic context might not be the most effective means of creating meaningful resolution of their complaints.

This chapter provides a conceptual framework for psychological intervention efforts with competitive recreational athletes. We begin by describing three competitive recreational athletes, their presenting problems, the complications that make their sport participation difficult, and how or why they chose to seek consultation from a sport psychologist. These athletes are quite similar to individuals we have treated. Some details about these individuals have been altered to protect their identity to accommodate the needs of this chapter. Next, we briefly discuss the literature on psychological skills training interventions, then place it in the broader context of each athlete's life. The interactions among athletic performance, individual dysfunction, family, workplace, and larger social and cultural issues are presented. Then, returning to our cases, we address assessment and intervention issues for our three athletes. In closing, we highlight some ethical issues of working with competitive recreational athletes. (Note that we use the labels *therapist* and *counselor* interchangeably throughout this chapter to refer to any professional who is adequately trained and credentialed to provide psychological services.)

■ THE CASE OF JULIO ■

Julio, a 42-year-old tenured associate professor in the computer science department of the local university, has been actively involved in masters swimming since his mid-30s. Recently he started to experience a disruptive amount of precompetition arousal and anxiety. After reading about sport psychology services available at the university's psychology clinic, Julio called and set up an appointment.

He described his problem as "nerves." Over the last year he had become increasingly anxious in the week before each swim meet. He had difficulty focusing on his workouts and often ended them early; he slept and ate poorly; and he regularly found himself distracted from his university responsibilities. The night before a meet was typically sleepless. By the time Julio's primary race (the 200-m backstroke) was called, he would have great difficulty remembering his race plan, and he either went

out too fast and died late in the race or went out too slowly and was out of contention by the last 50 m. In the big long-course meet that ended his summer competitive season, Julio was first at the halfway point of the race, but he faded to finish seventh in an eight-man field in a time slower than his best workouts.

Julio started in age-group swimming at age 7, and by junior high he was a budding star. In high school, at 6 ft, 4 in. and 170 lb (193 cm and 77 kg), he continued to improve, and in his senior year he was the 200-m backstroke state champion. These swimming achievements led to heavy recruitment by many colleges, and he chose an Ivy League school. His first problems appeared there.

Julio's parents and his club and high-school coaches had been easygoing. But his college coach seemed incredibly rigid. Practice workouts were more grueling than he had ever experienced, and there seemed no time for fun or camaraderie. Indeed, the coach appeared to foster an atmosphere of competition among team members. Halfway through his freshman season Julio began to experience "nerves" before competition. This led to increasingly poor practices and meet times and eventually to conflicts with the now-disappointed coach. The season ended with a stern warning from the coach that he "better come back tougher next year."

Julio had hoped that returning to his hometown swim club for the summer would energize him, but instead he found little motivation to work hard. Back at school in the fall he dreaded the beginning of regular practices and after just a few anxious weeks, Julio quit the squad. Then followed a 19-year period—through graduate school, his marriage, and his first academic job—where Julio swam only sporadically. Realizing one day that he weighed more than 230 lb (104 kg), Julio decided to start swimming for fitness and weight control.

Gradually, over the next 4-year period, Julio regained his long-lost physical skills. He eventually returned to competition in small local meets, and by age 40 he was approaching some of his best high-school times. At this point, Julio began to realize that he might be nationally competitive in masters age-group swimming. Later that year his "nerves" returned.

His training journal helped to detail the anxiety response. He described the initial physical experience as a "buzz," almost as if his body was perpetually vibrating. Cognitively, Julio tried to focus on winning, but he obsessed about losing after all the hard training and the compromises that he had to make at work and at home. The journal revealed a good deal of guilt about these sacrifices. He feared his university colleagues would soon realize his "lack of commitment" to his job. Similarly, he was concerned that he was not holding up his end of the marital and family relationships. He had come full circle; he was again considering giving up swimming.

Julio spent a good deal of time preparing for competitions. His daily journal detailed his workouts, his physical and emotional state, and other information that might prove valuable to his training and competitive efforts. The training regimen itself typically involved a gradual increase in training intensity followed by a tapering period before important competitions so that he would be both prepared and rested. Julio usually trained for about 2 hr each morning before work and often did some weight work in the afternoons. However, university or family commitments often forced training-schedule changes.

Julio was married to a 37-year-old lawyer, Maria, and they had a 2-year-old son, Ben. Maria's law career was demanding and involved long and irregular hours. She had no athletic involvement, and though she tolerated Julio's swimming, she was not fond of it. Although they had a housekeeper and relatives lived nearby, and although Ben was enrolled in a day-care center, home and child-care duties were often Julio's. Maria attended the second appointment with Julio, and she reported that

he was a devoted father and good companion. Though their career and family demands created a good deal of stress, she believed that the marriage was on solid ground. Maria also noted that she and Julio shared a group of friends with whom both enjoyed regularly socializing.

Although Julio was a tenured associate professor, his research career was at a pivotal point. Continued achievement in the academic community required much hard work and he clearly felt this pressure. Fortunately, his annual evaluations were very positive and he believed that his department chair and his peers valued his contribution. Given this relative stability and support from home and work, Julio viewed his current case of "nerves" as limited to competitive swimming.

■ THE CASE OF SHERRY ■

Sherry approached the therapist after the monthly meeting of the local bicycle club. Sherry, the 37-year-old manager of a local bank branch, said she was having difficulty getting motivated for the coming racing season and she wanted to talk. At a first appointment, Sherry reported that after several years of increasingly impressive performances and an eventual ranking as a Category II racer, she had hit a plateau during the past season. Although continuing to perform respectably in local races, she had failed to win any regional races and she had not obtained sponsorship. Even at the local level, her performance was somewhat more inconsistent than it had been in several years, and she was experiencing a number of small, nagging injuries.

Sherry reported feeling "distracted" from her racing and training. This was extremely surprising to her because both the camaraderie and the social world that surrounded racing and training as well as the racing itself were "the most enjoyable" parts of her life. She typically met a group of friends from the bike club for a long (3 hr or more) Saturday morning ride each week. Sherry also worked out with some members of this group on Sunday mornings and Tuesdays and Thursdays after work. On other days she usually worked out alone outdoors, weather permitting, or on an indoor trainer at home or at her health club. All told, Sherry spent 18 to 20 hr a week working out and averaged more than 300 mi (483 km) per week on the bike. Several of her riding buddies had commented that her intensity had been off lately. One even suggested that Sherry see a doctor, "or maybe even a shrink." The suggestion bothered her, so she increased her weekly distance and bought a few subliminal motivational tapes. When both her health and her motivation deteriorated further, her friends told her to give a sport psychologist a try.

She reported feeling lethargic and admitted to moments throughout the day of sadness and tears, all without any obvious explanation. She mentioned that she did not really want to talk to someone like a psychologist, but her husband had begun to insist on it. Sherry's husband, Robert, was a hospital executive, and they had two children, Suzan, 8, and Bobby, 11. Although generally positive about the relationship, Sherry offered little to substantiate the benefits of the marriage or the joys of motherhood. She was not sure what she and Robert had in common anymore. She seemed to find the day-to-day work at the bank enjoyable, but seemed unexcited by her future with the organization. She did not see much room for career advancement—and indeed Sherry had no lofty professional aspirations—but she was pleased that her current job gave her adequate time to train.

Sherry described herself as quiet and somewhat shy. She was the younger of two sisters and viewed her birth family as close but not overly affectionate. Her dominant memories of high school and college involved the struggle to keep her grades up and the challenge and pleasures of varsity cross-country and track.

Although her athletic career was not distinguished by titles or school records, Sherry lettered in cross-country and track in both high school and college.

She met Robert soon after taking a management-trainee position with the banking corporation, and they were married 18 months later. Bobby was born less than a year later. Sherry had run sporadically after college, but she hoped that a regular regimen of running after her pregnancy would "relieve some of the tension and lethargy" she was feeling. Unfortunately, an overuse knee injury after 3 months cut short this therapeutic effort. Upon recovering she took up cycling and almost immediately became "addicted." In addition to the pleasure she felt out on the road, alone and in the company of other cyclists, she was attracted to the hardware and technology of cycling. She described bicycles in romantic terms, as beautiful, graceful machines that soared almost silently over the road.

Robert joined a subsequent appointment. He too was puzzled by Sherry's recent behavior. Initially positive about the relationship, he became increasingly caustic and bitter as he described their home life. He was resentful about Sherry's cycling "addiction," and though he thought that Sherry was well-meaning, Robert angered as he detailed the burdens of caring for the children while Sherry was "riding around." He reported that over the last two years he had felt increasingly distant from Sherry and that their sex life had "been dropped from the back of the pack." Robert reported that he had even considered taking a job in another city. Sherry did not seem surprised by this information, but the couple had apparently not discussed these issues openly before.

■ THE CASE OF PETER ■

Peter, a 51-year-old lawyer and skilled recreational tennis player, was strongly urged to come in to see a therapist by a close friend and fellow lawyer who was concerned about Peter's explosions of temper on the tennis court. At the first meeting Peter noted that he had always engaged in "John McEnroe–like outbursts" on the court. However, during a recent match this escalated into first a verbal battle and eventually a physical confrontation with an opponent.

Peter appeared to realize the inappropriateness of his actions but saw the event as an isolated occurrence. He was more concerned with the effect his loss of emotional control was having on his tennis game. He reported a number of instances, especially in tournament play, where a close call or errant shot had set him off. Typically, after these eruptions Peter was unable to regain his composure, and he very often went on to lose the match. This was happening with increasing frequency over the past 5 years. He had read articles in the popular media on sport psychology and hoped that a sport psychologist could help him develop the skills necessary to handle these stressful moments.

Peter played tennis at least four times a week and often took a lesson from his club pro on the weekends. For years he had jogged to improve his endurance, but he had given this up to concentrate on tennis. Even at age 51 his tennis skills (though not his match performance) were still steadily improving.

A trial attorney for almost 25 years, he described himself as an intensely competitive and terribly proud man. He had grown up in a poor family; the situation at home had been "harsh." His concentration on his studies and later on high-school baseball was as much to buffer a combative relationship with his father and a somewhat distant relationship with his mother as it was for a sense of achievement. But even so, Peter was extremely proud of his accomplishments. He graduated 7th in his class of more than 200, started 3 years on the baseball team, and dated the captain of the cheerleaders. Peter was not gifted enough to play collegiate baseball, but he continued his academic achievement and eventually graduated from a prestigious Eastern law school. He married Ruth soon after completing his clerkship and taking his first job. They have one daughter, Randy, now 24, who lives more than 2,000 mi (3,218 km) away on the West Coast.

Peter described himself at work as "one tough son of a bitch." He seemed to take pride in his role as an intimidator of young lawyers in his firm and opposing attorneys in the courtroom. He argued that the tough guy image is an appropriate role model for his associate lawyers and the proper role in the courtroom on behalf of his clients.

As part of the assessment and before beginning the performance-related anger-management work, the therapist asked Peter to bring Ruth with him. Peter was adamant that this was not necessary and would not help the therapist to understand his athletic performance problems. In fact, he could not remember the last time Ruth had seen him play tennis. Peter missed his next appointment, and the therapist did not see him for approximately 3 months. He then made an appointment after a particularly embarrassing event at his racquet club. During mixed doubles he had shoved an opponent he said was verbally baiting him—a female opponent. He argumentatively justified his actions but admitted that others who witnessed the situation told him that he had seriously overreacted. Indeed, the club's governing board had given him a formal warning.

When the therapist informed him that any further work would require his wife's involvement, he tearfully admitted that he had regularly "lost my temper" with her. Finally, with a great deal of reluctance, he admitted to regular spouse abuse over the two and a half decades of their marriage. This typically involved slapping and pushing her during arguments that could be initiated by relatively innocuous events. Although he denied any drinking or drug problems, Peter drank regularly and heavily in the evenings. With a great deal of hesitancy and emotion, he agreed to bring Ruth to the next meeting.

VIEWING THE PERSON

Sport scientists compete vigorously for research time and opportunities with the rare, and often elusive, elite athlete. Obversely, the laboratories of sport scientists are filled with non-elite and maybe even nonathlete students from introductory psychology and introductory health, physical education, and recreation classes. Unhappily, we know very little about the psychology of the elite athlete. We know much more about how our clinical and educational interventions function with nonathletes or people who engage only infrequently in athletic endeavors (Whelan, Meyers, & Berman, 1989), but we must cope with the problem of generalizing these results to our athlete populations. The availability and intensity of competitive recreational athletes makes them a more promising test sample for our interventions than the population of first-year college students, yet surprisingly little is known about competitive recreational athletes.

Demographics

The population of competitive recreational athletes is extremely varied and for that reason is difficult to describe. However, we do have data on many athlete groups; this helps us develop an image of this citizen competitor. Perhaps the first such population of serious recreational athletes available to sport scientists came from the running boom of the 1970s, following Frank Shorter's 1972 Olympic marathon gold medal. Investigators have examined the demographics, personality characteristics, and psychological skills of these non-elite but often extremely committed runners.

According to data from the statistics division of The Athletic Congress (Honikman & Honikman, 1991), the average serious male runner is 38 years old, whereas the average serious female runner is 35 years old. Masters runners over age 40 are predominantly married, average 2.3 children, and run five times per week for a total of 27 miles (Okwumabua, Meyers, & Santille, 1987). Freischlag (1981), in a study of 55 marathoners, found that marathoners are usually from large families where boys outnumber girls, are typically first-born children, and rarely attribute their sport success to the influence of others. However, Freischlag reported that peers are most important to the runner's athletic achievement. Interestingly, coaches and parents received "neutral" influence ratings.

Meyers and Okwumabua (1985) found that marathon finishing time was related to many training variables, including the number of weeks spent training for the marathon, the runner's best past race performance, and the strength of the runner's self-efficacy, which in itself accounted for more than 40% of the variance in performance outcome.

Data from other studies suggest that these demographics are representative of competitive recreational athletes in many sports. More than half of triathlon participants are married, with 40% falling between ages 30 to 39. Forty-five percent are college graduates earning an average annual income of $50,100. These athletes reported spending approximately 16 hr per week training, and enter three to four triathlons a year (Whelan et al., 1987a, 1987b). More than half of masters swimmers are male (United States Masters Swimming, 1991), and the United States Tennis Association (1990) reports that a majority of the players in its recreational leagues are male. Most male participants are ages 25 to 34, whereas the highest percentage of female participants are ages 35 to 44. These players are also considered frequent participants, playing more than 30 days during a year. Bowling boasts the most equitable split between the sexes; there are approximately 3 million male and 3 million female sanctioned-league bowlers (National Bowling

Council, 1990). A significant majority of these athletes are married (74.6%) and most are ages 18 to 49. Nearly half of these bowlers have annual incomes greater than $35,000 and more than half attended college. A slightly different picture appears among volleyball players. The highest percentage of adult "frequent" volleyball players are age 18 to 34. More than half of these athletes are female; the majority have household annual incomes of $15,000 to $24,999 (Sporting Goods Manufacturers Association, 1990). This fairly low income figure is probably due to the younger age of the sample.

Personality

Ogilvie (1968) argued for the existence of "athletic" personality traits. This work was based on the assumption that athletes possess unique and definable personality attributes. These attributes are different from those of nonathletes, potentially different from one sport to another, and different across athletic skill levels. Some traits seem obvious: traits of endurance, ambition, and aggressiveness. Other traits that Ogilvie saw as characteristic of athletes include organization, dominance, and deference.

The late 1960s also saw Ogilvie and Tutko's (1966) attempt to integrate psychological assessment and personality theory into sport psychology. Their work marked the first contemporary meeting of clinical psychology and the study of athletic performance. Ogilvie and Tutko concentrated on the development of a personality test that they hoped would allow them to predict the performance of athletes. The success of such testing would facilitate athlete selection, coach-player interaction, and the design of training programs. Perhaps the most intense examination of the athlete personality has occurred with marathon runners. Sport scientists have reported that marathoners are typically more introverted, have lower anxiety levels, and better mood profiles than nonrunners (Clitsome & Kostrubala, 1977; Gondola & Tuckman, 1982; Gontang, Clitsome, & Kostrubala, 1977; Morgan & Costill, 1972; Morgan & Pollack, 1977; Silva & Hardy, 1986; Wilson, Morley, & Bird, 1980).

The work of Ogilvie and other sport "personologists" fell victim to the same problems and criticisms that general personality theory was receiving in the 1960s and 1970s. As Mischel (1968) eloquently argued, global personality traits have been poor predictors of behavior. This is in large part due to the failure of early personality theories to consider both situational contributions to behavior and the interaction among those situational demands and the individual behavioral and psychological skills. Those hunting for the athlete personality had returned empty-handed (Mahoney & Meyers, 1989; Meyers, 1980; Morgan, 1980; Rushall, 1972; Silva, 1984).

At the time personality views were foundering, evidence supporting the efficacy of *mental practice* or covert rehearsal on the acquisition and retention of complex motor skills began to appear (Corbin, 1972; Richardson, 1967a, 1967b). In their review, Feltz and Landers (1983) reported that covert rehearsal, compared to no practice, significantly improved skilled motor performance approximately one-half standard deviation. Then in 1972, Suinn applied a multicomponent cognitive-behavioral intervention to sport performance. He found that training in relaxation and imagery skills combined with a behavioral-rehearsal technique improved the race performances of skilled skiers. Based on Suinn's work, imagery-based mental-practice interventions for performance enhancement became more intricate and began to resemble the growing body of cognitively oriented clinical interventions that had come into favor in the 1960s (Bandura, 1969, 1977; Beck, 1976; Meichenbaum, 1985).

Psychological Skills

The movement away from personality-based approaches to athletic performance enhancement has largely adopted a cognitive-behavioral paradigm. Consistent with this learning-based perspective, investigators and practitioners have emphasized the assessment and development of sport-related psychological skills rather than invariant personality traits.

In a study focusing on collegiate racquetball players, Meyers, Cooke, Cullen, and Liles (1979) found that better athletes were more self-confident and possessed a more structured lifestyle. Imagery skills were also better developed in more skilled and successful racquetball players. Not only did more skilled players report images with more clarity than less skilled players, but the more skilled players also had less difficulty controlling the images. Importantly, the better players were also more skillful in dealing with competitive anxiety than were the less skilled players. The more skilled players reported anxiety at the beginning of matches, as did their less-skilled counterparts. The better players also reported a leveling of and eventual decrease in the amount of anxiety as the match progressed, whereas the less skilled players did not experience the same process. The existing evidence has generally supported the notion that successful athletes employ coping skills that positively influence motivation, preparation, arousal management, concentration, and self-confidence (Feltz & Ewing, 1987; Gould, Weiss, & Weinberg, 1981; Hemery, 1986; Mahoney, Gabriel, & Perkins, 1987).

In addition to these psychological-skill differences, sport scientists have also identified cognitive-strategy differences among competitive recreational athletes. In their work with masters runners over 40 years of age, Okwumabua et al. (1987) found that these athletes were more likely to use dissociative cognitive strategies during a race, concentrating on factors other than those associated with running the race. Younger runners were more likely to use associative strategies and to focus on race-related thoughts, such as performance time and pain level. Differences in strategy might be accounted for in part by differing motivations. Older athletes might run for health and social benefits, whereas younger athletes might focus on performance.

Although it is doubtful that competitive recreational athletes possess unique, sport-relevant psychological skills or cognitive strategies, this perspective presents us with both a framework for understanding the performance of these athletes and a model for psychological intervention. If psychological skills are indeed beneficial to the athlete, then programs to enhance those skills should improve performance.

VIEWING THE PERSON IN CONTEXT

We have described a group of adult athletes who must cope with the physical and emotional requirements of their competitive sports. However, competitive recreational athletes do not live in a sport vacuum; they exist in many worlds, all of which make demands on their time and energy. These various environments require a variety of physical, social, and mental skills for successful performance. Careers, marriage, and child rearing as well as larger community demands place heavy responsibilities on these people. They must meet their obligations and still find time for sport without the support systems sometimes available to elite athletes. Given these burdens or challenges, what motivates the competitive recreational athlete to continue to juggle potentially conflicting demands? As suggested in Figure 4.1, a variety

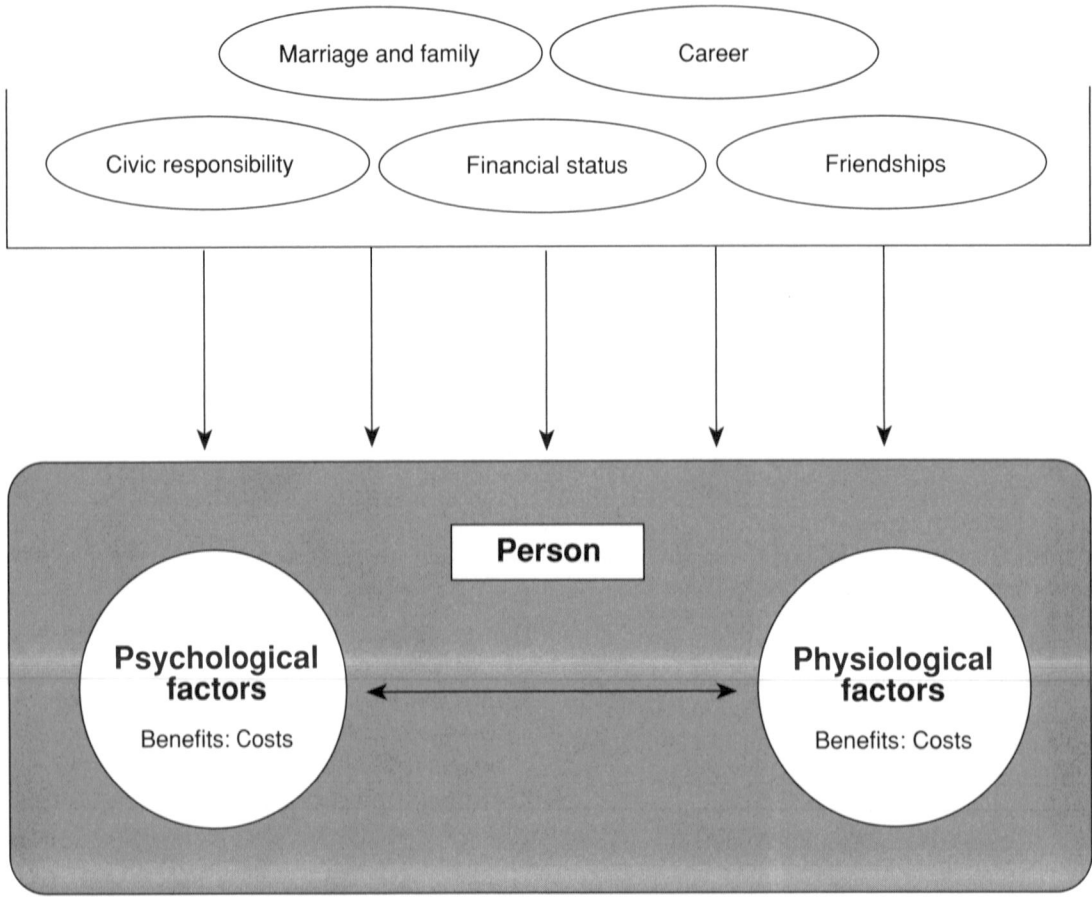

Contextual demands impacting sport involvement

Figure 4.1 Sport and exercise participation has specific psychological and physiological benefits and specific psychological and physiological costs to the person. These benefits and costs are directly impacted by the contextual demands that the person experiences.

of contextual demands can influence the individual athlete's psychological and physical well-being. Unfortunately, no intensive study of the competitive motivation of these athletes has been conducted. The sport literature does, however, detail several promising hypotheses concerning sport participation that may be applicable to the competitive recreational athlete.

Sapp and Haubenstricker (1978) have identified four primary motivators for children's sport participation. Fun is the reason most often given by children for their continued participation in sport, followed by (in descending order of importance) skill improvement, fitness benefits, and team atmosphere. Other motivators include sportspersonship, challenge and excitement, travel, and other extrinsic rewards (see also Gill, Gross, & Huddleston, 1981; Gould, Feltz, Weiss, & Petlichkoff, 1983; Griffin, 1978; Skubic, 1956; Wankel & Kreisel, 1985). These motivators either build self-efficacy or fulfill a social role.

The team as a motivating variable highlights the social and friendship aspects of sport participation. Team membership gives the child a sense of attachment, demonstrated by the team name emblazoned across the uniform. There is shared activity, celebration, and mourning. Success brings a sense of achievement, importance, and public admiration. Failure is often accompanied by the experience of camaraderie, an expression of mutual support in the face of defeat.

Although these motivational issues certainly operate for the competitive recreational athlete, they might not provide a complete picture. Several theoretical models attempt to explain the motivational benefits of exercise. Morgan (1985), in his *mental health model* of human athletic performance, suggested that adults might participate in athletics because of the positive mental-health benefits, increased levels of psychological well-being, and an increased sense of self-efficacy and competence provided by regular physical activity and competition (see also Weinstein & Meyers, 1983). Glasser (1976) has argued along similar lines that runners often manifest an addiction to their sport, albeit a positive one. Their athletic activities offer recreational competitors an element of controllability; athletes are in control of their exercise regime and, we hope, its place in their daily lives. Their developing athletic skills might well bring increased feelings of competence and physical and psychological well-being, the often reported "runner's high" (Sachs, 1984).

The psychological well-being supposedly related to all forms of regular physical exercise has received a considerable amount of research attention. Several investigators (Bahrke & Morgan, 1978; Folkins & Sime, 1981; Raglin & Morgan, 1985) have hypothesized about possible psychological benefits of exercise. Although the scientific debate

continues, exercise appears to provide some relief from stress and anxiety. Morgan (1987) has suggested that exercise produces stress reduction through distraction. The distraction model holds that exercise serves to move the person from negative ruminations to physical activity, thus reducing anxiety or depression (Brown, Ramirez, & Taub, 1978; Greist, Klein, Eischens, & Faris, 1978).

Along with the psychological benefits that might provide motivational bases for regular exercise and competition, other hypothesized mechanisms might account for positive addiction. Schildkraut, Orsulak, Schatzberg, and Rosenblum (1983) argued for the existence of a biological basis for the psychological well-being related to regular exercise. They contended that exercise alters one or all of the major brain monoamines. Briefly, when the neurotransmitter norepinephrine, a catecholamine, is experimentally injected into the ventricles of the brain, there is a marked increase in motor activity and other signs of behavioral arousal. Drugs used in the treatment of depression facilitate catecholaminergic transmission in the brain. The result of this facilitation is, among other things, an elevation in mood. These investigators hold that exercise works in ways similar to antidepressant medications by facilitating catecholaminergic transmission and thereby elevating mood.

Another possible biological moderator of the exercise–affect relationship concerns the elevation of body temperature produced during prolonged or intense physical activity. Elevated body temperature has been found to produce a variety of therapeutic effects, and there is clear evidence that deep body temperature is increased in proportion to the intensity of exercise a person performs (Morgan & O'Connor, 1988). This temperature elevation leads to a decrease in muscle tension (Morgan & O'Connor) and might influence the release, synthesis, or uptake of major brain monoamines (deVries, Wiswell, Bulbulian, & Moritani, 1981).

The final proposed biological mechanism for exercise effects on mood involves the relationship between endogenous opioids, such as the endorphins, and regular aerobic exercise (Steinberg & Sykes, 1985). Several studies have concluded that improved mood states following exercise might be stimulated by the release of endorphins, which have a morphinelike effect. However, other investigators examining the role of endogenous opioids in exercise-induced mood changes (Goldfarb, Hatfield, Sforzo, & Flynn, 1987; Williams & Getty, 1986) concluded that even though strenuous exercise stimulates the release of opioids, there is no clear empirical support that these substances are directly linked to exercise-associated mood changes.

From this work, it would appear that competitive recreational athletes might pursue exercise for a variety of reasons, most importantly physical and psychological well-being resulting from both exercise and competitive achievement as well as the social aspects of athletic involvement. Unfortunately, there is little convincing evidence that exercise is causal in improvements in either psychological well-being or the quality of social life. One reason for the dearth of evidence might be that our view of the athlete has failed to include the contextual variables that impact individual well-being, both physical and psychological.

INDIVIDUAL INTERVENTIONS

As we have noted, competitive recreational athletes often have been overlooked in investigations of clinical and educational sport-performance-enhancement interventions. However, we can derive some direction for this population from laboratory and field work with other athlete populations.

There is evidence that cognitive-behavioral interventions can positively impact athletic performance (Feltz & Ewing, 1987; Mahoney & Avener, 1977; Orlick & Partington, 1988; Whelan, Meyers, & Berman, 1989). These interventions have focused on goal setting, arousal management, and precompetition planning. Research in these areas, although not specifically geared toward the competitive recreational athlete, has been summarized by Whelan, Mahoney, and Meyers (1991).

Goal Setting

Locke and Latham (1985) speculated that the positive impact of goal-setting strategies could be applied to athletic contexts. According to Locke (1968), specific, difficult, and realistic goals, as compared to nonspecific, lenient goals or no goals, are associated with improved task performance. These findings have received both support (Barnett & Stanicek, 1979; Hall, Weinberg, & Peterson, 1987; Tu & Tothstein, 1979) and criticism, as many experiments have found no performance differences between no-goal, nonspecific-goal, and specific-goal conditions (Hollingsworth, 1975; Weinberg, Bruya, & Peterson, 1985).

Goal-setting research has also examined the motivational influence of goal orientation (Whelan et al., 1991). People whose achievement goals focus on task mastery rather than competitive superiority might be better prepared to cope more effectively with task demands (Csikszentmihalyi, 1990). Those who desire competitive superiority might seek less demanding tasks to showcase their abilities, whereas tasks that are difficult relative to skills might be perceived as threatening to self-esteem. People who hold task-mastery goals should view difficult tasks as challenges and learning opportunities (Nicholls, 1984; Orlick, 1986). The adoption of task-mastery goals should even serve to buffer the psychological and behavioral effects of task failure (Nichols, Whelan, & Meyers, 1991).

Arousal Management

Physiological and emotional arousal appear to be necessary for optimal response to most competitive demands (Mahoney & Meyers, 1989; Oxendine, 1970). What level of arousal enhances or debilitates performance depends on factors such as task characteristics and individual differences (Landers, 1980; Weinberg, 1989). Evidence indicates that across individuals and situations an athlete's performance can suffer from over- or underarousal (e.g., Fenz, 1975; Fenz & Jones, 1972; Mahoney & Avener, 1977). Arousal modulation, therefore, has become an important target for psychological interventions in sport (Hackfort & Spielberger, 1989).

Efforts to modify overarousal can rely on the anxiety-reduction and stress-management research of clinical psychology (Smith, 1980). Interventions such as relaxation training, biofeedback, and stress-management training (Meichenbaum, 1985; Woolfolk & Lehrer, 1984) have been employed effectively to control overarousal and anxiety in athletes (DeWitt, 1980; Murphy & Woolfolk, 1987; Smith, 1985; Ziegler, Klinzing, & Williamson, 1982). When used with athletes these interventions generally involve skill development, and most packaged skill-training interventions for athletes include at least one such anxiety-management component (Orlick, 1986; Suinn, 1987). In contrast, efforts to modify underarousal have relied on athletes' ability to psychologically ready themselves. The assumption underlying these "psyching-up" efforts is that mental preparation heightens arousal, thereby preparing the athlete to perform (Weinberg, Gould, & Jackson, 1980). The body of work on interventions designed to increase arousal is, however, much less developed than that to reduce arousal.

Precompetition Planning

Precompetition planning (Orlick, 1986) is used to help the athlete devise a general preparation plan for practice and competition. Orlick makes use of goal-setting and arousal-management strategies, but on a more basic level, his planning program enables the athlete to gradually build a process for applying psychological skills and strategies to the competitive task. The plan eventually allows the athlete to identify and refine approaches to preparation for travel; precompetitive routines; interaction with peers, coaches, and family; physical preparation; competitive tasks; the prediction of unexpected happenings; and the postcompetitive experience. It is in this framework that the athlete learns to employ goal-setting, arousal-management, concentration, and refocusing strategies.

MULTISYSTEMIC INTERVENTIONS

Competitive recreational athletes can use these cognitive-behavioral strategies to enhance their competitive performance. But what happens to the athlete plagued by sport performance problems that are influenced by nonsport factors? As we argued on pages 79-80, competitive recreational athletes juggle many responsibilities other than their sports. When family or career do not function smoothly, it is likely that one's sport performance will also be negatively affected. Cognitive-behavioral strategies directed solely at athletic performance issues might be effective, but we adopt the position that these other nonsport stressors must eventually receive attention. Assessment and intervention must consider the competitive recreational athlete's multiple worlds. Family, work, sport, and community demands must be recognized and evaluated. We hope the case studies presented here demonstrate that although sport-related mental-skills training can be useful in some situations, such programs do not completely address the range of presenting problems that competitive citizen athletes bring to the sport psychologist. The level of commitment that these athletes exhibit suggests the need to examine the reciprocal interaction between sport performance and other aspects of the athlete's life.

We do not argue that other athletes are immune to these systemic problems. Indeed, we believe that elite athletes share these same difficulties with competitive recreational athletes. However, elite athletes might have fewer nonsport career complications during their competitive lives (though perhaps more career complications after their athletic disciplines end; see chapter 14) and a more sophisticated support system for dealing with sport demands and life stress. But one of the premises of our argument in this chapter is that the competitive recreational athlete might serve as an appropriate analog for service issues with the elite athlete.

For all athletes, performance is not dependent simply on what happens in training or competition; it is contingent on events in the larger world. One need only to reflect on the tragic death during the 1988 Winter Olympics of the sister of American speed skater Dan Jansen, or the effects of the fall of communism in Eastern Europe on the athletes of formerly communist countries during the 1992 Olympic Games to understand this. What happens to a person in one context certainly and unavoidably influences behavior in other contexts.

This systemic approach to sport performance is equally important when working with competitive recreational athletes. The bridge between unidirectional cognitive-behavioral approaches to sport psychology and a systemic approach to athletic performance is Bandura's (1977) notion of reciprocal determinism (see Figure 4.2). From the unidirectional perspective, behavior is a

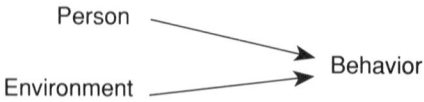

Unidirectional perspective

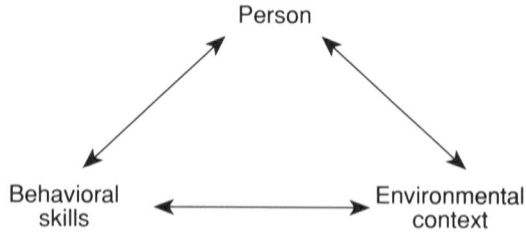

Reciprocal determinism perspective

Figure 4.2 Contrasting the relationship of behavior, mediating variables in the person, and environmental context for both unidirectional and reciprocal-determinism approaches.
Note. From "The Self-System in Reciprocal Determinism" by A. Bandura, 1978, *American Psychologist*, **33**, pp. 344-358. Copyright 1978 by the American Psychological Association. Adapted by permission.

function of two independent entities, the person and the environmental context. From the reciprocal-determinism perspective, Bandura argued that a person's behavioral skills, cognitive and other internal mediators, and environmental context are in a complex multidirectional interaction. Environmental happenings influence a person's actions and beliefs; beliefs affect behavior and the environment; and actions and their results influence the environment and subsequent beliefs. This interaction cannot be viewed as a linear sequence of events; rather it must be understood as a set of reciprocally interacting feedback and feedforward mechanisms (Mahoney & Meyers, 1989).

This notion of reciprocal determinism has been depicted graphically as a triangle in Figure 4.2 (Bandura, 1978). Behavioral skills, cognitive mediators, and the environmental context serve as the points of the triangle. The connecting lines demonstrate the reciprocal nonlinear influence that exists; the influence can start at any point and proceed in any direction, not necessarily following the same path in every situation a person might encounter. An event in the environment might influence an individual's behavioral skills, which in turn might impact the person's cognitive mediators. Just as easily, cognitive mediators might influence behavioral skills, which might bring about some environmental change. The key to reciprocal determinism is to remember that events do not occur in a linear sequence, and that an influence can arise from any point of the triangle and affect one or both of the other points.

When a competitive recreational athlete presents with environmental events that are restricted to the areas of training and competition, reciprocal determinism fits very nicely with the application of intervention strategies such as goal setting, arousal management, and precompetition planning, which are directed at enhancing the athlete's sport performance. By addressing the performance issues, which might result in changes in the level of the athlete's behavioral skills, these interventions should also influence both cognitive mediators and the environmental context. These changes should produce more successful sport performance outcomes. In situations where the treatment is limited to sport performance, the educational or cognitive-behavioral skill-building model that constitutes the foundation of current sport psychology intervention efforts should be beneficial. However, as is often the case, people who present with problem issues rarely fit easily into a neat package. When confronted with a person who also happens to be an athlete, limiting the scope of inquiry about environmental events to just those of the sport context might provide a restricted view of the person. This restricted view can lead to the application of interventions that,

although useful in some aspects, do not accurately address the broad issues and might result in a lack of progress in therapy.

To avoid the pitfalls of narrow vision, it is necessary to realize that, in reality, people operate in a variety of contexts and that the sport context is only one of many for the competitive recreational athlete. Although the theory of reciprocal determinism deals with only one particular situation at a time, the more accurate picture of influence is gained only when it is understood that environmental events from one situation or context often play a role in other contexts and that keeping the events of one context separate from other contexts is often impossible (see Figure 4.3). If a person has a stressful day at the office, this likely will have an effect on one's actions at home that evening. The person might have less patience for the children's roughhousing or become inappropriately angry with a spouse over trivial issues. Reciprocity not only occurs within a context, but also between contexts. Consequently, when attempting to understand the presenting problems of an athlete, we need to consider

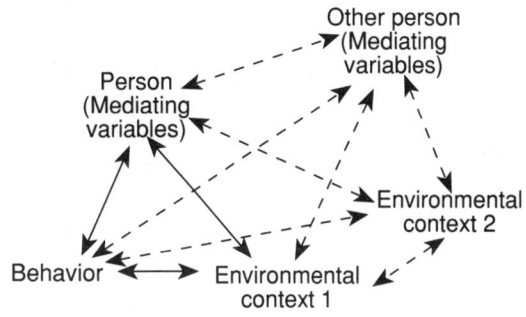

Figure 4.3 The bold lines indicate the reciprocal interaction between behavior, person, and environment when considering a single interaction. The addition of a second environmental context and a second set of person variables that impact immediately on behavior (as shown by the dashed lines) creates a significantly more complex view.

not only the happenings in sport, but also the happenings in other contexts of a person's life. In this example the sport context played no role in the drama, but therapists would not be aware of a stressful work environment if they restricted their inquiries to sport when assessing a presenting problem.

One model for thinking of these inter-related contexts is the multisystemic approach to conceptualizing problems and processes of change. The multisystemic approach (Henggeler & Borduin, 1990) might be seen as a more practical development of Bandura's reciprocal determinism. This approach takes into consideration all areas of a person's world before implementing any interventions. By assessing each of the areas in which the athlete is a participant, the issues causing poor sport performance can be addressed. Taking a systemic approach to the issues presented by athletes allows for a much more appropriately planned strategy for interventions, which should improve not only sport performance but also the level at which the athlete is functioning in other areas of life.

By adopting a multisystemic view of the person, therapists see presenting problems as attempts to handle demands in the contexts of sport, marriage, family, career, and social relations as well as the predictable and the unpredictable changes that occur in anyone's life. Increased marital conflict might be the result when the last child leaves home, leaving the spouses with the task of learning to readjust to being alone with each other. Alternatively, conflict might come about as a response to a career change that requires increased time commitments to work and corresponding decreases in time commitments to family. Not only are these problems attempts to handle stressors and changes, but they also demonstrate the influence contexts have on one another.

To gain a better understanding of the multisystemic perspective, we use a brief overview of systems theory suggested by Patricia Minuchin (1985):

• Systems are organized wholes, and elements within the system are necessarily interdependent. These elements are also bound by predictable relationships with one another. Applying this principle to people is similar to saying that behavior is best understood and predicted when considering as many contextual influences as possible.

• A system is circular, not linear. To conceptualize this principle, consider two people. The actions of Person A influence Person B, whereas the actions of Person B influence Person A, and so on. For example, in training for a triathlon, a woman might spend much time away from her family. Her husband might feel she is neglecting them and so might try to nag her into spending more time at home. She might respond by thinking that her husband is selfishly trying to keep her from accomplishing her goals. She becomes angry with him and spends more time training. He nags more, she trains more, and so on. Her actions influence him, his actions influence her; this feedback loop will continue until someone or something disrupts it.

• A system strives to maintain homeostasis, the status quo. The problem with a homeostatic goal is that evolution and change are also inherent in any system. These changes might be brought about by genetic or biological factors (like aging) or by environmental factors. They might be the result of psychological changes, such as confidence following a series of successes or failures. All potential stressors, be they developmental, predictable, or unpredictable, bring about evolution and change. Systems, however, attempt to minimize or resist the change. Although this resistance can be functional and adaptive, it might also have detrimental effects. The tendency to maintain stability, and therefore minimize helpful change, must be kept in mind when dealing with athletes.

• Complex systems are always composed of subsystems. Consider a family as an example. A family is a complex system, but when the family is examined, subsystems can be identified. These subsystems include a spousal subsystem, a parenting subsystem, a sibling subsystem, and perhaps a parent–child subsystem. The subsystems combine to form the system, and it is clear that there is no mutually exclusive membership in any one subsystem. Each subsystem has its own functions and boundaries (Henggeler & Borduin, 1990). The functions of a sibling are different from the functions of a child. Similarly, the functions of a parent are different from the functions of a spouse.

• Subsystems are separated from larger systems by boundaries, and there are implicit rules and structures that govern interactions across boundaries (Wood & Talmon, 1983). These boundaries affect the flow of information to and from systems (Henggeler & Borduin, 1990).

The idea of multiple contexts and the workings of multisystemic thought can be depicted as mutually interacting circles (see Figure 4.4). The fact that they do interact makes it clear that influences in one context can readily affect other contexts and can globally affect all contexts. Beyond the contexts depicted in Figure 4.4, or more appropriately the area in which these contexts are embedded, is the cultural context. Society, culture, politics, and economics all influence the athlete.

Stressors and demands impinge on the person in these multiple contexts or systems, affecting not only sport performance but also the ability to function successfully in the family and at work. These demands can be developmental, predictable, or unpredictable. According to Carter and McGoldrick (1988), developmental stressors are those events that, although expected during a normal life

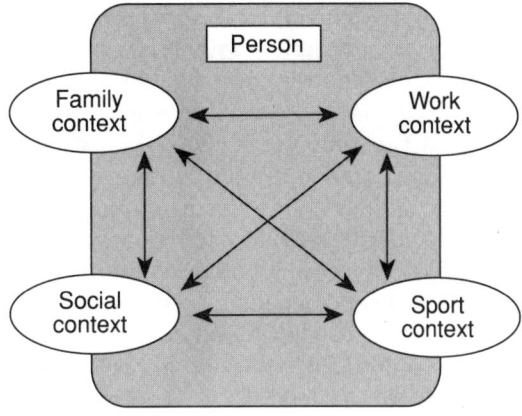

Figure 4.4 The multicontextual model of athletes highlights that individual functioning or performance is the product of reciprocal interactions between several influencing contexts.

span, are often intensely stressful to all members of a particular family system. These stressors usually occur at transitions in a family; that is, instances in which the role of a family member in the system changes dramatically or when a family member leaves the system. Some examples of these transition times include a divorce, the aging of a parent, the birth or death of a family member, or the departure of a child for college. Other developmental stressors can also occur in conjunction with a person's career. For example, a job promotion can significantly impact a person's work context; a new position might demand a significantly greater amount of time to maintain career success. The increased commitment to the work context might require the person to decrease commitment in other contexts, and this decrease might negatively affect performance in these contexts. A career demotion might also produce deteriorating performance in other contexts. Both of these situations carry with them potential for financial changes, and these changes can present additional stressors across many contexts.

These developmental stressors are, for the most part, predictable. However, there are other predictable stressors that are not developmental. An athlete's training season is one example. The training season requires the athlete to reduce the amount of time allotted to family or work. One's spouse must pick up the slack in the family system by assuming more of the caretaking, both of children and home, and both partners are left with less time to devote to their own relationship. In the work context, the athlete might be able to maintain previous levels of job performance, but in the more stressful situation of producing a similar quantity and quality of work in less time.

In addition to these predictable stressors, there are also unpredictable stressors, which might be even more problematic. The competitor has little time to prepare for these capricious stressors and must deal with them as they come. Such stressors might include athletic injuries that affect training or end a competitive season, major health problems experienced by a family member, a financial crisis, or conflicts that appear at work or at home. It is not difficult to imagine how any of these stressors would impact not only their immediate context but also other areas of the athlete's life. Again, understanding the overall impact of any stressor on multiple contexts is central to understanding the issues presented by the athlete. This understanding is necessary to plan useful interventions that target problematic issues, not merely act as bandages for one symptom. Taking a multisystemic approach when dealing with these athletes is possible only after understanding multiple contexts.

Before moving on to look at interventions used with competitive recreational athletes, several important points must be reiterated. Assessment and intervention must take into consideration the importance and influence of multiple systems. When gathering information from the client, it is insufficient to focus solely on sport issues. One must remember that valuable information can also be found in other areas in the athlete's life. The same holds true for interventions. Gearing them toward only a sport issue can lead to failure in treatment if the underlying causes of performance problems exist in other contexts. The interventions should be designed to address the conditions that maintain the problem, so that by positively influencing that area, all other areas will be affected as well. Just as problems reach out and affect other contexts, so will interventions. Elements in a system are interrelated; changing one results in effects throughout the system.

INTERVENTION ISSUES

Creating significant and lasting behavior change requires a clear picture of what needs to be changed, some ideas of how to precipitate that change, and the foresight to predict possible hindrances to the change process. One purpose of assessment is to collect the data to describe and specify the change process (Phares, 1992). The task of the therapist, therefore, begins with a definition of intervention goals. From our perspective, this is not a difficult task. Clients usually arrive with problems, complaints, or questions that they want resolved. Finding satisfactory solutions becomes the goal of therapy. These solutions involve changes in how the person thinks, feels, or behaves. For example, in the case of the anxious masters swimmer, Julio, his therapeutic goal was to overcome his "nerves" during the week preceding a meet and to concentrate on and implement his race strategy. For Sherry, the slumping cyclist, the therapeutic goal focused on developing her motivation to maximize her training and racing efforts.

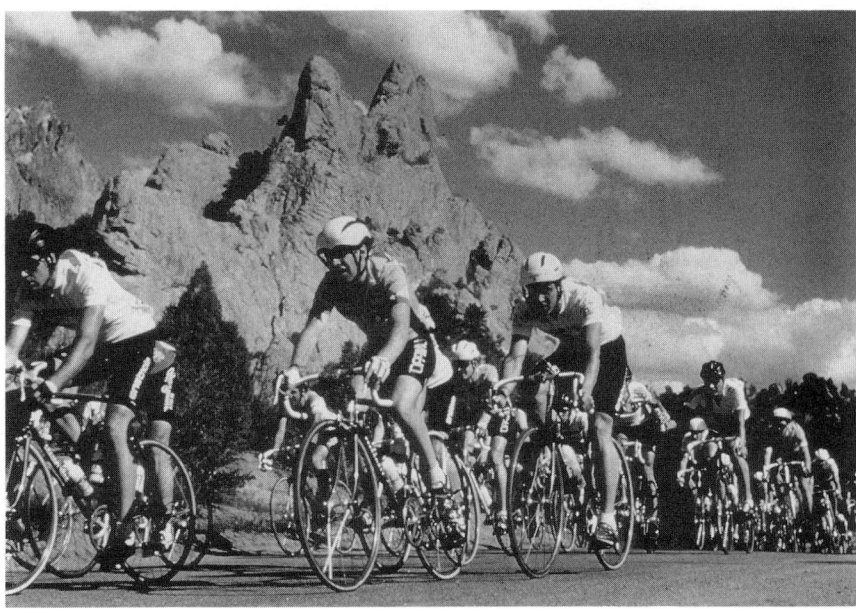

Courtesy USOC

Not all theories of psychological intervention propose such a direct definition of therapeutic goals. Some traditional approaches to psychotherapy necessitate that goals focus on more characterological or unconscious issues (Weiner & Bordin, 1983; Wolberg, 1967). Presenting problems are seen as symptoms of underlying pathological ways of organizing the world. These are the signs of a deficiency or disease. Resolving the pathology, not just removing the symptom, is seen as the only means of creating an enduring change in the person's life. Thus the pathology must be exorcised and then replaced with something healthier. This change often involves considerable time and money. This is a pathology-focused model of therapy.

Neither the cognitive-behavioral nor systemic theories that form the basis of the multisystemic model explained here view complaints as signs of psychopathology. Rather, problems are viewed directly without resorting to underlying hypothetical constructs (Guttman, 1991; Kanfer & Goldstein, 1986).

Problems result from the person's not possessing sufficient or appropriate skills to effectively cope with the present demands (Fisch, Weakland, & Segal, 1982; Kanfer & Goldstein, 1986). In addition, people are often entangled in reinforcing relationships with others that help maintain the problematic solutions or inhibit the implementation of more capable ways of coping. Sometimes the problems are context-specific; other times the problems seen in one context are the result of competent attempts to cope with demands and difficulties in another context. People are viewed as capable as well as vulnerable and as possessing the ability to learn. The goal of therapy is to develop skills or new ways of thinking, behaving, and interacting that will promote resolution of the complaint. This is a problem-focused model of therapy. Although the empirical evidence has suggested that pathology-focused and problem-focused models of therapy produce similarly effective outcomes, the problem-focused models are more economical and time efficient (Lambert et al., 1986).

The Assessment Process

Successful efforts to create change in an efficient and effective manner must depend on a thorough assessment of the person's complaints and primary contexts of life. We propose that the goal of the therapy effort is directly related to clients' complaints but believe that the selection of intervention methods for creating and maintaining change must consider all the factors that impact the individual target problem. The assessment process yields information that the therapist uses to generate hypotheses about the most efficient and effective methods for intervention (Kanfer & Goldstein, 1986; Nelson & Barlow, 1981; Nelson & Hayes, 1986). These hypotheses are based on the therapist's understanding of the client's complaints, awareness of the contextual cues that precipitate and follow the problem situation, knowledge of how the person functions in other contexts, and the interactions in and between contexts that support or promote the problem response.

Assessment begins with a clear statement of the presenting problem or complaint and the client's conceptualization of this complaint. Referred to as "pinpointing" (Patterson, 1974), the aim of this first step is to guide the client to unequivocally define what is wrong, its occurrence, its specific impact on the client's life, and its causes as conceived of by the client. In this way clients define their position about the problem and about change. The clients reveal, in their own language, their view of the world. Their perspective on the problem and expectations for both the therapy and the therapist provide an understanding of whether clients will cooperate with or accept various intervention strategies. Attempts to promote change that begin from the client's worldview and beliefs about potential change are thought to facilitate the therapeutic process (Fisch et al., 1982).

Simultaneously, a functional analysis of the problem can be completed. A functional analysis, in its most basic form, provides a temporal context for the occurrence of the problem by identifying its immediate antecedents and consequences (Kanfer & Goldstein, 1986; Nelson & Barlow, 1981). Antecedents are the discriminative stimuli that provide immediate triggers for the problem response. Consequences are the reinforcing stimuli that serve either to increase or decrease the probability of a future occurrence of the specific problem response. These stimuli can be comprised of thoughts, emotions, and behaviors of the client or interactions in the client's environment that have been found to cue the problem situation. As the therapist tracks the details of the client's problematic situations, antecedents and consequences are identified.

The therapist then assesses the client's functioning in the five primary contexts discussed in the previous section; individual, family, sport, work, and social functioning. The process is not a search for psychopathology, but rather an attempt to clarify how the person functions—successfully and unsuccessfully—in each context. Information pertaining to the strengths and weaknesses in each context helps the therapist develop a balanced understanding of how the person operates in different areas and how these areas interrelate. At the individual level, both psychological and physical functioning need to be considered. Are there any illnesses, injuries, or physical limitations that impact the current level of functioning? Does the person possess physical talent? What is the client's general health status? Similar questions about psychological functioning need to address issues such as intellectual capabilities, perceived ability, confidence, and motivation. Family functioning includes satisfaction and status of the marriage or primary relationship, the impact of the presence or absence of children, and relationships and interactions with the birth family. For the clients presented in this chapter, the strengths and weaknesses of the sport context and athletic performance receive considerable attention. Other contexts, such as work and social relationships, also play a vital role.

Once a clear conceptualization of client functioning in these differing environments is completed, patterns across contexts can be established and interactions between contexts will be more apparent. For example, in the case of Sherry, her submersion in cycling complements her dissatisfaction with her career and her avoidance of marital conflict. The purpose of assessing multiple contexts is to define the issues and generate a set of hypotheses about the causes that have precipitated and maintained the problem behaviors. These hypotheses should subsequently assist in identifying possible venues for change that will alleviate the complaints. Similarly, the information might reveal factors that would impede the process of change. Will the demands in the work setting and those made by family members interfere with an attempt to increase time or energy spent on sport performance?

A variety of methods can be used to complete the assessment. The specific methods used depend on the needs and questions of the particular client and creativity of the therapist. The basis of the assessment is a 1- or 2-hr interview with the client. In this time the primary presenting problems can be defined, a functional analysis initiated, and an understanding of the contextual functioning of the client can be obtained. A week or two of daily diary records of particular aspects of the client's life, such as training habits or cognitions, can help clarify questions and establish baselines. Typically, collateral sessions with significant others help clarify and correct for the client's biased conceptualization. Direct observation is often highly informative, particularly with clients who hesitate to disclose or are less verbally fluent. Pencil-and-paper measures of symptoms are used

to secure concrete evidence of particular strengths or weaknesses. The client's permission to complete any assessment that relies on information from others is required, especially with a potentially invasive assessment procedure such as direct observation (American Psychological Association, 1990; Pope & Vasquez, 1991).

Although assessment is emphasized in the first hours of contact, the assessment should be a continuous process (Nelson & Barlow, 1981; Nelson & Hayes, 1986). Regardless of the sophistication or the empirical support of our intervention efforts, verification of effectiveness is essential. At best, research provides a probabilistic statement on the effectiveness of interventions. Evaluation is necessary to identify whether a specific intervention was successful. In addition, continuous assessment provides clear indication to the client and the therapist about the targeted change.

The Intervention Process

The intervention phase of the therapy can begin when two criteria are met. The first is that the therapist is aware of the establishment of a cooperative working relationship. Often referred to as *the therapeutic relationship* or *rapport*, this relationship becomes the vehicle for the change (Frank, 1982; Frank & Frank, 1991; Goldstein & Myers, 1986). Traditionally, this relationship is based on the therapist's communication of empathy, support, and caring for the client. The client, in return, views the therapist as supportive and investing. This allows the client to self-disclose with greater intimacy and trust in the feedback and direction given by the therapist (Goldstein & Myers, 1986; Mahoney, 1991). As a result of this trust, power in the relationship becomes unbalanced, with the client believing in the therapist's intent to protect the client's best interest. The power provides the therapist maneuverability to begin to create change (Fisch et al., 1982). Before intervention begins, the therapist needs to understand these relationship issues to utilize them to promote the client's behavior change.

The second criterion is that the therapist must use the assessment phase to generate ideas about how to precipitate that change. This is accomplished by developing a set of viable hypotheses about the client's complaints and how change might most effectively and efficiently occur (Kanfer & Goldstein, 1986; Phares, 1992). The hypotheses must include a proposal for the change process, foresight to predict what might inhibit this process, and the long-term maintenance of change. There are parallels between being a good therapist and being a good scientist. Like the scientist, the therapist designs interventions to have measurable outcomes that support or disconfirm specific hypotheses. Confirmation of a hypothesis indicates that the interventions should be continued. Disconfirmation indicates the need to shift to a reassessment of the client's position and the selection of an alternate hypothesis. Consequently, the initial assessment phase ends when the therapist has collected enough data to propose a set of viable and testable hypotheses.

The therapist selects interventions that can be implemented by the client, that fit the client's expectations, and that generate information about the value of the therapeutic hypotheses. Although our approach is predominantly cognitive behavioral and systemic, we strive to broaden our intervention techniques beyond those traditionally associated with these approaches. For example, if the client believes in unconscious conflict, the intervention can involve using the language of unconscious processes to allow the client a degree of comfort with the intervention. To ensure a match between the client's view of change and the change strategies, the therapist uses the therapeutic relationship to continually solicit feedback about the acceptabil-

ity of the intervention (Fisch et al., 1982; Henggeler & Borduin, 1990).

The sessions with the client are used to maneuver the client into a position to accept the interventions and then to use the intervention to initiate change. The change itself begins in these sessions; enduring change depends on the execution of the intervention outside the therapy sessions. The client must enact the change strategy in the targeted context and then perceive that this change occurs. Therapy is terminated when changes have been successfully implemented in targeted contexts.

As evident in the three case studies described here, therapy appears considerably idiosyncratic. The prescriptions for change are tailored to the person's presenting needs. However, a number of similarities should be apparent across all three therapies. All these athletes present with a sport-related complaint. Assessment includes a functional analysis of the presenting problems and careful consideration of the person's functioning across the contexts. The assessment is used both to generate hypotheses about the presenting problem and to gauge progress. Interventions are introduced that consider the nature of the therapeutic relationship and are consistent with the primary hypothesis being tested. The therapist remains highly active throughout the therapy and brings other helping professionals into the treatment as necessary and as permitted by the client.

■ THE CASE OF JULIO ■

Julio, the 42-year-old university professor, complained that "nerves" in the week preceding masters swim meets interfered with his functioning at home and work and inhibited his ability to train or execute his race strategy. He believed that this anxiety significantly contributed to slower swimming times during the past 6 months. When asked to explain what "nerves" meant, Julio described physiological arousal cues that "oscillated with increasing amplitude" throughout the week. Symptoms primarily involved motor tension (jitteriness, inability to relax) and autonomic hyperactivity (heart pounding, tingling in hands, upset stomach). Furthermore, sleep and eating patterns were significantly disturbed. He said that he was "not scared, just nervous." When asked what he would do if this could not be remediated, he sighed, "I'd just quit."

A working relationship was easily established. Possibly because of the shared academic affiliation, Julio was immediately trusting and respectful. He seemed to view the therapist as a colleague, or collaborator. He was both receptive to new ideas and interested in understanding as much as he could. From the start, he requested readings that eventually facilitated the therapy work.

Assessment was simplified by Julio's attention to detail and by the training log. The log contained enough information to complete a functional analysis of the "nerves." It revealed that the "buzz" typically began as he started

to taper his training for the race, swimming fewer yards less intensely. Consequently, he usually felt that he had a bit more energy. He began to think about the meet, his competitors, how much time he would have between events, and what times he "needed" to swim. These thoughts would lead to growing concerns that he would fail, and failure would mean that all this swimming was a waste of time. As these ruminations escalated he would become irritable and isolated. The consequences included feeling disappointed that he would not swim as well as he knew he could. He would also return to ruminations about the neglect of research or his family. Self-report questionnaires—specifically the Hopkins Symptom Checklist (Derogatis, Lipman, Rickels, Uhlenhuth, & Covi, 1974), the State-Trait Anxiety Inventory (Spielberger, Gorsuch, & Lushene, 1970), the Psychological Skill Inventory for Sport (Mahoney et al., 1987), and the Sports Competition Anxiety Test (Martens, 1977)—supported his propensity to anxiety and concentration problems.

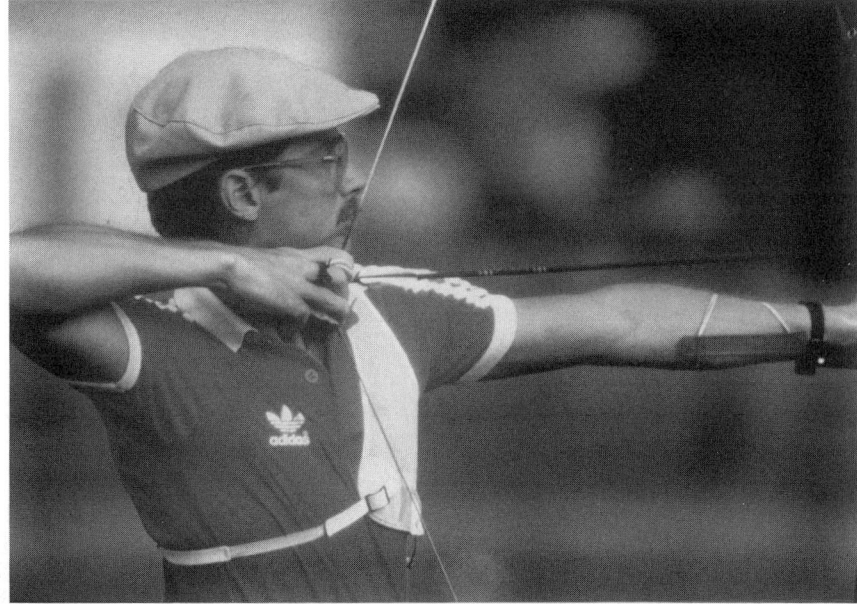

Courtesy USOC

In the second assessment session, Maria, Julio's wife, confirmed his report on the impact of the heightened arousal on his life at home and at work. She noted that although he typically was a good companion and father, these periods of anxiety drove everyone away. Her input placed Julio's self-critical presentation in perspective as she detailed her view of Julio as husband, father, and social companion. His attention to detail apparently often resulted in overly critical self-evaluation across life contexts. She noted that he had always been fairly uptight.

The information from Julio, Maria, and the training log yielded a fairly clear picture of Julio's functioning and his strengths and weaknesses across the various contexts (see Table 4.1). This assessment suggested that Julio is a dedicated, stable, and capable individual. He apparently achieved academically, was supported by family, and maintained a well-developed social network. In most situations, he successfully used his family and friends as a check for his overly harsh self-evaluation. The exception was swimming. Here Julio isolated himself from the relationships that helped him keep his worries in check. He had not developed supportive relationships with other swimmers or a coach. He continued to swim because of what quitting would say about him, not because he enjoyed it. His swim goals appeared diffuse and somewhat unreasonable. He generally lacked concentration.

Two hypotheses were then proposed. First, Julio was not psychologically equipped to manage the demands he faced. His arousal-management skills were severely overwhelmed. Although some arousal increase might be necessary for optimal performance, Julio reported an inability to control his physical response to competition. In turn, this arousal interfered with the execution of his

Table 4.1   Multicontextual Assessment: Julio

Presenting problems: "Nerves," high anxiety before meets, difficulty focusing
Related issues: Motivational lags (swimming; solution to problem is to work harder or get tougher); critical of performance in marriage, family, and job; few connections between swimming and other contexts in his life

---

	Strengths	Weaknesses
Individual		
Physical	—Healthy and injury free —Physically active life —Maintains nutritious diet	—Physiological arousal cues problematic
Psychological	—Motivated to achieve —Perceives self as capable —Intelligent	—Poor arousal-management skills —Arousal inhibits concentration —Overly self-evaluative —Diffuse, demanding outcome goals —Guilt feelings —Falters in presence of high demands —Anxiety promotes ruminations

	Strengths	Weaknesses
Family		
Marital/ significant other	—Wife says good companion —Wife reports solid marriage —Wife accepts swimming	—Feels he is neglecting marriage —Wife not involved in athletics —Restraints on time for ongoing development of marriage
Children, parents, and family issues	—One child —Wife says good father —Parenting responsibilities are satisfactory —Supportive birth family —Economically secure	—Critical of self as father
Sport	—Talented —Competitive in age group —Solid technical skills —Trains hard	—Competition cues an uncontrolled anxiety response —Diffuse swimming goals —No coach —Race strategy fails when anxious —Fun, camaraderie? —Regrets that he quit swimming
Work	—Tenured —Continued positive achievements —Flexible setting —Support of chair and colleagues	—Pivotal time in career —Wife works long hours
Social/peers	—Supportive friends who share interests with both Julio and Maria	—Peers isolated from his swimming —Undeveloped relationships with other swimmers

training and race strategies. In part, the lack of a coach or training partners placed the responsibility to follow through with a training regimen on him alone. In swim meets, the arousal undermined his ability to concentrate and attend to his race strategies. His personal goals and his strategies for preparing for competition were fueled by his fastidiousness and were consequently overly demanding.

The second hypothesis focused on how Julio separated swimming from the rest of his life. His anxiousness, his self-demanding style, and his attention to detail promoted successful coping in other contexts. He succeeded in a difficult and competitive work context. He capably managed primary child care responsibility. Fortunately, the very characteristics that plagued him in swimming benefited him in other areas. In part, success in these areas depended on feedback from his wife, colleagues, and friends. This feedback was unavailable in his swimming. Potentially, if the sport context were better integrated with his support systems, control would be enhanced.

Intervention

As these two hypotheses were complementary rather than competing, therapy was directed to testing both. Skill building first focused on arousal management. This skill was taught using a variation of David Barlow's integrated cognitive-behavioral treatment for anxiety and panic attacks (Barlow & Cerny, 1988). It is comprised of a rationale and education about anxiety, exposure, and attention to interoceptive or somatic cues; cognitive therapy to identify and challenge rumination or anxiety-producing cognition; and progressive relaxation training and respirator training. Designed for 14 one-hr sessions, this treatment has been found effective under a variety of controlled conditions (Barlow, Craske, Cerny, & Klosko, 1989; Klosko, Barlow, Tassinari, & Cerny, 1990).

The program was altered to highlight the potential value of physiological arousal and the importance of managing, rather than alleviating, this arousal. The treatment was also abbreviated and adapted to de-emphasize issues of psychopathology. In the first intervention session the relationship between anxiety, arousal, and performance was discussed. Julio's "buzz" was redefined as an appropriate bodily response to the need to be competitively aroused. Julio and the therapist discussed the goal of learning to use this response rather than fear it. Julio was encouraged to practice eliciting and controlling the "buzz." To promote understanding, he was given a set of readings about anxiety problems, the sport research on anxiety and on relaxation training (e.g., Lichstein, 1988; Mahoney & Meyers, 1989; Oxendine, 1970). Since Julio planned to race in 10 days, he was directed to monitor his somatic cues of arousal changes, conduct random ratings of the distressfulness of the anxiety, and identify the related cognitive reactions. The next appointment was arranged for the week following the swim meet.

In the subsequent session, Julio reported that he was "a mess" at the meet, but he did collect much data. He then produced a detailed diary of the anxiety response and demonstrated his ability to sense the physiological cues of anxiety and the related cognitive patterns. He had obviously mastered the ability to assess his anxiety response. Using this data, both relaxation training and cognitive therapy were initiated. He was given a daily practice tape of progressive relaxation and controlled breathing exercises, and he was instructed to monitor that practice. The diary provided data to construct a hierarchy of arousing stimulus situations. He was also taught to identify thoughts of catastrophe and use a set of self-statements to deal with the ruminations. Lastly, he agreed that he would find and enter a meet that was 2 to 3 months away.

During the next 6 weeks, Julio progressed through the arousal-management treatment, becoming more comfortable with arousal changes and gaining more control of arousal. Several mock swim meets were arranged to assess skill development and build confidence. His dedication to completing homework assignments made the assessment of progress easy. As gains were made, arousal-management issues received less attention and goal-setting and concentration skills received more. To establish a foundation for these skills, Julio purchased a copy of *Psyching for Sport* (Orlick, 1986). He was instructed to establish controllable effort goals, rather than outcome goals (Burton, 1989), and to strive for specific daily goals that he found challenging and fun. To enhance concentration, Julio's attention to detail was utilized to develop precompetition plans and similar prepractice plans (Orlick, 1986).

To test the validity of the second hypothesis concerning Julio's compartmentalization of his swimming, Maria joined Julio's sessions soon after therapy began. In the first joint meeting Maria's willingness to become more involved in Julio's swimming was assessed. She indicated that she had little interest in listening to the details—times, distances, stroke problems, interval training—but she would do what she could. Together with Julio, the therapist defined her role as "feedback from the real world" and began to involve her in Julio's weekly homework and self-monitoring exercises. Soon, Saturday morning became a family swim outing as Maria and Ben would join Julio toward the end of his workouts and then the family would go to breakfast together. Julio also began to talk with Maria more about his swimming; as long as he controlled the amount of swimming details, she seemed to enjoy providing support and feedback. Although Maria's involvement was only one connection between Julio's swimming and the rest of his life, her frankness and humor appeared to help Julio enjoy the experience and obsess less about his performance.

The outcome of this therapy was positive. Before the next swim meet, Julio still reported the "buzz," but he felt more in control of his week and able to moderate the physiological effects. He noted some ruminations about his performance while at the meet, but felt that the behavioral planning kept him on track. Maria did not attend the meet, which was about a 6-hr drive from their home, but they did talk on the telephone several times. These conversations were not focused on swimming. His performances did not meet his expectations and consequently he was somewhat disappointed. When the therapist asked about the implications of the disappointment, he joked, "Well, at least I don't want to quit."

Following this meet Julio attended two appointments, during which his sport-related psychological skills were honed and his course of treatment was reviewed. It was apparent in these sessions that Julio had a clear command of the skills related to arousal management, goal setting, and competition planning. Julio also realized the impact of encouraging Maria to be more involved in his swimming. The therapy was therefore terminated with the expectation that changes had been initiated and Julio was committed to continuing his efforts. Given

his motivation, his attention to detail, and the supportiveness of Maria, the planning for future sessions was left to Julio's discretion. Although he and the therapist never again met formally, the therapist had run into Julio several times on campus. On each occasion, Julio reported that he still was not swimming as well as he would like, but that he was enjoying both his workouts and his meets. In addition, he felt that the "buzz" was under control, and that Maria actually seemed to like her involvement in his swimming. He noted she had become friends with some of the masters swimmers and their families.

■ THE CASE OF SHERRY ■

Sherry's presenting problems were "feeling distracted" and "difficulty getting motivated." Furthermore, she related feeling emotional deterioration and fatigue. Although her present training consisted of long, easy "spinning" rides, she detailed a number of nagging injuries. She said that for the first time in years she was dreading the upcoming racing season. She provided details only after considerable hesitation. Finally, Sherry admitted that she was not sure that a therapist could help and that nothing much was really wrong with her.

Initially, relationship building appeared to be difficult. In addition to Sherry's quiet manner, she seemed reluctant, or afraid, to disclose. The therapist's initial impression, substantiated throughout the first few sessions, was that Sherry did not want to reveal any weaknesses or relinquish control. In order to maintain some flexibility as a therapist, the psychologist needed to carefully empower her by addressing her strengths and by deferring to her expertise. The hope was that if the therapist was careful not to fight for control and power, Sherry might begin to trust. Consequently, the therapist reframed the relationship establishing Sherry as the expert athlete and the therapist as an outside consultant.

This reframe proved productive. Sherry identified her main goal as overcoming her motivational slump. This slump included difficulty initiating and completing her workouts. After workouts, she felt feckless; sometimes just sitting in her car crying. Typically, her response to these occasions was to decide to push herself harder tomorrow. When asked about other antecedents or consequences, she said that the one positive consequence of the slump was that her husband left her alone. When asked what her husband would be like if she were to bounce out of this slump, she jokingly commented that he would probably start pestering her again.

Although she denied any problems in her family, work, and social contexts, the joke about her husband opened the door to the initial consultation with Robert. This meeting helped complete the multicontextual assessment (see Table 4.2). Robert related considerable anger toward Sherry and considerable frustration with the marriage. His answer to questions about Sherry's noncycling life was that she tended to avoid and ignore everything except cycling. He felt that he sometimes had to shame her into doing things with the family. He also noted that she hated her job and refused to associate with his friends. He believed that she was depressed. In contrast, Sherry verbalized some dissatisfaction with home and work, but did not relate the tension and conflict described by Robert. She said that she did not hate her job, she just saw it as a dead end. As for friends, she preferred being with people with whom she shared interests, that is, cyclists. Robert provided a better sense that serious problems existed in the marriage.

On the positive side, Sherry's strength, determination, investment in cycling, and supportive network of training partners strongly suggested her potential in other areas. She also seemed quite confident in her sport skills. The shyness she noted in other contexts was not apparent in cycling, suggesting that she possessed valuable social skills that tended to be underutilized.

A number of hypotheses were formulated. The first had already received considerable support, namely, that she was hesitant about seeking this consultation and therefore she was hesitant to trust. To confront the marital and work concerns would only frighten her away. Second, the marital discord was related to themes of control and dependence-independence. Conflict in the relationship pertained to a lack of interaction between spouses on a number of issues. Robert tended to pursue Sherry by confronting her on these issues. Her response was to withdraw in silence. Third, the motivational slump and training injuries resulted from overtraining. It is this third hypothesis that the therapist chose to focus on initially. It was anticipated that if addressed carefully Sherry would approach the marital issues once some confidence and trust was established.

Intervention

Before beginning any interventions, three referrals needed to be completed. Sherry needed to consult a physician. Although the nagging injuries and feelings of lethargy might be psychogenic in nature, a health clearance should be completed before intervention. Like many athletes, Sherry was hesitant to trust physicians because they tend to prescribe rest or greatly reduce the amount of exercise. In fact, she had consulted one physician who lectured her about trying too hard to be a teenager again. So Sherry was referred to a physician who was also an age-group competitive runner. He noted that she was in generally good health, except for a slightly anemic condition, and recommended that she consult a dietician and a coach. The therapist then helped her contact a dietician and the coach, a cycling guru. Sherry was so impressed with the physician that she immediately made appointments to have her diet evaluated and to visit the coach.

Meanwhile, the psychologist's role as a consultant was solidified, but Sherry did not indicate any reason to target issues other than

Table 4.2   Multicontextual Assessment: Sherry

Presenting problems: Difficulty getting motivated to train harder for upcoming season of bicycle racing

Related issues: Feeling distracted, nagging injuries, considerable distance in marriage

	Strengths	Weaknesses
Individual		
Physical	—Exercising regularly	—Small, nagging injuries —Lethargic, often tired —Pushes harder when fatigued —Health status unknown
Psychological	—Determined —Intellectually capable —Enjoys exercise and training	—Mood swings —Typically avoids confrontation —Generally, when the going gets tough, avoid and minimize
Family		
Marital/ significant other	—Married 13 years	—Husband bitter about relationship —Lack of communication on important family issues —Husband dissatisfied with sex life —Couple is disengaged —Unaware or ignoring husband's dissatisfaction
Children, parents, and family issues	—Two children —Reports close relationship with birth family	—Husband resents child care burden —Motherhood is not enjoyable —Minimal contact with sons
Sport	—Long history of running and cycling —Competitive locally —General self-efficacy positively influenced by sport success —Trains hard —Helps overcome shyness —Helps moderate mood and stress	—Recent inconsistent performances —Possibly overtrains —Difficulty maintaining motivation —No coaching
Work	—Job security —Good performance history	—Sees no room for advancement —Does not enjoy job —Works only for financial security

(continued)

Table 4.2 *(continued)*

	Strengths	Weaknesses
Social/peers	—Good camaraderie with training group —Historically has had a larger, more diverse social support network	—No shared social groups between spouses —Disconnected socially from noncycling peers

cycling performance. The focus, therefore, remained on motivation and distractions in training. The next few meetings involved the therapist's listening to the difficulties and frustrations of the last two racing seasons. Attention was drawn to the strength and importance of her drive to succeed despite these frustrations. She was directed to construct a retrospective training log for the last two seasons in an effort to identify her attempts to overcome her competitive plateau. The therapist predicted that she would find patterns of attempted solutions that she repeatedly implemented without success. She was also encouraged to keep a training log to document her pre- and postworkout thoughts and emotional responses. The goal was to reevaluate the problem and try to find a solution that she had not previously tried. Problem-solving skills were taught in session (D'Zurilla, 1988).

Although her meeting with the coach had not occurred, Sherry interpreted her logs as indicating that harder training was not the solution. She was still feeling fatigued and now decided that she needed rest. In order to utilize her general tendency to resist change, the therapist utilized the tactic of telling her not to change (Watzlawick, Weakland, & Fisch, 1974). In discussion the therapist agreed with her comments, noting the need to balance the risk of intense training with periods of recuperation. However, the therapist also expressed skepticism about any changes she might make

before consulting a coach, and she was asked to carefully consider the consequences of acting too quickly. She was reminded that if her performance improved Robert's criticisms would return. The psychologist then recommended that Sherry train more and ask Robert to attend the next session so that the therapist could help him to stop his harassment.

The session with Robert concentrated on convincing him to cease his pursuit of Sherry. Robert had again verbalized frustration with Sherry and the marriage. He saw her as disinterested in the family and he was tired of waiting for her to return from her ride so the family could eat together. He was told that he needed to take care of himself and the children and stop demanding that Sherry be a better wife and mother. He was to plan fun family activities, such as a trip to the zoo, during the time Sherry rode. Furthermore, he was not to wait for her at dinner and he was instructed to get a baby-sitter for the children one night per week. These nights he should spend with friends and explore new activities. The intention of these directives was to redirect his pursuit of Sherry. This would result in Sherry's no longer needing to distance herself from him.

In the next few weeks Sherry cut back on her mileage and began asking for ways to better plan her workouts. She was still fatigued but somewhat more motivated. She also became increasingly aware that Robert was acting differently. She stated that he stopped nagging her and that he appeared preoccupied. She speculated that he was having an affair, but knew that most of his time was being spent with the children. Obviously, Robert was complying with the directives given in the collateral session. Although Sherry was talking about the marriage, she had not yet identified it as a therapy issue.

During these sessions the therapist continued to express concern that Sherry was moving too quickly with the training changes, but agreed to discuss goal setting and the contingencies around successful training efforts that might be affecting her motivation. She was encouraged to expand her training log to include daily goals that focused on her effort rather than distance or speed. Stimulus control and contingency management (Rimm & Masters, 1979) were introduced to her preparations for workouts, and she also structured her post-workout time. The training log suggested that she no longer avoided going home but that she still isolated herself when there. The next week Sherry requested a joint session and arrived with Robert. Together they reported a series of conversations during the week. Sherry was riding better but was not any happier. In yet another attempt to do something different, she decided to skip her ride one day and find out what Robert was doing with the children. The afternoon together was tense yet enjoyable. That night Sherry began to cry and asked for Robert's support. This was the first of a series of discussions about the marriage. They realized that these conversations were just the beginning and they began to discuss marital therapy. Unlike many marriages seen in therapy (Guerin, Fay, Burden, & Kautto, 1987), Robert and Sherry presented with a low level of conflict. Their communication had been so severely restricted that any discussion was awkward.

Marital therapy initially targeted increasing the number and frequency of positive behaviors between Robert and Sherry. Behavior-exchange procedures (Holtzworth-Munroe &

Jacobson, 1991; Jacobson & Margolin, 1979) were introduced. This procedure involved spouses increasing the frequency of desired behaviors toward each other. The two basic steps involve having each spouse pinpoint specific desirable behaviors that they want from their partner and then increase the frequency of these behaviors. Variations of this exercise used with Sherry and Robert were for each person to identify behaviors the other desired and have each person make specific requests from the spouse. Following a successful week, the behavior-exchange exercises focused on sexual and nonsexual intimacy. Since some uncertainty about sexual intimacy was indicated, sensate-focus exercises were prescribed (Lazarus, 1988). These exercises involved the use of sensual massage to help the couple explore each other's bodies and learn, through verbal feedback, about the effects of this exploration.

As progress occurred, perspective taking and communication skills were discussed and role-played. Particular attention was directed at Robert's resentment over Sherry's spending so much time away from him and the boys. The content of the discussion was on how the couple could arrive at alternatives to overcome these resentments. This strategy for repairing hurt feelings has been described by Sherman, Oresky, and Roundtree (1991). As this discussion occurred, Robert and Sherry were individually interrupted so they could be coached and instructed on basic communication skills such as reflective listening, I-statements, and behavior descriptions of events (Holtzworth-Munroe & Jacobson, 1991). Whenever Sherry would begin to back away from the dialogue or Robert would begin to blame her, the couple were asked to sit apart and attempt to replicate the spouse's perspective on the problem. The couple was then brought back together to verify each of the perspectives.

After 2 months of marital sessions, Sherry and Robert requested an end to therapy. Sherry was racing again. Her performance had improved slightly but was still not at the level she desired. She trained fewer hours per week and spent more time in family activities. Robert reported that Sherry still tended to avoid stressors in the marriage but that he understood her reactions and felt better equipped when approaching her. The issue of Sherry's independence was never fully addressed in the therapy.

In general, this therapy was successful. Sherry's complaints centered on her cycling but were obviously issues in other contexts of her life, especially the marriage. The therapy accomplished several objectives related to the initial hypotheses. First, Sherry's stubborn resistance against change was undermined. By using her hesitation to trust, she was encouraged to examine her difficulties in a novel manner. This examination yielded her decision that training harder was not going to make her better or happier. She abandoned the overused solution of putting her head down and pushing harder. Secondly, by using Robert's frustration in the marriage, a change in how the family system functioned was initiated. Consistent with the homeostatic nature of a system, Sherry had to change to maintain the system. Lastly, as she abandoned the focus on training harder and directed some of her intensity toward the marital issues, she began to perform better. It might have been helpful for Sherry to continue in therapy but initiating the change was the goal.

■ THE CASE OF PETER ■

In the initial session Peter, the 51-year-old lawyer and tennis player, presented that his failure to control anger disrupted his tennis game. He disclosed that the anger outbursts were not limited to tennis, but he conceptualized this emotional reactivity as part of his competitive manner. He avoided most questions about his family, work, and social networks, and he refused to have his wife attend an assessment

session. The therapist was not surprised when he canceled the subsequent appointment.

The second session, 3 months later, provided a clearer picture of Peter's anger and his life. The warning by the club's board frightened him, which in turn promoted a greater degree of disclosure. Most of the information for the multicontextual assessment was obtained during this session. As is apparent in Table 4.3, angry and abusive outbursts and heavy drinking were the two key individual issues that permeated the problem situations in Peter's life. With the exception of these two behaviors, Peter presented as an intelligent, competent individual.

A functional analysis of these behaviors revealed that the anger and drinking were pervasive and essentially functionally autonomous. Peter noted that he would be angry, intimidating, rude, or demanding throughout a good part of each day. He saw these behaviors as a key part of his personality. It was also apparent that this anger was a key part of his success. When he barked, others tended to cower or react to his anger rather than to the content of his communication. In the adversarial world of law, this demanding, one-up position was adaptive. In addition, he said that most of the time he felt in control of his emotions and that he knew when to use and not use the ''personality.'' However, the cost of this style was considerable. In social, work, and sport contexts people with choices tended to avoid him. About once a month the anger would result in a physical altercation. He felt that his wife was frequently the undeserving target. Usually, he was frustrated about something that happened earlier in the day. Then after arriving at home, he would erupt at some incidental event. He admitted guilt in abusing his wife but was certain that she would not leave the marriage. He felt the marriage was strong. Drinking did not appear to be a reliable antecedent to the abuse.

Peter's drinking consisted of three or fewer drinks about 4 days a week, and about once every other week he would consume about 10

Table 4.3 Multicontextual Assessment: Peter

Presenting problems: Loss of emotional control affecting tennis game
Related issues: Explosion of temper, spouse abuse, alcohol consumption

	Strengths	Weaknesses
Individual		
Physical	—Physically active lifestyle —General good health	—Heavy drinking —Outbursts of anger —Strong potential for harm to others
Psychological	—Intelligent —Competitive and tough —Very achievement oriented	—Poor impulse control —Minimizes temper control problem —Is rewarded for aggressiveness
Family		
Marital/ significant other	—None revealed during assessment	—Physically abuses wife —Several separations
Children, parents, and family issues	—Wants to improve relationship with daughter	—Weak relationship with daughter —Aggression and violence in birth family (father as model) —No relationship with members of birth family
Sport	—Tennis skills improving —Plays frequently	—Angry outbursts have disqualified him for competition —Some trouble finding people to play with
Work	—Very successful lawyer —Economically secure —Drinking has not interfered —Toughness brings in clients	—Frightens and alienates most co-workers —Drinking part of unwinding with co-workers and peers
Social/peers	—Existing friendships are very loyal	—Small social network —Friends overlook aggressiveness

drinks. Other days he would abstain. He noted that drinking helped calm him down and helped him interact in a friendly manner. He thought that he tended to drink more when the demands at work were high or when he was bored. He would usually drink with others at bars or restaurants. Some peers who avoided him during the day would interact with him when he was drinking. He also believed that tennis gave him an alternative to drinking because drinking diminished his proficiency. He avoided alcohol until after he played. The evidence did not suggest that he was severely dependent on alcohol.

The therapeutic relationship with Peter was tenuous, at best. Although disclosing during the second interview, he obviously preferred to be in charge and in control. He wanted to set the agenda, and he was hesitant to deviate from it. As would be discovered later, Peter's information was not always reliable. He initially reported no marital difficulties other than the occasional abuse. Peter's wife, Ruth, later confirmed that they had separated several times and that her commitment to the marriage remained uncertain. Consequently, the therapy needed to be firm, but not confrontive. Although didactic presentation of ideas, especially rational scientific ideas, might be acceptable, Peter needed to make the decisions. He was currently receptive to counseling, but quick changes would be needed to keep Peter engaged and working in therapy.

Peter's descriptions of his drinking and his anger outbursts suggest problems in self-control or self-regulation (Kanfer & Phillips, 1970). He proficiently and successfully used both behaviors to gain control over his world. However, the control was not reliable. When demands were substantial, he tended to lose control over these behaviors. When control was lost, these behaviors became self-defeating and injurious. In such situations his repertoire of alternative coping responses appeared limited. Consequently, it was hypothesized that increased self-control of both the drinking and the anger were necessary.

Intervention

The initial task in therapy was to address Ruth's safety. Ruth accompanied Peter to the third session. Peter was seen first to obtain his consent and support for the therapist's agenda with Ruth. Then Ruth was seen alone, where she detailed both the drinking and the abuse history. Her report suggested that Peter tended to minimize his difficulties but confirmed that the drinking and the abusive anger appeared as separate issues. She was uncertain of her commitment to the marriage but consented to base her decision on Peter's commitment to making changes. Following recommendations

from the research on spousal abuse (Bagarozzi & Giddings, 1983; Steinfeld, 1989), Ruth was encouraged to attend therapy with another therapist. This therapy would be directed at empowering Ruth in the relationship, encouraging her to alter her interactions with Peter to further ensure her safety. She agreed to work with the second therapist for the next 6 weeks while Peter would work with the original therapist. At the end of the 6 weeks, both therapists met with Peter and Ruth to discuss the possibility of a series of marital-therapy sessions. Ruth was provided the name of a therapist who had previously agreed to provide this therapy.

Peter then joined the session and was informed about the specifics of the plan. He provided written consent so that his therapist could communicate with Ruth's therapist about his therapy. He also agreed to give written permission to inform Ruth's therapist if he terminated therapy. Peter and the therapist again discussed strategies to ensure Ruth's immediate safety. With her therapist Ruth was able to identify cues that indicated the potentially violent situations and her actions that tended to provoke Peter's anger. She was also able to plan ways of ensuring her safety, including staying with her sister if necessary.

Therapy with Peter then focused on cognitive-behavioral interventions to develop self-regulation skills (Karoly & Kanfer, 1982). The current trend in the treatment of heavy drinking is to view drinking as a disease requiring hospitalization and abstinence. However, the research evidence suggests that heavy drinkers are a heterogeneous group and that the disease model is not applicable to all heavy drinkers (Fingarette, 1985; Miller & Hester, 1986). An alternative treatment model (Sobel & Sobel, 1993) that has received empirical support is based on self-control principles and consequently fits well with Peter's presenting problems. In this treatment (controlled drinking versus abstinence) clients establish their drinking goals, which are reassessed each treatment session. Assessment then begins with the clients' completing a self-evaluation of drinking behaviors including frequency, amount, context, and consequences of drinking. In addition, clients begin self-monitoring drinking behavior and educating themselves about the medical contraindications and social contingencies of drinking. The self-monitoring helps identify particularly problematic or risky drinking situations. Treatment focuses on helping individuals identify and use their own strengths, resources, and preferred coping strategies to avoid excessive drinking. In addition to problem solving, treatment can also include assertiveness training, cognitive restructuring, relaxation training, and self-instructional training.

The most empirically supported treatment for anger has been Novaco's (1975; Bistline & Frieden, 1984) variation of Meichenbaum's (1985) stress-inoculation training. The rationale of this treatment closely fits with the self-control training intervention. The treatment consists of three stages: assessment and conceptualization, skill acquisition and rehearsal, and application and follow-through. Clients learn to think of their anger as controllable. They are asked to assess the parameters of the anger, including the physiological and cognitive antecedents of previously uncontrollable episodes. Working from self-monitoring forms, the anger is viewed as jointly determined by an initial provocation, mediating cognition, the somatic-affective state of the individual, and behaviors that might have the effect of escalating any potentially conflictual encounter. Treatment relies on the development of relaxation skills, coping skills, and use of self-instructional statements. These strategies are learned using imaginal rehearsal of stressful situations that are then applied to actual circumstances. Therapist and client need to be vigilant for interpersonal factors that inhibit the execution of these self-control skills. The application phase attends to feedback from others to alter intervention strategies to produce the most effective outcome.

Therapy with Peter blended these two treatment programs. Initial discussions focused on providing a general self-control model for these problem behaviors and an explanation of the transactional nature of his cognition, emotions, and behaviors. Incidences of both the drinking and anger outbursts were also tracked to educate Peter on how to identify the specific characteristics of provocative situations and interactions. Specific treatment goals were established by Peter. He identified the goal of controlling his drinking so that he would stop at two drinks on any given day. As for the anger outburst, Peter's goals included being aware of his angry reactions and being able to control his expression of anger to avoid "chewing people out" and to prevent physical altercations. Self-monitoring forms were then developed with the initial intention of more clearly defining the problematic contexts and toxic interactions.

Considerable gains were evident in the next two sessions. Using the self-monitoring forms, Peter related a considerably enhanced understanding of both behaviors and the contexts and interactions that precipitated these behaviors. He also appeared more aware of the adaptability of drinking and intimidating others. After the first week of monitoring, he proposed an experiment the following week to determine the effects of changing his drinking patterns. He proposed to go to the bar and drink considerably more some days and less on others while monitoring others' reactions to him. In the next session he seemed impressed by the relationship between his drinking and others' reactions to him. He still argued that the alcohol was a means of relaxing and that he felt somewhat socially isolated when not drinking with his friends. In an effort to provide alternatives to drinking, Peter began to learn progressive and imagery relaxation skills (Lichstein, 1988; Woolfolk & Lehrer, 1984), discuss social skills issues (Bellack & Hersen, 1979), and consider alternatives to socializing and relaxing at the bar.

During this period, Peter had become more aware of the cues that marked the onset of his anger. He was able to reliably identify somatic and cognitive indicators of relatively low levels of anger. He also successfully avoided high levels of anger during the second week of self-monitoring. However, he was frustrated in his attempts to avoid expressing anger. This frustration resulted from his attempt to alter his abrupt, demanding interpersonal style. Although he was warned that this style would evolve slowly, Peter's perception that he had made little progress bothered him. An alteration to the self-monitoring forms was made to help him differentiate angry responses and his intimidating style.

Unfortunately, Peter failed to keep the next appointment. Attempts to contact him failed; he did not return the therapist's telephone calls. Per the therapy agreement, the therapist contacted Ruth's therapist, who detailed that in their last session Ruth appeared on the verge of leaving Peter, at least temporarily. Ruth noted to her therapist that Peter was not drinking, but he was avoiding interaction with her. The lack of interaction bothered her. She felt she needed more support but that he was unwilling to provide it. In the therapy, continued uncertainty about the marriage led to the decision to separate. She thought that she needed time to make personal changes before dealing with the marriage. Ruth's therapist suggested that Ruth propose one conjoint session to discuss her decision. A week later, the therapist received a message that Peter had refused the conjoint session. No further contact with him occurred.

ETHICAL ISSUES

In these case studies we have proposed that competitive recreational athletes be approached from a multisystemic framework. However, we are not suggesting that basic athletic-performance-enhancement interventions are inappropriate—only that such interventions might ignore additional, nonsport factors that influence performance. We are also sensitive to the possibility that the competitive recreational athlete might not desire intervention beyond the sport context. This is the client's prerogative. But it is also the clinician's responsibility to offer the client the most appropriate intervention available.

This discussion brings us to the inevitable ethical issues that arise in work with competitive recreational athletes. Virtually every professional association with members who provide helping services has developed and maintained a set of ethical standards (American Association for Counseling and Development, 1988; American Association for Marriage and Family Therapy, 1988; American College Personnel Association, 1989; American Psychiatric Association, 1989; American Psychological Association, 1990; National Association of Social Workers, 1990). Ethical standards are made necessary by the potential conflict between the interests of the client (i.e., efficient, effective service) and the interests of the professional (i.e., income). These standards assist professionals in becoming aware of issues that might compromise their service delivery and guide their behavior in potentially conflictual situations (Lakin, 1991; Pope & Vasquez, 1991).

Confidentiality

Confidentiality (American Psychological Association, 1990, Principle 5) is perhaps the most obvious ethical issue germane to the multicontextual assessment and intervention described in this chapter. Confidentiality, ethically and legally, is the privilege of the client, not the therapist. The therapist is charged with protecting this privilege because clients are typically not in a position to regulate it and sometimes fail to understand the implications of confidentiality (Benson, 1984; Robinson & Merav, 1976). When nonclients are contacted and involved in assessment and treatment, the issue of confidentiality must be closely monitored. When treatment is directed at more than one person, as is the case in any marital or family therapy, the question of who is the client and who has the privileged and protected communication becomes more confusing (Zygmond & Boorhem, 1989). In each of our cases the therapist met with other family members and could have benefited from contacts with coaches and others (Henggeler & Borduin, 1990). In these situations the counselor must be extremely careful in defining who is the client, securing permission and limitations on communication with others, and clarifying issues of confidentiality with everyone involved.

In each case we defined the client as the individual who has requested assistance. It was the confidentiality of this person's communication that must be protected. Although we argued for permission to contact others, we also clarified with the client what would or would not be said to assess the client's understanding and gain consent for these contacts. When meeting with significant others, the counselor must begin with a clarification of the limits of confidentiality. Specifically, the counselor has a responsibility to alert the informants that promises to withhold information from the identified client cannot be made (though arguments for the value of disclosure can also be made). The paramount issue is the guaranteed confidentiality of the client and clarity of communication to all parties involved in the counseling process.

Competence

A second ethical issue evident in our case presentations was therapist competence.

Principle 2A of the American Psychological Association's ethical principles states that "psychologists accurately represent their competence, education, training, and experiences" (1990, p. 391). This principle implies a recognition of the power implicit in the counselor's role. Given this power, counselors must be aware of the limitations of their training and experience, and they adopt an obligation not to misrepresent themselves to their clients. Counselors must also build relationships with other professionals to be aware of available alternative competencies. Finally, counselors should continue training beyond their formal education to maintain the competencies identified by their credentials (Pope & Vasquez, 1991).

Competency limitations were evident in the treatment of both Sherry and Peter. With Sherry, three referrals to other professionals were made because of the possibility that her complaints might be related to issues outside the therapist's area of expertise. The referrals to the physician and dietician were made to address the possible physiological bases of Sherry's presenting problems. Although Sherry was not concerned about her general health or diet, existing evidence supported the possibility that her motivational and mood complaints might have been related to physical health issues.

The decision to refer her to a coach was less apparent but no less important. An examination of her workout log suggested that she was not basing her training plan on her performance or her fitness level. In fact, training was paradoxically related to her performance because indications of overtraining were met with efforts to train harder. Being a cyclist, the therapist fought a temptation to make training recommendations. The therapist was not trained as a coach and the relationship between Sherry and the counselor would have been altered if the counselor adopted both coach and therapist roles. Sherry, giving credence to the counselor's power as a helping professional, might acritically, and possibly dangerously, follow the counselor's advice.

In the treatment of Peter, the therapist was knowledgeable of the self-control treatment of alcohol consumption, but had no experience in providing this treatment. Consequently, to obtain consultative supervision before initiating this intervention, the therapist contacted a psychologist who regularly implemented such treatment. Although a referral was not thought to be necessary in this case, a method to ensure the competency of the treatment was. The supervisor was helpful in providing templates for the self-report assessment instruments, self-monitoring forms, and issues important to maintaining the integrity of the treatment.

Dual Relationships

A third ethical issue evident in the cases presented in this chapter involves the assessment and avoidance of dual relationships with clients (American Psychological Association, 1990, Principle 7). The greatest percentage of ethical complaints about mental health professionals concerns dual relationships (Lakin, 1991). Dual relationships are fairly easy to define; they are much more difficult to recognize. A dual relationship occurs when the counselor maintains another, significantly different relationship with the client that serves to confuse both roles (Pope & Vasquez, 1991). By far the most ethically troublesome exploitive dual relationships involve sexual contact with a client. More commonly, the dual relationship role is quite subtle and might be social, financial, or professional. These relationships frequently evade detection because they develop as purely secondary or appear as inconsequential. The problem with the addition of a second relationship is that it jeopardizes the professional relationship, the therapy process, and possibly the client's welfare (Borys & Pope, 1989; Keith-Spiegel & Koocher, 1985). The dual relationship creates a conflict of interest for the therapist and must be avoided (Lakin, 1991).

Julio's academic status presented an obvious potential for dual relationship. Both Julio and the therapist were employed by the same college in the same university. Although the two had never met previously, the potential for future interactions existed. For example, both client and therapist might be active on the same college or university committees. During the initial session the therapist explored Julio's reaction to this possibility and discussed the importance of carefully considering the impact of counseling on future interactions. Julio's understanding and sensitivity to the dual relationship issues does not alleviate the therapist's responsibility to ensure that future relationships are not negatively influenced by the nature of the therapeutic relationship.

Obviously, other ethical problems require our attention. All ethical issues, including confidentiality, competence, and dual relationships, are complex and often troublesome. They arise at moments when clients are vulnerable and therapists are lax. An understanding of these potential counselor-client conflicts is a necessary component of the counseling process, and a commitment to the highest ethical standards must accompany the therapeutic effort.

CONCLUSION

With the possible exception of high school athletes, there is no larger population of sport competitors than competitive recreational athletes. Their sheer numbers alone make competitive recreational athletes interesting to the applied sport psychologist, and their demanding lifestyles and competitive drive allow them to serve as valuable living laboratories for the sport scientist. Although competitive recreational athletes have traditionally been a relatively homogeneous group, dominated by middle-class males, subpopulations representing virtually all demographic categories can be identified. But common to almost all of these athletes is their voluntary participation in their sport in the face of heavy family and career responsibilities.

Given this, it is not surprising that competitive recreational athletes present to the therapist with psychologically heterogeneous problems and needs. Fortunately, our traditional sport performance enhancement interventions appear to be beneficial for them (Whelan et al., 1989). However, we have proposed here a multicontextual approach to the competitive recreational athlete. This holistic position acknowledges sport as one limited aspect of a person's extremely complex set of interacting spheres of influence. Based on this assumption, our model dictates specific multicontextual assessment and intervention activities that we believe offer the applied sport psychologist a richer, more comprehensive approach to the difficulties of the competitive recreational athlete.

REFERENCES

American Association for Counseling and Development. (1988). *Ethical standards.* Alexandria, VA: Author.

American Association for Marriage and Family Therapy. (1988). *Code of professional ethics for marriage and family therapists.* Washington, DC: Author.

American College Personnel Association. (1989). A statement of ethical principles and standards. Alexandria, VA: Author.

American Psychiatric Association. (1989). *The principles of medical ethics with annotations especially applicable to psychiatry.* Washington, DC: Author.

American Psychological Association. (1990). Ethical principles of psychologists. *American Psychologist,* **45**, 390-395.

Bahrke, M.S., & Morgan, W.P. (1978). Anxiety reduction following exercise and meditation. *Cognitive Therapy and Research,* **2**, 323-333.

Bagarozzi, D.A., & Giddings, C.W. (1983). Conjugal violence: A critical review of current research and clinical practices. *American Journal of Family Therapy,* **11**, 3-15.

Bandura, A. (1969). *Principles of behavior modification.* New York: Holt, Reinhart & Winston.

Bandura, A. (1977). Self-efficacy: Toward a unifying theory of behavioral change. *Psychological Review,* **84**, 919-925.

Bandura, A. (1978). The self system and reciprocal determinism. *American Psychologist,* **33**, 344-358.

Barlow, D.H., & Cerny, J.A. (1988). *The psychological treatment of panic.* New York: Guilford Press.

Barlow, D.H., Craske, M.G., Cerny, J.A., & Klosko, J.S. (1989). Behavioral treatment of panic disorder. *Behavior Therapy,* **20**, 261-282.

Barnett, M.L., & Stanicek, J.A. (1979). Effects of goal setting on achievement in archery. *Research Quarterly,* **50**, 328-332.

Beck, A. (1976). *Cognitive therapy and emotional disorders.* New York: International Universities Press.

Bellack, A.S., & Hersen, M. (Eds.) (1979). *Research and practice in social skills training.* New York, Plenum Press.

Benson, P.R. (1984). Informed consent. *Journal of Nervous and Mental Disease*, **172**, 642-653.

Bistline, J.L., & Frieden, F.P. (1984). Anger control: A case study of a stress inoculation treatment for a chronic aggressive patient. *Cognitive Therapy and Research*, **8**, 551-556.

Borys, D.S., & Pope, K.S. (1989). Dual relationships between therapist and client: A national study of psychologists, psychiatrists and social workers. *Professional Psychology: Research and Practice*, **20**, 283-293.

Brown, R., Ramirez, D., & Taub, J. (1978). The prescription of exercise for depression. *Physician and Sportsmedicine*, **6**, 35-45.

Burton, D. (1989). Winning isn't everything: Examining the impact of performance goals on collegiate swimmers' cognitions and performance. *Sport Psychologist*, **2**, 105-132.

Carter, B., & McGoldrick, M. (Eds.) (1988). *The changing family life cycle*. New York: Gardner Press.

Clitsome, T., & Kostrubala, T. (1977). A psychological study of 100 marathoners using the Myers-Briggs type indicator and demographic data. In P. Milvey (Ed.), The marathoner: Physiological, medical, epidemiological and psychological studies. *Annals of the New York Academy of Sciences*, **301**, 1010-1019.

Corbin, C.B. (1972). Mental practice. In W.P. Morgan (Ed.), *Ergogenic aids and muscular performance* (pp. 94-118). New York: Academic Press.

Csikszentmihalyi, M. (1990). *Flow: The psychology of optimal experience*. New York: Harper & Row.

Derogatis, L.R., Lipman, R.S., Rickels, K., Uhlenhuth, E.H., & Covi, L. (1974). The Hopkins Symptom Checklist (HSCL): A self-report symptom inventory. *Behavioral Science*, **19**, 1-15.

deVries, H.A., Wiswell, R.A., Bulbulian, R., & Moritani, T. (1981). Tranquilizer effect of exercise. *American Journal of Physical Medicine*, **60**, 57-66.

DeWitt, D.J. (1980). Cognitive and biofeedback training for stress reduction with university athletes. *Journal of Sport Psychology*, **2**, 288-294.

D'Zurilla, T.J. (1988). Problem-solving therapies. In K.S. Dobson (Ed.), *Handbook of cognitive-behavioral therapies*. New York: Guilford.

Feltz, D.L., & Ewing, M.E. (1987). Psychological characteristics of elite young athletes. *Medicine and Science in Sports and Exercise*, **19**, S98-S104.

Feltz, D.L., & Landers, D.M. (1983). The effects of mental practice on motor skill learning and performance: A meta-analysis. *Journal of Sport Psychology*, **5**, 25-27.

Fenz, W.D. (1975). Strategies for coping with stress. In I.G. Sarason & C.D. Spielberger (Eds.), *Stress and anxiety: Vol. 2* (pp. 305-336). New York: Wiley.

Fenz, W.D., & Jones, G.B. (1972). Individual differences in physiological arousal and performance in sport parachutists. *Psychosomatic Medicine*, **34**, 1-8.

Fingarette, H. (1988). *Heavy drinking*. Berkeley, CA: University of California Press.

Fisch, R., Weakland, J.H., & Segal, L. (1982). *The tactics of change*. San Francisco: Jossey-Bass.

Folkins, C., & Sime, W. (1981). Physical fitness training and mental health. *American Psychologist*, **36**, 373-389.

Frank, J.D. (1982). Therapeutic components shared by all psychotherapies. In J.H. Harvey & M.M. Parks (Eds.), *Psychotherapy research and behavior change* (pp. 9-37). Washington, DC: American Psychological Association.

Frank, J.D., & Frank, J.B. (1991). *Persuasion and healing: A comparative study of psychotherapy*. Baltimore, MD: Johns Hopkins University Press.

Freischlag, J. (1981). Selected psycho-social characteristics of marathoners. *International Journal of Sport Psychology*, **12**, 282-288.

Gill, D.L., Gross, J.B., & Huddleston, S. (1981). Participation motivation in youth sport. *International Journal of Sport Psychology*, **14**, 1-14.

Glasser, W. (1976). *Positive addiction*. New York: Harper & Row.

Goldfarb, A.H., Hatfield, B.D., Sforzo, G.A., & Flynn, M.G. (1987). Serum beta-endorphin levels during a graded exercise test to exhaustion. *Medicine and Science in Sports and Exercise*, **19**, 78-82.

Goldstein, A.P., & Myers, C.R. (1986). Relationship-enhancement methods. In F.H. Kanfer & A.P. Goldstein (Eds.), *Helping people change: A textbook of methods* (3rd ed.). New York: Pergamon Press.

Gondola, J., & Tuckman, B. (1982). Psychological mood states in "average" marathon runners. *Perceptual and Motor Skills*, **55**, 1295-1300.

Gontang, A., Clitsome, T., & Kostrubala, T. (1977). A psychological study of 50 sub-3 hour marathoners. In P. Milvey (Ed.), The marathoner: Physiological, medical, epidemiological and psychological studies. *Annals of the New York Academy of Sciences*, **301**, 1020-1046.

Gould, D., Feltz, D.L., Weiss, M., & Petlichkoff, L.M. (1982). Participating motives in competitive youth swimmers. In T. Orlick, J.T. Partington, & J.H. Salmela (Eds.), *Mental training for coaches and athletes* (pp. 57-58). Ottawa, ON: Coaching Association of Canada.

Gould, D., Weiss, M., & Weinberg, R. (1981). Psychological characteristics of successful and nonsuccessful Big Ten wrestlers. *Journal of Sport Psychology*, **3**, 69-81.

Greist, J.H., Klein, M.H., Eischens, R.R., & Faris, J. (1978). Running out of depression. *Physician and Sportsmedicine*, **6**, 49-56.

Griffin, L. (1978, April). *Why children participate in youth sports*. Paper presented at American Alliance for Health, Physical Education and Recreation Convention, Kansas City, MO.

Guerin, P.J., Fay, L.F., Burden, S.L., & Kautto, J.G. (1987). *The evaluation and treatment of marital conflict: A four-stage approach*. New York: Basic Books.

Guttman, H.A. (1991). Systems theory, cybernetics, and epistemology. In A.S. Gurman & D.P. Kniskern (Eds.), *Handbook of family therapy: Vol. 2* (pp. 41-62). New York: Brunner/Mazel.

Hackfort, D., & Spielberger, C.D. (Eds.) (1989). *Anxiety in sports: An international perspective*. Washington, DC: Hemisphere.

Hall, H.K., Weinberg, R.S., & Peterson, A. (1987). Effects of goal specificity, goal difficulty and information feedback on endurance performance. *Journal of Sport Psychology*, **9**, 43-54.

Hemery, D. (1986). *Sporting excellence: A study of sport's highest achievers*. Champaign, IL: Human Kinetics.

Henggeler, S.W., & Borduin, C.M. (1990). *Family therapy and beyond: A multisystemic approach to treating the behavior problems of children and adolescents*. Pacific Grove, CA: Brooks/Cole.

Hollingsworth, B. (1975). Effects of performance goals and anxiety on learning a gross motor task. *Research Quarterly*, **46**, 162-168.

Holtzworth-Munroe, A., & Jacobson, N.S. (1991). Behavioral marital therapy. In A.S. Gurman & D.P. Kniskern (Eds.), *Handbook of Family Therapy: Vol. II* (pp. 96-133). New York: Brunner/Mazel.

Honikman, B., & Honikman, L. (Eds.) (1991, September-October). *TAC times*. Santa Barbara, CA: The Athletic Congress.

Jacobson, N.S., & Margolin, G. (1979). *Marital therapy: Strategies based on social learning and behavior exchange principles*. New York: Brunner/Mazel.

Kanfer, F.H., & Goldstein, A.P. (Eds.) (1986). *Helping people change: A textbook of methods* (3rd ed.). New York: Pergamon Press.

Kanfer, F.H., & Phillips, J.S. (1970). *Learning foundations of behavior therapy.* New York: Wiley.

Karoly, P., & Kanfer, F.H. (1982). *Self-management and behavior change: From theory to practice.* New York: Pergamon Press.

Keith-Spiegel, P., & Koocher, G.P. (1985). *Ethics in psychology.* New York: Random House.

Klosko, J.S., Barlow, D.H., Tassinari, R., & Cerny, J.A. (1990). A comparison of Alprazolam and behavior therapy in treatment of panic disorder. *Journal of Clinical and Consulting Psychology,* **58**, 77-84.

Lakin, M. (1991). *Coping with ethical dilemmas in psychotherapy.* New York: Pergamon Press.

Lambert, M.J., Shapiro, D.A., & Bergin, A.E. (1986). The effectiveness of psychotherapy. In S.L. Garfield & A.E. Bergin (Eds.), *Handbook of psychotherapy and behavior change* (3rd ed.) (pp. 157-211). New York: Wiley.

Landers, D.M. (1980). The arousal-performance relationship revisited. *Research Quarterly for Exercise and Sport,* **51**, 77-90.

Lazarus, A.A. (1988). A multimodal perspective on problems of sexual desire. In S.R. Leiblum & R.C. Rosen (Eds.), *Sexual desire disorders.* New York: Guilford.

Lichstein, K.L. (1988). *Clinical relaxation strategies.* New York: Wiley.

Locke, E.A. (1968). Toward a theory of task motivation and incentives. *Organizational Behavior and Human Performance,* **3**, 157-189.

Locke, E.A., & Latham, G.P. (1985). The application of goal setting to sport. *Journal of Sport Psychology,* **7**, 205-222.

Mahoney, M.J. (1991). *Human change processes: The scientific foundations of psychotherapy.* New York: Basic Books.

Mahoney, M.J., & Avener, M. (1977). Psychology of the elite athlete: An exploratory study. *Cognitive Therapy and Research,* **1**, 135-141.

Mahoney, M.J., Gabriel, T.J., & Perkins, T.S. (1987). Psychological skills and exceptional athletic performance. *Sport Psychologist,* **1**, 181-199.

Mahoney, M.J., & Meyers, A.W. (1989). Anxiety and athletic performance: Traditional and cognitive developmental perspectives. In D. Hackfort & C.D. Spielberger (Eds.), *Anxiety in sports: An international perspective* (pp. 77-94). Washington, DC: Hemisphere.

Martens, R. (1977). *Sports competition anxiety test.* Champaign, IL: Human Kinetics.

Meichenbaum, D. (1985). *Stress inoculation training.* New York: Pergamon Press.

Meyers, A.W. (1980). Cognitive-behavior therapy and athletic performance. In C.H. Garcia Cadena (Ed.), *Proceedings of the First International Sport Psychology Symposium* (pp. 131-161). Monterrey, Mexico: Editorial Trillas.

Meyers, A.W., Cooke, C.J., Cullen, J., & Liles, L. (1979). Psychological aspects of athletic competitors: A replication across sports. *Cognitive Therapy and Research,* **3**, 361-366.

Meyers, A.W., & Okwumabua, T.M. (1985). Psychological and physical contributions to marathon performance: An exploratory investigation. *Journal of Sport Behavior,* **8**, 163-169.

Miller, W.R., & Hester, R.K. (1986). Inpatient alcoholism treatment: Who benefits? *American Psychologist,* **41**, 794-805.

Minuchin, P. (1985). Families and individual development: Provocations from the field of family therapy. *Child Development,* **56**, 289-302.

Mischel, W. (1968). *Personality and assessment.* New York: Wiley.

Morgan, W.P. (1980). The trait psychology controversy. *Research Quarterly for Exercise and Sport,* **51**, 50-76.

Morgan, W.P. (1985). Selected psychological factors limiting performance: A mental health model. In D.H. Clarke & H.M. Eckert (Eds.), *Limits of human performance* (pp. 70-80). Champaign, IL: Human Kinetics.

Morgan, W.P. (1987). Reduction of state anxiety following acute physical activity. In W.P. Morgan & S.E. Goldston (Eds.), *Exercise and mental health* (pp. 105-108). New York: Hemisphere.

Morgan, W.P., & Costill, D. (1972). Psychological characteristics of the marathon runner. *Journal of Sports Medicine and Physical Fitness*, **12**, 42-46.

Morgan, W.P., & O'Connor, P.J. (1988). Exercise and mental health. In R. Dishman (Ed.), *Exercise adherence: Its impact on public health* (pp. 91-121). Champaign, IL: Human Kinetics.

Morgan, W.P., & Pollack, M. (1977). Psychological characterization of the elite distance runner. In P. Milvey (Ed.), The marathoner: Physiological, medical, epidemiological and psychological studies. *Annals of the New York Academy of Sciences*, **301**, 382-403.

Murphy, S.M., & Woolfolk, R.L. (1987). The effects of cognitive interventions on competitive anxiety and performance on a fine motor skill accuracy test. *International Journal of Sport Psychology*, **18**, 152-166.

National Association of Social Workers. (1990). *Code of ethics*. Silver Spring, MD: Author.

National Bowling Council. (1990). *Profile of a dynamic market: Bowling*. Washington, DC: Author.

National Golf Foundation. (1991). *Golf participation in the United States*. Jupiter, FL: Author.

National Sporting Goods Association. (1990). *Sport participation in 1990*. Mt Pleasant, IL: Author.

Nelson, R.O., & Barlow, D.H. (1981). Behavioral assessment: Basic strategies and initial procedures. In D.H. Barlow (Ed.), *Behavioral assessment of adult disorders*. New York: Guilford.

Nelson, R.O., & Hayes, S.C. (1986). *Conceptual foundations of behavioral assessment*. New York: Guilford.

Nicholls, J.G. (1984). Achievement motivation: Conceptions of ability, subjective experience, task choice and performance. *Psychological Review*, **81**, 328-346.

Nichols, A., Whelan, J.P., & Meyers, A.W. (1991). Assessing the effects of children's achievement goals on task performance, mood and persistence. *Behavior Therapy*, **22**, 491-503.

Novaco, R. (1975). *Anger control: The development and evaluation of an experimental treatment*. Lexington, MA: Heath.

Ogilvie, B.C. (1968). Psychological consistencies within the personality of high level competitors. *Journal of the American Medical Association*, **205**, 780-786.

Ogilvie, B.C., & Tutko, K.A. (1966). *Problem athletes and how to handle them*. London: Pelham Books.

Okwumabua, T.M., Meyers, A.W., & Santille, L. (1987). A demographic and cognitive profile of masters runners. *Journal of Sport Behavior*, **10**, 212-220.

Orlick, T. (1986). *Psyching for sport: Mental training for sport*. Champaign, IL: Leisure Press.

Orlick, T., & Partington, J. (1988). Mental links to excellence. *Sport Psychologist*, **2**, 105-130.

Oxendine, J.P. (1970). Emotional arousal and motor performance. *Quest*, **13**, 23-30.

Patterson, G.R. (1974). Interventions for boys with conduct problems: Multiple settings, treatments, and criteria. *Journal of Clinical and Consulting Psychology*, **42**, 471-481.

Phares, E.J. (1992). *Clinical psychology: Concepts, methods, and profession* (4th ed.). Pacific Grove, CA: Brooks/Cole.

Pope, K.S., & Vasquez, M.J. (1991). *Ethics in psychotherapy and counseling: A practical guide for psychologists.* San Francisco: Jossey-Bass.

Raglin, J., & Morgan, W.P. (1985). Influence of vigorous exercise on mood state. *Behavior Therapy,* **8,** 179-183.

Richardson, A. (1967a). Mental practice: A review and discussion. Pt. I. *Research Quarterly,* **38,** 95-107.

Richardson, A. (1967b). Mental practice: A review and discussion. Pt. II. *Research Quarterly,* **38,** 263-273.

Rimm, D.C., & Masters, J.C. (1979). *Behavior therapy: Techniques and empirical findings* (2nd ed.). New York: Academic Press.

Robinson, G., & Merav, A. (1976). Informed consent: Recall by patients tested post-operatively. *Annals of Thoracic Surgery,* **22,** 209-212.

Rushall, B. (1972). Three studies relating personality variables to football performance. *International Journal of Sport Psychology,* **3,** 12-24.

Sachs, M.L. (1984). Psychological well-being and vigorous physical activity. In J.M. Silva & R.S. Weinberg (Eds.), *Psychological foundations of sport* (pp. 435-444). Champaign, IL: Human Kinetics.

Sapp, M., & Haubenstricker, J. (1978). *Motivation for joining and reasons for not continuing in youth sports programs in Michigan.* Paper presented at American Alliance for Health, Physical Education, and Recreation (AAHPER) Convention, Kansas City, MO.

Schildkraut, J.J., Orsulak, P.J., Schatzberg, A.F., & Rosenblum, A.H. (1983). Relationship between psychiatric diagnostic groups of depressive disorders and MHPG. In J.W. Maas (Ed.), *MHPG: Basic mechanism and psychopathology.* New York: Academic Press.

Sherman, R., Oresky, P., & Roundtree, Y. (1991). *Solving problems in couples and family therapy: Techniques and tactics.* New York: Brunner/Mazel.

Silva, J.M. (1984). Personality and sport performance: Controversy and challenge. In J.M. Silva & R.S. Weinberg (Eds.), *Psychological foundations of sport* (pp. 59-69). Champaign, IL: Human Kinetics.

Silva, J., & Hardy, C. (1986). Discriminating contestants at the United States Olympic marathon trials as a function of precompetitive anxiety. *International Journal of Sport Psychology,* **17,** 100-109.

Skubic, E. (1956). Studies of little league and middle league baseball. *Research Quarterly,* **27,** 97-110.

Smith, R.E. (1980). A cognitive-affective approach to stress management training for athletes. In C.H. Nadeau, W.R. Halliwell, K.M. Newell, & G.C. Roberts (Eds.), *Psychology of motor behavior and sport—1979* (pp. 54-72). Champaign, IL: Human Kinetics.

Smith, R.E. (1985). A component analysis of athletic stress. In M. Weiss & D. Gould (Eds.), *Competitive sports for children and youths: Proceedings of Olympic Scientific Congress* (pp. 107-112). Champaign, IL: Human Kinetics.

Sobel, M.B., & Sobel, L.C. (1993). *Problem drinkers: Guided self-change treatment.* New York: Guilford.

Spielberger, C.D., Gorsuch, R.L., & Lushene, R.E. (1970). *Manual for the state-trait anxiety inventory.* Palo Alto, CA: Consulting Psychologists Press.

Sporting Goods Manufacturers Association. (1990). *Volleyball: An emerging sport.* North Palm Beach, FL: Author.

Steinberg, H., & Sykes, E.A. (1985). Introduction of symposium on endorphins and behavioral processes: Review of literature on endorphins and exercise. *Pharmacology, Biochemistry and Behavior,* **23,** 857-862.

Steinfeld, G.J. (1989). Spouse abuse: An integrative interactional model. *Journal of Family Violence,* **4,** 1-23.

Suinn, R.M. (1972). Behavioral rehearsal training for ski racers. *Behavior Therapy*, **3**, 519-520.

Suinn, R. (1987). *The seven steps to peak performance: Manual for mental training for athletes* (2nd ed.). Ft. Collins, CO: Colorado State University.

Tu, J., & Tothstein, A.L. (1979). Improvement of jogging performance through application of personality specific motivational techniques. *Research Quarterly*, **50**, 97-103.

United States Cycling Federation. (1990). *United States Cycling Federation rulebook.* Colorado Springs: Author.

United States Masters Swimming, Inc. (1991). *Masters swimming: What's it all about.* Rutland, MA: Author.

United States Tennis Association. (1990). *USTA annual participation report for adult leagues.* Princeton, NJ: Author.

Wankel, L.M., & Kreisel, P. (1985). Factors underlying enjoyment of youth sports: Sport and age group comparisons. *Journal of Sport Psychology*, **7**, 51-64.

Watzlawick, P., Weakland, J.H., Fisch, R. (1974). *Change.* New York: Norton.

Weinberg, R. (1989). Anxiety, arousal and motor performance: Theory, research and applications. In D. Hackfort & C.D. Spielberger (Eds.), *Anxiety and sport: An international perspective* (pp. 95-115). New York: Hemisphere.

Weinberg, R.S., Bruya, L.D., & Peterson, A. (1985). The effects of goal proximity and goal specificity on endurance performance. *Journal of Sport Psychology*, **7**, 296-305.

Weinberg, R., Gould, D., & Jackson, A. (1980). Cognition and motor performance: Effect of psyching-up strategies on three motor tasks. *Cognitive Therapy and Research*, **4**, 239-245.

Weiner, I.B., & Bordin, E.S. (1983). Individual psychotherapy. In I.B. Weiner (Ed.), *Clinical methods in psychology* (2nd ed.). New York: Wiley.

Weinstein, W.S., & Meyers, A.W. (1983). Running as a treatment for depression: Is it worth it? *Journal of Sport Psychology*, **5**, 288-301.

Whelan, J.P., Mahoney, M.J., & Meyers, A.W. (1991). Performance enhancement in sport: A cognitive behavioral domain. *Behavior Therapy*, **22**, 307-327.

Whelan, J.P., Meyers, A.W., & Berman, J.S. (1989, August). Cognitive-behavioral interventions for athletic performance enhancement. In M. Greenspan (chair), *Sport psychology intervention research: Reviews and issues.* Symposium conducted at a meeting of the American Psychological Association, New Orleans.

Whelan, J.P., Meyers, A.W., O'Toole, M., Hiller, D., Stephens, M., Bryant, F.V., & Mellon, M. (1987a, September). *Psychological contributions to triathlon performance: An exploratory investigation.* Paper presented at the Association for the Advancement of Applied Sport Psychology, Newport Beach, CA.

Whelan, J.P., Meyers, A.W., O'Toole, M., Hiller, D., Stephens, M., Bryant, F.V., & Mellon, M. (1987b, September). *Triathlon performances: The role of experience in the athlete's psychological race preparations and responses.* Paper presented at the Association for the Advancement of Applied Sport Psychology, Newport Beach, CA.

Williams, J.M., & Getty, D. (1986). Effects of levels of exercise on psychological mood states, physical fitness, and plasma beta-endorphin. *Perceptual and Motor Skills*, **63**, 1099-1105.

Wilson, V., Morley, N., & Bird, E. (1980). Mood profiles of marathon runners, joggers and non-exercisers. *Perceptual and Motor Skills*, **50**, 117-118.

Wolberg, L.R. (1967). *The techniques of psychotherapy* (2nd ed.). New York: Grune & Stratton.

Wood, B., & Talmon, M. (1983). Family boundaries in transition: A search for alternatives. *Family Process*, **22**, 347-357.

Woolfolk, R.L., & Lehrer, P.M. (Eds.) (1984). *Principles and practice of stress management.* New York: Guilford.

Ziegler, S.G., Klinzing, J., & Williamson, K. (1982). The effects of two stress management training programs on cardiovascular efficiency. *Journal of Sport Psychology,* **4**, 280-289.

Zygmond, M.J., & Boorhem, H. (1989). Ethical decision making in family therapy. *Family Process,* **28**, 269-280.

Support for this chapter was provided by a Centers of Excellence grant from the State of Tennessee to the Department of Psychology at The University of Memphis.

CHAPTER 5

INVISIBLE PLAYERS: A FAMILY SYSTEMS MODEL

Jon C. Hellstedt, PhD
University of Massachusetts–Lowell

The family is the most important influence in an athlete's life. It is where the young athlete develops the life skills and coping mechanisms to meet the demands of competitive sport. The family provides the primary social environment where the athlete can develop an identity, self-esteem, and the motivation for athletic success. Successful athletes often credit their families for encouragement, discipline, valuing achievement, and, above all, love and support.

Unfortunately, a family can also have negative effects on an athlete's development. Parental demands can foster an atmosphere of rigid rules and unrealistic expectations. A poorly functioning or underorganized family system might engender substance abuse, inadequate interpersonal relationships, poor stress management skills, problems accepting authority from coaches, and a lack of internal controls and self-discipline. An athlete's performance can be negatively impacted by either excessive or ineffectual family influence.

The demands on athletes and their families have intensified in recent years. The wealth and glamour of professional sport and the proliferation of youth-sport programs have greatly affected the American family. Berryman, in a historical review of the rise of youth sports for children, states, "Children's sport organizations led to changes in the American family structure and, in many instances, added a new aspect to the socialization of children" (1988, p. 14).

This historical development provides a context for the scene described in the case of the Stanley family (see the case study that follows). This scenario occurs often in other families as well—after ski races, gymnastic events, hockey, and baseball games. The drama involves a talented youngster competing in an athletic event and not meeting parental expectations. The parents, who have put time, money, and emotional energy into their child's athletic development, are disappointed by their son's or daughter's performance. They appreciate the talent their child has but are frustrated by what they perceive as lack of effort. This family drama results in a young athlete's internal conflict (I can't please them so I must be a failure) or tension between parent and child (If they don't lay off, I am going to scream).

THE CASE OF
■ THE STANLEY FAMILY ■

Amy Stanley was ahead in the semifinal match for 14-year-olds at the regional tennis championships. She was leading, well into the match, when she seemed to get overconfident and she stopped playing aggressively. She lost in a third-set tiebreaker—a match, it seemed, she could have won.

Her parents, Fred and Betty, were watching. Betty was quiet and withdrawn. Fred was visibly upset at Amy's performance and mentioned to Betty, "Why does she always do this to herself? She's so good, yet she doesn't seem to want to win." In the car on the way home from the match, Fred turned to Amy and said, "You didn't seem to really want to win today." Amy was quiet, looked out the car window and said to herself, Maybe you're right.

Fred was concerned about Amy's erratic play and after the most recent match he discussed the situation with Amy's coach. The coach indicated to Fred that over the past year he has observed Amy questioning her commitment to tennis. He has noticed that she doesn't practice with as much intensity as before and lately often needs to be talked into workouts and competitions. The coach acknowledged Amy's considerable talents and told Fred that of all the juniors he has worked with, Amy has the most natural ability. The coach then suggested that Amy talk to Dr. Jane Hawthorne, a sport psychologist who has worked with many tennis players in the area. "She's very good, and she knows a lot about the sport," the coach said. Fred, though somewhat uncomfortable about the idea, talked it over with Betty and Amy and Fred called Dr. Hawthorne for an appointment.

Dr. Hawthorne has an interesting perspective as a clinical sport psychologist. In addition to her skills in using relaxation, visualization, and goal setting to help athletes improve their performance, she also has a background in family systems theory and intervention. During her graduate training she took courses in systems theory, and during her clinical internship she received supervision in family therapy. At many workshops and sport psychology conferences she has learned skills in working with individual athletes, but she is also interested in working with their families. She remembers attending a sport psychology conference where a psychologist who works with elite athletes said that overinvolved parents are often a problem. His policy was to "bar parents from the office" and to work only with the athlete. Dr. Hawthorne felt uncomfortable with that model of intervention. It overlooked an important reality. Parents can't be kept in the waiting room. Family influences are always present, visibly or invisibly, in the athlete's mind and performance.

The Stanley family (a hypothetical composite of several families I have worked with in my clinical practice) and the interactions that form their family system become invisible players and have a direct impact on Amy's performance on the court. As athletics at all levels become more professionalized and as elite athletes compete at increasingly younger ages, the assessment of family-based problems and interventions in the family system become essential skills for the sport psychologist.

REVIEWING THE LITERATURE

Since Rainer Martens (1978) first awakened the consciousness of parents, coaches, and psychologists about the potential emotional risk factors in youth sports, accounts of problems in athlete families have been common in the media. The image of the youth-league parent (or coach) who inflicts emotional (and sometimes physical) abuse on children who fall short of performance expectations is a common theme. Sport magazines, newspapers, and television documentaries have featured stories on young athletes who have been apparent victims of overbearing parents. This media attention raises an interesting question that needs to be addressed with empirical research: What are the positive and negative factors in families of young athletes? Unfortunately, few studies have addressed this issue.

Family Interactions

The research on athlete families underscores the major influence of the family on the developing athlete. For example, studies by both Greendorfer and Lewko (1978) and Sage (1980) found that parents are the major influence on introducing a youngster to youth sport. The role of the father is notable in both studies in that he appears to be the major influence on the sport participation of both male and female children.

Other studies document the major influence of parents. For example, McElroy and Kirkendall (1980) concluded that parents are the primary significant other in the formation of children's (especially males) attitudes toward winning and skill development. Melnick, Dunkelman, and Mashiach (1981) found in a study of Israeli athletes that parents of sport-gifted children held high expectations for their children's performance and offered more encouragement for sport participation than parents of a control group of non-athletic children.

The major influence of the parents is stronger in the early years of development. There is a shift in influence toward peers and other adults when a child reaches adolescence. Higgenson (1985) found that in preadolescent years the parents are the primary influence, but as the child reaches adolescence the influence shifts from parents to coach. During adolescence the influence of the parents is present but more subtle. For example, Berlage (1981), in a study of fathers' career aspirations for their hockey-playing sons, found that fathers of 11- and 12-year-old hockey players have pronounced aspirations for their children to continue in sport. Most of the fathers surveyed hoped their sons would play hockey in high school and college, and almost all fathers believed that continued participation would benefit their sons in adult life. An easy assumption to make is that this type of family environment has a major impact on the attitude of the developing athlete.

Parental stress and pressure are complex issues that are difficult to research. Attempts have been made, however, to determine what factors in the family create a stressful environment for the child. Gould, Horn, and Spreemann (1983) described many sources of stress in the youth-sport environment and indicated a major stressor is the young athlete's fear of failure. Although this fear of failure can emanate from other sources (self, peer, or coach), a major source appears to be parents. In his research on the development of competitive trait anxiety, Passer (1984) has concluded that negative performance evaluation from parents has a major role in the development of high trait anxiety. Conversely, in a study that looked at the other side of this issue, namely, the factors that support positive sport participation, Scanlan and Lewthwaite (1986) found that male wrestlers who experienced positive parental performance reactions and a high level of parental involvement in the sport experienced greater enjoyment than those who did not.

Research on family influences is complex and difficult. Quantitative methodology is often unable to explore the intricacies of the family processes that exist in athlete families. The subtle interactive factors that exist in family life lend themselves more to qualitative methods using interviews and content analysis. In recent years some studies have used this methodology to highlight some of the issues and processes that provide helpful insight into clinical assessment with these families. Among this research are the studies of Bloom (1985), Kesend (1991), and Scanlan, Stein, and Ravizza (1991).

Developmental Events

The work of a research team headed by Bloom studied the developmental events in the lives of exceptionally talented young people. Included in this study were samples of artists, musicians, mathematicians, and scientists, as well as athletes. Bloom's report included studies of Olympic-level swimmers (Kalinowski, 1985), professional tennis players (Monsaas, 1985), and an integrative analysis of their home environments by Sloane (1985). The results of this team of researchers is important to the model developed in this chapter, in that these results provide both a developmental perspective and the system qualities of the home environment.

The developmental process is similar for swimmers and tennis players. Three distinct phases of development occur beginning with early parental influence and ending with the family as an emotional support system for the independently functioning adult athlete.

- In the early years (ages 4 to 12) the child is introduced to a variety of sports mainly by the parents and mostly the father. The emphasis is on playfulness, fun, and family involvement in athletic activity. The parents provide early instruction but soon locate a coaching or instructional program that will expose the child to a higher skill level. Toward the end of this phase, the parents enjoy taking the child to entry-level competitions where the emphasis is on fun rather than on winning.

- In the middle years (ages 13 to 18) there is a shift from fun and playfulness to the development of sport specialization and a commitment to higher levels of training and competition. Both the athlete and the family center their leisure-time activities around the sport. The parents now provide transportation, structure practice time, arrange competitions, and secure the best coaching available. Some problems are reported with

parents' negotiating the transition as the coach assumes primary influence on skill development. Conflicts between parents and coaches often develop and coaching changes become frequent (Monsaas, 1985).

- In the later years (ages 19 to late 20s) the athlete separates from the family and moves on to college or independent living. The family is mainly a support system and an emotional refuge from the stress of competition. Monsaas (1985) reports that this stage is negotiated well by most of the parents. Some, however, "missed traveling to tournaments and felt a bit left out in these later years" (p. 265). It is also interesting to note that a few of the fathers continued in the role of coach and traveled with the athletes until they were in their late 20s.

There were similarities in the systemic composition of the families in the study. Sloane (1985) noted three main qualities of the home environment.

- The families shared a strong value system that emphasized success through hard work. This value system was clearly communicated by the parents to the children through verbal teaching and role modeling.

- The families valued the talent area. Both parents, but most clearly the fathers, valued athletic activity as a way to learn important character traits, such as a motivation to achieve and a dedication to hard work.

- The family system willingly organized itself around the athletic activities of the child athlete. Parents forfeited other activities to take the child to the pool or the tennis court. Family vacations were organized around training or competitions. Much time and money was devoted to sport, to the exclusion of other family activities.

Family: A Source of Support or Pressure?

In a study of the sources of stress in the lives of elite figure skaters, Scanlan and colleagues

(1991) demonstrated the multidimensional nature of stress and how the family system is paradoxically both a source of and a refuge from those pressures. They found family influences were a source of both valuable support and stress. On the positive side, most of the athletes reported that family support was essential in helping them cope with the pressures of being competitive athletes. Some athletes, however, reported stressful family interactions, such as performance criticism from parents, precompetition lectures, "backstabbing" from other competitors' parents, and guilt over the large sums of money spent on training. Financial pressures came from parents repeatedly and overtly reminding them of the costs and, covertly, from the athletes' observing their parents working hard to support them.

Another study using a similar methodology was conducted by Kesend (1991).

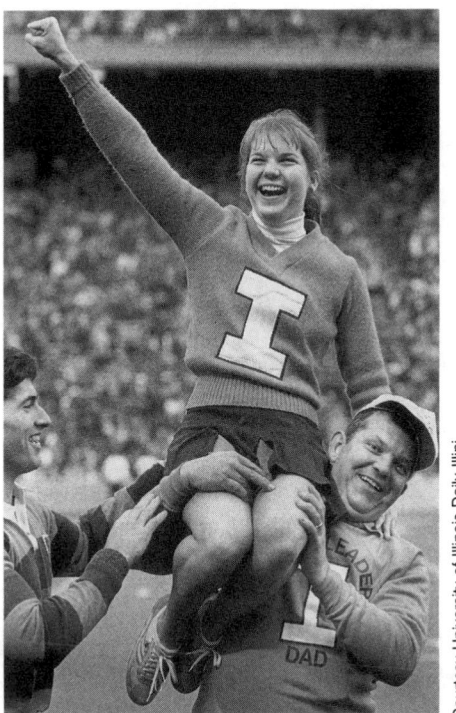

Courtesy University of Illinois Daily Illini

Using interview material obtained from 20 Olympic-level athletes (15 males and 5 females), Kesend examined sources of encouragement and discouragement in the athlete's development. The data showed that the family is the athlete's main source of encouragement. Parents and siblings were more widely cited for providing support than coaches, peers, and members of various sport organizations.

Specific mechanisms for family support were introduction to sport in the early years, support for sport participation, positive role modeling by parents, verbal and nonverbal approval of competitive accomplishments, and emotional acceptance of decisions and ideas about elite-level sport participation.

Parents and family, however, were also sources of discouragement. Parental behaviors interpreted by the athletes as discouraging were suggestions of pursuing alternative careers and parental worry over physical injury. Unrealistic parental expectations also were discouraging to some of the athletes (one athlete had scored 67 points in a basketball game and was criticized by a parent for not playing more aggressively). Overt parental "pushing," however, was not mentioned frequently.

Hellstedt (1990a, 1990b) investigated the parent–athlete interactions in a group of athlete families as they made the transition from the early to the middle stage of athletic development. In a longitudinal study of ski racers and their families, he found that the 12- and 13-year-old elite ski racers perceived their parents as having a strong influence on their athletic development. The specific mechanisms by which parents were influential are parental coaching (teaching and advice giving), off-season monitoring of conditioning and dry-land training, and support and expectations to continue participation in the sport (Hellstedt, 1990a).

In addition, he examined the changes in perceptions of parental pressure that developed between ages 13 and 15 (Hellstedt,

1990b). Parental pressure was measured along three dimensions: general participation in the sport, pressure to continue competing, and performance appraisal. At age 13 there was a substantial group that indicated they were "unhappy" with the amount of parental pressure, especially the pressure to continue participation in the sport. Two years later, however, the athletes perceived less parental pressure and were beginning to perceive the source of this pressure shifting away from parents (particularly the father) to their coach. Figure 5.1 indicates the changes in parental pressure ratings over the 2-year interval.

The data generally showed that these athletes felt positively about the contributions of their parents to their athletic development. However, at least two problem areas were apparent. There was a higher perception of parental pressure in the younger age group,

indicating that these years might be a time of higher sensitivity to this type of influence. As well, affective reactions of dissatisfaction were positively correlated with the amount of parental pressure in both age groups (Hellstedt, 1990b). This finding points toward the possibility that anger toward parents can be a factor in sport withdrawal or athlete burnout.

The Paradox of the Athlete Family

In summary, the research on athletes and their families suggests that though the family might be a source of stress to some athletes, in general the family is an indispensable source of support. Contrary to negative media images of the athlete family, studies on athlete families seem to indicate that for the majority of young athletes the family is a vital social support system that nourishes and encourages their development. The families of successful athletes appear to be tightly organized systems with very concerned, albeit competitive, parents with high expectations for their children. A common denominator in these families is strong parental role models that provide the energy and motivation for the young athlete. These families also value hard work and individual achievement.

It is because of these values that a paradox emerges. The strengths of these families can also be their weakness. What is perceived as a positive encouragement by some young athletes might be a negative, disabling, and damaging experience for others. There is a fine line between positive achievement motivation and excessive pressure. What some young athletes see as parental encouragement might feel like a lack of freedom and breathing space to others.

In addition, the research shows another problem area for families. Perhaps because of the tight organization that develops and

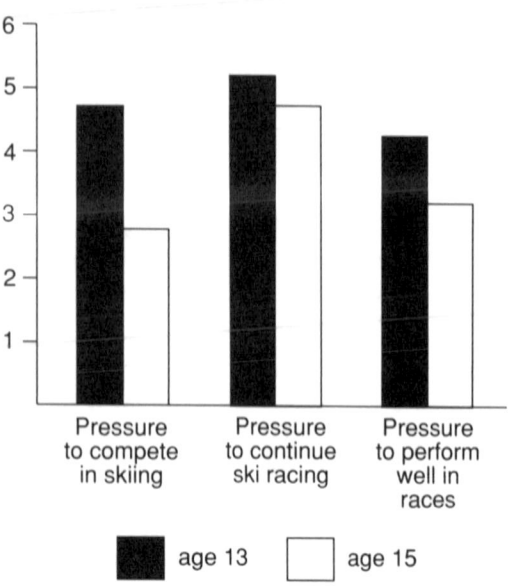

Figure 5.1 Changes in perceptions of parental pressure in a group (N = 67) of developing ski racers. Mean scores on scale of 1 (very little) to 9 (very much).

the close parent–child relationship, some of these families had difficulty negotiating the transition from one stage of family development to the next. For example, the transition from the parents as the dominant influence on the athlete's training to the teacher or coach was sometimes difficult. Parents and coaches often had conflict over what was necessary for the athletes' skill development.

There is also a developmental process that unfolds in a somewhat predictable course in athlete families. During the early years of sport involvement, the emphasis is on fun and skill development. There is a shift, however, in the commitment stage of development where both the athlete and the family system invest major levels of energy and financial resources in sport involvement. In the later stages of the athletes' development, the athlete separates from the parents and family and is influenced primarily by other adults, such as coaches, agents, and members of athletic organizations. For some families these transitions seem to be difficult and can result in conflict between extrafamilial adult influences and parents. In the next part of this chapter we will more closely examine transitions in the developmental processes of the families.

The balance between healthy encouragement and excessive parental involvement is precarious. When the parents cross over the line they are in danger of becoming too "child focused" (Bradt & Moynihan, 1971). In this process the spousal subsystem in the family loses its vitality, and children's success in sport becomes the emotional center of the family. The result can be marital conflict or family dysfunction during or subsequent to the period of children's active athletic involvement.

A DEVELOPMENTAL MODEL OF THE ATHLETE FAMILY

To fully understand the difficulties facing a young athlete like Amy Stanley, sport psychologists need a model for assessing the structural health and developmental maturity of the athlete family. In this section we will develop a model based on research on athlete families and concepts from family systems theory. We will apply this model to the Stanley family.

Family systems theory developed from the work of therapists and researchers who observed that symptom formation in a person is connected to developmental or structural problems in the family. Although there are many different perspectives and emphases among family theorists, there is basic agreement that the family is an interacting social system in which the component parts affect one another. A useful framework for understanding the structural properties of a family is found in the work of Minuchin (1974). According to this model, the main structural components of the family are the power hierarchy, rules, interactional patterns, subsystems, and types of boundaries between subsystems.

A family is more than structural components, however. A family system undergoes a constantly changing developmental process. A useful perspective on this process of change and the connections between generations as the family develops is provided by Bowen (1965, 1978). Bowen's insights have recently been enhanced by the developmental framework provided by Carter and McGoldrick (1989). This framework is basic to the model developed in this chapter. Following the stage theories of individual developmental paradigms such as Erikson's (1950), Carter and McGoldrick view the family as a social organism that, in much the same way a person does, passes through a life cycle. This is a series of stages in which certain tasks must be accomplished before the next stage of development can be successfully mastered. If these tasks are not completed during early stages there will be problems in later stages of development. The transitions from one stage to the next are particularly stressful for families and are often the interval of time when symptoms are present in individual members or in the family system as a whole.

The demands of athletic competition and training often present unique circumstances that are deviations from the normal family life cycle. For example, a young gymnast's family might experience premature separation brought on by the athlete's leaving home to receive specialized coaching. A swimmer or figure skater must train many hours a day and this absorbs family resources, with great impact on the entire family. A career-threatening injury after years of training will create a grief experience for an athlete and a family to resolve. Such developmental delays, barriers, or impasses can negatively affect the young athlete.

The first three columns of Table 5.1 present the stages and tasks of all families as developed by Carter and McGoldrick (1989). In the last column I have added my own formulation of the unique tasks of the athlete family. The model developed here is limited to intact, middle- to upper-class families, which demographically are no longer the norm in our society. Many athletes emerge from less organized families or families that experience major disruptions, such as abandonment or separation and divorce; these are not specifically addressed in this chapter due to space limitations. The general developmental tasks required of these families can be found in Peck and Manocherian (1989) and Fulmer (1989) and can be adapted to the athlete family system as it is presented in this chapter.

Although the following analysis will demonstrate how the Stanley family is having difficulty negotiating certain developmental transitions and tasks, it is not my intent to "pathologize" this family or athlete families in general. Even though this family is having some difficulty, it is a healthy family with many strengths. It is important to restate what was said earlier in the chapter: that in most cases (including this one) the family is the main source of support and encouragement for the developing athlete.

The Stanley Family: A Developmental Analysis

To an outside observer, the Stanleys are a model family. They are a successful, financially comfortable, professional family with two attractive children who are gifted athletes.

■ *Fred Stanley, age 43, is a lawyer and an avid recreational tennis player. His wife, Betty, 41, is a former school teacher who is currently enjoying her role as a full-time parent to their two daughters, Caroline, 17, and Amy, 14. Both Caroline and Amy are competitive tennis players, and since Caroline was 11 the Stanley family has organized itself around the tennis court. Both girls used to play other sports, but because of their potential and his own love of the game, Fred (with Betty's support) has encouraged them in tennis. At around age 12 each girl chose to specialize in tennis; they are now year-round competitors. Coaches, summer camps, indoor winter training, tournaments, travel, a racquet stringer in the garage, and a station wagon full of tennis gear are visible symbols of the family's avocation. The family used to go on family vacations, but now all family travel is for the girls' tennis tournaments. Fred goes to as many of the tournaments as he can, and both he and Betty attend the local matches.*

A closer look at the course of this family's development, however, reveals some unresolved developmental tasks that are affecting Amy's performance in tennis. We will begin our developmental analysis of this family at the time when Fred and Betty met, dated, and decided to marry.

Table 5.1 Stages and Major Tasks of Athlete Family Development

Stage of family development	Major transitional tasks	General changes needed to proceed developmentally	Athlete family changes needed to proceed developmentally
Single young adult	Differentiate self from parents and family of origin	• Become emotionally and financially independent from family • Develop intimate peer relationships • Establish work and career identity	• Attain psychological peace with own athletic successes, failures, and unfulfilled dreams • Resolve unfulfilled expectations from own parents • View present and future athletic involvement as a mode of self-fulfillment and physical well-being
New married couple	Commit and bond in a new relationship	• Develop internal relationship patterns in commitment, caring, communication, and conflict resolution • Perform external relationship tasks (such as work and recreation) to allow adequate space for marital relationship • Realign family of origin and peer relationships to include spouse	• Maintain boundary around athletic involvement to allow space for spousal relationship • Together with spouse, develop mutually fulfilling athletic and exercise activities
Family with young children (ages 4-12)	Accept children into the family system	• Adjust career and marital relationships to make space for children • Share parenting and household management tasks with spouse • Realign relationships with parents to include grandparental roles	• Introduce children to a variety of individual and team sport environments • Provide or secure quality coaching and safe sport environment for proper skill development • Emphasize fun and skill development and minimize competitive success • Maintain permeable boundaries to allow for nonathletic individual and family experiences

(continued)

Table 5.1 (*continued*)

Stage of family development	Major transitional tasks	General changes needed to proceed developmentally	Athlete family changes needed to proceed developmentally
Family with young children (*continued*)			• Demonstrate family value of hard work and goal attainment by parental example and role modeling rather than verbal persuasion
Family with adolescent children (ages 13-18)	Increase flexibility of family boundaries to allow for gradual independence of children	• Allow for gradual shift from parent to adolescent child in decision making • Develop permeable external family boundary to permit entrance and exits of adolescents and peers to and from family system • Maintain strength of spousal subsystem in the family • Refocus spousal subsystem on marital, midlife identity, and career issues	• Encourage and support commitment of child athlete to sport generalization or specialization, depending on child's skills and desires • Provide financial and emotional support without straining family financial and emotional resources • Encourage permeable boundaries for family and self to allow for nonsport social and intellectual involvement • Allow for increasing independence of child athlete in decision making • Secure safe and productive coaching environment for child athlete • Allow for shift of influence on child athlete from parents to teacher and coach • Encourage and support goal attainment and work ethic through both role modeling and verbal teaching • Maintain spousal identity and relationship apart from athletic activities of child athlete

Stage	Key principle	Family tasks	Athletic family tasks
Launching children (ages 18 to late 20s) and moving on	Accept children as adults and allow entries and exits from family system	• Refocus on spousal system as a dyad • Develop adult-to-adult relationships with grown children • Realign relationships with adult children to include spouses, in-laws, and grandchildren • Accept disabilities and death in grandparental generation	• Allow athlete to gain financial and emotional independence from parents • Continue emotional support and crisis intervention if necessary • Identify family as a refuge from the pressures and rigors of competition • Accept authority of coach and accept lesser role in coach–parent–athlete triangle • Reestablish spousal relationship in absence of direct involvement in athletic activity of children • Continue participation in recreational sport for personal fulfillment and health maintenance • Assist grown child athlete's retirement from competition and transition from competitive athletics to career and work
Family in later life (adult offspring ages late 20s to middle age)	Accept shift of generational roles	• Maintain spousal relationship in face of decline in physical strength • Support a central role in the family system of middle generation • Enjoy grandparental role with youngest generation • Engage in life review and integration • Prepare for and enjoy a fulfilling retirement • Prepare for loss of spouse, friends, and, eventually, one's own death	• Complete unresolved issues over athletic accomplishments of grown children • Assist adult athlete in retirement from competition and emotional resolution of the end of career • Focus on nonathletic activities with spouse and grown children • Participate in recreational sport and exercise for personal fulfillment and health maintenance

Note. From "The Changing Family Life Cycle: A Framework for Family Therapy" by B. Carter and M. McGoldrick. In *The Changing Family Lifecycle* (2nd ed.) by B. Carter and M. McGoldrick (Eds.), 1989, Needham Heights, MA: Allyn & Bacon. Copyright 1989 by Allyn & Bacon. Adapted by permission.

Stage One:
The Unattached Young Adult

A developmental analysis of the Stanley family begins with the life experience of Fred and Betty Stanley when they met in college as single, young adults. A genogram (McGoldrick & Gerson, 1985) of this period of the family's development appears in Figure 5.2.

■　*Fred and Betty met during college. Fred, a prelaw student, was a senior. Betty was a junior. Fred's stable, middle-class family encouraged his college education and his entering law school. But*

Fred had struggled throughout his life for his father's acceptance. His father was an emotionally closed person who had difficulty expressing positive feelings for his son. He owned his own manufacturing company, was a workaholic, and struggled financially at various times when the children were young. Fred's father was set in his ways and demanded a great deal from his children: Although he encouraged Fred to excel in sports and academics he gave him little verbal reward. Fred's mother, on the other hand, was nurturing to her three children. She was not a strong figure, however. She let her husband dominate most aspects of the family decision making. She avoided marital

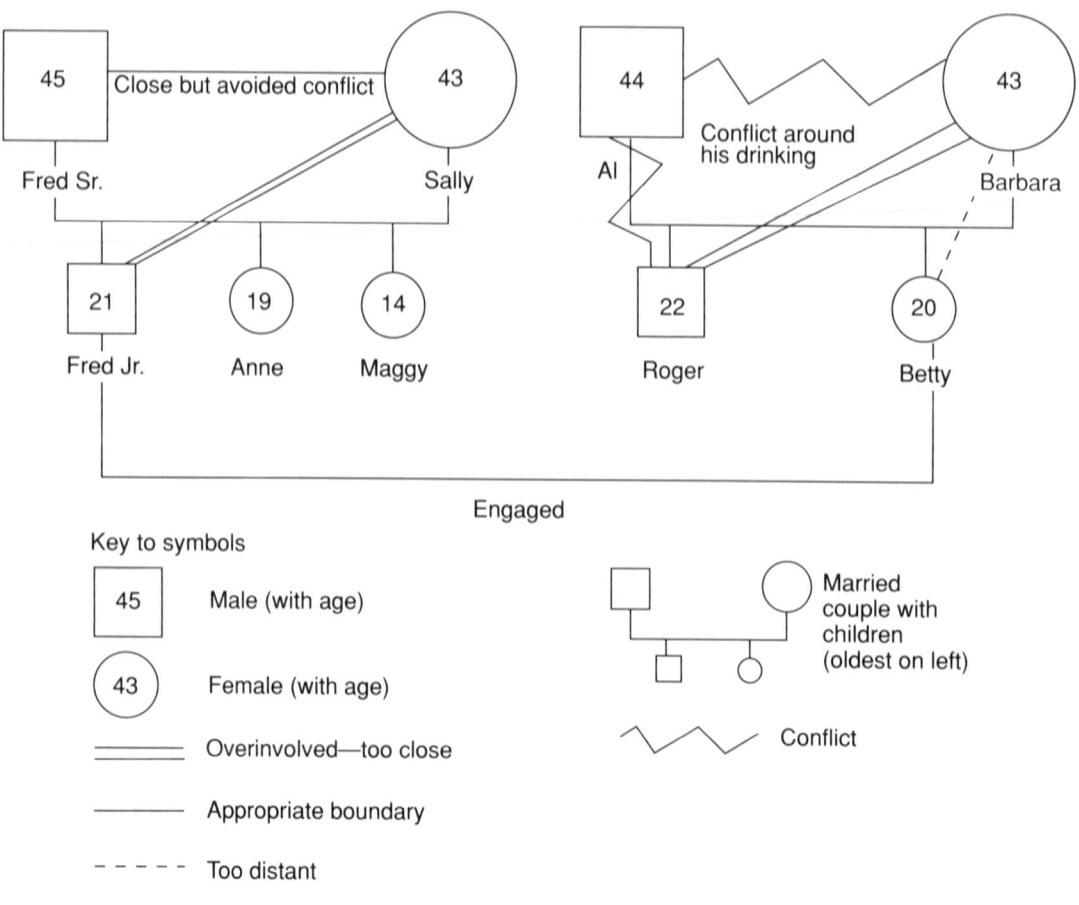

Figure 5.2　Genogram of Fred and Betty Stanley as single, young adults.

conflict and encouraged her children not to challenge their father.

Among the Stanley children, Fred was clearly the star. Throughout school he was a capable athlete and a good student. Fred played baseball, swam, and played tennis at the local club. In high school he played basketball, though he lacked height and often played in a backup role. He also played tennis and was elected team captain his senior year. Fred tried out unsuccessfully for the college tennis team—there were too many talented players at his school. He was frustrated by not making the team but continued to play recreationally.

In contrast to the Stanley family, which was tightly organized and devoid of conflict, Betty's family was quite different. There was open conflict between her parents, Al and Barbara, which centered on her father's drinking and her mother's anger at Al's irresponsibility. Betty's older brother, Roger, was the hero in this family and was often put in the responsible role of taking over many of Al's duties and becoming Barbara's helper. Betty took on the role of peacemaker in the family. The conflict between her parents bothered her, and she would mediate their disputes. Betty became emotionally controlled and internalized pain and sadness that she never expressed to others.

Betty was active in high-school sports. She ran cross-country and track and participated in gymnastics. She was also a solid, hardworking student. Because of her unhappy home life she enjoyed getting away from home, and when she met Fred she was immediately attracted to him.

To the casual observer, Fred and Betty were able to accomplish most of the developmental tasks of this stage of family development, which are

- to establish a sense of self in work and gain financial independence,
- to develop intimate peer relationships, and

- to differentiate themselves from their families of origin (Table 5.1).

At first glance, Fred and Betty looked and acted happy and self-confident. Some unresolved developmental tasks, however, were present that became problems in the development of their own family. Both failed to differentiate from their families of origin; Fred was and is still working to please his father. He is self-centered and fixated on being financially and professionally successful. Betty is a capable person, but she has low self-esteem and rigid emotional control. Her inability to differentiate from her family of origin manifested in a desire to avoid conflict and a need to establish a marital relationship in which Fred was the dominant player.

Athletically, the main task for the young couple was the development of an active and competitive lifestyle. This was relatively easy for both of them, because they were both active in sports. Fred taught Betty to play tennis, and she influenced him to enjoy running for exercise. During their courtship and early marriage they remained active in sport.

Stage Two: The Newly Married Couple

The major task for this stage of family development is to build a strong spousal relationship with an equal share of power. In addition, the couple must develop workable communication patterns, the ability to nurture and express affection for one another, and the mechanisms to resolve conflict (Nichols, 1988). Lastly, the newly married couple needs to establish itself as separate from their families of origin.

■ *Fred and Betty married. Both families were present, though Fred's father and Betty's mother seem to have been the major players in the wedding arrangements and events. Fred had finished his first year of law school, and Betty had graduated from college. They moved to an apartment at Fred's university and Betty began teaching in an elementary school in a nearby town.*

Betty taught school for the first 2 years of their marriage; this helped pay the bills while Fred went to law school. He graduated from school, passed the bar exam, and got an excellent job with a large law firm in the city.

Their marital contract was based on a complementarity of needs. The result was a marital system with an unequal balance of power. In choosing a partner, Betty sought stability; she chose a strong male figure, which she lacked in her own father. She also chose to avoid conflict as a way of making the marital relationship work. Fred, on the other hand, was comfortable with Betty, who was similar to his own mother. He was pleasing his father by being successful and having visibly successful children. He also followed his father's model by becoming a dominant and demanding father figure. Fred's fantasy when he met Betty was that they would create a close family of high achievers. Betty's fantasy was that they would be stable and free of conflict. Their marital roles were also influenced by their complementary sibling positions in their own families. Fred was the oldest and dominant male child, and Betty was the younger subordinate female child.

Fred remained on a successful career path. They were busy during these years. Tennis became a favorite pastime for Fred. He played at the club level and entered local tournaments. Their social life (mixed-doubles events and parties) centered on tennis. They also fell into a pattern of becoming active in activities outside their relationship and began to find little time for each other.

The major task that was not met at this stage was to establish mechanisms for resolving conflict. Betty's desire to avoid conflict and her collusion in the establishment of Fred's dominant role in the power hierarchy became a problem as the family developed.

Stage Three: The Athlete Family With Young Children

In athlete families the main task when the children are young is to introduce them to a variety of sports. In the families studied by the Bloom research team, this was a time of great excitement and playfulness. The excitement of seeing a child learn a sport skill is intense for parents. The child often loves the first encounter with sport because of the playful, noncompetitive nature of the environment.

■ *Soon after Fred began his career as a lawyer, they had their first child. Betty left her teaching position and became a full-time mother. Three years later their second child was born. The children developed without any major physical problems or illness. Fred and Betty stayed active in sports and gradually introduced the children to gymnastics, then soccer, swimming, and skiing. At age 6, Caroline began tennis lessons.*

The Stanleys are typical of athlete families at this stage of development. Parents introduce children to sport and spend time teaching their children sport skills. The family clearly values sport and the parents are willing to spend much family time with lessons and practice. For families who negotiate this stage well the playful and enjoyable quality of sport activity is not lost. Children enjoy the activity and the development of athletic skill.

There are potential problems at this stage of development for athlete families and they have begun to appear with the Stanleys. The main task of a family with young children is to make space for the children. The Stanleys had no problem with this; in fact, they made too much space for the children, who have become an enormous presence in the family.

Fred and Betty have grand expectations for their children and engage in what is called the family projection process (Bowen, 1965), in which one or both parents project their own unfulfilled wishes from their youth onto their children.

Many parents have grandiose fantasies about their children, but in the Stanley family these fantasies developed considerable intensity. Both Fred and Betty had images when their daughters were young (or perhaps even before they were born) that they would be exceptional children and top athletes. Fred's images were the strongest and derived from his relationship with his own father and his inability to be good enough to please him. The pattern of enmeshment with both Caroline and Amy stems from his own family experience. His two daughters have become involved in his need to achieve to please his father.

Another task of this developmental period is that the parents share in the nurturing and care of the children. In the Stanley family, however, these roles have become restrictive. Fred handles the sport role. Betty takes care of most other things.

■ *As the children grew, Betty did most of the parenting in the home and in relationship to school activities. Fred's parenting role largely centered on the girls' sport involvement. Evenings and weekends Fred threw a ball to the girls and took them to the tennis court to practice. As Caroline became more involved in tennis, Fred met her at the club after work and hit balls with her. He became disenchanted with the club pro and soon found another pro to work with her.*

Another unresolved issue at this stage is that Fred and Betty are not able to make adequate space in the family for their own spousal relationship. When too much space is made for the children, the family becomes child focused, and the boundaries in and around the family become rigid because most of the family involvement is in youth sport. They can become a tennis (or hockey, skiing, football, or equestrian) family. The children develop friendships with children in the same sport and don't meet others. The parents neglect their own relationship by focusing too much of their time and energy on the children. This is evident in Fred and Betty's relationship: they were unable to draw a boundary around their own relationship and the level of intimacy decreased.

Stage Four: The Family With Adolescent Children

For many families, adolescence can be the most difficult period of development. It is a time of great turmoil; the child begins to change from being dependent and compliant to being independent and more connected with peer group than family. The authoritative structure of the parental subsystem is challenged and the ability of the parents to adapt to this change is severely tested. If the parents are not able to adapt and retain the respect of the child, the ability of the family to function smoothly is diminished. The main tasks involve a realignment of the boundaries and power hierarchy of the family. The child must gradually be given more power in the family and more involvement in the decision-making processes. For example, Mom and Dad's saying no to a request to stay at a friend's house for the night changes to their asking the adolescent what is a reasonable hour to come home from a party and all agreeing to a mutually acceptable time.

Adolescence is also a difficult time for athlete families because it is during this stage that there is a transition from sports as fun to sports as serious business. Although adolescents in many families drop out of youth-sport programs to pursue other interests (Gould & Horn, 1984), in athlete families the pattern is reversed. The major task for them is to develop a commitment to sport and the role demands of the serious athlete.

Adolescence is also a time where the primary influence on the child athlete shifts from the parents to the coach. The parents' role changes. They become the athlete's support structure. The coach becomes the primary influence for skill and competitive development. Some parents have difficulty with this shift, and diffuse boundaries in the parent–athlete relationship result in conflicts in the coach–parent–athlete relationship (Hellstedt, 1987).

At the same time that the shift in influence is away from them, the parents continue to be influential in the child athlete's development by emphasizing a goal orientation and a strong work ethic. It is critical for parents to strike a workable balance between teaching discipline and determined effort while also fostering a sense of independence in the child athlete.

Adolescence is the stage when the first major derailment from the normal family life cycle occurs in the athlete family. For the child athlete, adolescence is a prolonged or substantially different period than for most of the child's peer group. The demands of athletic training and competition often result in a deprivation of free time, hanging out, and dating. Also, non-sport-related career issues are put on hold as the youngster focuses on the role of athlete. This prolonged adolescence is reinforced by the child's continuing to be dependent on the family for financial support during the early stage of competition. This derailment becomes a moratorium in which the athlete and the athlete's family does not share the experience of summer jobs, peer relationships, or decision making about college choice or career options. Instead, the family continues to concentrate on the young athlete's sport involvement. The result is a developmental impasse.

As shown in Table 5.1, the family can help the athlete through this period in several ways. One is to support, wherever possible, the athlete's sense of independence. A practical way of accomplishing this is for the parents to let the athlete travel and compete without their presence. Another is to let the athlete have major input into decisions about coaching, training programs, and competition schedules. Because they are often sheltered by coaches and sport organizations, some elite athletes need to find from their families the psychological permission as well as the necessary skills to establish independent thinking and decision-making patterns.

The parents' major task is to allow the influence shift from parents to coach by establishing a clear boundary between their roles as parent and coach to their child. This boundary will help the developing athlete view family as a safe and supportive refuge from the pressures of competition and training. Also, the family can encourage the adolescent's social maturity by supporting their efforts to have meaningful relationships with peers. Attending concerts, going to friends' homes for the weekend, and dating are important formative experiences and should be encouraged by parents. A life apart from sport is a healthy present and future resource for the athlete. It helps establish a permeable boundary to the extrafamilial social environment around both the athlete and the family.

The Stanley family has hit some snags at this stage of development (see Figure 5.3). Fred is overinvolved with the two girls. Betty is underinvolved and avoids conflict with Fred. Caroline has accepted the invitation to be overinvolved with her father. She has become so absorbed in competitive tennis that she has had limited peer relationships outside of the sport. She has rarely dated or partied; instead, she has devoted herself to competition and training. Her parents have collaborated in this delayed adolescence by

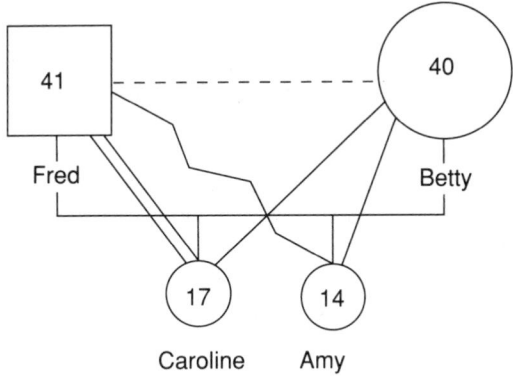

Figure 5.3 Genogram of the Stanley family with adolescent children.

continuing to monitor and supervise her decisions. Career decisions are not important for Caroline or her parents. She has a chance to be a professional tennis player and that has become their goal. She has been granted a college scholarship for her tennis, but the choice of school was made on the basis of the quality of the tennis program and not on academic factors.

Although this parenting approach seems to have worked with Caroline, it hasn't with her younger sister. Amy is uncomfortable with the family script. She wants more independence and is not sure she wants the life of a competitive athlete. Her individual desires are running into conflict with the family values. The crisis that is about to occur has its roots in the failure of the parents and their marital relationship to meet previous developmental tasks.

Amy is about to challenge the family's child-as-athlete focus. She wants more non-sport social involvement and generally more independence in decision making. In addition, Fred and Betty have not developed interests outside of tennis and will have difficulty if Amy pursues other directions. Lastly, Fred has problems with accepting other non-family adults as influences on Amy. This leads to conflict with her coaches.

Stage Five: The Launching of Children

The major tasks at the launching phase of family development involve the parents' letting go of their children, developing adult-to-adult relationships with them, and refocusing energy on their own marital relationship. These tasks produce a second major problem area or potential derailment of athlete families from the normal family life cycle.

The normal process is for the young adult (age 18 to 22) to attend college, move away from home, and begin career or graduate training. Marriage and the formation of the adult child's own family might soon follow. Although some young adult offspring will return home for brief periods of time, their goal is to establish independent living apart from the family.

In athlete families the prolonged adolescence of the previous stage results in a launching delay. These families might find they are "out of synch" with other families because their child has put off important life decisions in order to train and compete. There is a trend in many sports for athletes to delay or interrupt college or career preparation to allow them to train more intensively. The launching delay can also result from the parents' maintaining an overinvolved position by managing an abundance of the athlete's life decisions. The emotional separation and letting go of the young adult athlete is hindered by the overinvolvement that might have developed during the previous stages.

If the young adult athlete has committed to sport, the family needs to be aware of and tolerate this delay. Otherwise there will be additional stress or pressure on the young athlete. Athlete families might not have the empty nest that other families experience, so they must tolerate numerous entries and exits from the family caused by the young athlete's leaving home for periods of time to compete and then returning again.

The launching delay can present problems in families where the parents tend toward overinvolvement. The parents might gain emotional gratification from the young adult's delaying independent living, and this might work to the athlete's detriment. For example, in the tennis families studied by Monsaas (1985) two fathers were still actively coaching their young-adult-athlete-offspring well into their late 20s, a process which would likely inhibit the athlete's self-differentiation.

The major task for the athlete family during the launching phase is to perform a delicate balancing act between encouraging financial and emotional independence on the one hand and providing a source of emotional support and refuge from the stress of competition on the other. Finding and trusting a coach outside the family is an essential component in this process.

The Stanleys are in the transition to the launching phase. We can speculate that Fred and Betty will continue to manage Caroline's life and make decisions that will inhibit her growth. It is also possible that Fred and Betty will have difficulty adjusting their own marital relationship without Caroline's (and possibly Amy's) tennis as a focus. The process of separation will be a difficult one for this family.

Stage Six: The Family in Later Life

Later in life the athlete has finished the competitive phase, has retired from sport, and is making the transition to a new career and the establishment of a kinship family. The major issues for the parents are the completion of any unresolved issues about the athletic accomplishments of the adult offspring. It is a time for the parents to enjoy their own spousal relationship and retirement and feel a sense of dignity about their accomplishments as a family. The major issue for them relative to their offspring is to assist and support the athlete around retirement issues and the establishment of a new career and a separate family. A healthy, permeable boundary is appropriate here so that the parents are perceived as supportive but not fused with the adult offspring.

This phase is difficult to predict for the Stanley family. If Fred and Betty are not able to separate from their two daughters and establish their marital relationship as a distinct and valued subsystem, this stage will also be a difficult time for them.

This completes the developmental model. Now we will consider the Stanleys as a family with adolescent children and examine the assessment and treatment issues that emerge when a sport psychologist and family therapist becomes involved with the family.

CLINICAL ASSESSMENT AND TREATMENT

The assessment of the family system of the athlete is an important component to any sport-related assessment procedure. Family processes are often important factors in problems such as eating disorders (Minuchin, Rosman, & Baker, 1978), rehabilitation from injury (Rotella, 1985), burnout and overtraining (Odom & Perrin, 1985), substance abuse (Doherty & Baird, 1983; Krestan & Bepko, 1989), parental overinvolvement (Ogilvie, 1983), and problems in the coach–parent–athlete relationship (Hellstedt, 1987). Even though they present as individual problems, performance blocks or retirement from sport might involve family issues, and a family analysis should be included in the assessment and considered in treatment decisions.

Assessment of the Athlete Family

Based on the model presented in this chapter, two basic questions need to be answered in the process of doing a family-system-based assessment. The first question is, What are the developmental impasses? The second is, What are the structural and interactional strengths and weaknesses of the family?

The best procedure for collecting information is a cluster of interviews with key family members, but all family members do not need to be present for all assessment interviews. It is important, however, to have the principal players in the family together for at least one session to observe the patterns of communication and interaction. A suggested format is to see the athlete alone for a session, the parents together for another session, and the entire family together for one or two sessions. The order in which these sessions take place is interchangeable depending on the circumstances, motivation, and time schedules of family members.

To provide a framework for assessment of the family's developmental and structural characteristics, some assessment categories are helpful. Doherty and Baird (1983) present a succinct assessment formula based on four themes:

1. The level and the source of stress in the family
2. The degree of cohesiveness in the family
3. The ability of the family to adapt to change
4. The interaction patterns in the family

Brief examples from the Stanley family will illustrate these themes.

Levels of Stress

The first task of the clinician in family assessment is to determine the intensity and source of stress in the family.

■ *Fred Stanley called Dr. Hawthorne and asked for an appointment for Amy. "She's a promising young tennis player, but she is easily distracted. And since her last match, which she lost*

because she lacked the effort, she is talking about quitting tennis and giving up the opportunity to be a top-level player. Her coach suggested I give you a call in the hope that you can sit down and talk with her." Dr. Hawthorne explained to Fred that she likes to do a three- or four-session evaluation, at the end of which she will make treatment recommendations. She explained that the purpose of the evaluation is to get to know both Amy and the family so a treatment contract can be designed to meet everyone's particular needs. Because Caroline would be leaving soon for college, it was agreed that the family would come to the first session together.

Based on the tone of the telephone conversation, Dr. Hawthorne sensed that Fred Stanley sees the problem as Amy's. He had not defined the issue in a broader context. Dr. Hawthorne speculated that the Stanleys were in a moderate state of stress. No major life crisis faced any family member, but it is likely that feelings of anger, disappointment, and frustration were being felt but not expressed. Their intensity was not as elevated, however, as other athlete families Dr. Hawthorne was currently seeing, such as the family of an elite diver whose mother is dying from cancer during the peak of the diver's career or the family of a gymnast whose father is in the acute stage of alcoholism. Nevertheless, there seemed to be more stress in the Stanley family than Fred acknowledged.

In addition to the degree of stress in the family, it is important to identify the source of stress. Is the source in the family or outside the family system? Internal stressors such as parental pressure on a vulnerable adolescent athlete, financial strain due to a child's training and coaching costs, alcoholism or other substance abuse, death of a family member, or marital conflict and divorce are examples of stressors in the family. Examples of external stressors would be job loss, discrimination and racism, or conflict between the family and a coach or sport organization.

■ *Based on the brief phone conversation with Fred, Dr. Hawthorne formed her initial impression of the source of stress in the family. It seemed to be emanating from a developmental impasse in the Stanleys' transition from a family with young children to one with adolescent children. She also got the impression that Fred's dominance might be a problem in the family and that he might be an overinvolved parent. She would wait and see how they interacted in her office before forming any more impressions.*

Levels of Cohesion

A second dimension for assessing a family is cohesiveness. The main structural element in determining the level of cohesiveness is boundary formation. The rigidity or flexibility of boundaries in and around the family determines the level of cohesiveness in the family. A family that is too cohesive has diffuse boundaries and its members are overinvolved with one another. This would be apparent in a diagnostic interview in which family members think and speak for one another, sit close together, or try to mute the expression of affect. A family lacking in cohesion will have rigid boundaries, evidenced by an unwillingness to look at or speak to one another. This type of family will sit far apart, look distracted or recalcitrant, and not listen when a family member is talking about thoughts or feelings.

■ *In the waiting room Dr. Hawthorne observed that Fred spoke first and introduced the family members to her. Betty seemed quiet and soft-spoken, and Amy seemed sullen and moody. Caroline appeared pleasant and smiled frequently. When they came into the consulting room (with two love seats in an L-shape and the therapist's chair forming a triangle) Fred sat next to Caroline, and Amy sat next to her mother. After some pleasantries Dr. Hawthorne said, "I'd like to hear what each of you likes about your family." Fred was*

the first to respond by saying, "We have two really outstanding daughters."

Dr. Hawthorne's initial impressions were that Fred was overinvolved and controlling. He spoke for the other family members and controlled the flow of communication. The cohesion in this family seemed centered on Fred's efforts and agenda. Dr. Hawthorne wondered how the others responded to him.

Adapting to Change

All families need to be able to adapt to changes that are required as the family passes through the stages of the family life cycle. Adaptability implies flexibility in communication, problem solving, and resolving conflict, particularly when a family member asserts a need for change. The impetus for change can come from in the family, such as a developmental change in a member, or from outside the family, such as the death of a friend or relative. For example, the developmental task of the family with adolescent children is to begin to share the authority in the family. The children need to be given more power to make their own decisions. Many families find this difficult to negotiate and the Stanleys are no exception. They have difficulty changing the boundary and power arrangements in the family as the children become adolescents and young adults. A key indicator of the family's adaptability is how flexible the parents are when Amy asserts some independence. A hint of the parents' rigidity emerges early in the interview.

■ *Dr. Hawthorne asked Amy to describe what, if anything, she would like to see changed in her family. Her answer was, "I wish they would let me do more things with my friends and not always want me to be practicing tennis. My wishes don't seem to count." She went on to describe a situation where she wanted to go to a party at her friend's house and her parents wouldn't let her because she had what she described as a "minor" tournament that same weekend. "I don't see why I can't do both," she said in a sullen voice.*

Interaction Patterns

Recurring patterns of interaction form the fourth assessment dimension. Here the clinician looks for communication patterns, ability to tolerate closeness, decision-making processes, time structuring, conflict-resolution patterns, and the mechanisms by which the family accomplishes its daily tasks. Does the family have fun together? Do they spend time apart as well as together? Are they able to negotiate when they disagree on an important issue? Are they able to express intimacy to one another? How do they deal with conflicts between family members?

■ *Betty had been attentive but quiet for the first 15 min of the session. When asked what she liked about the family, she said, "I think we get along pretty well compared to a lot of families." Dr. Hawthorne agreed with her but then went on to ask, "What does happen in the family when you don't agree on something?" Betty indicated that she usually went along with the wishes of others, especially Fred. Amy said, "We don't ne-gotiate; they tell me what to do and I'm expected to do it." Caroline said, "The only two in the family that fight are Dad and Amy. I think they are too much alike. Mom and I get along with everyone just fine." Dr. Hawthorne then asked Fred and Betty what things they do for themselves without the children. They both indicated that right now they have very little time to do things as a couple because they are always going to the girls' tennis matches. They added that the travel and time involved make it difficult to do any-thing else.*

A week after the interview with the entire family, Dr. Hawthorne met with Amy. In that session she talked about her ambivalence about tennis—her love for the game and the people she had met through the sport but her occasional desire to quit and do other things. She expressed her frustrations about being pressured by her parents to stay with the sport.

■ *Amy told Dr. Hawthorne, "They want me to get a college scholarship just like Caroline did." Amy shared the fact that there are times when she didn't want to train any more but was afraid to say that because her father would be upset. She feels her mother is more understanding but is weak and will not stand up to her father.*

At the end of the session, Dr. Hawthorne asked Amy if she was willing to be involved in family therapy sessions to help improve the communication in the family and estab-lish herself in a more effective way than she had in the past. Dr. Hawthorne explained to her that she would also like to see Amy in some individual sessions to talk about her feelings about tennis, but by working to-gether the family can explore ways they can live together more productively. Amy agreed to participate.

As a final step in the assessment process, Dr. Hawthorne met with Fred and Betty alone. She asked them questions about their own parents and families, how they met, and what their courtship was like, and she ob-tained a brief picture of the development stages of their own family. She focused on their involvement with tennis, their stance around training, their attendance at matches, and their conversations with the girls before and after competition.

■ *Fred did a lot of the talking, but Dr. Haw-thorne skillfully drew Betty into the conversation at key times. For example, when Fred was describ-ing the scene in the car after Amy's last tennis match, Dr. Hawthorne turned to Betty and asked*

"Betty, how did you feel at the time?" Betty said she felt Fred was being a bit hard on Amy, but didn't say anything at the time. *"Do you often feel this way and not say anything?"* Dr. Hawthorne asked. *"Yes, I guess so,"* Betty replied. *"I don't like to have disagreements in front of the kids."* *"Did your parents fight in front of you?"* Dr. Hawthorne then asked Betty. *"All the time,"* said Betty. *"I couldn't stand it, and I vowed I would never do that in front of my own children."*

Treating Athlete Families

Though some therapeutic insight develops during the assessment phase, most of the change in perspective in the family takes place during and after a treatment contract is negotiated. It is important to involve the family in the treatment whenever possible, depending of course on the extent of family involvement in the level and source of stress and the definition of the problem from the athlete's perspective.

The Treatment Contract

The treatment contract often helps the family reframe a problem from an individual perspective to a broader family perspective. When Fred initially called for an appointment, he defined the problem as Amy's. Dr. Hawthorne's skillful assessment helped the family see Amy's difficulties on the tennis court in a broader perspective.

■ *At the end of the final evaluation session, Dr. Hawthorne explained to Fred and Betty that her experience with athletes has led her to see that the problems they face regarding competition have a direct impact on the family and vice versa. She explained that she believes the families of elite athletes experience unique pressures and stress that many other families do not. She also explained her belief that Amy is facing a personal crisis on two levels. One is her own self-doubt about her*

ability and desire to be an elite athlete. Another level is how her decisions about tennis impact the family.

Dr. Hawthorne suggested that treatment must take into account both these levels and asked Fred and Betty if they would be willing to be involved in some family sessions to explore how the family communication and decision-making patterns are related to Amy's feelings about her sport in general and her performance on the court.

Dr. Hawthorne recommended a series of 12 sessions with a mixture of individual, parental, and family meetings. She explained that in the individual work with Amy she will help Amy with competition-related problems of stress and will teach her relaxation and mental imagery skills that will help her performance. In addition, she will give Amy a chance to talk about some of the feelings she has about her self-image, her identity as an athlete, and her goals in the sport. The parental sessions will focus on their ways of dealing with the pressures and stresses of being athletes' parents. The goal of the family sessions will be to help all members of the family communicate with one another and feel that their own needs are being addressed. Fred and Betty agreed that the format makes sense and would be helpful. They began treatment together.

Goals of Treatment

Therapeutic intervention with athlete families has the following goals:

- Assist the family in resolving developmental impasses
- Improve the structural functioning of the family by strengthening boundaries, power hierarchies, communication patterns, and conflict resolution mechanisms
- Develop the support network, both inside and outside the family, necessary for the young athlete's achievement of goals.

To help set her treatment goals, Dr. Hawthorne drew a treatment genogram (see Figure 5.4). This genogram helps her develop strategies for her interventions with the family. She then begins to work with them using the following types of interventions: education and prevention, support, facilitation, and challenge (Doherty & Baird, 1983).

Education and Prevention

The interventions that are aimed at helping the family resolve developmental impasses are often educational interventions. The family needs help in understanding and adapting to the changes that are required as it negotiates the stages of the family life cycle. Educational interventions are geared toward helping the family resolve past and present impasses so they can better meet the challenges that lie ahead. A major impasse is Fred's inability to untangle himself from the drama that he played out as a young man with his own father. In one of the family sessions Dr. Hawthorne helped Fred to see the relationship between his inability to please his own father and his desire for his daughter's prowess in tennis.

■ *Dr. Hawthorne asked both Fred and Betty to talk with their daughters about their own athletic experiences when they were in high school. Betty talked about how little encouragement she received from her parents because they were always involved with her father's drinking. Fred recounted how he felt hurt when his father seldom watched him play. One year he won the high school district singles tournament, but his father hadn't come to see the match. Fred's eyes teared as he talked of how his father later said that he had been unable to get away from the office to attend the match.*

Dr. Hawthorne then asked Fred, "What did you decide at that time about how you would act when you became a parent?" Fred clenched his fist and replied, "I vowed that I would never miss one of my kid's matches. Never."

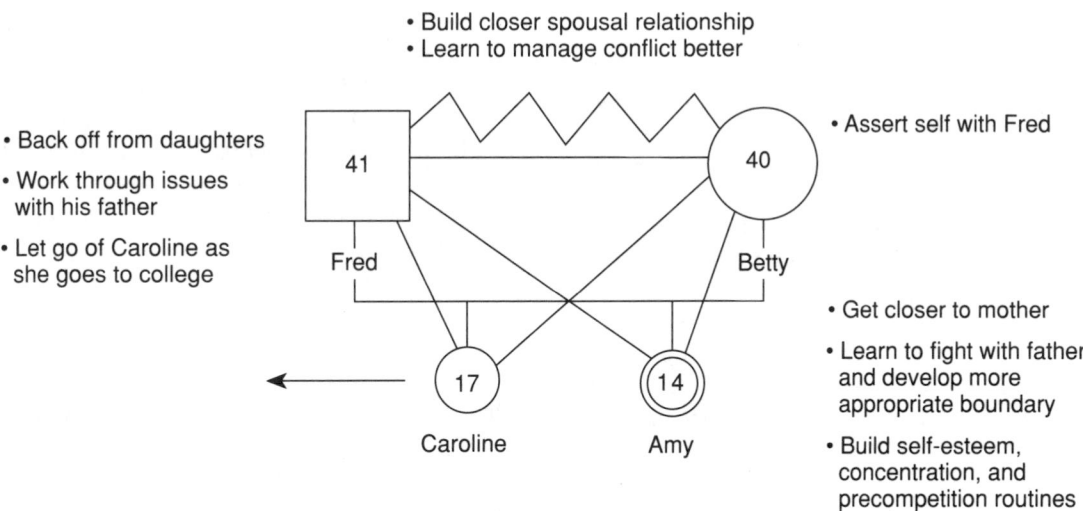

Figure 5.4 A treatment goals genogram of the Stanley family.

Dr. Hawthorne was able to use Fred's connection of past and present to help the family see the need for a change in the boundary between the parents and the adolescent children. She showed her appreciation for Fred's wanting to be at all of Amy's matches, but she was able to help him see the need for Amy to learn to deal with competition pressures without her parents being present. Dr. Hawthorne shared with Fred and Betty an article by a former champion tennis player (Smith, 1990) on how to be an effective tennis parent. One of Smith's suggestions is to attend no more than 75% of the child's matches. Dr. Hawthorne explained the reasons for this suggestion. Then she worked with Fred and Betty in setting up a behavioral change contract to practice during the coming week.

■ *The family agreed that Amy's parents will not attend her next match. When Amy returns home they will ask her, How did you feel about your performance today? Fred and Betty were helped to see that a question such as this shifts the focus from a concern about outcome to a concern for Amy's feelings about her performance. "I believe that the important thing for parents," Dr. Hawthorne said, "is that they not be so concerned about winning and losing, but rather how their child feels about the experience."*

This intervention is educational and preventive in that it helps the family resolve their present impasse and prepares them for the tasks of the next stage of family development. They are about to enter the launching phase; having more flexible boundaries is essential for the successful resolution of that phase.

Support

The athlete family faces a unique set of stressful events and conditions. The win-lose pressures of competitive sport as well as the demands on time and financial resources often contribute to tension in these families. However, these families also have a great deal of strength and their positive qualities need reinforcement. For example, their emphasis on goal attainment and the work ethic is a positive quality. They need to feel understood and supported in what they are seeking to accomplish. In meetings with subsystems of the family, the clinical sport psychologist affirms their struggle to develop the talent in the family.

■ *In one session Fred and Betty shared with Dr. Hawthorne the personal and financial sacrifices the two of them have made to further their daughters' tennis careers. They spoke of the pain that they sometimes felt when Amy didn't appreciate these sacrifices. They also shared how they felt that many of their friends had pulled away, both because of the time commitments to tennis and because they didn't think their friends could relate to the kind of intensity the family put into tennis. "I think many of our friends think we are crazy," Betty said at one point. Dr. Hawthorne listened empathically to these feelings and reinforced them. "You both have to understand that what you are working on is producing 'excellence' in your daughter's tennis, and with that comes a lot of pain and sacrifice. I am sure few people except for other tennis families understand the difficulties you face. Perhaps you need to share more of these feelings, both with one another and with some of your tennis friends."*

Facilitation

One of the main tasks of the clinician in working with athlete families is to open the communication process in the family. This can be done by encouraging the family members to communicate directly with one another. This openness produces meaningful changes in the boundaries and interactional patterns in the family.

■ *In the second session in which all family members were present, the incident that took place in the car after the regional championships was discussed. Dr. Hawthorne asked Fred to share with Amy what he was really feeling after the match. After some hedging he finally said, "I was angry and disappointed. I thought you could have won if you had played harder." Amy responded, "I knew you were angry. I was angry too. I felt like I tried hard [the tears begin to flow]. When I felt the match slipping away, I knew you were over there watching and getting upset. I thought of how you would be disappointed in me during the whole third set."*

Facilitation is more than simply allowing a catharsis to take place. It leads to positive behavioral change. Dr. Hawthorne was able to do this by first commenting that feelings are often communicated without words and that in this case Amy had sensed how Fred was feeling. Then Dr. Hawthorne pointed out that it is better to be direct, so the issue can be talked about and resolved.

■ *At the end of the session, Dr. Hawthorne helped the Stanleys establish a behavioral contract that involves Fred, Betty, and Amy. They agreed that the next time one of them felt anger they would acknowledge it and then state what they saw as the problem and how they would like it resolved.*

Challenge

The family structures that are not working well need to be challenged. A firm nudge often helps a family respond more creatively to the needs of its members. In designing challenging interventions the clinician hopes to rock the boat, shake up the system, and guide it toward reorganizing at a more adaptive level. One of the major areas where the Stanleys need to be challenged is in the area

of the power imbalance in the spousal system and the inability of Betty and Fred to deal openly with conflict in their own relationship. Betty needs to empower herself to the point where she is willing to challenge Fred's role in the family. Betty's softer and more understanding approach to problems is an undervalued source of energy in the family.

■ *In a session with Fred and Betty only, Dr. Hawthorne asked them about their fighting style. "We don't fight," said Betty. "What are some issues that you don't fight about?" asked Dr. Hawthorne. "Could you look at Fred and tell him some of the things you have been avoiding?" Betty went on to say that she was really upset with Fred during and after the regional championships, but she didn't say anything, because she "didn't want to start a fight." Dr. Hawthorne suggested they engage in a role play where the car scene is reenacted and the problem is discussed between them. She asked Betty to begin with a clear description of Fred's behavior that she is upset about, and her attendant feelings. Fred was asked to listen, and respond with his own feelings about what Betty has said. The role play went well. A contract was established that the next time Betty feels a strong disagreement with Fred about something she will tell him what the problem is. He will then respond with one of two statements Dr. Hawthorne taught him: either "I understand" or "I don't understand your feelings, please help me."*

Termination

At the end of the 12 sessions the Stanleys terminated their family sessions with Dr. Hawthorne. Amy is feeling better about her tennis and experiences less pressure from Fred and Betty. Betty believes that they are getting their own issues out on the table more openly with one another. Caroline has left for college and they have been able to let go of her. They miss Caroline, but they are not planning to visit her until the fall parents' weekend. Fred agrees with Dr. Hawthorne that he will let Caroline make her own decisions now about tennis and that he will support her choice of direction. Amy agrees, however, to come in for a session once a month to discuss her feelings about her tennis and her decisions about whether to continue or not. They will also continue working on imagery and concentration to enhance her tennis skills. The family also agrees to a follow-up session in three months with all members to assess the changes in the family.

ETHICAL ISSUES IN WORKING WITH FAMILIES

Certain ethical and value issues are more complex when intervening with a family than with an individual athlete. For example, the issue of confidentiality is more complicated when working with multiple family members. The question of whether and when to share information obtained in a separate interview is often a dilemma for the clinician. Corey, Corey, and Callanan (1988) present an excellent discussion of these general ethical issues. This section briefly discusses a few major guidelines that are important to follow when intervening in a family system.

Training and Competence

Working with the athlete's family system is more complex and more difficult than working with the individual athlete. It is important, therefore, that a clinician who takes a family-centered approach with athletes have specialized training in conducting family therapy. The clinician, however, also must have a background in sport psychology and a familiarity with the unique pressures that face a competitive athlete.

The Family as Client

There is a difference in value orientation with a family-centered approach to assessment and treatment. The goal of family treatment is to facilitate change in the whole family, not simply in an individual family member. A basic principle of family system theory is that anything that affects one family member impacts all other parts of the system. It is conceivable, for example, that an individually oriented clinician working with Amy on issues of self-differentiation might provoke a marital crisis between Fred and Betty. Amy might get stronger, but others might get worse in the process. The family-as-client approach allows all family members to negotiate the salient developmental task at the same time.

Avoiding Subsystem Alliances

The clinician must stay out of the triangles, alliances, and entanglements that develop in families as well as between families and coaches and sport organizations. In working with families it is important not to become an advocate of any one member of the family, but rather to remain neutral and be seen as an ally by all members. A basic rule when working with couples or families is that there are no villains and victims, but instead that everyone shares some responsibility for what goes on in the family. Had Dr. Hawthorne become only Amy's advocate (or Fred and Betty's) the family would not have been able to make the changes that it did.

Countertransference

In avoiding the entanglements and unhealthy alliances in families, it is essential that sport psychologists be aware of the role of their own families of origin so countertransference issues do not interfere in their work with client families. Just as we expect over-involved parents to see their own unresolved issues that they might be projecting onto their children, clinicians need to realize that they too engage in family projection. If a clinician empowers the adolescent athlete at the parents' expense or encourages parents to set limits on a rebellious adolescent because of residues of the clinician's own experience the family will not be helped.

A Model for the Healthy Family

Lastly, the sport psychologist who takes a family-centered approach should base interventions on a model for healthy family functioning that serves as a guide to the complexities of family life. In this chapter I have attempted to present a developmental model, and I hope that this model is a beginning for dialogue and refinement that will lead to an improvement in the quality of life for our young athletes.

An issue that did not come up with the Stanley family but that frequently presents itself in athlete families is whether a young athlete (under age 15) should leave the family home to train in a favorable geographical environment (e.g., warm climate for tennis or mountains for skiers) or with specialized coaching (e.g., tennis, gymnastics, and figure skating). This can be a dilemma for a family-oriented clinician because it presents a conflict between the value of family cohesion against the young athlete's training, coaching, or competition needs.

In keeping with the ethical guidelines of our profession, it is important for the clinician to help the family explore the issues involved in this decision and not impose a predetermined solution or answer. The developmental model can help the clinician and the family assess the developmental readiness of both the family and the young athlete. For example, in one family a dislocation of the young athlete might be appropriate; in another, it might be premature. The important questions for the clinician to help the family answer are What are the major developmental issues in the family now? How have they handled previous stages of family development? Is the young athlete developmentally ready for this kind of move? and How would it affect the various subsystems in the family such as the parents, the siblings, and the extended family? Once a decision is made, the family-oriented clinician can also help the family negotiate the separation so that the negative aspects of the separation are managed as well as possible. Also, during the period of separation the clinician can be of value to the family in helping solve various problems that develop, such as conflicts between the family and the coach or training academy. Lastly, the clinician can be helpful by consulting with sport organizations and academies for which this issue is a frequent problem. The consultant can help the organization both in managing these transitions and in rethinking training and competition philosophies so families can stay together and the athlete's needs can be met at the same time.

THE FINAL SESSION

About 3 months later, Dr. Hawthorne met with the Stanley family and discovered that the family had been able to maintain the changes they made earlier in treatment. They are communicating their feelings to one another; Fred and Betty are discussing their differences and even fighting occasionally. Amy is happier; she is still playing tennis but is taking more time away from the game to have fun with her friends. She is playing in fewer tournaments but with good results. Dr. Hawthorne gave them positive reinforcement for the changes they have made.

Dr. Hawthorne ended the session by asking Betty, Fred, Amy, and Caroline to create a "sculpture" of how they see the family now and the changes that have been made.

■ *Betty started by placing Fred and herself together so they can reach out and touch one another. She put Caroline near the door to the office, indicating her psychological departure for college. Amy is in front of them but standing sideways so she half faces them and half faces the*

door. When asked if anyone wants to change the sculpture, Amy said she would like to. She walked over to her parents, who faced toward her in the sculpture and moved their heads so they would look more at each other.

"This is a good place to end," Dr. Hawthorne said. After a family hug, Dr. Hawthorne said goodbye to the Stanley family. She is confident that Amy will be a better tennis player and a happier person as she continues her life's journey.

CONCLUSION

I hope that this chapter has demonstrated that the family is a key player in the athlete's development and performance. The practice of sport psychology is enriched by a family-based orientation to the assessment and treatment of athletes. Creating a workable family system is a challenge for parents, who have many difficult decisions to make and are often without support and direction in making those choices. Sport psychologists can help parents as well as athletes by using family-based assessments and treatment interventions that provide education, challenge, and support to negotiate the tasks and transitions in the family life cycle.

REFERENCES

Berlage, G. (1981, May). *Fathers' career aspirations for sons in competitive hockey programs*. Paper presented at the Regional Symposium of the International Committee for the Sociology of Sport, Vancouver, BC.

Berryman, J.W. (1988). The rise of highly organized sports for preadolescent boys. In F.L. Smoll, R.A. Magill, & M.J. Ash (Eds.), *Children in sport* (pp. 3-16). Champaign, IL: Human Kinetics.

Bloom, B. (Ed.) (1985). *Developing talent in young people*. New York: Ballantine Books.

Bowen, M. (1965). Family psychotherapy with schizophrenia in the hospital and in private practice. In I. Boszormenyi-Nagy & J. Framo (Eds.), *Intensive family therapy* (pp. 213-243). New York: Harper & Row.

Bowen, M. (1978). *Family therapy in clinical practice*. New York: Aronson.

Bradt, J., & Moynihan, C. (1971). Opening the safe—the child-focused family. In J. Bradt & C. Moynihan (Eds.), *Systems therapy*. Washington, DC: Groome Child Guidance Center.

Carter, B., & McGoldrick, M. (Eds.) (1989). *The changing family life cycle: A framework for family therapy*. Boston: Allyn & Bacon.

Corey, G., Corey, M., & Callanan, P. (1988). *Issues and ethics in the helping professions*. Pacific Grove, CA: Brooks/Cole.

Doherty, W., & Baird, M. (1983). *Family therapy and family medicine*. New York: Guilford Press.

Erikson, E. (1950). *Childhood and society*. New York: Norton.

Fulmer, R. (1989). Lower-income and professional families: A comparison of structure and life cycle process. In B. Carter & M. McGoldrick (Eds.), *The changing family life cycle: A framework for family therapy* (pp. 545-579). Boston: Allyn & Bacon.

Gould, D., & Horn, T. (1984). Participation motivation in young athletes. In J. Silva & R. Weinberg (Eds.), *Psychological foundations of sport* (pp. 359-370). Champaign, IL: Human Kinetics.

Gould, D., Horn, T., & Spreemann, J. (1983). Sources of stress in junior elite wrestlers. *Journal of Sport Psychology*, **5**, 159-171.

Greendorfer, S., & Lewko, J. (1978). Role of family members in sport socialization of children. *Research Quarterly*, **49**, 146-152.

Hellstedt, J. (1987). The coach/parent/athlete relationship. *Sport Psychologist*, **1**, 151-160.

Hellstedt, J. (1990a). Early adolescent perceptions of parental pressure in the sport environment. *Journal of Sport Behavior*, **13**, 135-144.

Hellstedt, J. (1990b, August). *The family pressure cooker: Reflections on parents, coaches and young athletes*. Paper presented at the 98th Annual Convention of the American Psychological Association, Boston.

Higgenson, D. (1985). The influence of socializing agents in the female sport-participation process. *Adolescence*, **20**, 73-82.

Kalinowski, A. (1985). The development of Olympic swimmers. In B. Bloom (Ed.), *Developing talent in young people* (pp. 139-192). New York: Ballantine Books.

Kesend, O. (1991). *The elite athlete's sources of encouragement and discouragement affecting their motivation to participate in sport: A qualitative study from a development perspective*. Unpublished doctoral dissertation, The Union Institute, Cincinnati, OH.

Krestan, J., & Bepko, C. (1989). Alcoholic problems and the family life cycle. In B. Carter & M. McGoldrick (Eds.), *The changing family life cycle: A framework for family therapy* (pp. 483-513). Boston: Allyn & Bacon.

Martens, R. (1978). *Joy and sadness in children's sports*. Champaign, IL: Human Kinetics.

McElroy, M., & Kirkendall, D. (1980). Significant others and professionalized sport attitudes. *Research Quarterly for Exercise and Sport*, **51**, 645-653.

McGoldrick, M., & Gerson, R. (1985). *Genograms in family assessment*. New York: Norton.

Melnick, M., Dunkelman, N., & Mashiach, A. (1981). Familial factors of sports giftedness among young Israeli athletes. *Journal of Sport Behavior*, **4**, 82-94.

Minuchin, S. (1974). *Families and family therapy*. Cambridge, MA: Harvard University Press.

Minuchin, S., Rosman, B., & Baker, L. (1978). *Psychosomatic families: Anorexia nervosa in context*. Cambridge, MA: Harvard University Press.

Monsaas, J. (1985). Learning to be a world-class tennis player. In B. Bloom (Ed.), *Developing talent in young people* (pp. 211-269). New York: Ballantine Books.

Nichols, W. (1988). *Marital therapy*. New York: Guilford Press.

Odom, S., & Perrin, T. (1985). Coach and athlete burnout. In L. Bunker, R. Rotella, & A. Reilly (Eds.), *Sport psychology* (pp. 213-222). Ithaca, NY: Mouvement.

Ogilvie, B. (1983). Psychology and the elite athlete. *Physician and Sports Medicine*, **11**(4), 195-202.

Passer, M. (1984). Competitive trait anxiety in children and adolescents. In J. Silva & R. Weinberg (Eds.), *Psychological foundations of sport* (pp. 130-144). Champaign, IL: Human Kinetics.

Peck, J., & Manocherian, J. (1989). Divorce and the changing family life cycle. In B. Carter & M. McGoldrick (Eds.), *The changing family life cycle: A framework for* family therapy (pp. 335-371). Boston: Allyn & Bacon.

Rotella, R. (1985). The psychological care of the injured athlete. In L. Bunker, R. Rotella, & A. Reilly (Eds.), Sport psychology (pp. 273-287). Ithaca, NY: Mouvement.

Sage, G. (1980). Parental influence and socialization into sport for male and female intercollegiate athletes. Journal of Sport and Social Issues, 49, 1-13.

Scanlan, T., & Lewthwaite, R. (1986). Social psychological aspects of competition for male youth sport participants: IV. Predictors of enjoyment. Journal of Sport Psychology, 8, 25-35.

Scanlan, T., Stein, G., & Ravizza, K. (1991). An in-depth study of former elite figure skaters: III. Sources of stress. Journal of Sport and Exercise Psychology, 13, 103-119.

Sloane, K. (1985). Home influences on talent development. In B. Bloom (Ed.), Developing talent in young people (pp. 439-476). New York: Ballantine Books.

Smith, S. (1990). Are you a good tennis parent? Tennis, 26(3), 42-44.

CHAPTER 6

THE COACH AND THE TEAM PSYCHOLOGIST: AN INTEGRATED ORGANIZATIONAL MODEL

Frank Gardner, PhD

Gardner Consulting Associates, Inc.

Applied sport psychology has undergone a rapid growth in recent years. Increasing membership in such organizations as the American Psychological Association's (APA) Division 47 (sport and exercise psychology) and the Association for the Advancement of Applied Sport Psychology (AAASP) reflects growth and acceptance of the profession. Sport psychology has experienced both increased recognition in print and electronic media and a rise in public acceptance. Individual athletes and sport organizations at the college, professional, and Olympic levels increasingly seek out the services of specialists in the psychology of sport to provide a variety of services in the sport milieu.

Often these services are sought in reaction to specific situations but with little understanding of what sport psychologists can and cannot do. This lack of understanding often leads to failed experiences when clients work with poorly trained professionals or when the team's or individual athlete's needs and the skills of the professional are poorly matched. Typically, the sport psychology literature has described specific services provided to athletes, either in one-on-one or group (team) format. With few exceptions, however, the literature lacks a discussion of the sport psychologist's overall role in the team setting.

One of my goals in this chapter is to clarify how organizational dynamics in team settings influence the way that psychological services are received and provided. A second goal is to give the psychologist a fuller understanding of the athletic environment and how sport psychology fits into this highly specialized and challenging setting. In addition, I present a model for sport psychologists to become integrated into the overall team structure, including relationships with the coaching staff, sports medicine team, and management personnel.

■ THE CASE OF TEAM BLUE ■

A Division I collegiate team begins the season expecting a conference championship and

147

hoping for a national ranking and success in the postseason tournament. From the outset of preseason training the coach, an intense, aggressive individual, pushes the team hard and repeatedly verbalizes his expectations. The team is young, having 25% freshmen and 25% sophomores. A year earlier the team had won its regular season conference championship and played consistently well, despite a disappointing (and unexpected) postseason tournament loss. A third of the starting lineup was lost to graduation. Halfway through this season, the team was unexpectedly hovering around .500 (win-loss percentage). At this point the head coach consulted with the team psychologist about what he perceived as "significant problems in team chemistry." The coach felt there was an absence of teamwork, a tendency toward finger-pointing, and a passive approach, both in games and practices.

THE SPORT PSYCHOLOGIST IN THE ATHLETIC ENVIRONMENT

The role of the sport psychologist differs markedly from one situation (i.e., team) to another. One has only to read the variety of descriptions of the role psychologists have in different organizations to realize this (Botterill, 1990; Ravizza, 1990; Smith & Johnson, 1990). That a psychologist's role differs across settings should not be surprising, given the diverse backgrounds of sport psychologists (Taylor, 1991). The relatively recent acceptance of sport psychology as a discipline has been hampered by some confusion as to who sport psychologists are and what they actually do.

Unfortunately, the various roles and job responsibilities that some psychologists have developed can reflect more the differences in their backgrounds and training than the needs of the organizations they serve. The danger is that this confusion about *role* often accompanies a lack of clarity about *goal*. Consequently, psychologists in the athletic arena are vulnerable to being seen as unnecessary, inept, and even as creating problems. As the field of sport psychology evolves and as its nature and purposes and its techniques and principles become clearer, this problem should abate. For now, however, we need to address the danger of sport psychology's being dismissed as trendy or superfluous. We can best accomplish this by staying informed of advances in basic psychological knowledge and technique, being aware of team and organizational dynamics, and by remaining cognizant of the job responsibilities of other professionals working alongside of us.

Organizational Dynamics

The athletic environment is highly complex, and a sophisticated understanding of it is critical for the would-be team psychologist's effectiveness. Nevertheless, little attention has been directed toward organizational dynamics awareness in the sport psychology literature. If the goal of organizational fit is attended to properly and ongoing efforts are made at educating athletic personnel about fundamental psychological principles and their relevance to athletic performance, the inevitable consequence will be more effective working relationships and greater respect for the sport psychologist's value.

It is critical that team psychologists understand that they are working in an organization and need to fully comprehend the organization's rules, administrative systems, goals, values, and reporting structure. These organizational dynamics, recently referred to in the business world as corporate or organizational culture (Schein, 1990), are critical to the success or failure of the team psychologist. Further, the psychologist must be aware that the circumstances of entry into the team and the person or people who brought the psychologist on board directly affect the psychologist's place in the group's organizational dynamics. For example, the psychologist whose entry into the team comes via contact with the coach has a different set of organizational issues than the one who is brought in by the general manager/athletic director. In addition, the previous successes and particular personal relationships of the coach or general manager/athletic director are additional elements necessary for a complete understanding of organizational dynamics. Prior experiences (both good and bad) that key personnel have had with sport psychologists further complicate organizational dynamics for the psychologist. Apart from these issues, the team psychologist must become aware of the roles and interactions of upper management, coaching staff, sports medicine team, media personnel, and so forth. Lastly, to fully appreciate the team culture, the psychologist needs to be clear about

- team goals and overall mission,
- relationship of the team to the larger organization,
- sources of particular pressures (e.g., fans, media), and
- history of the team or organization.

Identifying the Client

When working with an athlete in an individual sport, the dynamics involved are fairly simple. The athlete, possibly some family member(s), and quite probably a coach need to be consulted during the intervention. When these individual sports are at the professional level (e.g., tennis, golf), public relations or sport agents might also be involved and also might be consulted on occasion. This chapter's focus, however, will be on team settings. In the team setting, a multitude of people must be considered:

- The individual athletes who comprise the team—anywhere from 12 to upwards of 40, depending on the sport and type of organization (pro, college, etc.)
- A coaching staff comprised of a head coach and a number of assistants
- A sports medicine team consisting of training and physical therapy staff and team physician(s)
- Management, including general manager/athletic director and staff, scouting personnel, and public relations or sport information staff

Everyone's role must be evaluated and understood for the prospective team psychologist to become integrated into the organization. Figure 6.1 shows a sample organizational chart of a professional team. The team psychologist can realistically expect to be involved in three domains noted: sports medicine (directed by the team physician), team performance (directed by the head coach), and scouting and player development (directed by the director of player development).

In addition, the concept of team psychologist has many potential meanings (Halliwell, 1990; Neff, 1990). In some cases it implies working with athletes on the team for the express purpose of performance enhancement. In other situations it includes both performance-enhancement work (often referred to, incorrectly in my view, as educational service), more traditional clinical service (e.g., psychological counseling of non-performance-related issues, such as family problems, psychopathology, etc.), and even involvement in the player selection process (e.g., predraft psychological testing).

Qualities Necessary for Success

In a recent study evaluating the consulting effectiveness of sport psychologists (Gould,

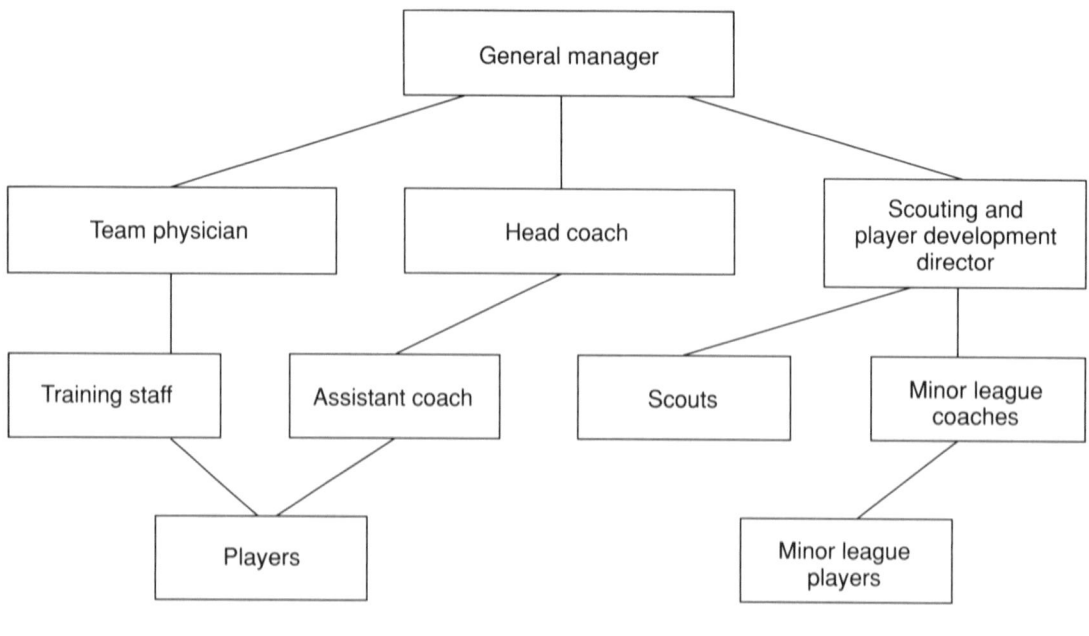

Figure 6.1   An organizational chart for a professional sport team.

Murphy, Tammen, & May, 1991), consultants achieved higher effectiveness ratings when working with individual athletes as opposed to working with teams. Further, consultants themselves reported that working in team situations was more difficult and involved significantly more variables. In addition, when a number of consultant characteristics were rated by coaches, the consultants were given their lowest ratings in ability to fit comfortably into the team environment. The authors suggest that this latter finding might imply a less-than-clearly-defined role for the sport psychologist in American amateur team sports. It might also be reflective of the difficulties in properly matching the skills and interests of the sport psychology consultant to the needs of the client organization. Recent studies have examined the views of coaches and athletes regarding necessary characteristics of effective sport psychologists. Canadian Olympic athletes cited the best sport psychology consultants as those

who were likeable, accessible, flexible, and professionally skilled (Orlick & Partington, 1987). In other words, both strong personal skills and sound mental-training skills were viewed as vital to successful sport psychology consultation. Conversely, poorly rated consultants lacked either of those two broad qualities. Similarly, when Canadian Olympic coaches were polled, highly rated sport psychology consultants were rated as positive, confident, capable of working in the sport environment without being intrusive, practical, and knowledgeable (Partington & Orlick, 1987). Once again, both personal and professional skills were implicated. These coaches identified desired services as mental-skills training with athletes as well as staff–athlete communication enhancement and direct consultation about coaching behaviors.

It has been my experience at the collegiate and professional levels that head coaches look to the sport psychologist for help in better understanding the individual athlete whom the coach needs to motivate and with whom the coach communicates regularly. This information (obtained from psychological assessment, observation, and interpersonal interaction) can allow coaches to more adequately perform their jobs. It has not been my experience after working with many coaches that they readily solicit strategies or techniques for team motivation. Coaches at elite competitive levels have their own methods and strategies for this task that they have developed over the years in keeping with their own personalities and experience. Coaches at lesser competitive levels, however, might have different needs and might turn to the team psychologist to help with numerous coaching issues, including team motivation. Further, assistant coaches often seek out the team psychologist for information that could be of value in their work with athletes. Assistant coaches are often more intimately involved in the nuances of the personalities of individual athletes, because these coaches frequently are given the responsibility of working with either one or a small group of players at a time.

Athletes, in my experience, have generally looked to the team psychologist for a variety of services that have included crisis intervention, psychological counseling, mental-skills training for performance enhancement, and relationship counseling. In keeping with the research findings noted previously, my experience suggests that over time the psychological services that athletes are likely to use most

will be based on both the interpersonal and the professional talents of the psychologist. The conclusion can readily be made that athletes consider as essential elements in effective consultation the trustworthiness of the psychologist and the psychologist's ability to easily fit into the team environment.

A must, however, for those choosing to work in team settings is a positive, professional relationship with the head coach and coaching staff. The development of a positive working relationship must begin with a full understanding of the team coach's roles and responsibilities.

THE COACH: ROLE, IMPACT, AND PRESSURES

Few jobs in sport, particularly professional sport, possess the pressures inherent in coaching. If we compare for a moment the job functions of a team coach to those of a business manager, there are striking similarities (see Figure 6.2). Traditionally, the business manager is seen as being responsible for personnel selection and utilization, personnel development and training, and strategic planning. This translates in the athletic domain into player selection and recruitment, athletic skills training, and game plan preparation and bench coaching. Another aspect

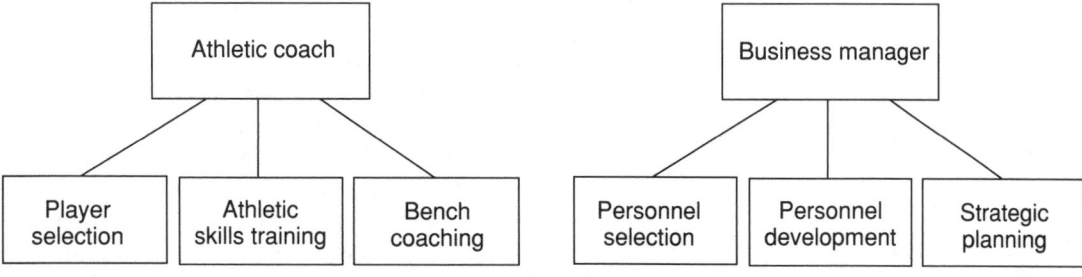

Figure 6.2 Similarities between the responsibilities of an athletic coach and a business manager.

of both jobs is in the development and maintenance of group (team) cohesion, often referred to popularly as chemistry. This is not considered a basic job function of a business manager or athletic coach because it is an indirect activity. That is, group cohesion occurs via a combination of coach and manager behavior, team members' personality mix, and situational variables. We will examine more thoroughly the topic of team cohesion and the role of the coach and psychologist later in this chapter.

Two goals most central to the perceived success of coaches are (a) winning and (b) participant enjoyment and education. The degree to which each one of these primary goals predominates depends on the level of sport participation (i.e., Little League, high school, college Division III, II, I, Olympic, or professional). One can view these two goals as inversely proportional to sport level (see Figure 6.3). As such, the degree to which a coach must focus on fostering enjoyment of sport involvement and is responsible for teaching values and contributing to the athletes' overall development as the primary objective—as opposed to maintaining a primary focus on winning—is similarly inversely proportional.

Some would probably argue that these two goals are not mutually exclusive and in fact can readily coexist—as might be the case in Ivy League sports. As shown in Figure 6.3, there is a point of intersection of these two goals occurring at the college sports level (e.g., Division I, II, or III). Although these two goals can equally coexist to a point, ultimately choices are made; this suggests that one might predominate. For example, Ivy League college teams are at a distinct competitive disadvantage, as they have decided to not offer athletic scholarships. Winning is secondary at these institutions. It is important to note that even as the primary goal of the job changes, the essential job functions of selection, development, and strategic planning remain the same, albeit with different prioritization.

Martens (1987) has a somewhat similar conceptualization. He considers coaching behavior as falling somewhere along a continuum between highly athlete-centered, where a coach places "the highest regard on the people being coached" (p. 11), and highly win-centered, where a coach places "the highest regard on the outcome of competition." In my view a coach sometimes is clear on the fit between primary personal goals and the primary organizational goals (e.g., organizations such as Ivy League or professional sports), and in other circumstances might not be. This incongruity of personal and organizational goals might be due to a poorly developed or poorly communicated vision about the mission of the organization, as is often the case in college sports. Sometimes a coach might not choose to align personal goals with the stated mission of the organization, as is sometimes the case in youth sports. The influence of these primary coaching goals on a coach's cognitive, emotional, and behavioral process is directly related to the concept of coach burnout (to be discussed in depth later in this chapter.)

It should be pointed out that the achievement of one of the two primary goals—

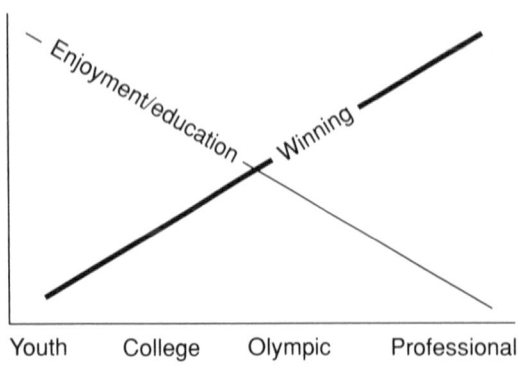

Figure 6.3   Importance at competitive levels.

winning or participant enjoyment and education—ultimately determines the perceived success of the team coach. Next, we must consider the question of which coaching functions contribute to the achievement of the team goal. In answering this question, we once again turn our attention to three general coaching functions: (a) player selection and utilization, (b) skill development, and (c) strategic planning and tactical decision making.

Player Selection

The job function of selection includes both initial selection (or recruitment in the case of college sports) and role determination. When winning is the primary goal, making decisions about team composition is critical. It is not a simple task to select players whose talent (or potential) is at a high enough level, who will fit into a particular style of play, who will interact comfortably with staff, and who can fit in with a particular group of personalities. In some situations (e.g., college sports), this responsibility lies almost exclusively with the coach, as does player utilization and role selection. Role selection involves decisions about playing time and starter–substitute status. At the professional level, player selection is typically the responsibility of the team general manager, often (but not always) with strong input from the coach. Player utilization is clearly the responsibility of the coach at all levels of sport. In situations where participant enjoyment and education is the primary goal, selection might be substantially less important. In youth sports, for example, it is not unusual for all who try out to make the team. Player utilization at this level is often the job function that forces a coach to remain focused on the primary objective. Making sure all players have an opportunity to play—even if doing so leads to a loss—is a difficult challenge for many involved in coaching youth sports.

When winning is the primary focus—in sport as in business—selecting the right people is the first step toward success. Correct selection ultimately simplifies the other tasks of developing both skills and strategic planning. Errors in selection invariably lead to more serious problems down the line. If one looks carefully, what at first glance is often viewed as coaching failure often is actually a failure in adequate player selection.

Athletic Development and Skill Training

Athletic development and skill training is often referred to as teaching. In this function the coach is responsible for developing players' sport-specific skills as well as their capacity to effectively use these skills in game conditions. Drills, practice schedules, and the like are coaching activities that are directed toward enhancing skill development. Included in this conceptualization of the players' skill development is the concept of motivation of players. Being able to get players to put forth maximum effort and to follow the game plan as prescribed is critical to the success of most coaches. Although a full discussion of motivation is well beyond the scope of this chapter, suffice it to say that a coach's effort at motivation has two components. That is, the coach is involved both in activating athletes (i.e., getting them up for athletic performance) and in focusing athletes on a given goal. Sport-specific skill development becomes somewhat less prominent as one moves up competitive levels, whereas efforts at player motivation typically become more central.

Strategic Planning

The last primary job function of the team coach considered here is what the business world calls strategic planning. In the athletic arena, this includes game preparation and analysis, tactical decision making, and so forth. This function remains fairly consistent whether the primary goal is winning or participant enjoyment and education. Of course, the relative importance of this function and thus the pressure coaches feel from their tactical decisions is based on the importance to their organizations of winning.

The nature of the relationship between coach and athlete depends on many factors. What is the primary goal of the organization and coach? Are these goals congruent and are they similarly held by the players? How effective is the coach in performing the basic job functions outlined above?

Does the coach utilize a directive or consensus-seeking style and does this style match correctly with the primary team goal? For example, an organization that holds a primary goal of winning is much more likely to accept (or even require) a more directive coaching style in which the coach is in nearly total control of decision making, whereas an organization that holds participant enjoyment and education as the primary goal might find a directive coaching style less tolerable and might be most comfortable with a coach employing a consensus-seeking coaching style.

How well does the coach understand the personalities of the players? Can the coach respond accordingly? Regardless of a coach's style and personality, the relationship between athlete and coach must be seen as dynamic and highly complex. The coach, in the role of an authority figure (especially for young athletes) must simultaneously

- motivate (i.e., focus the team on clear goals and elicit a consistently high level of intensity in working toward these goals),
- establish clear roles and responsibilities for team members,
- define and maintain team rules and regulations,

- oversee conditioning and injury rehabilitation,
- supervise assistant coaches, and
- be keenly aware of the emotional-behavioral needs, reactions, and problems of players.

An aspect of coach–athlete interactions typically neglected in the sport psychology literature is the athlete's responsibility for the development and maintenance of an adequate relationship with the coach. Although it is universally accepted that successful relationships require effort on the part of all parties involved, the burden for successful coach–athlete relationships is almost always placed exclusively on the shoulders of the coach.

The business world has recognized the duality of boss–subordinate relationships and sport psychology would be wise to incorporate some of the concepts currently used in the business area. For example, in a thoughtful paper written for the *Harvard Business Review*, Gabarro and Kotter (1987) present the notion that boss–subordinate relationships involve a mutual dependence between fallible human beings. They state that although people often place the burden of responsibility on their bosses for the success or failure of their relationships, the fact is that all parties involved need to recognize that both boss and subordinate (i.e., coach and athlete) require the help and cooperation of each other to perform their jobs effectively. Gabarro and Kotter use the term *managing your boss* to describe "the process of consciously working with your superior to obtain the best possible result for you, your boss, and the company" (p. 1).

Having defined the job of team coach and described the complexity of coach–athlete relationships, I now take up the issue of team cohesion.

Team Cohesion

Team cohesion, often popularly referred to as team chemistry, is an issue that all coaches at some time or another must consider. Carron (1982) defines team cohesion as a dynamic process that culminates in a group's tendency to remain united in pursuing its goals and objectives. The two key points in this definition are the phrases *dynamic process* and *united in pursuing goals and objectives.*

In his review of cohesion in sport teams, Carron (1984) suggests that cohesion is a dynamic process because the absolute amount of measurable cohesion fluctuates on an ongoing basis. Many variables appear to influence the development and maintenance of group cohesion. These include team selection, interpersonal attraction or conflict, role formation, acceptance or conflict, coach behavior, and team performance. For example, several studies have suggested that cohesion and performance are interrelated with no unidimensional causative relationship readily inferred (Landers, Wilkinson, Hatfield, & Barber, 1982; Ruder & Gill, 1982).

Studies of work-team effectiveness in industrial-organizational psychology have suggested that the relationship of team cohesion and performance might depend on group norms (Sundstrom, DeMeuse, & Futrell, 1990). Group norms can be defined as standards of work behavior and work output established by team members and managers on the basis of team mission and organizational goals. Stogdill (1972) studied a variety of different work groups and found that work-team cohesion amplified established norms, whether favoring high or low productivity. That is, cohesion can result in enhanced or diminished performance, depending on previously established levels of acceptable work output.

Unity of goal pursuit is also an important phrase in Carron's (1982) definition of team cohesion. Unity of goal pursuit refers to the need for clearly communicated team goals (Zander, 1971) as well as clearly defined individual roles, with the importance of each role in overall team success being understood.

Carron (1984) summarized his exhaustive review of the team cohesion literature with practical suggestions for coaches. These recommendations include

- establishing high norms for productivity through specific, measurable, challenging team goals;
- avoiding, wherever possible, excessively difficult early-season scheduling to promote cohesion via success;
- encouraging activities that enhance social cohesion, intragroup communications, and group identity (e.g., non-sport-related team activities);
- clearly defining individual roles and stressing the importance of those roles to team success; and
- avoiding excessive personnel turnover.

Team cohesion is a natural by-product of team activity and is influenced by factors both within and outside of a coach's direct control. Later in the chapter I will discuss many of these interventions in the context of the case study that was presented earlier. It appears that a coach can be a positive influence in the proper development and maintenance of team cohesion but cannot completely control it. For this reason, I do not list team cohesion here as a primary job function of coaches; rather, it is, at least in part, a consequence of overall coaching behavior.

It has been my experience that at the level of elite-professional team sports, role clarity and team success combine to yield optimal levels of team cohesion (see Figure 6.4). Although players need to understand their roles and how these contribute to ultimate team success, the reality is that elite athletes typically accept a reduced role (e.g., fewer shots, fewer minutes in the game, etc.) only when their team is winning.

Losing breeds unhappiness in several ways. It is difficult to accept the usefulness of a reduced role when you cannot see the

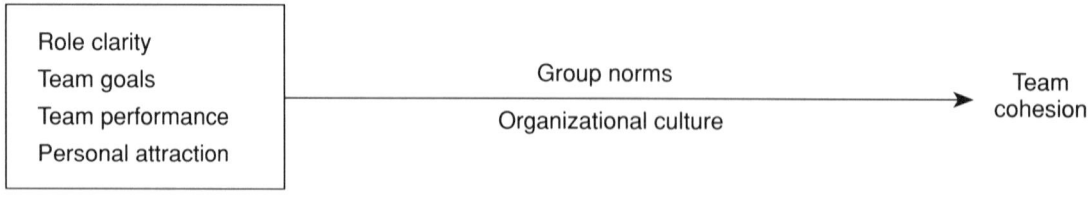

Figure 6.4   Factors affecting team cohesion.

role's leading to ultimate success (i.e., winning). Also, athletes that are competitive by nature naturally believe that the team would perform better if they had a greater role. Lastly, at the professional level athletes are paid for performance. They often (but not always) describe the importance of their roles in winning teams to make a case for higher salaries but cannot do so on losing teams. This increases the pressure for playing time and better statistics. "Playing for numbers," as this is often referred to, tends to have an additional negative impact on team cohesion, as players in losing environments become more and more focused on themselves.

The coach impacts on this process by being the central figure in creating a working environment that either accepts or does not tolerate a deviation from the commitment to team goals. In this environment numbers are viewed only in the context of the achievement of team goals. Thus what is created is an organizational culture that is demanding and challenging (i.e., high-productivity group norms).

In analyzing the job of team coach, we can draw the conclusion that success requires a high degree of sport-specific knowledge, analytic skills, interpersonal communication skills, an awareness of the differences between individual players, and a sensitivity to players' needs and feelings. In addition, the ability to create a vision that the team can strive for is of paramount importance (i.e., the ability to see how individual skills can connect in creating a cohesive team, thus

leading to an end product that achieves the established organizational goal). The coach must face the demands from management and administration, the particular requirements for successful performance in the chosen sport, and the emotional-behavioral reactions of individual players. Add to this equation the pressures typically found in high-level competitive athletics (professional, Division I collegiate, Olympic, etc.), such as fan and media pressure, and the job becomes even more difficult. It is therefore not surprising that the issue of coach burnout is often raised in high-level competitive sport.

Coach Burnout

Burnout is a catchword typically used to describe a person's reaction to chronic stress (Freudenberger, 1980). The pressures of coaching at an elite level, including organizational demands, constant expectation to win, frequent travel, maintenance of complex interpersonal relations, and the constant need for attention to a wide variety of detail, place great physical and psychological demands on any person working in this profession.

Smith (1986) brings together research from several areas and discusses the causes, nature, and consequences of burnout within a cognitive-affective model of stress. Taking essentially a social-learning perspective, Smith discusses how interactive situational, cognitive, physiologic, and behavioral components interact in stress and burnout. He places particular attention on an examination of burnout in the athletic arena, although the issue of coach burnout is not a direct focus. Smith suggests that burnout includes physical, mental, and behavioral components and occurs in response to a complex interaction between situational and personal characteristics. He further suggests that the most notable characteristic of burnout is a behavioral withdrawal from previously enjoyable pursued activity.

Burnout also has been described as including emotional exhaustion, depersonalization, and perceived lack of personal accomplishment (Caccese & Mayerberg, 1984). Research has implicated situational variables, such as organizational demands, role incongruence, and lack of social support (Shinn, Rosario, Morch, & Chestnut, 1984). Less attention has been paid to the role of individual (personality) characteristics, such as frustration tolerance, trait anxiety levels, and the like.

In an attempt to examine dispositional (i.e., personality), cognitive, and situational predictors of coach burnout within Smith's model, Vealey and associates (1992) studied 848 high-school coaches who completed self-report questionnaires. Trait anxiety emerged as the strongest predictor of burnout, although perception of role and reward were also predictive. The authors concluded that both dispositional and cognitive factors can be more predictive of burnout than situational and behavioral factors, thus offering some support for Smith's model.

Lastly, considering the literature as a whole, there has been a lack of systematic examination of the scope and magnitude of coach burnout, so this area appears to be fertile ground for future empirical study.

In attempting to understand coach burnout, Dale and Weinberg (1989), in one of the few empirical studies in this area, found that coaches exhibiting a giving, other-oriented, or considerate style of leadership scored higher in frequency and intensity of emotional exhaustion and depersonalization than those coaches displaying an initiating-structuring style of leadership. If this study is viewed as in the context of the winning–participation and education dimension of primary team goal noted earlier, it can be hypothesized that the high-school and college coaches utilized for this study were primarily focused on the participation end of the spectrum, and thus the emotional needs of their players were a high priority. As such, the coaching style utilized might have been particularly draining.

Capel, Sisley, and Desertrain (1987) studied the relationship in coach burnout between role ambiguity and role conflict. They found that although there was a statistically significant relationship between these variables, it accounted for only 14% of total variance. They did, however, suggest that role ambiguity and conflict can be reduced, thereby lowering the probability of coach burnout. Minimization of role ambiguity and conflict might be achieved by delineating the goals of the organization and the standards by which the coach would ultimately be evaluated.

In a study that directly asked 93 high-school and college coaches to describe the most stressful aspects of their jobs, nearly 50% listed player disrespect. Approximately 20% also listed not being able to "reach" their players, that is, not being able to effectively communicate with them (Kroll, 1982). It is noteworthy that 70% of those factors noted by these coaches as being major job stressors are issues relating to the coach–athlete relationship. Only 13% of the factors noted were related to performance issues.

The overview of the job of team coach presented here reveals numerous responsibilities, great pressures, and, from the perspective of the sport psychologist, many areas in which psychological expertise can be of value. However, before a coach can utilize these skills and talents, the psychologist must first fit comfortably into the team environment. In essence, what the psychologist can do is only part of the equation; knowing when and how to offer expertise, that is, knowing how the coach goes about the job, is the other often more crucial variable. Developing sound consulting skills and maintaining an awareness of the psychology of organizations are of paramount importance for the would-be team psychologist. An example of these pressures leading to coach burnout and an approach to intervention can be found in a case study presented later in this chapter.

THE TEAM PSYCHOLOGIST: ROLE DEVELOPMENT

Sport psychologists who desire to work in a team setting must first recognize that in many respects they are on foreign soil. The athletic community (as has been pointed out to me on numerous occasions) has survived for many decades without the need for psychologists. The first task of the psychologist, then, is to convince the organization that (a) applied sport psychology is a legitimate field that can make a real contribution to the achievement of organizational goals and (b) that the psychologist can comfortably fit into the team setting and not be a star-struck person who merely wants to be seen associating with athletes (especially those at the professional level).

Athletic Personnel Perceptions

There appear to be two components to the reluctance of athletic personnel to readily accept psychologists as having a useful contribution to make to the athletic organization. One is basically a lack of knowledge. Athletic personnel frequently do not see psychologists apart from their mental health–psychotherapy function and thus can see no role in sports for psychologists. If (and this is a big if) psychologists understand the sports world, if they can explain logically and without jargon the role of mental factors in athletic performance, if they are knowledgeable and experienced in the particular techniques of mental-skills training, if they are adept at functioning in an out-of-office consulting role and are able to work in the athletic milieu— often without suit, tie, and couch, going to athletes rather than having athletes come to them—then, and only then, do psychologists have a chance to be accepted and valued. The second component relates to the reluctance of athletic personnel, especially at elite and professional levels, to have excessive numbers of people involved with the team. There is often a sense of organizational paranoia as to which, why, and how people become involved with their team. Trust must be developed gradually. It must be pointed out here that as it relates to psychology, this organizational guardedness is particularly strong. The reason for this is understandable. Sports personnel lump all people who are licensed as psychologists, claim to be psychologists, infer themselves to be psychologists, or use titles such as *mental-training consultant*, *performance-enhancement specialist*, and so forth, into one group: psychologists. Many people in these groups are either improperly trained (and thus are at best ineffective and at worst harmful), or make outrageous claims (e.g., guarantee that they can predict who will be injured, or who will become an all-star). As such, professionals legally using the title *psychologist* must prove both their professionalism and their capacity to function in a team setting at a level often beyond that of other professionals. It also appears to be true that the connotation of the sport psychologist as a shrink is still widely held in the sport world, although this appears to be slowly changing.

Functioning in the Athletic Environment

How do psychologists enter and thrive in this seemingly hostile environment? Psychologists must first recognize that their role will in all likelihood evolve gradually and steadily over time as trust in their professional and interpersonal competence rises. As they spend more time around the team and are gradually seen as a natural part of the team, the likelihood of effective utilization increases. It is important to understand that a team is very much like an extended family; outsiders can be welcomed, but only time allows them to be fully accepted into the family. The impact of the psychologist attempting to do "too much, too soon" before the team has accepted the psychologist both personally and professionally can be negative to the long-term relationship with the organization. It is wise to view the development of a program of psychological service to a sport team as an evolutionary process rather than a revolutionary event. Even in the best of all situations, psychologists must remember that their roles are ever changing.

This evolutionary process is not necessarily a simple linear progression. Changes in administration and coaching staff can alter (or even end) psychologists' roles, suddenly and through no fault of their own. This is a fact of life in athletics. Team psychologists evolve from unproven rookies to contributing veterans over time. Their own experiences in this evolution can allow them to understand the hopes and frustrations of athletes, who must go through a similar process. Patience and an understanding that two steps forward might be followed by one step backward is essential. Correctly reading team readiness for advances in the role and responsibilities of the psychologist is critical.

To positively impact on this evolutionary process, sport psychologists must first be honest with themselves about whether or not they possess the necessary training, skills, and knowledge to function in this environment. As well, sport psychologists must be honest with the organization regarding skills, goals, and so forth. In a multidisciplinary field that has itself had some controversy over issues of credentialing, competence, and training (Brown, 1982; Gardner & Heyman, 1982; Silva, 1989), it is especially important that the athletic organization understand from the outset what the psychologist can and cannot do.

Merging Educational and Clinical Functions

I must stress one important point from my own experiences working at the professional level. Athletic personnel for the most part do not distinguish between educational and clinical sport psychologists. As such, there is an expectation that psychologists will be able to deal with not only issues relating to athletic performance, but also clinical issues such as family problems, bereavement and grief, depression, and so forth. If, by nature of training, practitioners of sport psychology cannot ethically, legally, or morally provide such services, they must make that clear from the beginning of employment or risk appearing dishonest or incompetent at best or negligent at worst. The role of a new team psychologist must of course be developed gradually in cooperation with administration and upper management, the coaching staff, the sports medicine team, and player personnel. Lack of clarity about the role of the team psychologist will inevitably lead to a variety of problems:

- Perceived failure of the team psychologist to "get the job done"
- Mistrust by players or staff
- Lack of true responsibility (thus blocking real opportunity)

- A perception that the psychologist has overstepped boundaries and created unnecessary problems for the team.

Defining the Job Function

The team psychologist role can best be conceptualized as an internal consultant. In this regard, my experiences are quite similar to those described by Murphy (1988). Murphy suggests that activities of the team psychologist are broad, involve numerous personnel, and are often difficult to categorize as educational or clinical. Interventions are often brief, informal, and intense. As a team consultant, the psychologist comes to be seen as the primary resource about human behavior, especially relating but not limited to sport. The team psychologist is a full member of the organization who functions as a professional with knowledge and skill that come to bear on a wide range of issues involving the entire scope of organizational personnel. Further, by seeing oneself as an internal consultant and in making an effort to make one's knowledge available to all, the team psychologist cannot easily be cast into the roles of management, coach, trainer, and so forth. This creates a unique positioning that allows for entry and availability all along the personnel continuum with full trust and confidence.

The internal consultant role fosters a positive relationship with all levels of organizational personnel. For example, the coaching staff can utilize the psychologist's knowledge while recognizing that players, administration, and the sports medicine team can also receive valuable service. Thus all members of all subgroups see the psychologist interacting with members of all other subgroups without fear or distrust. The psychologist is expected to consult with all levels of the organization openly and honestly. In establishing this role of internal consultant, issues such as confidentiality must be clearly defined and communicated to everyone early in the consultation process. This important issue will be discussed in greater detail later in this chapter.

The team psychologist potentially has numerous job functions and should have the position's role and job description defined based on personal training and the needs of the organization. The specific services provided by the team psychologist might include psychological testing, performance-enhancement counseling, relationship–team development work, clinical services, and other general consultative services. I will now briefly describe these various services, including to whom the service is most useful, the goal(s) of the service, the role of the coach in the service, the specialized knowledge and training that is required, and the potential obstacles and pitfalls.

THE TEAM PSYCHOLOGIST: SERVICES PROVIDED

One of the most controversial areas of applied sport psychology is the appropriate use of psychological testing. A complete discussion of psychological testing in sport is well beyond the scope of this chapter, and thoughtful discussions have previously been undertaken (Nideffer, 1981; Silva, 1984). Psychological testing has numerous functions in the sport world. Problem identification (i.e., assessment) and intervention planning are often aided by the use of psychometric instruments, such as the Sixteen Personality Factor Questionnaire (Cattell, Eber, & Tatsuoka, 1980), the Test of Attentional and Interpersonal Style (Nideffer, 1976), the Competitive State Anxiety Inventory-2 (Martens, Burton, Vealey, Bump, & Smith, 1990), and the Psychological Skills Inventory (Mahoney, Gabriel, & Perkins, 1987), to name a few.

Generally speaking, psychological testing used in conjunction with interview and behavioral observations can provide useful information for the team psychologist in developing a full understanding of interpersonal

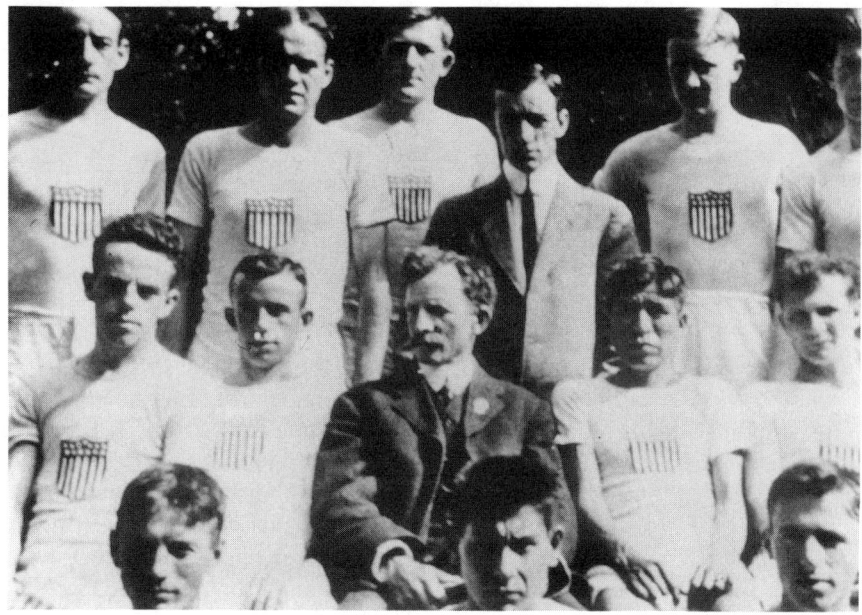

Courtesy USOC

dynamics, individual personality structure, and mental-skills development of player personnel. The information obtained from psychometric instruments can also be used in helping athletes more completely understand the rationale for various intervention efforts. For example, if the team psychologist determines that a player referred for inconsistent performance is experiencing exceptionally high levels of precompetitive anxiety and tends to readily lose necessary attentional focus during big games, it is often useful for the psychologist to see those results psychometrically, not only to possibly corroborate a hypothesis but also to objectively present conclusions to the athlete. As such, the suggested intervention, possibly relaxation training, mental rehearsal, and attention-control training, appear more rational to the athlete.

Although this use of psychological testing has benefits for both team psychologist and athlete, it can also be valuable to the coaching staff and the sports medicine team in allowing them to better understand their players and avoid misconceptions. For example, it can be helpful for medical personnel to recognize the need to more carefully monitor an athlete's injury rehabilitation in cases where the athlete tends toward a somewhat undisciplined approach to rules, structure, and so forth.

Similarly, it is not unusual for an athlete who has some difficulty in attentional focus to be misperceived as being lazy, disinterested, or nonmotivated. Providing a coaching staff with feedback about a player's psychological makeup (i.e., personality) and psychological skill strengths and deficits allows for a more accurate reading of the player and thus aids in coach-athlete relationship development. This team building function of psychological assessment has been described by nearly all the coaches I have worked with as the most useful aspect of having a sport psychologist on board. The testing of team personnel, with feedback first given to the individual players and later to the coaching staff, has been consistently valued by all participants and has consistently had a positive impact. A detailed example of the use of psychological testing in this manner is provided in a case-study presentation later in this chapter.

A few words of caution are necessary concerning the use of testing. First, only licensed psychologists are ethically, morally, and in most places legally able to administer and interpret most psychological tests. This fact is recognized by AAASP in its certification guidelines. Second, any psychologist providing this service should possess substantial specialized training and experience in the particular instruments being used and should have extensive experience in presenting test results to clients. Menu or simplistic score-by-score descriptions of test results or jargon-filled feedback are professionally unacceptable and in fact have contributed to negative attitudes about psychological testing in sports. Further, failure to fully educate the people receiving the feedback as to the nature, uses, and abuses of such information severely compromises the utility of the instruments and the function of assessment itself. The instruments used in psychological assessment often receive a great deal of criticism, whereas the fact that professionals often misuse the instruments typically receive very little. Some practitioners of sport psychology have maintained that athletes are "uncomfortable" about taking psychological tests (Halliwell, 1990). Some authors have suggested that the data obtained from psychological tests are unnecessary (Ravizza, 1990), and in some manner the administration of these instruments might interfere with the development of a personal relationship with players (Dorfman, 1990). Although I believe most people are uncomfortable with the thought of having their psyches explored, it has been my experience that players have not only accepted psychological assessment (if properly presented and utilized), but also that most players have been open to follow-up discussions about the results and their performance and interpersonal implications. Further, it has been my experience that these initial one-on-one feedback sessions are often the first close interaction between team psychologist and player. The sessions allow not only for relevant test results to be discussed but also for the psychologist and athlete to discuss numerous other issues—including the role of the sport psychologist. Thus this process allows for the beginning of both a personal and professional relationship. An adequate relationship between athlete and psychologist requires not only this type of one-on-one contact but also the opportunity for the psychologist to demonstrate professional skill and an approachable personality.

If the psychologist has strong skills in test administration and interpretation and fully understands the numerous issues surrounding test interpretation (Nideffer, 1981), psychometric instruments, particularly personality assessment inventories, are reliable and valid predictors of human behavioral characteristics. If used inappropriately for tasks for which they were not designed, such as predicting a player's likelihood of achieving all-star performance levels or of being injured, they are highly inaccurate (Davis, 1991). It is important to remember that these instruments were not designed to predict performance directly; they were designed for and are effective in describing and thus predicting normal human behavior. It is true that these tests are sometimes used as part of a selection process for professional teams, for example, prior to the yearly entry draft of college- or high-school-age players into the professional ranks. The use of personality tests for this purpose is not unlike testing often performed by psychologists in the business world as part of a corporate screening and selection process. Once again, the important fact to realize here is that the instruments should not be used to directly predict future athlete performance (although it is conceivable that empirical studies will one day make this feasible), but rather to predict how a person is likely to fit into a particular team, the likely interaction with particular coaches, and likely behaviors in a variety of situations (e.g., how athletes might best be motivated, how they are likely to handle criticism, how they are best disciplined, their likelihood of seeking leadership roles, their typical responses to frustration, etc.). This information can then be integrated into a selection process that includes scouting reports, face-to-face interviews, direct observation, and the feedback of former coaches, not unlike the typical selection process utilized in the business world.

An informal form of psychological assessment is often undertaken by scouts who provide reports describing athletic behavior and inferring personality variables such as dedication, heart, mental toughness, and so forth. Formal objective assessment allows for a more complete and accurate understanding of people who have already had their personalities informally evaluated.

The information obtained from psychological testing does not directly predict athletic performance, but is related to numerous performance-relevant characteristics and thus has value to the selection process.

Performance-Enhancement Counseling and Psychological-Skills Training

The function of the team psychologist most typically associated with the field of sport psychology and most often inquired about by students and interested professionals at conferences is performance-enhancement intervention, often referred to as psychological- or mental-skills training. Techniques used in athletic performance enhancement have been thoroughly discussed elsewhere (Williams, 1986), and an in-depth examination of these techniques is well beyond this chapter's scope. The goals of these techniques are typically to help people develop their athletic skills or use existing skills more effectively. These techniques are presented using a psychoeducational intervention model. Skills such as muscle relaxation, attention control, visualization and mental rehearsal, goal setting, and cognitive-control methods are systematically taught as part of a skill-training process. How performance-enhancement counseling and psychological-skills training is administered in a team setting varies across teams, but generally is provided in a lecture-educational type approach typically involving a group of players or in individual one-on-one sessions as needed.

As the team personnel begin to know the psychologist personally and begin to understand the concept of mental-skills training for performance enhancement, players will begin to openly discuss performance-related issues. These discussions are most often conducted in an informal manner, often just prior to or immediately following practice. These discussions may well make use of results previously obtained from psychological testing and will often lead to more formal performance-enhancement counseling. The coaches that I have worked with at first simply tolerated such interventions (it must be recognized that nothing is done with player personnel without full approval by the head coach). These individual sessions occurred when either a player sought out the aid of this psychologist or when a member of the coaching staff believed that an athlete's performance difficulties were frustrating or perplexing enough that they sought out psychological consultation. Later, as the personal relationship between head coach and myself matured and the staff appreciation and respect for the value of a sport psychologist evolved, the coaches began to allow more independence in working with players on my own initiative and finally to incorporate a series of structured mental-skills lectures during training camp. It cannot be stressed too strongly that without the support of the coaching staff, players are not likely to utilize the team psychologist in a performance-enhancement role. Once players see that the coaches value mental-skills training—possibly to the point of even using the language of sport psychology in their own interactions with players—they can feel free to consult the team psychologist without fear of negative reaction. Similarly, the longer the psychologist is involved with the team and the more the psychologist is perceived as a natural part of the environment, the greater the likelihood of adequate utilization of the psychologist's services.

Relationship Enhancement

Maintaining adequate relationships with players is critical to a coach's job. Using information from behavioral observation and psychological testing, the team psychologist can offer insights to the coach to more fully understand players' daily behaviors, motivational needs, and how they are likely to react to specific coaching techniques (e.g., public criticism, positive feedback). This information allows the coaching staff to proactively attend to the relationship with their players rather than to react with postproblem attention. One coach remarked that there is no information that he receives from this process that wouldn't become known to him over time but that the advantage is in being able to avoid the mistakes, confrontations, and misunderstandings that often lead to that knowledge. From this coach's perspective, the team psychologist gave him information that was easily used in enhancing his ability to effectively communicate with his players.

Similarly, understanding player and staff personalities allows the team psychologist to appropriately counsel players in developing effective communication with the coaching staff. Discussions as to how, where, and when

to communicate issues and concerns have been reported as valuable by numerous players. In addition, consultation about relationship issues between players has become necessary at times. The team psychologist can have an active role in promoting team chemistry by being a catalyst for effective communication between team members. It is important for would-be team psychologists to recognize that it is not their job to communicate roles, motivate, or impart strategy. Instead it is the psychologist's job to clarify thoughts and feelings and to aid in promoting open lines of communication. In keeping with the conceptualization of coach–athlete relationships noted previously, the team psychologist can aid in their developing a mutual understanding of each other as people as well as in recognizing their mutual dependence. This role is fraught with potential obstacles, and psychologists must continually be aware of the limitations of their roles. Prior organizational consulting experience is highly recommended for persons seeking to do team-building work in an athletic setting. Those interested in team building in organizational settings are referred to the article on effective work teams by Sundstrom and colleagues in the *American Psychologist* (1990), and the text *Building Productive Teams* by Varney (1990).

Clinical Services

The area of responsibility that psychologists are most closely identified with is that of clinical service. The identification, assessment, and treatment of clinical mental health issues such as anxiety, depression, family dysfunction, and so forth, are typical roles for psychologists and might well be expected of team psychologists if within their scope of training. In many respects, these job responsibilities are much like those found in the provision of an employee assistance program (EAP) in which short-term clinical services

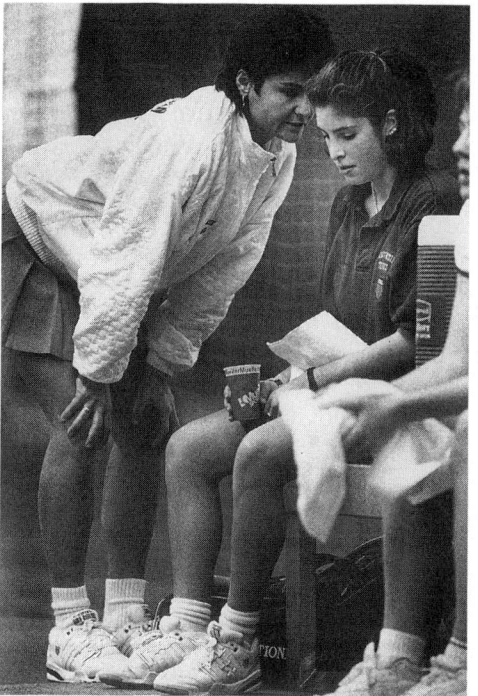

Courtesy University of Wisconsin Women's Sports Information

are readily available to members of the organization (and often their families).

This role may not, however, be required or desired in all settings. For example, in university settings, clinical needs of student athletes or staff are typically addressed by the university health counseling center. The team psychologist in these instances will serve to identify problem areas and assist in referring the person to the proper organizational resource. Further, the team psychologist might at times be required to make outside referrals. Referrals are usually required, for example, in situations requiring intensive or long-term care of drug or alcohol abuse. When outside referrals are necessary, the team psychologist would likely be required by the organization to coordinate or monitor outside treatment efforts. This job function is similar to that of the team physician, who often needs to refer to outside medical specialists while remaining actively involved in the ongoing medical care of the athlete.

In addition to the traditional role of psychological counseling for an athlete (or coach's) mental health needs, clinical services offered by the team psychologist should include active involvement with the sports medicine team concerning psychological aspects of athletic injuries. Injury to athletes is as much a part of sport participation as winning and losing. Psychological reactions to injury range from mild to severe. Variables such as premorbid personality factors, psychological coping mechanisms, severity of injury, level of athletic competition, playing status (starter or substitute, freshman or senior, etc.), and available social support, to name but a few, contribute to the intensity and direction of emotional-behavioral response to injury.

Before reviewing the basic clinical activities that sport psychologists employ in treating injured athletes, it is once again imperative to point out that the team psychologist's role and acceptance by the team will determine actual utilization. In the role of internal psychological consultant, the psychologist must effectively communicate to members of the sports medicine team, coaches, and athletes the psychological factors and reactions involved in the rehabilitation of the athlete's injuries (May & Sieb, 1987; Rotella & Heyman, 1986; Wiese & Weiss, 1987). This allows athletic trainers, coaches, physicians, and even teammates to recognize both expected and extreme psychological reactions to injury.

As the team psychologist becomes intertwined in the day-to-day functioning of the organization, ongoing contact between the athletic trainer and the psychologist will occur. It is most often trainers who not only deal with physical injuries but are first to notice mood and behavioral fluctuations and even hear about significant events in the athletes' personal lives. It is in close cooperation with the training staff that the psychologist truly becomes embedded in the fabric of the team.

As this relationship evolves, the psychologist becomes more intimately involved with the ongoing psychological care of the athlete. In reality, only through regular, direct involvement with the team physician will the psychologist truly be seen as a valued member of the sports medicine team. And only as a member of the sports medicine team can the psychologist be consistently involved, in a structured and meaningful manner, in the psychological care of the injured athlete.

As psychologists, we must again remember that we are in many respects outsiders in the broad area of sports medicine. Our knowledge base regarding psychological aspects of injury and rehabilitation is not typically well known in sports medicine circles. Thus we must be careful not to imply that all answers are within our discipline or that we can somehow predict who will be injured or that we can speed the recovery time for every injured athlete. We must recognize that injury treatment is primarily a physical–medical endeavor, and that psychology can make a unique contribution by offering useful adjunctive services in a consultative model. This will occur, however, only if the professionals offering such services are respected for their knowledge, skill, and interpersonal acumen.

Regular feedback to the trainer or team physician enhances the credibility of the psychologist and further develops trusting collegial relationships. The team psychologist can offer many specific services to the injured athlete and the sports medicine team:

- Assessment of psychological status (Lynch, 1988)
- Pain-control techniques (Singer & Johnson, 1987)
- Cognitive-behavioral interventions for medical treatment adherence and compliance (Meichenbaum & Turk, 1987)

- Stress-management and psychological counseling (i.e., psychological first aid)
- Imagery training and mental practice for facilitating the return to competition (Rotella & Heyman, 1986)
- Facilitation of social-team support (Wiese & Weiss, 1987)

By and large the clinical activities noted here focus on the maintenance and development of the athlete's psychological well-being. It must be pointed out that on occasion coaches or other staff or support personnel have psychological needs that might fit into the team psychologist's domain. There are, as noted previously, many pressures on coaches and administrators in competitive sports. As the previous discussion of coach burnout suggests, coaches and even administrative personnel are prone to severe emotional-behavioral reactions. Team psychologists can, if their personal relationship with the coach has matured properly, offer psychological support and counsel—typically in an informal manner—during periods of intense stress.

Whether or not this service can prevent burnout is essentially an empirical question. However, my own experience suggests that this support function can often allow an appropriate venting of built-up emotions and might not only aid in the coach's psychological well-being but also help insure continued team harmony by removing the need for the coach to act out his emotional reactions onto the team.

General Consultative Services

On occasion the team psychologist is asked to become involved in issues that are time limited and arise out of special circumstances. Examples of these might be

- crisis-intervention work immediately following a personal setback or a significant life event that has struck a team member and thus impacts the entire team;

- team meetings in the midst of a lengthy slump;
- helping to prepare a team to play against an opponent that it has not defeated for several years;
- helping to prepare motivational videos before the playoffs; and
- offering input as to the role of different practice scenarios on intrateam competitiveness and conflict.

Although the team psychologist can confront these issues with some aid from the literature, they often require creativity and a close working relationship with the coaching staff so that interventions can be developed by consensus. My experience suggests that early in the psychologist's tenure with the team, these issues will not be brought up by the staff. Only as the relationship matures does the staff become comfortable enough to ask for input about these matters. Being asked to become involved in such team issues is arguably a true measure of the psychologist's acceptance by and value to the coaching staff.

This overview of the services provided by the team psychologist presents many opportunities for the psychologist who is both trained in sport psychology and aware of the athletic environment (culture) to make a meaningful contribution. What must be stressed, however, is that the focal point of an athletic team is the coach. It is therefore critical that the team psychologist recognize that the relationship with this person to a large extent determines how or if the psychologist will operate. It safely can be said that without a positive, trusting relationship with the head coach, one cannot fulfill a team psychologist role.

Keeping the coach informed of your activities is necessary. This does not necessarily mean sharing all details of all interactions.

Rather, letting the coach know that players are seeking you out for mental-skills training, or that you are in contact with the assistant coach regarding a particular player, or letting the coach know that you are in contact with the sports medicine team regarding an injured player, or simply asking the coach if there is anything or anyone that you can help with goes a long way in building an exceptional working relationship.

There is one last point in this regard. I strongly suggest that new programs or ideas that the team psychologist would like to initiate, for example, the preparation and use of personal highlight videos, be discussed prior to training camp and thus implemented (if agreed upon) early in the year. Coaches at high competitive levels are not likely to initiate new ideas once their season gets under way, due in large part to the overall pressure and enormous day-to-day detail of coaching a team.

ETHICAL CONSIDERATIONS

The team psychologist has many aspects of day-to-day work that require careful attention to ethical principles. First and foremost is the use of the title *psychologist*. The issue of who can legally use the title of psychologist and what background sport psychologists must possess are complex issues that have been discussed in detail elsewhere (Gardner, 1991; Silva, 1989). Suffice it to say that those professionals wishing to function as team psychologists must first face the issue of their own training and credentials. Those practitioners of applied sport psychology that qualify to use the title *psychologist* under state and provincial law are already obligated to understand and follow the American Psychological Association's (APA) ethical standards (1981). Those practitioners who cannot legally use the title *psychologist* and whose educational backgrounds are for the most part in the areas of physical education and sport science have at present no clear ethical guidelines to follow, other than those of APA. Currently, the Association for the Advancement of Applied Sport Psychology (AAASP) is working toward constructing an ethical standard for all those classified by the organization as certified consultants. In understanding how ethical considerations impact on the applied sport psychologist working for athletic teams, I will briefly describe a number of areas mentioned in APA's ethical standards and comment on their relationship to the services previously reported.

Competence

The issue of competence in the area of sport psychology has been addressed in some detail (Gardner, 1991; Silva, 1989; Taylor, 1991). At this point in time it is the responsibility of psychologists seeking involvement in team sports to insure that they possess the necessary knowledge and skill to effectively work in the athletic environment. It is my opinion that organizations like AAASP must take a greater role in establishing guidelines on what training is required to offer what service.

At present the burden of determining competence falls squarely on the shoulders of the practitioner. One caution: In our society it is not unrealistic to believe that should professionals and their respective organizations disregard the need to carefully define issues of competence, the courts ultimately will be asked to make those determinations. I would suggest special caution to those non-psychologically-trained practitioners who offer treatment (i.e., counseling) of clinical problems masked as sport performance problems or utilize psychological (psychometric) assessment as part of their job descriptions.

Public Statements

Essentially, the principle on public statements requires psychologists to honestly and accurately represent their qualifications. This relates to competence, in that initially the psychologist naturally will try to sell services to the team that the psychologist wishes to work for. In all selling there is a temptation to focus on strengths and ignore limitations. Over time the team in question will undoubtedly look to the psychologist for most of the services mentioned in this chapter, so accurate presentation of one's limitations becomes critical to ethical practice. In addition, outlandish claims such as those mentioned earlier involving almost clairvoyant capacity to predict status, injury, and so forth, run contrary to this general principle.

Professional Relationships

As noted throughout this chapter, the team psychologist is required to interact with a variety of staff members responsible for a number of job functions. Maintaining these professional relationships by respecting boundaries and understanding roles and responsibilities of all members of an organization becomes an ethical mandate. Communicating regularly and following designated lines of administrative reporting similarly fall into this category.

Welfare of the Consumer and Confidentiality

Welfare of the consumer and confidentiality are presented as one principle, because in the athletic setting they in effect speak to the same issue. That is, psychologists working in team settings (or any organizational setting for that matter) must make clear to all parties involved the nature of their responsibilities, the purpose and nature of all assessment, treatment, and training procedures, and the limits (if any) of confidentiality. The role of team psychologist presented in this chapter places great demands on the psychologist to adequately fulfill a complex consultative role and simultaneously adhere to these ethical principles.

To walk this line, the psychologist must use judgment and forethought in establishing clear guidelines for all parties involved (administration, coaching staff, and athletes) at the onset of employment. Rules governing confidentiality in psychologist–athlete interactions must be established and understood by everyone involved. It then becomes the responsibility of the psychologist to insure that these rules are respected. What information is the coach going to get about performance-enhancement counseling with athletes or the psychological state of athletes following injury? When utilizing psychological assessment as part of team building and coach-athlete–relationship enhancement, the question arises as to who gets feedback, in what sequence, and toward what end. For example, when working with organizations, I typically establish a format that allows psychometric test feedback to first be given to the athlete. At that time, our discussion includes what information will be provided to the coach in addition to why and how it will be presented. This information is discussed fully until the athlete is comfortable with it. Then and only then do I review the testing material with the coach(es). It should be pointed out that these rules are explained to everyone before initiating the testing–feedback process. Despite the best intentions of the psychologist, not all potential ethical dilemmas can be foreseen. In such circumstances professional judgment, keeping in mind the basic ethical principles, allows the psychologist to effectively and professionally respond to any situation. I have found in my own experience that from top to bottom, athletic organizations respect the psychologist who incorporates ethical concerns into everyday practice. Honest, ethical, and professional behavior leads to trust and respect, which in turn lead to further acceptance.

INTERVENTION IN THE CASE OF TEAM BLUE

As a regular staff member, the team psychologist had an advantage of being involved in the everyday activities of Team Blue before the request for consultation by its coach.

The team psychologist had conducted a series of mental-skills-training lectures in preseason and conducted individual personality assessment utilizing the Sixteen Personality Factor Questionnaire and the Test of Attentional and Interpersonal Style. Detailed feedback, as previously outlined in this chapter, was provided to each athlete during the season. During the season about one third of the team chose to work individually on mental-skills training, one third consulted with the psychologist intermittently, and one third did not avail themselves of sport psychology consultation. Following much discussion with the coaching staff, individual meetings were held with each player, to whom confidentiality was guaranteed.

Based on these meetings, the following issues and problems became apparent:

• A significant portion of the team could not clearly identify their role on the team, did not feel as though they were significant contributors, and were more fearful of making errors than achieving success.

• The freshmen (a significant portion of the team), all former high-school stars used to receiving much attention and playing time, were adjusting poorly to their changed playing status.

• The team members felt they had failed to achieve the coach's preseason goals to that point, their perceptions of a failed season creating high levels of anxiety.

• The team generally felt little pride in its identity and members were more socially isolated from each other than is usual in college teams.

Without identifying particular players, these general themes were presented to the coach, as the athletes knew would be done. It was suggested that a series of meetings between the players and team psychologist be held to begin both a dialogue addressing issues of personal responsibility and commitment and an active effort to use goal setting and imagery training to prepare for practice sessions as well as games.

It was also recommended to the coach that roles and responsibilities might be communicated once again and presented more individually (the coach recalled that roles were discussed once in an early-season team meeting). In addition, to address the issue of mistake-avoidance behavior, it was suggested that discussion of season-long goals (outcome goals) at least temporarily be replaced by individual and team game-performance goals.

Lastly, it was suggested that some social non-sport-related activity involving the entire team be planned (preferably in a situation where the team could be introduced publicly) to help promote a greater social cohesion and sense of team. It was also advised that assistant coaches spend more time with the freshmen to aid in their adjustment to the realities of college sports.

After much discussion, often centering on how these suggestions fit into the coach's philosophy of coaching, all suggestions were implemented. The team psychologist and all players met in several group sessions, the coach arranged for individual meetings between himself and players for role clarification, goals were established on a game-by-game basis, assistant coaches became much more involved with freshmen and sophomores, and the team as a whole began scheduling social activities on a regular basis. Although the team did not achieve the original lofty goals, they did finish the season strongly, won their conference champion-

ship, and created a sound foundation for the following year.

■ THE CASE OF TEAM GREEN ■

Upon taking over the head-coaching job of a team with a reputation of having numerous difficulties in coach–player relationships, the new head coach consulted with the team psychologist about player personalities and their relevance to issues of communication and motivation.

In this case, a successful and experienced coach joined a team that had in recent years consistently demonstrated not only a losing record but also disharmony and interpersonal strife between players and coaches. The team psychologist brought into the organization by the administration joined the team just after the new coach was hired; after some initial resistance, the team psychologist was accepted by the coaching staff. Similarly, the players were slow to accept the value of the psychologist. Late in preseason, each player completed a psychological assessment battery that included the Sixteen Personality Factor Questionnaire and the Test of Attentional and Interpersonal Style. The assessment process was fully explained to the players in terms of

- its use to them in defining specific psychological strengths and weaknesses that might be further developed for enhanced athletic performance and
- its use in allowing the coaching staff better insight into the athletes' unique personalities.

It was explained that the athletes would receive feedback first and that no information would be presented to the coach without their knowledge and consent. Following these individual feedback sessions (which clearly helped develop the professional relationship between players and psychologist) discussions were held with the coaching staff. Discussed were each player's psychological makeup and how it might relate to previous difficulties as well as what areas and issues need to be remembered in interacting with each player (e.g., sensitivity, authority conflicts, distrust, etc.). Also discussed were specific suggestions as to motivational needs (e.g., praise, recognition, etc.) and suggestions for optimal communication (e.g., private discussion, repetition of verbal instruction due to attentional difficulties, etc.).

The head coach was open to this feedback and was able to readily integrate the information into his coaching style. During the course of the season, he frequently commented to the psychologist about the accuracy of the assessment results and ultimately gave much credit to the assessment process for a successful season that included no significant coach–athlete problems. This led to numerous consultations on a wide variety of issues and a close, long-term professional relationship.

■ THE CASE OF TEAM GRAY ■

A coach in the midst of a disappointing season, facing mounting criticism from both inside and outside the organization, and having experienced significant misfortune in his personal life (i.e., family illness), sought out the team psychologist for personal consultation after beginning to exhibit symptoms of burnout.

This head coach had successfully led the team for a number of years in a competitive, high-pressure environment, but at that time was in the midst of a season that had been highly disappointing in terms of wins and losses. As the losses mounted, he was faced with criticism from local print media and from within his own organization.

A hard worker who put in countless hours in preparing for each game and practice, he was confronted with the reality that his team, weaker than in previous years, was not re-sponding to his efforts with improved play. In addition, he had to face a serious family illness that had taken its toll mentally and physically. He had maintained a long-standing professional relationship with the team psychologist, who had provided service to this team for a number of years.

This request for a consultation followed a particularly difficult practice, during which the coach unleashed an intense verbal barrage on the team following a seemingly innocuous error by a player. The coach then ended practice and stormed out.

During the ensuing consultation, the coach reported psychophysiologic symptoms (headache and gastrointestinal distress), sleep disturbance, irritability, and lack of desire to continue coaching. The coach had had a recent physical checkup at which the physician recommended psychological counseling. The coach refused an outside referral at that point. After several meetings in which the psychologist, using a cognitive-behavioral approach, focused on numerous cognitive distortions that the coach exhibited about himself, his overall success-to-failure ratio, external criticism, and his career in general, the coach began reporting symptomatic relief.

Behavior change was accomplished through increased (enjoyable) noncoaching activities and the development of short-term coaching goals. Options for assertively confronting the internal criticism were discussed, as were psychological issues involved in his family crisis. Autogenic relaxation techniques were also taught.

Within 4 weeks (3 to 4 meetings per week) significant reduction of symptomatology occurred and his coaching behavior returned to normal. The coach began to more effectively handle both his team's difficulties and his personal life. By the end of the season the coach once again was committed to remain in coaching.

CONCLUSION

Few jobs in sport carry both the prestige and pressure of head coach. The coach is at the forefront of the team and might as a result get too much credit for producing winning teams and too much blame for losing ones. The coach's job is multifaceted and similar in basic function to that of the business manager. The coach is totally responsible for player development and training as well as strategic and tactical planning. In addition, player selection and recruitment is strongly influenced, if not totally controlled, by the coach. The coach must lead and motivate the team's players to function as a productive, cohesive unit while communicating roles, goals, rules, and strategy. In essence, the coach must understand, predict, and control the sport-related behavior of players.

It is no wonder coaches often exhibit intense emotional and behavioral symptomatology in response to stress. It is readily apparent that the applied sport psychologist has much to offer the coach. In fact, the goals of understanding, prediction, and control of human behavior have often been ascribed to the science of psychology. The sport psychologist can help coaches understand players and enhance communication and relationships with them. The psychologist can offer insights into motivation, group dynamics, and individual behavioral tendencies.

Sport psychology has developed a knowledge base in the psychological foundation of enhanced athletic performance that can benefit the athlete and can offer input into the effects of various coaching behaviors, understand elements of effective leadership, and convey principles of motor learning. The clinically trained sport psychologist can aid in the psychological care of the injured athlete and counsel those whose personal problems are impacting their athletic performance.

For sport psychologists to be given the opportunity to demonstrate their usefulness, they must first demonstrate interpersonal skill, comfort with the sport world, awareness of team culture and organizational dynamics, willingness to be flexible, ability to work informally, and sensitivity to ethical standards. In essence, the team psychologist must demonstrate social skills, knowledge, and professionalism. The model for the team psychologist presented here is that of an internal consultant offering expertise to a wide range of team personnel. The team psychologist must recognize that this role is evolutionary and dynamic, ever changing and slowly developing. There are many potential obstacles, but the successful team psychologist will be acutely aware that this job is a challenging and exciting venture requiring sound judgment, honesty, and an awareness of established standards of professional behavior.

It is my opinion that in the future sport psychology as a discipline must come to grips with the uncomfortable issue of who is trained to provide what services. Ignoring this issue makes it no less important. Confusion both within the field and in the consumer public as a whole requires strong leadership on the part of such organizations as APA Division 47 and AAASP. Failure to address this issue might ultimately have a devastating effect on the continued acceptance of this field. Similarly, these professional organizations must look to create an ethical standard for all practitioners of sport psychology.

For further development of the knowledge base of sport psychology, it is suggested that greater attention be paid to the literature in the field of organizational psychology. For example, a recent special issue on organizational psychology in the *American Psychologist* included the following articles, all of which have clear relevance for sport psychology.

- "Organizational Culture" (Schein, 1990)
- "Work Teams: Applications and Effectiveness" (Sundstrom et al., 1990)
- "Work Motivation: Theory and Practice" (Katzell & Thompson, 1990)
- "Designing Systems for Resolving Disputes in Organizations" (Brett, Goldberg, & Ury, 1990)
- "Power and Leadership in Organizations: Relationships in Transition" (Hollander & Offermann, 1990)
- "Developing Managerial Talent Through Simulation" (Thornton & Cleveland, 1990)
- "Women and Minorities in Management" (Morrison & Von Glinow, 1990)

If we begin to view athletic performance as in many ways analogous to work performance, coaching of athletes as a subset of personnel management, team cohesion as a subset of work team effectiveness, and so forth, we might begin to expand our knowledge base, suggest creative research opportunities, and potentially offer the athletic environment new and exciting insights.

In conclusion, the team psychologist and coach can offer much to each other. With the goals of the team clearly in mind, an effective relationship between the two can yield considerable return.

REFERENCES

American Psychological Association. (1981). Ethical principles of psychologists. *American Psychologist, 36,* 633-638.

Botterill, C. (1990). Sport psychology and professional hockey. *Sport Psychologist, 4,* 358-368.

Brett, J.M., Goldberg, S.B., & Ury, W.L. (1990). Designing systems for resolving disputes in organizations. *American Psychologist, 45,* 162-170.

Brown, M.J. (1982). Are sport psychologists really psychologists? *Journal of Sport Psychology, 4,* 13-18.

Caccese, T.M., & Mayerberg, C.K. (1984). Gender differences in perceived burnout of college coaches. *Journal of Sport Psychology, 6,* 279-288.

Capel, S.A., Sisley, B.L., & Desertrain, G.S. (1987). The relationship of role conflict and role ambiguity to burnout in high school basketball coaches. *Journal of Sport Psychology, 9,* 106-117.

Carron, A.V. (1982). Cohesiveness in sport groups: Interpretations and considerations. *Journal of Sport Psychology, 4,* 123-138.

Carron, A.V. (1984). Cohesion in sport teams. In J.M. Silva & R.S. Weinberg (Eds.), *Psychological foundations of sport* (pp. 340-352). Champaign, IL: Human Kinetics.

Cattell, R.B., Eber, H.W., & Tatsuoka, M.M. (1980). *Handbook for the Sixteen Personality Factor Questionnaire (16PF).* Champaign, IL: Institute for Personality and Ability Testing.

Dale, J., & Weinberg, R.S. (1989). The relationship between coaches leadership style and burnout. *Sport Psychologist, 3,* 1-13.

Davis, H. (1991). Criterion validity of the athletic motivation inventory: Issues in professional sport. *Journal of Applied Sport Psychology*, **3**, 176-182.

Dorfman, H.A. (1990). Reflections on providing personal and performance enhancement consulting services in professional baseball. *Sport Psychologist*, **4**, 341-346.

Freudenberger, H.J. (1980). *Burnout*. New York: Doubleday.

Gabarro, J.J., & Kotter, J.P. (1987). Managing your boss. In Harvard Business Review (Eds.), *People: Managing your most important asset* (pp. 1-9). Boston, MA: Harvard Business Review.

Gardner, F.L. (1991). Professionalization of sport psychology: A reply to Silva. *Sport Psychologist*, **5**, 55-60.

Gould, D., Murphy, S., Tammen, V., & May, J. (1991). An evaluation of U.S. Olympic sport psychology consultant effectiveness. *Sport Psychologist*, **5**, 111-127.

Halliwell, W. (1990). Providing sport psychology consulting services in professional hockey. *Sport Psychologist*, **4**, 369-377.

Heyman, S.R. (1982). A reaction to Danish and Hale: A minority report. *Journal of Sport Psychology*, **4**(1), 10-12.

Hollander, E.P., & Offermann, L.R. (1990). Power and leadership in organizations: Relationships in transition. *American Psychologist*, **45**, 179-189.

Katzell, R.A., & Thompson, D.E. (1990). Work motivation: Theory and practice. *American Psychologist*, **45**, 144-153.

Kroll, W. (1982). Competitive athletic stress factors in athletes and coaches. In L.P. Zaichkowsky and W.E. Sime (Eds.), *Stress management for sport*. Reston, VA: American Alliance for Health, Physical Education, Recreation and Dance.

Landers, D.M., Wilkinson, M.O., Hatfield, B.D., & Barber, H. (1982). Casualty and the cohesion-performance relationship. *Journal of Sport Psychology*, **4**, 170-183.

Lynch, G.P. (1988). Athletic injuries and the practicing sport psychologist: Practical guidelines for assisting athletes. *Sport Psychologist*, **2**, 161-167.

Mahoney, M.J., Gabriel, T.J., & Perkins, T.S. (1987). Psychological skills and exceptional athletic performance. *Sport Psychologist*, **1**, 181-199.

Martens, R. (1987). *Coaches guide to sport psychology*. Champaign, IL: Human Kinetics.

Martens, R., Burton, D., Vealey, R.S., Bump, L.A., & Smith, D.E. (1990). Development and validation of the Competitive State Anxiety Inventory-2 (CSAI-2). In R. Martens, R.S. Vealey, & D. Burton (Eds.), *Competitive anxiety in sport* (pp. 117-190). Champaign, IL: Human Kinetics.

May, J.R., & Sieb, G.E. (1987). Athletic injuries: Psychosocial factors in the onset, sequelae, rehabilitation and prevention. In J.R. May & M.J. Asken (Eds.), *Sport psychology: The psychological health of the athlete*. New York: PMA.

Meichenbaum, D., & Turk, D.C. (1987). *Facilitating treatment adherence: A practitioners guide*. New York: Plenum Press.

Morrison, A.M., & Von Glinow, M.A. (1990). Women and minorities in management. *American Psychologist*, **45**, 200-208.

Murphy, S.M. (1988). The on-site provision of sport psychology services at the 1987 U.S. Olympic festival. *Sport Psychologist*, **2**, 337-350.

Neff, F. (1990). Delivering sport psychology services to a professional sport organization. *Sport Psychologist*, **4**, 378-385.

Nideffer, R.M. (1976). Test of attentional and interpersonal style. *Journal of Personality and Social Psychology*, **34**, 394-404.

Nideffer, R.M. (1981). *The ethics and practice of applied sport psychology*. Ithaca, NY: Mouvement.

Orlick, T., & Partington, J. (1987). The sport psychology consultant: Analysis of critical components as viewed by Canadian

Olympic athletes. *Sport Psychologist*, **1**, 4-17.

Partington, J., & Orlick, T. (1987). The sport psychology consultant: Olympic coaches' views. *Sport Psychologist*, **1**, 95-102.

Ravizza, K. (1990). Sportpsych consultation issues in professional baseball. *Sport Psychologist*, **4**, 330-340.

Rotella, R.J., & Heyman, S.R. (1986). Stress, injury and the psychological rehabilitation of athletes. In J.M. Williams (Ed.), *Applied sport psychology: Personal growth to peak performance*. Mountain View, CA: Mayfield.

Ruder, M.K., & Gill, D.L. (1982). Immediate effects of win–loss on perceptions of cohesion in intramural and intercollegiate volleyball teams. *Journal of Sport Psychology*, **4**, 227-234.

Schein, E.H. (1990). Organizational culture. *American Psychologist*, **45**, 109-119.

Shinn, M., Rosario, M., Morch, H., & Chestnut, D.E. (1984). Coping with job stress and burnout in the human services. *Journal of Personality and Social Psychology*, **46**, 864-876.

Silva, J.M. (1984). Personality and sport performance: Controversy and challenge. In J.M. Silva & R.S. Weinberg (Eds.), *Psychological foundations of sport*. Champaign, IL: Human Kinetics.

Silva, J.M. (1989). Toward the professionalization of sport psychology. *Sport Psychologist*, **3**, 265-273.

Singer, R.H., & Johnson, P.J. (1987). Strategies to cope with pain associated with sport related injuries. *Athletic Training*, **22**, 100-103.

Smith, R.E. (1986). Toward a cognitive-affective model of athletic burnout. *Journal of Sport Psychology*, **8**, 36-50.

Smith, R.E., & Johnson, J. (1990). An organizational empowerment approach to consultation in professional baseball. *Sport Psychologist*, **4**, 347-357.

Stogdill, R.M. (1972). Group productivity, drive, and cohesiveness. *Organizational Behavior and Human Performance*, **8**, 26-43.

Sundstrom, E., DeMeuse, K.P., & Futrell, D. (1990). Work teams: Applications and effectiveness. *American Psychologist*, **45**, 120-133.

Taylor, J. (1991). Career direction development and opportunities in applied sport psychology. *Sport Psychologist*, **5**, 266-280.

Thornton, G.C., & Cleveland, J.N. (1990). Developing managerial talent through simulation. *American Psychologist*, **45**, 190-199.

Varney, G.H. (1990). *Building productive teams*. San Francisco: Jossey-Bass.

Vealey, R.S., Udry, E.M., Zimmerman, V., & Soliday, J. (1992). Intrapersonal and situational predictors of coaching burnout. *Journal of Sport and Exercise Psychology*, **14**, 40-58.

Wiese, D.M., & Weiss, M.R. (1987). Psychological rehabilitation and physical injury: Implications for the sports medicine team. *Sport Psychologist*, **1**, 318-330.

Williams, J.M. (Ed.) (1986). *Applied sport psychology: Personal growth to peak performance*. Mountain View, CA: Mayfield.

Zander, A. (1971). *Motives and goals in groups*. New York: Academic.

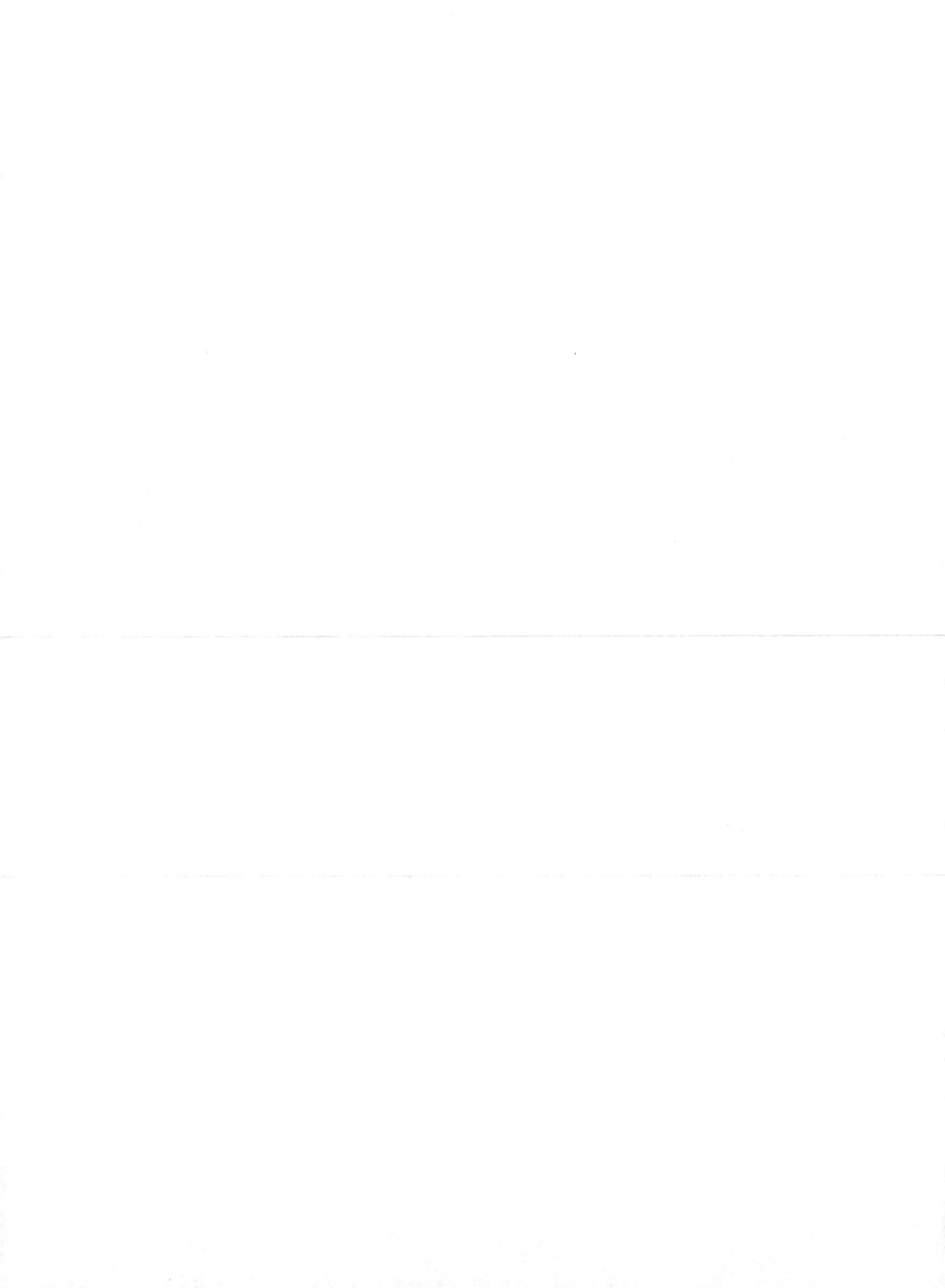

PROVIDING PSYCHOLOGICAL SERVICES TO STUDENT ATHLETES: A DEVELOPMENTAL PSYCHOLOGY MODEL

Michael Greenspan, PhD
Arizona State University

Mark B. Andersen, PhD
Victoria University of Technology

Student athletes in the 1990s face more pressure than those of earlier decades to perform well athletically, academically, and socially. Greater rewards as well as greater punishments make extraordinary demands of individual players. Placing so much pressure on people from 13 to 22 years old often causes performance and emotional difficulties. Such problems concern not only student athletes but also their teammates, coaches, physicians, trainers, instructors, advisers, friends, and family members.

The first psychologist to address the specific needs of student athletes from a clinical, or counseling, perspective was Bruce Ogilvie. While a staff member at the San Jose State University Counseling Center, he began in the early 1960s to provide performance enhancement and counseling services to members of several sport teams. Since that founda-

tional work (Ogilvie & Tutko, 1968), clinical sport psychology services for student athletes have developed greatly, with many enhancements both in technique and mode of delivery. Few university athletic departments currently employ psychologists full-time to address the mental health needs of student athletes, but over time psychologists likely will become more involved with university athletic departments as the stakes in major college sports continue to increase.

Although increasing attention is being paid to counseling collegiate athletes (Etzel, Ferrante, & Pinkney, 1991), similar attention to high-school athletes has been lacking. The literature about clinical sport psychology services in high schools is scant. Although some authors (Hellstedt, 1987; Hughes, 1990; Smoll & Smith, 1987) have proposed guidelines for performance enhancement services for younger athletes, to date only the areas of eating disorders and drug education have been addressed. Yet much of the present literature suggests that educational programs in such clinical areas as identity transitions, self-esteem and coping, drug usage, and eating disorders might be more successful at the high-school level than at the college level (Damm, 1991). Ideally, a program would offer developmentally appropriate and coordinated efforts for both the high-school and college levels.

This chapter presents an overview of the major developmental dilemmas facing student athletes and suggestions for the provision and structure of service. It addresses four separate topics: transitions that student athletes face, issues of psychopathology and medical concerns, existing resources at universities and high schools, and the professional and ethical dilemmas that might be encountered in providing services to student athletes.

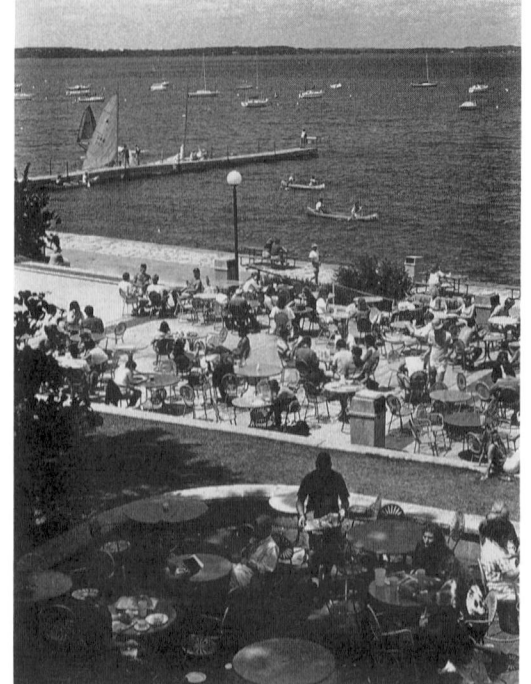

Courtesy University of Wisconsin Women's Sports Information

■ THE CASE OF THE PANTHERS ■

A consulting relationship between a university's counseling center psychologist and the women's golf team was emerging. The psychologist had provided a weekly series of performance-enhancement presentations and had attended practice once or twice weekly for 4 weeks. She had also met one team member for an initial intake regarding low self-esteem, which the golfer attributed primarily to conflict with the coaches and teammates.

After a particularly stormy team meeting, a number of the golfers and the head coach individually sought out the psychologist. Each expressed terrible frustration with others (athletes and coaches) on the team. It gradually became clear that three seniors were in conflict both with other team members (seven freshmen and sophomores) and with coaches. The seniors were clearly concerned with life beyond golf: Each had sustained at least one injury in the

last few years, each was involved in a long-term relationship with a nonathlete (one was married and two were engaged), and each planned to retire from golf at the end of the season. The younger team members, who were more openly enthusiastic and team oriented, were having difficulty relating to the seniors. Two of the freshmen were having to adjust to living far away from their parents and in an urban, fast-paced university. Their difficulty in adjusting manifested itself in excessive partying and poor academic performance. On the golf course, however, they were consistently strong. Most of the freshmen were quick to jump into the increasingly polarized situation on the side of the coaches and other younger golfers.

The head coach had always been exceptionally close with her team members, especially the golfers whom she felt worked hard and wanted "it" (success) more. She prided herself on the ability to keep her golfers motivated and "hungry." The coach was having a difficult time figuring out just how far to push the seniors. In turn the seniors believed that everyone was giving them a hard time, and they had difficulty seeing things from the others' perspectives. They reported anger toward certain coaches and team members for what they viewed as favoritism and preferential treatment.

TRANSITIONS FACING STUDENT ATHLETES

The transitions high-school athletes make are most likely to center on developmental tasks, such as identity formulation and developing self-esteem and social competence (Gould & Finch, 1991).

The transitions collegiate athletes face, however, usually can be grouped into one of four diverse categories:

- Making the transition onto a particular team at a particular university
- Making developmental transitions
- Experiencing conflict between the roles of student and athlete
- Making the transition out of competitive sport

Common Realizations

Making the transition to collegiate athletics can involve an awareness that there is much more at stake at the collegiate level than was anticipated. The realization is common that one will likely not play as important a role as previously. Such transitions include a star recruit at a major university who must adjust to all of the attention that comes with being a collegiate athlete or a high-school starter who gets to college and for the first time ever is faced with not starting.

Student athletes, like most other students, at times have a rough semester in school and have to drop a course or two or take an incomplete. They might also, like many young adults, occasionally embarrass themselves in public and possibly even receive a citation from a campus police officer. When it concerns the student athlete, however, such news might appear on the front page of their university's newspaper or on the evening television news. Such heightened visibility is often experienced as tremendous pressure, both on and off the playing field.

A related type of transition is experienced by student athletes who leave a familiar environment to attend college. A college campus might seem a very unfamiliar and confusing environment in terms of size, location, climate, off-campus activities, resources, costs, and social and racial relations. The degree to which a geographical or cultural transition is felt as stressful depends typically on the student athlete's personal resources (self-esteem, ego strength, coping skills), support system (family, friends, advisers, coaches), and experiences as a student athlete (academic and athletic history). A poor combination of these factors can lead to an isolated and troubled person. For example, a basketball player from a low socioeconomic area of a northern city might thrive at a rural southern university if he has a high level of self-esteem, the ability to cope with stress effectively, and the ability to trust and relate to coaches. A high-school teammate with few consistent and effective coping resources and strategies, however, might struggle at a nearby campus, believing coaches do not understand her.

Ethnic and Cultural Transitions

Transitions into college might be even further complicated by issues of ethnicity and culture. Although little research exists on the cultural transitions faced by student athletes,

Anshel (1990) provided an interesting view of the unique needs of black intercollegiate football players in terms of their sport experiences. Although his research was based solely on the experiences of members of one team at one university under one white head coach, Anshel's research is consistent with earlier research by Evans (1978) and Anshel and Sailes (1990) suggesting that black athletes trust white coaches less than they trust black coaches. Research by Cashmore (1982) suggested this mistrust might be due to white coaches' misinterpretation of black athletes' supposed lack of demonstrated intensity (e.g., "virtual absence of verbal assertiveness" before game) as laziness and as reflecting a lack of motivation. Anshel suggested black football players might "take in and respond to environmental demands in a less intense and emotionally demonstrative manner." Anshel's research also suggested clear differences in how black and white football players prepare for competition:

> Rather than demonstrate the proper psychological state with boisterous vocal responses in the locker room, the black players in this study preferred to behave in a calm, low-key manner.

Differences were also noted in black and white football players' degree of affiliation with team goals, in terms of need for individual recognition, motives for participation, and responsiveness to certain coaching communication styles and strategies. For a black student athlete who has rarely or never played for a white coach, a substantial adjustment period might be necessary. Although one might hypothesize that the same is true for white athletes playing for black coaches, no research evaluating that hypothesis exists. We must caution against stereotyping, however, even in the name of cross-cultural sensitivity.

Role Conflict: Student Versus Athlete

Conflict between the roles of student and athlete is not uncommon and is well summarized by Chartrand and Lent (1987). For many people, the conflict seems like a choice between two drastically different sets of expectations, demands, and, most importantly, rewards. Students often see academic studies as demanding, irrelevant, and time consuming, with only moderate potential for reward in the distant future. Athletic participation, on the other hand, is often seen as more enjoyable and as providing more consistent, tangible, immediate, and potentially greater rewards.

According to Chartrand and Lent (1987), conflict occurs when the demands of one role are incompatible with the requirements of another. For those participating in athletics as a means of preparing for professional sports, the role of student might be a perfunctory one that leads mainly to stress and overcommitment (Sack & Thiel, 1985). However, as the research by Mueller and Blyth (1984) shows, many more collegiate athletes expect to play professional sports than reach that level. Much of the conflict between roles typically revolves around time-management and social-development limitations and restrictions.

As commitment to one's sport increases, one's range of possible social and professional options is usually restricted. This reduction in exploratory behaviors contributes to Pearson and Petitpas's (1990) notion of identity foreclosure. Some athletes, as they grow and develop, begin to identify themselves more and more with the athlete role to the exclusion of other potential roles or identities. In a sense, they have foreclosed, or shut out any other identity possibility. Such identity foreclosure places individuals in a tenuous position if their athletic goals are not attained, are interfered with (e.g., by injury), or are not as satisfying as the athlete expected. The role of athlete might be incompatible with many specifics of the student role. Such role conflict has the potential to be academically, interpersonally, and athletically disruptive. It has been our experience, however, that such conflict is typically not a primary presenting problem. More common are academic problems, coach complaints of low motivation, or stress management difficulties. Whenever a referral for such concerns is made, it is important that the issue of role conflict be explored.

Retiring From Competitive Sport

Retiring from competitive sport is usually a difficult transition for student athletes. The degree to which the process is experienced as stressful is likely mediated by a number of factors. Probably most important is how unidimensional the student athlete's identity is. The less one has considered other possible social and professional roles and options, the more likely one is to struggle with the transition. In cases where retirement is due primarily to injury, the severity, acuity, and expectedness of the injury are certain to influence one's coping. The more severe, acute, and unexpected an injury, the less likely the student athlete will have prepared emotionally.

In contrast, a student athlete who has had to deal with a chronically injured and deteriorating knee might resist retirement but should be more prepared for other roles in life. A high-risk situation exists (as it also can in other circumstances) when a student athlete with little in life (present or anticipated future) except sport suffers a sudden, career-ending injury. Most athletes retiring from sport would benefit from a program like the United States Olympic Committee's Career Assistance Program for Athletes (CAPA) program (Petitpas, Danish, McKel-

vain, & Murphy, 1992); some student athletes, however, need counseling to deal with grief over the loss of a major part of their identity. For those people, the grief process is likely to be remembered vividly for decades.

Intervention in the Case of the Panthers

The case of the Panthers illustrates a number of transitions faced by student athletes that can have profound effects on both their athletic and academic performance as well as on their social relationships. Some younger team members were struggling not only with separation and individuation from their families but also with role conflict (athlete versus student), peer influence (excessive partying and further polarization of the team), sexuality, and the transition from rural areas to an urban university.

The three seniors on the team, however, were struggling with totally different though equally age-appropriate developmental concerns. Their identities were more multidimensional, and they were struggling with identity transitions out of competitive sport and into careers and long-term relationships. Though they had a difficult time recognizing it, these seniors very badly wanted the approval of the coach they reported disliking. Essentially, they were looking for an emotional relationship with a peer, but their coach tended to distance herself when a relationship became too intimate. The seniors then interpreted that as rejection and so viewed the coach as not being there for them when they struggled both on and off the course.

Further exploration suggested that the coach's tendency to get very close to her players fostered a dependency early in the relationship that became a problem when the coach had to discipline her golfers or when the golfers wanted too much intimacy or equality. In the past this pattern of relationships with her athletes had rarely caused the coach problems. These particular seniors, however, were developmentally different than the typical collegiate athlete in that they viewed themselves as women in stable relationships looking for support from a colleague and friend (the coach). Though well intentioned, the coach's managerial style had the potential to exacerbate this situation; thus intervention was important to the team's and the coach's well-being.

The psychologist's interventions involved weekly group meetings with the team and individual meetings with the head coach and some of the players. Continually aware of the fact that she was at times acting as both therapist and team consultant (and constantly processing this seemingly unavoidable situation with her supervisor), the psychologist tried to help those involved understand the validity of others' views without undermining the validity of their own. This, in addition to team process meetings, was intended to reduce some of the conflict and factionalism on the team.

At the same time, support was offered to the coach in de-enmeshing from the team and looking to meet her emotional needs in other ways. This was intended more as an intervention for the coach's present as well as the team's future well-being. Trying to help the coach feel more comfortable with conflict was intended to foster a healthy, appropriate emotional distance from her golfers and to lessen the potential for golfers' becoming too dependent on her. It was agreed that such strategies made actual coaching conflictual at times. Helping the coach with conflict became even more important because some of the sophomores began to sense the distancing and reported feeling like they were losing a friend. Without becoming too enmeshed herself, the psychologist then tried to help those golfers and the coach understand some of the relationship dynamics and the fact that in the long run the changes initiated by the coach were best for the team as a whole.

■ THE CASE OF NIKKI ■

Nikki, a female diver at a small southern university, had been attending a process group for athletes composed primarily of swimmers and divers. Group discussions had covered many topics, including adjustment to college life, communication issues, weight control, and appearance concerns. Participation in the group provided part of the impetus to seek individual treatment. The diver was also a nutrition major and in time confided to her favorite professor that she believed she might be developing a problem with her eating behavior. She was referred by the professor to the university's counseling center. She expressed reservations about seeing someone who was not involved in athletics because she felt her problems would not be understood by a nonathlete. The professor eventually was able to locate a counseling center staff member who was a former collegiate swimmer and who had experience treating athletes.

During the initial intake assessment, Nikki revealed that she was the captain of the university's team, and her high GPA showed her to be an excellent student. She had struggled all of her competitive years with perfectionism in and out of the pool and was never satisfied with her athletic and academic performances. Nikki gradually became aware that her mother would subtly withdraw affection if she was not pleased with her daughter's performance. This was a major factor in Nikki's extreme perfectionism.

Nikki reported that she was concerned with her appearance, which she believed correlated highly with her diving scores, and had been restricting her caloric intake. She also used excessive exercise as a means of controlling her weight. She was afraid that she might begin using more drastic measures to control weight, such as vomiting after meals. She had been battling with her weight for several years but stated that her eating-disorder-like symptoms disappeared at the end of each season when she took a break from diving. A brief medical history revealed a recent stress fracture of the ankle, the onset of menses at age 17, and amenorrhea for the last 6 months. She was eating only a small salad and drinking only water at most meals (including team functions), and she was exhibiting increased emotional instability during practices, resulting in several blowups with the coach and other team members.

Nikki's case was discussed at a weekly meeting of the university eating disorders team, which was composed of psychiatrists, psychologists, physicians, and nutritionists. The psychologist from the counseling center presented the case. It was decided to have Nikki see a physician for a complete physical and gynecological exam along with a thorough blood analysis. In addition, the diver was to meet with one of the nutritionists for dietary counseling. It was agreed that because good rapport seemed to have been established between the intake psychologist and Nikki, she should begin exploratory psychotherapy with this psychologist. Psychotherapy focused on helping the athlete gain a better understanding of her perfectionism, her relationship with her mother, and how that relationship influenced her present relationships and behaviors. Counseling progressed favorably over a 9-month period. Despite her emotional progress, Nikki continued to exercise excessively as a means of weight control and experienced another stress fracture in her shin.

PSYCHOPATHOLOGY IN STUDENT ATHLETES

Although we know of no sound epidemiological data, we believe severe psychopathology among student athletes, at least at the university level, is rare. This is most likely due to a type of natural selection process that over time screens out many lower-functioning persons from sport. When difficulties arise, they tend to be mild to somewhat-severe adjustment, mood, eating, and substance-abuse disorders.

Pathogenic Weight Control

One area of pathology with clearly greater incidence among athletes is eating disorders and pathogenic weight-control behavior (see chapter 13). Pathogenic weight control behaviors are more common in sports that stress appearance than in other sports (Borgen & Corbin, 1987). They are also more common among athletes in general when compared to the nonathlete college population (Black & Burckes-Miller, 1988; Borgen & Corbin, 1987) and seem to be more prevalent when coaches tell athletes they are too heavy (Rosen & Hough, 1988). Interestingly, one can apply similar criteria and speculate (sound research does not exist yet) that prevalence differences might be similar for the abuse of anabolic steroids. In other words, steroid use is higher among athletes than nonathletes, is higher in sports emphasizing size and appearance, and is higher when coaches tell athletes they are too small or too weak. Research is sorely needed in this area, however. Because eating disorders are covered thoroughly in chapter 13, we will not go into further detail here except to advocate a university-wide team approach to the treatment of eating disorders.

Injuries and Overtraining

Besides eating disorders, issues arising from injuries and overtraining are the most common problems faced by student athletes. As described previously, transitions due to

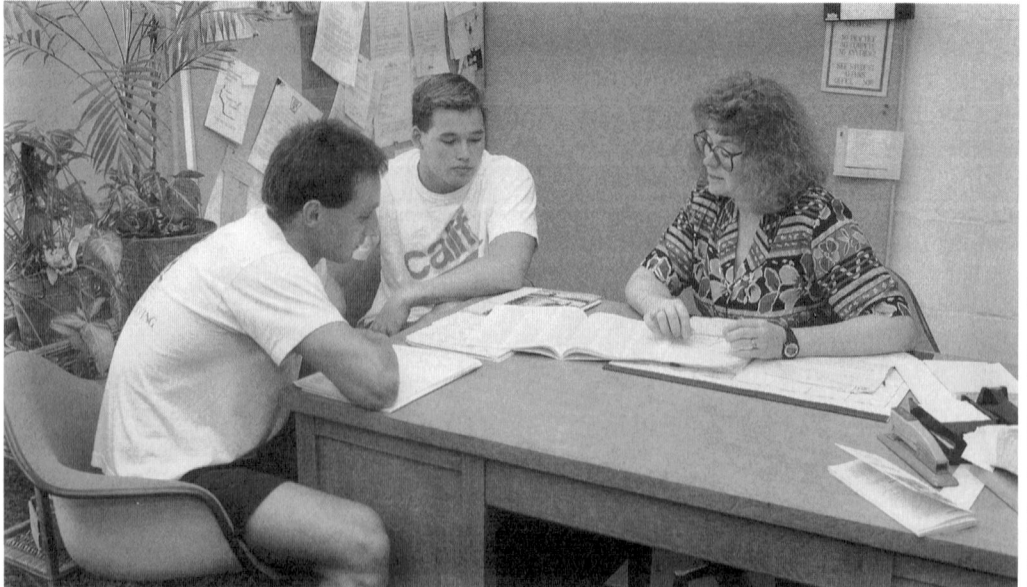

Courtesy University of Wisconsin Women's Sports Information

career-ending injuries can be terribly stressful and depressing. Non-career-ending injuries, however, might also have an emotional impact and people with such injuries might benefit from support, validation, or stress management throughout the rehabilitation process.

Our experience suggests it is important for injured athletes to maintain a performance-goal orientation. In other words, athletes must be helped to view rehabilitation as a process of small but steady increases and to not try too rapidly to regain preinjury performance levels, because this can lead to recurring or overuse injuries.

The symptoms of severe overtraining, like career termination due to injury, can parallel those of depression. Although the pain of overtraining is primarily of physiological etiology, intervention in both the physiological and psychological realms is suggested. The assessment of overtraining and burnout (presented in chapter 15) is crucial, for if these go undiagnosed, their course is often insidious and destructive.

Effects on the Team

No research exists studying the effects of an individual member's pathology on the team as a whole. The effects can depend on the impaired person's role, the degree to which that person influences teammates, and the type and degree of pathology. We believe pathology such as depression is likely to have little lasting effect on the team beyond temporary impairment of the depressed person's performance and perhaps the team's to a lesser extent. If severe enough (see "The Case of Steven," which follows), though, a team's performance can be drastically altered and teammates can be significantly affected emotionally. Other pathologies, such as eating disorders and substance abuse, have the strong potential to affect other team members if the affected person is an influential team member. Burnout, if present in an influential team member, might slightly affect morale and intensity, but we see little risk of its seriously affecting a team. Until sound research exists, however, we can only speculate about such processes.

■ *THE CASE OF STEVEN* ■

Steven, a freshman football player at a large northeastern university, shot and killed himself at a party attended by some of the other members of the football team. Early the next morning the head coach contacted the athletic department's psychologist and described to the best of his knowledge what had transpired. Other members of the team were informed of Steven's suicide as they arrived for practice.

The head coach asked the psychologist to speak to the team once it was assembled. The psychologist spoke about normal responses to highly abnormal situations, about how emotions are likely to be a mix of sadness, anger, and guilt (among other feelings), that even emotional numbness was a normal response, and that it is OK to have these feelings. The psychologist also discussed what might occur emotionally to the team members over the next several days and weeks. The wisdom of talking with others about what had happened was strongly emphasized. Suggestions were made to speak to teammates, coaches, family, academic advisers, counselors, or psychologists. The team was given information on where services are available on campus.

The psychologist then solicited comments and feelings from team members he knew well and believed would not be uncomfortable disclosing and sharing some personal reactions. The head coach and the head trainer also talked about how they were reacting. The team was then told that the psychologist would be available if they wanted to talk one-on-one or along with a few teammates.

The psychologist had never dealt firsthand with the suicide of a team member and so prior to meeting with the team called in a senior psychologist from the university employee assistance program (who personally knew the head coach) to consult on what might be the best approaches. The senior psychologist made some suggestions and within an hour was on the scene and helped by talking individually to athletes and coaches.

Members of other mental health agencies on campus were then informed of the situation (i.e., the mental health division of the student health center and the university's counseling center). The next day, counseling center personnel intervened in the dormitory where the student had lived and spoke with residents about responses to tragedy, grief processes, and the availability of campus services. Student life and residence life personnel were also debriefed. A memorial service was arranged by the player's academic adviser. Less than one week later, in the conference championship game, the football team played far below par and was easily defeated despite being a 15-point favorite.

The last campus agency to become actively involved in this case was the student mental health center, more than a month after the incident. Three of the teammates who had been at the party where the death occurred were experiencing insomnia, anxiety, confusion, and depression, which significantly impaired their academic functioning. With the cooperation of the head coach, the eligibility coordinator for the athletic department, the athletic department psychologist, and a student mental health psychiatrist, a medical withdrawal from school was arranged that left the players' academic standing and team eligibility unaffected. The players then left the university with the mutually agreed plan to seek counseling at home (future contact confirmed that each player did enter counseling). If they decided to return to the university, they were to meet with the athletic department psychologist and the head of the student mental health center. One of the three reenrolled the following fall and began counseling on an as-needed basis with a counseling center psychologist.

The case of Steven illustrates the widespread effects a tragedy can have on an athletic team and a university community as a whole. It also reveals the extensive resources available at a large university for the management of a critical incident. At small colleges and high schools, such resources are rarely available, but other avenues of crisis management exist. For example, high schools have academic counselors who might have some training in dealing with crises, and many school districts employ a school psychologist who in such a situation should be contacted for consultation. Most school districts also have referral lists of mental health professionals in their areas. Small colleges have at least one advantage over high schools in that there is typically a clinical or school psychologist on the faculty.

Information on the resources available for crisis management or for any other counseling, psychological, or psychiatric concern should be made available to all faculty and staff and be a part of new employees' orientation. The experiences of the psychologists at Steven's university suggest that most educational institutions should have a designated crisis management team with a predetermined procedural plan for use in emergencies.

UNIVERSITY-WIDE RESOURCES

The academic culture of a university or college and the culture of the athletic department, though housed on one campus, constitute two different worlds. Unfortunately, in many cases communication and cooperation between these two worlds are attenuated. Athletic departments take care of their own and athletes often feel uncomfortable going over to the "other" (academic) side where service providers might not understand the special needs, pressures, and concerns of student athletes. Athletic departments usually supply much of the medical and academic counseling services; for scholarship athletes, housing and nutritional needs might also be met. One area, however, in which athletes are underserved is in the realm of psychological services. Only a handful of university athletic departments in the United States offer in-house psychological services to athletes who need them. At other schools the athletes must pursue services on campus but that are on the academic side, something many athletes are reluctant to do. Thus many psychological concerns, some with serious consequences (e.g., severe depression, eating disorders) go untreated for long periods of time.

What is the solution? Most athletic departments are conservative and tend to change slowly, so there is a responsibility for university service delivery organizations (e.g., student health centers, counseling centers, clinical and counseling psychology training centers, exercise science departments) to initiate contact and become involved in a two-way educational process with athletic department personnel. This could involve a wide spectrum of presentations to administrators, coaches, sports medicine personnel, academic advisors, and athletes concerning the different services available, the medical, psychological, and legal aspects of treatment and nontreatment, and ways to help the athletic program become better integrated into the university community.

As one can see from the case study of Steven, the athlete who committed suicide, many university agencies were mobilized, and we hope this will always happen in such exceptional cases. This case, however, is an example of reactive mobilization. The future calls for a proactive, preventive model of interaction between university agencies and athletic department staff, coaches, and athletes.

■ *THE CASE OF KENNY* ■

Kenny, a swimmer at a small midwestern college, came to a psychology professor who was known to have an interest in sport psychology. Ostensibly, the athlete was seeking performance-enhancement services, but it soon became obvious that the athlete had another agenda. Kenny stated that he wanted to improve his performance but would spend whole sessions talking about personal concerns, such as his relationships with his girlfriend and his overbearing father. Kenny felt a combination of ambivalence and fear of engulfment with his current (and first) girlfriend, and he was very resentful of his father's demanding and psychologically abusing nature. This swimmer presented as a very lonely person with low self-esteem who was looking for a loving surrogate parent.

Kenny began making requests of the psychologist for attention outside the sport psychology sessions. The psychologist had attended some swim meets and this greatly pleased the athlete. In addition, Kenny's times appeared to be improving, and he tended to swim particularly well when the psychologist was in attendance. After one particularly good performance that the psychologist witnessed, the coach gave the psychologist some swim team attire (shirts, sweatshirt, and a bag) while discussing how well Kenny was doing. Kenny wanted more attention, however, and began to invite the psychologist out to lunch or dinner and would offer to pay. The psychologist knew that accepting might be in violation of the APA standards on multiple relationships (American Psychological Association, 1992) but temporarily acquiesced with the stipulation that they each pay their own way. Upon further thought, the psychologist tried to cancel the lunch date and attempted to get counseling on a more appropriate track. This led to Kenny's expression of anger through stories about being rejected and abandoned by those he thought close to him.

The psychologist hypothesized that Kenny was likely looking for an ally in his struggles with both his girlfriend and father and that the psychologist had made the mistake, albeit only temporarily, of getting pulled into a therapeutic misalliance (Basch, 1980). In addition, one must wonder if the coach was rewarding the psychologist with team attire for being helpful or, instead, for providing results. Unfortunately, the break in the counseling relationship was severe. Kenny soon left sport psychology services.

ETHICAL AND PROFESSIONAL DILEMMAS

Ethical dilemmas in the practice of applied sport psychology in academic settings might arise in several situations. The two most obvious are working with the student athletes themselves and with coaches. Other likely situations where ethical dilemmas might arise exist in working with parents, administrators, instructors, and recruiters. Ultimately, though, the psychologist is responsible for identifying ethical concerns and preventing negative consequences. We would like to address some of these problem areas and offer some suggestions.

Working With Athletes

A common pitfall in working with athletes is falling into their advocacy too easily. At times athletes will seek out a psychologist to help them with their problems with a coach. The coach might be portrayed as demanding, unreasonable, punishing, and abusive. The psychologist might be too quick to take the athlete's side, an act that easily could backfire. A better approach is to examine the communication patterns of coach and athlete and make suggestions on how to improve coach–athlete interaction. In chapter 6, some useful suggestions are presented for helping athletes take responsibility for managing their relationship with their coach in a positive and direct manner. If possible, it is usually best to meet both the coach and athlete separately at first and then together for clarification of the problem and conflict resolution. Advocacy for the athlete is wonderful, but zeal for protecting the client should not blind the psychologist to the viewpoint, needs, and concerns of another party, in this case the coach.

Working With Coaches

Another common source of ethical problems concerns attempts by coaches to obtain confidential information. There are two main approaches to deal with requests for information. The first is preventive education. A thorough talk with the coaches, at the beginning of a working relationship, about how crucial confidentiality is and the psychologist's code of professional ethics can avoid many future problems. Another path is to ask the athlete, "What would you like me to say if the coach asks me about what we are doing?" For example, the athlete might feel comfortable having the psychologist talk about performance issues but not about family issues.

Another dilemma with coaches is that they might try to enlist the psychologist in selection processes. We believe these practices are questionable and ultimately will backfire. We know of no evidence that psychology can help predict athletic success of student athletes. Only in rare cases might a psychologist's opinion be of value, such as in screening out people with psychopathology. It is seductive for the psychologist to get involved in important decisions like selection, but in general we advise against such involvement.

There are those who advocate that sport psychologists should become members of the coaching team, and in many cases this seems like a good idea. For a psychologist, however, some problems can arise in the form of dual-role conflicts. The psychologist might be an athlete's mental-skills trainer, clinician, companion, and on-site intervention coach. In most clinical situations, this overfamiliarity would constitute a therapeutic misalliance and would be cause for terminating the relationship. This overexposure of the sport psychologist can look suspiciously like dependency fostering. It is not the sport psychologist's job to make him or herself indispensable to the athlete. The answer to the question, "Who is being served?" is "the sport psychologist" and that is the wrong answer. The sport psychologist's job with an athlete is to help empower and encourage independence in the athlete and ultimately to terminate therapy.

Sport psychologists must also carefully manage their public exposure around athletes. Our own preference, developed over time, is for the sport psychologist to actively deflect as much publicity as possible and refuse to talk about any specific athlete-client with any outside sources. The greatest temptation is probably when others, such as the media, are willing to give the sport psychologist credit for an athlete's performance gains. It is essential, however, that sport psychologists continue to encourage the media to attribute such progress to the athletes themselves.

Countertransference

Another source of problems can be countertransference issues. Athletes are in general a very attractive group (socially and physically) and a psychologist's own positive (or negative) countertransference is likely to influence some interventions, just as the athlete's positive or negative transference to the sport psychologist will have an effect on the learning process. This idea is troubling in that only recently has it begun to be addressed in the sport psychology literature (Ogilvie & Harris, 1990).

Working With Administrators

The sport psychologist might also face pressure from administrators and athletes for special academic treatment. An administrator might want a star athlete diagnosed as learning disabled to receive special attention (e.g., more time for tests, testing in special environments, deadline delays). It might be that the athlete has no specific learning disability but is intellectually just slightly below average. An athlete or coach might ask the psychologist to intercede on behalf of the athlete in gaining special consideration for retaking a course or receiving an incomplete. Determining when such requests are legitimate because of extenuating circumstances and when they are just stopgaps for poor preparation may be difficult. Awareness of exploitation should be of concern to a sport psychologist; it is easy to see how the psychologist can be seduced into such misalliances. Our own experiences suggest that guidelines need to be established and clearly communicated early in the relationship and then followed as diligently as possible.

Preventing Dilemmas

The training of sport psychologists in ethical decision making and professional practice needs greater attention. It is not enough merely to know that it is not a good idea to break confidentiality or to become sexually involved with your client. Much more subtle pressures and cues from athletes and others can place psychologists in precarious situations. One dilemma we have encountered is coaches offering us team clothing (shoes,

shirts) as an expression of gratitude for our consultation. Little was made of this initially. When we realized the equipment was offered only after athletes we were working with performed well, it became a concern. Although the coaches might have merely intended to thank us or were not aware of any relationship to performance, we still struggle with this topic. Another is the making public of consulting relationships with sport teams. Are consultation clients not to be treated as counseling clients with respect to confidentiality? We never make public statements about our work with individual clients, but sometimes a coach or client may say something even though we encourage them to keep our names out of the media.

More frequently than we would like, the practitioner is put in a double bind. For example, many practitioners of sport psychology services have been trained in physical education or exercise science departments and rightly have been taught that if a client presents with a clinical concern they should refer the client to a qualified professional. What often occurs, however, is that an athlete seeks out a sport psychologist for performance enhancement and then later might bring up more clinical concerns. It might have taken 2 months for the athlete to feel comfortable enough to bring up a sensitive subject, only to be referred to another person. This proper procedure might make the athlete feel rejected. The message, no matter how gently handled, might still be You trusted me with this, but I can't deal with it, and I have to reject you. The athlete might understand the referral on a conscious, rational level but on a deeper level might be hurt. This unavoidable situation argues not against the current role of physical-education–trained sport psychologists but for more broad-based training (assessment, counseling skills, etc.) of future sport psychology practitioners. Andersen (1992) has suggested that in such situations, the sport psychologist refer *in*, that is, bring a clinician into the sport psychology sessions and do tandem treatment. Such an arrangement might help avoid feelings of abandonment and could provide some professional development for both the clinician and the sport psychologist.

CONCLUSION

A psychologist working in an athletic department is often a "stranger in a strange land." Intercollegiate athletics today is often not in the business of education, much less of therapy. It is primarily an entertainment business that is *terra incognita* for most psychologists. The best place to start, as with most newly evolving relationships, is through mutual education. Psychologists need to educate themselves about the structure and function of the athletic organization. Questions such as Who are the key players in the organization? Where might I find allies? Who are the successful innovators? Who is resistant? and What do these people really want? are important to consider. In many cases, the athletic directors and coaches might not know the answer to this last question, and that is where it becomes the psychologist's role to educate the organization as to what services might be offered and what benefits might accrue from the practice of sport psychology and clinical psychology.

For some coaches and organizations, this may be a tough sell. It would behoove most psychologists to wage a campaign of gradually earning the respect of effective internal champions in the organization. In selecting an internal champion, one would be wise to select someone who has successfully introduced and championed an innovative and controversial program. Although it is important to have support at the top of the organization, it has been our experience and is our belief that true innovation more typically happens at a system's lower levels.

This chapter has emphasized that provision of effective services to student athletes requires an understanding of both the developmental issues of the athletes and the systemic issues of the academic organization. Sport psychology consultants working in academic settings will help athlete-clients most if they further their own education and experience in both areas.

REFERENCES

American Psychological Association. (1992). Ethical principles of psychologists and code of conduct. *American Psychologist*, **47**, 1597-1611.

Andersen, M.B. (1992). Sport psychology and procrustean categories: An appeal for synthesis and expansion of service. *Association for the Advancement of Applied Sport Psychology Newsletter*, **7**(3), 8-9.

Anshel, M.H. (1990). Perceptions of black intercollegiate football players: Implications for the sport psychology consultant. *Sport Psychologist*, **4**, 235-248.

Anshel, M.H., & Sailes, G. (1990). Discrepant attitudes of intercollegiate team athletes as a function of race. *Journal of Sport Behavior*, **13**, 68-77.

Basch, M.F. (1980). *Doing psychotherapy*. New York: Basic Books.

Black, D.R., & Burckes-Miller, M.E. (1988). Male and female college athletes: Use of anorexia nervosa and bulimia nervosa weight loss methods. *Research Quarterly for Exercise and Sport*, **59**(3), 252-256.

Borgen, J.S., & Corbin, C.B. (1987). Eating disorders among female athletes. *Physician and Sports Medicine*, **15**(2), 89-95.

Cashmore, E. (1982). *Black sportsmen*. Boston: Rutledge & Kegan Paul.

Chartrand, J.M., & Lent, R.W. (1987). Sports counseling: Enhancing the development of the student-athlete. *Journal of Counseling and Development*, **66**, 164-167.

Damm, J. (1991). Drugs and the college student athlete. In E. Etzel, A. Ferrante, and J. Pinkney (Eds.), *Counseling college student athletes: Issues and interventions* (pp. 151-176). Morgantown, WV: Fitness Information Technologies.

Etzel, E., Ferrante, A., & Pinkney, J.P. (Eds.) (1991). *Counseling college student athletes: Issues and interventions*. Morgantown, WV: Fitness Information Technologies.

Evans, V. (1978). A study of perceptions held by high school athletes toward coaches. *International Review of Sport Sociology*, **13**, 47-53.

Gould, D., & Finch, L. (1991). Understanding and intervening with the student athlete to be. In E. Etzel, A. Ferrante, and J. Pinkney (Eds.), *Counseling college student athletes: Issues and interventions* (pp. 51-69). Morgantown, WV: Fitness Information Technologies.

Hellstedt, J. (1987). Sport psychology at a ski academy: Teaching mental skills to young athletes. *Sport Psychologist*, **1**, 567-568.

Hughes, S. (1990). Implementing psychological skills training in high school athletics. *Journal of Sport Behavior*, **13**(1), 15-22.

Mueller, F.O., & Blyth, C.S. (1984). Can we continue to improve injury statistics? *Physician and Sportsmedicine*, **12**(9), 79-84.

Ogilvie, B.C., & Harris, D. (1990, August.). *Intervention discussion hour: Sexuality in sport*. Paper presented at the 5th Annual Meeting of the Association for the Advancement of Applied Sport Psychology, San Antonio, TX.

Ogilvie, B.C., & Tutko, T.A. (1968). *Problem athletes and how to handle them*. London: Pelham Books.

Pearson, R.E., & Petitpas, A.J. (1990). Transitions of athletes: Developmental and preventive perspectives. *Journal of Counseling and Development*, **69**, 7-10.

Petitpas, A., Danish, S., McKelvain, R., & Murphy, S. (1992). A career assistance program for elite athletes. *Journal of Counseling and Development*, **70**, 383-386.

Rosen, L., & Hough, D. (1988). Pathogenic weight control behaviors of female college gymnasts. *The Physician and Sports Medicine*, **16**(9), 141-144.

Sack, A.L., & Thiel, R. (1985). College basketball and role conflict: A national survey. *Sociological Abstracts*, **33**(5), 1743.

Smoll, F.L., & Smith, R.E. (1987). *Sport psychology for youth coaches: Personal growth to athletic excellence*. Washington, DC: National Federation of Catholic Youth Ministry.

CHAPTER 8

RELATIONSHIP ISSUES IN SPORT: A MARITAL THERAPY MODEL

David B. Coppel, PhD
University of Washington Medical School

This chapter covers the bidirectional association between relationships and athletic performance or involvement. Athletes are involved in relationships both in and outside the sport world. Nonsport relationships—marital, familial, or other—can play important roles in determining emotional adjustment, mood, and, ultimately, athletic performance. Likewise, athletic involvement or performance can influence the quality or outcome of human relationships. General relationship issues, such as independence, identity, security, intimacy, power, control, and communication, can become even more complex in the structure and demands of sport involvement.

Although recognition of the importance of relationships to athletes is not new, little focus has been placed on it in sport psychology. This has been discussed in the context of the role that significant others (e.g., family members) play both in influencing sport involvement (Greendorfer & Lewko, 1978) and in the development of professionalized sport attitudes (McElroy & Kirkendall, 1980) in children; however, little has been written on how relationships impact sport perfor-

mance or how sport involvement impacts close relationships.

Each of the following case studies illustrates only one direction of this bidirectional relationship. In the first, Mike and Denise deal with how Mike's professional sport involvement has impacted their married life, their moods, and the way they think about or perceive each other. It is clear that Mike feels the distress in the relationship affects his sport performance. In the second case study, Sandra focuses on how her relationship with Dan impacts her training and sport performance; Dan, on the other hand, focuses on how her training and sport involvement detracts from their relationship.

■ THE CASE OF MIKE ■

Mike, a professional athlete, and his wife, Denise, are having marital difficulties. Mike and Denise have been married for about two and a half years. They have no children but would like to start a family soon. Mike is in the middle of his second season; he is struggling this year and believes that he is not playing up to last year's level. This disappointment and frustration has caused Mike to experience

193

sleep difficulties, anxiety, depressed moods, and social withdrawal. He is concerned about the possible reduction of playing time and even about his future with the team. He has increased his personal training in hopes of improving his performance. Denise met Mike in college through a mutual friend; over several months of dating they found they had many interests in common and began an exclusive relationship. Denise has been pursuing her interest in a career in interior design by taking courses at a local university. She expresses anger and dissatisfaction with the marriage. She claims that communication is poor and says she does not feel special in the relationship. There is no time for fun together. She has a clear sense of being a lower priority, behind Mike's sport involvement. She has attempted to discuss her feelings with Mike, but this has not helped; it made her feel more frustrated, and Mike believed she was not being supportive of him in his difficult time—in other words, he believed she was adding to his stress. Mike initially told Denise to go to individual counseling to deal with *her* problems; he finally agreed to marital counseling as a couple on two conditions: confidentiality from their families and friends, including other teammates' wives, and an appointment time arranged around his travel and training schedules.

■ *THE CASE OF SANDRA* ■

Sandra is an 18-year-old figure skater who has performed well over the past 2 years and appears to be on the verge of breaking into the top senior women's competition at the national level. Sandra currently lives with her mother, who has been divorced for 4 years. Sandra has a younger sister who is also showing some promise as a skater. Sandra's mother has been intensely involved in Sandra's 8 years of skating. Sandra has also had the same coach for 8 years. Sandra is currently in training for skating, about 6 hr daily at the ice rink. Most of her

friends are fellow skaters from the rink. She takes correspondence courses to complete her high-school education. Sandra has been involved with Dan, a 21-year-old ex-skater, for about 1 year. Their relationship has been a source of concern for both Sandra's mother and her coach. They both believe Dan is a bad influence and a distraction. Sandra has altered her training schedule around Dan's schedule to maximize their time together. She has been looking for him during her practices and has even skipped practice to spend time with him. Sandra's training has become quite variable in intensity and motivation, and clean programs have been infrequent (in contrast to her usual skating and training regimen over the years). At times, Sandra appears to be hurrying through jumps, programs, and practice to spend time with Dan. This is Sandra's first boyfriend relationship. Dan has just recently asked Sandra to cut back on her skating and spend more time with him. This occurred as her training for an important skating competition intensified. This request weighs heavily on Sandra, causing her to be distracted and ambivalent. She is torn between her strong feelings for Dan and her desire to compete as a skater. Dan cannot understand her feelings about continuing with skating and focuses instead on the lack of time they spend together. Sandra believes that whatever choice she makes, people will be hurt, and she is confused about what she wants to do. Sandra has been working with a sport psychologist individually for about 8 months, focusing mostly on concentration, enhancing performance, and reducing the stress associated with her sport. At this point in time, Sandra asked Dan to attend a sport psychology consultation session with her to talk about their relationship and its impact on her skating performance.

REVIEWING THE LITERATURE

Research in sport psychology concerning athletes and relationship issues has been almost nonexistent. As sport psychology has become somewhat more aware of the relationship of social supports or resources to mood (Golding & Ungerleider, 1991), to adjustment to retirement from sports (Baillie & Danish, 1992), or to the life stress–injury relationship (Hardy, Richman, & Rosenfield, 1991; Rosenfield, Richman, & Hardy, 1989), the importance of relationships in sport psychology consultation has increased. Significant others and social support are included in some form in most models of sport stress and adjustment, including burnout and sports injury (Smith, 1986; Smith, Smoll, & Ptacek, 1990); thus they should have some place in most intervention strategies. Strategies to enhance social support or minimize marital or relationship distress appear to have the potential to positively impact the athlete in terms of sport performance and personal emotional adjustment. Botterill (1990) included spouses and friends in his consultation program with a professional hockey team, indicating that "these significant others are usually the most important support people in the lives of professional hockey players."

Sport psychology has tended to focus most extensively on athletic performance, with relationship issues in sports, both positive and negative, typically emerging in images created by the media. On the positive side, there might be the supportive friend or spouse during training or recovery from injury, the rock and inspiration during hard times, and the spouse behind the athlete. However, on the negative side, relationships of athletes might be portrayed in the media with images of the angry cuckolded spouse, domestic violence incidents, promiscuity, and insensitivity.

Athletes and the media have also described how social entrances and exits in athletes' lives, such as divorce, remarriage, death, or even a new coach, appear to impact performance and general adjustment. One can observe media reports of inspired and dedicated successful performances traced to relationship factors; likewise, the media also connects relationship factors to performances

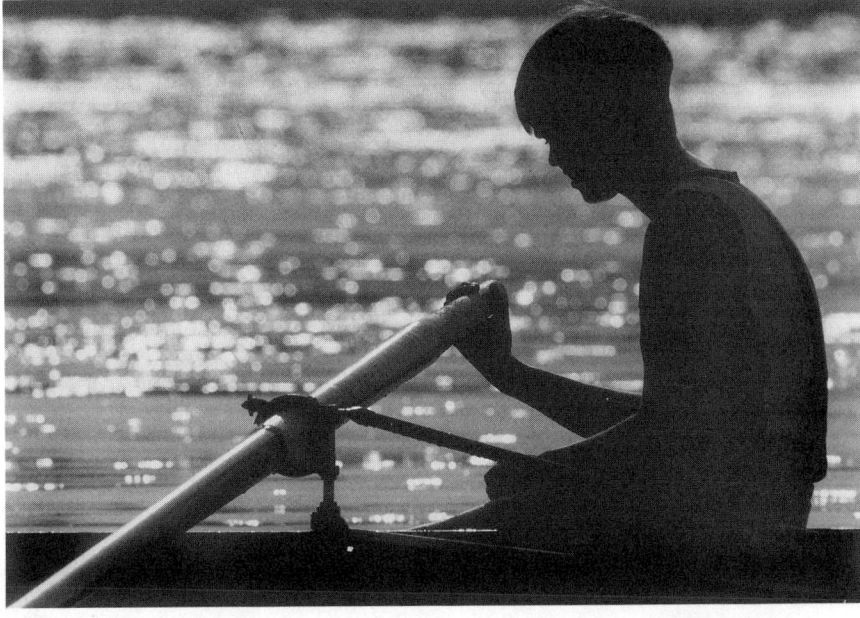

Courtesy University of Wisconsin Women's Sports Information

described as lackluster, unfocused, and pre-occupied.

Athletes, like most people, have attributions and perceptions about how changes in their relationships have (or will) impact their athletic performance. In working with athletes, understanding their perceptions or models of how relationships impact their thoughts, feelings, and behaviors as well as their athletic performance can be important. This might involve breaking through the often tough shell of self-focus and self-involvement that has typically been adaptive and successful for them in their sport involvement but has become dysfunctional in a relationship. From an early age athletes are primed to engage in self-focus and, to some degree, block out concerns of others. This focus, this drive, this all-consuming eat-drink-sleep-your-sport attitude, is associated with success; thus for some athletes, focusing on interrelationships can be difficult and is sometimes resisted. This different "other-focus" can be seen as threatening, because it might disrupt or break the focus they feel is necessary to achieve success.

Mike expresses some of these concerns. He feels that the focus on discussions of his marriage and the upset that might ensue or already be present is a distraction that is likely to interfere with achieving his athletic goal. He expresses this feeling to Denise by claiming that she is being unsupportive of him.

Most athletes must deal with relationship issues like anybody else, but in some cases media coverage makes this more difficult. With some high-profile professional or Olympic athletes, the human-interest factor can focus more media attention on relationship issues and less on athletic performance. How many times have aspects of athletes' personal or interpersonal lives been used as lead-ins to or commentary during their athletic performances? Recent Olympic athlete examples include death of a family member, estrangement or divorce from a spouse, and

conflicts with teammates or coach. Unfortunately, athletes often end up dealing with not only the actual relationship issues, but also the impact of media reports of their relationships. This situation can occur at the same time they are trying to focus on training or competitive performance.

Athletes show significant variation in how they respond to public discussion of their personal or interpersonal lives. Some athletes find it extremely distracting, disorienting (the focus is not on athletic performance as they are used to), and intrusive; it might lead other athletes to increase their focusing efforts to a higher level.

Resistance to or denial of the existence of interpersonal difficulties is fairly common in athletes. Athletes can find themselves battling others' perceptions that athletes have no emotional, personal, or interpersonal problems. In professional sports the money, fame, and general prestige are thought to make athletes immune to adversity. As is becoming clearer, athletes might be, at the least, just as vulnerable to insecurities and interpersonal difficulties, drug abuse, and diseases as nonathletes. However, the possibility that highly competitive athletes are more at risk for interpersonal difficulties because of the nature of their intense training and focused lives must be considered. Heyman (1987) cites the misunderstanding of training demands, sport-related travel away from home, jealousy, infidelity possibilities, and identity questions of the spouse as possible problem areas for athlete relationships. He suggests that in some cases "the role of athletics and sport can play a unique role in maintaining the patterns that will be dysfunctional to the marriage."

DEVELOPMENTAL CONSIDERATIONS

Relationship issues have developmental differences based on factors such as age and level of athletic involvement. Sandra and Dan's relationship concerns are different in many ways from Mike and Denise's. The stage of the relationship (e.g., dating vs. marriage) is an important factor, as it often reflects the different levels of commitment and role expectation. Couples who are dating are likely to have different implicit and explicit expectations about interactive behaviors than couples who are married. Relationships that have endured over time have typically made some attempts to cope with the integration of two people and the formation of a relationship; the degree to which these attempts and strategies are functional to both the couple and the individuals generally relates to relationship satisfaction and helpfulness.

Identity Development

Different levels of personal development in the couple can yield relationship difficulties, as the developmental issues being confronted might be very discrepant. At the core of many developmental stages is the ongoing issue of identity in one's self and in connection to others and the world (Erikson, 1959). Athletes often generate identities based primarily on their athletic performance and potentially face different life crises at each stage of development (Heyman, 1987). For example, issues of intimacy or isolation face those in early adulthood (Erikson, 1963); these issues are seen in our two case studies. Sandra is struggling with her identity as a figure skater, which at this time appears to be at conflict with her developing identity as a caring person in a relationship. Mike and Denise are dealing with identities at different levels. They are trying to maintain and sustain their identity as a couple while trying to do the things they need to do to establish more secure individual identities. For Mike, a more secure personal identity emerges directly from successful athletic performance and to a lesser degree from a successful relationship.

Priorities and Sacrifice

To achieve success, athletes typically place sport training and related activities as their number-one priority. They often sacrifice social lives and experiences to pursue athletic success. Often, as mentioned earlier, they focus on themselves, rather than being other focused, except to please others by successful performances. The most negative consequences and sequelae of these sacrifices can often be seen in relationship difficulties. Age-related social immaturity, significant emotional difficulties with low self-esteem, and social evaluative anxiety are prominent factors.

With some athletes, an intense involvement in sport has deprived them of typical adolescent, young adult, or school experiences; these players might display a sort of developmental gap in the ability to relate to others. In some cases, athletes relate to others almost exclusively by using their physical bodies, leaving other relating skills to develop more slowly. For other athletes the physical (often intimidating) skills that have served them well in sport are brought or generalized to their relationship interactions. Perhaps, on a speculative note, the focus on using the physical body in highly stressful and competitive environments even desensitizes athletes or lowers the threshold to physical action during, for example, marital arguments.

Social Life and Relationships

May and Veach (1987) indicate that interpersonal issues such as relationships with girlfriends, boyfriends, spouses, and parents are frequent focuses in their work with the United States Alpine ski team. Some of the emotional symptoms seen in athletes might be associated with their efforts to maintain meaningful personal relationships.

Harris (1987) suggests that the lack of opportunity for a social life creates "conflict and discontentment among the female athletic population." She also states that sustaining a relationship with another person is problematic due to travel demands and training; this parallels Sandra's situation as she experiences the conflicts between her relationship with Dan and the time and concentration demands of her training.

Like most people in marital or relationship counseling, athletes can bring a wide range of family-of-origin issues to their adult relationships. Sometimes the intense involvement of the parents and family in the athlete's support over the years can delay the onset of individuation and independence activities. The relationships that athletes are involved in often reflect the expectations and behaviors found in their own family-of-origin experiences. From a clinical standpoint, it is probably extremely helpful, if not crucial, to explore and gain information about the families of origin in relationship counseling. This allows one to look for systems factors (Aylmer, 1986) as well as origins of socially learned behavior and cognitions (Jacobson & Holtzworth-Munroe, 1986).

POTENTIAL PROBLEM AREAS IN ATHLETES' RELATIONSHIPS

The most common problem areas athletes must face in their relationships are related to sport demands, priority issues, and power.

Sport Demands

Sport demands have been mentioned earlier in this chapter as being a significant detriment, not only to the establishment of relationships but also to their maintenance. In some instances, spouses or significant others might not realize the time required for training as well as competing; they might hope for a change over time or, in some cases, that their presence will create change in these training patterns. Some athletes use sport demands as a way out of confronting relationship issues.

Priority Issues

Priority issues are usually expressed by spouses, girlfriends, and boyfriends in the statement, You care more about the sport than me. This is a corollary to the sport-demand issue, but typically goes deeper, because it relates to how loved, how special, or how important a partner feels in the relationship. Spouses can feel rejected if most energy, enthusiasm, and excitement is oriented to sport, with very little experienced in relationship time. Sometimes athletes are preoccupied with a coming competition and are not as attentive to the communications of others; this further contributes to the feelings of lower priority or even devaluation.

Power

Athletes' relationships often emerge out of their athletic status or prestige; people relate to them because of who they are athletically. It should be noted that this can also be the origin of many athletes' insecurities about others' motives and their own abilities to relate (Why can't people like me for me, not just me the athlete?). It also establishes, for some, the belief that relationships are dependent on successful athletic performance; thus after a perceived poor performance some athletes fear rejection.

Power and control can be exerted by the degree to which relationships are centered on the athlete's sport involvement. These power and control (and probably priority) issues are seen in the conditions Mike put on his involvement in therapy, namely, that it not interfere with his training and travel. Athletes who are used to getting what they want (they set goals and achieve them) and getting special allowances or accommodations because of who they are typically enter into relationships with a sense of entitlement and expectation. This can create difficulties in communication, activities, and problem solving. A sense of equality in the relationship might be further undermined if income discrepancies are a factor.

INTERVENTION STRATEGIES AND CONSIDERATIONS

There are many models and approaches to working with relationships (Jacobson & Gurman, 1986), each generating intervention strategies focused on how relationship problems are conceptualized. A social-learning–cognitive-behavioral framework (Jacobson & Holtzworth-Munroe, 1986) focuses primarily on interventions designed to impact the couple's behavior together: perceptions, expectations, communication skills, and problem-solving skills. Systems-oriented approaches see relationship conflict emerging out of "interactive influences in the self-system, extended-family system (families of origin), and the couple–nuclear family system" (Aylmer, 1986).

Recognition of the influence of family-of-origin experiences on current relationship interactions and emotional patterns can make a significant impact for couples in distress (Framo, 1981). Other approaches and models emphasize emotional expression experiences, which allow for vulnerability and acceptance sequences, followed by new solutions and responses (Greenberg & Johnson, 1987).

Social learning approaches tend to focus on social or environmental determinants and patterns of behavior in marital interaction (the idea that action and reaction successively influence each other). Behavior marital therapy (Jacobson & Margolin, 1979) focuses on behavior exchange principles and the notion that spouses can change behaviors of their partners by changing their own behaviors and achieving some reciprocity arrangements. In this way they can create new behavior patterns that are more satisfying to each person and the relationship.

Beck (1988) presents a marital therapy model based on his cognitive therapy. In this model the nature of marital problems is found in the self-defeating and dysfunctional attitudes and distortions in thinking and communicating of the couple. Examining the couple's negative or distorted thinking and generating alternative, more accurate thinking is one way to improve communication. Communication based on distorted thinking produces greater distortion and more negativity in the relationship. For example, the assumptions that Mike and Denise have about each other's motives in the relationship provide a negative lens for each of them to interpret subsequent behavior and comments.

GENERAL STRUCTURE AND PROCEDURES

Relationship, or marital, therapy often consists of an initial joint consultation session, then an individual session with each person, followed by a return to joint sessions. Some therapists collect information in the form of questionnaires or inventories; this helps specify problem areas or aspects of the partners or the relationship that might impact the process or course of therapy. It is important that the therapist know about high-risk behaviors, such as spouse abuse, domestic violence activity or threats, alcoholism, or drug abuse. For example, in the athletic world relationship difficulties are often found in athletes involved in steroid abuse due to the "roid rage" responses, general irritability, and aggressiveness that can be present.

Creating a Safe Environment

As with most therapy approaches, creating a safe environment for couples becomes a crucial component. In the cognitive-behavioral models (Beck, 1988; Jacobson & Holtzworth-Munroe, 1986), focusing on positive aspects of the relationship can be important. This shifts and changes the generally negative focus of distress and might offer some cognitive perspective for the couple. Helping the couple to generate behaviors and pleasant activities they can do together is also a component. Some couples have gotten out of the habit of doing what they enjoyed together or have forgotten about common interests; thus returning to some of the patterns that contributed to mutual attraction earlier in the relationship can be helpful.

Changing Behavior

Jacobson and Holtzworth-Munroe (1986) discuss behavior exchange as a way to overcome the negative perceptual bias and counteract the feelings of helplessness that the couple might express. It also serves to show the couple's connectiveness and might restructure their efforts to improve their relationship. Typically, the couple is told to focus on their own individual behaviors, i.e., what each can do to improve the relationship, and increase the frequency of these behaviors. Effort in changing or increasing behaviors can be appreciated by partners and provide a more positive platform to explore the interactive and process aspects of the relationship.

Teaching Communication Skills

Helping couples to improve communication is usually a large component of relationship work. Communication-skills training allows couples to become more aware of their communication process (both functional and dysfunctional). Learning more about the way words, tone, volume, or body language are used and the way these aspects are perceived by the couple can be revealing. For example, understanding that being loud might not mean that one is angry or on the verge of violence can change the feeling of threat and escape that might occur in a communication exchange.

Often couples' communication behavior patterns have become so presumptive (mind reading or, I know what they are thinking) that partners feel unheard or misunderstood. The teaching of basic communication skills such as listening, paraphrasing, and clarifying is extremely useful. These communication-skills training components have been used with great success in my consultation with doubles tennis partners, ice dancers, and pair skaters to improve their ability to communicate and to reduce chances of misunderstanding that would directly impact their tandem performances.

Developing Problem-Solving Skills

In addition to communication skills, specific problem-solving skills are typically included in therapy to aid couples in communication about conflict areas and help them engage in some structured attempts at problem solving and resolution. Briefly, couples are asked to spend time on problem definition so that they are ultimately solving the same problem. Problems are discussed in specific, behaviorally referenced terms, which include direct expression of feelings. Most important in the process of problem definition and solution is the validation of the problem (hearing and understanding) and the assumption of a collaborative problem-solving set.

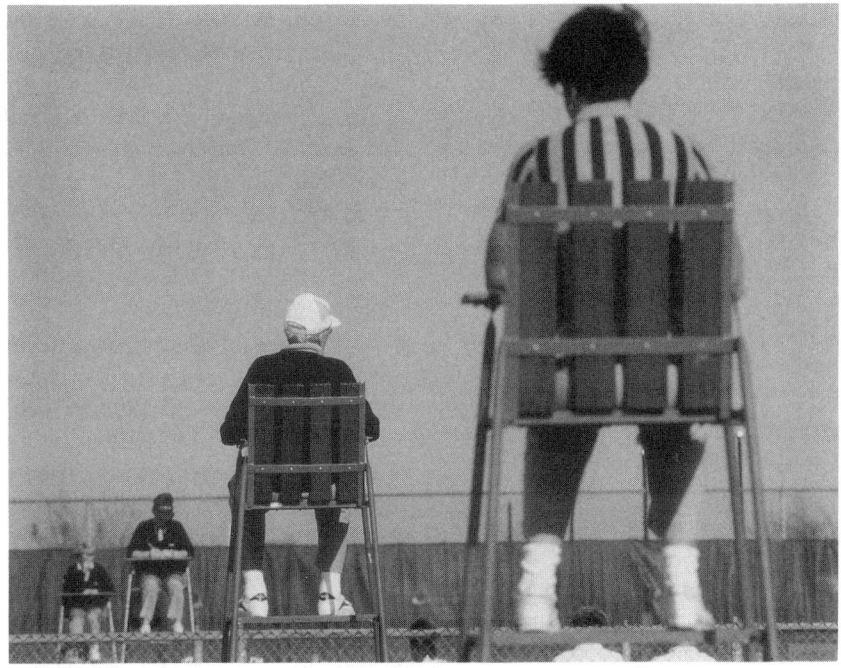

Courtesy University of Wisconsin Women's Sports Information

Problem solution involves generating solutions in a brainstorming procedure and forming *contracts* or agreements to attempt to solve the defined problem. For a detailed description of problem-solving and communication-skills training, see Jacobson and Margolin (1979).

Providing Neutrality

For some couples, it is important that they have a neutral place to discuss and express their feelings. They have typically been focused on blaming each other for the problems and have strong beliefs and ideas about how the other person can change to improve the relationship. If the relationship difficulties have continued over a long time, couples have usually developed patterns in their thinking and behavior that perpetuate both their positions and the distress. Interventions in relationship therapies are aimed at increasing awareness or bringing about better

understanding of these patterns. With this new understanding, along with generating and trying alternative approaches (interpersonally and intrapersonally), a different and more mutually-satisfying relationship can emerge.

CASE STUDIES FOLLOW-UP

Mike and Denise entered into couples therapy after several cancellations due to Mike's sport commitments. Their communication skills and problem-solving attempts were based on blame and apparent misunderstanding, which further alienated each of them. Structured communication training and problem solving gave them a common language and structure to connect with each other. Over the course of therapy, Mike and Denise began to share some of the assumptions and beliefs they had about each other and about marriage that related to their frustrations.

Denise expressed concern over her feelings of helplessness and dependency in the relationship. She revealed feeling that she was repeating her mother's marital experience. She was also able to express her own anxiety and insecurity about pursuing a career. She assumed Mike would reject her if she failed as an interior designer. Mike was initially quiet and absorbed Denise's anger and upset. When he finally shared his feelings with Denise about failing as a professional athlete and his sense of having nothing else he could do in life, Denise's anger was reduced.

They worked out agreements concerning time together and began to plan activities they both enjoyed. They appeared to achieve an increased sense of mutual understanding and support. They reaffirmed their basic acceptance of each other, not as an athlete or interior designer, but as people. In addition, they were able to support each other in changing some of the basic assumptions concerning their self-worth, confronting their fears of rejection, and forging a new comfort and nurturance in their relationship.

Reframing—suggesting to Mike that if his marital and home life is more positive, he is more likely to improve his sport performance and would be less distracted—was an important shift. Mike could now commit to working on the marriage and still feel he was working on his performance. Denise and Mike were seen for approximately 7 months; over that time their marital relationship improved, Mike's sport performance reached last year's strong level, and Denise successfully completed several interior design courses.

Sandra and Dan were seen for five sessions. A time-limited structure was established to preserve the individual consultative relationship initially started with Sandra. If further relationship work was needed a referral would have been given. Sandra and Dan

were quite apprehensive about the first meeting. Dan felt it was a cut-and-dried issue of Sandra having to choose skating or him; Sandra felt that a compromise should be reached. In the background, mother and coach felt more aligned with Dan's either-or approach but could not let go of their investment and entitlement issues. Sandra and Dan were able to talk about what they liked about each other.

It was noted that communication about disagreements and conflicts was very frustrating for Dan, and anxiety provoking for Sandra. Dan was challenging of Sandra's goals and dreams in skating; this attitude was apparently rooted in his negative experience in the sport. Rather than being a source of empathy and commonality for the relationship, his skating history became the venue for his frustrations. Sandra expressed her belief that if she focused on her skating she would lose Dan and, as she later revealed, her chance to be happy in a relationship. Skating was Sandra's main source of self-esteem, and she held it tightly. Dan backed away from his threatened breakup as he heard Sandra becoming more focused on wanting to make her "wholehearted" skating efforts.

When Sandra realized Dan would not break up with her, she felt even more confident about her choice to skate. Dan's threat and ultimatum had made her think that perhaps he wasn't as sensitive or supportive as she expected in a relationship partner. Sandra and Dan had to come to some understanding and arrangement concerning time together, so some problem-solving techniques were implemented. Agreements were reached that limited time together, and skating demands were designated as the top priority. Sandra and Dan eventually concluded that they were too young for their relationship to be top priority. Sandra's skating immediately improved and she described that a "weight was off my shoulders" (a weight that apparently had been throwing off her double axel). Following the competitive season, Sandra and Dan continued to date, but 3 or 4 months later, as training for the new season was about to begin, they broke up with only short-lived upset for Sandra.

ETHICAL ISSUES

When working with athletes and their relationships, one can be faced with numerous ethical or practice-related issues. Sometimes the exploration of an important relationship issue is likely to have an emotional or distracting effect on the athlete, who might be in the middle of training or competing. Do you pursue the issue for the benefit of the relationship or wait until the competition is over? Generally, this is an issue that can be brought up to the couple so that choices to explore or not explore are explicit, not implicit; in this way, you also protect yourself as a therapist from alienating the nonathlete spouse as you would by seeming to buy into the idea that the relationship is a lower priority than sport involvement is.

It is also important to be clear about confidentiality issues and policies in relationship therapy. This is especially important if an individual consultative relationship previously had been established. If you want to maintain the individual consultative relationship, it seems prudent to either limit the number of sessions with a collateral or make a referral to another therapist.

Awareness of cultural and sex-role issues is important, as ethical issues can arise out of these factors. Further discussion of ethical issues in marital therapy can be found in Margolin (1986).

CONCLUSION

Relationships play an important role in the lives of most people, including athletes. The bidirectional arrow between relationships and sport performance and involvement seems well established but has been explored only minimally. On an anecdotal basis, relationships among athletes are seen as sources of support as well as sources of upset and distraction.

Little research is available on relationship issues among athletes. This appears to be an area that warrants exploration. Relationship enrichment might indeed prove to be a strong influence on level of performance or effort. The other arrow direction deals with the impact of both sport and sport-related behavior and attitudes on the development of relationships—in terms of quality and quantity, problem areas, and suggestions for enrichment. Retrospective interviewing of athletes might explore how they came to understand the role of relationships in their sport goals. These perceptions might be helpful in understanding current relationship patterns or problems.

Monitoring aspects of social networks and relationship functioning among athletes might prove to be important in suggesting focuses for interventions designed to improve general personal adjustment, sport adjustment, and sport performance.

Further research into the relationship difficulties facing athletes is crucial. Exploring how their involvement in sport influences their relationship behavior patterns, both positive and negative, would make a significant contribution to sport psychology.

REFERENCES

Aylmer, R. (1986). Bowen family systems marital therapy. In N. Jacobson & A. Gurman (Eds.), *Clinical handbook of marital therapy* (pp. 107-148). New York: Guilford Press.

Baillie, P., & Danish, S. (1992). Understanding the career transition of athletes. *Sport Psychologist*, **6**, 77-98.

Beck, A.T. (1988). *Love is never enough*. New York: Harper & Row.

Botterill, C. (1990). Sport psychology and professional hockey. *Sport Psychologist*, **4**, 358-368.

Erikson, E. (1959). Identity and life cycle. *Psychological Issues*, **1**, 1-171.

Erikson, E. (1963). *Childhood and society* (2nd ed.). New York: Norton.

Framo, J. (1981). The integration of marital therapy with sessions with family of origin. In A. Gurman & D. Kniskern (Eds.), *Handbook of family therapy* (pp. 133-186). New York: Brunner/Mazel.

Golding, J., & Ungerleider, S. (1991). Social resources and mood among masters track and field athletes. *Journal of Applied Sport Psychology*, **3**, 142-159.

Greenberg, L., & Johnson, S. (1987). Emotionally focused couples therapy. In N. Jacobson & A. Gurman (Eds.), *Clinical handbook of marital therapy* (pp. 253-276). New York: Guilford Press.

Greendorfer, S., & Lewko, J. (1978). Role of family members in sport socialization of children. *Research Quarterly*, **49**, 146-152.

Hardy, C., Richman, J., & Rosenfeld, L. (1992). The role of social support in life stress/injury relationship. *Sport Psychologist*, **5**, 128-139.

Harris, D. (1987). The female athlete. In J. May & M. Asken (Eds.), *Sport psychology: The psychological health of the athlete* (pp. 99-116). New York: PMA.

Heyman, S. (1987). Counseling and psychotherapy with athletes: Special considerations. In J. May & M. Asken (Eds.), *Sport psychology: The psychological health of the athlete* (pp. 135-156). New York: PMA.

Jacobson, N., & Gurman, A. (Eds.) (1986). *Clinical handbook of marital therapy*. New York: Guilford Press.

Jacobson, N., & Holtzworth-Munroe, A. (1986). Marital therapy: A social learning-cognitive perspective. In N. Jacobson & A. Gurman (Eds.), *Clinical handbook of marital therapy* (pp. 29-70). New York: Guilford Press.

Jacobson, N., & Margolin, G. (1979). *Marital therapy*. New York: Brunner/Mazel.

Margolin, G. (1986). Ethical issues in marital therapy. In N. Jacobson & A. Gurman (Eds.), *Clinical handbook of marital therapy* (pp. 621-638). New York: Guilford Press.

May, J., & Veach, T. (1987). The U.S. Alpine ski team psychology program: A proposed consultation model. In J. May and M. Asken (Eds.), *Sport psychology: The psychological health of the athlete* (pp. 19-39). New York: PMA.

McElroy, M., & Kirkendall, D. (1980). Significant others and professionalized sport attitudes. *Research Quarterly for Exercise and Sport*, **51**, 645-653.

Rosenfield, L., Richman, J., & Hardy, C. (1989). Examining social support networks among athletes: Description and relationship to stress. *Sport Psychologist*, **3**, 23-33.

Smith, R. (1986). Athletic stress and burnout: Conceptual models and intervention strategies. In D. Hackfort & C. Spielberger (Eds.), *Anxiety in sports: An international perspective* (pp. 183-201). New York: Hemisphere.

Smith, R., Smoll, F., & Ptacek, J. (1990). Conjunctive moderator variables in vulnerability and resiliency research: Life stress, social support and coping skills, and adolescent sport injuries. *Journal of Personality and Social Psychology*, **58**, 360-370.

CHAPTER 9

GENDER ISSUES: A SOCIAL-EDUCATIONAL PERSPECTIVE

Diane L. Gill, PhD
University of North Carolina at Greensboro

Gender as an issue in sport psychology is relatively recent. Gender was not an issue in the sport psychology of Coleman Griffith's day. From Griffith's time in the 1920s up to the 1970s when sport psychology emerged as an identifiable area, *athlete* meant *male athlete*. Women were active in sport and physical activity much earlier, as historians of women's sport note (e.g., Spears, 1978), but women entered the modern athletic world in significant numbers only with the passage in 1972 of Title IX of the Educational Amendments Act and the related social changes of the early 1970s. Modern sport science, particularly sport psychology, also emerged in the 1970s, with the more professionally oriented applied sport psychology following in the 1980s. Given the short history of women's sport participation, we should not be surprised to find that the history of gender issues in sport psychology is short. What is surprising, though, is that despite the tremendous influx of females into athletics over the past 20 years and the increasing popularity of applied sport psychology over the last 10 years, we have little research or professional writing on gender issues in applied sport psychology.

This is a particularly striking void because even a moment's reflection or a glance at the popular media reveals many gender issues. The Billie Jean King–Bobby Riggs Battle of the Sexes tennis match captured public attention in the early 1970s. Women athletes gained prominence through Olympic coverage in the 1970s and 1980s; in the 1992 Winter Olympics, the female contingent of the United States team garnered most of the country's medals. In the 1990s the NCAA, the major governing body of intercollegiate sports, grapples with the issue of gender equity. Sport psychologists have contributed little to these discussions, and we seldom consider the implications of gender in our work.

By definition, psychology focuses on individual behavior, thoughts, and feelings. But we cannot fully understand the person without considering the larger world, that is, social context. Social context is important for all our work—no behavior takes place in isolation—and social context is critical in gender issues. Thus this chapter's title contains the word *social*. I follow a social approach easily, as nearly all my sport and exercise psychology work takes a social-psychological perspective. The second part of the title, educational, is a bigger stretch for me. I have reviewed the sport psychology work on gender elsewhere (Gill, 1992a), but not with the applied emphasis of this chapter.

As noted in the introduction, this book is intended for practicing sport psychologists. I purposely used *educational* rather than *clinical* in this chapter's title for several reasons. I do not have clinical training or experience and could not legitimately claim that perspective. Indeed, I do little educational sport psychology practice, although I have consulted with teams in the past on psychological skills. Primarily, I am an academic sport and exercise psychologist researching and writing on social-psychological aspects of physical activity and attempting to draw implications for those who work more directly with men and women, girls and boys, as teachers, coaches, or practicing sport psychologists.

For this chapter's topic, gender, this social-educational approach seems appropriate. Gender is not a special issue; it is an issue for everything we do in sport psychology. Gender is not a psychological disorder or problem that calls for therapy. Rather, gender influences all other issues, practices, problems, and experiences that are discussed in other chapters of this book. This chapter's point is that gender makes a difference. Sport psychologists who are aware of gender influences on athletes, the athletic world, and sport psychology practice will better serve athletes and society.

To better understand this issue, consider the following cases. These are not clinical cases, and I will not offer a solution to them either here or later in this chapter. Instead, these brief scenarios represent situations that a practicing sport psychologist might encounter. At the end of the chapter we will return to these cases to discuss gender implications. But for now, consider how you would interpret the situation and respond as well as what approaches you might take if you were to encounter these situations. If you have already encountered such cases, consider your reactions.

■ *THE CASE OF TERRY* ■

Terry, a 16-year-old figure skater, has been referred to you because the coach is concerned about a possible eating disorder. Terry says, "There's no problem. I need to stay trim to keep that 'line' the judges look for. I've always had trouble keeping extra pounds off, but I need to work at it to be at my best, make it to nationals, and eventually get endorsements."

■ *THE CASE OF A.J.* ■

A.J. is an 18-year-old freshman on the intercollegiate soccer team. A.J. is given to angry outbursts and temper tantrums and has already been thrown out of two games. A.J. says, "I know I need to stay in the game for my coach and teammates, but I play better when I'm on the edge. I need to be really up for the game and sometimes I just lose it." The coach is concerned about A.J.'s lack of control and further reports that A.J. shows a similar lack of control by skipping the team study hall to drink and party.

■ *THE CASE OF CHRIS* ■

In contrast to A.J., Chris, starting forward on the basketball team, never gets angry or loses control. Chris has talent and size but plays tentatively and seems to lack confidence. The coach not only wants 100% from Chris but also is concerned that the other players, who look to Chris for leadership, might be affected. Chris says, "I can't do what the coach wants. I can't get mad at my opponent, and it doesn't seem right to me to throw elbows or try to hurt someone. And I'm no good at being a leader, I don't like telling others what to do; I want to be a teacher, not a coach."

■ THE CASE OF PAT ■

Pat's the third-ranked singles player on the tennis team. Normally a solid, consistent player, lately Pat's play has been off. After some discussion Pat says, "I'm worried about the assistant coach. Although nothing has been said or done directly, I think the coach likes me and hints at wanting more of a relationship. I'm not at all interested, but I don't want to hurt the coach's feelings. I used to stay after practice and do extra work, but now I don't hang around or ask for any help because I'm avoiding the coach. I want the extra practice and coaching, and I know I'm not concentrating, but I don't know what to do."

Consider how gender influences your interpretations and responses. I did not identify the athletes by gender, but in imagining the scenarios you probably did. (To develop a vivid image you probably also imagined athletes of a particular race and with other characteristics; we'll get back to some of those issues later.) Consider the gender implications. Terry could be a male figure skater, but chances are much greater that a female skater would exhibit those behaviors. Perhaps you were tuned in to gender issues by the title and introduction and tried to be non-sexist, assuming that you should treat females and males the same way. But if you tried to do that, you likely had difficulty. Gender indeed makes a difference. Take any of the scenarios and try to imagine the situation with the other gender (e.g., if you imagined a male A.J., imagine a female and see if you still have the same interpretations and responses). Does athlete gender influence your immediate reactions, your expectations, or the options and approaches you would consider? I suspect that gender influences all of these and, moreover, I believe that gender *should* have an influence. If you try to assume a gender-neutral approach and treat everyone the same, I believe you'll do a disservice to the athletes. Again, gender makes a difference.

Of course I am not arguing for an approach based on biases and stereotypes. Indeed, the literature indicates that even trained therapists and educational professionals hold many stereotypes and that we should consciously try to avoid acting on such biases. However, misguided attempts to treat everyone the same go against current practice in sport psychology. Specifically, one of the strongest guidelines in most discussions of educational and clinical sport psychology is individualization. Each athlete has individual characteristics, experiences, and preferences, and gender is a salient individual characteristic.

However, in this chapter I do not wish to emphasize gender as an individual characteristic, but rather as a social characteristic and one of the most salient and powerful aspects of the social context. For example, Terry is more likely to be a female figure skater not simply because females are more likely to have eating disorders but because society expects and values thinness more in women than in men and communicates that message in many ways. You might consider different options for Christine or Christopher, not because of gender biases or stereotypes but because you know that their situations are different because of gender. For example, media coverage, social support systems, future opportunities, and teammate and coach expectations all vary with gender, even if both are talented players in competitive programs. Pat's scenario seems the most directly tied to biological sex. Yet even here with a change of gender of Pat or the coach your responses might change dramatically because of the social connotations of gender and sexuality.

Before continuing with a review of the literature related to gender and sport, go back through the scenarios and try to imagine each one with both male and female athletes. Consider how your reactions, interpretations, or approaches might change. Consider how a change of gender for others (e.g., coaches, parents) might influence you. Lastly, consider how your own gender influences your views and approaches. When you are actually dealing with cases such as these, does your gender have an influence? Do you do anything, or not do anything, because you are a man or a woman? No doubt you can think of some ways that gender influences your behavior. Still, it's probably impossible for any of us to really identify all the ways that gender affects us. From birth our world has been shaped by gender. Our parents, teachers, peers, and coaches reacted to us as girls or boys. Our images of athletes have been shaped by gendered media portrayals. Gender is such a pervasive influence in society that it's nearly impossible to pinpoint. Sport is no exception, and sport psychologists should be aware of gender influences in the larger society and in the sport world.

REVIEWING
THE LITERATURE

Neither psychology nor sport and exercise science provides conclusive answers to our many questions about gender, but we can draw on both areas to develop our sport psychology literature. Gender is a recent topic for sport and exercise science, but some scholars are beginning to build a knowledge base. Given that most research has been done with men, the phrase *considering gender* implies that issues specific to women will now be incorporated. For example, exercise physiologists have studied specific training responses, injury patterns, and nutritional issues for women, and journals often include articles on exercise during pregnancy, athletic amenorrhea, and other issues of special

concern to women (see Wells, 1991, for a review). As some of the biological scientists in sport and exercise are examining gender issues, the most prominent gender scholarship is being conducted by sociocultural sport scholars (see Birrell, 1988, for a review). Sport has a social and historical context; individual differences and psychological processes operate in this context, and to understand gender and behavior sport psychologists should be aware of this sociocultural scholarship as well as biological research.

The sociohistorical context of competitive athletics for women, the setting most sport psychologists work with, is particularly relevant. Sport psychologists today will find a vastly different athletic world than they themselves might have experienced 25, 15, or even 5 years ago. In 1967, Kathy Switzer created a stir when she defied the rules barring women and sneaked into the Boston Marathon; today (after much prodding) we have an Olympic marathon for women. I grew up as an avid backyard baseball player, but was left with few options when most of my teammates moved into Little League; today two girls are the star players on my 9-year-old nephew's soccer team.

The landmark beginning for this turnaround in women's sports was the 1972 passage of Title IX of the Educational Amendments Act. This law emerged from the civil rights and women's movements, when actions such as those of Switzer and several young women who tried to break into all-male athletic programs helped highlight larger discrimination issues. Title IX is a broad ban on sex discrimination in all educational programs receiving federal assistance, including educational sport programs. Most educational programs quickly moved to eliminate discrimination, but athletic programs took a defensive posture. Discrimination persists and Title IX challenges continue today, but women and girls have taken giant steps into the sport world.

The number of girls in interscholastic athletics and women in intercollegiate athletic programs has increased about 6- to 10-fold from pre-Title IX days. Mariah Burton Nelson illustrates some of these changes in describing her experiences at Stanford:

Between 1974 and 1978, I played varsity basketball at Stanford. Those years bridged the transition from female-controlled to male-controlled women's sports. For the first two years, we played in the "women's" (read: old, tiny) gym. We wore plain red shorts and white blouses; over those we tied "pinnies," a word only women seem to know. My teammates and I spent our spare time in the athletic department, begging the male athletic director to enforce Title IX. In my junior year, we finally received uniforms, a more experienced coach, and playing time in the men's gym. In 1978, my senior year, Stanford offered its first women's basketball scholarship. In 1990, Stanford won its first national championship. (Nelson, 1991, p. 6)

Women have gained a place in the sport world and now constitute about a third of high-school, college, and Olympic athletes. But, a third is not a half, and in other ways women have failed to gain or actually have lost a place. Most noticeably, the competitive sport world is hierarchical, and women are clustered at the bottom. The glass ceiling is lower and more impervious than in other domains, and women have not broken through in significant numbers to become coaches, administrators, sports writers, or sports medicine personnel. Vivian Acosta and Linda Carpenter have followed the status of women in athletics for several years, and the trends are clear. Before Title IX (1972) nearly all (more than 90%) women's athletic teams were coached by women and had a

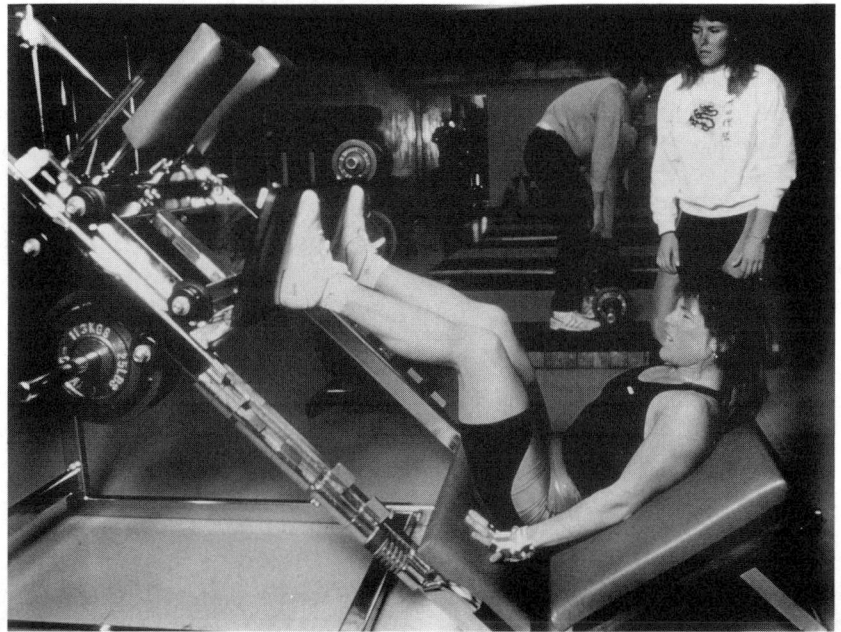

Courtesy USOC

woman heading the program. Today less than half of women's intercollegiate teams are coached by a woman and just 16% of women's programs have a woman director, usually as an associate athletic director (e.g., Carpenter & Acosta, 1993; Nelson, 1991; Uhlir, 1987). Of course, no parallel change has occurred for men's athletics, which were and continue to be coached and administered nearly entirely (more than 99%) by men.

Other changes are less noticeable—but just as notable—for gender implications. Although women have moved into previously all-male competitive athletic programs, other sport programs with more emphasis on participation, skill development, cooperation, and recreation have been lost to both men and women. And the implications extend beyond participation numbers. Safrit (1984) noted declining numbers of women in university physical education and exercise science departments, particularly in research-oriented programs, and a continuing low percentage of women as authors and editors in the professional literature. Duda (1991) specifically noted that most articles in the *Journal of Sport & Exercise Psychology*, our main research journal, from 1979 to 1986 were by male authors, about male athletes, and focused on competitive sports. In summarizing the journal's articles during my editorial term (1985 to 1990), I (Gill, 1992b) noted that most samples included both males and females and that although we had more male than female authors, proportions were closer to equal. Still, my observations of conferences, journals, and organizations suggest that males (definitely white males) dominate research and professional practice in sport psychology as well as competitive athletics, and sport psychologists should be aware of potential gender bias because of this pattern.

Like sport and exercise science, psychology is male dominated, although the numbers are not as striking. Psychology programs attract more female than male students, and the

American Psychological Association (APA) has a task force exploring the implications of this gender shift. Still, as with other fields, organizational leadership, research journals, and university faculties are male dominated. The psychology of women and gender is more peripheral than central to psychology, but the area is active and sport psychologists can look to that literature to help understand gender and sport.

As with sport and exercise science, psychologists have approached gender by studying women and women's issues. Division 35 (psychology of women) is active in the APA, and several journals focus on the psychology of women. Psychologists as well as women's studies scholars are beginning to focus more on gender rather than on women, recognizing that gender issues apply to both women and men and that *gender* means more than simply *gender differences*. In the following review I focus on this work from psychology and incorporate the related sport-specific psychology work.

Sex Differences

Generally, psychology work on women and gender has progressed from a sex-differences approach, to an emphasis on gender role as a personality orientation, to more current social-psychological models that emphasize social context and processes. Before reviewing that work, though, I should clarify terminology. Typically, *sex* differences refers to biologically-based differences between males and females, whereas *gender* refers to social and psychological characteristics and behaviors associated with females and males. The early sex-differences work assumed dichotomous biologically-based psychological differences that paralleled and, indeed, stemmed from biological male–female differences. Today, consensus holds that psychological characteristics and behaviors associated with females and males are neither dichotomous nor biologically based. Indeed, even most biological factors that are relevant to sport and exercise are not dichotomously divided between males and females, but are normally distributed in both females and males. For example, considering NCAA tournament basketball teams, the average male center is taller than the average female center, but the average female center is taller than most men. For social-psychological characteristics and behaviors, average differences are elusive, no evidence supports a biological basis, and no dichotomous sex-linked connections are evident.

The most widely cited sex-differences work is Eleanor Maccoby and Carol Jacklin's 1974 compilation of the existing research. Although they cautioned that few conclusions could be drawn, most subsequent discussions ignored that caution and their suggested "possible" sex differences quickly became accepted as established fact. Most people assume that males are more aggressive and have greater math and visuospatial ability, whereas females have greater verbal ability; these sex differences are sometimes cited as a reason for males' presumed superiority in sport.

Despite many attempts to identify sex differences and their biological correlates, the bulk of the research casts doubt even on the possible differences cited by Maccoby and Jacklin (1974). Several reviews, and most notably the meta-analytic reviews by Eagley (1987) and Hyde and Linn (1986), indicate that sex differences in ability are minimal, inconsistent, and not biologically based and that interactions are common. For example, boys might complete a timed math test faster than girls, but do no better on math accuracy with unlimited time. In general, overlap and similarities are much more apparent than differences.

Ashmore (1990) summarized the meta-analyses and research on sex differences and concluded that sex differences are large for certain physical abilities (e.g., throwing velocity, body use, posturing), more modest for other abilities and social behaviors (e.g., math, aggression), and negligible for all other domains (e.g., leadership, attitudes, such physical abilities as reaction time and balance). Even the larger sex differences are confounded with nonbiological influences. Ashmore as well as Maccoby (1990) and Jacklin (1989) advocate abandoning sex-differences approaches for more multifaceted and social approaches. Jacklin states that although researchers have been preoccupied with the search for sex differences, the tentative 1974 conclusions cannot be supported. Maccoby suggests that behavioral sex differences emerge mainly in social situations and vary with the gender composition of the group. Most psychologists who have reviewed this topic suggest that a sex-differences approach assumes an underlying, unidimensional cause (biological sex) and ignores the rich and complex variations in gender-related behavior.

In response to criticisms of the sex-differences approach and its failure to shed any light on gender-related behavior, psychologists turned to personality and individual differences for explanations.

Personality and Gender-Role Orientation

Psychologists have focused on gender-role orientation as the relevant personality construct to explain gender-related behavior. Specifically, Sandra Bem's (1974, 1978) work and her Bem Sex Role Inventory (BSRI) served as the major impetus for a large body of research and brought the constructs of masculinity, femininity, and androgyny to public attention and debate. Janet Spence and Bob Helmreich (1978) developed their parallel measure of gender-role orientation, the Personality Attributes Questionnaire (PAQ).

Both the BSRI and PAQ assess masculinity (or instrumentality) and femininity (or expressiveness) as separate, independent constructs. Most sport psychology research on gender uses the constructs and measures developed by Bem or by Spence and Helmreich. Helmreich and Spence (1977) sampled intercollegiate athletes and reported that most female athletes were either androgynous or masculine, in contrast to their nonathlete college female sample, who were most often classified as feminine.

Several subsequent studies with female athletes yielded similar findings. Harris and Jennings (1977) surveyed female distance runners and reported that most were androgynous or masculine. Both Del Rey and Sheppard (1981) and Colker and Widom (1980) found that most intercollegiate athletes were classified as androgynous or masculine. Myers and Lips (1978) reported that most female racquetball players were androgynous whereas most males were masculine.

Many more studies have surveyed women athletes using the BSRI or PAQ, but listing them would not tell us more about women's sport and exercise behavior. Moreover, both the methodology and underlying assumptions of this line of research have been widely criticized (e.g., Locksley & Colten, 1979; Pedhazur & Tetenbaum, 1979; Taylor & Hall, 1982). Most investigators accept the separate masculinity–instrumentality and femininity–expressiveness dimensions but question the meaning of the underlying constructs and the implications for other gender-related constructs and behaviors. Deaux (1985) concluded that the BSRI and PAQ seem to measure self-assertion and nurturance and do predict specific assertive and nurturant behaviors but do not relate very well to other gender-related attributes and behaviors.

Overall, then, the sport and exercise psychology research on gender-role orientation suggests that female athletes possess more masculine–instrumental personality characteristics than do female nonathletes. This is not particularly enlightening. Sport, especially competitive athletics, is an achievement activity that demands instrumental, assertive behaviors. Both the BSRI and PAQ include *competitive* as a masculine item, and the higher masculine scores of female athletes probably reflect an overlap with competitiveness. Competitive orientation can be measured directly (e.g., Gill & Deeter, 1988; Gill & Dzewaltowski, 1988), so we need not invoke more indirect, controversial measures.

Perhaps even more important, athlete–nonathlete status is an indirect and nonspecific measure of behavior. If instrumental and expressive personality characteristics predict instrumental and expressive behaviors, we should examine those instrumental and expressive behaviors in sport. Even in highly competitive sports, expressive behaviors might be advantageous. Creative, expressive actions might be the key to success for a gymnast; supportive behaviors of teammates might be critical on a soccer team; and sensitivity to others might help an Olympic coach (not to mention a sport psychologist) communicate with each athlete.

Even if we recognize cautions and limits, gender-role orientation raises concerns. Ann Hall (1988), one of the first sport sociologists to take a feminist approach, charges that using the gender-role constructs and measures reifies abstract masculine–feminine dichotomous constructs. Hall (1990) also cautions that this gender-role approach encourages a focus on "role conflict," (i.e., that the role of athlete conflicts with the female role.) Del Rey (1978) and Harris (1980), for example, discussed the conflicting demands of sport and femininity as problems for athletes. Today that role-conflict approach has been largely discounted. Female athletes typically do not express role conflict as defined in this literature, and both Hall (1990) and Allison (1991) summarize this work by concluding that the notion of role conflict has not been helpful and should be abandoned.

Although this early role-conflict work is not credible today, athletes might experience role conflict in which gender plays a role. Blinde and Greendorfer (1992) summarized five previous studies and concluded that athletes experience four types of conflict:

- Value alienation (conflict of athletic values with personal values)
- Role strain (difficulty meeting others' varied expectations of the athlete role, such as coach and professor expectations of the athlete)
- Role conflict (difficulty meeting expectations of multiple roles, such as athlete and student)
- Exploitation (dominance of the athlete role such that other roles cannot be fulfilled)

Although both male and female athletes might experience any of these conflicts, they might be gender-related. For example, values of intercollegiate coaches and programs might well be more alien to a freshman female recruit than to her male counterpart, or the demands of the male-athlete role in a big-time basketball program might more likely lead to exploitation. Blinde and Greendorfer (1992) noted fewer conflicts for female athletes in pre-Title IX and post-Title IX Division III programs than for post-Title IX female athletes in Division I who are moving into the male sport model. Importantly, for most female athletes the sport experience was not negative but worthwhile and challenging. Thus sport psychologists should not assume role conflict for female athletes, but should be aware that some female or male athletes might experience conflicts in which gender might play a role.

Overall, the sport and exercise psychology research on gender-role orientation has all the drawbacks of early sport personality research wrapped up with limiting gender

stereotypes and biases. Most psychologists now recognize the limits of the earlier sex-differences and gender-role approaches and look beyond the simple male–female and masculine–feminine dichotomies.

Gender and Sport Achievement

For example, research on achievement has progressed from early sex differences through gender roles to more current social-cognitive models. Achievement is a prominent topic in the psychology research on gender, as well as a clear concern of sport psychologists. Most sport and exercise activities involve achievement behavior and particularly competitive achievement. Gender differences were ignored in the early achievement research (McClelland, Atkinson, Clark, & Lowell, 1953), and researchers simply took male behavior as the norm until Matina Horner's (1972) doctoral work focused attention on gender. Horner suggested that success has negative consequences for women, because success requires competitive achievement behaviors that conflict with the traditional feminine image. This conflict arouses a motive to avoid success, popularly termed the fear of success (FOS), and leads to anxiety and avoidance. Horner provided some evidence, and her work was widely publicized, but critics (e.g., Condry & Dyer, 1975; Tresemer, 1977) noted that FOS imagery was prevalent in men as well as women, the FOS measure confused stereotyped attitudes with motives, and the research failed to link FOS directly to achievement behaviors. McElroy and Willis (1979), who specifically considered women's achievement conflicts in sport contexts, concluded that no evidence supports a FOS in female athletes and that achievement attitudes of female athletes are similar to those of male athletes.

Current scholars have replaced global achievement motives with multidimensional constructs and an emphasis on achievement

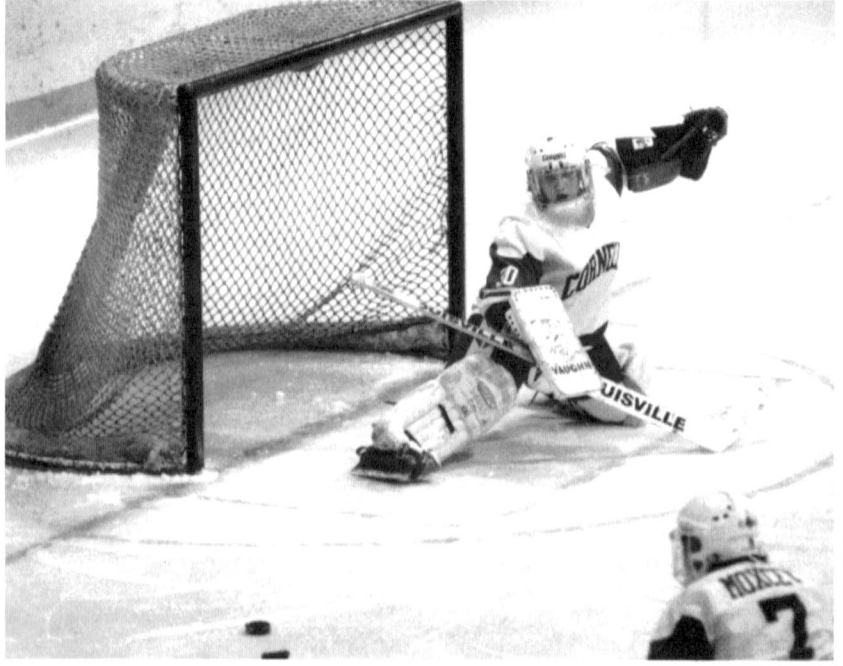

Courtesy Tim McKinney

cognitions. Spence and Helmreich (1978, 1983) developed a multidimensional measure with separate dimensions of mastery, work, and competitiveness; they found that males score higher than females on mastery and competitiveness, whereas females score higher than males on work. Gender differences on mastery and work diminish for athletes, but males score higher than females on competitiveness. Also, masculinity scores relate positively to all three achievement dimensions, whereas femininity scores relate slightly positively to work and negatively to competitiveness. Generally, gender influence is strongest and most consistent for competitiveness.

My work (Gill, 1988, 1993) with the Sport Orientation Questionnaire (SOQ) (Gill & Deeter, 1988) that assesses competitiveness (an achievement orientation to enter and strive for success in competitive sport), win orientation (a desire to win and avoid losing),

and goal orientation (an emphasis on achieving personal goals) also suggests that gender influences vary across dimensions. Males typically score higher than females on competitiveness and win orientation, whereas females typically score slightly higher than males on goal orientation. Comparing females and males who participated in competitive sport, noncompetitive sport, and nonsport achievement activities revealed that, overall, males consistently scored higher than females on sport competitiveness and win orientation, and males also reported more competitive sport activity and experience. However, females were just as high as males, and sometimes higher, on sport-goal orientation and general achievement. Also, females were just as likely as males to participate in noncompetitive sport and nonsport achievement activities. Thus the gender differences do not seem to reflect either general achievement orientation or interest in sport and exercise activities per se. Instead, gender is related to an emphasis on social comparison and winning in sport.

Other researchers report similar gender influences on reactions to competitive sport. When McNally and Orlick (1975) introduced a cooperative broomball game to children in urban Canada and in the Northwest Territories, they found girls were more receptive to the cooperative rules than boys were. They also noted cultural differences, with northern children more receptive, but the gender influence held in both cultures. Duda (1986) similarly reported both gender and cultural influences on competitiveness with Anglo and Navajo children in the southwestern United States. Male Anglo children were the most win oriented and placed the most emphasis on athletic ability. Weinberg and Jackson (1979) found that males were more affected by success and failure than were females, and in a related study Weinberg and Ragan (1979) reported that males were more interested in a competitive activity whereas females preferred a noncompetitive activity.

Although several lines of research suggest gender influences on competitive sport achievement, the research does not point to any unique gender-related personality construct as an explanation. Instead, most investigators are turning to socialization, societal influences, and social-cognitive models for explanations.

Cognitive approaches currently dominate research on achievement. The concept underlying these approaches is that what the person *thinks* is important, *is* important. For example, if you expect to do well at volleyball, you probably will. Research consistently indicates that expectations are good predictors of achievement behavior and performance (e.g., Bandura, 1977, 1986; Crandall, 1969; Eccles et al., 1983; Feltz, 1988), and research also suggests gender influences. Typically, females report lower expectations of success and make fewer achievement-oriented attributions than males do. However, gender differences are not completely consistent. In her

review of the self-confidence literature, Lenney (1977) concluded that gender differences in confidence are more likely to occur in achievement situations that

- involve tasks perceived as masculine,
- provide only ambiguous feedback or ability information, and
- emphasize social comparison.

In sport and exercise psychology, Corbin and his colleagues (Corbin, 1981; Corbin, Landers, Feltz, & Senior, 1983; Corbin & Nix, 1979; Corbin, Stewart, & Blair, 1981; Petruzzello & Corbin, 1988; Stewart & Corbin, 1988) have conducted a series of experimental studies that confirm Lenney's propositions. Specifically, Corbin and his colleagues demonstrated that females do not lack confidence with a gender-neutral, non-socially-evaluative task and that performance feedback can improve the confidence of low-confidence females; the researchers also suggested lack of experience as an additional factor affecting female self-confidence. In our lab (Gill, Gross, Huddleston, & Shifflett, 1984) we matched female and male competitors of similar ability on a pegboard task. Males were slightly more likely than females to predict a win, but performance expectations were similar; females performed slightly better in competition than males did, and females generally had more positive achievement cognitions (higher perceived ability, more effort attributions).

Thus females and males display similar levels of confidence when tasks are appropriate for females, when females and males have similar experiences and capabilities, and when clear evaluation criteria and feedback are present. Importantly, though, the confirming research involves experimental studies in controlled settings. We cannot so easily equate task appropriateness, experience, and social influence in the real world of sport. We must consider socialization and social context.

Jacquelynne Eccles's (1985, 1987; Eccles et al., 1983) model incorporates such socio-cultural factors along with achievement cognitions. Eccles recognizes that both expectations and importance or value determine achievement choices and behaviors. As discussed earlier, gender differences in expectations are common, and gender also influences the value of sport achievement. Eccles further notes that gender differences in expectations and value develop over time and are influenced by gender-role socialization, stereotyped expectations of others, and socio-cultural norms, as well as individual characteristics and experiences. Recently, Eccles and Harold (1991) summarized existing work and provided new evidence showing that her model holds for sport achievement, that gender influences children's sport achievement perceptions and behaviors at a very young age, and that these gender differences seem to be the product of gender-role socialization.

Physical Activity and Self-Perceptions

Before moving away from personality and individual differences I want to consider the role of sport and exercise on self-perceptions, particularly body image and self-esteem. As just noted, females tend to lack confidence in their sport and exercise capabilities. Thus sport has a tremendous potential to enhance women's sense of competence and control. Many women who begin activity programs report such enhanced self-esteem and a sense of physical competence that often carries over into other aspects of their lives. A few studies add some support to these testimonials. Holloway, Beuter, and Duda (1988), Brown and Harrison (1986), and Trujillo (1983) all report that exercise programs, particularly weight and strength training, enhance the self-concepts of women participants.

As well as developing feelings of physical strength and confidence, sport offers the opportunity to strive for excellence, the chance to accomplish a goal through effort and training, and the psychological challenge of testing oneself in competition. Marathon swimmer Diana Nyad expressed this:

> When asked why, I say that marathon swimming is the most difficult physical, intellectual, and emotional battleground I have encountered, and each time I win, each time I reach the other shore, I feel worthy of any other challenge life has to offer. (1978, p. 152)

The values expressed by Nyad should be gained in competitive athletics, but too often we lose these real benefits when we focus on competitive outcomes. Research clearly shows that overemphasizing extrinsic rewards detracts from intrinsic interest, other psychological benefits, and even performance achievements. Focusing on intrinsic standards for both performance and nonperformance goals should benefit all athletes and especially help women enhance their sense of physical competence and confidence.

Sport psychologists should take particular note of the work on gender and the relationship of body image to individual perceptions and attitudes about physical activity and to participation and behavior in sport and exercise settings. For example, *The Bodywise Woman* (Melpomene Institute, 1990) and Rodin, Silberstein, and Streigel-Moore's (1985) symposium contribution "Women and Weight" provide excellent reviews and discussion. This information clearly points to a strong sociocultural influence on body image. Our images of the ideal body, and particularly the ideal female body, have changed through history and across social contexts. Today's ideal is a slender, lean female body, and most women recognize and strive for that ideal—which is much less than ideal in terms of physical and mental health. Boys and men also have concerns about body image, but the literature indicates that girls and women are much more negative about their bodies. Moreover, these concerns are gender related. Girls are particularly concerned with physical beauty and maintaining the ideal thin shape, whereas boys are more concerned with size, strength, and power. Research indicates that most adult women perceive an underweight body as ideal and tend to see themselves as overweight even though most fall within normal weight ranges. We could simply encourage young women to ignore media images, but unfortunately our obsession with body image and particularly weight loss has justification in our society. Studies indicate that people who don't match the ideal, especially overweight, obese people, and more especially overweight, obese women, are evaluated negatively and discriminated against. Thus society shapes body image; this societal pressure for a body image that is not particularly healthy nor attainable for many women likely has a negative influence on self-esteem and psychological well-being as well as on physical health.

We must also note here that biology plays an important role in body image, particularly when we consider overweight and obese women. Obese people do not necessarily lack willpower, and they cannot lose weight merely by "really" wanting to. Metabolic rates and processes vary greatly among people and are largely genetically determined; some of the assumed links between obesity and health might reflect psychological and social problems rather than medical problems; and the constant dieting, especially with a yo-yo pattern of weight gains and losses, might be more detrimental to health than remaining consistently overweight.

Concerns about body image affect all women, but we should be especially mindful of how such body concerns influence women in sport. Athletes are just as susceptible as other women to the general societal pressure toward eating disorders and unrealistic, unhealthy thinness. Sport psychologists need to be aware of this possibility. Pressures toward thinness, and thus unhealthy eating behaviors, are of most concern in the thin-body sports, such as gymnastics, dance, and running. Coaches in such sports should be especially sensitive to what they communicate about ideal and realistic body shapes to their athletes. For example, one athlete reported:

> At age 14 my cycling coach told me I was "fat" in front of my entire team . . . At 5 ft, 5 in., 124 lb [56 kg], I was not fat, but my self-esteem was so low that I simply believed him. After all, he was the coach." (Melpomene Institute, 1990, p. 36)

Coaches and teachers should know that pressuring an athlete, who already has tremendous societal pressure to lose weight, is not a desirable approach. Most enlightened coaches and instructors follow nutritional guidelines and emphasize healthy eating rather than weight standards.

Gender and Social Processes

As Deaux (1984) reported, gender research in the 1980s moved away from studying sex differences and individual differences to regarding gender as a social category. Even Bem moved away from her early focus on personality to a broader, more social gender-schema theory (1985). Gender-schema theory suggests that sex-typed people (masculine males and feminine females) are more likely than non-sex-typed people to classify sports as gender-appropriate and to restrict their participation to gender-appropriate activities. Matteo (1986, 1988) and Csizma, Wittig, and Schurr (1988) confirmed that sports are indeed sex-typed (mostly as masculine). Matteo further reported that sex-typing influenced sport choice and that sex-typed people did not participate in gender-inappropriate sports.

Gender Beliefs and Stereotypes

Deaux (1984, 1985; Deaux & Kite, 1987) focuses on social categories and social context, suggesting that how people think males and females differ is more important than actual differences. As discussed earlier, psychological differences between females and males are small and inconsistent. Nevertheless, we maintain our beliefs in gender differences. Deaux proposes that our gender stereotypes are pervasive and exert a major influence on social interactions. Considerable evidence supports the existence of gender stereotypes. From their often-cited research, Broverman, Rosenkrantz, and their colleagues (Broverman, Vogel, Broverman, Clarkson, & Rosenkrantz, 1972; Rosenkrantz, Vogel, Bee, Broverman, & Broverman, 1968) found that people believe males and females differ on a large number of characteristics and behaviors (e.g., women are more emotional and sensitive, whereas men are more forceful and independent). More relevant to clinical practice, I.K. Broverman and her colleagues asked therapists to judge the healthy man, healthy woman, and healthy adult on these characteristics. Therapists held gender stereotypes, and their ratings of the healthy adult more closely resembled their ratings of the healthy man than of the healthy woman.

More recent work (Deaux & Kite, 1987; Deaux & Lewis, 1984; Eagley & Kite, 1987) suggests that bipolar stereotypes persist and that gender stereotypes have multiple components. We not only hold gender stereotypes about personality traits but also about role behaviors, occupations, physical appearance, and sexuality. For example, we tend to picture construction workers as men and secretaries as women; if women are construction workers we picture them as looking like men in physical appearance. Deaux suggests that these multiple components are interrelated and that the relationships and implications for gender-related behavior might vary with the social context. For example, Deaux and Lewis found that people weigh physical appearance heavily and infer other gender-related traits and behaviors (e.g., personality, sexuality) from physical characteristics. Such multidimensional gender stereotypes certainly have counterparts in sport. We expect men with athletic body types to be athletes and, moreover, to be aggressive, competitive, independent, and of course heterosexual. Coaches seldom encourage a smaller young man, or one with artistic talents, to try out for football. We also tend to assume that women with athletic body builds or talents are aggressive, competitive, independent, and lesbian. Such stereotypes are prominent and have far-reaching implications for women and men in sport.

Considerable research suggests a gender bias in the evaluation of female and male performance. In a provocative study, Goldberg (1968) reported a bias favoring male authors when women judged articles that were equivalent except for sex of author. Subsequent studies confirmed a male bias, but suggest that the bias varies with information and situational characteristics (e.g., Pheterson, Kiesler, & Goldberg, 1971; Wallston & O'Leary, 1981). A series of studies that adopted the Goldberg approach to examine gender bias in attitudes toward hypothetical female and male coaches (Parkhouse & Williams, 1986; Weinberg, Reveles, & Jackson, 1984; Williams & Parkhouse, 1988) revealed a bias favoring male coaches. However, Williams and Parkhouse reported that female basketball players coached by a successful female did not exhibit the male bias, suggesting more complex influences on gender stereotypes and evaluations.

Although sport psychologists have not examined multidimensional gender stereotypes and interrelationships, gender stereotypes and gender bias in evaluations certainly exist in sport. Eleanor Metheny (1965) identified gender stereotypes in her classic analysis of the social acceptability of various sports. For example, Metheny concluded that it is not appropriate for women to engage in contests in which

- the resistance of the opponent is overcome by bodily contact,
- the resistance of a heavy object is overcome by direct application of bodily force, or
- the body is projected into or through space over long distances or for extended periods of time.

According to Metheny, acceptable sports for women (e.g., gymnastics, swimming, tennis) emphasize aesthetic qualities and often are individual activities in contrast to direct competition and team sports. Although Metheny offered her analysis more than 25 years ago, our gender stereotypes have not faded away with the implementation of Title IX. Gender stereotypes persist, and they seem more persistent in sport than in other social contexts. For example, Kane and Snyder (1989) recently confirmed gender stereotyping of sports, as suggested by Metheny, and more explicitly identified physicality as the central feature.

Not only do gender beliefs persist in sport and exercise, but socialization pressures toward such gender beliefs are pervasive, strong (although often subtle), and begin early (e.g., see Greendorfer, 1987). Gendered beliefs and behaviors are apparent even in infants, and parents, schools, and other socializers convey gendered beliefs in many direct and indirect ways. For example, in a text on women and gender, Unger and Crawford (1992) summarized the literature by noting that toys (boys have more vehicles and active toys, whereas girls have more dolls), clothes (colors, ruffles even on play suits of girls), and play (stories, activities) are powerful sources of gender stereotyping in early childhood and that by school age children's social

networks are sex-segregated. Overall, differential treatment is consistent with producing independence and efficacy in boys and emotional sensitivity, nurturance, and helplessness in girls. Pressures for gender-role conformity are stronger for boys, and, of particular interest for this chapter, many girls resist typing to be active in sports. Although both girls and boys participate, sport psychologists should expect subtle but pervasive gender pressures; an understanding of gender socialization provides the basis for understanding individual gender-related behavior in sport and exercise.

One prominent source of gender stereotyping that has been investigated by sport scholars is the media. Investigations of television, newspaper, and popular magazine coverage of female and male athletes reveal clear gender bias (e.g., Kane, 1989; Kane & Parks, 1992; Messner, Duncan, & Jensen, 1993). Females receive little media coverage (less than 10%) whether considering TV air time, newspaper space, feature articles, or photographs. Moreover, female and male athletes receive different coverage that reflects gender hierarchy. Generally, athletic ability and accomplishments are emphasized for men, but femininity and physical attractiveness are emphasized for women athletes. Kane (1989) described one graphic example with a photograph on the cover of the 1987-88 Northwest Louisiana State women's basketball media guide showing the team members wearing Playboy bunny ears and tails, captioned "These girls can Play, boy!" Gender bias in the sport media also occurs in more subtle ways. Eitzen and Baca Zinn (1993) reported that a majority of colleges had sexist nicknames or symbols (e.g., adding "elle" or "ette," Lady) that gender marked the women athletes as different from and less than the men athletes.

In a study of 1989 NCAA basketball tournaments and U.S. Open tennis coverage, Messner et al. (1993) noted less stereotyping than in previous studies, but still found considerable

- gender marking (e.g., *Women's* Final Four but Final Four for men), and
- gendered hierarchy of naming (e.g., females referred to as *girls, young ladies,* or *women*; men never referred to as *boys*).

Gender marking might be appropriate and useful when it's symmetrical or similar for women and men, as it was for most of the tennis coverage, but asymmetrical marking labels females as other than the norm or real athletes. Gendered language was also apparent in comments about success, failure, and strength. Comments about strength and weakness were ambivalent for women, but clearly about strength for men, and emotional reasons for failure (e.g., nerves, lack of confidence) were cited more often for women. Messner et al. noted that "dominants" in society typically are referred to by last names and subordinates by first names. They found first names used more than 50% of the time to refer to females but only 10% of the time to refer to males. Also, the few male athletes referred to by first names were black male basketball players. No race differences were observed for females; gender seemed to be more prominent.

My own observations of the most recent Olympic and NCAA tournaments suggests improvement with less stereotyping and trivialization of female athletes, but institutional change is slow and the sports media does not reflect current female sport participation. Overall, gendered beliefs seem alive and well in the sport world. Sport activities are gender stereotyped, and the sex-typing of sport activities seems linked with other gender beliefs (e.g., physicality). Gender beliefs influence social processes, and the research on gender bias in evaluation of coaches suggests that influence is at least as likely in sport as in other social interactions. Overt discrimination is unlikely, and participants might not recognize the influence of gendered beliefs in themselves or others. For example, many sport administrators and participants fail to recognize gender beliefs operating when athletic programs developed by and for men, stressing male-linked values and characteristics, are opened to girls and women.

Gender and Social Context

Not only should we consider gender stereotypes and beliefs, but as Deaux and Major (1987) state, we must consider the immediate social context and understand gender-related behavior in a given situation. Like Deaux, who has moved from her earlier gender work on attributions and individual characteristics to emphasize social context, Bem (1993) has moved beyond gender-schema and strictly psychological approaches to a more encompassing gender perspective. Bem now offers a more comprehensive analysis and proposes that the three gender lenses of

- gender polarization (the view that male–female differences are an organizing principle for social life),
- androcentrism (the view that the male is the norm), and
- biological essentialism (the view that these differences are the inevitable consequence of biological nature)

interact in historical context to perpetuate male dominance, particularly wealthy, white, heterosexual male dominance.

Deaux and Major, as well as Bem, advocate moving beyond traditional psychology boundaries to incorporate broader sociocultural perspectives on gender. Those recent calls echo Carolyn Sherif's (1976, 1982) earlier prolific and provocative social psychology work and her early advocacy for women and gender issues in psychology. Sherif, a persistent advocate for social psychology, emphasized social context and process in all her work and extended her discussions to sport and competition (e.g., Sherif, 1976). Unfortunately, sport and exercise psychologists have not adopted Sherif's suggestions or other current social-psychological approaches. Indeed, our research and practice seems narrower and more oblivious to social context and process than ever before. To break out of this isolation, sport psychologists might incorporate some of the sociology work on gender.

In *The Female World*, Jessie Bernard (1981) points out that social experiences and contexts for females and males are different, even when they appear similar on the surface. Indeed, male and female worlds are different. In the early days of organized sport, from the 1920s to Title IX in 1972, we intentionally established and maintained separate sport worlds for females and males. These separate sport worlds have not disappeared with legal and organizational changes. The social world differs for female and male members of intercollegiate basketball teams, for male and female joggers, and for girls and boys pitching a youth baseball game. In sport and exercise science, sport psychologists can look to the work of sport sociologists, who are doing the most prominent and innovative work on gender. Sport psychologists familiar with the work of such scholars as Ann Hall (1988), Susan Birrell (1988), Alison Dewar (1987), Nancy Theberge (1987), and Michael Messner (1992) could develop a fuller understanding of gender and sport. I particularly recommend Helen Lenskyj's (1986) coherent and provocative analysis of sexuality and gender, which emphasizes the historical and sociocultural pressures toward compulsory heterosexuality that influence women's sport and exercise participation and behaviors.

The work of these feminist sport scholars suggests that gender is pervasive in society, and specifically in sport society; that gender beliefs, relations, and processes are multifaceted; and that an understanding of the historical–cultural context and immediate social context is necessary to understand women's sport and exercise experiences.

Diversity in Social Context

Not only should we adopt more encompassing conceptual frameworks, but we should look into a wider range of issues and behaviors with more diverse women and men. Gender influences are just as prominent in youth sports, physical education classes, and exercise settings as in competitive athletics. Moreover, sport is not only male, but white, middle class, and heterosexual. Gender is one of several social identities and we should consider gender relations across varying social groups.

Duda and Allison (1990) point out the striking void in the field of sport and exercise psychology on race and ethnicity. Most of the issues raised for gender have parallels in race and ethnicity. That is, stereotypes are pervasive and multifaceted; racial and ethnic socialization, self-perceptions, and social context influence sport and exercise behavior; and a grounding in sociocultural history would enhance our understanding of race and ethnicity in sport. Although parallel issues arise, race and class are qualitatively different from gender; moreover we do not even have the limited work on racial or ethnic stereotypes and individual characteristics to parallel the gender research. More important for this chapter, gender likely interacts with race and class in many complex ways. For example, the experiences of a black, female tennis player are not simply a combination of the experiences of white female and black male players. Althea Gibson (1979) described her experiences in a personal account that highlights some of the complex interactions of race and gender and illustrates some of the influences of both social history and the immediate social situation in her development as a tennis player and as a person.

Significant numbers of athletes are not white and middle class, yet power in sport remains solidly white and middle class. As noted earlier for women, sport's glass ceiling keeps all but white middle-class athletes clustered at the bottom. The popular media and some sport scholars have discussed such practices as "stacking" (e.g., playing African-Americans in certain positions such as football running back or baseball outfield but not in central quarterback or pitching roles) and the nearly exclusive white male dominance of coaching and management positions. To date, few of these reports have included in-depth or critical analysis of race or socioeconomic class in sport.

Thus the sport experience varies with race and socioeconomic class, as it does with gender. Majors (1990) added more critical analysis to the literature with his discussion of the "cool pose" (a set of expressive lifestyle behaviors) used by black males to counter racism. Majors noted that although a few black males escape limits and express pride, power, and control, the emphasis on the cool pose in sport is self-defeating for the majority because it comes at the expense of education and other opportunities for advancement. Moreover, Majors notes that the cool pose uses sexist oppression to counter racist oppression, rather than encouraging more empowering strategies. Majors's discussion begins to tie together analyses of race and gender, but few others have done so. Smith (1992) drew together literature on women of color in sport and society with the primary conclusion that we have a deafening silence on diverse ethnic women in sport.

Recently, Brooks and Althouse (1993) edited a volume on racism in college athletics focusing on the African-American athlete's experience. Not only does this volume draw together needed scholarship on race and sport, but it includes a welcome section on gender and race. In one chapter Corbett and Johnson (1993) drew on the limited research

and their own insights to focus on African-American women in college sport. They noted that society holds different stereotypes and treats African-American women differently than white women. African-American women in America have a social-historical context of sexual exploitation, low wages, and substandard education; they are stereotyped as independent, loud, and dominating. Also, Corbett and Johnson noted that our popular myth that African-American women gravitate to track is not supported. African-American women have had more opportunities in track than in some other activities, and some talented athletes from Wilma Rudolph to Jackie Joyner-Kersee are widely recognized, but the limited survey data indicates that track is not a particularly popular activity for African-American students, and both formal and informal opportunities likely are limited by social stereotypes and constraints. In another chapter Tina Sloan Green (1993) optimistically discusses such opportunities as Girls Clubs, YWCA, PGM golf and the NCAA's national Youth Sport Program as strategies that might help overcome barriers and encourage more young African-American women to participate and develop their full potential in sports and athletics.

We can extend considerations further to incorporate other ethnic groups and other social categories such as socioeconomic class, age, and physical attributes. The lack of sport and exercise research on any such categories precludes conclusions. Clearly, though, we should move to consider diversity within gender in our gender research.

Not only should we consider greater social diversity within gender, but we should consider gender issues for both men and women in sport and exercise. Given that most sport and exercise psychology research (like most research) focuses on men, research aimed at understanding women's sport is essential. The recent influx of women into the traditional male sport world has brought gender issues to light for men as well as for women. Messner and Sabo (1990) edited a volume on sport, men, and gender, and Messner (1992) has followed that with an insightful analysis of sport and masculinity in *Power at Play*.

As discussed by Messner (1992), sport is a powerful force that socializes boys and men into a restricted masculine identity. Messner cites the major forces in sport as

- competitive hierarchical structure with conditional self-worth that enforces the must-win style and
- homophobia.

Messner describes the extent of homophobia in sport as staggering, and states that homophobia leads all boys and men regardless of sexual orientation to conform to a narrow definition of masculinity. Real men compete and, above all, avoid anything feminine that might lead one to be branded a sissy. Messner interviewed one successful elite athlete who noted that he was interested in dance as a child, but instead threw himself into athletics as a football and track jock. He reflected that he probably would have been a dancer except that he wanted the athlete's macho image. Messner ties this masculine identity to sport violence, because using violence to achieve a goal is acceptable and encouraged in this identity. Notably, female athletes are less comfortable with aggression in sport. Messner further notes that homophobia in athletics is closely linked with misogyny; that is, sport bonds men together as superior to women.

Messner's linking of homophobia and misogyny reflects Lenskyj's (1986, 1991) analysis citing compulsory heterosexuality as the root of sexist sport practices and Bem's (1993) contention that sexism, heterosexism, and homophobia all are related consequences of the same gender lenses in society. We expect to see men dominate women, and we are uncomfortable with bigger, stronger women who take the active, dominant roles that we expect in athletes.

Homophobia in sport has been discussed most often as a problem for lesbians, with good reason. Nelson (1991), in her chapter "A Silence So Loud, It Screams," illustrates restrictions and barriers for lesbians by describing one LPGA tour player who remains closeted to protect her status with friends, family, sponsors, tour personnel, and the general public. A few years ago Penn State women's basketball coach Renee Portland made headlines by declaring that she did not allow lesbians on her team. Few other coaches or administrators are as blatantly discriminatory, but more subtle discrimination is widespread. In a *Village Voice* article, Solomon (1991) cites several incidents of athletes or coaches losing jobs, positions, or roles on teams, as well as the use of accusations of lesbianism as scare tactics in recruiting or to keep women in line. Not surprisingly, those involved with women's athletics often go out of the way to avoid any appearance of lesbianism, like the golfer in Nelson's chapter, or deny a lesbian presence in sport. Pat Griffin, who has written and conducted workshops on homophobia in sport and physical education, describes this state as people "tip-toeing around a lavender elephant in the locker room and pretending that it's just not there." As Griffin notes (1987, 1992), lesbians are not the problem; homophobia is the problem. Homophobia manifests itself in women's sports as

- silence,
- denial,
- apology,
- promotion of a "heterosexy" image,
- attacks on lesbians, and
- preference for male coaches.

We stereotypically assume that sport attracts lesbians (but not gay men); however, there is no inherent relationship between sexual orientation and sport (no "gay gene" will turn a woman into a softball player or a man into a figure skater). No doubt, homophobia has kept more heterosexual women than lesbians out of sports, and homophobia restricts the behavior of all women in sport. Moreover, as the analyses of Messner (1992) and Ponger (1990) suggest, homophobia probably restricts men in sport even more than it restricts women.

Homophobia is not likely to bring gay or lesbian athletes to sport psychologists. As Rotella and Murray (1991) note in their discussion of the ramifications of homophobia for sport psychology practice, most problem issues are brought up by heterosexual athletes. Homosexual athletes are more reluctant to trust and discuss sexual issues. Sport psychologists would do well to check themselves for homophobia or heterosexist assumptions and approach sexuality as an issue of diversity calling for education rather than therapy. As with race and other gender-related issues discussed earlier, sexuality and sexual orientation are largely socially constructed and context-dependent. Sport psychologists must look beyond the individual and immediate issue to understand and deal with diversity and gender-related issues with a social-educational approach.

A Note on Biology

Now that I've taken a giant step in the social direction, I'll drag my feet just a bit to caution that sport psychologists should not dismiss biology. Sport and exercise are physical activities. Biological factors are not unidirectional determinants of behavior, and we should not fall into the old trap of assuming that biological factors necessarily dominate or underlie social and behavioral influences. As Birke and Vines (1987) suggest, biological factors are not static and absolute, but rather are dynamic processes that can interact with social-psychological influences in varied,

complex ways. Thus we should incorporate biology into our social psychological models to develop a *biopsychosocial* perspective. Consideration of physical characteristics along with related social beliefs, self-perceptions, and social processes might add insight to research on youth sport and health behavior, body image, exercise behavior, and competitive sport behavior. Now, after a lengthy discussion of the literature, let's return to the cases presented at this chapter's beginning to try to more directly tie some of this work to sport psychology practice.

INTERVENTION ISSUES AND CASE DISCUSSION

Before considering specific gender-related cases and issues, let's consider how gender affects sport psychology practice in general. Given the pervasiveness of gender influence and the inextricable linking of gender with everything we do, as illustrated by the previous review, an understanding of the gender literature is likely to lead sport psychologists to adopt more feminist or at least more enlightened nonsexist approaches.

A great deal has been written and discussed in clinical psychology about feminist approaches to practice. Psychoanalysis and other more popular current approaches have been criticized for sexist assumptions and practices. Current clinical and counseling literature typically advocates nonsexist practice, but we still find considerable gender bias in diagnosis, labeling, prescriptions, and treatment strategies (e.g., Travis, 1988; Unger & Crawford, 1992). A sizable contingent of (mostly) women in clinical psychology have moved beyond nonsexist practices to advocate more actively feminist approaches. In general, feminist practice incorporates gender scholarship, emphasizes neglected women's experiences (e.g., sexual

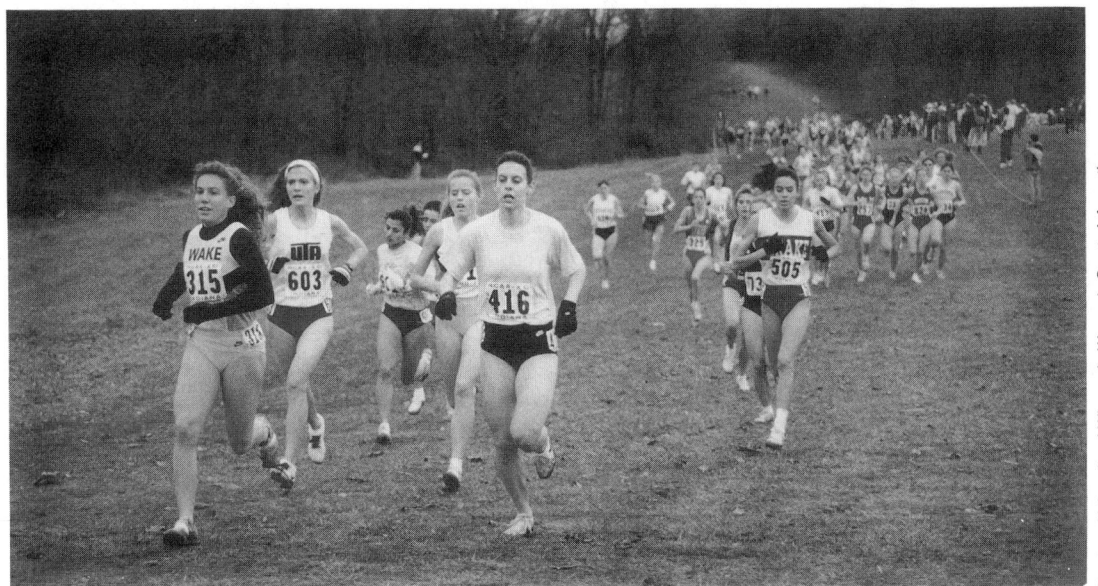

Courtesy University of Wisconsin Women's Sports Information

harassment), and takes a more nonhierarchical, empowering, process-oriented approach that shifts emphasis from personal change to social change. Because sport is more sexist, heterosexist, and homophobic than the larger society, I'm not optimistic that sport psychology, as a field, will turn to a feminist approach—but if some sport psychologists adopt a feminist approach, both individual athletes and sport will be better off. At the least all sport psychologists can educate themselves about gender, look beyond superficial gender differences, and stay aware of gender in the social context of their practice.

First, sport psychologists might consider gender influences on interactions with athletes. A recent special issue of the *Sport Psychologist* highlighted gender issues for female consultants working with male athletes (Yambor & Connelly, 1991), male consultants working with female athletes (Henschen, 1991), and issues for consultants working with other diverse groups. Considerable research (e.g., Hall, 1987; Tannen, 1990) indicates that gender influences communication

and interaction, and this may affect sport psychology practice. For example, although we stereotype females as more talkative, men talk more, interrupt more, and take more space and dominant postures. Tannen proposes that women and men speak different languages, and that suggests special concern for cross-sex consulting. Moreover, when a male sport psychologist consults with female athletes, the situation reflects the sexual power hierarchy of society, raising further potential barriers. Sport psychologists with training in communication and interpersonal skills, as well as in gender issues, might adjust. Still, the larger world is different for female and male athletes, and gender influences both the issues athletes present and their options.

Gender influences clinical disorders, as categorized in DSM-III-R (American Psychiatric Association, 1987), because women are more likely to present certain disorders, such as anxiety and depression, whereas men are more likely to exhibit antisocial or substance-abuse disorders. The largest gender gap, by far, appears for eating disorders, with females nine times more likely than males to exhibit either anorexia or bulimia. Terry, the 16-year-old figure skater in the case study who was referred because of a possible eating disorder, is much more likely to be a female, particularly a white, middle- to upper-class adolescent female, than a male. The relevant psychology literature not only indicates that females are more likely to exhibit eating disorders, but also that body image plays a major role. Eating disorders might also pose unique concerns with athletes. Female athletes are not necessarily more prone to identified associated factors of dysfunctional family background or compulsive desire for control, but female athletes in certain sports might be more prone to body-image concerns related to appearance and performance in their sports. Indeed, many poor eating behaviors in athletes might not be clinical eating disorders but misguided attempts to improve performance. For such cases an educational approach stressing proper nutrition without discounting the athlete's understandable concern for body image might be effective. A team approach including medical and nutritional experts as well as psychologists is preferable if an athlete lacks information and critical if an athlete presents more pathological eating behaviors. Perhaps most important for feminist sport psychologists would be to educate the coach and significant others and to try to change the system that leads athletes to pursue an unhealthy body image.

The case studies of both A.J. and Chris represent cases more likely to fall in the realm of the educational sport consultant focusing on performance enhancement. Both could be either male or female, but given gender socialization and context, A.J. is more likely a male athlete who has grown up in a world that reinforces aggressive behavior. Moreover, a male athlete is more likely to continue to have such behaviors reinforced (e.g., teammates cheer; the coach encourages related

behaviors only slightly less dramatic than those that draw penalties).

Chris presents a less aggressive, more tentative approach generally typical of female athletes. Even talented, competitive female athletes are socialized to keep quiet, be good, and let others take the lead. Moreover, chances are good that a female athlete will have a male coach, trainer, athletic director, and professor and that she will see males in most other power positions. To be sure, overly aggressive, uncontrolled behavior is not exclusively male, nor is a tentative style exclusively female. Still, sport psychologists will work more effectively with such athletes if they recognize gender influences in the athlete's background and situation.

Pat's case study reflects sexual harassment, an issue with clear gender connotations that's prevalent and likely to emerge yet one that's been neglected in sport psychology. Research and writing on violence toward women has expanded greatly in the past few years, and this is a major contribution of the gender scholarship to the field of psychology. Given the prevalence of sexual harassment and sexual assault (discussed in following paragraphs), especially for college women, female athletes are much more likely to present problems related to these issues than eating disorders or any other potentially clinical issues. Yet, despite the relevance of sexual harassment and assault for female athletes, and the growing related psychology work, I have seen virtually nothing in the sport psychology research or professional literature on this topic.

Recently, several studies as well as more public attention have demonstrated the prevalence of sexual harassment and assault (e.g., Matlin, 1993 or Unger & Crawford, 1992). In mid-1993 a media release reported a study on sexual harassment in Grade 8 through 11 students indicating that the majority of both boys and girls reported being harassed. Girls reported more harassment in all categories except being called gay or lesbian; however, boys reported being called gay or homosexual more often. Also, girls were much more likely to report negative emotional impact. About one third of college women report being sexually harassed, and when jokes and discriminatory remarks are included, the number goes to more than 50%. Recent work also indicates that sexual assault is much more prevalent than previously assumed, and recent attention to acquaintance rape reveals that most assaults are not committed by strangers. Koss (1990; Koss, Gidycz, & Wisniewski, 1987) has done considerable research on sexual assault, and her findings indicate that 38 of 1,000 college women experience rape or attempted rape in one year, that 85% of sexual assaults are by acquaintances, and that men and women define and interpret sexual situations and behaviors differently. All women are at risk, and no particular psychological pattern characterizes victims, although college students are more at risk and alcohol is often involved. Given that most sport psychologists work with college athletes, we should be particularly familiar with this work. Sexual harassment can be a tremendous barrier to educational and athletic achievement, and rape can be a devastating experience. Many rape victims remain anxious and depressed months later, and some experience severe substance abuse, eating disorders, major depression, or other symptoms, in some cases years later (e.g., Gordon & Riger, 1989; Koss, 1990; Murphy et al., 1988).

Although I know of no sport research, some authors have started to discuss these issues for athletes. Nelson (1991), in her aptly titled chapter "Running Scared," notes (and any woman jogger can confirm) that harassment is almost routine and expected by women runners. Women cannot run without harassment any time, any place. Lenskyj (1992) recently discussed sexual harassment in sport, drawing ties to power relations and ideology of male sports. Lenskyj notes that sexual harassment raises some unique concerns for female athletes, in addition to the concerns of all women: sport (as a nonfeminine activity) might elicit derisive comments; clothes are revealing; male coaches are often fit and conventionally attractive; female athletes might have spent much time training and less in general social activity; coaches are authoritarian and rule much of athletes' lives; for some sports, merit is equated with heterosexual attractiveness.

Of course, the gender socialization and social context that holds for everyone else also holds for athletes, and Pat is much more likely to be a female athlete harassed by a male coach than any other combination. Given that virtually no females coach male athletes, we can eliminate that, although with that combination the social male-over-female hierarchy could counter the coach-over-athlete hierarchy. Sexual harassment could occur with same-sex athletes and coaches. Writings on homophobia suggest that fears of lesbian harassment are often invoked, but reality clearly is otherwise. Overwhelmingly, sexual harassment is males harassing females, even in less gender-structured settings than sport. As Lenskyj (1992) notes, and earlier discussions of homophobia suggest, lesbians and gay men are more likely to be the targets than perpetrators of sexual harassment. Lenskyj notes that allegations of lesbianism might deter female athletes (regardless of sexual orientation) from rejecting male advances or complaining about harassment. A student in my women and sport class interviewed female coaches about lesbianism and to her surprise found the married female coach more open and willing to discuss these issues than single coaches (lesbian or heterosexual). Given the sport climate, we should not be surprised that female coaches are so worried about charges of lesbianism that they refrain from complaining about harassment or seeking equity for their programs. Sexual harassment (heterosexual or homophobic harassment) intimidates women and maintains traditional power structures.

Sexual harassment and assault have recently been brought to public attention as a concern for male athletes as well as female athletes. Recent accounts (e.g., Neimark, 1993) suggest that male athletes are particularly prone to sexual assault. These popular media reports, as well as more theoretical work (e.g., Lenskyj, 1992; Messner, 1992), suggest that male bonding, the privileged status of athletes, and the macho image of sport are contributing factors.

Pat's case probably occurs much more often than we recognize, and many athletes in Pat's situation would not discuss the problem with a sport psychologist or anyone else. Sport psychologists who are aware of the sport and gender dynamics that can lead to such situations might be quicker to recognize such issues and help athletes deal with the situation. As well as educating athletes, sport psychologists can take steps to change the situation by educating coaches and administrators. Most universities have developed counseling and educational programs on sexual harassment and assault and have established policies and procedures to deal with incidents. Sport psychologists can use these resources (e.g., refer victims, incorporate workshops) but also can develop programs targeted to athletes. As previously noted, some female athletes might be more susceptible to harassment or assault because of the situation unique to sport. Athletes often train both in isolated locations and during late hours; they also travel and might be placed in vulnerable situations more so than other students. Female athletes must be aware of sexual harassment and assault and concerns related to the particular demands of athletes.

Male athletes must also be aware of these issues, and male administrators must support such educational efforts. As Guernsey (1993) reports, several rape-prevention programs have been designed for male athletes. Such programs as those now operating at Cornell University and The University of Arkansas are supported by athletic coaches and administrators and aim to prevent the aggression needed on the field from affecting personal lives. With carefully planned programs developed with the athletic administration and relevant university resources, sport psychologists could educate female and male athletes, coaches, and others and go far toward preventing sexual harassment and assault. Again, to take a more feminist approach, sport psychologists could attempt to change the social situation as well as educate individuals—perhaps by demanding safe lighting, secure facilities, and clear, enforceable policies.

CONCLUSION

Gender makes a difference. Gender is a pervasive social force in society, and the sport world reflects in the extreme society's gender hierarchy. Gender is so ingrained in our sport structure and practice that we cannot simply treat all athletes the same. But neither can we assume that male and female athletes are dichotomous opposites and thus treat all males one way and all females another. Gender is a dynamic influence that varies with the individual, situation, and time. Sport psychologists should be aware of the many overt and subtle ways that gender affects athletes, the sport setting, and sport psychologists themselves and attempt to turn that awareness into action in their practice.

REFERENCES

Allison, M.T. (1991). Role conflict and the female athlete: Preoccupation with little grounding. *Journal of Applied Sport Psychology, 3*, 49-60.

American Psychiatric Association. (1987). *Diagnostic and statistical manual of mental disorders* (3rd ed., rev.). Washington, DC: Author.

Ashmore, R.D. (1990). Sex, gender, and the individual. In L.A. Pervin (Ed.), *Handbook of personality theory and research* (pp. 486-526). New York: Guilford.

Bandura, A. (1977). Self-efficacy: Toward a unifying theory of behavior change. *Psychological Review, 84*, 191-215.

Bandura, A. (1986). *Social foundations of thought and action*. Englewood Cliffs, NJ: Prentice Hall.

Bem, S.L. (1974). The measurement of psychological androgyny. *Journal of Consulting and Clinical Psychology, 42*, 155-162.

Bem, S.L. (1978). Beyond androgyny: Some presumptuous prescriptions for a liberated sexual identity. In J. Sherman & F. Denmark (Eds.), *Psychology of women: Future directions for research* (pp. 1-23). New York: Psychological Dimensions.

Bem, S.L. (1985). Androgyny and gender schema theory: A conceptual and empirical integration. In T.B. Sonderegger (Ed.), *Nebraska Symposium on Motivation, 1984: Psychology and Gender* (pp. 179-226). Lincoln, NE: University of Nebraska Press.

Bem, S.L. (1993). *The lenses of gender*. New Haven: Yale University Press.

Bernard, J. (1981). *The female world*. New York: Free Press.

Birke, L.I.A., & Vines, G. (1987). A sporting chance: The anatomy of destiny. *Women's Studies International Forum, 10*, 337-347.

Birrell, S.J. (1988). Discourses on the gender/sport relationship: From women in sport to gender relations. In K. Pandolf (Ed.), *Exercise and Sport Science Reviews: Vol. 16* (pp. 459-502). New York: Macmillan.

Blinde, E.M., & Greendorfer, S.L. (1992). Conflict and the college sport experience of women athletes. *Women in Sport and Physical Activity Journal, 1*, 97-113.

Brooks, D., & Althouse, R. (1993). *Racism in college athletics: The African-American athlete's experience*. Morgantown, WV: Fitness Information Technology.

Broverman, I.K., Vogel, S.R., Broverman, D.M., Clarkson, F.E., & Rosenkrantz, P.S. (1972). Sex role stereotypes: A current appraisal. *Journal of Social Issues, 28*, 59-78.

Brown, R.D., & Harrison, J.M. (1986). The effects of a strength training program on the strength and self-concept of two female age groups. *Research Quarterly for Exercise and Sport, 57*, 315-320.

Carpenter, L.J., & Acosta, R.V. (1993). Back to the future: Reform with a woman's voice. In D.S. Eitzen (Ed.), *Sport in contemporary society: An anthology* (4th ed.) (pp. 388-398). New York: St. Martin's Press.

Colker, R., & Widom, C.S. (1980). Correlates of female athletic participation. *Sex Roles, 6*, 47-53.

Condry, J., & Dyer, S. (1976). Fear of success: Attribution of cause to the victim. *Journal of Social Issues, 32*, 63-83.

Corbett, D., & Johnson, W. (1993). The African-American female in collegiate sport: Sexism and racism. In D. Brooks & R. Althouse (Eds.), *Racism in college athletics: The African-American athlete's experience* (pp. 179-204). Morgantown, WV: Fitness Information Technology.

Corbin, C.B. (1981). Sex of subject, sex of opponent, and opponent ability as factors affecting self-confidence in a competitive situation. *Journal of Sport Psychology, 3,* 265-270.

Corbin, C.B., Landers, D.M., Feltz, D.L., & Senior, K. (1983). Sex differences in performance estimates: Female lack of confidence vs. male boastfulness. *Research Quarterly for Exercise and Sport, 54,* 407-410.

Corbin, C.B., & Nix, C. (1979). Sex-typing of physical activities and success predictions of children before and after cross-sex competition. *Journal of Sport Psychology, 1,* 43-52.

Corbin, C.B., Stewart, M.J., & Blair, W.O. (1981). Self-confidence and motor performance of preadolescent boys and girls in different feedback situations. *Journal of Sport Psychology, 3,* 30-34.

Crandall, V.C. (1969). Sex differences in expectancy of intellectual and academic reinforcement. In C.P. Smith (Ed.), *Achievement-related motives in children* (pp. 11-45). New York: Russell Sage.

Csizma, K.A., Wittig, A.F., & Schurr, K.T. (1988). Sport stereotypes and gender. *Journal of Sport & Exercise Psychology, 10,* 62-74.

Deaux, K. (1984). From individual differences to social categories: Analysis of a decade's research on gender. *American Psychologist, 39,* 105-116.

Deaux, K. (1985). Sex and gender. *Annual Review of Psychology, 36,* 49-81.

Deaux, K., & Kite, M.E. (1987). Thinking about gender. In B.B. Hess & M.M. Ferree (Eds.), *Analyzing gender* (pp. 92-117). Beverly Hills, CA: Sage.

Deaux, K., & Lewis, L.L. (1984). The structure of gender stereotypes: Interrelationships among components and gender label. *Journal of Personality and Social Psychology, 46,* 991-1004.

Deaux, K., & Major, B. (1987). Putting gender into context: An interactive model of gender-related behavior. *Psychological Review, 94,* 369-389.

Del Rey, P. (1978). The apologetic and women in sport. In C. Oglesby (Ed.), *Women and sport: From myth to reality* (pp. 107-111). Philadelphia: Lea & Febiger.

Del Rey, P., & Sheppard, S. (1981). Relationship of psychological androgyny in female athletes to self-esteem. *International Journal of Sport Psychology, 12,* 165-175.

Dewar, A.M. (1987). The social construction of gender in physical education. *Women's Studies International Forum, 10,* 453-465.

Duda, J.L. (1986). A cross-cultural analysis of achievement motivation in sport and the classroom. In L. VanderVelden & J. Humphrey (Eds.), *Current selected research in the psychology and sociology of sport* (pp. 115-132). New York: AMS Press.

Duda, J.L. (1991). Editorial comment: Perspectives on gender roles in physical activity. *Journal of Applied Sport Psychology, 3,* 1-6.

Duda, J.L., & Allison, M.T. (1990). Cross-cultural analysis in exercise and sport psychology: A void in the field. *Journal of Sport & Exercise Psychology, 12,* 114-131.

Eagley, A.H. (1987). *Sex differences in social behavior: A social-role interpretation.* Hillsdale, NJ: Erlbaum.

Eagley, A.H., & Kite, M.E. (1987). Are stereotypes of nationalities applied to both women and men? *Journal of Personality and Social Psychology, 53,* 451-462.

Eccles, J.S. (1985). Sex differences in achievement patterns. In T. Sonderegger (Ed.), *Nebraska Symposium of Motivation, 1984: Psychology and Gender* (pp. 97-132). Lincoln, NE: University of Nebraska Press.

Eccles, J.S. (1987). Gender roles and women's achievement-related decisions. *Psychology of Women Quarterly, 11,* 135-172.

Eccles, J.S., Adler, T.F., Futterman, R., Goff, S.B., Kaczala, C.M., Meece, J.L., & Midgley, C. (1983). Expectations, values and academic behaviors. In J. Spence

(Ed.), *Achievement and achievement motives* (pp. 75-146). San Francisco: Freeman.

Eccles, J.S., & Harold, R.D. (1991). Gender differences in sport involvement: Applying the Eccles expectancy-value model. *Journal of Applied Sport Psychology*, **3**, 7-35.

Eitzen, D.S., & Baca Zinn, M. (1993). The de-athleticization of women: The naming and gender marking of collegiate sports teams. In D.S. Eitzen (Ed.), *Sport in contemporary society: An anthology* (4th ed.) (pp. 396-405). New York: St. Martin's Press.

Feltz, D.L. (1988). Self-confidence and sports performance. In K. Pandolf (Ed.), *Exercise and Sport Sciences Reviews: Vol. 16* (pp. 423-457). New York: Macmillan.

Gibson, A. (1979). I always wanted to be somebody. In S.L. Twin (Ed.), *Out of the bleachers* (pp. 130-142). Old Westbury, NY: Feminist Press.

Gill, D.L. (1988). Gender differences in competitive orientation and sport participation. *International Journal of Sport Psychology*, **19**, 145-159.

Gill, D.L. (1992a). Gender and sport behavior. In T.S. Horn (Ed.), *Advances in sport psychology* (pp. 143-160). Champaign, IL: Human Kinetics.

Gill, D.L. (1992b). Status of the *Journal of Sport & Exercise Psychology*, 1985-1990. *Journal of Sport & Exercise Psychology*, **14**, 1-12.

Gill, D.L. (1993). Competitiveness and competitive orientation in sport. In R.N. Singer, M. Murphey, & L.K. Tennant (Eds.), *Handbook on research in sport psychology* (pp. 314-327). New York: Macmillan.

Gill, D.L., & Deeter, T.E. (1988). Development of the Sport Orientation Questionnaire. *Research Quarterly for Exercise and Sport*, **59**, 191-202.

Gill, D.L., & Dzewaltowski, D.A. (1988). Competitive orientations among intercollegiate athletes: Is winning the only thing? *Sport Psychologist*, **2**, 212-221.

Gill, D.L., Gross, J.B., Huddleston, S., & Shifflett, B. (1984). Sex differences in achievement cognitions and performance in competition. *Research Quarterly for Exercise and Sport*, **55**, 340-346.

Goldberg, P. (1968). Are women prejudiced against women? *Transaction*, **5**, 28-30.

Gordon, M.T., & Riger, S. (1989). *The female fear: The social cost of rape.* New York: Free Press.

Green, T.S. (1993). The future of African-American female athletes. In D. Brooks & R. Althouse (Eds.), *Racism in college athletics: The African-American athlete's experience* (pp. 205-223). Morgantown, WV: Fitness Information Technology.

Greendorfer, S.L. (1987). Gender bias in theoretical perspectives: The case of female socialization into sport. *Psychology of Women Quarterly*, **11**, 327-340.

Griffin, P.S. (1987, August). *Homophobia, lesbians, and women's sports: An exploratory analysis.* Paper presented at the APA convention, New York.

Griffin, P. (1992). Changing the game: Homophobia, sexism, and lesbians in sport. *Quest*, **44**, 251-265.

Guernsey, L. (1993, February 10). More campuses offer rape-prevention programs for male athletes. *Chronicle of Higher Education*, pp. A35, A37.

Hall, J.A. (1987). On explaining sex differences: The case of nonverbal communication. In P. Shaver & C. Hendrick (Eds.), *Sex and gender* (pp. 177-200). Newbury Park, CA: Sage.

Hall, M.A. (1988). The discourse of gender and sport: From femininity to feminism. *Sociology of Sport Journal*, **5**, 330-340.

Hall, M.A. (1990). How should we theorize gender in the context of sport? In M.A. Messner & D.F. Sabo (Eds.), *Sport, men, and the gender order* (pp. 223-239). Champaign, IL: Human Kinetics.

Harris, D.V. (1980). Femininity and athleticism: Conflict of consonance? In D.F. Sabo & R. Runfola (Eds.), *Jock: Sports and male identity* (pp. 222-239). Englewood Cliffs, NJ: Prentice Hall.

Harris, D.V., & Jennings, S.E. (1977). Self-perceptions of female distance runners. *Annals of the New York Academy of Sciences*, **301**, 808-815.

Helmreich, R.L., & Spence, J.T. (1977). Sex roles and achievement. In R.W. Christina & D.M. Landers (Eds.), *Psychology of motor behavior and sport—1976: Vol. 2* (pp. 33-46). Champaign, IL: Human Kinetics.

Henschen, K. (1991). Critical issues involving male consultants and female athletes. *Sport Psychologist*, **5**, 313-321.

Holloway, J.B., Beuter, A., & Duda, J.L. (1988). Self-efficacy and training for strength in adolescent girls. *Journal of Applied Social Psychology*, **18**, 699-719.

Horner, M.S. (1972). Toward an understanding of achievement-related conflicts in women. *Journal of Social Issues*, **28**, 157-176.

Hyde, J.S., & Linn, M.C. (Eds.) (1986). *The psychology of gender: Advances through meta-analysis*. Baltimore: Johns Hopkins University Press.

Jacklin, C.N. (1989). Female and male: Issues of gender. *American Psychologist*, **44**, 127-133.

Kane, M.J. (1989). The post Title IX female athlete in the media. *Journal of Physical Education, Recreation and Dance*, **60**(3), 58-62.

Kane, M.J., & Parks, J.B. (1992). The social construction of gender difference and hierarchy in sport journalism—Few new twists on very old themes. *Women in Sport & Physical Activity Journal*, **1**, 49-83.

Kane, M.J., & Snyder, E. (1989). Sport typing: The social "containment" of women. *Arena Review*, **13**, 77-96.

Koss, M.P. (1990). The women's mental health research agenda. *American Psychologist*, **45**, 374-380.

Koss, M.P., Gidycz, C.A., & Wisniewski, N. (1987). The scope of rape: Incidence and prevalence of sexual aggression and victimization in a national sample of higher education students. *Journal of Consulting and Clinical Psychology*, **55**, 162-170.

Lenney, E. (1977). Women's self-confidence in achievement settings. *Psychological Bulletin*, **84**, 1-13.

Lenskyj, H. (1986). *Out of bounds: Women, sport and sexuality*. Toronto: Women's Press.

Lenskyj, H. (1991). Combatting homophobia in sport and physical education. *Sociology of Sport Journal*, **8**, 61-69.

Lenskyj, H. (1992). Unsafe at home base: Women's experiences of sexual harassment in university sport and physical education. *Women in Sport & Physical Activity Journal*, **1**, 19-33.

Locksley, A., & Colten, M.E. (1979). Psychological androgyny: A case of mistaken identity? *Journal of Personality and Social Psychology*, **37**, 1017-1031.

Maccoby, E.E. (1990). Gender and relationships. *American Psychologist*, **45**, 513-520.

Maccoby, E., & Jacklin, C. (1974). *The psychology of sex differences*. Stanford, CA: Stanford University Press.

Majors, R. (1990). Cool pose: Black masculinity and sports. In M.A. Messner & D.F. Sabo (Eds.), *Sport, men, and the gender order* (pp. 109-114). Champaign, IL: Human Kinetics.

Matlin, M.W. (1993). *The psychology of women* (2nd ed.). Fort Worth: Harcourt Brace Jovanovich.

Matteo, S. (1986). The effect of sex and gender-schematic processing on sport participation. *Sex Roles*, **15**, 417-432.

Matteo, S. (1988). The effect of gender-schematic processing on decisions about sex-inappropriate sport behavior. *Sex Roles*, **18**, 41-58.

McClelland, D.C., Atkinson, J.W., Clark, R.A., & Lowell, E.C. (1953). *The achievement motive*. New York: Appleton-Century-Crofts.

McElroy, M.A., & Willis, J.D. (1979). Women and the achievement conflict in sport: A preliminary study. *Journal of Sport Psychology*, **1**, 241-247.

McNally, J., & Orlick, T. (1975). Cooperative sport structures: A preliminary analysis. *Mouvement*, **7**, 267-271.

Melpomene Institute. (1990). *The bodywise woman*. Champaign, IL: Human Kinetics.

Messner, M.A. (1992). *Power at play: Sports and the problem of masculinity*. Boston: Beacon Press.

Messner, M.A., Duncan, M.C., & Jensen, K. (1993). Separating the men from the girls: The gendered language of televised sports. In D.S. Eitzen (Ed.), *Sport in contemporary society: An anthology* (4th ed.) (pp. 219-233). New York: St. Martin's Press.

Messner, M.A., & Sabo, D.F. (1990). *Sport, men, and the gender order*. Champaign, IL: Human Kinetics.

Metheny, E. (1965). Symbolic forms of movement: The feminine image in sports. In E. Metheny (Ed.), *Connotations of movement in sport and dance* (pp. 43-56). Dubuque, IA: Brown.

Murphy, S.M., Kilpatrick, D.G., Amick-McMullen, A., Veronen, L., Best, C.L., Villeponteaux, L.A., & Saunders, B.E. (1988). Current psychological functioning of child sexual assault survivors: A community study. *Journal of Interpersonal Violence*, **3**, 55-79.

Myers, A.E., & Lips, H.M. (1978). Participation in competitive amateur sports as a function of psychological androgyny. *Sex Roles*, **4**, 571-578.

Neimark, J. (1993). Out of bounds: The truth about athletes and rape. In D.S. Eitzen (Ed.), *Sport in contemporary society: An anthology* (4th ed.) (pp. 130-137). New York: St. Martin's Press.

Nelson, M.B. (1991). *Are we winning yet: How women are changing sports and sports are changing women*. New York: Random House.

Nyad, D. (1978). *Other shores*. New York: Random House.

Parkhouse, B.L., & Williams, J.M. (1986). Differential effects of sex and status on evaluation of coaching ability. *Research Quarterly for Exercise and Sport*, **57**, 53-59.

Pedhazur, E.J., & Tetenbaum, T.J. (1979). BSRI: A theoretical and methodological critique. *Journal of Personality and Social Psychology*, **37**, 996-1016.

Petruzzello, S.J., & Corbin, C.B. (1988). The effects of performance feedback on female self-confidence. *Journal of Sport & Exercise Psychology*, **10**, 174-183.

Pheterson, G.I., Kiesler, S.B., & Goldberg, P.A. (1971). Evaluation of the performance of women as a function of their sex, achievement, and personal history. *Journal of Personality and Social Psychology*, **19**, 114-118.

Ponger, B. (1990). Gay jocks: A phenomenology of gay men in athletics. In M.A. Messner & D.F. Sabo (Eds.), *Sport, men, and the gender order* (pp. 141-152). Champaign, IL: Human Kinetics.

Rodin, J., Silberstein, L., & Streigel-Moore, R. (1985). Women and weight: A normative discontent. In T.B. Sonderegger (Eds.), *Nebraska Symposium on Motivation, 1984: Psychology and Gender* (pp. 267-307). Lincoln, NE: University of Nebraska Press.

Rosenkrantz, P., Vogel, S., Bee, H., Broverman, I., & Broverman, D.M. (1968). Sex-role stereotypes and self-concepts in college students. *Journal of Consulting and Clinical Psychology*, **32**, 286-295.

Rotella, R.J., & Murray, M. (1991). Homophobia, the world of sport, and sport psychology consulting. *Sport Psychologist*, **5**, 355-364.

Safrit, M.J. (1984). Women in research in physical education: A 1984 update. *Quest*, **36**, 104-114.

Sherif, C.W. (1976). The social context of competition. In D. Landers (Ed.), *Social problems in athletics* (pp. 18-36). Champaign, IL: Human Kinetics.

Sherif, C.W. (1982). Needed concepts in the study of gender identity. *Psychology of Women Quarterly*, **6**, 375-398.

Smith, Y.R. (1992). Women of color in society and sport. *Quest*, **44**, 228-250.

Solomon, A. (1991, March 20). Passing game. *Village Voice*, p. 92.

Spears, B. (1978). Prologue: The myth. In C. Oglesby (Ed.), *Women in sport: From myth to reality* (pp. 3-15). Philadelphia: Lea & Febiger.

Spence, J.T., & Helmreich, R.L. (1978). *Masculinity and femininity*. Austin, TX: University of Texas Press.

Spence, J.T., & Helmreich, R.L. (1983). Achievement-related motives and behaviors. In J.T. Spence (Ed.), *Achievement and achievement motives: Psychological and sociological approaches* (pp. 7-74). San Francisco: Freeman.

Stewart, M.J., & Corbin, C.B. (1988). Feedback dependence among low confidence preadolescent boys and girls. *Research Quarterly for Exercise and Sport*, **59**, 160-164.

Tannen, D. (1990). *You just don't understand*. New York: Morrow.

Taylor, M.C., & Hall, J.A. (1982). Psychological androgyny: Theories, methods and conclusions. *Psychological Bulletin*, **92**, 347-366.

Theberge, N. (1987). Sport and women's empowerment. *Women's Studies International Forum*, **10**, 387-393.

Travis, C.B. (1988). *Women and health psychology: Mental health issues*. Hillsdale, NJ: Erlbaum.

Tresemer, D.W. (1977). *Fear of success*. New York: Plenum Press.

Trujillo, C. (1983). The effect of weight training and running exercise intervention on the self-esteem of college women. *International Journal of Sport Psychology*, **14**, 162-173.

Uhlir, G.A. (1987). Athletics and the university: The post-women's era. *Academe*, **73**, 25-29.

Unger, R., & Crawford, M. (1992). *Women and gender: A feminist psychology*. New York: McGraw-Hill.

Wallston, B.S., & O'Leary, V.E. (1981). Sex and gender make a difference: The differential perceptions of women and men. *Review of Personality and Social Psychology*, **2**, 9-41.

Weinberg, R.S., & Jackson, A. (1979). Competition and extrinsic rewards: Effect on intrinsic motivation. *Research Quarterly*, **50**, 494-502.

Weinberg, R.S., & Ragan, J. (1979). Effects of competition, success/failure, and sex on intrinsic motivation. *Research Quarterly*, **50**, 503-510.

Weinberg, R., Reveles, M., & Jackson, A. (1984). Attitudes of male and female athletes toward male and female coaches. *Journal of Sport Psychology*, **6**, 448-453.

Wells, C.L. (1991). *Women, sport, and performance: A physiological perspective* (2nd ed.). Champaign, IL: Human Kinetics.

Williams, J.M., & Parkhouse, B.L. (1988). Social learning theory as a foundation for examining sex bias in evaluation of coaches. *Journal of Sport & Exercise Psychology*, **10**, 322-333.

Yambor, J., & Connelly, D. (1991). Issues confronting female sport psychology consultants working with male student-athletes. *Sport Psychologist*, **5**, 304-312.

CHAPTER 10

CONSULTATIONS WITH SPORT ORGANIZATIONS: A COGNITIVE-BEHAVIORAL MODEL

Frank Perna, EdD, Megan Neyer, PhD, Shane M. Murphy, PhD
United States Olympic Committee

Bruce C. Ogilvie, PhD
Los Gatos, California

Annemarie Murphy, PhD
AimCare Clinic, Colorado

The psychology professional wishing to consult for a sport organization faces an often daunting and confusing task. There are few areas where psychological consultation presents the challenges that are to be found in the sport world. The goal of this chapter is to describe a process that clarifies the consultation role with a sport organization and offers a model of consultancy that has proven effective in a variety of situations.

As Gardner points out in chapter 6 of this book, one of the principal challenges that often faces the potential sport psychology consultant is an unfamiliarity with the milieu of the professional sport world (see also Ravizza, 1990). Typically, sport psychology consultants have come from academic institutions and clinical settings but are asked to function in a business atmosphere. Also, members of the professional sport world are not accustomed to having psychologists, psychiatrists, or educators interact with their teams on an ongoing basis. Thus the partners in the prospective consultation relationship are unfamiliar with their respective roles, responsibilities, and generally accepted rules of interaction. This unfamiliarity can contribute to mutual uncertainty and the potential for a perceived lack of consultant credibility. This chapter emphasizes that a critical aspect of all sport consultations is the process of clarifying expectations on the part of clients, so that consultation can proceed with both parties agreeing on the criteria by which the efficacy of consultation will be evaluated.

At present, no standard model exists to guide interactions between professional sport teams and the sport psychology consultant (McKelvain, 1988). However, it is crucial for consultants to develop a philosophy of service delivery defining the scope of practice, structure of interaction, and professional limits. By addressing these issues consultants will be in a better position to decrease ambiguity and to clarify expectations of consultation. This chapter presents the currently prominent philosophies and approaches of sport psychology consultation, identifies critical issues in the sport consultation process, presents a comprehensive cognitive-behavioral model for consultation in sport psychology, and demonstrates the model through a case-study illustration.

■ *THE CASE OF LI-WU* ■

Li-Wu is a 16-year-old elite gymnast. At the end of the last competitive season, Li-Wu was seriously injured while performing on the vault. Her hands slipped on the horse, and she landed on her neck, causing a minor concussion and temporary numbness throughout her body. She was removed from the competition site on a backboard and taken to the hospital, where she was admitted for neurological testing and observation. It was determined that she had sprained ligaments and strained muscles in the cervical region of the spinal cord. Li-Wu was instructed to take a month off from gymnastics and report for injury rehabilitation three times a week.

After diligently following the prescribed regime of the sports medicine team for 2 months, Li-Wu was permitted to return to full training. Although she seemed to be progressing well with the floor exercise and with her difficult moves on the uneven bars and the balance beam, it was clear she was reluctant to attempt her difficult vaulting exercises. Li-Wu was frustrated with herself; she was unable to manage her fear of vaulting and considered quitting gymnastics. At this point she was referred to a sport psychology consultant by her coach.

CHOOSING A CONSULTATION MODEL

Two important questions must be answered in choosing a consultation model that will best fit the philosophy and training of the consultant: (a) Who is the client? and (b) What services are provided? Identifying the client clarifies the consultant's primary allegiance, which in turn determines the limits of confidentiality existing in the consultation relationship. Deciding which services will be offered clarifies expectations and helps define the boundaries of the consultation relationship. Leading sport psychology consultants vary in their opinions both as to whom they view as the primary client and as to the scope of services they provide to professional and elite sport organizations (see the December 1990 special issue of the *Sport Psychologist*). The consultant must decide these issues prior to initial contact with the sport organization. By comprehensively answering these initial questions, the consultant is in the best position to clarify client expectations.

Identifying the Client

The primary client potentially includes the coach(es), general manager, sports medicine staff, athletes, and parents (in situations where the athlete is a minor). Unlike in some other consulting relationships, the party requesting and paying for services is not necessarily the client. The sport organization typically pays the consultant's salary, although, as will be seen, the sport organization is often not the client in the consulting relationship (Biddle, Bull, & Seheult, 1992). This situation most closely resembles one that often exists in corporate settings, where the corporation pays for the consultant's services but the employees are the primary clients.

Although the range of potential clients is wide, the essential decision is to identify the athlete(s) or a member of the sport organization as the primary client. Defining the primary client is essential for two reasons.

- For psychologists, legal and professional obligations regarding limits of confidentiality are determined by the client's identity.

- Defining the client is essential for clarifying expectations and the professional role of the consultant with the sport organization.

One potential model is that all services, decisions, and interventions must first be processed with the head coach, thus defining a sport organization official as the primary client (Ogilvie, 1977). Ogilvie contends that the commitment to the head coach can be maintained without diminishing the professional responsibilities to others in the organization. Adherence to this model places the consultant in the role of deciding what information will or will not be shared about inter-actions with players. This model also carries the expectation that coaches and management are privy to discussions and information pertaining to the athlete. In this model the consultant has the burden of notifying the athlete that a coach or team official might request information from the consultant (e.g., case summaries and test result interpretations). Operating from this philosophy, the consultant might more readily be granted access to players but might not find athletes to be totally forthcoming.

Other consultants view the athlete(s) as the primary client and seek assurances from coaches and management that the consultant will not be expected to disclose information without the athlete's permission (Ravizza, 1990; Rotella, 1990). The materials (e.g., notes or test results) derived from consultation are the property of the athlete rather than the organization. A subtle but important shift from the first model has occurred that directly influences the services that ethically can be offered. For example, testing or interview

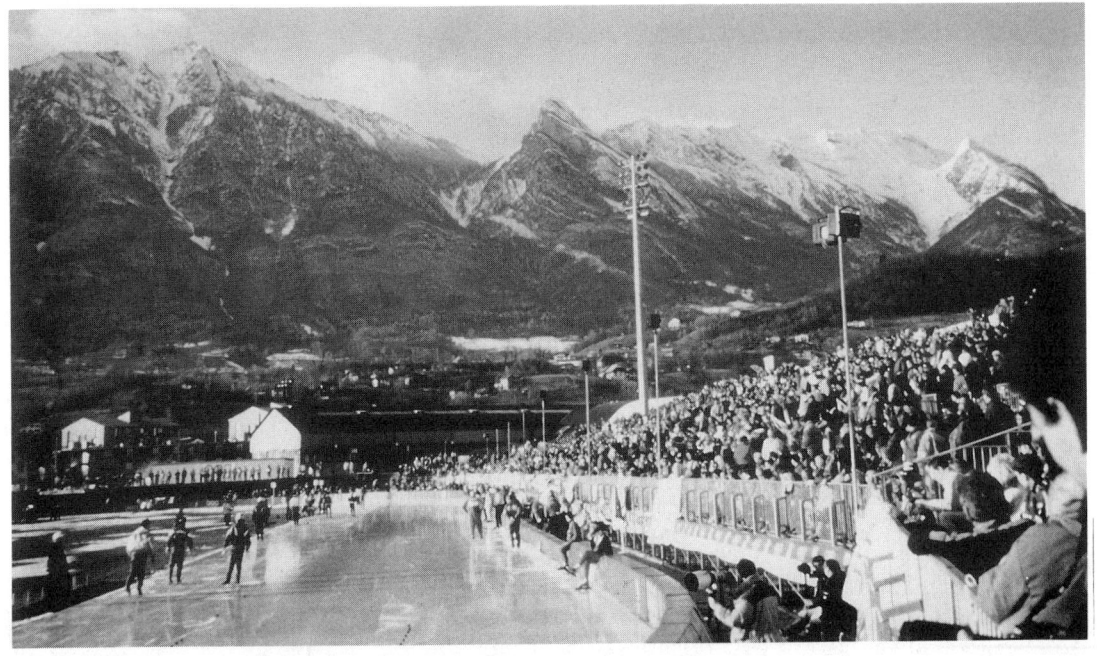

Courtesy USOC

information regarding an athlete ethically could not be provided to the organization unless an athlete releases the information. To facilitate the strongest client-consultant bond, some consultants who identify the athlete as the primary client either specify that they will not become involved in player selection (Rotella) or clarify the conditions by which athlete information can be released.

When working with adult athletes the consultant has a choice in specifying who is the primary client, the athlete or an outside agent (e.g., coach or management). However, in cases where the athlete is a minor, consultant psychologists are obligated to obtain permission from parents, who are the legal clients, since minors are legally incapable of providing informed consent (American Psychological Association, 1990). In this situation another shift in the right to information has occurred. When working with minors, the consultant psychologist is obligated to protect the minor's best interests; however, case summaries and written test interpretations must be provided to parents on request.

Three important points emerge from a discussion of identifying the client in sport psychology consultation.

- Identifying the primary client in the consultation process determines the flow of information and concomitantly restricts the range of services that may be ethically provided.

- The consultant has a responsibility to communicate to sport organization officials and to athletes at the outset the conditions of consultation. By clarifying client status and limits of service delivery, consultants can avoid misperceptions as well as provide guidelines to direct behavior. For example, the sport organization, having been provided a clear statement of what to expect from the consultant, may not expect nor ask for confidential player information; thus the consultant and the sport organization are saved from potentially awkward situations.

- Although recent debate continues regarding appropriate practice requirements of sport psychology consultants (Anshel, 1992; Gardner, 1991; Silva, 1989; Zaichkowsky & Perna, 1992), consultants who are psychologists have clear legal and professional responsibilities. Sport psychology consultants who are psychologists must align their consultation practice to conform with state licensing and American Psychological Association guidelines (Gardner). It appears, however, that non-psychologist-consultants will also be encouraged by major sport psychology bodies such as the Association for the Advancement of Applied Sport Psychology (AAASP) to incorporate APA ethical guidelines into their practice.

Consultation Models

Four models of consultation are examined in this section: educational, clinical, supervisory, and cognitive-behavioral.

The Educational Consultation Model

Educational approaches to sport psychology consultation conceptualize the purpose of consultation as optimizing the use of mental skills by the athlete client (Botterill, 1990; Halliwell, 1990; LaRose, 1988; Loehr, 1990; McKelvain, 1988; Ravizza, 1990; Rotella, 1990). This approach seeks to teach people how to further develop existing skills or to teach athletes new skills appropriate for managing performance in competition. Frequently used mental skills in training or actual competition include goal-setting strategies, arousal control techniques, visualization procedures, attention and refocusing training, and cognitive restructuring (self-talk). A typical consultation might include a series of group presentations by the consultant, who explains and demonstrates the potential of mental-skills training, followed by individual conferences, on request, with athletes and coaches. Crucial to the educational approach is the sport specificity of examples and an explanation of how skills can be applied in a competitive pressure situation or built into a precompetitive routine (Ravizza, 1988). Additionally, LaRose (1988) highlights that the success of the educational approach with athletes largely hinges on reinforcement of techniques by coaches. That is, although some success might accrue to athletes using mental-skills training, maximal benefit occurs when coaches become thoroughly versed in and reinforce the use and development of these skills in the practice setting.

The educational approach requires the consultant to spend considerable time at the practice field observing situations and implementing on-the-spot interventions. Ravizza (1988) comments that immediate interventions and visibility of the consultant on the field hastens rapport, facilitates "teachable moments," and lowers barriers to effective consultation.

The Clinical Consultation Model

The clinical approach to consultation (Dorfman, 1990; Neff, 1990; Nideffer, 1981; Ogilvie, 1979), in contrast to the educational approach, focuses on the special stressors affecting athletes in elite sports and does not automatically assume that athletes possess all the coping resources necessary to deal with these. The clinical consultation model involves interventions designed to help athletes function more effectively in their special roles and can involve interventions at the organizational, team, or individual level. However, interventions at the individual level have most commonly been described in the literature (Murphy, 1988; Murphy and Ferrante, 1989). In the clinical approach, the organization often approaches the consultant with a specific issue, and the consultant's main task is to assess the problem and recommend a solution (McKelvain, 1988).

The clinical model stresses that cost effectiveness is the standard by which all services are measured in professional and elite sport (Ogilvie, 1992; Ravizza, 1988, 1990; Rotella, 1990). Some clinical consultants contend that identifying athletes with serious emotional reactions that could intrude upon their performance is the service most valued by the elite sport organization (Ogilvie, 1992). Consultants using the clinical approach argue that early recognition and design of an appropriate support system for the athlete is a service that receives high priority and increases the consultant's credibility with players and management, because these services are intended to prevent loss of talent that was acquired at considerable cost to the organization.

Dorfman (1990) draws an analogy between traditional employee assistance programs (EAP) and his clinical consulting approach with professional sports teams. In an employee assistance program, direct services are offered, but the consultant's primary role is to provide diagnostic services and coordinate appropriate interventions. Dorfman suggests offering a range of services to the team, including traditional diagnostic assessment and mental-skills training as well as educational presentations. However, assessment and intervention-planning skills are highlighted as those most valued by organizations.

Consultants using the clinical approach can function in a manner similar to their educational colleagues, operating from an outreach perspective and maintaining frequent contact with the team throughout the preseason and the regular season. It is also possible to use a consultation approach that is more typical of mainstream clinical psychology, involving a very low profile with the team and serving primarily as a referral source for athletes identified as needing services. In either mode the consultant must determine whether a performance problem is confined to the athletic field or also affects other life spheres. When problems occur, clinical consultants might intervene directly, but they often refer when long-term or inpatient treatment is required, such as for substance abuse counseling and eating disorders. The consultant then assumes the role of liaison between the sport organization and the primary treatment provider (Thompson & Sherman, 1993). Depending on training, it is possible for educational consultants to also perform liaison functions. However, identification and management of clinical concerns is not the primary focus of consultation, and some consultants who use the educational model specify at the outset that they will not become involved in any clinical matters (Rotella, 1990).

As a caution, consultants wishing to use the clinical approach with elite sports teams should be aware that the clinical approach has been criticized by clinical as well as educational consultants as being at times inappropriate and contributing to a negative stereotype of sport psychology (Halliwell, 1990; Murphy & Murphy, 1992; Rotella, 1990; Smith & Johnson, 1990). Additionally, Ravizza (1988) and Gordon (1990) have claimed that even identifying oneself as a clinical consultant raises barriers to effective consultation with elite sport organizations.

The Supervisory Consultation Model

A third approach used with competitive sports teams involves the consultant acting as a supervisor to a staff member of the organization (Smith & Johnson, 1990). In this paradigm, the consultant and the management officers of the team select a trainee—ideally a former player or coach with a counseling background in the organization—to receive specific training and ongoing supervision from the consultant. Although the consultant initially spends a large block of time on-site teaching and demonstrating mental-skills

training applications to the trainee, the consultant steadily decreases on-site involvement with the team. The trainee, however, maintains regular contact with the supervisor and daily contact with the team.

The supervisory approach addresses many of the barriers that arise for a consultant initially gaining access to the sport organization (Ravizza, 1988). Because trainees are selected from existing sport organization personnel, they have sport-specific experiences to draw on and understand the political climate of the team environment. Smith and Johnson (1990) recommend that the trainee be instructed in a cognitive-behavioral orientation to counseling that meshes well with an educational-skills-building approach.

The supervisory model is an appealing consultation approach offering many benefits to the sport organization as well as minimizing potential barriers to effective entry and intervention. However, few teams have available potential trainees with adequate counseling or sport-science backgrounds to receive supervision. In addition, those trainees who have the requisite background might not wish to change their current status with the team. Trainees who do make a shift into a sport-psychology role with their teams might find difficult the adjustment to new roles and changing relationships with players and coaches.

The Cognitive-Behavioral Consultation Model

Murphy and Murphy (1992) have outlined a comprehensive eight-step cognitive-behavioral consultation model that they use to structure initial contacts and subsequent interactions with the national governing bodies or administrative organizations of various sports. Murphy and Murphy highlight the importance of the initial contact with the sport organization. The primary objective of the initial contact is to determine if consultation is desirable and possible and to derive an agreement outlining consultation parameters. Coaches' and athletes' needs and expectations are identified before beginning consultation, and the philosophy of the cognitive-behavioral model is explained to the client. Murphy and Murphy recommend drawing up a contract that specifies client and consultant behaviors and expectations and includes a prearranged evaluation meeting after a specified period to determine if consultation should be continued.

The cognitive-behavioral consultation model espouses an educational approach with a focus on mental-skills training; however, evaluation and assessment of the athlete's functioning in multiple contexts is crucial. An emphasis is placed on viewing the athlete as a person, not just a performer, and assessments of the athlete's functioning in sport, in relationships, and in work and academic settings are all part of a comprehensive evaluation. A comprehensive view of the athlete's experience is emphasized.

The cognitive-behavioral model represents a hybrid of the educational and clinical approaches. Assessment, diagnosis of problems, and intervention planning, characteristic functions of a clinical approach, figure prominently. Sport familiarization and mental-skills training—elements of an educational approach—are also key characteristics of the cognitive-behavioral approach. Essential to the consulting process is establishing a "collaborative empiricism" so that the athlete and consultant (or coach and consultant) experience assessment as a process in which they are involved rather than one in which they are passive. The assessment process is focused primarily on determining the pertinence of specific mental skills to the sport situation, the mastery level of mental skills, the use of skills, and obstacles that interfere with the use of mental skills. The assessment and evaluation process drives interventions that are carried out in both group and individual settings.

Athletes and coaches supply data regarding both baseline and postintervention functioning; therefore, they determine their needs and evaluate the efficacy of interventions. Furthermore, there is no assumption of pathology. Collaborative assessment helps athletes and coaches identify specific areas that they determine would benefit from improvement.

The eight steps of the Murphy and Murphy (1992) model are

1. consultation orientation,
2. sport familiarization,
3. evaluation and assessment,
4. goal identification,
5. group intervention,
6. individual intervention,
7. outcome evaluation, and
8. reassessment of goals.

These steps are presented here in some detail to help professionals working in a sport setting or with athletic populations. A great amount of trial-and-error learning has gone into the development of this model, and it is hoped that the suggestions that are offered will help others avoid making some of the mistakes made in developing the model. Figures 10.1 through 10.8 present the cognitive-behavioral model in an easily accessible graphic manner. In each step, the objective of that phase of consultation is described, followed by a list of bullet points describing the methods developed to reach that objective.

A CONSULTATION PROCESS FOR LI-WU

A comprehensive description follows of a consultation process for Li-Wu using the cognitive-behavioral model. This case is presented in sufficient detail to clarify the issues and steps involved in working with an athlete in the framework of the cognitive-behavioral

Objective

To determine if consultation is desirable and possible; to come up with an agreement outlining the parameters of the consultation

Methods

- Set up initial meeting with coach; determine coach's expectations; clarify nature of consultation relationship
- Meet with athlete and determine athlete's wants and needs; is consultation appropriate?
- Meet with appropriate parties; explain philosophy and approach; set realistic expectations
- Set up preliminary contract specifying only *parameters* of the consultation. Specify
  - Goals of consultation
  - Amount and length of consultation (suggest evaluation of progress after a specific time)
  - Payment

Figure 10.1 Step 1. Consultation orientation.

model described above. The case material has been altered to represent a composite person.

Assessment of Li-Wu

The BASIC ID format (see Figure 10.3), designed by Lazarus (1981), was used to evaluate Li-Wu to determine the most effective intervention plan. Following is a description of the assessment in each of the key component areas.

Behavior

An examination of Li-Wu's behaviors revealed an absence of vaulting behavior during her practice sessions. In particular, it was noted that she avoided her difficult vaulting

Objective

To become familiar with athlete's sport so effective communication is possible; to identify key sport-specific factors impacting athlete's performance

Methods

- Attend practices and competitions to learn about sport and build trust with athlete
- Ask many questions; don't let technical details go over your head
- Talk to athlete; ask athlete to explain the sport
- Read up on athlete's sport (both technical and historical details will aid in consultation)
- Try out athlete's sport yourself; if possible, participate in an event to learn about performance demands but don't become a fan to clients
- Go to a competition; talk to competitors (other than clients)

Figure 10.2 Step 2. Sport familiarization.

skills, such as the one that resulted in her injury. Instead, she spent more time practicing other events.

Affect

Li-Wu's affect included anxiety, frustration, fear, anger, and a loss of pleasure in activities that previously produced enjoyment. Li-Wu was administered the Competitive State Anxiety Inventory-2 (CSAI-2) (Martens, Burton, Vealey, Bump, & Smith, 1990) to assess the dimensions of her anxiety. Although the results indicated she was experiencing high levels of cognitive and somatic anxiety, it was determined that most of Li-Wu's anxiety originated in cognitive concerns.

Sensations

Li-Wu reported experiencing nervousness, sweaty palms (a particular concern given the

Objective

To obtain all information necessary to identify

- Key mental skills for sport
- Reasons for performance blocks
- Potential intervention targets

Methods

Assess	*By*
B Behavior (performance)	Self-report, observation, video
A Affect	Self-report, observation, testing
S Sensations (attentional focus)	Self-report, testing, self-monitoring
I Imagery	Self-report, testing, guided imagery
C Cognitions (self-talk)	Self-report, self-monitoring, video (watch with client)
I Interpersonal (coach, team, family)	Self-report, interviews
D Drugs (training, diet)	Self-report, medical evaluation

Testing Instruments

SAS: Trait anxiety scale (Smith, Smoll, & Schutz, 1990)

CSAI-2: State anxiety scale (Martens et al., 1990)

SIMS: Sports inventory of mental skills (Murphy, Hardy, Thomas, & Bond, 1993)

POMS: State emotional inventory (McNair, Lorr, & Droppleman, 1971)

Note. In Step 3, Lazarus's (1981) BASIC-ID assessment paradigm has been adopted for sport settings and guides the evaluation process.

Figure 10.3 Step 3. Evaluation and assessment.

circumstances of her accident), feeling "sick to her stomach," and an inability to focus her attention. An interview revealed that Li-Wu did not believe she had the confidence or correct frame of mind to perform on the vaulting apparatus.

Imagery

Li-Wu's imaging involved seeing herself slip and land on her neck again. Although she had tried to visualize herself successfully completing the vault, she was unable to do so.

Cognitions

Li-Wu's self-talk was dominated by negative beliefs about herself, her abilities, her future as an Olympian, and specifically her ability to complete the vaulting routine that resulted in her injury. For example, she reported she was "certain" she could not perform the vault and that there was "no way" she could make the Olympic team.

Interpersonal

Li-Wu and her coach reported having a positive working relationship. However, Li-Wu

Objective

To identify in specific terms the nature of the mental–performance relationship; to suggest specific interventions based on this analysis to improve athlete's coping skills

Methods

- For team education
  - Describe key mental skills for sport
  - Identify interventions to enhance skills
  - Generate curriculum; explain key skills and set agenda for how relevant techniques will be taught
- For individual consults
  - Generate summary of athlete's current mental strategies; identify strengths and weaknesses
  - Identify the critical areas appropriate for intervention
  - Map out the mental–performance relationship in detail for critical areas
  - Devise plans for improving athlete's coping skills in weak areas; use athlete's strengths if possible; identify intervention techniques, using approaches taught in group sessions
  - Discuss plans with athlete: get feedback from the athlete and use in your plans
  - Devise method for evaluating progress toward goals (in what specific areas do you expect to see change?)

Figure 10.4   Step 4. Goal identification.

stated that her coach's anxiety about her difficulties performing on the vault have not helped her in coping effectively with her fears. Although Li-Wu does not live with her family (she moved away from home to train at an elite gymnasium), the relationship appears to have been appropriately supportive.

Objective

To expand and strengthen coping resources of athlete with respect to sport performance

Methods

- Adopt an educational approach; explain rationale of techniques to athlete; teach athlete how to apply techniques in relevant contexts
- Encourage use of mental skills in athletic situations; if needed, visit appropriate facility (gym, pool, track, rink, etc.)
- Be systematic in developing a rationale for importance of mental skills and showing how these assist in developing sport skills; this involves
  - Course curriculum
  - Teaching exercises
  - Methods for encouraging athlete participation
  - Follow-up and feedback strategies
  - Coach feedback

Experience indicates that athletes learn more and derive more enjoyment from participatory learning rather than didactic exercises.

Figure 10.5   Step 5. Group intervention.

Drugs and Biology

Li-Wu must spend a considerable amount of time caring for her injury. For example, she must thoroughly warm up and stretch her neck muscles before each workout and apply ice to these same muscles afterwards to prevent swelling. Additionally, she continues to take anti-inflammatory medication although she reports it makes her feel groggy and upsets her stomach.

Li-Wu appears to be inappropriately concerned about her weight. She reported that she worries about her weight a great deal and believes she is not thin enough for her

Objective

To help individuals develop and practice a mental routine for performance that will help with consistency and self-control. This routine will use coping techniques learned in group sessions. Individual sessions allow athlete to share unique ideas, thoughts, perspective; to discuss personal issues athlete brings up.

Methods

- Stick to plan developed in Step 4; be flexible and adjust where necessary

- Devise a mental routine for competition; include specific preparations day before, morning of, 30 min before, immediately before, during, and after competition, if necessary; include cues for use of coping skills

- Have athlete practice mental routine during workouts and at competitions

- Identify potential obstacles and ways to refocus if encountered

- Build toward problem resolution; don't try to take care of everything at once; prioritize interventions

- Deal with athlete's personal issues (this is important, and in many cases counseling will be appropriate); be aware of any limitations in your own expertise, make these clear to athlete, and have support available if athlete wants to discuss issues outside of your expertise; be firm in limiting inappropriate discussion of such issues

- If counseling and mental skills training are concurrent, give separate time to each; help athlete focus on single issues

Figure 10.6 Step 6. Individual intervention.

sport. To determine if her diet was too restrictive, Li-Wu was referred to a nutritionist. It was reported that she had no indications of an eating disorder, but several further consultations with the nutritionist were scheduled

Objective

To assess how well goals of Step 4 (goal identification) have been met; if goals not met, to identify reasons

Methods

- Use evaluation method devised when intervention plans were made. Evaluation should include

  - Feedback from athlete regarding satisfaction with consultation

  - Measurable feedback regarding relevant performance goals

  - Feedback from coach

- Include a variety of criteria in the evaluation, such as

  - Performance

  - Attitude

  - Commitment to sport

  - Life balance

  - Personal development

- Provide feedback on mental-skills training progress to both coaches and athletes

Figure 10.7 Step 7. Outcome evaluation.

to help her select and maintain a more well balanced diet that would meet her nutritional and caloric needs.

Conceptualization of the Case

A cognitive-behavioral approach suggested that each of the affective, cognitive, and behavioral systems be addressed to most effectively help the client. According to Mahoney and Meyers (1989), the experience of anxiety creates an interaction among systems (muscular, respiratory, cardiac, attention, etc.) in anticipation of danger or pain, which in turn leads to an attempt to avoid or control the

Objective

To reassess goals if necessary; to modify plans as needed

Methods

- Be prepared for the unexpected; especially in group sessions, group dynamics can change dramatically

- Be prepared to focus on new issues as they arise; a team might unexpectedly fail to qualify for a competition, an athlete might be severely injured, a coach might be fired—all can greatly impact the program

- Use athlete's progress in individual sessions as an indicator of pace you should maintain with athlete

- Use constructive feedback in an effort to improve your program (our programs have placed more and more emphasis on individual sessions based on feedback from coaches and athletes; also, we have tried harder to get the teaching out of the classroom and into the gym)

Figure 10.8   Step 8. Reassessment of goals.

experience. Anxiety is the result of the memories or anticipation of an experience and whether that experience was good or bad. Anxiety is also determined by the sense of efficacy the individual has about the experience (Bandura, 1977, 1982, 1986; Beck, Emery, & Greenberg, 1985).

Ellis's (1975) Rational-Emotive Therapy (RET) approach was utilized in the management of Li-Wu's worries. His A-B-C principle can be applied with Li-Wu.

- The activating event is the difficult trick on the vault.
- The consequence is Li-Wu's anxiety level.
- Her belief about the vault is what causes Li-Wu anxiety, not the difficult vault itself.

The intervention suggested is that by utilizing positive self-statements, Li-Wu must dispute her irrational belief that she is definitely going to be injured again and instead create new emotional affects, such as confidence, strength, and positive feelings that she will, indeed, be able to efficiently do the difficult vault.

Intervention With Li-Wu

Intervention began with teaching Li-Wu some relaxation exercises to help manage her anxiety. Progressive relaxation (Jacobson, 1974) is based on the notion that the body responds with muscle tension to anxiety-provoking thoughts and events. This physiological tension then increases the subjective experience of anxiety. Deep muscle relaxation reduces physiological tension and is incompatible with anxiety. By alternately tensing and relaxing her muscles, she learned where she "holds" her tension and how to release it and relax. Li-Wu had a high level of shoulder tension, preventing her from moving her arms freely when she was anxious. Deep diaphragmatic breathing was also incorporated in this exercise, as it is an easy-to-use way to produce a relaxed state.

The positive effects of these exercises help the consultant build trust with the client. At the same time, the consultant teaches the client about both anxiety and self-control of anxiety. After some practice, progressive relaxation can be a 10-second exercise that can be done at any time, even during a competition.

The next intervention step with Li-Wu was cognitive restructuring (Davis, Eschelman, & McKay, 1988). This treatment method is based on the assumption that emotional problems result from maladaptive thought patterns (Ellis, 1975). The task of therapy is to alter these faulty cognitions (Wilson, 1984). An assumption of cognitive restructuring is that reorganizing and restructuring verbal statements about oneself and one's world will result in a corresponding reorganization of behavior with respect to one's world (Risley & Hart, 1968). Li-Wu was taught to become aware of her maladaptive thoughts and learn to modify them with more positive, rational ones. Several frequently expressed self-statements, identified through self-monitoring, such as I'm going to wipe out on the vault and get injured again or I can't do this vault, were increasing her anxiety levels. A list of positive, coping self-statements were then developed to replace these negative cognitions:

- I am calm and at peace.
- I am a good gymnast.
- I am able to do difficult tricks.
- I am able to do difficult tricks on the vault.
- I am confident and strong.
- I am in control of my body and mind.
- I can meet this challenge.

Li-Wu was able to transform her self-talk through practice with these self-statements, which resulted in increased self-confidence and more adaptive coping behaviors in the gym.

Another problem identified in the assessment phase was that Li-Wu was unable to imagine herself successfully completing the vault trick and consistently saw herself getting hurt again. The first step to enabling Li-Wu to visualize completing the vault trick was to find some videos of her doing the trick successfully. Her coach had some footage of her doing the vault well. Li-Wu was instructed to watch these successful vaults repeatedly to gain a clear image of herself doing that vault effectively. The goal was to readopt a vision of herself performing the behavior successfully (a self-modeling exercise). Bandura (1977) suggested that modeling is effective in changing behaviors, as it teaches new skills and assists in disinhibiting the anxiety associated with the feared behavior. Rushall (1988) has suggested that covert

modeling can progress from imaging others to imaging oneself. This self-modeling procedure enabled Li-Wu to start imaging herself completing the trick without anxiety.

However, Li-Wu found that she could begin the image appropriately but then suddenly see herself crashing to the floor, injured once again. Li-Wu was instructed to utilize a "freeze-frame" technique to control the image. When imaging the difficult trick, Li-Wu was told to stop the image by using the "freeze-frame buttons, just as if you were watching it on a VCR." She could then move the image frame by frame in order to see herself complete the image successfully. Li-Wu was encouraged to visualize the element from an internal perspective, although the research literature suggests that both internal and external imagery can be used effectively for mental rehearsal (Murphy & Jowdy, 1992).

Suinn's (1980) visuomotor behavior rehearsal (VMBR) combines several coping skills that involve total reintegration of experience, including visual, auditory, tactile, kinesthetic, and emotional cues (Murphy, 1990). When Li-Wu was told to visualize "vividly," she was encouraged to use all of her senses to more closely assimilate the actual experience of doing the vault. Li-Wu was asked to visually put herself in the gym, smell the chalk in the air, hear the music of someone else doing a floor routine, hear her coach giving her instructions, feel the chalk on her hands, feel the horse under her hands when attempting the skill, taste the dryness in her mouth and chalk particles floating in the air, feel her body running down the runway and flying through the air to and over the vault, and experience landing the skill successfully. If she is able to recreate this experience and manage her anxiety about it, she will be more likely to feel self-efficacious and, therefore, more likely to attempt the skill without balking.

A variant of systematic desensitization (Wolpe, 1958) was used to help Li-Wu start approaching the actual vault with conviction. A stimulus hierarchy was constructed in which the aspects of the situation the client fears (in Li-Wu's case, approaching the vault on her difficult trick) are ordered along a continuum from mildly stressful to very threatening. The client is instructed to conjure a clear and vivid image of each item on the hierarchy while deeply relaxed (Wilson, 1984). Progressive relaxation can be used to produce deep relaxation. As Li-Wu moved through the levels of the hierarchy, she was instructed to cease visualization and utilize progressive relaxation whenever she began to feel anxious. The item was then repeated until Li-Wu could visualize doing that behavior on the hierarchy without feeling anxious. The entire hierarchy was completed in this fashion until Li-Wu was able to successfully imagine the difficult vault without fear. Then Li-Wu was taken into the gym to complete an in vivo experience similar to the one she was able to achieve by visualization. A new step in the hierarchy was completed each day until she was able to execute the skill. This hierarchy was used by Li-Wu:

- Go to the gym and sit by the vault.
- Walk down the runway to the vault.
- Turn around at the end of the runway to the vault.
- Look down the runway to the vault.
- Visualize doing a simple vault at the end of the runway.
- Run down the vault runway.
- Run down the runway and execute a simple vault.
- Visualize a difficult vault at the end of the runway.
- Run down the runway toward the vault.
- Run down the runway and execute the difficult vault.

It is important to be aware that elite athletes might want to rush the desensitization

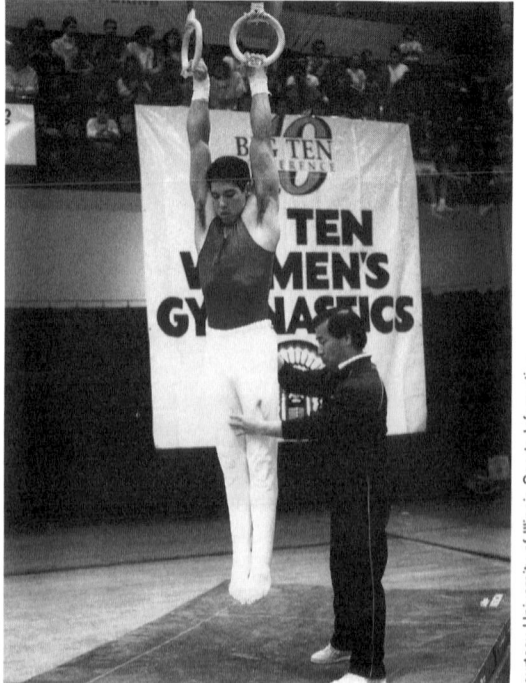

Courtesy University of Illinois Sports Information

process, but this can lead to setbacks. Encourage the athlete to be patient and take only one step at a time.

A meeting was conducted with Li-Wu, her coach, and the sport psychology consultant to encourage Li-Wu to share her feelings about the coach's behaviors and how they were affecting her. A separate meeting between the coach and sport psychology consultant involved discussion of the coach's feedback style and ideas to more effectively work with a fearful gymnast. The coach was receptive to the meeting with the consultant and was willing to make changes.

The case of Li-Wu demonstrates that even a specific, well-defined athletic issue (in this case, return from injury) can involve a variety of interventions in several modalities. The consultant must be flexible to be able to adapt to the specific needs of the athlete and the sport situation. There are several combinations of cognitive-behavioral interventions that can be used effectively with athletes experiencing anxiety-related or confidence problems. The combination could include a relaxation exercise (see Davis et al., 1988 for a variety of both relaxation and cognitive restructuring ideas), cognitive restructuring, and imagery. A review of the literature on psychological interventions with competitive athletes by Greenspan & Feltz (1989) indicated that educational relaxation-based interventions and remedial cognitive-restructuring interventions with individual athletes are generally effective.

Additional Case Management Considerations

Li-Wu's case demonstrates how traditional cognitive-behavioral interventions can be successful with managing many performance issues. However, there are several other issues in such cases to which the sport psychology consultant must be sensitive. In any case involving athlete injury, the consultant must obtain information from medical and other personnel concerning the likely postinjury level of athletic functioning, which is often extremely difficult to predict. Even if the injury is not career ending, it is possible nevertheless that the athlete will be unable to return to the previous training and competition level. Preparing in advance for such issues can help the athlete's adaptation to rehabilitation. For many athletes, rehabilitation can be a long and arduous process, often accompanied by depression. Injuries can have a profound impact on an athlete's sense of identity and self-esteem, particularly if it is likely that the athlete will not be able to perform at the previous level. Athletes often derive a certain amount of their identity from sport and athletes at any level can experience an identity crisis when forced to relinquish their sport. Elite athletes generally structure their lives to be compatible with athletic advancement (Brewer, Van Raalte, & Lindner, 1993; Ogil-

vie & Howe, 1986). Injuries can completely alter an athlete's lifestyle and socialization patterns, so there is a need to be sensitive to the potential problems that can occur when working with this kind of situation.

The coach also plays a critical part in managing such a situation as Li-Wu's. Li-Wu's coach was amenable to consultation and implemented suggestions made by the consultant, but this does not always happen. Coaches can feel threatened by consultants, whom they might view as coming in to tell them what to do with their athletes. Good rapport with the coach is necessary to provide the most effective intervention with an athlete. It is important for the sport psychology consultant to get out of the office and into the gym to become familiar with the sport and its jargon, the training and competition environment, and the dynamics between the athletes and coach. It is best to observe the environment before offering any interventions. If a consultant does not become familiar with the sport (see Figure 10.2), know the coach, and learn about the training and competition environment, the probability of success with the consultancy is low.

Transfer of Cognitive-Behavioral Skills to Nonsport Areas

Cognitive-behavioral interventions teach skills to the client that can be generalized across a broad variety of situations, which means that once the client has learned the skills specifically for one area of life, the skills can be adapted to other life areas. For instance, goal setting, stress management, and cognitive restructuring can be used in academic or work environments to manage many anxiety-provoking situations. Behavioral medicine has utilized many cognitive-behavioral techniques over the years in an attempt to facilitate preventive medicine efforts in patients and to help the chronically ill manage their illnesses and reduce pain (see Turk, Meichenbaum, & Genest, 1983). Therefore, these techniques are not situation specific, but can be viewed as techniques that facilitate healthy and effective coping behaviors in life (see the discussion of this issue by Danish and colleagues in chapter 2).

CONSULTATION AND INTERVENTION GUIDELINES

Adopt an educational, coping-skills approach.

Performance enhancement is achieved in personal development.

Never take credit for the athlete's performance. Adopt the approach, Look at what you can do with your new skills!

Set realistic expectations. If the coach or athlete has unreasonable expectations, educate them right at the beginning as to what you can and can't do.

Be careful of boundaries in the sport consultation setting. By the nature of the process, it is easy to become friendly with your clients (going to practices, going to competitions, etc.). However, you need to retain consultant–client boundaries.

Help athletes realize that they must practice skills for them to be effective. Athletes should not try out a new mental skill for the first time in competition. Skills and mental routines must be gradually built into the repertoire.

CONCLUSION

In this chapter we have examined existing models of psychology consultancy with sport organizations and offered a cognitive-behavioral model that has been effective in a variety of sport situations. The cognitive-behavioral approach presented here offers the advantages both of being based on educational and coping skills and also of viewing the athlete in the context of her life situation. It thus avoids the medical-model drawbacks often associated with the clinical approach and minimizes the overly narrow emphasis on performance concerns typically associated with the educational model.

We close this chapter with some important guidelines for sport consultants, no matter what the level of assistance offered sport organizations. By observing these principles, helping professionals can avoid common pitfalls in their work as consultants. A key to successful interventions is a coherent outlook, and this chapter has shown you how to develop such a model.

REFERENCES

American Psychological Association. (1990). Ethical principles of psychologists. *American Psychologist*, **45**, 390-395.

Anshel, M. (1992). The case against the certification of sport psychologists: In search of the phantom expert. *Sport Psychologist*, **6**, 265-286.

Bandura, A. (1977). Self-efficacy: Toward a unifying theory of behavior change. *Psychological Review*, **84**, 191-215.

Bandura, A. (1982). Self-efficacy in human agency. *American Psychologist*, **37**, 122-147.

Bandura, A. (1986). *Social foundations of thought and action*. Englewood Cliffs, NJ: Prentice Hall.

Beck, A.T., Emery, G., & Greenberg, R.L. (1985). *Anxiety disorders and phobias: A cognitive perspective.* New York: Basic Books.

Biddle, S.J.H., Bull, S.J., & Seheult, C.L. (1992). Ethical and professional issues in contemporary British sport psychology. *Sport Psychologist,* **6,** 66-76.

Botterill, C. (1990). Sport psychology and professional hockey. *Sport Psychologist,* **4,** 358-367.

Brewer, B., Van Raalte, J., & Lindner, D. (1993). Athletic identity: Hercules' muscle or Achilles' heel? *International Journal of Sport Psychology,* **24,** 237-254.

Davis, M., Eschelman, E.R., & McKay, M. (1988). *The relaxation and stress reduction workbook* (3rd ed.). Oakland, CA: New Harbinger.

Dorfman, H.A. (1990). Reflections on providing personal performance enhancement consulting services in professional baseball. *Sport Psychologist,* **4,** 341-346.

Ellis, A. (1975). *Humanistic psychotherapy: The rational-emotive approach.* New York: McGraw-Hill.

Gardner, F.L. (1991). Professionalization of sport psychology: A reply to Silva. *Sport Psychologist,* **5,** 55-60.

Gordon, S. (1990). A mental skills training program for the Western Australian cricket team. *Sport Psychologist,* **4,** 386-399.

Greenspan, M.J., & Feltz, D.L. (1989). Psychological interventions with athletes in competitive situations: A review. *Sport Psychologist,* **3,** 219-236.

Halliwell, W. (1990). Providing sport psychology consulting services in professional hockey. *Sport Psychologist,* **4,** 369-377.

Jacobson, P. (1974). *Progressive relaxation.* Chicago: University of Chicago Press.

LaRose, B. (1988). What can the sport psychology consultant learn from the educational consultant? *Sport Psychologist,* **2,** 141-153.

Lazarus, A.A. (1981). *The practice of multimodal therapy.* New York: McGraw-Hill.

Loehr, J.E. (1990). Providing sport psychology consultation services to professional tennis players. *Sport Psychologist,* **4,** 400-408.

Mahoney, M., & Meyers, A. (1989). Anxiety and athletic performance: Traditional and cognitive-behavioral perspectives. In D. Hackfort (Ed.), *Anxiety in sports: An international perspective* (pp. 77-94). Washington, DC: Hemisphere.

Martens, R., Burton, D., Vealey, R., Bump, L., & Smith, D. (1990). Development and validation of the Competitive State Anxiety Inventory-2 (CSAI-2). In R. Martens, R. Vealey, & D. Burton (Eds.), *Competitive anxiety in sport* (pp. 117-190). Champaign, IL: Human Kinetics.

McKelvain, R. (1988, October). *Consulting effectively with national governing bodies.* Paper presented at the Annual Conference of the Association for the Advancement of Applied Sport Psychology, Nashua, NH.

McNair, D., Lorr, M., & Droppleman, L. (1971). *Profile of mood states manual.* San Diego: Educational and Testing Service.

Murphy, S.M. (1988). The on-site provision of sport psychology services at the 1987 U.S. Olympic Festival. *Sport Psychologist,* **2,** 337-350.

Murphy, S.M. (1990). Models of imagery in sport psychology: A review. *Journal of Mental Imagery,* **14,** 153-172.

Murphy, S.M., & Ferrante, A.P. (1989). Provision of sport psychology services to the U.S. Team at the 1988 Summer Olympic Games. *Sport Psychologist,* **3,** 374-385.

Murphy, S.M., Hardy, L., Thomas, P., & Bond, J. (1993). *The Sports Inventory of Mental Skills.* Unpublished manuscript, U.S. Olympic Committee, Colorado Springs.

Murphy, S.M., & Jowdy, D. (1992). Imagery and mental practice. In T. Horn (Ed.),

Advances in sport psychology (pp. 221-250). Champaign, IL: Human Kinetics.

Murphy, S.M., & Murphy, A.I. (1992, August). *Sport psychology: Performance enhancement for athletes*. Workshop presented at the Annual Meeting of the American Psychological Association, Washington, DC.

Neff, F. (1990). Delivering sport psychology services to a professional sport organization. *Sport Psychologist*, **4**, 378-385.

Nideffer, R. (1981). *The ethics and practice of applied sport psychology*. Ithaca, NY: Mouvement.

Ogilvie, B.C. (1977). Walking the perilous path of the team psychologist. *Physician & Sportsmedicine*, **5**(4), 63-67.

Ogilvie, B.C. (1979). The sport psychologist and his professional credibility. In P.H. Klavora & J.V. Daniel (Eds.), *Coach, athlete, and the sport psychologist* (pp. 45-55). Toronto: University of Toronto Press.

Ogilvie, B.C. (1992). *Consultation issues within professional sport*. Unpublished manuscript, U.S. Olympic Committee, Colorado Springs.

Ogilvie, B.C., & Howe, M. (1986). The trauma of termination from athletics. In J.M. Williams (Ed.), *Applied sport psychology: Personal growth to peak performance* (pp. 365-382). Palo Alto, CA: Mayfield Press.

Ravizza, K. (1988). Gaining entry with athletic personnel for season-long consulting. *Sport Psychologist*, **2**, 243-254.

Ravizza, K. (1990). Sportpsych consultation issues in professional baseball. *Sport Psychologist*, **4**, 330-340.

Risley, T., & Hart, B. (1968). Developing correspondence between the nonverbal and verbal behavior of preschool children. *Journal of Applied Behavior Analysis*, **1**, 267-281.

Rotella, R.J. (1990). Providing sport psychology consulting services to professional athletes. *Sport Psychologist*, **4**, 409-417.

Rushall, B. (1988). Covert modeling as a procedure for altering an athlete's psychological state. *Sport Psychologist*, **2**, 131-140.

Silva, J.M. (1989). Toward the professionalization of sport psychology. *Sport Psychologist*, **3**, 265-273.

Smith, R.E., & Johnson, J. (1990). An organizational empowerment approach to consultation in professional baseball. *Sport Psychologist*, **4**, 347-357.

Smith, R.E., Smoll, F.L., & Schutz, R.W. (1990). Measurement and correlates of sport specific cognitive and somatic trait anxiety: The Sport Anxiety Scale. *Anxiety Research*, **2**, 263-280.

Suinn, R. (1980). Psychology and sports performance: Principles and application. In R. Suinn (Ed.), *Psychology in sports: Methods and applications* (pp. 26-36). Minneapolis: Burgess.

Thompson, R., & Sherman, R. (1993). *Helping athletes with eating disorders*. Champaign, IL: Human Kinetics.

Turk, D.C., Meichenbaum, D., & Genest, M. (1983). *Pain and behavioral medicine: A cognitive-behavioral perspective*. New York: Guilford Press.

Wilson, T.E. (1984). Behavior therapy. In R.J. Corsini (Ed.), *Current psychotherapies* (3rd ed.). Itasca, IL: Peacock.

Wolpe, J. (1958). *Psychotherapy by reciprocal inhibition*. Stanford, CA: Stanford University Press.

Zaichkowsky, L.D., & Perna, F.M. (1992). Certification of consultants in sport psychology: A rebuttal to Anshel. *Sport Psychologist*, **6**, 287-296.

PART II

SPECIAL ISSUES IN COUNSELING ATHLETES

CHAPTER 11

CARING FOR INJURED ATHLETES

Al Petitpas, EdD
Springfield College

Steven J. Danish, PhD
Virginia Commonwealth University

Traditionally, physicians and sports medicine professionals have focused most of their attention on the physical aspects of athletic injuries. This emphasis has spurred others to develop marked improvements in sports equipment, conditioning, and training methods, yet incidence of athletic injury have at best remained constant (Yaffe, 1983). With the recent emphasis on psychobiological relationships, it is not surprising that researchers have turned their attention to the impact of psychological variables on the sports injury process. In fact, several practitioners have suggested that adverse psychological factors are instrumental in predicting sports injury, prolonging the rehabilitative process, and causing subsequent performance decrements, emotional problems, and even suicide in certain athletes.

This chapter examines some psychological factors that affect athletes with injuries, emphasizing the psychological rehabilitative process. The chapter's five sections explore the following questions:

- How do sports injuries affect athletes psychologically?

- What are some warning signs of a potentially difficult adjustment?
- What are some psychological factors to consider in treatment planning?
- What would be a typical treatment protocol?
- What are some practical and ethical issues sport psychologists face in the sports medicine setting?

Critical psychological considerations can be present in the full range of athletic injuries. From sprains and strains to overuse and knee injuries, many athletes have found psychological interventions a necessary component of their rehabilitation. The following case studies might help to illustrate some of the psychological dynamics to be explored and underscore material that will be presented later in the chapter. The outcome of these cases will be presented in the chapter's conclusion.

■ *THE CASE OF JANE* ■

Jane is a 30-year-old mother of two children. She met her husband while competing in the NCAA National Gymnastics Championships.

They married shortly after her graduation 3 years later. After a 2-year stint as an assistant gymnastics coach, Jane decided to open her own gymnastics school. With her reputation as an all-American collegiate athlete and excellent coach, her school thrived.

Jane's injury problems began with a stress fracture of her left foot. This was quickly followed by a badly sprained neck, sustained while demonstrating a dismount, and a back injury resulting from a car accident. After more than 2 years of hard work in physical therapy and a demanding home rehabilitation program, Jane was able to resume a full work schedule. However, within a month she began to experience pain in her heel. Her physician explained it as pain referred from her neck and suggested that she stop working and refrain from exercise. Within 2 days, Jane reported that she had lost most of the stability she had gained during the previous 2 years of physical therapy. She quickly found another physician who gave her the green light to resume physical therapy and light exercise. Jane decided to stop working and concentrate on her rehabilitation. She returned to work two months later only to find herself becoming "extremely fatigued and feeling overwhelmed" each time she attempted to demonstrate her routines to her students. She has since had three additional setbacks with chronic pain, numbness, and tingling. She has crying spells, depression, difficulty sleeping, and is unable "to feel my body working correctly." A complete neurological workup proved negative.

Jane's husband has been very supportive as she has struggled with each successive injury. However, recently he has begun to lose his patience with her crying spells and inability to do anything around the house.

■ *THE CASE OF MIKE* ■

Mike, an 18-year-old straight-A high-school senior, was a two-time captain and all-state performer on the state championship football team. He had been contacted by more than 200 colleges with various scholarship offers and was the odds-on favorite to win the prestigious scholar-athlete award for his region.

Mike had always stood out. From youth league through high school, he was the biggest, fastest, and toughest player. His father, a highly successful college player, had been grooming Mike to follow in his footsteps. Mike had not been a disappointment.

After a preseason scrimmage game, Mike complained of discomfort in his stomach and lower back. The pain grew progressively worse and Mike went to his physician for a complete examination. To everyone's amazement, it was discovered that Mike had only one kidney, located in the abdominal area. He underwent surgery to extract the kidney stone that had caused his discomfort.

Although Mike was declared healthy, he was advised to avoid contact sports. Mike could not believe it. He and his father spent the next few weeks contacting sports medicine professionals from around the country about special protective gear, but the risk of serious injury was too great. After a couple of weeks of angry outbursts and moodiness, Mike was forced to accept the decision to terminate his football career. He appeared to handle the loss of football remarkably well. In fact, he was the first person to admit that "football is only a game." He seemed more concerned with how his father was handling the situation and suggested that his father "needs some help in dealing with it."

Mike continued to stay active with the team. He went to every practice and every game. He represented his team at the coin toss before every game and was appointed as an unofficial coach to assist the underclassmen during practices. Academically, Mike decided to work even harder on his studies in the hope of getting an academic scholarship. Instead of socializing with his teammates after practice as he had been accustomed, he went directly home and hit the books.

As a tribute to Mike's courage and dedication, he was awarded a trophy at the annual December football dinner. This trophy recognized his inspiration, courage, and contributions to the team. Mike accepted the trophy by honoring his coaches and most importantly his father "for making me what I am today."

PSYCHOLOGICAL EFFECTS OF ATHLETIC INJURY

For many people physical injury and the accompanying treatment and rehabilitation process can be extremely stressful. For athletes who might derive significant amounts of self-esteem and personal competence from their ability to perform, the injury process can be emotionally devastating.

The impact of athletic injury is dependent on a number of factors, including the nature and severity of the injury, the importance of sport in the athlete's life, and the reaction of the athlete's support network to the injury. The complexity of these and other factors makes predicting individual reactions difficult at best. To complicate matters, research efforts have concentrated on injury prediction rather than the rehabilitation process. Thus most of what is reported about psychological effects of athletic injury is based on the experience of a small number of practitioners. Despite these limitations, a few reactions have been reported consistently enough to warrant further discussion.

Grief Reaction

Suinn (1967) was one of the first sport psychologists to suggest that athletes cope with injuries in essentially the same manner as any person faced with disablement or significant loss. He proposed a sequence of reactions including shock, denial, depression or anxiety, and partial or complete acceptance. Others (Astle, 1986; Rotella, 1984; Rotella & Heyman, 1986; Weiss & Troxel, 1986) have suggested that athletes frequently undergo a grieving process for the temporary or permanent loss of athletic self. This process follows Kubler-Ross's (1969) familiar stages of denial, anger, bargaining, depression, and acceptance.

Recent studies have suggested that these stage models might not accurately reflect athletes' affective responses to injuries that result in temporary impairment. It appears that athletes experience a brief period of mood disturbance (increased tension, depression, and anger with decreased levels of vigor) following an injury but return to normal when they perceive they are making progress toward recovery (McDonald & Hardy, 1990; Smith, Scott, O'Fallon, & Young, 1990). It might be that a grief reaction occurs in athletes who experience career-ending injuries, but so far we have only anecdotal evidence for this assumption.

It is clear that the severity of emotional reaction is dependent on numerous factors, not the least of which is the athlete's own coping skills. However, awareness of these possible reactions can help professionals identify potential warning signs for those athletes who might need more specialized assistance. In some situations the lack of an emotional reaction can signal potential problems. This might be seen in the case of Mike, the high-school football player, where his denial and anger were not as surprising as the suddenness of his public acceptance of the loss of football. Based on the centrality of sport in Mike's life, a longer and more emotional adjustment period might have been expected.

Identity Loss

Injured athletes might also experience a threat to personal identity. Elkin (1981) contends that athletes who have made premature or exaggerated commitments to sport are most vulnerable to ego-identity loss and subsequent depression. Little (1969) labeled this syndrome *athletic neurosis* and described it as

> a bereavement reaction to the loss of a part of the self, the overvalued physical prowess. Athleticism may not be neurotic in itself; but, like exclusive and excessive emotional dependence on work, intellectual pursuits, physical beauty or any other overvalued attribute or activity, athleticism can place the subject in a vulnerable pre-neurotic state leading to manifest neurotic illness in the event of an appropriate threat, or actual enforced deprivation, especially if it is abrupt or unexpected. (p. 195)

If Little's observations are accurate, overidentification with athletics could lead to emotional upset in people who are forced to disengage from sport roles. This notion has received some support in the literature (Chartrand & Lent, 1987; Haerle, 1975; Hill & Lowe, 1974; Ogilvie & Howe, 1986). Others (Orlick, 1980; Svoboda & Vanek, 1982) view disengagement from sport roles as a life transition similar to leaving a job or becoming a parent. (See chapter 14, where Murphy discusses at length transition issues faced by athletes retiring from sport.) Each transition offers an opportunity for self-evaluation and growth. The levels of emotional upset would be a function of people's coping abilities coupled with the quality and availability of their social supports (Pearson & Petitpas, 1990).

Kleiber and Greendorfer (1983) conducted one of the few studies of the impact of sport participation on college athletes. Their survey of former Big Ten Conference athletes found that most of their sample expressed some

sense of loss over the termination of the college athletic experience. For most, the bereavement centered on either a loss of identity and friendship or regrets about unmet goals and lost opportunities. The disengagement process was not as traumatic as some other writers (Haerle, 1975; Ogilvie & Howe, 1986) would have predicted. Kleiber and Greendorfer suggested that the athletes might have been able to adjust their priorities by moving sport to a lesser status or that perhaps these athletes were not unidimensional and had other activities in which they were invested.

Kleiber, Greendorfer, Blinde, and Samdahl (1987) reexamined these same athletes to learn about their level of life satisfaction 3 to 8 years after college graduation. Those athletes who suffered a career-ending injury expressed significantly lower levels of life satisfaction than their noninjured counterparts.

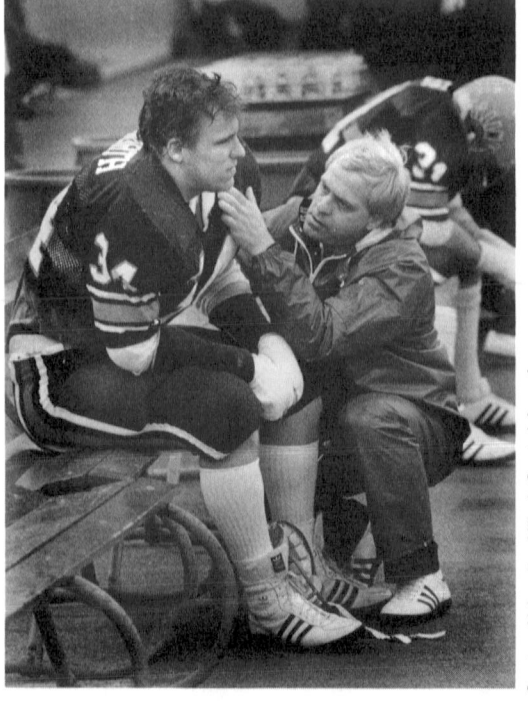

Courtesy University of Illinois Sports Information

The authors speculated that this reaction could be a result of "unfinished business" or unfulfilled dreams. Regardless of the reason for the feelings, injuries are significant events in the lives of athletes. This link has received some empirical support from Brewer (1991), who found that a strong and exclusive athletic identity is a risk factor for depressive reactions among injured athletes.

Numerous cases of college, Olympic, and professional athletes who have suffered acute depression or abused alcohol or other drugs as a result of a sudden career-ending injury have been described in the literature (Hill & Lowe, 1974; Mihovilovic, 1968; Ogilvie & Howe, 1986). Recreational runners have been found to experience guilt, irritability, and depression after they stop exercising for a few days (Sacks & Sachs, 1981). Danish (1986) cited several other effects of athletic injury including threats to self-concept, belief systems, values, commitments, emotional equilibrium, and social and emotional functioning. All of these reactions could be influenced by the level of personal identification with sport roles. The potential impact of injuries on role identity should not be underestimated.

Separation and Loneliness

Sport psychologists have suggested that feelings of separation and loneliness can also result from athletic injury (Crossman & Jamieson, 1985; Lewis-Griffith, 1982). If injured athletes can no longer practice or participate on the team, they can lose an important element of their social support system. Many sport psychologists recognize the importance of social interactions with teammates and encourage injured players to remain actively involved with the team in some capacity. Some athletes, however, will purposely avoid contact with the team when they are unable to play because they feel guilt at letting down their teammates and coaches. Others find

watching practice or a game highly stressful and "a painful reminder of all I'm missing."

Some injured athletes find it easier to withdraw from their support system rather than deal with their feelings. At the same time, some teammates might ignore injured athletes because they feel they are bad luck. Other teammates and friends might not know how to respond to the injured athlete. This is particularly true if their primary connections and identifications are through athletic roles and the injury is severe. Feeling inadequate to help, friends might avoid the athlete (Rotella & Heyman, 1986). The result of this interaction can be a withdrawal of social support at a time when it is most needed.

Injured athletes are also faced with a dramatic increase in their amount of unstructured time. The 3 to 5 hr per day of practice or game time is now devoid of activity. As one injured athlete put it, "I used to go down to the gym and get my fix every day; now I sit in my room staring at my books or daydreaming of what it used to be like."

Helping athletes plan strategies to cope with their unstructured time is often critical to the success of the psychological intervention. Some athletes need continued active involvement with the team through activities such as scouting, charting, or practice coaching. Other athletes need to get their exercise "fix" through alternative sports or activities. Still others might need assistance in coping with coaches or teammates who do not want injured players hanging around the team for fear that they might distract players or encourage less aggressive play. Helping professionals need to be aware of these individual differences in planning appropriate interventions.

Fear and Anxiety

Injured athletes face uncertain futures and potentially diminished social support. Many athletes begin to question their ability to cope with everything that is happening to them. The loss of a daily routine, the pain and discomfort of the injury, and the threats to future plans all can lead to anxiety and fear.

With more free time and uncertainty about the immediate future, it is not surprising that many athletes begin to have self-doubts. They question: Will I recover? What if I am reinjured? Will I be strong enough to regain my starting position? What if I can never play again? In many cases these doubts lead to behaviors that adversely affect the healing process (Rotella & Heyman, 1986). Athletes push too hard. They attempt shortcuts in their rehabilitation programs. They lose hope if they do not make continuous progress. In each of these examples, an athlete's behavior can become self-defeating and prolong the recovery process. As rehabilitation time increases, so does the fear and anxiety.

The emotional reactions to injury can consume a person's life. Feeling helpless in the face of stress and uncertainty, athletes can become externally controlled by the injury itself (Weiss & Troxel, 1986). This occurred in the case of Jane, which began the chapter. The multiple injuries and protracted rehabilitation eroded her confidence and increased her self-doubt. Soon the injury assumed an existence of its own. Even Jane's language reflected this, as she would insist that her "foot would not allow her to participate" or "I have to wait to see how the pain is before I go out." Helping injured athletes regain a sense of control often becomes the primary counseling goal.

Loss of Confidence and Performance Decrements

With all the physical and emotional changes with which some injured athletes must cope, it is not surprising that many of them lose confidence in their athletic skills as well. Athletes often feel that they are indestructible

(Rotella, 1984). They learn to push their bodies to the limit, often taking major physical risks.

Once hurt, they begin to question their invulnerability, and many return to competition before they are psychologically ready. This is seen in athletes who become much more tentative in their play or protective of the injured area. They often lose the spontaneity and assertiveness that allowed them to excel. Their cautious play translates into performance decrements, which can further erode their confidence and lead to more stress and frustration. The end result of this process can be reinjury, injury to another area of the body, temporary or permanent performance problems, or emotional upsets that further drain motivation and the desire to compete (Rotella & Heyman, 1986).

Athletes can be affected by injuries in numerous ways. Depending on the severity of the injury, ego-involvement with sport, and the person's and support network's coping skills, athletes can experience significant psychological trauma, including emotional upheaval, identity loss, fear, anxiety, and decrements in athletic performance and self-confidence. Health-care professionals need to be sensitive to these potential psychological reactions to insure an optimal recovery process. Failure to do so can lead to tragic consequences.

WARNING SIGNS OF A POOR ADJUSTMENT

Health-care professionals can be in an excellent position to identify those athletes who are having difficulty adjusting to an injury. Ryde (1977) suggested that physicians and other professionals need to spend more time understanding what the injury means to the athlete. Without an understanding of the psychological aspects of the injury, there is a greater risk of missing important diagnostic material; this could lead to prolonged recoveries or greatly exacerbated symptoms.

Professionals who are able to establish rapport with injured athletes are better able to recognize potential warning signs of a poor adjustment. If athletes feel understood, there is a much greater chance that they will share their fears and insecurities. Based on our clinical experience, some of the signs of a potential problematic adjustment are

- evidence of anger, depression, confusion, or apathy;
- obsession with the question, When will I be able to play again?;
- denial, reflected in remarks such as, "Things are going great," "The injury is no big deal," or other remarks that lead you to believe that the athlete is making an extraordinary effort to convince you that the injury does not really matter;
- a history of coming back too fast from injuries;
- exaggerated storytelling or bragging about accomplishments in or out of sport;
- dwelling on minor somatic complaints;
- remarks about letting the team down or feeling guilty about not being able to contribute;
- dependence on the therapist or the therapy process or "just hanging around the training room" too much;
- withdrawal from teammates, coaches, friends, family, or therapist;
- rapid mood swings or striking changes in affect or behavior; and
- statements that indicate a feeling of helplessness to impact recovery.

The presence of several of these warning signs might indicate that the athlete is in need of assistance in adjusting to the injury. Attending simultaneously to both the physical and psychological aspects of the injury can greatly enhance the establishment of therapeutic rapport and facilitate the development of a comprehensive treatment plan.

In those facilities where a sport psychologist or athletic counselor is a member of the treatment team, psychological aspects of injury are addressed routinely as part of intake and evaluation. In other cases, various health-care professionals could assess the situation and where appropriate enlist the services of a trained counselor or psychologist.

Much care is needed in making psychological referrals. Face-saving is important for most people. For athletes, it might be even more critical (Kane, 1984). For people who are already questioning their own abilities, being told that they need to see a psychologist can be harmful. It might be more therapeutic to introduce psychological services as education or skill-building activities. More will be said about this later in the chapter.

Attending to the person and not just the injury should be the goal of the intervention. Once initial trust is established and the athlete feels somewhat understood, it might be easier to detect areas of concern and plan more appropriate multimodal treatments.

PSYCHOLOGICAL FACTORS IN TREATMENT PLANNING

The adage that you need to understand a problem before you can fix it is clearly indicated when treating injured athletes. In these situations professionals are faced with a complex picture of psychological factors (see Figure 11.1). Their initial goals should be to understand the athlete, build rapport, and assess the specifics of the case. Assessment requires consideration of a number of intrapsychic, interpersonal, and situational factors.

Ego-Involvement in Sport

The threat of identity loss for athletes with severe injuries has been discussed earlier. In

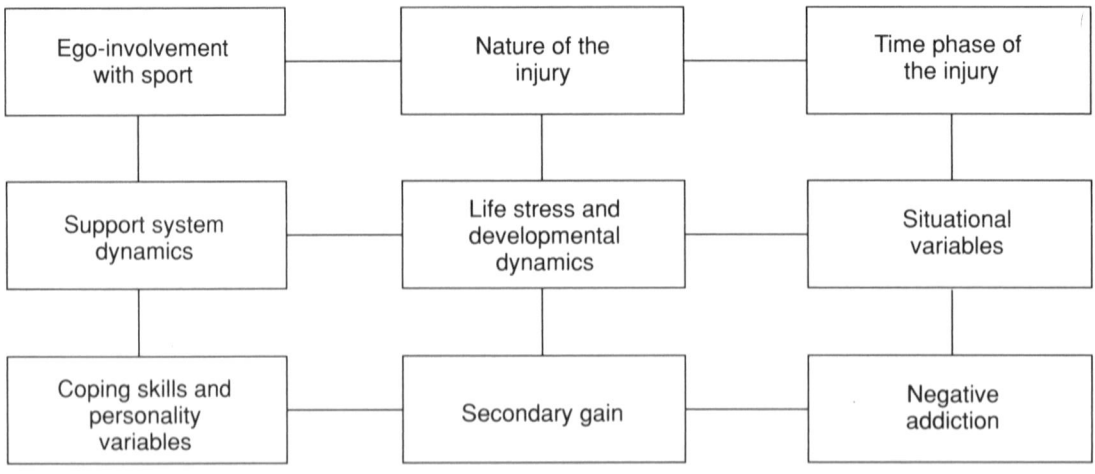

Figure 11.1   Factors in treatment planning.

assessment it is important to evaluate the degree to which players' identities are tied up in their sport roles.

Studies have suggested that involvement in high-level athletics might require athletes to focus their energies on a limited number of activities (Blann, 1985; Petitpas, 1981; Sowa & Gressard, 1983). Danish has called this process *selective optimization* and contends that "athletes invest maximal effort both physically and emotionally on behaviors judged to be essential for optimal athletic performance because this is where they believe their skills lie" (1983, p. 13). The more they continue through the sport system, the more committed athletes become to that role (Chartrand & Lent, 1987). For some athletes, sport can become the prime source of their identity.

Commitment to sport roles has the potential to be both positive and negative. It provides athletes with numerous opportunities to demonstrate their skills, interact with others, and measure their personal abilities. This is particularly valuable for young athletes who need to develop a sense of industry and competence. Sport experiences can enhance self-esteem and build confidence (Danish, Petitpas, & Hale, 1990). However,

these experiences can also be harmful to young athletes, especially in situations where winning is promoted as the only measure of personal success. For example, Kozar and Lord (1983) found that a large number of overuse injuries were found in children and young adolescents who participated on teams that stressed winning rather than learning and fun. Emphasis on winning has also been cited as the chief cause of burnout in young athletes (Feigley, 1984; Henschen, 1986; Rowland, 1986).

The pressure to win can come not only from coaches and the sport system but also from parents. Noakes and Schomer (1983) found that parental pressure to win resulted in fictive injuries in some young athletes. They labeled this process *eager parent syndrome* and suggested that some young athletes found injury their only escape from the pressures imposed on them.

Sport participation can also impact the developmental process of college-age athletes. At a time when these athletes should be exploring career and ideological alternatives, many find themselves caught up in a system that demands exclusive devotion to their sport (Petitpas & Champagne, 1988; Remer,

Tongate, & Watson, 1978). The conflict between student versus athletic expectations often causes role strain (Chartrand & Lent, 1987). Many athletes will opt to forgo opportunities to expand the student role and commit more to sport as a source of identity. The process of making role commitments without adequate experimentation has been labeled *identity foreclosure* (Marcia, 1966).

It is important to understand that premature foreclosure is not in itself harmful. Many of our most respected careers necessitate early commitments of exclusive time and energy. Foreclosure becomes problematic only when people fail to develop adequate life skills. In bypassing the exploration of alternatives, foreclosed people miss opportunities to learn about their strengths and weaknesses. They avoid an identity crisis, but they do so at the expense of self-knowledge. The ultimate cost of foreclosure might become apparent only when people are faced with the threat of role loss due to a career-ending injury, the selection process, or other forced disengagement from sport (Petitpas, 1978).

In treatment planning, it is necessary to evaluate the degree to which a person's identity is based solely on athletic roles. If foreclosure is present, it is important to distinguish between psychological and situational types (Henry & Renaud, 1972). (See the highlight box on this page.)

Athletes in a state of psychological foreclosure typically require more intense treatment options than those in the situational type. For this reason, it is important to give athletes opportunities to disclose what sport means to them and what part it has played in their lives. In situations where the injury is career threatening, the psychologically foreclosed athlete is more likely to display denial and hostility.

Athletes' Coping Skills

There is some evidence that athletes with fewer coping skills tend to have more injuries

---

Psychological and Situational Foreclosure

Psychological Foreclosure

In psychological foreclosure people rigidly adhere to their identities to maintain security or to cope with intrapsychic anxiety. This might be seen in athletes who are adult children of an alcoholic parent. They may be resistant to change and more vulnerable to threats of identity loss because their method of coping with their life situations is to seek approval through their athletic successes. The loss of their athletic role would compromise their entire defensive structure.

Situational Foreclosure

In situational foreclosure people might initially appear resistant to change, but this is due to a lack of exposure to new ideas and options. Their commitment to athletic roles is not defensive but rather a function of selective optimization. In the words of one situationally foreclosed athlete, "I went to college because that was the next league, not to get an education."

---

and more difficulty during the rehabilitation process (Williams, Tonyman, & Wadsworth, 1986). In assessing coping skills, it is critical to differentiate practical (problem-focused) and affective (emotion-focused) problem-solving skills (Smith, Scott, & Wiese, 1990). Some athletes can manage all the practical aspects of treatment. They keep all their medical appointments and adhere to their physical therapy and home exercise programs. However, they might have difficulty dealing with their anger or loss. Their interpersonal relationships might become strained, and they might isolate from their support system.

Other athletes become so involved in putting up a good emotional front that they neglect the practical aspects of treatment. They do not adhere to their therapy protocols. They push themselves beyond prescribed physical therapy limits or fail to comply with treatment at all.

Related to coping skills is the athlete's belief system concerning the injury and the rehabilitation process. One of the effects of injury outlined earlier was the loss of a sense of control. Athletes who feel powerless to impact their own recovery can impede rehabilitation. They often blame themselves for the injury, citing a careless warm-up or their own "stupid mistake" as the cause. Now filled with guilt, they fail to invest in their own recovery and, instead, rely solely on external agents, such as God or physicians.

It is also important to determine the athlete's attitudes before the injury. Some athletes have adopted sport-specific learning that can sabotage their physical or psychological recovery. Rotella and Heyman (1986) have suggested that such learned attitudes ("Injured athletes are worthless," "Act tough and give 110%") can sabotage the athlete's recovery. Many athletes feel that they can never allow themselves to be vulnerable; this attitude prevents them from using available sources of social support.

Assessment of the coping skills and the belief system of injured athletes provides insight for planning cognitive interventions. These interventions might be required to assist athletes in gaining confidence in their own ability to impact their recovery or adjust to their level of disability.

Life Stress and Developmental Dynamics

A growing body of research shows a correlation between life stress and athletic injury (e.g., Coddington & Troxell, 1980; Cryan & Alles, 1983). Although this relationship might account for only a small portion of the injuries (Lysens, VandenAuweele, & Ostyn, 1986), it

remains an important consideration in treatment planning. It is obvious that a person who is coping with large amounts of life stress might be more susceptible to breaking down under the additional weight of an injury. The amount of life stress experienced is affected by the personal meaning that a person places on the event. For example, a divorce can be stress reducing for some and catastrophic for others.

Investigating other sources of stress in an injured athlete's life can uncover potentially exacerbating situations and provide insight into the athlete's coping skills. It also provides opportunities to teach stress management techniques in life areas that might be less sensitive to the athlete. For an athlete who is presenting a brave front, indirect intervention might be the only viable course of action.

In addition, individual and family-life-cycle tasks and dynamics warrant consideration. The college football player who is undergoing a developmental identity crisis might be feeling additional pressure from a father in mid-life transition. A young gymnast reported that injury was her only escape from the incredible family pressures she felt to exceed the athletic accomplishments of her recently deceased older sister. Developmental and family-life-cycle dynamics can significantly affect rehabilitation. In some cases, these considerations demand primary therapeutic emphasis.

Secondary Gain

As with other injuries, it is important to consider whether the athlete seems to derive any benefits from the injury. Sanderson (1977) outlined a number of these potential benefits, including face-saving, escape, passive-aggressiveness against parental pressure, and avoidance of training. An injury can provide struggling athletes with a socially acceptable reason for leaving a team or for playing poorly. Rather than quit or accept a reserve role, some athletes find injury a face-saving mechanism.

The number of athletes who use injury to avoid competition has been reported as small (Kane, 1984). Some athletes discover the benefits of being injured while dealing with minor ailments. While hurt, they may receive extra attention from friends, teammates, coaches, or trainers. If this occurs at the same time that their playing time is diminishing or they are not performing well, they might find a prolonged recovery period an attractive escape route.

The adage "Never underestimate the power of secondary gain," often used in conjunction with conversion reactions, may also hold true for injured athletes. In planning treatment, it might become necessary to acknowledge the benefits of the injury and develop a strategy that will provide the same advantages without some of the ensuing costs. Exploring transferable skills and building self-confidence are examples of these strategies (Danish et al., 1990).

Social Support Systems

As with the athlete, it is important to explore the practical problem-solving skills and emotional responses of a person's support system. Family, friends, and teammates can have difficulty dealing with an injured athlete's affect. If the injury is severe enough to threaten full recovery, support system members might feel uncomfortable talking about sport. They often focus on the practical aspects of rehabilitation and avoid the athlete's feelings. In these cases, the athlete is denied the support needed to facilitate psychological adjustment.

In addition there is evidence that the attitudes and beliefs of a person's social support system can have considerable impact on the recovery process (Rolland, 1984). If significant others have doubts about an athlete's

ability to get well, they can unconsciously sabotage rehabilitation. This has been shown in studies of males recuperating from uncomplicated heart attacks. O'Leary (1985) found that if the patients' wives took treadmill tests along with their spouses, they were less likely to misinterpret fatigue or heavy breathing as heart attack related. Convinced that the patients have sturdy hearts, their spouses were more likely to encourage normal physical activities, which in turn strengthen the heart.

Family and friends can unwittingly foster doubts in an injured athlete's mind by overprotecting, acting frightened, or purposely avoiding all talk about either the injury or sport. Coaches and teammates can impact rehabilitation by indirectly causing stress or guilt if they apply pressure to return too quickly or threaten playing status.

Often, social support system members play a substantial role in the recovery process. For example, working with a coach on an athlete's psychological readiness to return to competition can help avoid reinjury, injury to another body part, or performance decrements (Rotella & Heyman, 1986). For instance, an athlete's reentry into game situations might need to be a gradual process. This might be indicated in situations where an athlete is experiencing internal or external pressure to rescue the season. Rushed back into a starting position, an athlete can force action at the expense of injury or poor performance.

In treatment planning it is often necessary to understand the types of support an injured athlete might be receiving. Rosenfeld, Richman, & Hardy (1989) identified six distinct types of social support:

listening
technical appreciation
technical challenge
emotional support
emotional challenge
shared social reality

They also found that coaches, parents, friends, and teammates differed in the types of support they offered. For example, coaches and teammates were not good sources of emotional support. This could present a major deficit to athletes who are physically separated from their families; for example, college athletes and athletes attending Olympic training centers who are too proud to share emotional issues with friends.

Another area of concern is the density of the social support network. In the sport environment, athletes tend to be highly interactive with a limited set of similar peers. This can be problematic because it tends to restrict the range of information, skills, and knowledge available to assist people in developing alternative coping responses (Mitchell, 1974; Pearson & Petitpas, 1990).

Assessment of social support concerns is often necessary to plan the concurrent interventions that are often required. For example, the helping professional might need to work with parents or coaches on how to cope with an athlete's withdrawal or intense emotions.

The Nature of the Injury

At least five main considerations describe the nature of the injury. These are severity, onset, course, history, and type.

Severity

Whether an injury causes permanent or temporary impairment is clearly a fundamental consideration in treatment planning. Athletes with high levels of ego-involvement in sport might face a perceived total loss of identity in the face of a career-ending injury. Their reactions might be more severe and protracted than those of athletes whose prognosis for full recovery is more favorable. The same might be true for injured athletes who face an extended or uncertain rehabilitation (Smith et al., 1990). A protracted recovery process with an unpredictable outcome can seriously test the coping resources of an athlete who is used to a highly regimented, structured life. Severity is often linked with control and predictability, two factors that clearly impact on the levels of anxiety experienced.

Onset

Athletes can experience the onset of an injury in either an acute or gradual manner. This differentiation does not reflect biological onset, but rather the athlete's subjective experience of the injury. A sudden, unexpected injury can find a person's social support system as well as the person ill prepared to cope. Yet crisis management skills are typically quickly mobilized and support becomes readily available. This can contrast markedly from the more solitary experience of an injured athlete coping with a gradual onset.

The emotional process for an athlete with a gradual-onset injury can take a much different form from that of an athlete with an acute injury. Athletes often live with physical discomfort. They learn to manage or ignore pain. Yet for some a nagging injury might gradually progress to a point where they can no longer tough it out. These athletes reach pain levels where they must give in. For an athlete who has learned to act tough and give 110%, admitting that the pain is affecting performance can add guilt or anxiety and further erode self-confidence.

Course

Rolland's (1984) typology of illness suggests that chronic diseases essentially follow three general courses: progressive, constant, or episodic. The same holds true for athletic injuries.

In a progressive-course injury, there is a continual stepwise progression toward either recovery or permanent disability. The speed of the progression might vary, but the course

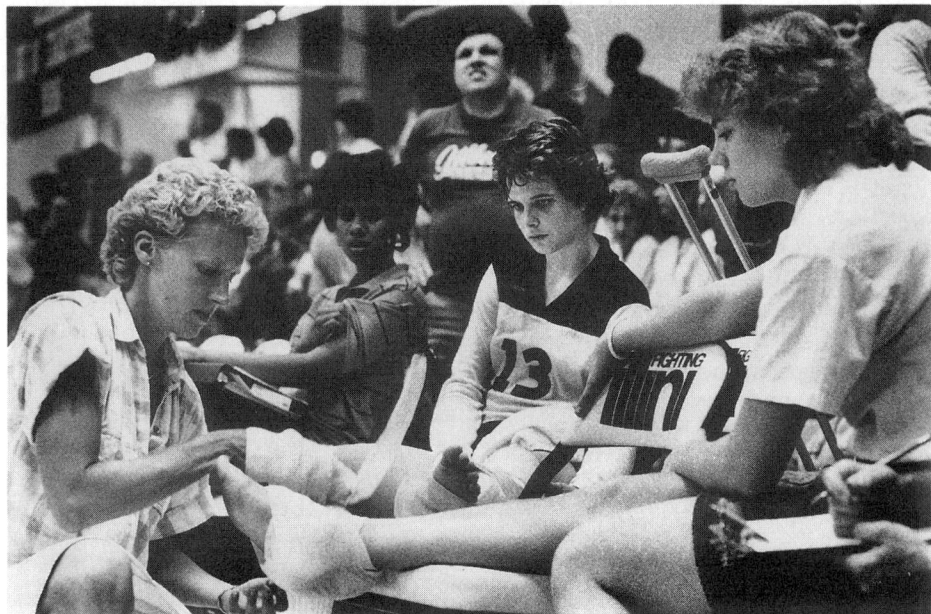

Courtesy University of Illinois Sports Information

would be predictable and gradual, with few surprises or unknowns. Athletes and their support systems would need to make a series of adaptations and role changes in response to the different levels of health or incapacitation.

For example, Thomas, an intercollegiate basketball player, had suffered an ankle injury that was to sideline him for 3 to 4 weeks. He was the only black player on the team and was the leading scorer and assist man. He was described as "a cocky kid who did everything his way." During the first week of physical therapy, Thomas's athletic trainer was surprised by his openness and self-disclosures of fear that he would not recover. The trainer assured him that his injury was common and full recovery was a sure bet, but Thomas continued to express doubts and spent considerable time sharing his concerns with the trainer.

As he began to see himself make measurable progress during the latter part of the second week, Thomas returned to his pre-

injury interpersonal style. His initial dependence on his athletic trainer was replaced by arrogance and disdain. The athletic trainer was not prepared for this sudden turnaround in behavior. He felt used and stated that he was "not thrilled to have to treat that jerk."

In the previous example, the sports medicine professional had difficulty adapting to the changing needs of the injured athlete. In progressive-course injuries, where full recovery is expected, it is not uncommon for athletes to return to their preinjury personality style after a brief period of fear, self-doubt, or confusion. In cases where permanent disability is evident, athletes are much more likely to experience the grief process outlined previously.

In constant-course injuries, athletes are required to adapt to a biological condition that remains stable. Athletes are faced with a clear-cut prognosis of permanent physical change. Although the course of the injury is stable and predictable, athletes and their support systems need to adapt to and accept a new level of physical ability. This may mean adjusting to life without sport, changing sports, or adjusting one's game based on physical limitations. The latter can be seen in examples of baseball players who had to learn to be pitchers instead of just throwers because of an arm injury that inhibited their throwing velocity.

Injuries can also be characterized as episodic-, or relapsing-course injuries. In these cases, athletes are faced with adapting to physical conditions that can flare up at any time, as in the cases of a golfer with a back problem or a tennis player with tendinitis. Symptom-free periods alternate with relapses. Athletes and their support systems are constantly faced with the uncertainty of when the injury will flare up again. Being overcautious when competing can cause declines in performance; this can lead to additional stress. These situations require adaptation to the unpredictability of the injury. Athletes often need assistance in accepting their condition without abandoning the physical style that gave them their competitive edge.

History

An exploration of the history of previous injuries can provide insight into the athlete's coping skills, beliefs about injury, levels of stress, and supports from their social network. Athletes who are injured for the first time might require much more initial information and understanding. Without a track record, injured athletes might not know what to expect. They might be too frightened or too proud to ask for help. In these cases, it is often more difficult to predict an athlete's response to the injury or the types of support that might be required.

Type

Injuries that require a cast or other visible sign of impairment often involve a much different experience for an athlete when compared to injuries that are not obvious. For example, in the case of Mike, the high-school football player, his internal injury did not provide him with a visible badge of courage. He was forced to field numerous questions as to why he was not playing. If he had a cast on his leg or arm, there would have been no question as to why he was not playing, and he would probably have received more support from his social system.

Phases in the Injury Process

Athletic injuries have three distinct phases that necessitate consideration in treatment planning. These can be described as the crisis period, the rehabilitation phase, and the recovery target date.

The crisis period includes the time immediately after a sudden onset or the point at which an athlete becomes concerned with the nagging injury that won't go away. It is important to initiate treatment as soon as possible following the onset of the injury to alleviate fears and handle denial (Danish, 1986; May & Seib, 1987; Rotella & Heyman, 1986). During this phase it is important to help an athlete feel understood and evaluate an injury in a realistic manner.

The rehabilitation phase follows the crisis period; the athlete has accepted the reality of the injury and is now focused on the recovery process. This phase can last from a few weeks to several years and is distinguished by feelings of resignation, calm, mood swings, relief, or growth. During this phase it is essential to help the athlete cope with the ups and downs of rehabilitation, teach new coping skills, and support and encourage an athlete's efforts to manage frustrations.

The recovery target date is the phase during which an athlete must test the injured area under game conditions or accept the loss of that valued activity because of the permanency of the impairment. It is often a time marked by a reactivation of earlier fears and doubts. This period is characterized by the need to assist the athlete to work with coaches, parents, spouse, or teammates in preparing for the reentry process or to help the athlete readjust to life without sport.

Rolland (1984) suggests that movement from one phase of the injury process to the next can be similar to a life transition. In such situations, unfinished business from an earlier phase can hinder the adaptation to the new time period. For example, individuals who deal with the crisis of an athletic injury by using denial might have difficulty taking responsibility for their own recovery during the rehabilitation process.

Situational Variables

A number of situational variables also come into play in developing a treatment plan. Among these are the type of sport, the duration of the sport season, the amount of playing time the injured athlete is receiving, the performance of the athlete, the team or individual record at the time of the injury, and the player's age or career stage. For example, an Olympic-medal-winning athlete, who was in the midst of preparation for the 1994 Winter Olympics, expressed initial relief when he experienced a potential career-ending injury. He said "winning the medal in 1992 was my goal, but competing in 1994 was for everyone else." Helping him cope with his injury required a different emphasis from working with two other similarly injured athletes who had not yet reached their goals. One needed to "get back in control of my life." He had to decide if competing was something that he wanted to do, or, instead, was doing for family, friends, and the media. The other felt cheated out of the opportunity to reach a goal. In these cases, treatment focused much more on managing anger and depression.

Situational variables often play into face-saving concerns. A senior collegiate football player who is not getting much playing time is likely to cope with an injury quite differently than a freshman superstar player.

In treatment planning, it is important to understand how these situational factors are interpreted by an injured athlete. One athlete who was "finally living up to my potential" experienced an early-season injury as "Murphy's Law—just when things are going well I get hurt, and I'm never going to make it now." This athlete had struggled for years to prove her abilities. She was a classic practice superstar who could never produce in a game. Just as her play was coming all together, she injured her shooting hand. Her initial reaction of frustration and anger quickly turned to despair and hopelessness. Ironically, 2 years earlier this same athlete had described a similar injury as "a godsend, I needed to get away from the game to get my head on straight."

Negative Addiction

The last psychological factor in treatment planning that we address in this chapter is negative addiction. Morgan contends that an increasing number of people have become addicted to exercise and manifest many negative physical and psychological symptoms. "A hard-core exercise addict can't live without daily running, manifests withdrawal symptoms if deprived of exercise, and runs even when his physician says he shouldn't" (1979, p. 57). What begins as a positive and healthy endeavor for the vast majority of exercisers can become a negative addiction. The classic symptoms of this syndrome might best be illustrated by the following case.

■ THE CASE OF RICHARD ■

Richard is a 40-year-old regional sales manager for a large northeastern company. In high school he was an outstanding basketball player and continued in the sport until 8 years ago, at which time the "roughness of the city-league games'' and his lack of playing time led him to seek an alternative activity. Richard always had run to stay in shape for basketball, but now decided to take running more seriously. He quickly progressed from 2 to 6 mi per run. He entered local road races. Eventually, basketball became no match for the competition, the trophies, the positive feelings, and ''the cardio-vascular rush and endorphin highs'' that running provided. He was now averaging 85 to 95 mi a week. Often he ran twice a day. He purchased a treadmill and an exercise bike for home. He ''never felt better.''

At work, Richard was extremely successful. He became the youngest regional sales manager in the company's history. His social life ''could be a little better'' since he broke up with his long-time girlfriend about a year ago, but his style had always been long-term relationships (2 to 4 years) with highly successful women. ''Unfortunately, things never seemed to work out,'' he commented.

Although Richard reported that his life was going well, he had become increasingly more frustrated with the nagging foot, ankle, and back problems that he had suffered through over the last 3 years. He often found himself struggling to run through the pain, only to find it worse the next day. On the advice of a friend, Richard decided he needed to cross train for triathlons. He enrolled in an individualized fitness program, purchased an expensive racing bike, and took advanced swimming lessons. The resulting 3.5 to 5 hr of exercise per day put Richard in ''the best shape of my life.''

Unfortunately, the increased time commitment to working out began to affect Richard's work productivity and his social life was ''at an all-time low.'' On the advice of his fitness instructor, Richard decided to consult an athletic counselor for some life-work planning so he could ''fit in everything.''

Initially, running had served many positive functions for Richard. It had given him a replacement for basketball. It gave him a new source of competence, feelings of fitness, and filled a void created by his slumping social life. Unfortunately, Richard increased his workouts to a point where overuse injuries and work decrements began to take a toll.

In treatment planning it is helpful to understand the dynamics of negative addiction. For example, direct challenges to the efficacy of intensive exercise are usually ineffective. Often indirect strategies prove to be more viable. More will be said about this when a suggested treatment protocol is examined.

PSYCHOLOGICAL TREATMENT FOR INJURED ATHLETES

Much of the literature on psychological treatment for injured athletes focuses on specific techniques (see a list of some of these techniques in the highlight box on page 271). Rather than reiterate these approaches, we will now outline a protocol for managing psychological treatment. The protocol suggests progressing through four phases and concurrently working with the injured athlete's social support network. Although these phases are presented as discrete, in practice they are interdependent and not absolutely differentiated.

Rapport-Building Phase

The initial task is to understand the injury from the athlete's perspective. Use basic attending skills to gather information in a manner that allows an athlete to feel understood. The goal is to explore also the various intra-psychic, interpersonal, and situational variables related to an athlete's injury. Although emotional support is often needed during this process, it is critical to insure that the

Psychological Treatments for Injured Athletes

1. *Attention control training* (Nideffer, 1983)
2. *Biofeedback* (Gordon, 1986; Nideffer, 1983)
3. *Cognitive strategies*—modification of self-talk, rational-emotive psychotherapy, reframing, restructuring, time projection, thought stoppage (Gordon, 1986; Rotella, 1984; Wiese & Weiss, 1987)
4. *Communication-skills training* (Wiese & Weiss, 1987)
5. *Crisis intervention* (Rotella & Heyman, 1986)
6. *Goal setting* (Danish, 1986; Wiese & Weiss, 1987)
7. *Grief counseling* (Astle, 1986; Wehlage, 1980)
8. *Imagery*—coping rehearsal, emotive rehearsal, mastery rehearsal, task-oriented rehearsal, visual rehearsal (Gordon, 1986; King & Cook, 1987; Rotella, 1984; Rotella & Heyman, 1986; Samples, 1987)
9. *Progressive relaxation* (Gordon, 1986; Nideffer, 1983; Weiss & Troxel, 1986)
10. *Psychological-skills training* (Ievleva & Orlick, 1991; Weiss & Troxel, 1986)
11. *Psychotherapy* (Eldridge, 1983; Scott, 1984)
12. *Stress inoculation training* (Meichenbaum, 1985)
13. *Systematic desensitization* (King & Cook, 1987; Rotella & Campbell, 1983)
14. *Support system interventions* (Wiese & Weiss, 1987)

often feel out of control and confused as to how to react to their injuries. In some cases they turn to potentially self-defeating methods, such as withdrawal or substance abuse, in an attempt to cope. It is critical to validate the intent of these attempts at self-cure. Acknowledging the short-term efficacy of withdrawal can allow an athlete to maintain self-respect and may enhance the rapport between athlete and helper. Conversely, premature confrontations over these behaviors might jeopardize the counseling relationship and further erode the athlete's confidence. Confrontations about self-defeating behaviors are often better addressed under the guise of skill acquisition, which occurs later in the counseling process. In the example of Richard, the negatively addicted runner, direct confrontations of the efficacy of running would test the strength of the counseling relationship and probably would lead to premature termination of therapy.

Once initial rapport is established, enlist the injured athlete as a collaborator in the planning and implementation of the treatment strategy. This usually enhances the athlete's sense of control and continues the process of rebuilding the athlete's confidence in being able to impact recovery.

Education Phase

The counselor should insure that an injured athlete has as much accurate information as possible about the injury and the recovery process. This helps the athlete become a collaborator in the treatment and reduces exaggerated worry or fear of the unknown. Danish (1986) suggests that injured athletes want information on specific topics:

- The nature of the injury and the medical reasons for initiating particular treatments
- The goals of treatment

athlete feels understood and accepted. Premature attempts at encouragement can cause an athlete to feel discounted.

Many athletes feel particularly vulnerable during the initial time after an injury. They

- Details of medical procedures that will be performed
- Possible sensations or side effects
- Coping strategies for adjusting to the upcoming treatment

This phase is also an appropriate time to discuss the change process. Athletes, especially those who have been injured for the first time, might not be aware that change—whether psychological or physical—usually does not occur along a smooth continuum. This knowledge can help athletes cope with setbacks or plateaus in rehabilitation.

Educating athletes about their injuries and the change process can eliminate some surprises that might otherwise occur during treatment. This educating process also sets the stage for athletes to acquire new coping skills during the next phase of treatment.

Skill-Development Phase

The goals of the skill-development phase are to help athletes acquire new coping strategies and build confidence in their problem-solving abilities. It is important to assess and utilize the athlete's learned coping skills before introducing any new strategies. Many athletes have learned to use goal setting, relaxation techniques, guided imagery, deep breathing, and other strategies to enhance athletic performance. Building on proven skills enables athletes to gain confidence and feel more in control.

When an injury raises fear and self-doubts, an athlete may "catastrophize" about the future (Gordon, 1986). Introducing complicated treatment options at this time can exacerbate the feelings of worry and of being overwhelmed. Counselors who adopt a philosophy of using the least-involved intervention possible can better help to quell these exaggerated fears by creating some doubts in the doubts of the athlete.

Counselors and athletes should evaluate possible advantages and disadvantages of various self-help strategies, concentrating on those skills already familiar to the athlete. Once the most promising primary options have been identified, an implementation plan should be agreed on. While determining the appropriate choices, evaluate both the strategies and the implementation plan. In some cases, athletes report that a selected strategy did not help, even though in reality the failure developed from an implementation plan that did not allow sufficient time to practice new skills or did not provide ways in which to measure (and note) progress.

Establishing short-term and long-term goals greatly facilitates measuring skill attainment levels and planning implementation strategies. Although many goal-setting formats are available, Danish (1986) has developed a model (Life Development Intervention, or LDI) that is readily adaptable to injury rehabilitation. This approach begins with a three-part goal assessment: goal identification, goal importance, and goal roadblocks.

In goal identification, injured athletes are assisted in specifying intended actions in positive, behavioral terms. This helps an athlete avoid focusing on negative thoughts and provides observable criteria for measuring progress. This process also allows a counselor to sense how realistic an athlete is concerning physical aspects of rehabilitation and the recovery target date.

Investigating goal importance helps to determine whether goals are more important to the athlete or to coach, teammates, family, or friends. The Olympic athlete who felt initial relief after a potential career-ending injury (outlined earlier in this chapter) was not achieving his early rehabilitation goals because they were not his own. It was only when the goals became important to him that he was able to put out the commitment and concentration necessary to recover fully.

The final stage in the goal-setting model is to identify potential roadblocks to goal attainment. Four major blocks to goal achievement identified by Danish (1986) are

- lack of knowledge,
- lack of skill,
- lack of risk-taking ability, and
- lack of social supports.

Consideration of the level of importance for each of these roadblocks is critical to establishing the implementation plan.

If the selected strategies were already part of the athlete's repertoire, short-term goals need to be established to measure progress. If new skills are to be introduced, they should be taught systematically. Such a format might include these steps (Danish & Hale, 1983):

1. Describe the skill in behavioral terms
2. Give a rationale for the new skill
3. Specify a skill-attainment level
4. Demonstrate effective and ineffective uses of the skill
5. Provide opportunities to practice the new skill with supervision and feedback
6. Assign homework to promote generalization of the skill
7. Evaluate the skill-attainment level

Although building confidence and learning new coping strategies are the stated goals of the skill-development phase, the importance of the interaction between counselor and athlete should not be underestimated. By initially limiting the number of strategies to test out and enlisting the athlete as a collaborator in the helping process, adherence to the treatment regimen is greatly enhanced (Genest & Genest, 1987). It also places greater responsibility for a successful rehabilitation in the athlete's hands. Once injured athletes have assumed some ownership for their role in the recovery process and have learned some coping skills, the stage is set for the next phase of treatment.

Practice and Evaluation Phase

The goals for the practice and evaluation phase are

1. to provide opportunities for injured athletes to practice their coping skills with continuous feedback,
2. to evaluate goal-attainment levels,
3. to plan strategies to cope with setbacks in rehabilitation,
4. to prepare for the recovery target date, and
5. to terminate the counseling relationship.

The success of this phase is dependent on the counselor's proficiency during the rapport-building, education, and skill-development phases of treatment.

During the practice phase, injured athletes test out their coping skills in vivo. The counselor monitors progress and provides feedback and encouragement to help the athletes stay actively involved with their own recovery process. As goal-attainment levels are evaluated, the athlete is assisted in coping with plateaus or setbacks in rehabilitation. At times athletes might become impatient with the speed of recovery and begin to question the effectiveness of the coping skills they are employing. In these situations, a counselor who has established good rapport can assist athletes in facing realistic barriers and encourage them to allow adequate time for their coping skills to work. A well-developed short-term-goal-setting plan would allow athletes to see measurable progress and help lessen their doubts. At other times, situational problems or outside stressors might make it necessary to recycle through the skill-development phase to further expand the range of coping skills available to the athlete.

Beyond the monitoring process that takes place during this phase, it is also important to assist the athletes in developing a strategy to deal with setbacks in rehabilitation. This process serves two functions. It enables the athletes to understand that both physical and psychological setbacks are common during the recovery process. This can help prevent the athletes from interpreting setbacks as failures due to their own inadequacies (Meichenbaum, 1985). This is particularly important for athletes who display a tendency toward self-doubt and hopelessness during the initial crisis period of the injury experience. In addition, developing a strategy to deal with setbacks reinforces the concept that the counseling process is directed at teaching injured athletes to become more self-reliant. It provides a plan to directly utilize coping skills at a time when many athletes can get bogged down in negative self-talk or other self-defeating behaviors.

Another goal of this phase is to help injured athletes prepare for their recovery target date. As mentioned earlier, this is the period of time when athletes must test out their rehabilitation in game situations or else face the fact that they will not be able to continue to participate in their sport at their preinjury ability level. This period can be extremely anxiety provoking for athletes even though most do not show their concerns outwardly. It can also come at the heels of a relatively uneventful rehabilitation period in which the athlete seems to have everything under control. The sudden resurgence of doubts and fears can catch an athlete and the treatment team off guard. The athlete can be prepared for this transitional period by examining the reentry into competition from both intrapsychic and interpersonal perspectives. Once an athlete has received the OK to return to competition, counselors can be in a position to assess the athlete's readiness from a psychological standpoint. An athlete who is filled with exaggerated fears might benefit

more from a slow, gradual reentry into competition than from being thrust directly into a starting role (Rotella & Campbell, 1983).

It is more difficult to prepare athletes to cope with the loss of their ability to perform. Ideally, regular contact with athletes is planned throughout the entire recovery period. As a result, contact with athletes is maintained at a time when they still might be denying or grieving the loss of sport. If an athlete continues to deny the permanency of an injury, it might be more helpful to develop contingency plans than to challenge the denial head-on.

The final goal of this phase is the termination of the counseling relationship. For those few athletes who become highly dependent on their counselors, this is the most critical part of treatment. It is not unusual for these athletes to hold on to the counseling relationship by developing new symptoms as the termination date approaches. In these situations, a modified time-limited psychotherapy model (Mann, 1973) has proven helpful by teaching athletes how to separate from relationships and find their own unique identities. This situation is most likely to occur with career-ending injuries or when athletes lack the physical skills to compete at their desired level.

In all counseling relationships with injured athletes, the termination phase is an opportunity to review and reinforce the range of skills that have been learned, to self-disclose what the relationship has meant, to share ambivalence about ending, and to discuss the transferability of acquired skills and knowledge to other areas of life. For some athletes this process can be critical to the success of the entire treatment and can take many sessions.

Social Support System Interventions

So far, the treatment protocol has focused on the individual athlete. In practice, successful treatment often necessitates concurrent work with the athlete's social support (family, friends, teammates, coaches) and sports medicine systems (athletic trainers, physical therapists, physicians).

Without presenting a long discourse on confidentiality, it must be noted that an athlete's permission must be obtained before information can be disclosed to others. This important caveat notwithstanding, involving significant members of the injured athlete's support system can create a positive environment to facilitate the recovery process. For example, family members can be instructed on how to listen to the athlete's concerns rather than trying to fix them. Coaches can be informed about the athlete's psychological readiness to return to competition and alternative methods of reentry can be explored. Physical therapists can be assisted in individualizing treatment programs to enhance adherence.

Helping the support network understand the importance of listening to the athlete when feelings are being expressed cannot be overstated. If social support and sports medicine systems are skillful at helping an injured athlete feel understood, the physical and emotional rehabilitation process will be greatly enhanced.

Working with the social support network can also help lessen an athlete's tendency to isolate or withdraw following a severe injury. Whether it is a problem with members of the support system not knowing how to interact with an injured athlete or an athlete's own attempt at getting away from the hurt, withdrawal will be less likely to occur if the support system understands what to expect and how to respond.

Incorporating a family systems perspective, in which the entire family becomes the treatment unit, is often indicated in situations where face-saving inhibits the recovery process. This would be the case in situations like the eager parent syndrome outlined earlier.

Family-life-cycle dynamics and interactions might dictate a systemic counseling approach.

Whatever the case, developing a positive social support system can become an important aspect of the intervention. A counselor can help athletes understand what types of support are provided by their support network and what types are lacking. Learning to identify support needs and to develop new sources of support are important life skills.

THE PSYCHOLOGIST IN THE SPORTS MEDICINE CLINIC

Although the importance of psychological factors in athletic injury rehabilitation has been well documented (Crossman, 1985; Eldridge, 1983; Feigley, 1984; Hair, 1977; King & Cook, 1987), the inclusion of sport psychologists on sports medicine treatment teams has been slow to develop. Some of the probable reasons for this are a lack of understanding of the role of sport psychology in injury rehabilitation, financial considerations, insurance reimbursement policies, and issues of medical or psychological hegemony.

Not all people who identify themselves as *sport psychologists* have the training or the interest to function on a sports medicine team. In general, the ideal professional would have a background in both psychology and the sport sciences, possess an understanding of the sport experience, and have solid counseling skills. Throughout the chapter, the term *counselor* has been used in place of *sport psychologist* to signify such a professional.

Involving sport psychologists as integral members of the sports injury team is gaining increased support in the medical literature (Lombardo, 1985; Murphy, 1991; Samples, 1987; Yukelson & Murphy, 1992). Utilization of a sport psychologist often allows an injured athlete to bypass additional losses in self-confidence and control. Sports medicine teams that include a sport psychologist provide athletes with an opportunity to be introduced to sport psychology skills as a normal part of rehabilitation. The connection between mind and body healing is reinforced and the athlete learns additional life skills as part of the treatment process.

Some sports medicine clinics have chosen to use a different title to describe the sport psychologist to spare athletes any stigma or loss of face as a result of needing to see a psychologist. Titles such as athletic counselor, self-help skills specialist, and mental training specialist are being used to get around the word *psychologist*. Whatever the title, the key is to provide quality services.

Beyond providing direct services to injured athletes, sport psychologists must also spend considerable time and energy building credibility with the sports medicine staff. This is accomplished through educating the medical team about the services that are available and documenting progress through well-designed evaluation and follow-up studies. Great care must be exercised to avoid "stepping on the toes" of the medical staff during this process. The sport psychologist must be perceived as an ally, not an adversary or competitor.

Clinics that choose to utilize sport psychology services on a consultant basis must devote ample time during in-service training to educate staff members on how to make effective referrals. For example, referring to the sport psychologist as the "person who teaches self-help skills" sends a different message to injured athletes than telling them they "need to see a psychologist."

Sport psychologists can train sports medicine personnel to use basic counseling skills. This can help the staff create psychologically safe environments where injured athletes feel free to express their fears or concerns. Patients who feel understood are more likely to

adhere to both physical and psychological treatments (Genest & Genest, 1987).

In addition, sport psychologists who have expertise in process consultation can provide a sports medicine clinic with valuable resources to handle communication problems, conflict management, problem solving, motivation, burnout prevention, or other employee concerns. It is important for a sport psychologist to be particularly sensitive to the frustrations and politics of a sports medicine clinic. Direct services to staff members assist in building credibility and demystifying the helping process. Indeed, sport psychologists can make major contributions to a sports medicine clinic in direct patient care, consultation with the medical staff, or employee assistance.

Along with playing multiple roles in a sports medicine clinic comes the potential burden of ethical problems. It is imperative to always be clear about who is the client and who is the patient. For example, if a softball coach contacts you about a player, the coach is the client. Ethically, the coach should also be your patient. You can assist the coach in managing the situation, but you must be clear that changing the coach's behavior is the focus of your interventions, not changing the player.

In addition, confidentiality and record-keeping practices should be addressed early in staff training, and it is advisable to maintain a separate record-keeping system. Often sport psychologists in the sports medicine clinic setting get caught up in the dilemma of needing to justify their existence based on the number of contacts, while at the same time maintaining the confidentiality of athletes, coaches, and support system members. Evaluation procedures, confidentiality, and record keeping are but a few of the concerns that should be addressed before a sport psychologist accepts a position in a sports medicine clinic.

CONCLUSION

Before closing, we think it helpful to follow up on the three cases presented earlier in the chapter. Jane, the gymnastics instructor, eventually came to understand that she had allowed her pain to control her life. Early in her injury process she was able to "tough it out," but the cumulative effects of the stress and frustrations surrounding her injuries eroded her confidence and prompted depressive episodes. The final straw was her husband's refusal "to cover for me anymore." His withdrawal of emotional and physical support forced her to seek psychological help.

In counseling, the therapist assisted Jane in getting back in control of her life. This was accomplished through building on her experience with mental imagery to distinguish between "injury" pain and "getting into shape" pain. The ability to differentiate the two elements placed the responsibility for choosing to perform in Jane's control. Other sport skills that she had learned, such as goal setting and progressive relaxation, were utilized to help her gain confidence in her own coping behaviors. Family counseling allowed her husband to continue to refrain without guilt from enabling behaviors. Jane's ability to manage the psychological aspects of her injury soon translated into physical and emotional gains. Her symptoms dissipated and she was able to resume her demonstrations. Ironically, Jane now has less need to demonstrate and spends more time on staff training and motivation.

Mike was the high-school football star who suffered a career-ending diagnosis. Unfortunately, Mike's story does not end on a positive note. Following his award at the football dinner, Mike committed suicide. The case material came from Mike's father, who sought counseling to deal with "guilt over not recognizing Mike's pain." Although this is an extreme case, it is an important reminder of the significance of sport in the identity of some people. For a few athletes, sport becomes more than just a game and disengagement from it can be traumatic. Greater sensitivity to the importance of football in Mike's life might have raised some concerns about his rather cavalier attitude toward not being able to play. His withdrawal from his social supports and projections about his father's needs might have been warning signs. Whatever the case, professionals need to pay particular attention to the psychological aspects of athletic injuries.

Richard, the runner who illustrated some of the classic symptoms of negative addiction, continued to push himself until the frequency of his injuries and work-related problems prompted him to seek professional counseling for stress management. The therapist was clear not to challenge the efficacy of Richard's physical activities. Instead, the initial meetings focused on building rapport and exploring the range of Richard's coping skills. This process validated Richard's physical efforts and set the stage for more in-depth exploration of potential sources of job, interpersonal, and physical stress.

Eventually, Richard was able to identify his level of diminishing physical returns and acknowledge that his increased time commitments to working out had allowed him to avoid certain fears, such as "being alone for the rest of my life."

The therapist worked with Richard and his exercise trainer to find a comfortable and appropriate level of physical activity and time involvement for workouts. Richard began to address his fears of social rejection and was better able to "just be myself" and "focus on enjoying" when he went out socially.

This chapter's purpose has been to focus on the psychological aspects of athletic injuries and to offer suggestions for designing and implementing comprehensive rehabilitation strategies. The most important consideration is to understand injured athletes as individuals. Numerous intrapsychic, interpersonal, and situational variables impact the recovery process. We hope the information outlined in this chapter provides a departure point for researchers to investigate the weight of these factors and the effectiveness of various intervention strategies.

REFERENCES

Astle, S.J. (1986). The experience of loss in athletes. *Journal of Sports Medicine and Physical Fitness, 26,* 279-284.

Blann, F.W. (1985). Intercollegiate athletic competition and students' educational and career plans. *Journal of College Student Personnel, 26,* 115-119.

Brewer, B.W. (1991). Athletic identity as a risk factor for depressive reactions to athletic injury. Unpublished doctoral dissertation, Arizona State University, Tempe, AZ.

Chartrand, J.M., & Lent, R. (1987). Sports counseling: Enhancing the development of the student-athlete. *Journal of Counseling and Development, 66,* 164-167.

Coddington, R.D., & Troxell, J.R. (1980). The effect of emotional factors on football injury rates: A pilot study. *Journal of Human Stress, 6*(4), 3-5.

Crossman, J. (1985). Psychosocial factors and athletic injury. *Journal of Sports Medicine and Physical Fitness, 25,* 151-154.

Crossman, J., & Jamieson, J. (1985). Differences in perceptions of seriousness and disrupting effects of athletic injury as viewed by athletes and their trainers. *Perceptual and Motor Skills, 61,* 1131-1134.

Cryan, P.D., & Alles, W.F. (1983). The relationship between stress and college football injuries. *Journal of Sports Medicine, 23,* 52-58.

Danish, S.J. (1983). Musings about personal competence: The contributions of sport, health, and fitness. *American Journal of Community Psychology, 11,* 221-240.

Danish, S.J. (1986). Psychological aspects in the care and treatment of athletic injuries. In P.E. Vinger & E.F. Hoerner (Eds.), *Sports injuries: The unthwarted epidemic* (2nd ed.). Boston: Wright.

Danish, S.J., & Hale, B. (1983). Teaching psychological skills to athletes and coaches. *Journal of Physical Education, Recreation, and Dance, 54*(8), 11-12, 80-81.

Danish, S.J., Petitpas, A.J., & Hale, B.D. (1990). Sport as a context for developing competence. In T. Gullotta, G. Adams, & R. Montemayor (Eds.), *Developing social competence in adolescence: Vol. 3* (pp. 169-194). Newberry Park, CA: Sage.

Eldridge, W.D. (1983). The importance of psychotherapy for athletic related orthopedic injuries among adults. *Comprehensive Psychiatry, 24,* 271-277.

Elkin, D. (1981). *The hurried child.* Reading, MA: Addison-Wesley.

Feigley, D.A. (1984). Psychological burnout in high level athletes. *Physician and Sportsmedicine, 12,* 109-114.

Genest, M., & Genest, S. (1987). *Psychology and health.* Champaign, IL: Research Press.

Gordon, S. (1986). Sport psychology and the injured athlete: A cognitive-behavioral approach to injury response and injury rehabilitation. *Science Periodical on Research and Technology in Sports, 3*, 1-10.

Haerle, K.K. (1975). Athletic scholarships and the occupational career of the professional athlete. *Sociology of Occupations, 2*, 373-403.

Hair, J.E. (1977). Intangibles in evaluating athletic injuries. *Journal of the American College of Health, 25*, 228-231.

Henry, M., & Renaud, H. (1972). Examined and unexamined lives. *Research Reporter, 7*(1), 5.

Henschen, K.P. (1986). Athletic staleness and burnout: Diagnosis, prevention, and treatment. In J.M. Williams (Ed.), *Applied sport psychology: Personal growth to peak experience* (pp. 327-342). Palo Alto, CA: Mayfield.

Hill, P., & Lowe, B. (1974). The inevitable metathesis of the retiring athlete. *International Review of Sport Sociology, 9*, 5-29.

Ievleva, L., & Orlick, T. (1991). Mental links to enhanced healing: An exploratory study. *Sport Psychologist, 5*, 25-40.

Kane, B. (1984). Trainer counseling to avoid three face saving maneuvers. *Athletic Training, 18*, 171-174.

King, N.J., & Cook, D.L. (1987). Helping injured athletes cope and recover. *First Aider, 3*, 10-11.

Kleiber, D.A., & Greendorfer, S.L. (1983). *Social reintegration of former college athletes: Male football and basketball players from 1970-1980.* (Report No. 3). Unpublished manuscript.

Kleiber, D.A., Greendorfer, S.L., Blinde, E., & Samdahl, D. (1987). Quality of exit from university sports and subsequent life satisfaction. *Sociology of Sport Journal, 4*, 28-36.

Kozar, B., & Lord, R.M. (1983). Overuse injuries in the young athlete: Reasons for concern. *Physician and Sportsmedicine, 11*, 221-226.

Kubler-Ross, E. (1969). *On death and dying.* New York: Macmillan.

Lewis-Griffith, L. (1982). Athletic injuries can be a pain in the head too. *Women's Sports, 4*, 44.

Little, J.C. (1969). The athletic neurosis: A deprivation crisis. *Acta Psychiatrica, 45*, 187-197.

Lombardo, J.A. (1985). Sports medicine: A team approach. *Physician and Sportsmedicine, 13*, 70-74.

Lysens, R., VandenAuweele, Y., & Ostyn, M. (1986). The relationship between psychosocial factors and sports injuries. *Journal of Sports Medicine and Physical Fitness, 26*, 77-84.

Mann, J. (1973). *Time-limited psychotherapy.* Cambridge, MA: Harvard University Press.

Marcia, J.E. (1966). Development and validation of ego-identity status. *Journal of Personality and Social Psychology, 3*, 551-558.

May, J.R., & Seib, G.E. (1987). Athletic injuries: Psychosocial factors in the onset, sequelae, rehabilitation, and prevention. In J.R. May & M.J. Asken (Eds.), *Sport psychology: The psychological health of the athlete* (pp. 157-186). New York: PMA.

McDonald, S.A., & Hardy, C.J. (1990). Affective response patterns of the injured athlete: An exploratory analysis. *Sport Psychologist, 4*, 261-274.

Meichenbaum, D. (1985). *Stress inoculation training.* Elmford, NY: Pergamon Press.

Mihovilovic, M.A. (1968). The status of former sportsmen. *International Review of Sport Sociology, 3*, 73-96.

Mitchell, J.C. (1974). Social networks. *Annual Review of Anthropology, 3*, 279-300.

Morgan, W.P. (1979). Negative addiction in runners. *Physician and Sportsmedicine, 7*(2), 57-70.

Murphy, S.M. (1991). Behavioral considerations. In R.C. Cantu & L.J. Micheli (Eds.), *ACSM's guidelines for the team physician* (pp. 252-265). Malvern, PA: Lea & Febiger.

Nideffer, R.M. (1983). The injured athlete: Psychological factors in treatment. *Orthopedic Clinics of North America*, **14**, 373-385.

Noakes, T.D., & Schomer, H. (1983). The eager parent syndrome and schoolboy injuries. *South African Medical Journal*, **63**, 956-968.

Ogilvie, B.C., & Howe, M. (1986). The trauma of termination from athletics. In J.M. Williams (Ed.), *Applied sport psychology: Personal growth to peak performance* (pp. 365-382). Palo Alto, CA: Mayfield.

O'Leary, A. (1985). Self efficacy and health. *Behavior Research and Therapy*, **23**, 437-441.

Orlick, T.D. (1980). *In pursuit of excellence.* Champaign, IL: Human Kinetics.

Pearson, R., & Petitpas, A. (1990). Transitions of athletes: Pitfalls and prevention. *Journal of Counseling and Development*, **69**, 7-10.

Petitpas, A. (1978). Identity foreclosure: A unique challenge. *Personnel and Guidance Journal*, **56**, 558-561.

Petitpas, A. (1981). The identity development of the male intercollegiate athlete (Doctoral dissertation, Boston University, 1981). *Dissertation Abstracts International*, **42**, 2508A.

Petitpas, A., & Champagne, D.E. (1988). Developmental programming for intercollegiate athletes. *Journal of College Student Development*, **29**, 454-460.

Remer, R., Tongate, R.A., & Watson, J. (1978). Athletes: Counseling the overprivileged minority. *Personnel and Guidance Journal*, **56**, 616-629.

Rolland, J.S. (1984). Toward a psychosocial typology of chronic and life threatening illness. *Family Systems Medicine*, **2**, 245-251.

Rosenfeld, L.B., Richman, J.M., & Hardy, C.J. (1989). Examining social support networks among athletes: Description and relationship to stress. *Sport Psychologist*, **3**, 23-33.

Rotella, R.J. (1984). Psychological care of the injured athlete. In L. Bunker, R.J. Rotella, & A.S. Reilly (Eds.), *Sports psychology: Psychological considerations in maximizing sport performance* (pp. 273-288). Ithaca, NY: Mouvement.

Rotella, R.J., & Campbell, M.S. (1983). Systematic desensitization in the psychological rehabilitation of the injured athlete. *Athletic Training*, **18**, 140-142.

Rotella, R.J., & Heyman, S.R. (1986). Stress, injury, and the psychological rehabilitation of athletes. In J.M. Williams (Ed.), *Applied sport psychology: Personal growth to peak performance* (pp. 343-364). Palo Alto, CA: Mayfield.

Rowland, T.W. (1986). Exercise fatigue in adolescents: Diagnosis of athletic burnout. *Physician and Sportsmedicine*, **14**, 69-75.

Ryde, A. (1977). The role of the physician in sport injury prevention: Some psychological factors in sport injuries. *Journal of Sports Medicine and Physical Fitness*, **17**, 187-194.

Sacks, M.H., & Sachs, M.L. (1981). *Psychology of running.* Champaign, IL: Human Kinetics.

Samples, P. (1987). Mind over muscle: Returning the injured athlete to play. *Physician and Sportsmedicine*, **15**, 172-180.

Sanderson, F.H. (1977). The psychology of the injury prone athlete. *British Journal of Sports Medicine*, **11**, 56-57.

Scott, S.G. (1984). Current concepts in the rehabilitation of the injured athlete. *Mayo Clinic Proceedings*, **59**, 83-90.

Smith, A.M., Scott, S.G., O'Fallon, W., & Young, M.L. (1990). The emotional responses of athletes to injury. *Mayo Clinic Proceedings*, **65**, 38-50.

Smith, A.M., Scott, S.G., & Wiese, D.M. (1990). The psychological effects of sports injuries coping. *Sports Medicine,* **9**(6), 352-369.

Sowa, C.J., & Gressard, C.F. (1983). Athletic participation: Its relationship to student development. *Journal of College Student Personnel,* **24**, 236-239.

Suinn, R.M. (1967). Psychological reactions to physical disability. *Journal of the Association for Physical and Mental Rehabilitation,* **21**, 13-15.

Svoboda, B., & Vanek, M. (1982). Retirement from high level competition. In T. Orlick, J. Partington, & J. Salmela (Eds.), *Mental training: For coaches and athletes* (pp. 166-175). Ottawa, ON: Coaching Association of Canada and Sport in Perspective.

Wehlage, D.F. (1980). Managing the emotional reaction to loss in athletics. *Athletic Training,* **15**, 144-146.

Weiss, M.R., & Troxel, R.K. (1986). Psychology of the injured athlete. *Athletic Training,* **2**, 104-109, 154.

Wiese, D.M., & Weiss, M.R. (1987). Psychological rehabilitation and physical injury: Implications for the sportsmedicine team. *Sport Psychologist,* **1**, 318-330.

Williams, J., Tonyman, P., & Wadsworth, W. (1986). Relationship of life stress to injury in intercollegiate volleyball. *Journal of Human Stress,* **12**, 38-43.

Yaffe, M. (1983). Sports injuries: Psychological aspects. *British Journal of Hospital Medicine,* **29**, 224-230.

Yukelson, D., & Murphy, S. (1992). Psychological considerations in the prevention of sport injuries. In P. Renstrom (Ed.), *Sport injuries: Basic principles of prevention and care* (pp. 321-333). Cambridge, MA: Blackwell Scientific Publications.

CHAPTER 12

ALCOHOL AND DRUGS IN SPORT

Chris M. Carr, PhD
Washington State University

Shane M. Murphy, PhD
United States Olympic Committee

Alcohol and drug use in athletics has been present since the 3rd century B.C., when Greek athletes experimented with many types of psychoactive substances to improve performance (Chappel, 1987). The saga of drug use for performance enhancement has continued into the modern Olympic Games, most notably with Canadian sprinter Ben Johnson's disqualification and loss of a 1988 Olympic gold medal because of his anabolic steroid use. The role of alcohol in sport, although less identified in the media, has been just as significant. The alcohol-related driving death of Philadelphia Flyer goalie Pelle Lindbergh represents the often tragic consequences of excessive alcohol use. Ryne Duren, a former New York Yankees pitcher and recovering alcoholic, describes his experience combining alcohol use with athletic performance:

> . . . Alcohol was bombarding my central nervous system to the point where I was never able to control my eye/hand coordination sufficiently. I was lucky to be there. . . . I was a very vulnerable person on the mound, in spite of the fact that I put together some pretty impressive innings pitched. (Wholey, 1984).

All drugs, including alcohol, represent a risk of danger for athletes. From the Little Leaguer to the major leaguer, participants in all levels of age and competition in sport suffer consequences from the use and abuse of alcohol and other drugs. This chapter defines the various types of drugs used in the athletic community. An examination of some possible sociological explanations for alcohol and drug-using behaviors will be presented. Specifically for the clinical sport psychologist who might provide counseling services for athletes, we discuss assessment, intervention, and prevention measures in cases of substance use and abuse. This information is intended to provide an overview of the sociological and psychological issues related to the use and abuse of alcohol and other drugs in sport. The following case example might be typical of identification and intervention issues confronting the clinical sport psychologist in an athletic setting.

■ *THE CASE OF SHEILA* ■

Sheila first sought professional help at the insistence of her partner, Mary. Sheila, a bright, outgoing 25-year-old, had been a world-class synchronized swimmer for 4 years. She and Mary were the current world champions in the pairs event. But with the Olympics just 11 months away, Mary refused to practice with Sheila unless she sought counseling. Sheila visited a clinical psychologist in a nearby city, someone recommended by the sport psychology consultant who worked with her coach.

In the initial sessions Sheila revealed a long history of drinking, although she attempted to minimize the seriousness of the problem. She first experimented with alcohol in junior high with some friends, but began to get drunk on an "occasional basis" during high school. Sheila said she drank to forget about her "worries"— including her parents, who were constantly fighting, and school, which she found difficult and boring. She was a good high-school swimmer and became involved in synchronized swimming through a friend who took her to some coaching sessions at an area pool.

In synchronized swimming, Sheila found the success and excitement that had eluded her in other life areas. She had great talent, and after 18 months in the sport her coach paired her up with Mary, a successful competitor who had recently broken up with a partner. They trained long and hard together, and after 3 years broke into the national rankings. Now rewarded with international trips and competitions, they performed well at the world level and soon became the second-ranked pair in the U.S. They came in second at the U.S. Nationals three years in a row, until the first-ranked pair broke up after a series of injuries. Last year they not only won the U.S. title for the first time but the world championship as well. Now they are aiming at the Olympics.

Sheila reported her drinking became less of a problem once she attained success in synchronized swimming. Her main problems apparently occurred on trips to competitions, when she hung out with friends after competition and "occasionally had a few too many." Sheila's partner, Mary, requested to come to the next session, and Sheila agreed. The clinical psychologist first met alone with Mary and heard a very different account of Sheila's situation. According to Mary, Sheila showed up drunk to morning practices at least three times a week. Mary always knew if Sheila had drunk heavily the previous night by the smell of alcohol on Sheila's breath. Sheila's drinking had seemingly become more frequent over the past year, since the world championship. Mary believed that Sheila was hanging out with "a bad crowd," and that she was getting too much attention for their recent successes. Practices were going poorly because of Sheila's poor coordination. Mary felt totally frustrated and eventually coerced Sheila into counseling by refusing to practice with her until counseling was initiated. When Sheila joined Mary in the session, she did not refute Mary's accusations, but instead began complaining about Mary's "weight problem," saying that Mary had gained 10 lb (4.5 kg) over the past 2 years. Sheila told the psychologist that performing routines with Mary was difficult because of Mary's weight.

Realizing that many issues were involved and that Sheila was still in some denial about the severity of her problem, the psychologist arranged to meet with both athletes in the next session to discuss some inpatient treatment possibilities for Sheila. Only 3 days later, the psychologist received an urgent phone call from Mary. Sheila had missed a morning practice session, and when she visited Sheila's apartment, Mary found the door locked and was unable to get an answer to the doorbell. She called the police, and when they entered the apartment they found Sheila on the bedroom floor in a drunken stupor. The psychologist arranged for Sheila to be admitted that afternoon to a 30-day inpatient residential treatment program for alcoholics.

SOCIOLOGICAL ISSUES

For the practitioner working with athletes, a relevant question is: Do athletes (at various levels of participation) use alcohol more often than their nonathletic peers? Previous research by Hayes and Tevis (1977) found that high-school athletes used less alcohol than nonathletes. Rooney (1984) found that there were no differences at the secondary level between athletes and nonathletes. More recent survey data suggests that athletic involvement might reinforce the social use of alcohol for males at the high-school level. In a survey of 1,700 high-school students, Carr, Kennedy, and Dimick (1990) found that male athletes reported significantly more alcohol use behaviors as compared to male nonathletes. In the same study, it was found that there were no differences between female athletes and female nonathletes. In an NCAA study of collegiate student athletes in 1985, it was found that 88% of respondents reported alcohol use in the past year, with 37% reporting marijuana use and 17% reporting cocaine use (National Collegiate Athletic Association Drug Education Committee, 1985). Table 12.1 demonstrates the reported use of alcohol by

Table 12.1 Use of Alcohol by Athletes

Athletic level	Used alcohol during past year	N
Secondary and high school (Carr et al., 1990)	92.3%	1,713
Collegiate (College of Human Medicine, Michigan State University, 1985)	88.0%	2,048
Elite (Carr, 1992)	90.4%	70

athletes at the secondary, collegiate, and elite level.

In a nonscientific poll of professional athletes by *USA Today*, 50.7% of 278 respondents surveyed indicated that they believed that alcohol and drug abuse problems with professional athletes had worsened. Just 10.4% believed that the problem had gotten better (*USA Today*, 1992). The facts remain inconclusive; however, these data indicate that the risk for potential problems with alcohol and drug abuse might exist in the athletic population. In a survey of 1,713 high-school students, Carr et al. (1990) found that male athletes not only consumed more alcohol than male nonathletes, but also drank to intoxication significantly more often. The data in this study also supported Duda's findings (1986), which indicate no differences between female athletes and female nonathletes. These findings suggest that male athletes might be one of the greatest at-risk groups for alcohol abuse problems at the high-school level.

Very few universities offer specific alcohol and drug education to combat this problem. In a review of 71 university athletic departments, Tricker and Cook found that athletic trainers reported that most college programs do not offer drug education as a drug-abuse prevention strategy. The results of the study, according to the authors, "strengthened the assumption that drug education programs for college athletes continue to remain largely unexplored" (1989, p. 45).

The data in Table 12.1 reflect the alcohol usage patterns of a specific social group: athletes. Denial might play a major role in the abuse of alcohol in this social microcosm. Athletes represent a distinct social group in local high schools, on university campuses, and in major communities. In order to understand alcohol abuse by athletes, it is essential to understand the norms and standards of the athletic social group. An understanding of the unique stressors experienced by athletes is also important in designing interventions for athletes.

Peer Pressure and Sensation Seeking

Heyman (1986) suggests that there are two social factors that might be relevant to the use of alcohol and other drugs by athletes: peer pressure and sensation seeking. Pressure from peers to engage in experimental risk-taking behaviors is common in the developmental stages of adolescence and early adulthood. When the association between alcohol use and athletics is so strongly identified in the print and electronic media (e.g., beer commercials in sport contexts), the external pressure might be transmitted even more strongly by the sport group. Males might be at greater risk to engage in macho drinking behaviors, such as chugging beer or having contests to see who can drink the most alcohol in a certain period of time. The study by Carr et al. (1990) found that male athletes drank to intoxication significantly more often than male nonathletes; this might suggest that male athletes engage in the previously mentioned behaviors.

Sensation-seeking behaviors might be represented by the use of cocaine or other illicit stimulants to heighten stimulation and sensory input (Heyman, 1986). The nature of sport, where the athlete stretches the physical limitations of endurance, might promote similar nonsport behaviors. The use of anabolic steroids (discussed later in this chapter) among athletes at all levels suggests pushing the limits of the human body. Both of these factors, in addition to other sport-related social norms, must be studied by clinical sport psychology researchers to ascertain the relevance for effective prevention and treatment of potential problems.

Clinical sport psychologists must not only be able to identify and provide intervention and counseling for the athlete abusing alcohol and other drugs but also must be aware of the social pressures and norms demonstrated by the athletic group they serve. It is advisable before beginning consulting with any sport team to discuss with coaches, trainers, and athletes themselves the social climate regarding the use of alcohol and other drugs. This information will allow the consulting sport psychologist to provide complete and effective education, intervention, and treatment recommendations for the sport team. Thomas Griffin (1985), a substance-abuse specialist with the Hazelden Foundation, identifies several key societal variables that might place risks on the student athlete.

One of these issues is the social demands that fans might place on athletes in addition to the athletic demands. At all levels of competition (high school, collegiate, and professional), athletes are expected to be available to the public via the media, public appearances, or speaking engagements. An athlete who might be too tired or unwilling to commit to these due to family or other relationships might be perceived as snobbish or too egocentric. These expectations are often unrealistic and place additional stressors on the athlete. Another societal pressure includes the media, which monitor the movements and activities of athletes, especially at the professional level. Most people from the general population who experience substance abuse problems will impact only a limited number of others and will most likely obtain confidential treatment. However, when an athlete, whether it be at the collegiate or professional level, experiences a problem with alcohol or drugs, many people become involved. The much-publicized substance-abuse treatments of athletes such as Dwight Gooden, Dexter Manley, Steve Howe, and Chris Mullin lent little room for confidentiality. Societal expectation is a stressor that today's athlete must acknowledge. Both personal and athletic endeavors are likely to be evaluated and judged by the wide audience reached by today's media.

The Advertising Media Influence

Another societal factor that must be identified is a clear connection between sports and alcohol use (Griffin, 1985). It is difficult to observe a televised sporting event without also seeing advertisements for alcohol (usually beer). As a billion-dollar industry, the sale of alcoholic beverages is clearly connected with sport. Sport teams, sporting events, and even individual athletes are sponsored by brewing companies. It is not just alcohol that is problematic, because a person must first make the choice to drink alcohol before any problems can develop. However, this connection can be confusing in the development of coping skills and stress-reduction techniques for the student athlete. The study of advertising media influence on individual drinking behaviors has received little attention in the literature. It is important, however, that clinical sport psychologists be attentive to the messages that are heard by the athletes they consult with. Providing athletes with alternative methods of coping and stress management, for example, might replace the belief that one or two beers before bed helps one relax. In and of itself, such alcohol use might not be harmful. Yet the message that alcohol must be consumed to relax is wrong. Open and knowledgeable communication with athletes regarding the societal messages they receive about drugs and sport must be facilitated by the consulting sport psychologist. Beyond the societal norms and expectations that must be identified, specific assessment and intervention skills must be addressed. The next section addresses clinical issues relevant to substance-abuse assessment, intervention, and treatment.

CLINICAL ISSUES

As a consultant for a high school, college, or professional sports team, coaches, trainers, managers, teachers, or athletes themselves might be referred to you with the question: Do I have any alcohol [and/or drug] problem? This section identifies diagnostic symptoms of alcohol and other drug abuse and dependence according to the *Diagnostic and Statistical Manual of Mental Disorders* (3rd Edition, Revised) (American Psychiatric Association, 1987). Familiarity with the criteria specified by the DSM-III-R is essential in the diagnosis of abuse of alcohol and other drugs. In addition, the specific sport-related context of alcohol-abuse symptoms is presented. It is important to note that not all classes of drugs will be discussed; for further review, readers should refer to the DSM-III-R.

This chapter will present relevant symptoms and diagnostic categories regarding abuse of and dependence on various substances. The focus of this section is to familiarize clinical sport psychologists with information related to observing symptoms of substance abuse and substance dependence among people whom they might consult with in an athletic arena.

Substance Abuse

According to the DSM-III-R (American Psychiatric Association, 1987), the prevalence of drinking alcohol is highest and abstention is lowest in people ages 21 to 34. Among all ages, males are two to five times more likely than females to be heavy drinkers. Among athletes, particularly at the high-school level, male athletes have been found to drink to intoxication significantly more often than female athletes (Carr et al., 1990). The consulting sport psychologist should be aware of this information, especially if working with an all-male team. On an individual level, it is important for the psychologist to be able to recognize and intervene with patterns of abusive drinking or drugging behaviors.

The consulting sport psychologist should be aware that the DSM-III-R provides a list of identifying behaviors that might be observed when a person is abusing substances, including alcohol and other drugs. The DSM-III-R criteria serve as the reference for clinical diagnosis and intervention or treatment recommendations in many substance-abuse treatment agencies. The diagnostic criteria for psychoactive substance abuse is as follows:

A. A maladaptive pattern of psychoactive substance use indicated by at least one of the following:
   (1) continued use despite knowledge of having a persistent or recurrent social, occupational, psychological, or physical problem that is caused or exacerbated by use of the psychoactive substance
   (2) recurrent use in situations in which use is physically hazardous (e.g., driving while intoxicated);
B. Some symptoms of the disturbance have persisted for at least one month, or have occurred repeatedly over a longer period of time;
C. Never met the criteria for Psychoactive Substance Dependence for this substance. (American Psychiatric Association, 1987, p. 169)

Any psychoactive substance, including alcohol, marijuana, cocaine, amphetamines, and hallucinogens, can be included in this diagnostic criteria. For example, if a college athlete demonstrates continued use of alcohol despite academic difficulties due to drinking behavior and this has been prevalent since high school, the clinical sport psychologist can substantiate an evaluation of alcohol abuse and seek appropriate referral and intervention.

Abuse Symptoms With Athletes

Maladaptive patterns of drinking or drugging behaviors might lead to a diagnosis of psychoactive substance abuse. In the athletic community some of these symptoms might be readily visible, and some might be more covert. The clinical sport psychologist must be attentive to the persistent and recurring issues present in the assessment of a student athlete for alcohol or drug abuse. For example, if an athlete has identified repeatedly driving while intoxicated, the criteria for "recurrent use in situations in which substance use is physically hazardous" would be met. It is also important to assess the length and persistence of the symptoms, particularly if the athlete has identified specific symptoms lasting longer than a few months.

Social problems due to alcohol and drug abuse are often more visible and easily identified. For example, if an athlete has been involved in a physical confrontation at a social gathering, a coach is likely to be informed, particularly if the police are involved. Assessing the athlete's social support system will also help to identify potential problems. The team itself represents a significant social network, and internal confrontations often take place when a team member demonstrates inappropriate behaviors that reflect on the team as a whole. For example, such a confrontation might take place when an athlete involved in a social altercation is identified in the media. The resulting messages from fans, peers, faculty, and family members might be negative and indicting. The clinical sport psychologist should be aware of and attentive to the team dynamics if such an incident were to occur; in particular, observation of locker-room, practice, and team-meeting behaviors can often detect interpersonal conflicts. These conflicts might be focused on one specific athlete who might have a substance-abuse problem.

If a student athlete is being seen for individual counseling, another area of assessment should be the person's academic progress. Student athletes face stress in balancing academics and athletics; however, as identified by Finn and O'Gorman (1989), decreased academic performance (particularly among adolescents) is often attributable to the abuse of alcohol and other drugs. Sudden declines in such academic markers as grades are special warning signs.

Assessing the individual athlete's coping and stress management skills is crucial. Athletes at all levels of competition might turn to the use of alcohol and other drugs to cope with the stress of pressures from athletic injury, dejection, exhaustion, and other related stressors (Ogilvie, 1981). Given the frequent media messages that alcohol is a great relaxant and social elixir, it is not surprising that some young athletes learn to manage stress and self-confidence through chemical use (Ryan, 1984).

As a clinical sport psychologist, identifying how the athlete copes with the stress of academics, friends, and rejection (e.g., losing starting position, being yelled at by coaches) is important. If an athlete has experienced an injury, particularly one that prohibits further sport activity, assessment of coping strategies is again relevant. Research on athletes and injury (May & Seib, 1987) has identified frustration and impatience as specific emotional consequences of injury. The use of alcohol and other drugs might be deemed by the athlete as an effective release of pressure, anxiety, and depression associated with lack of sports participation due to injury.

Specific symptoms of psychoactive substance abuse that may be observed in the athlete population include

- drinking or drugging in secrecy (either alone or with others);
- feelings of guilt about drinking or drugging;
- lying about drinking or drugging behavior when confronted by others;
- needing increased intake to produce the desired effects (i.e., increased tolerance); and

- the experience of alcohol-induced amnesia or blackouts (Carroll, 1989).

In the athletic environment, specific team rules often regulate the use of alcohol and other drugs. Violation of these rules can lead to suspension or removal from the team. It is most likely that when confronted, athletes will not risk their future participation if they have violated team rules regarding substance use or abuse. The clinical sport psychologist must be attentive to this complex dynamic and must be aware of confidentiality issues during the assessment process. If athletes believe that reports of alcohol use will be shared with coaches, they most likely will not report such behavior. However, if the athletic policy includes a supportive condition for self-referral, the chances for acknowledgment of symptoms might be enhanced. Later in this chapter we will discuss the role of the clinical sport psychologist as a policy consultant.

Symptoms of alcohol and drug abuse are often difficult to detect. If, as a consulting sport psychologist, you assess your own knowledge of substance-abuse issues as limited, a referral to a chemical dependency agency or specialist is warranted. Being aware of local agencies that provide assessment of substance-abuse problems is ethical and competent consultant behavior, particularly considering the psychological welfare of the athletes. Once abuse symptoms are identified, appropriate interventions must be implemented. We will discuss these later in this chapter.

Substance Dependence

The issue of psychoactive substance dependence, whether it concerns alcohol, cocaine, or amphetamines, is of great importance for the clinical sport psychologist involved with the individual counseling of athletes. The DSM-III-R identifies that 13% of the adult population has had alcohol-abuse or dependence problems at some time in their lives (American Psychiatric Association, 1987). That 10% of the total population experiences problems with alcohol abuse and dependence is frequently referenced (e.g., Carroll, 1989; Finn & O'Gorman, 1989). If this means that only one member of a team of 15 has a problem, there will surely be residual effects on each team member and individual intervention will be a necessity. The issue of dependence on substances is indeed a touchy subject, for the label *drunk, addict, alcoholic,* or *doper* often seems permanent. What must be identified is the insidious aspect of the problem of psychoactive substance dependence and, yet, the treatable nature of this disorder.

The DSM-III-R (American Psychiatric Association, 1987) identifies the following diagnostic criteria for psychoactive substance dependence:

A. At least *three* of the following:
   (1) substance often taken in larger amounts or over a longer period than the person intended
   (2) persistent desire or one or more unsuccessful efforts to cut down or control substance use
   (3) a great deal of time spent in activities necessary to get the substance (e.g., theft), taking the substance (e.g., chain smoking), or recovering from its effects
   (4) frequent intoxication or withdrawal symptoms when expected to fulfill major role obligations at work, school, or home (e.g., does not go to work because hung over, goes to school or work "high," intoxicated while taking care of his or her children), or when substance use is physically hazardous (e.g., drives when intoxicated)
   (5) important social, occupational, or recreational activities given up or reduced because of substance use
   (6) continued substance use despite knowledge of having a persistent or recurrent social, psychological, or physical problem that is caused or exacerbated by the use of the substance (e.g., cocaine-induced depression, or having an ulcer made worse by drinking)
   (7) marked tolerance: need for markedly increased amounts of the substance (i.e., at least a 50% increase) in order to achieve intoxication or desired effect, or markedly diminished effect with continued use of the same amount

Note: The following items may not apply to cannabis, hallucinogens, or phencyclidine (PCP):

   (8) characteristic withdrawal symptoms
   (9) substance often taken to relieve or avoid withdrawal symptoms

B. Some symptoms of the disturbance have persisted for at least one month, or have occurred repeatedly over a longer period of time.

These criteria assist in establishing the baseline symptoms in assessing whether or not an athlete might be dependent on any psychoactive substance, including alcohol. Whether or not treatment should be differential for abusers and for those who are dependent will be discussed later in the chapter. It is important that the clinical sport psychologist be either competent in the assessment of psychoactive substance abuse and dependence or knowledgeable about the local referral sources that we will discuss later in this chapter. The bottom line is ultimately the responsibility of the clinical sport psychologist whose assessment must provide the athlete with the optimal treatment intervention to alleviate this debilitating disorder.

Dependence Issues With Athletes

Specific symptoms related to alcohol dependence include

- preoccupation with drinking behavior;
- rapid intake behaviors, such as gulping and guzzling;
- an inability to abstain from alcohol use;
- the loss of control phenomenon, where the individual is unable to control the use of alcohol once it has begun;
- withdrawal symptoms, including involuntary shakes, insomnia, loss of appetite, mental confusion, and restlessness; and
- an inability to predict behavior once drinking has begun (for example, people who are alcohol dependent go to a social event unable to predict if they will have only a couple of drinks) (Carroll, 1989).

Most of these symptoms will be observed outside of the athletic arena. If an athlete comes to a practice or competition under the influence of alcohol or other drugs, however, it is important that immediate intervention take place. My (CC) previous assessment experience has found that substance-abuse behaviors observed at practice or competition are always symptomatic of more severe abuse or dependence issues. Although the signs and symptoms of psychoactive substance dependence vary greatly among people, the most common and shared features include psychological dependence (e.g., alcohol use as stress management), tissue tolerance, physical dependence, loss of control over use, and withdrawal symptoms (Carroll, 1989). Referral to a chemical dependency treatment program is the intervention of choice for an athlete who demonstrates symptoms of alcohol or drug dependence. In most cases, the clinical sport psychologist will serve as the catalyst for referral for the addicted athlete.

Other Assessment Issues

The previous sections focused on the essential diagnostic features of psychoactive substance abuse and dependence. As discussed in other chapters in this book, a key factor in being an effective clinical sport psychologist is the skill of observational analysis. Being able to observe the athlete's environment is essential to understanding that person's view of life as an athlete, whether it be at the collegiate level or at the elite level (e.g., Olympic). Each level of athletic participation presents a variety of external stressors and situations where the symptoms of alcohol and drug abuse or dependence might be observed.

Perhaps most relevant to understanding potential substance abuse problems is that most athletes begin using alcohol and drugs, with the exception of cocaine, in high school or earlier (College of Human Medicine, Michigan State University, 1985). This fact bears direct relevance for the clinical sport psychologist who may be consulting with a local high-school team. The attainment of age 21 appears to have little relevance as to whether athletes will or will not use alcohol or any other drug. If the clinical sport psychologist is working in a university setting or with an older group of athletes, the second diagnostic criterion for psychoactive substance abuse (repetition of symptoms over time) might already be met. Persistence of symptoms might be more marked if the athlete began use of substances in high school or earlier. A thorough assessment of the athlete's previous substance-use history is warranted. This history should include an examination of the athlete's peer group and peer-group activities. There is a social factor to alcohol and drug use; the literature indicates that most athletes use these substances with other teammates in a social setting (College of Human Medicine, Michigan State University; Heyman, 1986). The consulting sport psychologist should be aware of the social affiliations where alcohol or other drugs appear to be the main source of interest.

Another nonperformance factor to consider is the athlete's family history of psychoactive substance abuse and dependence. The literature in chemical dependency research demonstrates a familial pattern of substance-abuse tendencies (Ward, 1980). Research has demonstrated a familial pattern of alcohol dependence; for example, studies have found that people whose biological parents (one or both) display alcoholism and who were adopted as children by nonalcoholic parents have a significantly higher incidence of alcoholism than adoptees whose biological parents were not alcoholics (Cloninger, 1987; Vaillant & Milofsky, 1982). Readers interested in assessment and treatment of dependence should familiarize themselves with the literature regarding substance abuse and family dynamics, such as the book *Another Chance* by Sharon Wegscheider (1981).

Gender Differences: Issues in Assessment

As indicated on page 285, high-school male athletes were found to consume alcohol significantly more often than male nonathletes (Carr et al., 1990). Among collegiate athletes, no differences have been observed between males and females in the usage patterns of alcohol and other drugs, except that males were more likely to use steroids (Bell & Doege, 1987; College of Human Medicine, Michigan State University, 1985). There were no observed differences between female athletes and female nonathletes; however, research has shown that at the high-school level male athletes drink to intoxication significantly more often than female athletes (Carr et al.).

In our society, there are differences in the perceived social acceptance of alcohol use behavior by men or women. For example, women tend to drink alone or in the privacy of their homes more often than men (Sandmaier, 1980). The stigma of drinking secretly or alone often encourages females to hide

their problems rather than to seek help (Carroll, 1989). This stigma plays itself out in relationships, as research has found that men are more likely to leave their alcoholic spouses than are women (Bourne & Light, 1979).

Some specific gender differences in alcohol dependence are that women usually begin both drinking and problem drinking at a later age than men; women progress from abuse to dependence more rapidly than men; females more often than males cite a specific stressor or traumatic event as the beginning reason for problem drinking; and alcohol-dependent women more often than alcohol-dependent men are described as feeling guilty, anxious, or depressed (Bourne & Light, 1979; Sandmaier, 1980). These differences are important to acknowledge, especially in sport psychology consulting. Often, clinical sport psychologists consult with both men's and women's teams and therefore must be attentive to the gender differences regarding not only performance issues but also psychological development issues.

The Team-as-Family Dynamic

Theories identifying family systems dynamics have proven to be extremely useful in the assessment and treatment of family dysfunctions, including substance abuse. The literature on the dynamics of alcoholism in families includes work by such authors as Claudia Black, Sharon Wegscheider-Cruise, and John Bradshaw, to name a few. This section provides a brief analysis of the athletic team as a family. The resultant dynamics of health and dysfunction in teams can be examined utilizing this analogue.

Wegscheider identifies four broad functions of the family system:

1. To establish attitudes, expectations, values, and goals for the family
2. To determine who will hold the power and authority, how they will be used,

and how members are expected to respond to them

3. To anticipate how the family will deal with change—in itself as a unit, in its members, and in the outside world

4. To dictate how members may communicate with one another and what they may communicate about (1981, p. 47)

Similarly, an athletic team might be observed to maintain similar functions. There are certain attitudes (1979 Pittsburgh Pirates theme We are Family), expectations (e.g., practice attendance, NCAA rules, grade point average), values (e.g., team unity, discipline in training, etc.), and goals (e.g., conference championship, Olympic medal) that are demonstrated in the athletic realm. The role of power and authority is clearly represented by coaches, administrators, and team captains. As well, all athletic teams are confronted with change. Each athletic season represents the potential for change, whether it be the first winning season or defense of a national championship. With team members changing consistently, change is a constant in athletics and sport. Lastly, each team develops communication lines and style. Viewing the team as a family and examining the team (family) functions can help us understand the effect of substance abuse and dependence on the team system.

When family system rules are rigid, enforced, and closed, they are often unhealthy and facilitate dysfunction (Wegscheider, 1981). In alcoholic families, symptoms shared by family members include denial of the problem, acute pain and stress regarding the family pattern, highly developed defenses to protect family members from even greater pain and lower self-worth, a predictable and fixed pattern of defensive roles, limited access to healthy communication, and lack of trust in members of the family (Wegscheider). The clinical sport psychologist might see patterns of enmeshment, detachment, and dysfunction with athletic teams

in which members have substance abuse problems.

An unhealthy behavior manifested in alcoholic (dysfunctional) families is *enabling*. One can enable an alcoholic (or drug dependent person) by preventing the person from understanding the consequences of dysfunctional behaviors. For example, teammates may continually bail out a team member who has a pattern of getting drunk at social events. Although motivated by care, the enabling behaviors allow the dependent person to become more pathological. Although there are benefits to this enabling behavior (e.g., coach doesn't find out, so there is no threat to status on the team), the potential damage is more severe. The goal of intervention is to ensure that the dependent person not only receives help but also understands individual responsibility. In addition, it is important that the enablers receive help in understanding the process of healthy and nonenabling communication and behavior. Helping team members understand how they might unwillingly be playing enabling roles can be a primary goal of preventive education programs.

Specific interventions are required when a member of an athletic team suffers from alcohol or other drug problems. Effective sport psychology consultants will utilize extra resources when their own seem limited. The key feature is understanding the complex dynamics of the team as a family. Recent work by Oglesby and Hill (1990) explores sport psychology interventions, utilizing family systems theory. Regarding the intervention of abuse and dependency issues among athletes, it is important to recognize the role of the team in conjunction with the individual. As an effective clinician and consultant, one should be able to identify dysfunctional family behaviors and implement or suggest alternative methods of communication and intervention. This requires that the entire family is treated; thus it is recommended that when an athlete is treated or counseled for substance-abuse or dependence issues, the whole team (e.g., coaches, teammates, trainers) also receive some type of intervention.

For example, in the case study presented at this chapter's beginning it would be helpful to involve Mary (Sheila's partner) and their coach for follow-up counseling on Sheila's discharge from the treatment center. (The psychologist should obtain a release from Sheila approving such an intervention.) In this manner both Mary and the coach (and other teammates who have been involved) can learn about the process of recovery and aftercare for Sheila. They can be taught what to expect and how to react and, most importantly, they can be given an opportunity to seek counsel to discuss how Sheila's drinking behavior had affected them. If this type of intervention were not provided, resentment and frustration might develop among the family. This can jeopardize the individual's recovery from abuse or dependence problems. Although the focus of intervention and treatment is on the athlete who is abusing or dependent on alcohol and other drugs, it is important to consider intervention at a systems level. This allows for all affected members to have an opportunity to discuss their own feelings and learn about how to best support their teammate on return. Specific interventions for the athlete who is abusing

alcohol and other drugs are discussed in the following section.

TREATMENT ISSUES

Once an athlete has been identified as having a substance-abuse or dependence problem, it is important that appropriate intervention and treatment steps be implemented. The goal of the initial intervention is for the person to acknowledge the possibility of having a substance-abuse problem and of further treatment proving helpful. The focus of this section is to identify specific types of treatment and briefly discuss the implications of treatment for the athlete with a substance-abuse or dependence problem (see Figure 12.1). The following treatment modalities are discussed: inpatient treatment, aftercare, outpatient treatment, and Alcoholics Anonymous (AA).

Inpatient Treatment

When an athlete is diagnosed with psychoactive substance dependence (whether alcohol or other drugs), it is important that inpatient treatment be explored. It is often necessary for a person who has demonstrated symptoms of dependency to be removed from the current environment so that the recovery process can begin. If detoxification is

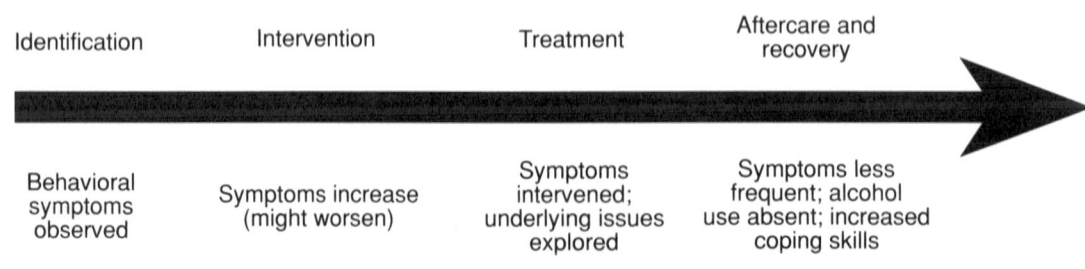

Figure 12.1 Symptoms change during the course of treatment.

necessary, inpatient programs often provide the environment to monitor for withdrawal symptoms and provide medical assistance. During the 4- to 6-week inpatient stay, the patient usually receives both individual and group psychotherapy. The groups and assigned counselors remain intact throughout treatment, and the patient experiences learning and growth via exploration of emotions, cognitions, and behaviors related to the drug-use pattern (Mann, 1979).

Typically, individuals are introduced to Alcoholics Anonymous during their inpatient stay. In addition, family members are usually involved in the treatment process by attending their own family treatment and receiving education on the salient issues of alcohol and drug addiction. Most inpatient programs involve family members from the beginning to end of treatment, due to family members' significant role in the recovery process.

Aftercare

Aftercare is a program of outpatient care for people who have completed inpatient treatment. This program usually lasts anywhere from 3 months to 2 years after treatment (Mann, 1979). Aftercare usually focuses on reentry into the person's environment; this includes family, occupation, and social network and, for athletes, their teams. The clinical sport psychologist must be attentive to the dynamics that occur when an athlete returns to the team from chemical dependency treatment. Often, teammates are unsure as to how to respond or what to say to their teammate. By facilitating normal communication and honest disclosure (e.g., "I'm not sure how to respond—can you help me?"), the clinical sport psychologist can assist the difficult process of reentry for the recovering athlete.

Typically, involvement in AA is an essential component of aftercare. In addition, family members usually attend aftercare sessions for their own recovery (from enabling behaviors) and transition. The focus of aftercare is to provide support and encouragement for personal responsibility and change.

Outpatient Treatment

The purpose of outpatient therapy is to provide intensive substance abuse treatment while at the same time allowing continuation of other occupational, family, and personal pursuits. This type of treatment is often unsuccessful if the patient continues to use alcohol and other drugs. St. Mary's Adult Chemical Dependency Center, Minneapolis, requires that the patient comply with three conditions to be admitted to outpatient therapy: (a) the maintenance of sobriety (abstinence from mood-altering substances), (b) the ability to continue employment without disruption, and (c) the ability to sustain home life and personal life (Mann, 1979). A patient's inability to comply with these conditions is seen as loss of control necessitating a recommendation for inpatient therapy.

It is important that the clinical sport psychologist be aware of local substance-abuse treatment agencies that provide both inpatient and outpatient care. Arranging tours and meeting personnel can help consultants to increase not only their own understanding, but often that of coaches, trainers, and sports-medicine personnel who might be able to attend. These local treatment groups can often serve as a resource for speakers for educational and prevention programs, discussed later in this chapter.

Alcoholics Anonymous

I never believed I was an alcoholic. I never believed I couldn't handle my alcohol. All the problems I had—bankruptcy, loss of career, the end of my first marriage after 13 years, the fact that my current wife was going to divorce me—were just a part of my life, I thought. I never attributed it to my alcoholism. . . . Eighteen years ago, I didn't know anything about AA, and I wasn't ready to admit that I was an alcoholic. . . . Now I do what Don Newcombe wants to do. . . . You've got peace of mind when you are in control of your own well-being. . . . (Newcombe, in Wholey, 1984)

One of the most widely accepted approaches to recovery from alcoholism is Alcoholics Anonymous (AA), a fellowship of problem drinkers who together seek help in maintaining abstinence from alcohol and other drug use. Voluntary membership in AA involves the admission that a person, alone, is powerless over alcohol. Using the "Twelve Steps" of AA, members strive to maintain their sobriety through emotional self-exploration and a philosophy of basic goals including a searching personal moral inventory, a public admission of personal wrongs, a willingness to make amends to those who have been harmed by one's drinking behavior, and an attempt to carry AA's message to alcoholics who are still suffering (Carroll, 1989).

Various groups have been patterned after AA, including Al-Anon (for family members of alcoholics), CA (Cocaine Anonymous, for those who have abused cocaine), NA (Narcotics Anonymous, for those whose drug of abuse is heroin, opium, or morphine), and Alateen (for children of alcoholics). All of these groups operate without therapists as facilitators and are true self-help groups, in that the only membership requirement is a desire to quit using alcohol or other drugs.

For the clinical sport psychologist, a listing of local AA and other support group meetings is usually available through local mental health agencies. There are both open and closed meetings; open meetings are typically designed for people who might be struggling with whether or not they have a problem, whereas closed meetings are usually attended by persons who identify themselves as alcoholic and are in the day-to-day process of recovery. AA is a recommended referral option, as research has shown that a supportive social network is an essential element of long-term behavior change (Carroll, 1989). At the same time, by listening to others share their history, the people can confront their own denial systems and pursue further counseling.

Treatment Goals

The development and course of psychoactive substance abuse and dependence are based largely on unique individual and family processes. Treatment goals can be selected based on the therapist's specific theoretical orientation (e.g., client-centered, gestalt, behavioral, etc.). Additional treatment goals will be influenced by the focus of treatment (individual, group, or family).

The following three goal areas must be addressed in the treatment of the chemically abusive or dependent athlete client.

Awareness

Clients must become aware of not only the chronic and damaging effects of mood-altering drugs (basic drug education), but they must also be aware of how their own use has disrupted such life areas as

- family (including spouse, children, parents, siblings, and other nuclear-family members);
- social life, including relationships with peers;
- employment or academic performance;

- athletic performance (which may be the least-recognized effect);
- and, most importantly, their sense of self-esteem.

Clients should be informed about the disease concept of alcoholism so they can begin to formulate recovery philosophies.

Implementation of Change

Awareness should lead to action. This concept usually works well with people who develop an athletic lifestyle of practice, practice, practice, and performance. Often, practice time is spent in developing awareness of an opponent's abilities. This awareness helps the athlete to develop a more proficient game plan for success. If this plan is practiced successfully, the chances for performance success are optimized. Using this metaphor with the chemically dependent athlete might enhance implementation of treatment goals. Once athletes are aware of the dynamics of their addiction, they must practice the following skills: (a) increase self-knowledge through therapy by examining personal strengths and attributes that can assist in developing a healthy lifestyle; (b) learn skills of stress management, decision-making, and assertiveness to facilitate independence (vs. dependence); and (c) develop healthy communication skills that can be practiced with supportive family members and friends. Family therapy is often a necessary adjunctive process to reestablish positive relationships and to explore the damaging effects of the client's behaviors. Especially in chronic cases, there is considerable anger toward the abusing person, often expressed indirectly.

Process of Healing

For the chemically dependent person to heal and fully recover from alcoholism and drug dependency, self-esteem enhancement and self-awareness must continue over the long term. In fact, this must become a lifelong goal. It is important for the client to recognize that recovery happens one day at a time. Many athletes must confront this same dynamic as they prepare for a long competitive season leading to a higher goal, such as NCAA competitions or the Olympic games. Again, relevant sporting metaphors may assist in adherence to treatment goals. The therapist must continue to help people recognize their personal strengths and limitations.

The following factors should be considered by the therapist and client in the treatment of a substance-abusing athlete:

- The effect of the clash of self-images between that of the healthy athlete and the sick patient
- The impact of public exposure on the treatment process (Some athletes are celebrities and their entire treatment will be open to public scrutiny.)
- The role of exercise in treatment (There has been some debate as to whether exercise can serve as a positive replacement addiction for the client.)
- The effect of organizational policy on treatment (Many sports organizations react to substance abuse with a punishment, rather than a treatment, philosophy.)
- The likelihood of a return to competition (Often the high stress levels associated with the sport contributed to the abuse problems, and return to competition must be considered in a context of an athlete's developing the coping skills necessary to survive in a stressful environment.)

This is not an exhaustive description of the treatment process. It does not take into consideration the unique individual issues that confront the athlete with a substance-abuse or dependence problem. However, it provides a basic guide to the process of recovery and attainment of a chemical-free lifestyle.

An important goal for the sport psychology consultant involved in alcohol education is to create a supportive and receptive attitude towards treatment within the athletic community. In an interview with *USA Today*, Thomas "Hollywood" Henderson, a former NFL player with the Dallas Cowboys and recovering alcoholic, responded to the question of how sports administrators should attend to helping athletes with alcohol and drug problems:

> They need to understand, rather than be understood. They need to understand the disease. . . It's not just willpower. They need to believe in treatment (*USA Today*, 1992).

The sport psychologist is in a unique and influential position in providing such information not only to athletes, but to coaches, trainers, sports medicine personnel, and administrators. The team physician is an important potential ally in this process. The next section of this chapter will discuss the education and prevention issues related to substance abuse and dependency with athletes. Ryan (1984) emphasized the need for athletes to have a better awareness of the myths and risks associated with alcohol and drug use than they have received from many drug education programs.

PREVENTION AND EDUCATION ISSUES

The role of the sport psychology consultant in substance-abuse education has received increased attention in recent years. Tricker, Cook, and McGuire (1989) identify the significant role of the sport psychologist in the planning, preparation, facilitation, and presentation of substance-abuse education. Chappell (1987) identifies education as the cornerstone of drug abuse prevention programs for athletes. Yet the frequency and quality of drug education programs for athletes at all levels of competition might be inadequate. In a survey of 71 collegiate athletic departments, Tricker and Cook found that 95% of respondents identified their drug education programs as infrequently organized and holding from no meetings at all to one or two per year. The most frequent substance-abuse education meetings for athletes occurred once a month and were primarily informational (1989). With the high incidence of reported alcohol use by athletes at the secondary, collegiate, and elite levels, it appears that substance-abuse education would be a priority; rather, at the collegiate level the incidence of this type of programming is minimal, based on the literature.

It is premature to say that all athletic systems are negligent in providing substance-abuse education programs for their athletes; however, some data suggest that more extensive education is warranted. The clinical sport psychologist might be able to facilitate substance-abuse education through contacts with local chemical-dependency treatment centers, university counseling center staffs, and other outreach contacts. This section reviews the essential components of substance-abuse education for athletes. Literature on effective and ineffective methods of prevention are discussed, and a model of substance-abuse education used with resident athletes at the United States Olympic Training Center will be presented. This model is not intended to represent the ideal program; rather, it is presented as a demonstration of a multimodal education program specifically designed for athletes.

What Works in Education?

The effectiveness of substance-abuse education has been debated for the past 20 years.

In most education and prevention literature, the stated goal for substance-abuse education is to decrease substance-abuse behaviors and to facilitate more healthy and nonusing attitudes and beliefs. It is at this cognitive and behavioral level of functioning that substance-abuse education with athletes must minimally be targeted. In a large meta-analytic study of 143 adolescent drug prevention programs, Tobler (1986) was able to ascertain the significant and nonsignificant factors related to outcome. She found that peer programs (drug prevention facilitated by same-age peers) were the most effective substance-abuse education models; these peer programs produced the most significant decrease in drug use behaviors from pretest to posttest measures. Results in the same study indicate that the least effective programs at changing drug use attitudes and behaviors are information-only and affective-only (experiential) programs. Information-only programs focus on the sharing of drug abuse statistics and symptoms, whereas affective programs focus on role plays and self-awareness (e.g., values clarification). Subsequent research has demonstrated that effective substance abuse prevention programs must be multimodal to assist the transfer of knowledge to attitudes and to subsequent behavior changes (e.g., Botvin, Baker, Renick, Filazzolla, & Botvin, 1984; Rozelle, 1980).

Utilizing a multimodal substance-abuse education model, Marcello, Danish, and Stolberg (1989) assessed the efficacy of such a program with university-student athletes. The program, developed out of the life skills training model designed by Botvin et al. (1984), incorporates four separate components; education, decision-making skills, interpersonal and communication skills, and alternative coping methods. Presented over a 6-hr format, the results demonstrated no differences between the treatment group and the control group. Due to questions concerning the motivation of the participants, limited time, and the small sample size, the researchers viewed the study as exploratory. However, it represented the first study of multifaceted substance-abuse education specifically for athletes to be presented in the literature.

Chapter 2 discusses the utility of counseling athletes via a life skills through sport model. This model emphasizes the various facets of athletic involvement at the cognitive, behavioral, and affective level of the athlete. In the same manner, an effective substance-abuse education model with athletes must incorporate a multifaceted approach to the athlete as a person; such a model stresses substance abuse information as integrally, but not solely, connected to the athlete's physical and psychological well-being. Tricker et al. (1989) postulate that individual progress can be achieved by developing the precursors to behavior change, including heightened awareness, improved attitudes, and decision-making skills.

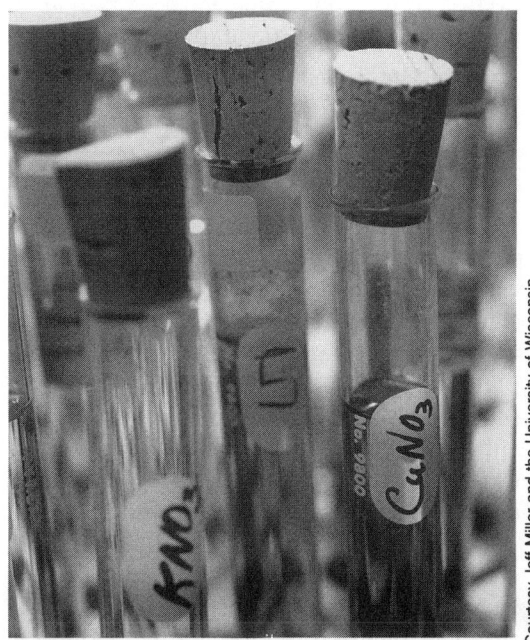

Courtesy Jeff Miller and the University of Wisconsin

Performance-Enhancing Versus Social Drug Use

The focus of this chapter has not been on the identification of pharmacological components of various classes of drugs (e.g., depressants, narcotics, stimulants) or on the specific differences between recreational drug use and performance-enhancing drug use. Rather, the focus has been on identifying the psychological symptoms, treatments, and prevention modalities of psychoactive substance abuse and dependence. It is assumed that health-care professionals who read this chapter will seek additional references when implementing their own intervention, prevention, or education strategies. However, there are some differences between the recreational use of drugs, such as alcohol and marijuana, and the use of performance-enhancing drugs, such as anabolic steroids and growth hormone. This section identifies some factors related to differences between the use of drugs to enhance performance and for recreational purposes.

A truly comprehensive substance-abuse education program will include information on performance-enhancing drugs such as steroids. Tricker and Cook (1989) found that 66% of surveyed collegiate athletic departments tested athletes for anabolic steroid use. In a survey of 2,048 collegiate student athletes, 4% reported steroid use (College of Human Medicine, Michigan State University, 1985). The sports medicine community has become increasingly aware of the harmful effects of steroid use among young athletes, and physicians are being encouraged to refrain from prescribing steroids unless medically warranted (Bell & Doege, 1987). Wagner (1989) identifies that athletes seeking a competitive edge might turn to drugs that risk serious adverse effects; he encourages other pharmacists to work toward ensuring that athletes do not abuse drugs, whatever the reason.

Although athletes might recognize that the use of alcohol and other illicit drugs does not enhance performance, the fact is that some performance-enhancing drugs (e.g., anabolic steroids) increase strength and performance (Wagner, 1989). The athlete's ego-involvement often has been identified as strongly attached to athletic performance (Ogilvie, 1987). Involvement of ego and self-worth in athletic success might blind the athlete to negative effects of performance-enhancing drug use. Effective substance-abuse education must address this conflict; the athlete works many hard and long hours to achieve success and might view drug use as an adjunct of training. Particularly if the family system enables this type of behavior, the athlete might not view steroid use as negative. Jay Coakley and Robert Hughes, sport sociologists at the University of Colorado in Colorado Springs, have identified this type of behavior as "positive deviance" (Hughes & Coakley, 1991).

In brief, positive deviance involves over-compliance to the norms and values embodied in the sport ethic, such as Win at all Cost, No Pain, No Gain, and Sacrifice for the Team (Hughes & Coakley, 1991). This sport ethic emphasizes positive norms; however, the ethic itself might become the vehicle by which athletes participate in deviant behaviors (e.g., steroid use) as a means of over-conformity. Some of Hughes and Coakley's recommendations in addressing this issue include trying to develop team norms emphasizing an awareness of one's limits (physical and psychological), not allowing athletes to play while injured, and a reframing of sport science goals to emphasize the growth and enhancement of the athlete through the expansion and continuation of the sport experience for athletes at all levels.

Additional information on performance-enhancing drugs is available in much of the sports medicine literature. Including a physician or pharmacist who is knowledgeable about anabolic steroids, growth hormone, and blood doping can be valuable in a multi-faceted substance-abuse education program for athletes. The significant point is acknowledging and discussing decision-making skills when athletes examine performance-enhancing drugs.

United States Olympic Committee's Alcohol Education Model

Based on the literature concerning the efficacy of substance-abuse education among adolescents and young adults, combined with a study of previous programs used with athletes, a multimodal substance-abuse program was developed for resident athletes at the United States Olympic Training Center in Colorado Springs. The program was administered in three separate sections, each representing the essential components of substance-abuse education for athletes, based on the existing literature. The sections included (a) an education component; (b) a decision-making and coping skills component; and (c) a social skills and self-esteem component (Carr, 1992). As we present this program, we will discuss each section both theoretically and pragmatically.

Each separate component of the model includes lecture presentations, group discussions, role-play exercises, and written materials. The program uses a cognitive-behavioral framework. As a theoretical construct, this framework represents the most empirically supported prevention model. This theoretical approach suggests that substance-use behavior, like other behaviors, is learned through a process of modeling and reinforcement and is mediated by intrapersonal factors, such as cognitions, attitudes, expectations, and personality attributes. Each of the components of this model were presented based on this

theoretical paradigm, and examples were demonstrated in a similar manner.

Education Component

The purpose of the education component was to present factual and updated information on the prevalence of alcohol and drug abuse in athletics, as well as to provide information on the pharmacological effects of alcohol and other drugs on the human system. Today's athlete is much more attuned to the effects of nutrition and physical preparation on the physiological processes of training. Therefore, it is important that relevant and updated information on the effects of alcohol, performance-enhancing drugs, and other drugs be included.

Definitions of the terms *use, abuse,* and *addiction* were presented and discussed. The DSM-III-R guidelines were used to define abuse and dependency (addiction) with various drugs, including alcohol. Symptoms of abuse and dependency were discussed and various treatment alternatives were presented. A group discussion on responsible attitudes and drug use behaviors was facilitated; included in this process were ethical dilemmas confronted by athletes who use psychoactive substances.

Decision-Making and Coping Skills Component

As indicated by various researchers (e.g., Botvin et al., 1984; Tobler, 1986), peer-resistance training is essential in effective substance-abuse education programs. The focus of this component was on discussing stress-management techniques as alternatives to alcohol and drug use, communication-skills (assertiveness) training, and general decision-making strategies using a cognitive-behavioral approach. Identifying sport-specific stressors was extremely relevant in this section, and subsequent group discussion focused on stressors similar to those discussed earlier in this chapter. Role-play scenarios allowed for the participants to demonstrate alternative coping responses to stressful situations. An example of a scenario related to coping behaviors and alcohol use follows:

> An athlete does not make the final selection for a national team. He/she goes out with friends and drinks to intoxication. Is it OK for him/her to get drunk this night? The next two nights? Why or why not? (Carr, 1992)

The work of Finn and O'Gorman (1989) assisted in the development and creation of athlete-specific scenarios that facilitated group discussion among participants. This specific component also allows for the clinical sport psychologist to discuss psychological techniques such as relaxation training and imagery training as alternative interventions for stress (e.g., competitive training stress). Trained sport psychologists might find this opportunity significant in identifying the utility of mental training techniques as necessary components for optimal performance. Concurrently, these techniques can assist the athlete in coping with stressors that might otherwise be managed through the use of alcohol and other drugs.

Social Skills and Self-Esteem Component

During the program for resident athletes at the Olympic Training Center, the theme of social responsibility was adopted by the participants in group discussion. The athletes identified the incongruent societal values attached to alcohol and sport (e.g., in the media). Regarding responsibility for self and the team, small groups discussed the choices of alcohol- and drug-use behavior during preseason, in-season, and postseason time frames.

A discussion of the positive benefits of sports participation was used in this component. Values clarification exercises were used to explore the role of drug use and the personal conflicts that arise when drug-use consequences interfere with self-selected personal values. One area of discussion that would have benefited from more time was the influence of others on usage behaviors and attitudes. As identified by Marcello et al. (1989), substance-use behaviors and attitudes are influenced by parental modeling, media advertising, cultural, ethnic, and religious factors, and peer influence prior to an athlete's arrival at college (or even high school, or the Olympic Training Center).

Upon completion of the 8-hr program (three separate components about 2-1/2 hr long), the participants evaluated the program contents. In addition, pretest (before beginning the program), posttest (immediately following completion of the program), and follow-up (7 weeks after completion of the program) data were collected on both participants and control-group athletes (who were offered the opportunity to attend the substance-abuse program that was scheduled after collection of follow-up measures). Although the evaluation of the program by participants was positive—participants rated the organization, presenter receptivity, participation allowed, and presentation style as good to excellent—the outcome data was disappointing.

The outcome results of this program (Carr, 1992) demonstrated no posttest or follow-up differences between the initial participants and control-group members on measures of substance-abuse knowledge, attitudes, or self-esteem. The author submitted some possible reasons for consideration. Perhaps the longitudinal effects of substance-abuse education are difficult to measure with current inventories; in the future, we hope that more sensitive attitudinal and self-report measures will be developed. Another potential problem with analyzing this type of study is the low baseline of reported use of other drugs (besides alcohol). This might make any actual changes in behavior and attitudes difficult to measure due to the lack of statistical sensitivity. Future research efforts will benefit from studies using such models as the Olympic Training Center's and other sport-specific models (e.g., Marcello et al., 1989).

Education and Prevention Recommendations

Again, the multifaceted model we have discussed is not all inclusive. It is intended as representative of a multidimensional (cognitive-behavioral-affective) prevention program for athletes. Clinical sport psychologists might be able to creatively implement similar programs; however, the literature indicates that inclusion of the previously mentioned components is essential. Perhaps of even more impact, particularly based on the results of Tobler (1986), would be the development of a peer-based prevention model.

The clinical sport psychologist involved with secondary or collegiate student athletes might be in a unique position to develop a peer model of substance-abuse prevention. After requesting volunteers, specific substance-abuse prevention training that includes presentation style, group facilitation, and role-play skills could be developed for potential peer leaders. For example, a list of volunteer athletes from the resident training program was developed. Athletes who participated in the training were asked to speak at local high schools. This experience was both challenging and rewarding, according to reports of the athletes involved. The potential benefits of peer programs with athletes as a group have yet to be studied in the literature; however, the previous literature on peer programs in substance-abuse education in general is promising.

We hope the roles of the clinical sport psychologist as consultant, counselor, and educator with substance-abuse issues have been made clearer during this chapter. An additional component of effective consultation includes policy (substance abuse and dependence) consultation and implementation in athletic organizations.

Policy Issues

The guiding force for substance-abuse education in athletic communities is athletic policy. Overall, such policies dictate the athlete's required grade point average, practice hours, athletic eligibility status, rules concerning recruitment, and other external variables. The adoption of substance-abuse education as a policy issue ensures its implementation and effective growth. Often, a consulting sport psychologist might have the opportunity to suggest policy changes or adoptions. Given this potential, the role of the sport psychologist in enhancing the potential for effective substance-abuse education is encouraging.

The NCAA Drug Education Committee has developed a set of minimum guidelines for policy consideration at its member institutions. These guidelines might be successful for athletes at the secondary as well as the elite (national governing body) level. A partial description of the program guidelines follows:

1. Schedule at the beginning of the school year a course on drug and alcohol awareness for all men and women athletes. It is suggested that each institution utilize the expert resources available on its campus or in its community. . . .

2. Each member institution should develop and have in place a plan for treatment of student-athletes with drug or alcohol-related problems. Such plans might utilize treatment centers and programs available in the local community and should emphasize

rehabilitation rather than punishment. It obviously is more prudent to have such a plan in place before rather than after a problem develops.

3. Coaches should become more aware of potential drug-related problems in student-athletes, and specifically should be an available source of support in the identification and treatment of such problems.

4. In relation to Recommendation #3, the athletics department at each member institution should schedule training sessions for all coaches, trainers, and team physicians as to how to recognize and handle drug and alcohol-related problems. (NCAA Drug Education Committee, n.d.)

Although clearly not all inclusive, these guidelines provide support for the process of identification, treatment, and prevention of substance abuse in athletes. The NCAA recommends a minimum of three sessions, but based on a review of the literature, we recommend more sessions of a longer format and with more specific content material guidelines. The goal of effective policy implementation is to reinforce intervention, treatment, and education; even in its brief form, the NCAA guidelines identify each of the essential issues. The clinical sport psychologist might serve as a catalyst to ensure the implementation of effective and realistic programs.

CONCLUSION

This chapter focused on substance-abuse and dependence issues relevant to the assessment of, intervention with, treatment of, and education of athletes at various levels of competition. Specific stressors for athletes were identified; the subsequent risk factors associated with alcohol and other drug use were discussed. Although pharmacological information on various drugs, including performance-enhancing drugs, was not presented here, there are many references for this information.

The authors do not expect that, having read this chapter, readers will feel proficient enough to be chemical dependency counselors; rather, we hope that previously unidentified clinical issues are now salient. More importantly, issues of treatment options and suggestions for educational alternatives have been presented. As a reference guide, this chapter is intended to answer questions that might arise for a sport psychologist in any athletic setting, be it with high-school, collegiate, or elite-level teams.

The authors suggest that additional resources be consulted for information on the disease concept of alcoholism and other specific concerns regarding behavioral pharmacology. In addition, local chemical dependency hospitals might be able to provide sport psychologists with handouts, assessment materials, or speakers for substance-abuse education programs. A complete copy of the model presented in this chapter is available directly from the first author. A key component of effective consulting is knowing where local resources exist; often, substance-abuse specialists can be found in mental health directories. For sport psychologists in university settings, contact the university student-counseling center and student health service for information. At some universities, substance-abuse counselors or coordinators exist through the division of student affairs. Sport psychologists who consult with national governing bodies or other national sport organizations can contact the sports medicine and sport science programs of the United States Olympic Committee in Colorado Springs.

The multifaceted role of the clinical sport psychologist requires basic knowledge about alcohol and drug abuse and dependence. The psychological concerns of athletes can be exacerbated by the abuse of alcohol and other psychoactive substances; appropriate intervention and treatment referral is necessary and can be facilitated by the sport psychologist. In addition, the sport psychologist can share insights and techniques that help athletes to deal with the pressures of sport. Non-clinicians can play a valuable role in promoting and coordinating substance-abuse education programs with sport organizations. Although not the most popular subject to discuss, the devastating effects of alcohol and drug abuse and dependence can create permanent consequences for the athlete, the coach, teammates, and the family. The effective sport psychology consultant will be able to assist athletes in recognizing, treating, and preventing substance-abuse problems, thereby allowing each athlete to strive for and achieve their optimal performance potential as athletes and as people.

REFERENCES

American Psychiatric Association. (1987). *Diagnostic and statistical manual of mental health disorders* (3rd ed. rev.). Washington, DC: Author.

Bell, J.A., & Doege, T.C. (1987). Athlete's use and abuse of drugs. *Physician and Sportsmedicine*, **15**(3), 99-108.

Botvin, G.J., Baker, E., Renick, N.L., Filazzola, A.D., & Botvin, E.M. (1984). A cognitive-behavioral approach to substance abuse prevention. *Addictive Behaviors*, **9**, 139-147.

Bourne, P.G., & Light, E. (1979). Alcohol problems in blacks and women. In J.H. Mendelson & N.K. Mello (Eds.), *The diagnosis and treatment of alcoholism* (pp. 110-115). New York: McGraw-Hill.

Carr, C.M. (1992). *Substance abuse education with athletes*. University Microfilms: Ann Arbor, MI.

Carr, C.M., Kennedy, S.R., & Dimick, K.M. (1990). Alcohol use and abuse among high school athletes: A comparison of alcohol use and intoxication in male and female high school athletes and non-athletes. *Journal of Alcohol and Drug Education*, **36**(1), 39-45.

Carroll, C.R. (1989). *Drugs in modern society* (2nd ed.). Dubuque, IA: Brown.

Chappel, J.N. (1987). Drug use and abuse in the athlete. In J.R. May & M.J. Asken (Eds.), *Sport psychology: The psychological health of the athlete* (pp. 187-211). New York: PMA.

Cloninger, C.R. (1987). Neurogenetic adaptive mechanisms in alcoholism. *Science*, **236**, 410-416.

College of Human Medicine, Michigan State University. (1985, June). *The substance use and abuse habits of college student-athletes*. Presented to NCAA Drug Education Committee, Michigan State University.

Duda, M. (1986). Female athletes: Targets for drug abuse. *Physician and Sportsmedicine*, **14**(4), 142-146.

Finn, P., & O'Gorman, P.A. (1989). *Teaching about alcohol*. Dubuque, IA: Brown.

Griffin, T.M. (1985). *Paying the price*. Hazelden Foundation: Minneapolis, MN.

Hayes, R.W., & Tevis, B.W. (1977). A comparison of attitudes and behavior of high school athletes and non-athletes with respect to alcohol use and abuse. *Journal of Alcohol and Drug Education, 23*(1), 20-28.

Heyman, S.R. (1986). Psychological problem patterns found with athletes. *The Clinical Psychologist, Summer,* 68-71.

Hughes, R., & Coakley, J.J. (1991). *Positive deviance among athletes: The implications of overcommitment to the sport ethic.* Unpublished manuscript.

Mann, G.A. (1979). *Recovery of reality: Overcoming chemical dependency.* New York: Harper & Row.

Marcello, R.J., Danish, S.J., & Stolberg, A.L. (1989). An evaluation of strategies developed to prevent substance abuse among student-athletes. *Sport Psychologist, 3,* 196-211.

May, J.R., & Seib, G.E. (1987). Athletic injuries: Psychosocial factors in the onset, sequelae, rehabilitation, and prevention. In J.R. May & M.J. Asken (Eds.), *Sport psychology: The psychological health of the athlete* (pp. 157-187). New York: PMA.

National Collegiate Athletic Association. (n.d.) Drug Education Committee. *Drugs, the coach, and the athlete*: Author.

Ogilvie, B.C. (1981). The emotionally disturbed athlete: A round table. *Physician and Sportsmedicine, 9*(7), 68-74.

Ogilvie, B.C. (1987). Counseling for sports career termination. In J.R. May & M.L. Asken (Eds.), *Sport psychology: The psychological health of the athlete* (pp. 213-230). New York: PMA.

Oglesby, C.A., & Hill, K. (1990). *Family systems approaches: A new methodology for work with athletic teams.* Colloquium presentation at Association for the Advancement of Applied Sport Psychology Annual Conference, San Antonio.

Rooney, J.F. (1984). Sports and clean living: A useful myth. *Drug and Alcohol Dependency, 13,* 75-87.

Rozelle, G.R. (1980). Experiential and cognitive small group approaches to alcohol education for college students. *Journal of Alcohol and Drug Education, 26*(1), 40-54.

Ryan, A.J. (1984). Drugs and self-confidence. *Physician and Sportsmedicine, 11*(1), 42.

Sandmaier, M. (1980). *The invisible alcoholics: Women and alcohol abuse in America.* New York: McGraw-Hill.

Staff. (1992, January 23). Drugs, alcohol and professional athletes: Special article. *USA Today.*

Tobler, N.S. (1986). Meta-analysis of 143 adolescent drug prevention programs: Quantitative outcome results of program participants compared to a control or comparison group. *Journal of Drug Issues, 16,* 537-567.

Tricker, R., & Cook, D.L. (1989). The current status of drug intervention and prevention in college athletic programs. *Journal of Alcohol and Drug Education, 34*(2), 38-45.

Tricker, R., Cook, D.L., & McGuire, R. (1989). Issues related to drug abuse in college athletics: Athletes at risk. *Sport Psychologist, 3,* 155-165.

Vaillant, G.E., & Milofsky, E.S. (1982). The etiology of alcoholism. *American Psychologist, 37,* 494-503.

Wagner, J.C. (1989). Abuse of drugs to enhance athletic performance. *American Journal of Hospital Pharmacy, 46,* 2059-2067.

Ward, D.A. (1980). *Alcoholism: Introduction to theory and treatment.* Dubuque, IA: Kendall/Hunt.

Wegscheider, S. (1981). *Another chance: Hope and help for the alcoholic family.* Palo Alto: Science and Behavior Books.

Wholey, D. (1984). *The courage to change.* Boston: Houghton Mifflin.

CHAPTER 13

EATING DISORDERS AND WEIGHT MANAGEMENT IN ATHLETES

Robert A. Swoap, PhD and Shane M. Murphy, PhD
United States Olympic Committee

It is likely that most competitive athletes have been concerned with weight control at one time or another. There are many reasons why serious athletes self-monitor weight and diet, such as making weight, appearing attractive in front of judges, or trying to reach ultimate performance potential. Weight management is a necessary part of most athletes' training. For some athletes, however, weight management goes awry and becomes a serious problem. These athletes, having become obsessed about their weight, begin using harmful methods, such as severe dehydration, to lose weight; some cases progress to clinical eating disorders. Because weight management is a prevalent issue in competitive sport and because there can be severe consequences for eating-disordered people, it is critical for the helping professional working with athletes to understand how to recognize and treat eating disorders. More generally, it is greatly beneficial for the helping professional in sport to be able to inform athletes about safe and effective methods of weight management.

Why so much concern about weight management in sport? From a purely perfor-mance perspective, athletes can experience compromised competitive ability due to poor weight-management practices. For example, rapid weight reduction often results in loss of lean-body mass but unsustained weight loss (Blackburn et al., 1989; Stuart, Mitchell, & Jensen, 1981). The loss of lean-body mass and carbohydrate stores can be exceptionally harmful to athletes who participate in a de-manding athletic training regimen (Porcello, 1984). The rapid weight loss associated with some techniques (e.g., fasting, long steam baths) comes primarily from water depletion, and dehydration is an unfavorable state in which to compete. The American College of Sports Medicine (ACSM) has recognized that female athletes might be at special risk for a triad of related health issues: eating dis-orders, amenorrhea, and osteoporosis (Otis, 1993; Yeager, Agostini, Nattiv, & Drink-water, 1993).

In addition to the deleterious effects that poor weight-management techniques have on performance, it is probably the case that when athletes engage in medically unsafe weight-loss practices, they place themselves at higher risk for developing eating disorders. The following case history illustrates how a focus on weight loss in sport can become unhealthy and self-destructive.

■ *THE CASE OF KARL* ■

The following case is from the second author's files. It represents elements of case histories of several athletes and does not portray any one person.

I first met Karl at a multisport competitive event in Florida. He was a competitor in the diving competition. I was a sport psychologist assigned to the medical team providing services at the event. Karl asked to see me before his competition, and we met in an office in the medical center. He was worried about his upcoming competition and described symptoms of lack of sleep and disturbed appetite. Only 2 years before, at age 25, Karl had won a bronze medal in a World Cup competition in his event. He had appeared destined for a stellar career, but the 2 years after his win were described by Karl as "a nightmare." His competitive performances had deteriorated, his confidence was low, and he was struggling just to make international teams. Karl asked for help in dealing with his nerves. He described a pattern of losing focus in the moments leading up to his dive. He described being distracted and feeling physically weak as he stood on the board. Karl attributed his poor performances to predive anxiety. We worked on finding a way to deal with his anxiety; I taught Karl a simple relaxation method to use a few minutes before his dives. He tried to identify his negative precompetition cognitions (e.g., If I mess up on this dive, I'll drop out of the top five) and constructed positive coping statements to substitute (I'm nervous, but I only need to focus on a good takeoff and good position on the board. The rest will follow). We met twice before Karl's competition began.

Karl finished fourth in his competition. The top three divers qualified for an overseas trip to compete in several world competitions. I did not see Karl the next day but encountered him at breakfast in the competitor's dining hall the following morning. I asked Karl if he wished to meet again, and he set up an appointment for that afternoon. As we began, Karl stated that his career was "finished." He seemed greatly upset and began crying as he struggled to describe his competition. He mentioned that his "starvation diet" had left him feeling so weak that he felt physically unable to perform his best. I asked Karl about this diet, and he began to describe a pattern of self-injurious eating behaviors that spanned 7 years.

Karl began his diving career at age 17. Over the next 3 years he progressed steadily, and at age 20 he was offered a chance to train with one of the country's top coaches. This coach was famous for his strict work ethic, which Karl eagerly embraced. All athletes on the team weighed in twice a week and their levels of body fat were closely monitored. Karl became obsessed with his weight and with the idea that losing 15 lb (about 7 kg) was the key to his becoming a top diver. At this time he began the habit of purging, forcing himself to vomit after any meal he regarded as self-indulgent. He used laxatives regularly in an attempt to control his weight, especially before competitions. After 2 years with his new coach, Karl had tried a variety of weight-control approaches, including many different diets, subliminal tapes, fasting before competitions, and using diuretics. His weight frequently fluctuated, but he could never seem to keep that 15 lb off for any length of time.

After finishing college, Karl left his coach to train in a new program near where his girlfriend lived. His new coach soon took him aside for a frank discussion about Karl's weight-loss efforts. He told Karl that his current weight was acceptable and that he wanted Karl to stop dieting. "You need to be strong to be a great diver," he told Karl. Over time, Karl began to gain confidence in his body image and stopped his purging and fasting behaviors. Two years later, he broke onto the world scene with his third-place finish in a major international competition. Karl made the United States team to go to the world championships. The national coach was his old college mentor. When Karl arrived, the coach commented that he looked "heavy" and asked Karl if he had gained weight recently. The coach told Karl that weight control was essential for diving success and suggested that Karl drop a few pounds. Karl was devastated. His confidence plummeted, and he had a miserable competition. When he returned home, Karl found himself returning to his old habits. Scared that his coach would find out, Karl became extremely secretive about his dieting and eating. He noticed that his mood fluctuated rapidly, from exhilaration one day to deep depression the next. Over the next 2 years his good performances became more and more infrequent. His coach tried to talk to him about it, but Karl felt that he had to work things out on his own. After finishing his story, Karl began crying again. "I tried to tell my parents about this last Christmas," said Karl, "but they just told me that I was a great athlete and that things would work out. I feel like nobody cares."

This chapter has two main goals: (a) to promote an understanding among helping professionals of the special issues related to weight management in the sporting community and (b) to educate those concerned people in the sporting community about major issues in identifying and treating eating disorders and to encourage healthy weight-management behaviors. It is not necessary in this chapter to deal extensively with the literature on eating disorders in general, as this has been done thoroughly in other texts. Indeed, two excellent texts dealing with eating and weight-loss issues in sport have been published recently (Brownell, Rodin, & Wilmore, 1992; Thompson & Sherman, 1993). This chapter is organized to examine

and provide information on the prevalence of eating disorders in the athletic population, promote an understanding of predisposing factors to the development of eating disorders in sport, indicate how to recognize an eating or weight-loss problem, discuss treatment issues with athletes, and provide a brief guide to the prevention of eating disorders in sport, with an emphasis on healthy weight-management techniques for athletes and their coaches.

PREVALENCE

Some basic definitions and classifications are necessary to examine the prevalence of eating disorders in athletes. According to the *Diagnostic and Statistical Manual of Mental Disorders* (3rd Edition, Revised) (American Psychiatric Association, 1987), the diagnostic criteria for anorexia nervosa include the following:

- Refusal to maintain body weight over a minimal normal weight for age and height, e.g., weight loss leading to maintenance of body weight 15% below that expected; or failure to make expected weight gain during period of growth, leading to body weight 15% below that expected
- Intense fear of gaining weight or becoming fat, even though underweight
- Disturbance in the way in which one's body weight, size, or shape is experienced (e.g., the person claims to "feel fat" even when emaciated, believes that one area of the body is "too fat" even when obviously underweight)
- In females, absence of at least three consecutive menstrual cycles when otherwise expected to occur (primary or secondary amenorrhea) (A woman is considered to have amenorrhea if her

periods occur only following hormone, e.g., estrogen, administration.)

The DSM-III-R diagnostic criteria for bulimia nervosa include these:

- Recurrent episodes of binge eating (rapid consumption of a large amount of food in a discrete period of time)
- A feeling of lack of control over eating behavior during the eating binges
- The person regularly engages in either self-induced vomiting, use of laxative or diuretics, strict dieting or fasting, or vigorous exercise in order to prevent weight gain
- A minimum average of two binge-eating episodes a week for at least 3 months
- Persistent overconcern with body shape and weight

An accurate assessment of the prevalence of bulimia and anorexia nervosa in any population is difficult to achieve, due to the secretive nature of these disorders. In the athletic domain, discovery might lead to serious repercussions for an athlete who has this type of problem, including being dropped from a team or program. Jack Wilmore states that "even the roommates and parents of those who have a problem often don't know what's going on. Sometimes they don't find out until it becomes almost catastrophic and professional help is a necessity. So we may be seeing just the tip of the iceberg" (Thornton, 1990, p. 118). Researchers and clinicians who examine eating disorders in sport must take into account the perceived threat of their assessments.

The accuracy of most studies purporting to measure the prevalence of eating disorders in sport is uncertain. Part of this uncertainty is due to the secretive nature of the disorder. However, part of the lack of confidence in current findings is due to the assessment techniques (paper-and-pencil self-report surveys) used in the majority of these studies.

As Brownell, Rodin, and Wilmore point out, ". . . self-reports have questionable validity, at least with certain athletes under some circumstances [therefore] prevalence figures from existing studies might underestimate the extent of the problem" (1992, p. 138). Alternative methodologies, such as clinical interviews, randomized telephone surveys, admission records in sports medicine clinics, and representative population sample surveys with follow-up interviews, have been used infrequently. In addition, many investigators have not specifically determined the prevalence of clinical eating disorders but instead have focused on describing the frequency of eating-disordered behaviors. Although the prevalence of subclinical eating problems (i.e., pathogenic weight loss techniques) in athletics is also very important to determine, it should not be construed as an estimate of eating disorders. Because of these assessment problems, current prevalence findings must be interpreted cautiously.

Burckes-Miller and Black (1988b) surveyed 695 male and female athletes and reported that 3% met DSM-III-R criteria for anorexia nervosa (4.2% female, 1.6% male), and that 21% met the criteria for bulimia nervosa (39.2% female, 14.3% male). They also found that several techniques were used to lose weight (see Figure 13.1). Dick (1991) found that there is a sport-specific prevalence for eating disorder conditions, but cautioned that no sport should be considered "exempt" from having individuals susceptible to eating disorders (p. 139) (see Figure 13.2.).

To ascertain the prevalence of subclinical eating problems, Rosen, McKeag, Hough, and Curley (1986) surveyed 182 female collegiate athletes and reported that 32% practiced at least one pathogenic weight-control behavior (e.g., self-induced vomiting; use of laxatives, diet pills, or diuretics). They also found these behaviors to be sport-related, as 74% of gymnasts and 47% of distance runners

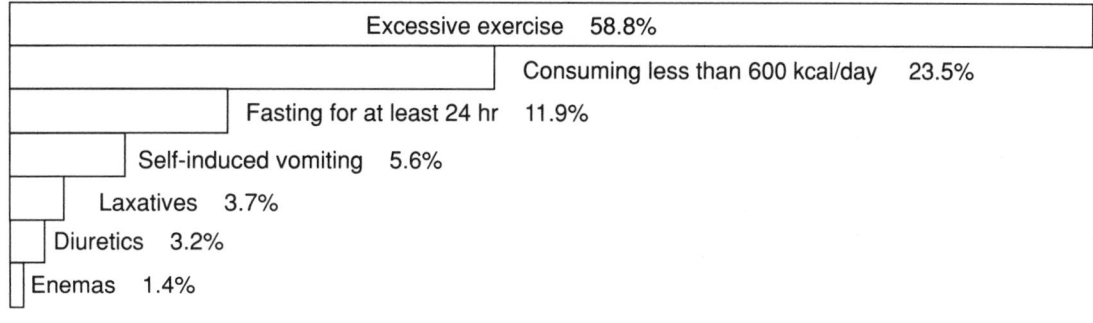

Figure 13.1 Common weight-loss techniques used by athletes.

Note. From "Male and Female College Athletes: Prevalence of Anorexia Nervosa and Bulimia Nervosa" by M.E. Burckes-Miller and D.R. Black, 1988, *Athletic Training,* **23** (pp. 137-140). Copyright 1988 by the National Athletic Trainers Association. Adapted by permission.

practiced pathogenic weight-control behavior. A subsample of the athletes (*N* = 30) indicated that 83% used pathogenic weight-control behavior to improve athletic performance and only 7% did so to improve appearance. In a follow-up study, Rosen and Hough (1988) found that of 42 gymnasts, all were attempting to lose weight and 62% used at least one pathogenic method. Furthermore, of the 42 gymnasts, 67% reported that they had been told by coaches that they were too heavy, and 75% of these then resorted to pathogenic weight-control behavior. Gustafson (1989) examined attitudes and behaviors about weight in surveying 227 female collegiate athletes. Of these, 71% believed they were at least 5 lb (about 2 kg) overweight, 53% were not satisfied with their body weight, and 37% reported bingeing behavior. In these studies, athletes with some of these behaviors might or might not meet the DSM-III-R criteria for diagnosis of eating disorders. In any event, it is important to remember that these studies did not use clinical interviews and standardized reports to determine prevalence according to current diagnostic standards.

These and other prevalence studies (Black & Burckes-Miller, 1988; Burckes-Miller & Black, 1988a; Clark, Nelson, & Evans, 1988; Klesges,

1983; Pasman & Thompson, 1988; Thornton, 1990; Zuckerman, Colby, Ware, & Lazerson, 1986) demonstrate a number of patterns in the prevalence of eating disorders in athletes.

- Clinical eating disorders appear to occur more often in athletes than in the general population.
- A significant percentage of athletes engage in pathogenic eating or weight-loss behaviors, which, although subclinical, are important to examine.
- Eating disorders and use of pathogenic weight-loss techniques in athletics tend to have a sport-specific prevalence (e.g., they occur more frequently in gymnastics and in wrestling than in archery and football).

Brownell and Rodin (1992), in their review of the prevalence of eating disorders in athletes, call for more epidemiological research to identify prevalence rates in the athletic population. Such research is required, and we propose that it address critical questions for athletes and coaches. Such questions include the following:

- Do the conditions in which athletes participate in sports make it more likely that

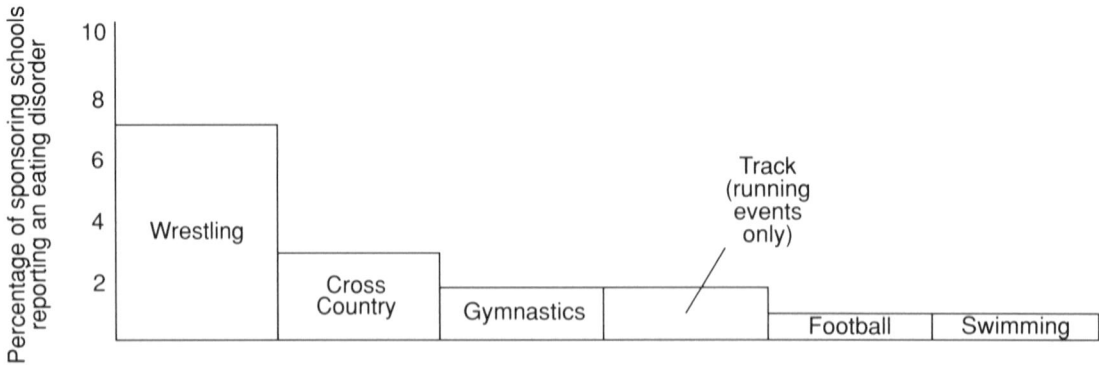

Figure 13.2a   Prevalence of eating disorders in men's collegiate sports.
Note. From "Eating Disorders in NCAA Athletics Programs" by R.W. Dick, 1991, *Athletic Training,* **26** (pp. 137-140). Copyright 1991 by the National Athletic Trainers Association. Adapted by permission.

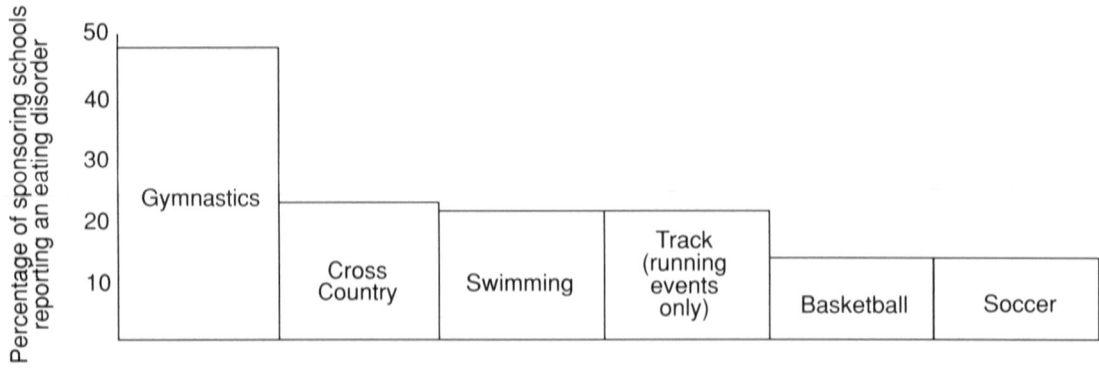

Figure 13.2b   Prevalence of eating disorders in women's collegiate sports.
Note. From "Eating Disorders in NCAA Athletics Programs" by R.W. Dick, 1991, *Athletic Training,* **26** (pp. 137-140). Copyright 1991 by the National Athletic Trainers Association. Adapted by permission.

they might resort to eating-disordered behaviors?

• If a person is predisposed to an eating disorder (family history, metabolic rate), does athletic participation increase the disorder's risk of occurring?

• Are the behaviors of sport personnel (coaches, officials, judges) sometimes instrumental in the onset of an eating disorder? Can such behaviors be changed?

• If an athlete adopts pathogenic weight-loss techniques while participating in sport, do such behaviors persist when competitive participation has ended?

These issues have received little attention in the literature, but experience indicates that they are critical to a complete understanding of the sport–eating disorders relationship. Answers to these questions have crucial implications for prevention and treatment efforts.

PREDISPOSING FACTORS

As emphasized at this chapter's beginning, one of the potential problems in modern sports is that leanness has become equated with performance to such a degree that there is an almost obsessive preoccupation with maintaining low body weight. The following accounts from the *Austin American-Statesman* illustrate how serious the ramifications of an unhealthy focus on weight in a sports program can be.

During the past 18 months, more than a dozen university women athletes, including some of the best swimmers in the world, have been diagnosed as having severe eating disorders traceable in most cases to the pressures of their sport and the training method of their coaches. One of every 10 female athletes at the university has been diagnosed as having an eating disorder and referred to a specialist for treatment, according to university documents and officials. Another 20 to 30% show signs of a disorder. (Halliburton & Sanford, 1989b, D1)

She did not want to come into workouts overweight, so she started resorting to drastic measures. Her swimming began to falter, so she would try to forget her sorrows by indulging in food. But that made more of the drastic measures necessary to keep the pounds off. Soon she was trapped in the bulimic cycle of binges and purges. . . . "It was hard for me to tell him [coach]," she said. "He said 'You have to take care of it.' That was it. He never brought it up again. It was still real hard. I still felt pressure. And he would say to me, 'Work on your weight.'" (Halliburton & Sanford, 1989a, D8)

It was indicated that the coach emphasized weight in training and competition and insisted that his swimmers remain under maximum weight limits. Those who failed to do so were required to participate in special workouts. According to current and former university swimmers . . . the pressure to meet those guidelines was so intense that many routinely fasted, induced vomiting, used laxatives and diuretics, or exercised in addition to workouts. They did not want to be relegated to the group they called "The Fat Club." "Primarily the pressure came from the coach, until you started to internalize it. Then it became self-inflicted—torture almost—where some people would weigh themselves three or four times a day." (Halliburton & Sanford, 1989c, D1, D7)

"Weighing in is a constant reminder of your weight," [a former swimmer] said. "I remember being at the swim center at 5:30 in the morning and being on that stupid freight scale and looking at everybody else and looking at . . . the reaction on their faces, and it was just non-stop. You became obsessive with it. I'm talking to the pound—that's how fanatical it makes you." (Sanford & Halliburton, 1989, D7)

The sports environment does not necessarily facilitate an unhealthy focus on weight concerns, but as shown in this section, many aspects of various sports promote a focus on weight. This can be especially dangerous to a person who, for whatever reason (genetic or familial factors or unusual stress level), is predisposed to an eating disorder or weight-management problem. It is plausible that the extra pressure of such an intense focus on weight might precipitate an eating disorder in a predisposed person.

Factors commonly encountered in sport that encourage this strong focus on weight issues are as follows:

- Weight restrictions
- Judging criteria that emphasize thin and stereotypically attractive body build
- Performance demands encouraging very low percent body fat
- Coach-applied pressure to lose weight
- Peer pressure to try pathogenic weight-loss techniques

Weight Restrictions

The following sports in the Olympic program have weight classifications that determine in which group an athlete competes:

- Boxing
- Wrestling (Greco-Roman and freestyle)
- Weightlifting
- Judo
- Tae kwon do

Other sports, such as rowing, also commonly use weight classifications, such as *lightweight*, to subdivide competitors based on body weight. In professional sports, jockeys always perform under weight restrictions and have been identified as a high-risk group (Thompson & Sherman, 1993). Weight classifications become a problem when a desire to perform and win at high levels influences athletes to compete at below their natural body weight, hoping that by competing against lighter opponents they will be more successful. Often, this results in athletes resorting to unusual and dangerous practices in an effort to drop several pounds immediately before competition and weigh-in (the practice of "cutting weight"). Weight-loss techniques typically encountered in such sports as boxing and wrestling are

- dehydration (sauna, sweat box, heat-restrictive clothing),

- use of laxatives,
- use of diuretics,
- use of diet pills,
- fasting,
- crash dieting,
- purging (self-induced vomiting), and
- fluid restriction.

Rapid dehydration is the end result of many of these practices; paradoxically, the athlete intent on winning typically does not have sufficient time to fully rehydrate before competition and thus competes in a weakened state. Although the practice of cutting weight has the goal of improving performance, two factors militate against improvement: (a) Many other athletes of larger body type are also losing weight to compete at lower weight classes and (b) the dehydration experience weakens the athlete and typically results in poorer performance.

In addition to such performance concerns, the medical literature shows that rapid dehydration is a dangerous behavior in terms of impact on the body, particularly if carried out repeatedly (Webster, Rutt, & Weltman, 1990). In addition, as mentioned previously, concerns are growing over long-term health effects, including osteoporosis, for female athletes who maintain low body weight and suffer chronic amenorrhea.

Judging Criteria

The following Olympic sports depend on judging to determine performance outcome; physical attractiveness, especially for women, is considered by participants to be a determining factor in the final score.

- Diving
- Figure skating
- Gymnastics (artistic and rhythmic)
- Synchronized swimming

It is difficult to describe the powerful influence that perceived judging biases have on the attitudes of young athletes participating in such sports. Research in this area is lacking, but our personal experience with divers and figure skaters indicate that there is frequently open communication between judges, coaches, and athletes about the perceived body weight (and often, the need to lose weight) of the competitors. An athlete might receive feedback such as, "If you lose ten pounds, you will do much better in competition this year." Such a message has a powerful influence on the competitive adolescent who fiercely desires success in sport and whose parents may have spent between $30,000 and $50,000 in the previous year to support training. Helping professionals working with athletes in this area must be alert to the variety of pressures on the athlete and to the gender-specific issues often involved (see chapter 9). Education of all those involved in the process, including athletes, coaches, judges, parents, and administrators, is essential.

An unknown is whether losing weight to meet stereotypic notions of attractiveness results in higher marks from judges. At this time, no research on this topic exists. Observation, however, indicates that frequently such weight losses have either no effect or a deleterious effect on performance, particularly when weight loss comes at the expense of muscle development. Strong muscular development is a necessity among both male and female athletes in these sports to accomplish the difficult maneuvers that result in high scores.

Performance Demands

One of the consequences of the increasing application of science to sport performance (Wilmore, 1992) is that coaches and athletes have become increasingly aware of the statistical relationship between various physical factors and sport performance. In some sports, research has indicated that there is a correlation between low percent body fat and high levels of performance (swimming, speedskating, long-distance running, cross-country skiing). Problems arise when this information is applied in individual cases without a full understanding of the body type–performance relationship. For example, a male runner might assume that if he is able to lower his percent body fat from 10% to 8%, he will increase his running times. But if such a change proves beneficial, is it possible to predict that lowering percent body fat from 8% to 5% will have a similar effect on performance? In the sports under discussion, a commonly encountered belief is that Lean Equals Mean, or that the leaner the body, the better the performance. Research, however, provides no evidence for such an all-encompassing relationship.

Problems can begin when the desire for success is married to the perceived need to lose weight to achieve success. Unhealthy weight-management practices are often employed because young athletes have no knowledge of effective and safe nutrition and exercise principles. If coaches also lack knowledge of nutrition and exercise principles, young athletes have few options for sources of information. A runner stated that

> she went to the coach and said, "How can I improve my times?" And he said, "Well, I think you have to knock off some weight." He was right. She was overweight. And she said, "It's really very difficult for me." And he said, "Well, a lot of the kids vomit after they eat and use that as a means of weight control." She took him up on this suggestion. ("Eating disorders," 1985, p. 96)

Coach-Applied Pressure

In the situations discussed, in which the perception exists that weight loss results in more athletic success, the coach can play a critical role in shaping the attitude and behaviors of athletes. The greatest danger to an athlete's health exists when pressure is applied to lose weight in the absence of knowledge concerning safe and effective weight-management procedures. Harris and Greco (1990) studied 28 female gymnasts who believed that their current weight was significantly more than they or their coach would like. Fifty-six percent experienced pressure from the coach to lose weight. Team weigh-ins averaged 6 a month and individual weigh-ins, 14 a month. Also, it has been suggested that some coaches might suspect that an athlete working with a therapist for treatment of an eating disorder might either be encouraged to abandon the sport or return to their event with a lower competitive drive ("Eating disorders," 1985).

Peer Pressure

Another factor in many sport situations that is not as common in other life areas is the close and shared experience of people who train together, compete together, and often travel together on competitive trips. This increases the possibility of peer modeling of pathogenic weight-loss techniques. Chiodo and Latimer (1983), for example, found that most bulimic patients could identify specific incidents associated with the onset of vomiting and that many developed the problem after learning from someone else or the media about the behavior. To the extent that athletes are likely to spend a greater amount of time than their nonathletic peers in close proximity to other people who might have an intense focus on weight and might be using pathogenic weight-loss techniques, this is likely to be a greater problem in sport than in other life areas.

These sport-specific factors, then, must be understood by the helping professional intervening in a case involving an eating-disordered athlete or, indeed, when educa-

tion efforts are called for. In a survey of 384 intercollegiate athletes, Guthrie (1986) found that their top self-reported reasons for weight loss were as follows:

1. Required for performance excellence
2. Required to reach aesthetic ideals of beauty
3. Remark by a member of athletic staff concerning need to lose weight
4. Required to meet a lower weight category

Guthrie also found that other contributing factors were identified by the athletes:

- Peer pressures (e.g., engage in bingeing and purging as a form of ritualistic behavior after a meet)
- Poor travel diets
- Public ridicule of overweight athlete's body
- Fear of not being able to participate in a particular match if weight loss did not occur (1986)

RECOGNIZING EATING DISORDERS IN ATHLETES

Although athletes might use pathogenic weight-loss methods frequently and experience eating disorders occasionally, these problems are not always obvious, and many cases are unrecognized and untreated. How does one recognize and identify a problem? With clinical eating disorders in athletes, early detection (and early intervention) is associated with better outcome (Thompson, 1987). For a sport psychologist or consultant, the ability to identify both the eating-disordered and at-risk athlete is vital. In some situations, e.g., life-threatening anorexia nervosa, there is a need for immediate treatment. In other cases, especially with bulimia nervosa, the athlete's problems are not so readily observed. This section discusses the signs and symptoms that might indicate the presence of an eating problem.

Standardized Assessment

It is important to take a multimodal approach to the assessment of eating disorders in athletes. Standardized assessment tools should be used in initial assessment stages. For example, the Diagnostic Survey for Eating Disorders—Revised (DSED) (Johnson & Pure, 1986) can be used as a self-report inventory or in a semistructured interview. It provides information in eight areas: demographic factors, weight history and body image, dieting behavior, binge eating and purging behavior, related behaviors, menstruation and sexual functioning, medical and psychiatric history for patient (athlete) and family, and life adjustment. Additional self-report inventories often of use are (a) the Eating Disorders Inventory (EDI) (Garner, Olmsted, & Polivy, 1983), a self-report scaled instrument that provides information regarding individual eating attitudes and behaviors (i.e., drive for thinness, bulimic tendencies, body dissatisfaction, ineffectiveness, perfectionism, interpersonal distrust, interoceptive awareness, and maturity fears), and (b) the Eating Attitudes Test (EAT) (Garner & Garfinkel, 1979), a test of disordered eating symptoms associated with anorexia nervosa. It should be stressed that for diagnostic purposes, these tools should be administered and interpreted by a licensed psychologist and followed up with a clinical interview as indicated.

Behavioral and Personality Assessment

Another important source of information is behavioral observations, either directly or as reported by the athlete's coaches or teammates. The use of behavioral assessment to validate self-report or test data can help to clarify the nature of the problem. Some behavioral signs of eating disorders include weight loss, eating alone, preoccupation with food, mood changes, and body distortion statements. Weight loss is by definition a characteristic of the anorexic, i.e., at least 15% below expected body weight. Individuals with bulimia can be normal weight, overweight, or somewhat below expected weight. Thus, body weight is an inadequate predictor of bulimia. However, frequent fluctuations in weight might be an indication of bulimia or a bulimic-type weight-management style.

Eating alone might be a sign of either anorexia nervosa or bulimia. Anorexics are often involved in food preparation, but might only eat their small portion after everyone else has finished. Bulimics might eat alone, making it easier to engage in purging after the meal. However, in a bulimic athlete who is required to attend team training meals, other signs might emerge (e.g., frequent trips to the bathroom; returning from the bathroom with bloodshot eyes, due to the strain of vomiting; much talk of and preoccupation with the composition and caloric content of the meal).

Changes in mood and personality styles are additional factors helpful in detecting eating disorders. For example, depression, irritability, and wide fluctuations in mood are often associated with the eating-disordered athlete (Thompson, 1987). Self-worth issues might be salient, with some athletes using "athletics as a vehicle to be accepted" (Bickelhaupt, 1989, p. 80). An intense drive for being thin, dissatisfaction with one's body, feelings of ineffectiveness, interpersonal distrust, maturity fears, and perfectionism are also factors associated with many eating-disordered people (Garner et al., 1983).

It is important to note both that an eating-disordered athlete might have some or none of the personality characteristics previously described and that a non-eating-disordered athlete might have some of these characteristics. For example, although perfectionistic tendencies are a hallmark of anorexic patients, perfectionistic tendencies are also common in many athletes, eating-disordered or not. Indeed, the emerging consensus appears to be that "there is no one personality structure characteristic of either anorexia nervosa or bulimia. . . . [instead these] are multi-determined and multidimensional syndromes; they develop in different people at different times for different reasons" (Garner, Rockert, Olmsted, Johnson, & Coscina, 1985, p. 561). This might be true especially in athletes where, as discussed in the section on predispositions, a variety of environmental factors might contribute to the onset of a disorder. However, if taken with other information, emotional and personality characteristics can be useful in understanding and treating the eating-disordered athlete.

Medical Assessment

A thorough medical evaluation is a necessary part of the detection and diagnosis of an eating disorder. Recognition of the common medical symptoms of eating disorders can assist the sport psychology consultant in understanding the nature of the disorder. Medical symptoms of eating disorders might include the following: anemia, leukopenia, osteopenia, renal and liver problems, peripheral edema, electrolyte imbalance, cardiac problems (e.g., bradycardia), dental problems, and gastrointestinal problems. Some medical problems (e.g., anemia, leukopenia) have overt signs (e.g., fatigue, increased susceptibility to infection) that a coach or psychologist can detect and use for additional validation of a suspicion of an eating problem.

In attempting to identify eating disorders in athletes, it is important to distinguish between dieting and anorexia nervosa. Many researchers believe that anorexia is not simply an extreme point in a continuum of dieting, but is qualitatively different (e.g., psychological manifestations such as ineffectiveness and interpersonal distrust occur more frequently in eating-disordered people than in dieters). "In a weight-preoccupied culture, this distinction is important in distinguishing illness from overvalued social attitudes" (Garfinkel, Garner, & Goldbloom, 1987, p. 627). This is especially important in assessing athletes, because effective weight control (including reasonable diets) is essential in sport. Often, a distorted body image is a sign that a more serious problem exists. Self-critical references to one's body (e.g., "I think my stomach is too big," or "My hips are much too large") can be associated with eating disorders or weight-management problems. Evidence of a body image that is widely discrepant with an objective viewpoint is cause for serious concern; for example, a very thin, 90-lb (41 kg) 19-year-old woman saying that she is "a fat blob."

Treatment Referral Issues

Knowing when and how to refer an athlete for treatment is crucial. As mentioned previously, early referral and intervention is associated with better outcome. In such cases as an 80-lb (36 kg) anorexic, immediate referral and treatment is vital. For coaches and staff, when a serious question exists as to the presence or the absence of an eating disorder, referral for a more extensive assessment is necessary. Athletes in general, and in particular those with eating disorders, often have perfectionistic tendencies (including considerable desires to please others) and thus often have difficulty admitting that a problem exists. This perfectionistic tendency, along with the fear of possibly losing a spot on the team or suffering reduced playing time, contributes to the athlete's resistance to any referral. Tact, respect, and awareness of these issues is paramount to a successful referral.

Because many athletes might be hesitant to seek treatment for their problem, certain guidelines can be helpful. Thompson (1987) recommends that the coach or sport psychologist approach the athlete with an emphasis on feelings, rather than directly focusing on eating behaviors. Focusing on eating behaviors and attempting to exert control in this area can be counterproductive, because eating is often the only thing over which the athlete feels control. Targeting feelings might facilitate the athlete to confide in the referring person. In the case of Karl, presented at the chapter's beginning, the initial focus of assessment was on performance, and a strong message was sent to the athlete that the psychologist cared about Karl and his diving. Karl was able to describe his eating and weight problems at a subsequent session.

We also suggest that referrals be made to specific persons or clinics. A clear and explicit referral will more likely produce compliance with seeking treatment than will a vague

"you should seek help." Thompson suggests that "if the athlete is hesitant about seeking professional assistance, suggest to her that she see the referral person for an 'assessment' to determine if there is a problem" (1987, p. 118). This request is often easier for the athlete to comply with than is going to "therapy." It is additionally recommended that as soon as the referral is accepted the athlete be encouraged to call immediately to schedule the initial consultation. In all cases, a concerned, not confrontational, style is advisable.

TREATMENT ISSUES

Although there is an abundance of information on treating the eating-disordered patient, there is little information on treating the eating-disordered athlete. Furthermore, some of the information addressed to coaches and other athletic staff is incorrect. For example, an assistant athletic director wrote that the coach should provide the primary

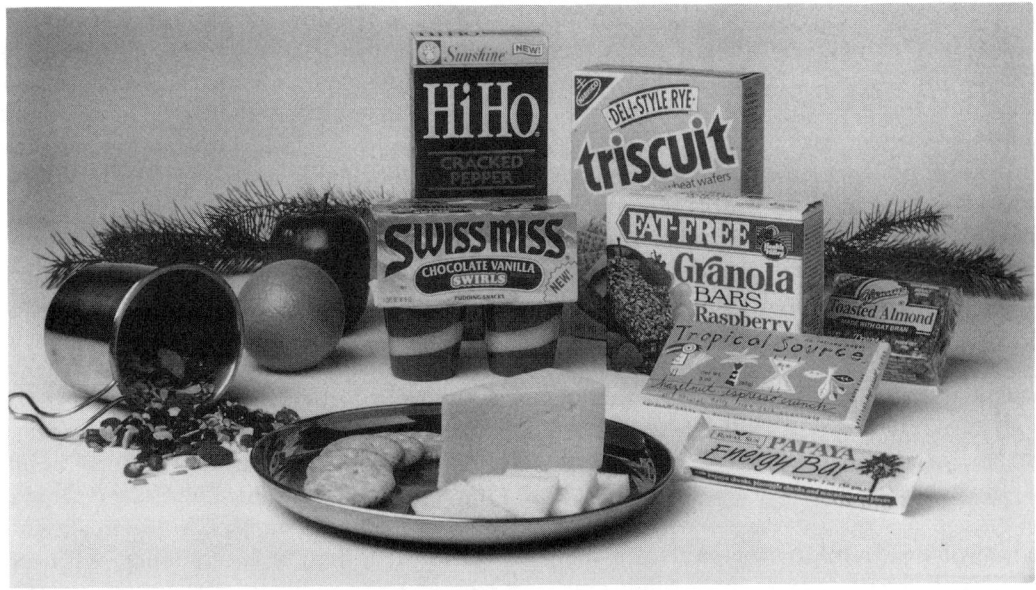

Courtesy K R Maier

assistance to the athlete and "make up a diet and a schedule of workouts. He/she should explain the balance of caloric intake and expenditure, set a specific weight goal, and coordinate the intake and expenditure to meet that goal in a specific time frame" (Bickford, 1990, p. 87). This is simply not appropriate or feasible in most cases. Few coaches have the training, knowledge, or time to be nutritional counselors and dieticians. In fact, some athletes have reported that unreasonable weight goals set by their coaches contributed to their eating disorders (Guthrie, 1986; Halliburton & Sanford, 1989c).

This section gives an overview of treatment for the eating-disordered athlete. A general guide to treatment modalities in the management of eating disorders or pathogenic weight-loss techniques is provided. In this context, the special needs of an athlete undergoing treatment are addressed. The reader interested in a more detailed presentation of treatment is referred to the *Handbook of Psychotherapy for Anorexia Nervosa and Bulimia* (Garner & Garfinkel, 1985). This edited book has discussions of cognitive, behavioral, and cognitive-behavioral therapy, response prevention treatment, group therapy, family therapy, inpatient and residential treatment, self-help and support groups, and psychoeducational therapy. Additional guides that address treatment issues are also widely available (Blinder, Chaitin, & Goldstein, 1988; Brownell & Foreyt, 1986; Gross, 1986; Johnson, 1991; Johnson & Connors, 1987; Reece & Gross, 1982; Thompson & Sherman, 1993).

Individual Therapy

Some therapists suggest that during individual therapy, the focus should be on the patient as a person and not on eating habits or weight. It has been suggested that "if the therapist gets stuck on issues of weight or food, it will only reinforce the patient's game and allow the patient to avoid dealing with the underlying causes of the disorder" (Gross, 1986, p. 4). This may or may not be true with the athlete client. In some cases the athlete in individual therapy may need an outlet to discuss the pressure to compete at a low body weight. Thus the therapist might well focus on weight issues, in an educational and supportive manner.

In addition to educating and supporting an athlete in individual therapy, other aspects of treatment might include reality-oriented cognitive feedback (to challenge all-or-nothing thinking, personalization, superstitious thinking, and underlying assumptions). Also, improving affective expression—guiding the patient to identify a range of feelings to learn how to tolerate uncomfortable affect—will often prove useful. Similarly, enhancing body image perception (e.g., through movement therapy, relaxation) might assist in the task of freeing self-esteem from weight, shape, and familial or societal expectations.

Group Therapy

Group therapy is a mode of treatment that has been effective for eating-disordered patients, usually as an adjunct to other therapies (Davis, Olmsted, & Rockert, 1990; Fernandez, 1984; Huerta, 1982; Maher, 1984). Although there has been little information regarding its efficacy with athletes, a group setting appears to provide advantages with this population. A group setting could provide support, for example, by allowing the opportunity for members to share their experiences of competitive pressure, demanding coaches, perfectionistic strivings, and so forth. It would also provide a forum for the sharing of information, interpersonal learning, instillation of hope, and development of socializing techniques (Yalom, 1985). Group therapy should primarily be used in the treatment of eating disorders in combination with other treatment modalities. Group interventions might be the most useful in education efforts, which will be discussed later in this chapter.

Family Therapy

In working with athletes, traditional family therapy is a viable treatment option (cf. Miller, 1984; Minuchin & Fishman, 1981). Interestingly, family therapy in sport might be conducted by bringing together the athlete's "family" (i.e., athlete, coach, nutritionist, and closest teammates) and working with them as a family structure. In this setting, the members of the athlete's family would be encouraged to share in a supportive fashion their concern for the athlete. In addition, educational information could be imparted to the whole competitive group in a consistent way. Lastly, understanding the influences that the behaviors of these people have on one another (e.g., interpersonal relationships) can be examined in this context. According to Garfinkel (1991), family therapy is especially useful with patients under age 19 who have had an eating disorder less than 3 years.

Inpatient Treatment

Ideally, pathogenic weight-loss behaviors in athletes are discovered and addressed before the problem becomes severe. However, if the eating disorder has become critical, inpatient hospitalization might be necessary. Inpatient treatment must always be carefully considered as an option and will usually be chosen if the medical risk to the athlete is great. The factors that suggest consideration of inpatient treatment for anorexia and bulimia are shown in Table 13.1.

Due to factors related to sports participation issues or to interpersonal factors, an athlete might resist hospitalization. However, a joint and cooperative decision with the athlete and the athlete's family, physician, and coaches is most productive for treatment success.

Table 13.1   Major Considerations in the Decision to Provide Inpatient Treatment for Anorexia and Bulimia

Anorexia nervosa
- Weight loss of more than 25% of ideal body weight
- Weight loss of more than 15% with a lack of control
- Failure of outpatient treatment
- Medical and psychiatric complications (e.g, gastrointestinal consequences, suicidal ideation)
- Persistent substance abuse

Bulimia nervosa
- Failure of outpatient treatment
- Medical complications
- Uncontrolled insulin dependent diabetes mellitus
- Pregnancy
- Concomitant depression
- Persistent substance abuse

Note. From "Treatment Issues in Eating Disorders" by P. Garfinkel (paper presented at the Second Annual Rocky Mountain Conference on Eating Disorders, Colorado Springs, CO); and from "Multidisciplinary Approach to Treatment and Evaluation" by P.S. Powers, in *Current Treatment of Anorexia Nervosa and Bulimia* by P.S. Powers and R.C. Fernandez (Eds.), 1984, New York: Karger. Table 13.1 is adapted from both sources with permission.

Psychoactive Medication

Medication has a secondary but often useful role in the treatment of eating disorders. Because of drug-use standards and restrictions in sports, the physician who is considering pharmacological treatment of an athlete must be extremely sensitive to and knowledgeable of these issues. Medications to avoid include thyroid hormones, insulin, diuretics, laxatives, or benzodiazepines (for bulimics who might abuse this class of potent psychotropic drugs). Benzodiazepines for the nonbulimic anorexic restrictor might be useful if given premeal. Tricyclic antidepressants might be indicated as an adjunct treatment for bulimics.

In all modes of psychotherapy (e.g., group, family, individual therapy), a multimodal approach is recommended. Components of an effective intervention might include a combination of psychoeducation, cognitive therapy (e.g., challenging irrational beliefs), behavior therapy (e.g., response prevention), and interpersonal and individual therapy (cf. Johnson, 1991). Also, the assistance of a dietician or nutritionist is recommended. In each case, keeping the athlete's coach generally informed as to the progress of treatment is vital. Many coaches might fear that treatment providers are steering the athlete in an unproductive direction. It is the sport psychologist's duty to reassure the coach that you both have the athlete's best interests in mind and that the athlete will continue to participate in sport if it can be done safely and the athlete so desires. Lastly, an overall goal is to sequence and individualize treatments. This involves starting with the least intrusive intervention and working up as necessary and as appropriate for the individual athlete.

Many athletes might not have any idea that help is available. The pressures to maintain or lose weight can be intense, and attempts at seeking help might be viewed as a sign of weakness. In all cases, the issue of sensitivity to the athlete's fears (real or imagined) is significant in a successful intervention. An athlete may fear that disclosing the problem is a sure way of losing a spot on the team. This is not an unfounded fear because, as we have seen, extreme weight-loss methods are often not only tolerated, but encouraged.

Lastly, it is helpful to keep in mind that the course of recovery from anorexia is gradual. Current estimates are that approximately one third recover in the first 3 years after onset, one third by 6 years, and one third do not recover. Treatment outcome for bulimics,

whose symptoms often wax and wane throughout and beyond the treatment period, is more difficult to assess. However, there are some factors related to prognosis:

- Age of onset—A younger onset is associated with a better outcome.

- Gender—There is some evidence that males do worse in treatment. They might have more severe underlying pathology, because cultural factors are less involved. This might be less true in sports, where pathogenic weight-loss behavior in male athletes is often culturally determined (e.g., the wrestling culture).

- Marriage—Onset after marriage is related to poorer prognosis.

- Chronicity—Delay of treatment carries a poor prognosis.

Treatment in the Case of Karl

Karl, the diver described earlier, illustrates a typical pattern or course in the development of an eating disorder. Several factors common in the sport context are evident, including a history of self-initiated efforts to overcome the eating disorder followed by a relapse, the critical role of coaches in promoting healthy or unhealthy attitudes and behaviors, and the severe negative impact of the disorder on performance. This section on treatment issues concludes with a discussion of a treatment scenario for Karl.

Treatment in this case involved several subsequent sessions between the sport psychologist and Karl that helped Karl identify the fact that he was suffering from bulimia. Reading materials were provided that described the similar experiences of other athletes. When he understood more about the nature of his problem, he was more committed to taking the necessary steps to return to an optimal state of functioning.

Next, Karl identified for the psychologist his whereabouts during the upcoming summer training and competition season. Athletes often live a semi-nomadic existence, and their busy travel schedules often increase the difficulty in arranging for consistent outpatient treatment. Fortunately, Karl was planning to stay in a large West-Coast city for 4 months over the summer, and Karl was referred to a weight-management and eating-disorder treatment program there. He signed a release of information so the sport psychologist was able to contact the program staff, make the referral, and provide background information on Karl's situation. Karl entered into treatment in the program and was exposed to an interdisciplinary intervention approach that involved a medical evaluation, individual counseling, group therapy, nutritional counseling, and behavioral contracting involving homework assignments and extensive self-monitoring. After 4 months of intensive intervention, Karl had made considerable progress and was asked to regularly attend a self-help group. He also received further individual counseling every 2 months. At follow-up a year after the referral, Karl was still attending the self-help group and had made excellent progress toward adopting and maintaining a healthy lifestyle and a balanced and productive approach toward weight management. He had cut back on his diving involvement, although he still competed and had even won a national-level meet. But the majority of his efforts were devoted toward establishing the business career he had always dreamed of, and he was attending night school while working at a financial-management company.

PREVENTING EATING DISORDERS IN ATHLETES

Perhaps one of the most important services we can provide as health care professionals is promoting the prevention of a problem. This is the case with eating disorders and pathogenic weight-loss techniques in sports. Communicating knowledge about eating, weight, health, and sport performance to the appropriate populations is vital. This can be done through educational workshops (e.g., through a university counseling center), interviews with the media, discussions with coaches, and consultations with teams or individual athletes. Because of the high incidence of eating disorders in adolescents, an efficient prevention program might target high-school or junior-high athletes. The factors that should be considered in proactive sport education programs include de-emphasizing body weight, providing nutritional education, promoting sensitivity to weight issues, and facilitating healthy weight management.

De-Emphasize Body Weight

One concept to emphasize is fitness rather than body-weight ideals. Many athletes and coaches become obsessed with setting and obtaining a certain weight. However, body weight is often insignificantly related to athletic outcome. Despite many efforts to alter athletes' and coaches' beliefs about ideal weights in sport, many athletes at all competitive levels continue to rely on pathogenic weight-loss methods, which are both dangerous and deleterious to performance. It is important to discuss with coaches and athletes that there is no ideal body composition or weight for an athlete. Guidelines exist for sports and participants, but these can fluctuate greatly, depending on the athlete's specialty (e.g., long-distance vs. sprinter); natural variations in both body composition (e.g., lean-body vs. fat mass) and metabolic rate; and patterns of eating and exercise. For an analysis of metabolic and health effects of weight-regulation practices in athletes, see Brownell, Steen, and Wilmore (1987). Ultimately, the decision to strive for an ideal range must be individually determined, preferably with the assistance of an exercise physiologist and the coach.

Provide Nutritional Education

Similarly, nutritional education and counseling are important aspects of athletes' training. This knowledge has been improving among the athletic world such that most competitors no longer eat steak and eggs a few hours before a competition. However, there is much more to be learned: "It has been said that there is no area of nutrition where faddism, misconceptions, and ignorance are more obvious than in athletics" (Leaf & Frisa, 1989, p. 1066). An abundance of research indicates that many athletes and coaches have limited or incorrect views on proper sport nutrition (Bedgood & Tuck, 1983; Benadat, Schwartz, & Wertzenfeld-Heller, 1989; Clark et al., 1988; Douglas & Douglas, 1984; Koszewski & Strong, 1991; Perron & Endres, 1985; Tilgner & Schiller, 1989; Wolf, Wirth, & Lohman, 1979).

Although accurate and useful information can be obtained from a variety of sources (e.g., nutritionists, dieticians, and written materials), Koszeski and Strong (1991) found that most athletes unsuccessfully turn to their peers or coaches for nutritional advice. It is imperative that the consulting sport psychologist working with eating and weight-management strategies be knowledgeable of general nutritional principles, sport nutrition, and weight management and, as well, have a good working relationship with a qualified nutritionist. The sport psychologist should not be expected to work with the individual athlete to plan dietary intake. However, the consultant should be able to refer a coach or athlete to the proper source for this information; for example, a nutritionist or the

Coaches Guide to Nutrition and Weight Control (Eisenman, Johnson, & Benson, 1990). Athletic personnel and athletes would also benefit greatly from attending a workshop on sport nutrition and weight control. This could include such topics as carbohydrate loading, precompetition meals, water and electrolyte replacement, and so on.

Promote Sensitivity to Weight Issues

In the prevention of pathogenic weight-loss practices and eating disorders in athletes, it is important to help athletic personnel become more sensitive to issues of weight control and dieting. This might involve working with them to be more tactful about weight issues (e.g., eliminating statements such as "You're looking a little heavy today"). The coach and staff must understand that they have a powerful influence on athletes: Some athletes will go to extremes to please coaches. Therefore, it is useful to present to the coach and staff some examples of unhelpful and potentially dangerous weight-management practices, including

- group weigh-ins,
- arbitrary weight or body-composition goals,
- punishment for not making weight,
- careless or unfeeling remarks about weight issues,
- always associating weight loss with enhanced performance, and
- minimizing the detrimental and unhealthy effects of rapid weight gain or loss.

Facilitate Healthy Weight Management

Attention has increased recently on eating disorders in sport, and there has been a corresponding increase in the availability of educational resources. For example, the NCAA has produced an informative set of three videos and supporting educational information on eating disorders in sport (National Collegiate Athletic Association, 1989). Ron Thompson and Roberta Sherman from the Bloomington Center for Counseling and Human Development recently wrote a volume on *Helping Athletes with Eating Disorders* (1993), and other authors have presented a variety of model systems for managing eating problems in athletic settings (Grandjean, 1992; Ryan, 1992). Much has been learned about behavioral approaches to the management of weight and the effectiveness of a variety of weight-management strategies (Kirschenbaum, 1992). Perhaps most important for education efforts aimed at changing attitudes, much has been learned about

the effects of unhealthy weight-loss methods on sporting performance (Thompson & Sherman, 1993, chapter 4).

It will probably take some time to change ingrained and perhaps institutionalized attitudes toward weight in the sport setting (Lopiano & Zotos, 1992), but health-care professionals must take the lead in emphasizing the relationship between body type and weight, the realities of optimal body composition and weight for effective performance, and the nature of healthy and effective weight-management strategies that can be employed by athletes and coaches. Only through such efforts will negative examples (like the cases of Karl and the university team described earlier) become rarities rather than all-too-common encounters.

CONCLUSION

Eating disorders and their subclinical manifestations exist all too frequently in the sport environment. Given this fact, in-service training regarding eating disorders is essential for athletic personnel. In the case of Karl, many problems might have been prevented if his coach had displayed more awareness of the impact of his weight-related comments on the athlete. Because early detection and referral is associated with a more successful treatment outcome, the importance of increasing the awareness of sport personnel concerning these issues cannot be overemphasized. It might be particularly important for male coaches of female athletes to understand the relevant issues that have been raised in this chapter. The training program should be for the entire athletic and support staff (coaches, trainers, physicians, weight coaches, psychologists, and all other associates), and should have as its emphasis prevention, recognition, and referral. As Murphy (1991) has described, a critical ingredient for successful interventions in the sport world is the presence of a clear plan of action and the readiness of a team of qualified personnel to respond to problems. The coach's active involvement is, from experience, probably the most critical ingredient in the success of any such program. The coach's influence in the sport environment is such that a clear communication to athletes that "this is important" will result in active participation, whereas the opposite message that "this should be ignored" will ensure the program's failure. Education and prevention efforts should also include a realization that information alone will probably not change attitudes or behaviors. The inclusion of other behavior-change methods (such as athlete involvement in education, mentor programs, and peer counseling involvement) should be considered in efforts to prevent eating disorders in sports.

There is still much that is not known about the development and maintenance of eating disorders in the sport setting. We hope that research efforts will continue to address these issues as a matter of urgency for the health, well-being, and safety of athletes everywhere.

REFERENCES

American Psychiatric Association. (1987). *Diagnostic and statistical manual of mental disorders* (3rd ed., rev.). Author: Washington, DC.

Bedgood, B.L., & Tuck, M.B. (1983). Nutrition knowledge of high school athletic coaches in Texas. *Journal of the American Dietetic Association*, **83**, 672-677.

Benadat, D., Schwartz, M., & Wertzenfeld-Heller, D. (1989). Nutrient intake in young, highly competitive gymnasts. *Journal of the American Dietetic Association*, **89**, 401-403.

Bickelhaupt, S. (1989, September 13). The thin game. *Boston Globe*, 73.

Bickford, B. (1990). Eating disorders: Treatment and prevention. *Scholastic Coach*, **59**, 86-88.

Black, D.R., & Burckes-Miller, M.E. (1988). Male and female college students: Use of anorexia nervosa and bulimia nervosa weight loss methods. *Research Quarterly for Exercise and Sport*, **59**, 252-256.

Blackburn, G.L., Wilson, G.T., Kanders, B.S., Stein, L.J., Lavin, P.T., Adler, J., & Brownell, K.D. (1989). Weight cycling: The experience of human dieters. *American Journal of Clinical Nutrition*, **49**, 1105-1109.

Blinder, B.J., Chaitin, B.F., & Goldstein, R. (1988). *The eating disorders: Medical and psychological bases of diagnosis and treatment*. New York: PMA.

Brownell, K.D., & Foreyt, J.P. (1986). *Handbook of eating disorders: Physiology, psychology, and treatment*. New York: Basic Books.

Brownell, K.D., & Rodin, J. (1992). *Prevalence of eating disorders in athletes*. In K.D. Brownell, J. Rodin, & J.H. Wilmore (Eds.), *Eating, body weight, and performance in athletes* (pp. 128-145). Malvern, PA: Lea & Febiger.

Brownell, K.D., Rodin, J., & Wilmore, J.H. (Eds.) (1992). *Eating, body weight, and performance in athletes*. Malvern, PA: Lea & Febiger.

Brownell, K.D., Steen, S.N., & Wilmore, J.H. (1987). Weight regulation practices in athletes: Analysis of metabolic and health effects. *Medicine and Science in Sports and Exercise*, **19**(6), 546-556.

Burckes-Miller, M.E., & Black, D.R. (1988a). Eating disorders: A problem in athletics? *Health Education*, 22-25.

Burckes-Miller, M.E., & Black, D.R. (1988b). Male and female college athletes: Prevalence of anorexia nervosa and bulimia nervosa. *Athletic Training*, **23**, 137-140.

Chiodo, J., & Latimer, P.R. (1983). Vomiting as a learned weight-control technique in bulimia. *Journal of Behavior Therapy and Experimental Psychiatry*, **14**, 131-135.

Clark, N., Nelson, M., & Evans, W. (1988). Nutrition education for elite female runners. *Physician and Sportsmedicine*, **16**, 124-136.

Davis, R., Olmsted, M.P., & Rockert, W. (1990). Brief group psychoeducation for bulimia nervosa: Assessing the clinical significance of change. *Journal of Consulting and Clinical Psychology*, **58**, 882-885.

Dick, R.W. (1993). Eating disorders in NCAA athletics programs: Replication of a 1990 study. *NCAA Sports Sciences Education Newsletter*, 3-4.

Douglas, P.D., & Douglas, J.G. (1984). Nutrition knowledge and food practices of high school athletes. *Journal of the American Dietetic Association*, **84**, 1198-1202.

Eating disorders in young athletes: A round table (1985). *Physician and Sportsmedicine*, **13**, 88-106.

Eisenman, P.A., Johnson, S.C., & Benson, J.E. (1990). *Coaches guide to nutrition and weight control* (2nd ed.). Champaign, IL: Leisure Press.

Fernandez, R.C. (1984). Group therapy of bulimia. In P.S. Powers & R.C. Fernandez (Eds.), *Current treatment of anorexia nervosa and bulimia* (pp. 277-291). New York: Karger.

Garfinkel, P. (1991, May). *Treatment issues in eating disorders*. Invited address presented at the Second Annual Rocky Mountain Conference on Eating Disorders, Colorado Springs.

Garfinkel, P.E., Garner, D.M., & Goldbloom, D.S. (1987). Eating disorders: Implications for the 1990's. *Canadian Journal of Psychiatry*, **32**, 624-631.

Garner, D.M., & Garfinkel, P.E. (1979). The eating attitudes test: An index of the symptoms of anorexia nervosa. *Psychological Medicine*, **9**, 273-279.

Garner, D.M., & Garfinkel, P. (1985). *Handbook of psychotherapy for anorexia nervosa and bulimia*. New York: Guilford Press.

Garner, D.M., Olmsted, M.P., & Polivy, J. (1983). *Eating Disorders Inventory*. Odessa, FL: Psychological Assessment Resources.

Garner, D.M., Rockert, W., Olmsted, M.P., Johnson, C., & Coscina, D.V. (1985). Psychoeducational principles in the treatment of bulimia and anorexia nervosa. In D.M. Garner & P.E. Garfinkel (Eds.), *Handbook of psychotherapy for anorexia nervosa and bulimia* (pp. 513-572). New York: Guilford Press.

Grandjean, A.C. (1992). The dilemma of making weight. *The U.S. Olympic Team Experience: A Model for Sports Medicine*. Brochure published by the United States Olympic Committee, Colorado Springs, CO.

Gross, M. (1986). Anorexia nervosa: Treatment perspectives. In F.E. Larocca (Ed.), *Eating disorders: Effective care and treatment* (pp. 1-10). St. Louis: Ishiyaku Euro-America.

Gustafson, D. (1989). Eating behaviors of women college athletes. *Melpomene*, **8**(3), 11-13.

Guthrie, S.R. (1986). The prevalence and development of eating disorders within a selected intercollegiate athlete population (Doctoral dissertation, Ohio State University, 1985). *Dissertation Abstracts International*, **46**, 3649A.

Halliburton, S., & Sanford, S. (1989a, July 30). Battle with bulimia tarnishes Cohen's golden world. *Austin American-Statesman*, pp. D1, D8.

Halliburton, S., & Sanford, S. (1989b, July 30). Being thin turns grim at Texas. *Austin American-Statesman*, pp. D1, D8.

Halliburton, S., & Sanford, S. (1989c, July 31). Making weight becomes torture for UT swimmers. *Austin American-Statesman*, pp. D1, D7.

Harris, M.B., & Greco, D. (1990). Weight control and weight concern in competitive female gymnasts. *Journal of Sport and Exercise Psychology*, **12**, 427-433.

Huerta, E. (1982). Group therapy for anorexia patients. In M. Gross (Ed.), *Anorexia nervosa: A comprehensive approach* (pp. 111-118). Lexington, MA: Collamore Press.

Johnson, C. (1991). *Psychodynamic treatment of anorexia nervosa and bulimia*. New York: Guilford Press.

Johnson, C., & Connors, M. (1987). *The etiology and treatment of bulimia nervosa: A biopsychosocial perspective*. New York: Basic Books.

Johnson, C., & Pure, D.L. (1986). Assessment of bulimia: A multidimensional model. In K.D. Brownell & J.P. Foreyt (Eds.), *Handbook of eating disorders: Physiology, psychology, and treatment* (pp. 405-449). New York: Basic Books.

Kirschenbaum, D.S. (1992). Elements of effective weight control programs: Implications for exercise and sport psychology. *Journal of Applied Sport Psychology*, **4**, 77-93.

Klesges, R.C. (1983). An analysis of body image distortions in a nonpatient population. *International Journal of Eating Disorders*, **2**, 35-41.

Koszewski, W.M., & Strong, D. (1991). *Dietary beliefs and practices among college student athletes*. Unpublished manuscript.

Leaf, A., & Frisa, K.B. (1989). Eating for health or for athletic performance. *American Journal of Clinical Nutrition*, **49**, 1066-1069.

Lopiano, D.A., & Zotos, C. (1992). Modern athletics: The pressure to perform. In K.D. Brownell, J. Rodin, & J.H. Wilmore (Eds.), *Eating, body weight, and performance in athletes* (pp. 275-292). Malvern, PA: Lea & Febiger.

Maher, M.S. (1984). Group therapy for anorexia nervosa. In P.S. Powers & R.C. Fernandez (Eds.), *Current treatment of anorexia nervosa and bulimia* (pp. 265-276). New York: Karger.

Miller, S.G. (1984). Family therapy of the eating disorders. In P.S. Powers & R.C. Fernandez (Eds.), *Current treatment of anorexia nervosa and bulimia* (pp. 92-112). New York: Karger.

Minuchin, S., & Fishman, M. (1981). *Family therapy techniques*. Cambridge, MA: Harvard University Press.

Murphy, S.M. (1991). Behavioral considerations. In R.C. Cantu & L.J. Micheli (Eds.), *ACSM's guidelines for the team physician* (pp. 252-265). Malvern, PA: Lea & Febiger.

National Collegiate Athletic Association. (1989). *Nutrition and eating disorder in collegiate athletics* (Video). Author: Kansas City, MO.

Otis, C.L. (1993, March). *The active woman: Special concerns*. Paper presented at the American College of Sports Medicine Team Physician Course, Lake Buena Vista, FL.

Pasman, L., & Thompson, J.K. (1988). Body image and eating disturbance in obligatory runners, obligatory weightlifters, and sedentary individuals. *International Journal of Eating Disorders*, **7**, 759-769.

Perron, M.S., & Endres, J. (1985). Knowledge, attitudes and dietary practices of female athletes. *Journal of the American Dietetic Association*, **85**, 573.

Porcello, L.A. (1984). A practical guide to fad diets. *Clinical Sports Medicine*, **3**, 723-729.

Powers, P.S. (1984). Multidisciplinary approach to treatment and evaluation. In P.S. Powers & R.C. Fernandez (Eds.), *Current treatment of anorexia nervosa and bulimia* (pp. 166-179). New York: Karger.

Reece, B.A., & Gross, M. (1982). A comprehensive milieu program for treatment of anorexia nervosa. In M. Gross (Ed.), *Anorexia nervosa: A comprehensive approach* (pp. 103-109). Lexington, MA: Collamore Press.

Rosen, L.W., & Hough, D.O. (1988). Pathogenic weight-control behaviors of female college gymnasts. *Physician and Sportsmedicine*, **16**, 141-144.

Rosen, L.W., McKeag, D.B., Hough, D.O., & Curley, V. (1986). Pathogenic weight-control behavior in female athletes. *Physician and Sportsmedicine*, **14**, 79-86.

Ryan, R. (1992). Management of eating problems in athletic settings. In K.D. Brownell, J. Rodin, & J.H. Wilmore (Eds.), *Eating, body weight, and performance in athletes* (pp. 344-362). Malvern, PA: Lea & Febiger.

Sanford, S., & Halliburton, S. (1989, July 31). Rhodenbaugh's path winds through secret world of bulimia. *Austin American-Statesman*, pp. D1, D7.

Stuart, R.B., Mitchell, C., & Jensen, J.A. (1981). Therapeutic options in the management of obesity. In L.A. Bradley & C.K. Prokop (Eds.), *Medical psychology: A new perspective* (pp. 321-353). New York: Academic Press.

Thompson, R.A. (1987). Management of the athlete with an eating disorder: Implications for the sport management team. *Sport Psychologist*, **1**, 114-126.

Thompson, R., & Sherman, R. (1993). *Helping athletes with eating disorders*. Champaign, IL: Human Kinetics.

Thornton, J.S. (1990). Feast or famine: Eating disorders in athletes. *Physician and Sportsmedicine*, **18**, 116-122.

Tilgner, S.A., & Schiller, M.R. (1989). Dietary intakes of female college athletes: The need for nutrition education. *Journal of the American Dietetic Association*, **89**, 967-969.

Webster, S., Rutt, R., & Weltman, A. (1990). Physiological effects of a weight loss regimen practiced by college wrestlers. *Medicine and Science in Sports and Exercise*, **22**, 229.

Wilmore, J.H. (1992). Body weight and body composition. In K.D. Brownell, J. Rodin, & J.H. Wilmore (Eds.), *Eating, body weight, and performance in athletes* (pp. 77-93). Malvern, PA: Lea & Febiger.

Wolf, E.M., Wirth, J.C., & Lohman, T.G. (1979). Nutritional practices of coaches in the Big Ten. *Physician and Sportsmedicine*, **7**, 112-124.

Yalom, I.D. (1985). *The theory and practice of group psychotherapy*. New York: Basic Books.

Yeager, K.K., Agostini, R., Nattiv, A., & Drinkwater, B. (1993). The female athlete triad: Disordered eating, amenorrhea, osteoporosis. *Medicine and Science in Sports and Exercise*, **25**, 775-777.

Zuckerman, D.M., Colby, A., Ware, N.C., & Lazerson, J.S. (1986). The prevalence of bulimia among college students. *American Journal of Public Health*, **76**, 1135-1137.

CHAPTER 14

TRANSITIONS IN COMPETITIVE SPORT: MAXIMIZING INDIVIDUAL POTENTIAL

Shane M. Murphy, PhD
United States Olympic Committee

The issue that helping professionals most commonly encounter in the sport setting is how athletes will plan for and cope with life after competitive sport. Unlike such issues as injury or drug use, which many athletes avoid, all athletes must consider the prospect of ending their competitive athletic careers. The helping professional might encounter this issue in a variety of forms, often depending on the athlete's developmental stage. A teenage athlete might face the decision of whether to enter college or to put academic aspirations on hold while spending 2 intensively athletic years trying to make an Olympic team. A young adult might struggle with a relationship, facing conflicting input from his spouse, who wants to begin a family and structure some stability in their relationship, and from his own desires to chase his dream of professional baseball, even though it means an almost nomadic existence with a low income level. A young tennis player might be faced with a variety of choices about what career path to follow after a knee injury forces abandonment of a lucrative career as

a tennis professional on the tour. Difficult choices in the career area are universally encountered by athletes, but they are not always acknowledged and they are not dealt with in the same way by everyone. The following case examples offer two styles of coping with career transition issues.

■ *THE CASE OF DARIUS* ■

Darius grew up in a suburb of Los Angeles, the son of middle-class parents who encouraged his natural athletic interests. Blessed with great speed and excellent hand-eye coordination, Darius excelled at a variety of sports, but his lack of size prevented him from a long career in his two favorite activities, football and basketball. By age 16, he had played competitive baseball, basketball, football, tennis, and soccer and had tried out such sports as surfing, golf, bowling, cycling, and skiing. In his junior year at high school, a friend of his father encouraged him to attend a local field hockey club, where Darius's rapid skill development brought him to the attention of a national-level development coach. Darius was offered a spot at a national coaching clinic on the East Coast and subsequently was selected for a national junior development squad.

In his senior year, Darius was offered the chance to enroll in an exchange program with an Australian high school; this included a place on a local Australian hockey-club team. He made the trip, played a lot of field hockey, and made many contacts in the Australian field-hockey community. When he returned to the United States, he again attended a national training camp, and this time the national coach selected him for one of four scholarship spots with the national team, whose members lived and trained at the Olympic Training Center in San Diego. Once again, Darius took advantage of the opportunity and moved to San Diego. He enrolled part-time in a local college, studying engineering, and in his second year got a part-time job as an assistant with a local construction firm.

From the time he moved to San Diego, Darius impressed coaches and officials with his aggressive approach to career development. As he traveled around the country on competition trips, Darius handed out his personal card to many people he came in contact with, including sponsors, supporters, and sport officials. The inexpensive card simply read Darius McKee, Member of the U.S. National Field-Hockey Team, and gave his address and telephone number. He also collected hundreds of business cards from these contacts and stored them alphabetically in a plastic folder. Those who met him at after-game dinners or sponsor-related functions remember that he was never afraid to ask questions and that he showed a great interest in the careers of those he met, often questioning them at length about the type of work they did and how they got started in their businesses.

After 3 years of hard work, Darius won a spot on the United States Olympic team, one of just 18 athletes to earn that honor in field hockey. The team played hard at the Games, but lost four matches and tied one, finishing 11th in the field of 12. The coach, full of praise for Darius, who scored four goals in the tournament, told the press that "if I had another 10 who worked as hard as Darius, we would have won a couple of those close games." Taking 2 months off after the Olympics, Darius, after a long talk with the national coach, decided to end his national team career in field hockey. Darius believed that he had reached the level of excellence he had aimed for in the sport and that his Olympic experience had been a tremendous bonus for him. His coach asked him to stay on for 4 years, but supported Darius's decision to go back to school full-time and complete his engineering degree.

The job market was tight when Darius finished his degree, but he landed a good job with the second company he interviewed with. A deciding factor in his final interview with the company was his response to a question posed to all three final candidates. Minutes before a meeting with the selection panel, Darius was given a blank piece of paper and asked to "fill up this sheet by writing down as much about yourself as you can." After completing sections about his education, job experience, and career goals, Darius was still faced with a blank two inches at the bottom of the paper. For a moment he was stuck, but then he wrote down the name of every state and country he had visited during his extensive field-hockey tours. When he sat down to meet with the panel, the first questions they asked were about some of the more exotic locales he had mentioned on his interview sheet.

After 6 productive years with that firm, Darius, now married, left to start his own consulting business with a colleague in Los Angeles. After a rough start-up year, they experienced great success and Darius displayed many of the hard-work skills he had shown in field hockey years before. He was very proud of his hockey career and at the bottom of his business card was a line that read Member of the USA 1976 Olympic Team, Field Hockey.

As he and his partner expanded their business, many of the contacts Darius had made in his field-hockey years and had kept in touch with proved to be valuable sources of information about a variety of business opportunities. Darius became a well-known, active member of his local community, and after the birth of his first child he successfully ran for mayor of the suburb in which he lived, becoming the first black mayor of that community. When young people ask him for advice on how to get started in a career, he tells them to "pay attention to all the great lessons you learn in sport. My sporting career helped me out a great deal, and it can help you out, too, if you keep your eyes and ears open."

■ THE CASE OF ELEANOR ■

Eleanor began her figure skating career at age 6, after she had watched a graceful young American win the gold medal at Grenoble. She showed remarkable aptitude on the ice, and her coach encouraged her parents to enroll her in individual lessons in addition to the group classes in which she had started. By age 10, she was competing successfully at the national level in novice competitions, and her coach admitted to her parents that for Eleanor's skating career to advance, she would need a more experienced coach. Eleanor and her mother moved to a city in the Rocky Mountains that was home to a prestigious international figure skating coach, while her father and two siblings stayed in the large midwestern city she had grown up in.

In high school, Eleanor's skating goals took precedence over everything else. Her school allowed her to design a special school day so she could practice in the morning, attend 3 hours of concentrated schooling, and get 4 hours of practice in during the afternoon. Because Eleanor could not take enough credits on this schedule, she fell behind her age-group peers in grade level, but her skating career

continued to rocket. At age 15, she became national junior champion, and the next year found her competing with the other senior women for a spot on the Olympic team in two years.

The year before the Olympics, Eleanor stopped going to school completely and kept up her education with only some correspondence classes. She had very few friends outside of skating, but her national success had taken her on trips to such faraway places as Australia and Belgium, and she was very satisfied at the outcome of her choices. Then, in the first major international competition of the Olympic season, she fell on a triple axel and broke a bone in her ankle. She had to undergo extensive rehabilitation to make it back on the ice for the Olympic trials 4 months later, but she showed her usual tenacity and entered the competition. She was in first place after the figures section of the competition, but in the short program, she fell to sixth place after falling on her weak ankle three times. Devastated, Eleanor withdrew from competition and scarcely noticed the Olympics 3 weeks later as her competitors proudly represented their country at the brand-new Olympic skating facility.

After 6 months of indecision, Eleanor turned professional, deciding that 4 years was too long to wait for the uncertainty of another chance at an Olympic team. As an attractive and exciting skater, Eleanor was popular at ice shows across the country, and she earned more than $100,000 in her first year as a professional. Yet 2 years after breaking her ankle, she still felt confused and depressed. She experimented with a variety of drugs and often used cocaine at the parties following the ice shows. Because she had gained 10 lb (4.5 kg) over the 2 years, she underwent liposuction to restore her "original" figure. Eleanor believed that she might be attracted to a career as a professional in law or health care, but without even her high school diploma she didn't know where to begin. When she confided in her old coach at a tour stop in her city, the coach recommended a local psychologist who had helped several skaters in the community. It took Eleanor another 6 months before she telephoned the psychologist and made her first appointment.

These two case studies illustrate how the same basic process, transferring from a competitive sport career to another career area, can be experienced in different ways. Many of the issues raised in these case studies will be addressed later in this chapter. The case of Darius, in particular, shows how high-level sports participation can play an important role in optimizing career opportunities. This chapter examines from a number of perspectives the transition process when leaving high-level competitive sport and analyzes ways in which helping professionals can assist athletes in making such transitions effectively.

The chapter is organized into four main sections. First, an attempt is made to understand the motivation of elite athletes. To help athletes who are leaving elite competition, it is necessary to understand what this transition means to them and what they feel they are leaving behind. Next, the nature of the transition process in sport is examined, and typical transition scenarios are presented. Then, factors related to optimal transition are presented. Lastly, several alternatives for assisting athletes in making effective transitions in sport are offered.

PARTICIPATION MOTIVATION IN ELITE ATHLETES

Elite athletes have an extensive history of socialization into the sport role (Ames, 1984), and during their competitive careers most have as their central identity the role of athlete. Leaving competitive sport means that they must adapt to viewing themselves in other roles and realizing that they will no longer be identified as athletes (although many develop an identity of ex-athlete). In helping athletes who are undergoing transition from sport, it is important to understand the athlete identity and the changes that result when this identity is altered.

A large part of the athlete identity can be understood in terms of the motivation of elite athletes. That is, what reasons lead athletes to devote so many resources to developing excellence in sport, and what factors continue to encourage them to participate in high-level sports when many of their cohort have left competition? A large literature exists on participation motivation in sport, and a consistently clear picture has emerged of the motivation of athletes (Gould, 1987a). One of the more thorough studies of elite athletes and their participation motivation was conducted by Kesend and Murphy (1989). They studied athletes in training for the Olympic Games and used an interview-and-qualitative-analysis methodology to identify the major motivational themes expressed by these elite athletes (Kesend, Perna, & Murphy, 1993). These are the main motives these athletes identified as encouraging them to participate in sport during their careers:

1. Perceived competence
   - Measurement of skill
   - Improvement of skill
2. Intrinsic motivation
   - Fun
   - Drive to achieve
3. Recognition
4. The sport
5. Self-development
6. Affiliation and life opportunities
7. Health, fitness, and activity
8. Overcoming adversity
9. Turning points in life
10. Altruism or idealism

Similar participation motivation themes have been identified in other research studies (Scanlan, Stein, & Ravizza, 1989). An examination of these themes indicates the central place of sport in the elite athlete's life and suggests the difficulty in leaving this high-level participation behind. If sport is satisfying because it enables a person to develop and demonstrate competence, because it provides a high level of intrinsic motivation, because it offers the athlete opportunities for social recognition, because is it fun, and because it provides many opportunities to develop satisfying social relationships, then it is likely that the athlete will seek to satisfy these motivational needs in other life areas, including work, on cessation of competitive sport involvement. People who can plan career alternatives that are also motivating are likely to better adjust to competitive sport cessation than those who cannot find ways to replace the role of sport in their lives.

A large literature exists on career counseling (Bolles, 1992; Sinetar, 1987), but much less has been published on the career counseling that might be provided to athletes in transition (Baillie, 1993; Petitpas, Danish, McKelvain, & Murphy, 1992). The career counselor or helping professional who is assisting athletes in transition must first understand the athletes' perspectives and the role sport has played in their lives. Motivational issues that are likely to impact the transition process must be identified. A rich literature exists to help the consultant understand the drives and motivations of elite athletes, but each individual has unique issues in the transition process.

Society has an ambivalent attitude toward the superstar gymnast who retires at age 18 with lucrative endorsement opportunities, or the professional athlete who retires at age 30 after earning many millions playing a sport that most people participate in for fun. Until recently, there has been little to guide us in understanding these unique experiences. The next section examines the literature that has attempted to describe the nature of the transition experience for athletes.

THE NATURE OF THE TRANSITION PROCESS

Two extremes of the reaction to leaving sport are provided in a study by Baillie (1992), who surveyed 260 elite and professional athletes concerning their experiences in leaving sport. The responses of two United States Olympians clearly demonstrate the wide range of possible responses to leaving high-level competition:

. . . you assume that once the athlete has retired from *their* sport they have retired from *all* sport. I haven't touched an oar since retirement, but I do a zillion other sports, some competitively, and I work on a program that takes athletes overseas to coach in black townships in South Africa. I doubt any athlete ever retires from sport, just from *their* sport.

Retirement from competition was . . . frustrating because 1988 was to be my best year, but illness prevented that (and an injury). . . . The only thing I truly regret is that I did not jump off the building in Seoul as I had contemplated every night. All I had to do was slide six inches further forward, but didn't. (Baillie, 1992, p. 157)

On the one hand, leaving high-level competitive sport can be an experience that opens up many avenues for athletes, allowing them to try new career paths and explore new opportunities. As the first athlete points out, sport can still play an important role in the athlete's life even when elite competition has ended. On the other hand, leaving elite competition can be a confusing and depressing experience, especially when the athlete has unfinished business in sport or when the future is filled with doubt and uncertainty. Sinclair and Orlick (1993) surveyed 200 retired Canadian athletes and found that athletes who had achieved their sport-related goals tended to feel more satisfied with their present life than those who had not accomplished their goals. Pearson and Petitpas (1990) examined the transition process and predicted that six factors would make the process most difficult for athletes:

- identity strongly and exclusively based on athletic performance
- a great gap between level of aspiration and level of ability
- little experience with the same or similar transitions
- behavioral or emotional deficits that limit the ability to adapt to change
- limited supportive relationships
- the need to deal with the transition in a context that lacks the emotional and material resources that could be helpful

Other writers who have tried to predict the natural course of the transition experience from elite sport have had a difficult time because the experience is unlike other experiences to which it has commonly been compared, such as the retirement from work or the experience of loss from a death (Rosenberg, 1981). Unlike the typical retirement from work, the athlete who retires from competitive sport still has many productive career years left. And although the loss of the athlete identity might be compared to the loss of someone close through death, the athlete still has time to forge a new identity by building on the old one, a process dissimilar to the experience of loss through a death. Such differences have led theorists to criticize attempts to use social gerontological or thanatological theories to describe the sport transition process (Blinde & Greendorfer, 1985). They argue that such theories are too limiting

and that attempts to explain the sport transition process must be developmentally based, focusing on the socialization experience of the athlete, the nature of the transition, the reaction of others, the development of coping resources to handle the transition, and the development of new individual roles.

The effects of the transition out of sport on elite or very competitive athletes have been examined in many studies. If this process is indeed difficult for athletes, then it can be hypothesized that they will show signs of psychological distress after retiring from sport or that their adjustment to new careers will not be effective. One of the first studies to examine this question was conducted by Mihovilovic (1968). He surveyed 44 former first-league players from the Yugoslavian soccer league about the end of their soccer careers and subsequent adjustment. His results indicated that 95% of the athletes ended their careers involuntarily, due to age, injury, or other factors. In 52% of cases, players reported that their career end was sudden. Mihovilovic found that if a player had no other profession on retirement, then the career ending was painful, marked by feelings of frustration and conflict. He also found that for many of the players, their circle of friends diminished after retirement. Mihovilovic concluded with several suggestions from these players as to how their retirement process could have been structured to lessen the negative aspects. These include giving players increased responsibilities during their playing careers and continuing to participate in sports on a recreational basis.

A variety of other researchers since Mihovilovic have studied other groups of athletes undergoing transition out of sport (Allison & Meyer, 1988; Blann & Zaichowsky, 1986; Haerle, 1975; Koukouris, 1991; Reynolds, 1981). Ogilvie and Taylor (1992) provide an excellent summary of the literature on career transitions in sport. Several of these studies demonstrate that the transition process is not automatically distressing. Allison and Meyer, for example, found that 50% of the 28 retired female tennis professionals they surveyed expressed relief at being off the tour. All the studies, however, indicated that at least some of the elite athletes experienced difficulties at some stage of the transition process, such as Allison and Meyer's finding that 30% of the tennis professionals described feeling a loss of identity after cessation of tour play. Most of the researchers described changes that the athletes would like to see in the transition process, such as more organizational support from the sporting body involved (Blann & Zaichowsky, 1986) or a more gradually phased retirement process, such as that described by Mihovilovic (1968). In the comprehensive study mentioned earlier of 260 elite and professional athletes (Baillie, 1992), adjustment to the transition from competition was measured by such variables as level of family disruption, feelings of loss, acceptance of the situation, valuing new pursuits, and self-rated satisfaction with the transition process. Using these criteria, Baillie found that athletes tended to adjust better to the end of their sports career when they had

- retired by choice,
- accomplished their goals,
- been able to remain as involved in their sports as they would like,
- completed college undergraduate programs, and
- been able to disengage from their sports at or shortly after the peak of their careers (1992, p. 78).

These factors suggest that certain aspects of the way the transition is structured have a large impact on the adjustment of the athlete. Some of the ways in which the transition process is structured are examined next.

STRUCTURAL FACTORS IN SPORT TRANSITIONS

A variety of circumstances might initiate the athlete's transition out of elite-level competitive sport. Some of the most common reasons for leaving high-level sport are choice, being cut, injury, and age.

Choice

Although the Mihovilovic (1968) study found that just 5% of the sample retired "voluntarily" (no desire to continue sport practice), the present author has found that many athletes make a decision at some stage of participation that the expected benefits of pursuing some other life activity outweigh the advantages of continued sporting involvement and so decide to leave. In a study of British teenagers participating in a fitness and sports campaign, White and Coakley (1986) argue that the term *dropout* is an inaccurate one when applied to youth sports participants. Instead of dropping out, most teenagers have simply decided that they want to do other things with their limited time than play sports. Elsewhere, Coakley has suggested that "one should not assume that retirement from competitive sport automatically creates problems until the experiences of former athletes are compared with the experiences of similar nonathletes" (1983, p. 9).

The case of Darius shows that making the choice to leave high-level sports participation can lead to great satisfaction and fulfillment in other areas. On the other hand, however, the case of Eleanor shows that a voluntary decision to make the transition out of elite sport can be a confusing and troubling one. Two important factors, gender and ethnicity, must be considered by the helping professional working with athletes in transition. Experience and preliminary research suggest that both factors can have a significant impact on the experience of the transition process, but little research exists clarifying the role of either factor.

The findings of Lee (1983) suggest that there are differences in the career expectations of athletes with different ethnic backgrounds. Specifically, Lee found that a significantly higher percentage of black high-school athletes than white high-school athletes expected to pursue a career in sports. Such differences might be a reflection of the promotion of different role models by society for blacks, whites, Asians, Hispanics, and others. Insufficient research exists to understand possible differences in career expectations for athletes from varying ethnic and cultural backgrounds, but such differences in this area should be kept in mind by the helping professional.

Gender issues also undoubtedly impact the transition experiences of athletes, particularly women. As documented by Diane Gill in chapter 9, many fewer professional career opportunities exist in sport for women than for men. Far fewer women than men are employed in intercollegiate athletic programs as coaches or administrators. This inequitable situation impacts women even earlier during their athletic careers, because there are many fewer athletic roles for women in sport, despite the passage of Title IX. As an example, an elite male basketball player can expect to make a financially rewarding career from basketball, but few opportunities exist in her sport for the elite female basketball star graduating from college. The issue of gender equity is being seriously examined by the NCAA and might have far-reaching consequences for collegiate and high-school athletics. The dearth of female coaches in elite coaching positions is so severe that the United States Olympic Committee is exploring institutional changes that might be implemented to enhance the quality and status of coaching, encouraging more female athletes to enter the coaching profession upon completion of their sport careers. Consultants working with female athletes should be especially aware of these issues concerning transition processes in sport.

Being Cut

In this author's experience, a common reason for an athlete to leave sport is being cut from

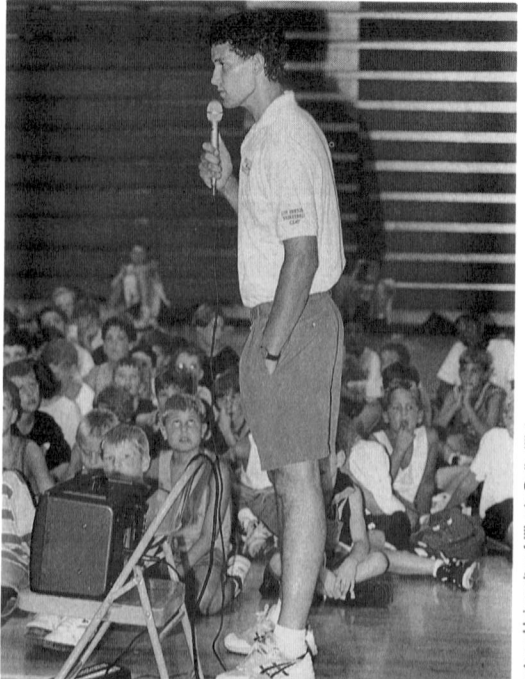

Courtesy University of Illinois Daily Illini

a team or failing to progress to the next higher level of competition. Studies have indicated that the loss rate of young athletes from organized sport is about 35% in any one year (Gould, 1987b). It is probable that the greatest problems arise when high expectations for continued athletic success clash with the reality of not moving forward to the next level of participation. For example, in the study mentioned earlier, Lee (1983) found that 36% of black and 14% of white high-school starting team athletes expected a career in sport. Contrast this figure with findings that in football, for example, less than 5% of high-school players receive college scholarships to play and, of these, only 1% ever have a chance to play in the National Football League (Ogilvie & Howe, 1986). If alternative plans are not made for the development of a career in an area other than sport, transition problems are likely to arise.

Athletes who have been unexpectedly cut and whose performance goals were never met in the sport are most likely to have negative emotions toward the transition process and perhaps develop bitterness or frustration toward the sporting groups with which they were involved. Such attitudes of frustration toward the political system in sport have been a common encounter in my experience with athletes who are having trouble adjusting to a transition. Another athlete from the Baillie study describes this attitude well:

> The most difficult part of retirement was the strange way your sport treats you. One minute everyone involved loves you and includes you. Then, you make a decision to leave the team and they don't even say goodbye. At least at university, they have a graduation ceremony. As an athlete we give a lot to the sport. They dictate all you do. . . . A happy retired athlete does a lot more good than a bitter one! (1992, p. 152)

Injury

Another factor that might lead to the unexpected and sudden transition out of sport for an athlete is illness or injury. Chapter 11 in this book describes the experience of injury for an athlete and discusses in some detail the possible emotional ramifications of the injury experience. If the injury is severe enough to force the athlete out of high-level competition or to raise doubts about the possibility of continued participation, then the athlete must begin to deal with the transition from sport in addition to coping with the process of rehabilitation from the injury. Unless the athlete has excellent coping resources, this dual challenge is likely to tax the athlete's ability to adjust. In a follow-up study of elite-level college athletes, Kleiber, Greendorfer, Blinde, and Samdahl (1987)

found that athletes who had left sport as the result of an injury had significantly lower ratings of current life satisfaction than other athletes.

Although in the case of Eleanor her injury did not lead directly to her retirement from skating, we can hypothesize that if she had had a chance to fulfill her Olympic dream her subsequent decisions and experiences might have been different. Thus injuries can impact later career adjustment in a variety of ways, not merely through sports cessation.

Age

The final reason to be considered here for sport termination is the decline in sport skills and capabilities that inevitably accompanies advancing years. Depending on the sport, this point might occur at a wide variety of ages. In women's gymnastics, for example, the onset of maturation and the rigors of years of training usually lead top-level competitors to quit around age 20 or earlier. International competitors can still be found achieving great success in their 40s in some sports, such as shooting or golf. Again, the reason for career transition is not as important as a person's reaction to that situation. Some athletes accept the decline in skills as obvious, make other plans, and complete a successful transition to another career. Others, however, fight the process, perhaps by training harder or more scientifically and, feeling that they have been betrayed by officials and coaches who do not recognize their continued skill level, might eventually be forced out of the sport by younger competitors.

Helping professionals should understand the transition experience from the athlete's viewpoint and recognize the variety of transition experiences commonly encountered by athletes. To help athletes achieve optimal transitions, it is also important to understand the change process in human behavior. Methods for achieving positive change are discussed next.

HELPING ATHLETES ACHIEVE OPTIMAL TRANSITIONS

As professional sports leagues have grown in size and popularity, as opportunities for elite athletes have increased, and as popular participation in many forms of organized sport has grown, there has been a development of interest in helping athletes refocus their lives in other areas once their competitive careers are finished. A variety of perspectives has been offered to help athletes in transition (Baillie, 1993; Chartrand & Lent, 1985; Danish, Petitpas, & Hale, 1990; Pearson & Petitpas, 1990; Skovholt, Morgan, & Negron-Cunningham, 1989). The perspective taken in both this chapter and in this book is that athletes can manage their sporting experience to achieve optimal satisfaction and that the role of helping professionals is to assist athletes maximize their potential and help those who are having difficulty with some aspect of the sport experience.

The author has had the opportunity to be involved in the process of helping elite athletes at all stages of transition through his participation in the United States Olympic Committee's Career Assistance Program for Athletes (CAPA), which has been described elsewhere (Petitpas et al., 1992). The author has participated in more than 20 career-planning workshops offered by CAPA and has personally counseled several hundred athletes struggling with transition in his role as sport psychologist at the Olympic Training Center in Colorado Springs. These experiences have led to the formulation of the model of transition assistance that is offered here. This model draws on the thoughts of

many career guidance experts who have been involved in CAPA and has as its basic philosophy the goal of enabling athletes to develop the skills necessary to gain a feeling of control over the transition process. Effective strategies to help athletes with transition are described next.

Career Planning Assistance

Athletes differ from most of their college-age peers in that their career planning must involve sports participation as their primary focus, whereas most of their cohort are focused primarily on education or work. As discussed previously, elite-level sports participation usually lasts a decade or less (although in some sports, such as golf, top-level participation can be lifelong) and can be abruptly terminated through injury or selection decisions. Thus education and work-related decisions are often put on hold until the sporting career is completed. This often leads athletes to feel that they have fallen behind their peers in the career development area, as they are often making critical education and work decisions in the mid-20s or later.

> Unfortunately, hockey was what I knew best, am most competent at, my 'job' since ten years old. To be like a 21-year-old entry-level business person with 34-, 35-, 36-year-olds is very difficult. The lack of preparation, training to succeed in difficult economic environments is a problem I am still overcoming. (Baillie, 1992, p. 166)

A common theme expressed by many athletes is that they desire to somehow make use of their sport experiences in their future careers. In a survey of career needs of 531 Olympic athletes, Hilliard (1988) found that 67% of respondents endorsed the statement, I would like to learn how to emphasize my special qualifications obtained through sports, whereas only 24% endorsed the statement, I need help preparing my resume. Athletes realize that they are special in their career needs and they desire this to be acknowledged in the transition process. The basics of career guidance planning are the same for athletes as for nonathletes, but the issues both of active sports participation interfering with education and work planning and of athletes' special experiences must be taken into account in helping athletes with career planning. The five major steps in career planning assistance are briefly described next.

Understanding the Career Process

At any point in their athletic careers, athletes can benefit from an understanding of the career process and the necessary steps involved in making well-informed career decisions. During many CAPA seminars, the concern has been expressed that planning for a life after sport will somehow distract the athlete from a focus on high-level achievement. Instead, many athletes have told us that planning for another career after sport lessens their anxiety about the transition process and allows them to concentrate more fully on sporting goals. As the case of Darius illustrates, such simple steps as making contacts throughout a sport career, making up business cards, and taking advantage of corporate sponsorship opportunities can set the stage for an easier transition when sport involvement ends.

Developing Job-Relevant Skills

A common concern heard from athletes at CAPA seminars is, "I'm just an athlete, I don't know how to do anything else." Actually, athletes learn many job-relevant skills during their years of sports participation. Skills learned in one area that can be used in another are called *transferable skills* by career

counselors. A large segment of the CAPA seminars is devoted to helping athletes realize the variety of skills they have learned through sports participation and how these skills can be targeted at potential employers in new career areas. Some examples of transferable skills commonly gained by playing sports are as follows:

- Performing optimally under pressure
- Communicating effectively with a team to reach group goals
- Setting weekly goals that lead to long-range goal attainment
- Accepting criticism and using it effectively
- Adhering to a strict schedule
- Competitiveness

Identifying Personal Career Needs

Self-knowledge is emphasized by career counselors as a critical aspect of developing a satisfying career (Bolles, 1992). Elite athletes often realize the special nature of their passionate involvement in sport and wonder about replacing it with another career.

- . . . The toughest part of the transition was finding a replacement for the challenge and the stimulation, not to mention financial security, that baseball afforded (Baillie, 1992, p. 162).

- . . . I really do believe that it's hard for all athletes to retire from a pro sport because [you miss] the thrill of playing in front of large crowds and the ego strokes of people wanting your autograph. It's very difficult to replace that rush of scoring a goal, blocking a shot to save a goal, or just being part of a winning team. It would be very difficult to replace that, no matter what we did afterwards (Baillie, 1992, p. 166).

Like others dealing with transition, athletes must identify their own skills and interests, the values they hold most strongly, and understand the influence their personality would have on a job. Then they can plan to develop new skills or try to find a career that they will find satisfying and fulfilling. It might be important to emphasize to elite athletes in transition that a job alone might not replace sport in satisfying all their needs, but that a career is made up of many elements besides a job (e.g., family, recreation, friends, community service). The combination of these various elements should provide the satisfaction and fulfillment athletes seek after transition.

Identifying Job-Related Opportunities

A critical reason that many people seek help from professional career counselors is that they do not understand the job marketplace or the many opportunities that exist there. Some athletes, like Darius, make use of their sporting careers to widen their exposure to various jobs and career possibilities. Others, like Eleanor, are so focused on their sport career that when it ends they feel ignorant about other opportunities that might exist. A critical ingredient of the CAPA seminars is providing training to athletes in such skills as informational interviewing, which they can apply in seeking information about new career possibilities.

Setting Career Goals

At some point, career guidance offered to athletes must move from the advice-giving stage to the action-oriented stage. Athletes are, in general, very goal oriented, so it is natural for them to set career-related goals that help them follow through on their objectives. However, because athletes are often very results-oriented, it can be helpful to emphasize that career management is a gradual process, and that often many opportunities must be pursued before a satisfying career after sport is developed. Some of the individual counseling strategies discussed in the next section can help in dealing with the common frustrations encountered in the job-finding or career-building stage of the transition.

Individual Counseling

Along with the special career needs of athletes just described, an optimal transition experience might depend on dealing with some of the emotional issues described earlier in this chapter. Athletes not only need to know how to find and get a job after sport, but they must also develop the skills and resources to manage the transition experience effectively. The helping professional working with the athlete in transition can be a great support by providing individual counseling concerning the following four issues.

Expansion of Self-Identity

The process of making an early commitment to a career identity and not exploring other alternatives has been called "identity foreclosure" by some writers (Marcia, 1978). Identity foreclosure can cause problems in adjustment if that identity is lost and the person has few alternatives for structuring a new identity. This process might be a common one for athletes, who are often rewarded for athletic excellence at an early age and are sometimes encouraged to de-emphasize educational and work opportunities in favor of developing athletic excellence. The case of Eleanor illustrates how confusing the end of a high-level career can be when a person has invested a great deal in developing an identity that is no longer functional. Eleanor thought of herself almost exclusively as a figure skater and found it difficult to even begin the sort of career planning (described above) necessary to move on to a new stage of her life.

When counseling the athlete who has a strong investment in the athlete identity, emphasizing the special qualities that the person has developed through sports experiences is a good way of building rapport and understanding. Counseling with Eleanor, for example, was a gradual process, as she saw herself as an overachiever who accomplished things on her own, without much support. It was, therefore, difficult for her to see herself as in need of counseling. Instead, it was emphasized that Eleanor had been a star in one field and would need to plan just as carefully and work just as hard to achieve success in another area. This approach paid off, as Eleanor became committed to the development of a new career and got her high-school diploma and enrolled in night school. Although she still skated occasionally to earn money, she felt confident enough to start a serious relationship and was able to kick the drug habit that she had found so egodystonic.

Emotional and Social Support

As is the case when dealing with other sources of stress, having support during the transition period can be the key to a successful career change. Athletes experiencing transition have emphasized the importance of support from their family and friends.

> Retirement is not an easy experience but I truly believe that my family and close friends made the difference for me. They really supported me. (Baillie, 1992, p. 152)

> Getting married sure made retirement easier for me. (Baillie, 1992, p. 157)

Some authors have argued that the very nature of sport makes it unlikely that athletes will seek emotional support themselves (Petitpas et al., 1992). This viewpoint contends that the athletic system reinforces individuals who can tough it out, so many athletes do not disclose their fears or vulnerabilities to others. Emotional support is often a major lack for such people. A counselor who encourages these people to share their feelings, providing a safe and supportive environment for the disclosure of emotions, can be a great source of support. In the CAPA seminars conducted by the USOC, it is striking how many participants commented on the relief they felt when they heard other athletes disclose feelings of insecurity and doubt about the transition process. Many athletes said they felt "alone" or "unique" in experiencing negative emotions associated with the transition.

There is often such a strong social network connected with sports participation that the athlete contemplating transition might be drawn back to sport because such social support exists. Many athletes interviewed by the author say they have retired several times during their sport career before making a final break with elite-level participation. The counselor can help the athlete identify and develop other sources of social support away from the sporting area. From the author's experience, athletes often feel better about their posttransition career if they have at least had the chance to explore other nonsport career possibilities.

Enhancement of Coping Skills

A person-environment relational view of stress sees the amount of stress experienced by a person as a product of the severity of the stressor and the extent of coping resources possessed by the person (Lazarus & Folkman, 1984). People high in coping resources will experience less stress than people with few coping strategies. Thus, whatever the cause of the transition experience, for elite athletes, the greater the variety of coping strategies at their disposal the less stress they will experience. An important part of the assistance the helping professional can provide athletes in transition is identifying athletes' coping skills, helping athletes apply their skills to the transition situation, and teaching athletes appropriate new coping skills.

Development of a Sense of Control

The major reasons identified for the cessation of an elite sport career are often outside the athlete's control (selection, injury, age). Even when they have voluntarily decided to retire from high-level sport, athletes might feel that the process is one over which they have little control. This sensed loss of control can be a frightening impediment to an optimal transition.

> Suddenly my life went from a structured, organized lifestyle where goals were predetermined to no structure and feeling at a loss as to which way to turn—a support system of guidance would have been very helpful. The decision to retire was my own and I have NO regrets. Nevertheless, there was a profound sense of loss and a feeling of being forgotten quickly. (Baillie, 1992, p. 150)

The feeling that you are in control of events, rather than events controlling you, has been called having an internal locus of control (Rotter, 1975), a feeling of competence (White, 1959), or having a sense of self-efficacy (Bandura, 1977). Experience with the CAPA seminars indicates that athletes who perceive themselves as having control are more likely to initiate actions that are likely to help their posttransition career development (e.g., prepare a resume, go on job interviews, actively build a network). The counselor can promote this sense of control in athletes by explaining the career development process, showing them the variety of transferable skills they possess, and helping them develop a plan for managing the transition process.

CONCLUSION

In this chapter I examined in detail the transition experience for the elite athlete. Helping professionals who offer guidance to athletes in this situation are encouraged to understand what sports participation and the transition out of sport mean to the elite athlete. The causes of transition from sport were described, as were the factors that have been identified as relating to optimal transition experiences. Lastly, ways were suggested to help athletes achieve optimal transitions to new careers.

Many athletes make the transition from high-level sport to the next stage of their lives with few problems and little distress. However, the opportunity to make an effective and satisfying transition to a new career should be afforded to all athletes. It is hoped that this chapter will help those professionals working with athletes to assist them in structuring an optimal transition experience. We can all benefit from helping such a high-achieving group of people use their extraordinary capabilities to the fullest.

REFERENCES

Allison, M.T., & Meyer, C. (1988). Career problems and retirement among elite athletes: The female tennis professional. *Sociology of Sport Journal, 5*, 212-222.

Ames, N.R. (1984, Winter). The socialization of women into and out of sports. *Journal of NAWDAC*, pp. 3-8.

Baillie, P. (1992). *Career transition in elite and professional athletes: A study of individuals in their preparation for and adjustment to retirement from competitive sports.* Unpublished doctoral dissertation, Virginia Commonwealth University, Richmond, VA.

Baillie, P. (1993). Understanding retirement from sports: Therapeutic ideas for helping athletes in transition. *The Counseling Psychologist, 21*, 399-410.

Bandura, A. (1977). Self-efficacy: Toward a unifying theory of behavioral change. *Psychological Review, 84*, 191-215.

Blann, W., & Zaichowsky, L. (1986). *Career/life transition needs of National Hockey League players.* Report prepared for the National Hockey League Players Association, Boston.

Blinde, E., & Greendorfer, S. (1985). A reconceptualization of the process of leaving the role of competitive athlete. *International Review of Sport Sociology, 20*, 87-94.

Bolles, R.N. (1992). *The 1992 what color is your parachute.* Berkeley, CA: Ten Speed Press.

Coakley, J. (1983). Leaving competitive sport: Retirement or rebirth? *Quest, 35*, 1-11.

Chartrand, J., & Lent, R. (1985). Sports counseling: Enhancing the development of the student-athlete. *Journal of Counseling & Development, 66*, 164-167.

Danish, S., Petitpas, A., & Hale, B. (1990). Sport as a context for developing competence. In T. Gullota, G. Adams, and R. Monteymar (Eds.), *Adolescent development: Interpersonal competence.* Elmsford, NY: Plenum Press.

Dubois, P.E. (1981). The youth sport coach as an agent of socialization: An exploratory study. *Journal of Sport Behavior, 4*, 95-107.

Gould, D. (1987a). Promoting positive sport experiences for children. In J. May & M. Asken (Eds.), *Sport psychology: The psychological health of the athlete.* New York: PMA.

Gould, D. (1987b). Understanding attrition in youth sports. In D. Gould & M. Weiss (Eds.), *Advances in pediatric sport sciences: Vol. 2. Behavioral issues* (pp. 61-85). Champaign, IL: Human Kinetics.

Haerle, R. (1975). Career patterns and career contingencies of professional baseball players: An occupational analysis. In D.W. Ball & J.W. Loy (Eds.), *Sport and social order* (pp. 461-519). Reading, MA: Addison-Wesley.

Hilliard, N. (1988). *The career counseling needs of Olympic and Pan-American athletes: A needs assessment survey.* Unpublished survey conducted for the United States Olympic Committee, Colorado Springs.

Kesend, O., & Murphy, S.M. (1989, August). *Participation motivation in elite athletes: A developmental perspective.* Paper presented at the 7th World Congress in Sport Psychology, Singapore.

Kesend, O., Perna, F., & Murphy, S. (1993). *The development of participation motivation in elite athletes.* Paper submitted for publication.

Kleiber, D., Greendorfer, S., Blinde, E., & Samdahl, D. (1987). Quality of exit from university sports and subsequent life satisfaction. *Sociology of Sport Journal, 4*, 28-36.

Koukouris, K. (1991). Disengagement of advanced and elite Greek male athletes from organized competitive sport. *International Review for the Sociology of Sport, 26*, 289-306.

Lazarus, R.S., & Folkman, S. (1984). *Stress, appraisal and coping*. New York: Springer.

Lee, C. (1983). An investigation of the athletic career expectations of high school student athletes. *Personnel and Guidance Journal*, **61**, 544-547.

Marcia, J.E. (1978). Identity foreclosure: A unique challenge. *Personnel and Guidance Journal*, **56**, 558-561.

Mihovilovic, M. (1968). The status of former sportsmen. *International Review of Sport Sociology*, **3**, 73-96.

Ogilvie, B., & Howe, M. (1986). The trauma of termination from athletics. In J.M. Williams (Ed.), *Applied sport psychology: Personal growth to peak performance* (pp. 365-382). Palo Alto, CA: Mayfield.

Ogilvie, B., & Taylor, J. (1992). Career termination issues among elite athletes. In R.N. Singer, M. Murphy, & L.K. Tennant (Eds.), *Handbook of research on sport psychology* (pp. 761-775). New York: Macmillan.

Pearson, R., & Petitpas, A. (1990). Transitions of athletes: Developmental and preventive perspectives. *Journal of Counseling & Development*, **69**, 7-10.

Petitpas, A., Danish, S., McKelvain, R., & Murphy, S. (1992). A career assistance program for elite athletes. *Journal of Counseling and Development*, **70**, 383-386.

Reynolds, M.J. (1981). The effects of sports retirement on the job satisfaction of the former football player. In S.L. Greendorfer & A. Yiannakis (Eds.), *Sociology of sport: Diverse perspectives* (pp. 127-137). Champaign, IL: Leisure Press.

Rosenberg, E. (1981). Gerontological theory and athletic retirement. In S.L. Greendorfer & A. Yiannakis (Eds.), *Sociology of sport: Diverse perspectives* (pp. 119-126). Champaign, IL: Leisure Press.

Rotter, J. (1975). Some problems and misconceptions related to the construct of internal versus external control of reinforcement. *Journal of Consulting and Clinical Psychology*, **43**, 56-57.

Scanlan, T.K., Stein, G.L., & Ravizza, K. (1989). An in-depth study of former elite figure skaters: II. Sources of enjoyment. *Journal of Sport and Exercise Psychology*, **11**, 65-83.

Sinclair, D.A., & Orlick, T. (1993). Positive transitions from high-performance sport. *The Sport Psychologist*, **7**, 138-150.

Sinetar, M. (1987). *Do what you love, the money will follow*. New York: Dell.

Skovholt, T.M., Morgan, J.I., & Negron-Cunningham, H. (1989). Mental imagery in career counseling and life planning: A review of research and intervention methods. *Journal of Counseling and Development*, **67**, 287-292.

White, A., & Coakley, J. (1986). *Making decisions: The response of young people in the Medway towns to the "Ever Thought of Sport?" campaign*. West Sussex Institute of Higher Education Sports Council, Greater London and Southeast Region, London.

White, R.W. (1959). Motivation reconsidered: The concept of competence. *Psychological Review*, **66**, 297-333.

CHAPTER 15

OVERTRAINING AND BURNOUT

Sean McCann, PhD

United States Olympic Committee

Virtually every issue facing a sport psychologist working with elite athletes in today's sport environment involves questions of training. Diverse problem areas (such as sport performance difficulties, coach-athlete conflicts, drug use, emotional stress, and athlete career-choice anxiety), are all intensified by the incredible training pressures and demands facing the modern elite athlete. Although much attention is paid to competition performance, little in the sport psychology literature focuses on the preparation leading to competitions. This emphasis on competition performance is often misplaced, because in many cases, most of the sport psychologist's job is to help athletes successfully cope with training—getting them to, rather than through, competition.

This less-than-glamorous truth is old news for elite athletes themselves. Practices and training sessions always have accounted for most of the time a top athlete works at a sport. What has changed, however, is the nature of training time. At the elite sport level, in response to increasing rewards for success and increasing pressures on athletes and coaches, there has been a marked increase in the stress of training. In attempts to maximize performance at competitions, many athletes

and coaches have experimented with increases in the duration and intensity of training time. Many of these experiments have been organized attempts to capitalize on knowledge gained from recent studies in sport science, whereas others have been based on the simple notion that more is better. These studies suggest that large increases in training stress can have both obvious and subtle effects, many of which are detrimental to athlete performance. This chapter focuses on the negative psychological and physiological responses, collectively referred to as *overtraining*, that result from overwhelming training stress. After defining terms and briefly reviewing the literature on overtraining and athlete burnout, I discuss intervention and ethical issues for the consulting sport psychologist.

■ *THE CASE OF CINDY* ■

Cindy is an elite bicycle racer in her late teens. She quickly rose in earlier years to elite status, showing talent and, even more markedly, an amazing work ethic and an ability to train harder than everyone else. Cindy felt more confident when she knew she had ridden more miles and had done more high-intensity training than her competitors. Now at the senior elite level, she has found that her improvement has slowed considerably, to only gradual, incremental increases in performance. Even more disturbing, Cindy has discovered that everyone trains hard at this level. Unsatisfied with her rate of progress and fearful that her lack of rapid improvement might threaten her national-team status, she began extra evening training rides without her coach's knowledge to gain an edge over other competitors.

Despite Cindy's efforts to hasten her improvement, she and her coaches began noticing significant negative changes in her performance during the current training season. Cindy appeared sluggish and slow to respond to attacks in training rides. Always an aggressive rider in the past, Cindy began to ride defensively and cautiously. In sprint and interval sessions, Cindy was losing ground to riders she had earlier beaten easily. She began to complain of chronic knee pain and developed a cough that wouldn't go away. Perhaps even more disturbing to the coaches were changes in Cindy's personality. Always the first to arrive at training sessions, she often arrived late and appeared sleepy. Previously a positive and exuberant athlete, Cindy began to complain about minor equipment problems and other team members. As the training season progressed, Cindy began expressing doubts about her ability and on two occasions quit training sessions in tears. After she missed an important training race due to oversleeping and missing a ride, her coaches called a conference to discuss Cindy's attitude and to determine if she belonged in the elite cycling program. The team's consulting sport psychologist was asked to attend.

DEFINITIONS

A clear definition of terms is essential to reviewing work in overtraining. One difficulty encountered when reviewing the literature is a tendency for authors to use a variety of terms to describe similar concepts. *Overtraining* refers to a maladaptive response to training stress, often due to chronically high training stress levels without periods of lower training loads. The end result of this chronic stress can be an *overtraining syndrome* with a variety of psychophysiological signs and symptoms. *Staleness* is another term used to describe the negative results of excessive training stress (Morgan, Brown, Raglin, O'Connor, & Ellickson, 1987), and authors have variously described it as the end result of overtraining (Hackney, Pearman, & Nowacki, 1990) or a stage in the development of the overtraining syndrome (Silva, 1990). In this chapter I will not distinguish staleness from overtraining.

In addition to using different terms for similar concepts, authors have also used similar terms to convey different concepts. Some reasons for this inconsistency are that training stress can impact athletes both positively and negatively and that terms describing training stress have been used to describe both positive and negative results. In contrast to *overtraining*, the terms *overload* or *overwork* typically refer to a short-term increase in an athlete's training load that can result in a short-term performance decrease. Overload, often a well-planned phase of an athlete's training program, is based on sport physiology research showing that this short-term decrease in performance can be followed by increased future performance. This phenomenon is often used in a program of *periodization* (Bompa, 1983; Matveyev, 1981), in which a period of lower training loads (known as the rest or taper stage) follows the overload phase, ideally resulting in a peak physical state at competition.

OVERTRAINING RESEARCH

The search for an ideal training approach is not new; it has always been the central focus

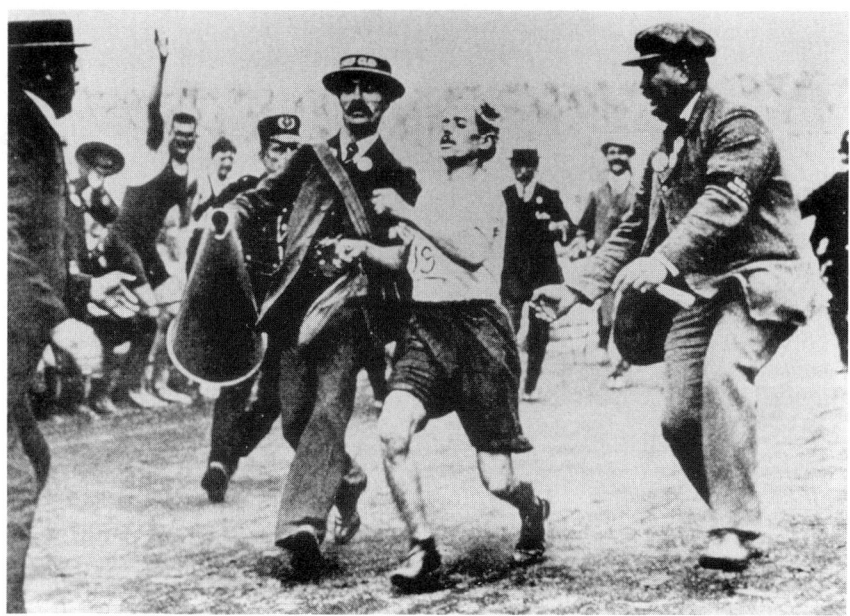

Courtesy USOC

for coaches and athletes attempting to improve competitive performance. At the elite level, even the most gifted athletes cannot afford to be undertrained. The fear of being undertrained and unprepared often produces a more-is-better training philosophy. Where athletes are free to make sport a full-time occupation, significant increases in training load length and intensity have been attempted. In many cases, these have been at a significant cost. Just as undertraining can spell defeat for athletes, too-high and too-long training loads can negatively impact performance (Levin, 1991). The impact can be seen in physiological and psychological effects or, perhaps more accurately, in a combined *psychophysiological* effect.

Many studies of athletes' responses to high training loads use methodologies developed in generalized studies of response to stress. Following the early work of Hans Selye (1946), who saw stress as the body's reaction to a noxious stimulus, many researchers studied hormonal and other physiological changes in humans and other organisms in response to *stressors*. As stress research expanded from purely physiological studies to the study of psychological stress, researchers developed a growing awareness of the interaction between psychological and physiological stress reactions (Lazarus & Folkman, 1984). A similar realization recently occurred in overtraining research, but for the purpose of review, I will discuss research findings on the physiological effects of overtraining separately from the psychological effects before considering the interconnection of the psychological and physiological effects.

Specific Areas of Physiological Impact

Physiological research on overtraining has built on Selye's early work on hormonal changes in response to increased training stress, and additional studies have included cardiovascular changes, neuromuscular changes, performance changes, and immune system changes (Hackney et al., 1990). A common theme throughout much of the recent literature is the search for a physiological marker indicating the approach of overtraining (Callister, Callister, Fleck, & Dudley, 1989; Kuipers & Keizer, 1988; Levin, 1991).

The efforts to search for a physiological marker, or warning sign, of overtraining have generally begun with a recognition that athletes who have reached a full-blown overtraining syndrome exhibit characteristic physiological symptoms. These include hormonal changes (such as increased serum cortisol levels and decreased testosterone), higher resting heart rates and blood pressure (according to some reports), loss of body weight and percent body fat, and chronic muscle soreness (Callister et al., 1989; Costill et al., 1988; Dressendorfer and Wade, 1983; Hackney et al., 1990; Kirwin et al., 1988). In addition, athletes experiencing an overtraining syndrome appear to be at significantly greater risk for injuries and illnesses, with concomitant changes in the immune system (Costill, 1986; Hackney et al., 1990). Most applied research has monitored one or more of these physiological signs while tracking or modifying training loads.

Unfortunately, short-term physiological studies, using varying methods, have produced inconsistent findings (Hackney et al., 1990). Also, individual differences in ability to tolerate increased training stresses might mask results in studies using group designs (Levin, 1991; Morgan, 1991). As well, individual differences might exist in symptom expression of an overtraining syndrome. Lastly, comparing results from studies with athletes of various abilities is difficult, because elite athlete programs might, by their very nature, select for athletes who can tolerate higher training loads (Callister et al., 1989). Thus, despite some interesting and suggestive findings, early physiological markers for overtraining have not been clearly established. It

appears that physiological symptoms accompanying overtraining are evident primarily after a fully developed overtraining syndrome exists (Hackney et al.; Levin); at this point, rest or greatly reduced training load is the preferred intervention.

Psychological Impact of Overtraining

Much of the work on the psychological impact of overtraining has focused on emotional and mood states in response to large training demands. The most comprehensive efforts to document this impact have been by Bill Morgan and his co-workers at the University of Wisconsin (Morgan et al., 1987; Morgan, 1991). Much of this work has utilized the Profile of Mood States (POMS), (McNair, Lorr, & Droppleman, 1971), a measure of mood states with six subscales, to characterize the psychological functioning of athletes across time and various training and competitive situations.

Early in Morgan's work, he found that active individuals and elite athletes have a positive mood profile on the POMS, which he labeled the *Iceberg Profile* (1985). This name was derived from the shape of this characteristic profile: a higher than average score on the *Vigor* scale, and lower than average scores on the five other negative mood scales (*Tension, Depression, Anger, Fatigue,* and *Confusion*). The strength of the relationship between POMS scores and elite-athlete status led to a theoretical hypothesis that elite athletes might be emotionally healthier than non-elite athletes and that mental health is correlated with sport success (1985, 1991).

In addition to Morgan's characterization of the iceberg profile, his research team performed a 10-year longitudinal study of competitive college swimmers, using the POMS and other means to monitor the swimmers' psychological states during training periods of various intensity (Morgan et al., 1987). The researchers found that with ever-increasing training levels, the iceberg profile disappeared and that an overall negative mood disturbance increased in conjunction with increased training levels. The authors described the relationship as following a *dose–response* pattern, with training levels being the dosage level and mood disturbance being the response. At the highest training levels, the iceberg profile actually inverted, with the *Vigor* subscale falling below negative mood subscale levels. Morgan (1991) notes that, despite the clear group results, there were significant individual differences in response to various training loads.

In a companion study, which monitored the physiological status and performance levels of the swimmers (Costill et al., 1988), there was a correspondence between mood disturbance and physiological signs of lower functioning. This pattern of psychological and physiological disturbances in response to higher levels of training was described as a state of "staleness," the product of intense training levels (Morgan et al., 1987). Interestingly, mood disturbances on the athlete's POMS scores fell to a preovertrained baseline following a period of rest or reduced training load (tapering).

Interaction of Psychological and Physiological Effects

Recent research on overtraining has focused on the interaction of psychological, physiological, and general performance effects in response to training. This focus is due to two major factors, one being recognition on a theoretical level of the problems of attempting to separate mind from body when describing the effects of stress (Lazarus & Folkman, 1984; Yukelson & Murphy, 1993). Another factor in the trend toward studying physiological and psychological effects together is the need

for cross-validating data on the impact of overtraining (Levin, 1991; Murphy, Fleck, Dudley, & Callister, 1990).

On the theoretical level, recent work from the field of psychoneuroimmunology (PNI) has influenced thinking on the connections between physiological and psychological systems (Ader, 1981). The work in this area has interesting implications for overtraining research as well as for sport psychology in general. PNI research focuses on the interaction of the body's three major information systems: the nervous system, the endocrine system, and the immune system (Hall, 1989). Although molecular connections between these systems have been charted, research on their mechanisms of communication is just beginning. Perhaps PNI's greatest utility at this time is its use as a theoretical model to explain what has been suspected for some time: that behavioral factors as well as environment and genetic predisposition have an impact on disease and health (Borysenko, 1984). PNI research might also be useful as a heuristic for understanding the relationship between training levels, mood states, and immune-system functioning in overtrained athletes.

In addition to increasing the research's theoretical sophistication, monitoring the interaction of psychological and physiological effects when studying overtraining increases the ability to accurately document the impact of very high training levels (Morgan, Brown, et al., 1987). For example, considering physiological and psychological data simultaneously has shown that the impact of overload can occur at different times for different systems (Murphy et al., 1990). Thus the timing of an overload training period and accompanying taper for competition might be appropriate for maximizing physical capacity for competition, but not for maximizing emotional readiness for competition.

An interdisciplinary study with elite judo athletes at the United States Olympic Training Center systematically controlled training levels over a 10-week period while monitoring psychological states, physical performance variables, and physiological markers of overtraining, such as resting heart rates and resting blood pressure levels (Callister et al., 1989; Murphy et al., 1990). Following a protocol suggested by Matveyev (1981) to optimize performance at the end of the training period, the athletes in the study participated in baseline, increased conditioning, and increased sport-specific skill-training periods, in that order.

Interestingly, the results of the Murphy et al. (1990) study differed in some respects from earlier studies. The performance data indicated that decreases in strength and speed occurred despite the absence of physiological markers. Psychological results revealed (unlike those of earlier studies also using the POMS) a lack of overall mood disturbance on the POMS, but the POMS *Anger* scale was significantly higher at the end of the 10-week period. In addition, general anxiety and somatic competitive anxiety also increased over the course of the study. Psychological indices and performance measures showed similar patterns in response to training load, despite the absence of physiological markers. These results as well as other studies showing a link between psychological state and performance in the absence of clear early physiological markers (Morgan, Costill, Flynn, Raglin, & O'Connor, 1988) have led some authors to advocate that coaches pay closer attention to individual athletes' self-reports of effort and psychological state when there is a concern about a potential overtraining syndrome (Levin, 1991; Morgan, 1991). This emphasis on a person's psychological state might be even more important in the burnout syndrome, which is of recent interest to sport psychologists studying training stress.

BURNOUT RESEARCH

Burnout is a psychological term that first appeared in the 1970s but is now a frequent subject of popular-magazine articles and television talk shows. Like many popularized terms or phrases that originated as psychological constructs, the word *burnout* now means many things to many people. Much of the early research on burnout focused on the stress and stress reactions of people working in "helping professions." From an initial focus on a job-related syndrome (Maslach, 1976), the definition of burnout syndrome has now been broadened to include many situations where characteristic signs of burnout are present. In a recent review, Dale and Weinberg (1990) summarize the classic characteristics of burnout: exhaustion, negative responses to others, and low self-esteem and depression. In addition, most definitions of burnout emphasize the presence of chronic stressors (Dale & Weinberg; Silva, 1990; Smith, 1986).

Based on these definitions, the characteristics of burnout are in some ways similar to those of an overtraining syndrome. For this reason, overtraining and burnout are often included together in discussions of athlete stress. Before discussing burnout in further detail, it is useful to determine how these concepts differ and how they overlap. Some authors have argued that overtraining and burnout are on a continuum, burnout being the product of chronic overtraining (Silva, 1990), whereas others have noted parallels and interactions between these syndromes (Dale & Weinberg, 1990; Henschen, 1986; Smith, 1986).

Perhaps the most obvious overlap between the overtraining and burnout syndromes is that stress appears to play a major role in the etiology of each. A salient difference between the two syndromes as typically defined is the specific theoretical role of cognitive factors posited for burnout (see Figure 15.1). As in Selye's early stress studies, research on overtraining has generally focused on a stressor (training load) and a reaction (overtraining

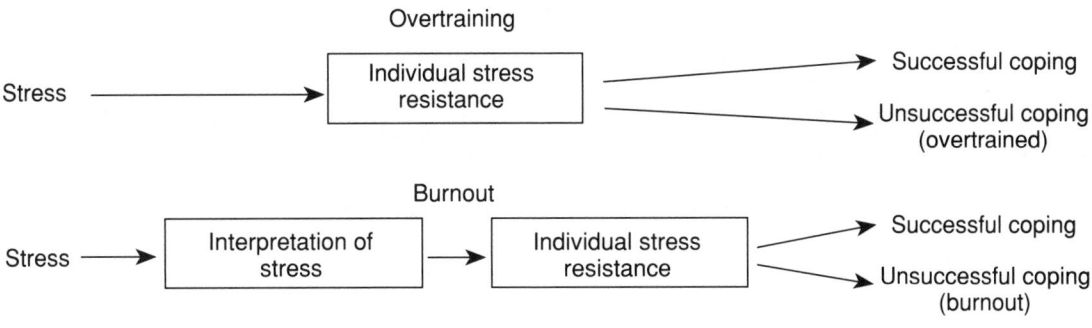

Figure 15.1 The role of stress in overtraining and burnout models.

symptoms), omitting an athlete's interpretation of the stressor. Research on burnout, begun in the midst of the cognitive-behavioral era, pays a great deal of attention to the cognitions of persons suffering from burnout. This introduction of cognitive factors in burnout research mirrors developments in the stress-coping literature (Lazarus & Folkman, 1984), and adds a level of complexity and subtlety that might also be an important part of future overtraining research.

The application of burnout concepts to the sporting world is a fairly recent development, and the earliest work focused on burnout in coaches (Caccese & Mayerberg, 1984; Dale & Weinberg, 1990; Wilson & Bird, 1984) and athletic trainers (Capel, 1986; Gieck, Brown, & Shank, 1982). One reason for the focus on these populations is the similarity of job requirements of previously studied helping professions (nurses, teachers, mental health workers) and those of coaches and trainers.

The topic of burnout in athlete populations was advanced and given a theoretical focus in an article by Smith (1986), who proposed a model to explain athlete burnout. Smith used the social exchange model of Thibault and Kelly (1959), which suggests that humans behave logically to maximize or approach positive experiences and minimize or avoid negative experiences. Smith emphasizes that

burnout is a kind of withdrawal and that athletes with burnout syndrome withdraw, either physically or psychologically, from sport participation.

Smith (1986) makes many theoretical points that have relevance for both research on and intervention in athlete burnout. He notes that sport might have distinct causal burnout factors and cautions against over-reliance on work-based models. He argues, as well, for development of sport-specific burnout scales and behavior-based ratings of burnout effects and causal variables. Another important observation is Smith's distinction between dropping out of sport versus burnout; he makes the point that people stop participating in sports for many reasons other than burnout.

For sport psychologists, perhaps the most important contribution of Smith's article was its integration of ideas from the general stress-coping literature into the study of burnout and overtraining. In particular, the addition of individual cognitive factors and individual differences in personal resources suggests that burnout and overtraining are not simple and inevitable responses to stimuli like increased training load or competitive stress. By emphasizing the importance of individual interpretation, Smith's model of burnout suggests avenues of intervention for sport psychologists. Because addressing the levels of training load might not be possible or appropriate for a consulting sport psychologist, working to develop the personal resources or choices of an athlete might at times be the only viable avenue of clinical intervention.

INTERVENTION ISSUES

Before proceeding with an intervention in burnout or overtraining, the sport psychologist must be clear about role and value issues. As is emphasized in chapter 7 with respect to student athletes, a lack of specificity of roles can lead to uncomfortable and occasionally untenable positions for a sport psychology consultant. Clarity of roles is especially critical in overtraining, where role conflicts can be exacerbated by value clashes over training practices and philosophy. Consultants must know whether they are acting as psychologists or whether their opinions are straying into the areas of coaching, competitive career planning, physiological consulting, nutritional consulting, or even athlete decision making.

Although these roles initially might seem clear, exposure to training issues reveals the complexity and value-laden nature of consulting in this area. Consider these examples:

- How does the sport psychologist feel about a 12-year-old gymnast's chronic use of ice packs and anti-inflammatory medicine?
- Should a figure skater compete in the national championships with stress fractures in one leg?
- Is a coach ignoring signs of overtraining due to a desire for a world-championship medal?

When the responsibilities and potential limits of a consultant role are clear, questions of boundaries are less frequent. By communicating these boundaries to coaches, organizations, and athletes, the consultant should be able to impact the complex subject of overtraining by working cooperatively with other disciplines. Difficult moral and ethical decisions will, however, inevitably be encountered.

Diagnosing Overtraining

Recognizing or diagnosing an overtraining syndrome is one role in which the sport psychologist might be particularly useful. As with other interventions discussed in this book, not all problems are immediately apparent to athletes and coaches, so a psychologist's training in assessment can be invaluable. In diagnosing overtraining, the consultant should use multimodal assessment methods wherever possible. As in the case example of Cindy, the young cyclist, at the beginning of this chapter, indications of overtraining can come from a variety of data. Sources of information for the sport psychologist include

- physiological symptoms,
- psychological symptoms,
- decreased performance indicators,
- results of medical testing,
- athletes' reports,
- psychological test data, and
- the reports of coaches and significant others.

Overtraining Symptoms

A first step for consultants wishing to assess overtraining syndrome is to be familiar with the symptoms documented in the literature. As previously described, symptoms can be divided into physiological, psychological, and general performance effects, although authors generally agree that these symptoms interact (Morgan, Costill, et al., 1988). Physiological symptoms described in the literature include

- elevated resting heart rate and blood pressure,
- muscle soreness,
- weight loss and loss of body fat,
- changes in serum hormonal levels,
- sleep disturbance, and
- increased incidence of sickness and injury (Callister et al., 1989; Costill et al., 1988; Hackney, et al., 1990).

Given the importance of these symptoms, developing a good working relationship with physicians or exercise physiologists for teams or athletes can be critical to a consultant's successful interventions. Trainers for athletes or teams are useful but often neglected sources of information. The degree to which ice-packs, aspirin, and ultrasound are used might give a good indication of athlete stress levels. Often trainers are the first to hear of physical and emotional complaints from athletes. Developing a working relationship with athletic trainers can be a key step in prevention of training-stress-related problems (Heil, 1993).

The search for a purely physiological marker for overtraining has met with mixed success, due to individual differences and to the appearance of most physiological signs late in the course of a syndrome (Hackney et al., 1990; Levin, 1991). There is recent evidence that performance measures might reflect signs of overtraining before physiological signs appear (Callister et al., 1989). Close communication with a coach can help a consultant be aware of important performance areas, including strength and speed measures, longer recovery times after exertion, and decreasing performance despite increased training (when this is an unplanned consequence of the training load).

Psychological symptoms might be the most sensitive measures of overtraining (Levin, 1991). Signs of apathy, fatigue, anger, and depression should be carefully monitored. When working with teams, it should

be emphasized that individual differences might result in these signs appearing in some athletes and not others. Occasionally, these individual differences can result in an overtrained athlete's being perceived as having an attitude problem, as was the case with Cindy in the case example at the beginning of this chapter. When present, however, these signs should prompt a consultant to gather further information, such as physiological and performance data.

Athlete Report

Perhaps the most powerful source of information about overtraining is an athlete's direct report to a consultant. An athlete's self-report of feelings of overtraining should always be taken seriously. In this author's experience, athletes in a proper state of training are generally the most positive and energetic of clients. Thus, athlete reports of fatigue, feelings of amotivation, increases in perceived exertion, anger, or distress are unusual and should be carefully heeded. In addition to anecdotal and subjective evidence of the novelty of athlete self-reports of negative mood, the body of Morgan's work at the University of Wisconsin is strongly supportive of the notion that successful competitive athletes generally possess greater energy and less negative affect than the population as a whole (Morgan, 1985, 1991; Morgan and Pollock, 1977; Morgan et al., 1987). As has been noted in many recent articles, athletes are often aware of the affective and behavioral symptoms of overtraining before the physiological signs of overtraining are present (Levin, 1991). Thus an athlete's self-report might be the only early-warning signal of an impending overtraining syndrome.

When listening to an athlete's self-report, a consultant can gain a great deal of information about an athlete's interpretation of the training environment. As mentioned previously in the discussion of Smith's (1986) model of burnout, the introduction of a cognitive-behavioral perspective to the problems of burnout and overtraining emphasizes the importance of an athlete's perspective. Subjective self-reports of stress might reflect individual differences in the ability to cope with certain training pressures and might be much more informative than objective reports of training loads. These individual interpretations of the training environment might also provide a critical opportunity for psychological intervention.

One very practical method for gathering athletes' self-report data is through the use of training logbooks (see Figure 15.2) that record an athlete's thoughts, feelings, and behaviors in training and competition. The structure and use of this method can vary greatly across settings. Many athletes use logbooks as a private method of better understanding their reactions to various training and competition settings. Other athletes might feel comfortable using logbooks as a method to communicate with their coach or sport psychologist about mental training issues. Physical training logbooks are used by athletes in a number of sports, and space for recording moods, self-talk, goals, and behaviors can be easily added. After a brief period of monitoring these factors, an athlete can more directly see the interaction of mental and physical states and more easily spot early signs of overtraining.

Psychometric Devices

The psychological research data on overtraining collected by Morgan and his coworkers (1987) is a convincing argument for the use of psychometric testing to identify overtraining problems. In addition, the classic work by Meehl (1954) on the increased accuracy of clinical decision making when using psychometric testing is a reminder of the importance of using the science of psychology whenever possible. The question for

the consulting sport psychologist, therefore, should be, Is it possible to effectively use psychometric testing in the competitive sport setting? In some sport settings, the use of any formal psychological test data can meet with resistance, whereas in other settings coaches and athletes welcome psychological data. This is especially true when feedback from the testing is rapid and useful.

Using the POMS as a specific tool for monitoring athlete training responses generally requires the cooperation of a coach who is interested in psychological feedback and who will not feel threatened by this method. A theoretical discussion of overtraining and the POMS might be a useful part of early discussions with a coaching staff. At this time, the consultant might suggest specific nonintrusive data collection and feedback points throughout a season. Also important is a clear understanding among athletes as to the use of the POMS and the level of confidentiality or disclosure to coaches. Cooperative efforts with coaches and athletes toward the goal of preventing overtraining will reduce the likelihood that a consultant will identify an overtraining problem through the use of testing, only to find out that the athlete does not want this information shared.

Coaches Report

Although the case example of Cindy suggested that her coaches were unaware of her overtraining problem, coaches often are in the best position to identify potential overtraining situations. At elite sport levels, there appears to be a growing awareness of the problems of overtraining (Levin, 1991). In endurance sports in particular, programs designed to produce peaking for major races typically are monitored carefully by coaches and are often individualized based on athletes' differences in response to planned training stress (Carmichael, 1992). Most elite coaches in endurance sports have worked

Training Logbook for Cycling

Date _____

Hr sleep _____   Resting pulse _____

Appetite _____   Muscles feel _____

———————————————————————— **Preride plan** ————————————————————————

Miles _____

Pace _____

Specific tasks _____

Preride attitude: How motivated are you?

1	2	3	4	5
Don't want to ride		Average motivation		Can't wait to get riding

Mental goals for the ride

1 _____

2 _____

———————————————————— **Postpractice comments** ————————————————————

Energy level: How much energy did you have?

1	2	3	4	5
Very low energy				Very high energy

Why? _____

Performance: How was your riding, recovery from effort, sense of how hard it was?

_____

_____

Self-talk: What were you saying to yourself during the ride?

_____

Goals: Did you meet your mental goals for the ride?

1	2	3	4	5
Met no goals		Met 50% goals		Met 100% goals

Name at least **one positive accomplishment** from today's ride:

_____

_____

Figure 15.2 A training logbook for cycling.

with overtrained athletes and understand how devastating the impact on performance can be. In these situations, coaches often have a keen eye for early signs of overtraining and can also act as powerful change agents when problems are identified.

Goals of an Overtraining Intervention

The potential goals of an overtraining intervention are

- performance focus,
- psychological well-being,
- education of coaches and athletes,
- protecting the physical health of the athlete,
- increasing coach–athlete communication, and
- developing athlete resources to cope with training.

Although at first glance the goals of intervention in overtraining might seem obvious—eliminate or prevent it—in reality the intervention goals for a consulting sport psychologist can be varied, subtle, and potentially conflicting.

One reason for this is the contrast between the role of a sport psychologist and the role of a psychologist not involved in working with athletes. For example, when a clinical psychologist works with a person who has a stress-related disorder, one goal might be to eliminate or reduce the level of the stressor. A sport psychologist, however, is typically asked to optimize the level of the stressor for the athlete's benefit. As mentioned previously, determining optimal stress and determining optimal benefit are value questions and at times might become ethical questions. This will be discussed more fully later in this chapter. Because stress is a fact of life at elite levels of sport, a sport psychologist

working at elite levels needs to be attentive to the goals of any overtraining intervention.

Performance Focus

One potential goal for an overtraining intervention is improved performance. Athletes and coaches are comfortable with performance as a focus, and thus discussing the problems of overtraining as a performance issue might allow a consultant to have immediate access to participants and information about their training levels. Ability to effect change might also be aided by a performance focus. There are, however, potential pitfalls.

One potential problem with a performance focus is a consultant's lack of expertise and credibility. Consider the consultant's answers to the following questions:

- What does the consultant know about planned overload and periodization?
- Does the consultant understand the importance of peaking for particular meets or competition?
- Which performance is the focus, short-term or long-term?

These legitimate questions are critical to athletes whose entire career might be significantly affected by one performance in a single competition. Unless a consultant has established a strong working relationship with an interdisciplinary group that can monitor and plan for performance (coach, athlete, exercise physiologist, trainer, team physician), intervening solely with the goal of performance enhancement not only is difficult but is likely inappropriate.

A second problem with making performance enhancement a goal of intervention is a general issue in applied sport psychology. Should a consultant take credit or blame for an athlete's performance? Although the temptation to take pride in the performance of a client athlete is great, are consultants also willing to take responsibility for poor performance? It is important to note that there are many valid goals for overtraining interventions besides performance enhancement. An alternative focus, based on developing an athlete's coping resources, can also take performance-enhancement goals into account; this will be described later in this chapter.

Psychological Well-Being

Unlike in performance issues, sport psychologists typically have special expertise and training in psychological assessment and treatment. This knowledge can be usefully shared during an intervention and can give a consulting sport psychologist a special and important role in an athletic context, even though the psychological health of an athlete might not always be a priority or focus in an athletic setting.

Even in this more familiar area, it is necessary to consider the importance of temporal and sport-specific factors. One question might be whether the level of negative emotional response to a current period of planned overload is worth it if it means that athletes will compete at their best and succeed at a critical competition 1 month later. Another relevant question might be whether coaches are ignoring the human need for short-term reinforcement in an effort to concentrate solely on peaking for a later competition. By emphasizing the importance of enjoyment of sport by athletes and coaches, even in the high-stress world of elite athletics, a consultant can help contribute an awareness of the need for balance in training.

Educating Coaches and Athletes About Overtraining

In addition to special training in psychological assessment and treatment, many consulting sport psychologists have expertise as educators and information specialists. Although more and more elite coaches and athletes in endurance sports are highly knowledgeable about overtraining, many less-experienced coaches and athletes are not. Often, the sport psychologist might have the most current information available about overtraining, thanks to access to current sport science journals. Providing general knowledge about overtraining and specifying the potential impact for individuals being consulted can be useful.

Occasionally, a prime benefit of this education can be the relabeling of a "bad attitude" as simply one facet of an overtraining syndrome. This might be true in the chapter's case example of Cindy, where overtraining symptoms might have been mislabeled.

In addition to the potential benefits of education for a specific individual or situation, the education process can work as a proactive mechanism to prevent further cases of overtraining. For athletes, this education might be their first detailed discussion of overtraining, and it might give them an explanation for present or past performance and training problems. For some coaches, education on overtraining might act to challenge long-held More is Good—Much More is Very Good notions about training.

Physical Health

Although physical health is not often thought to be a focus of psychological consultation, one goal of an overtraining intervention can be to indirectly impact the physical health of athletes. Advances in health psychology or behavioral medicine as well as the PNI research described previously provide evidence that behavior can have a significant impact on health. By discussing the research on overtraining, with specific mention of the relationship between overtraining and increased potential for injury and illness, a sport psychologist can add a useful and unique voice in discussions about training levels. By using connections with team physicians and athletic trainers and coaches, a consultant with an understanding of health and behavior can sometimes recognize patterns of overtraining behavior that might otherwise be missed.

Increasing Coach-Athlete Communication

Although more communication might seem to be a particularly indirect method of addressing overtraining, communication enhancement can be a critical intervention goal. In the case example of Cindy, her lack of openness about actual training levels and the resultant lack of coaching awareness was a prime factor in her development of overtraining symptoms.

Cindy's story is common in endurance sports, where highly motivated young athletes who have seen benefits from increased training add private workouts in an attempt to increase these benefits. Even at the national-team level, athletes might sometimes choose not to disclose actual training levels to coaches for a variety of reasons.

Athletes also might be unwilling to disclose symptoms of overtraining to coaches in situations where training levels are fairly well controlled and uniform, for fear of losing playing time or losing the coach's respect. This might be especially true in team sports where individual differences in the ability to tolerate increased training stress can result in the labeling of some athletes as tough and others as weak. A sport psychology consultant who can facilitate structured discussions about training levels and athlete responses can provide a useful service for a team that needs all its athletes to be fit and ready to play a long season. Ideally, this sort of structured discussion would allow athletes to understand coaching philosophy and coaches to understand athletes' differing resources in response to increased training stress. This information is critical, given the growing awareness that individualized training regimens are critical, even in team sport settings (Levin, 1991).

Developing Athlete Resources

A good deal of the sport psychology services provided at the United States Olympic Training Center in Colorado Springs falls into the category of stress-management work with athletes. This work attempts to develop an athlete's resources in managing the stress of elite athletics. Of all the intervention goals in overtraining, building an athlete's resources might be the most universally applicable. One advantage of this intervention goal is that it focuses on elements potentially in the athlete's control. Many of the stressors involved in elite athletics are simply not controllable by the participants, athletes, or coaches. In Olympic sport, training levels inevitably are high, competition is intense, and public and private pressures to perform are unavoidable. By developing resources, or "inoculating" against stress (Meichenbaum, 1985), a consultant shifts focus to those elements athletes and coaches can purposefully work on. The development of personal coping skills is the focus of a number of recent applied sport psychology studies.

As Smith's (1986) article on athlete burnout suggests, variations in personal cognitive and affective resources can result in greatly differing responses to similar stressors. In developing personal resources, a consultant can help athletes determine areas of strength and weakness, including time-management skills, relaxation ability (Davis, 1991), personal social-support networks (Smith, Smoll, & Ptacek, 1990), useful goal setting for training (Yukelson & Murphy, 1993), and self-reinforcing ability (Heiby & Campos, 1986).

Recent work by Davis (1991), who taught athletes relaxation skills to impact injury rates, is an example of proactively building personal resources in anticipation of training stress. This research and clinical trend is encouraging, as often the ability to relax is addressed in the context of enhancing competition performance, although the vast majority of an athlete's time, which is spent training, is ignored.

Another area receiving much research attention is social support and its relationship to injuries and illnesses. Many researchers have found evidence to argue for a model of social support as a "buffer" to reduce the impact of stress on injury rates (Andersen & Williams, 1988; Billings & Moos, 1981; Hardy, Richman, & Rosenfeld, 1991; Sarason, Sarason, & Pierce, 1990). These studies suggest that helping athletes identify, build, and utilize social-support systems might help reduce the impact of training-stress problems.

Borysenko (1984) argues for a model of disease susceptibility with three factors acting alone and in concert: genetic predisposition, environmental factors, and behavioral factors. This model, developed from research in PNI, might be usefully applied as well to susceptibility to overtraining and burnout (see Figure 15.3). In the case of overtraining, behavioral factors can encompass the range

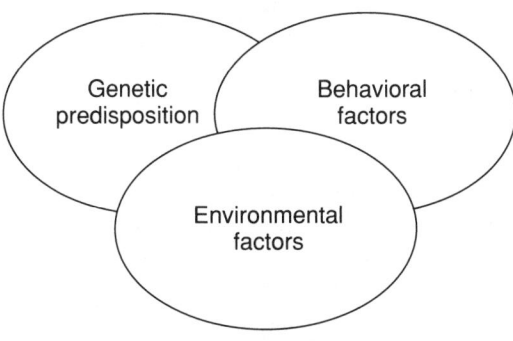

Figure 15.3 Factors that can impact vulnerability to overtraining.

of personal resources and stress-coping responses available to an athlete. Building an athlete's resources for dealing with training stress might help reduce the tendency in elite athlete selection to rely on a survival-of-the-fittest test (with fittest being those most genetically hardy rather than most talented).

Determining the Success of Interventions

Determining the success of any psychological intervention can be difficult, and the large literature on evaluating the success of therapy suggests that the process can be controversial as well (Eysenck, 1979; Smith & Glass, 1981). Having specific intervention goals, as previously discussed, can be helpful in the determination of success. If intervention goals are well specified, then the measurement of outcome becomes clearer.

- Are athletes performing better?
- Do athletes feel psychologically stronger?
- Are athletes and coaches better educated about overtraining?
- Are athletes healthier and less injury-prone?
- Do coaches and athletes communicate more completely about training issues?
- Do athletes have more resources to cope with the stress of training?

The measurement of coping resources in athletes to determine the success of an intervention is not well developed, and measurement accuracy will likely benefit from a standardized psychometric device. Hardy, Richman, and Rosenfeld (1991) describe the use of the Support Functions Questionnaire (SFQ) (Pines, Aronson, & Kafry, 1981), a social support questionnaire modified for use with athletes, as one formal measure of athletes' social support resources.

In an athletic context where participants' performances are measured regularly and

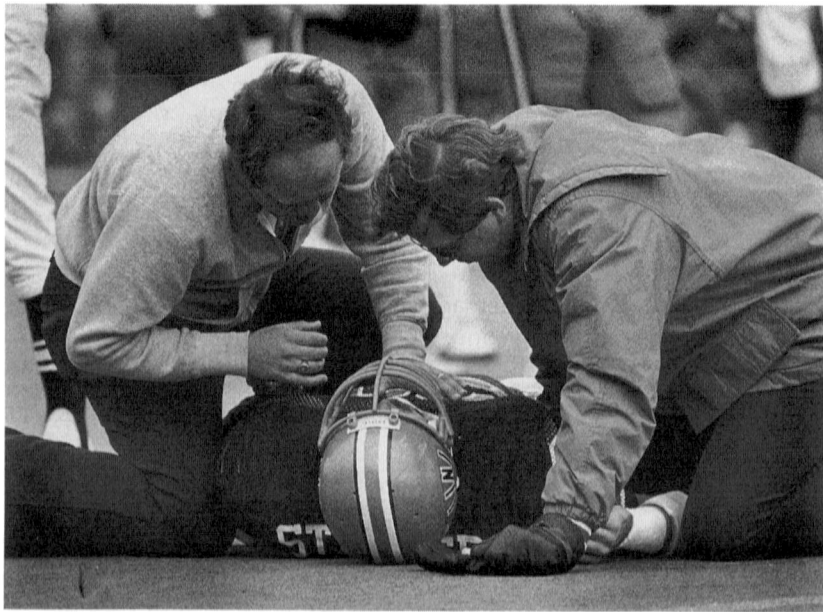

Courtesy University of Illinois Sports Information

objectively, sport psychologists should objectively review their own effectiveness. As the field is still developing a basic research base, there is a need for applied data, and a number of creative dependent variables are available for use by applied researchers (Murphy, 1991). For the practitioner, these same variables can be used as documentation of practitioner effectiveness for employers (e.g., coaches, professional and amateur sport organizations). The need of practitioners and researchers for an objective review of effectiveness is especially apparent with training stress, which is often neglected due to emphasis on competition outcomes.

Intervention in the Case of Cindy

Cindy, the young bicycle racer described at this chapter's beginning, had many characteristics of an overtraining syndrome, apparently a result of her self-imposed extra training rides in addition to an already intense team-training schedule. Her case highlights many issues this chapter discusses. Cindy's

coaches called a meeting at which a consulting sport psychologist was asked to attend. The first step for a sport psychologist in addressing overtraining issues is to establish a role that allows the opportunity to intervene. Building a clearly defined role and relationships with coaches, athletes, and administrators was the crucial first step in Cindy's case.

Once at the meeting, the psychologist's expertise in assessment was very important. Recognition of the signs and results of overtraining, collected from the various areas of Cindy's performance, physical condition, and psychological condition, were used to suggest that Cindy's problems might stem from something other than a bad attitude. A psychologist aware of the overtraining symptoms might suggest psychological testing and further interdisciplinary assessment, including physiological testing.

In Cindy's case, the intervention included individual work to increase her understanding of overtraining issues. Through discussion of the psychological impact of an overtraining syndrome, Cindy was able to reinterpret her own feelings and behavior and move productively toward recovery. Individual sessions also focused on other issues that might have contributed to her desire to speed up her rate of progress, such as unrealistic expectations for competitive progress.

Additionally, Cindy needed to understand that training stress results from more than just physical training load. Teaching her a model of stress that describes the interaction of psychological and physical factors allowed her to recognize that training levels are not independent of the rest of her life. Cindy used a logbook to record both physical and psychological factors in her training, giving her a better understanding of her reactions to various training loads. A review of this logbook with a sport psychologist was combined with periodic use of the POMS to provide Cindy with more data about herself. Although not necessary in Cindy's case, another area of individual intervention could be a referral to the team physiologist or team physician to detail the physiological manifestations of an overtraining syndrome.

An especially important area in Cindy's case is communication between coaches and athlete. If the expectations of Cindy and her coaches regarding her performance were made clear to each other, Cindy might not have initiated the secret workouts on her own. With a better understanding of training theory and the underlying physiological theory, Cindy was better able to understand her training program as designed by her coaches. Perhaps the most useful intervention the psychologist arranged was a facilitated discussion between Cindy and her coaches to clarify future training and competitive goals.

ETHICAL ISSUES

In applied sport psychology, some ethical issues that arise are common to other areas of psychology, whereas others are particular to sport consultation. Using the latest revision of the American Psychological Association's Ethical Principles (American Psychological Association, 1992), issues can be grouped under three of the APA's general principles: competence, professional and scientific responsibility, and integrity (see Figure 15.4).

Competence
- Experience with sport-training issues
- Adequate access to information
- Awareness of diagnostic issues

Professional responsibility
- Relationships with experts

Integrity
- Role clarity—who is the client?
- Awareness of own values

Figure 15.4 Ethical issues the sport psychologist must consider.

Competence

Competence in the area of overtraining comprises many factors that address the central question: Is the sport psychologist qualified to give consulting advice about training issues? Although there are no established guidelines, efforts of the Association for the Advancement of Applied Sport Psychology (AAASP) to set educational and training guidelines for certified consultants have helped clarify this issue. A specific element especially important for the area of overtraining is education in exercise physiology and modern training methods. Specialized knowledge of planned overwork, periodization of training cycles, and planned peaking also are particularly useful.

The potential for misdiagnosis of overtraining and burnout should be recognized as a significant issue. Due to overtraining's impact on multiple facets of an athlete's life, it is important to rule out differential diagnoses. The question of potential depression should be addressed, as a number of symptoms of a major depressive episode listed in the DSM-III-R (American Psychiatric Association, 1987) have also been used to describe symptoms of overtraining (e.g., depressed mood, weight loss, sleep disturbance, fatigue, inability to concentrate). Of course, one might argue that overtraining could be an etiological factor in depression; this is an interesting counterpoint to the literature on the beneficial impact of moderate exercise on mood.

Another obvious and important possible alternative diagnosis is a physical disorder. If an athlete has not seen a physician about feelings of fatigue, muscle soreness, or the need for more sleep, for example, then a referral to rule out any physical problem should be a part of any planned intervention. As previously described, PNI research suggests that overtraining might have a role in the etiology of illnesses. Because vulnerability to injury and illness can be a sign of overtraining, awareness of an athlete's physical condition and contact with team health personnel is important.

Professional and Scientific Responsibility

The responsibility to "consult with, refer to, or cooperate with other professionals and institutions" (American Psychological Association, 1992) falls under APA's general principle of professional and scientific responsibility. Perhaps even more important than the psychologist's acquisition of knowledge about training and overtraining is ongoing access to experts. Given the interaction of physiological, psychological, and performance factors in overtraining, contact with trainers, coaches, and team physicians is critical in making responsible decisions. Interdisciplinary resources appear to be a necessary condition for successfully intervening in overtraining.

Integrity

The need for interaction with other experts brings up the issue of professional relationships. As was emphasized in the section on role issues, consulting sport psychologists must be clear regarding their place in the sport environment to maintain boundaries and avoid uncomfortable and unethical relationships. APA's general ethical principle of integrity specifically calls for psychologists to clarify the roles they are performing and to identify their own value systems.

One specific question that might arise is, Who is the client—athlete, coach, or team? Although in some situations (such as in the professional sports world) where the consultant is clearly hired by the team organization, there might be less clarity in other consulting environments.

At the United States Olympic Training Center in Colorado Springs, for example, an athlete might come to the sport psychology department singly and present indications of overtraining to the psychologist. Should the psychologist work individually with the athlete to build personal resources to deal with the training load or should the psychologist attempt to intervene with the coach (within the bounds of confidentiality)? What if large numbers of athletes all present with symptoms of overtraining? Does the psychologist have a responsibility to intervene at the team or national governing body level to eliminate the overtraining? These systemic or professional relationship issues are highly relevant in training. Ideally, consultants should establish good relationships with all levels of an organization to ensure maximum freedom to intervene as appropriate.

Personal values about sport participation might be the most difficult ethical issue for a consulting sport psychologist. In particular, a consultant needs to recognize personal values about playing with injury or training under severe stress. When a consultant sees that training stress is having a negative impact on other facets of an athlete's life (whether or not the athlete has an overtraining syndrome), the dilemma of choosing an appropriate course of action exists. If the training load is necessary for a long-term goal of national or international success, should the consultant attempt to continue to build an athlete's personal resources, or does there come a point when the consultant recommends that an athlete avoid the stress? Does it matter how old the athlete is? Does it make a difference whether daily ice packs are used by a 30-year-old professional baseball player or a 13-year-old figure skater?

Most sport psychologists have a positive orientation toward sport and despite the stress of elite sports see genuine benefits for participants. Given this viewpoint and the organizational and social pressures for continuing in sport when success at an elite level is near, consultants must be aware of their own biases when attempting to help an athlete concerned about training stress. One possible bias is the tendency to treat star athletes differently. Does a realistic opportunity at a professional contract or an Olympic gold medal outweigh the risk of altered moods, chronic fatigue, loss of family support, loss of life outside of sport, and loss of positive marital interactions that might result because of the training time required for success? These questions might need to be addressed individually, based on personal circumstances, but they are not merely philosophical queries. They are real issues likely to be faced by a sport psychologist involved with athletes in training.

Although athletes make personal choices about sport participation, does a sport psychology consultant have a professional obligation to advise against sport participation based on the negative impact of training stress? I believe that a sport psychologist can and should give this advice at times. Although the development of psychological conditions, such as depression, disordered eating, or anxiety disorders might be obvious signals that training stress can be a negative moderator or etiological variable, other impacts of training stress might be more subtle.

CONCLUSION

This chapter's major premise is that sport psychologists must understand the stress of training for elite athletic competition. This understanding begins with the recognition that the elite athlete's life is dominated by training as well as by competition and that an athlete's ability to master intense training loads is a necessary step in reaching elite status. Currently, however, sport psychology consultations typically focus more on competition preparation than on training issues. Increasing the attention given to and research on training issues remains a challenge for the field.

There are some encouraging signs of greater interest in the area of training and overtraining. For example, there is an increase in psychological research in the area of overtraining and burnout. A recent special issue of the *Journal of Applied Sport Psychology* was devoted entirely to studies of training stress (Association for the Advancement of Applied Sport Psychology, 1990) and summary literature reviews have appeared in other recent publications (Morgan, 1991).

Individual sport psychologists face the challenge of becoming familiar and comfortable with basic knowledge in exercise physiology. Recent reviews of overtraining suggest that psychological and physiological elements are clearly interrelated and that both should be considered in assessment and interventions in this area (Callister et al., 1989; Morgan, 1991). Currently, sport psychologists might have greater familiarity with the psychological signs of overtraining than with physiological signs or symptoms. For psychologists to better recognize physiological warning signs of an overtraining syndrome, it is important to understand and recognize a well-planned training program. For sport psychologists without a background in exercise physiology, obtaining knowledge in this area might greatly increase their ability to understand the training stress of elite athletes. An encouraging trend for the future of the field is a strong emphasis on physiological aspects of psychology in the proposed certification criteria for AAASP consultants (Association for the Advancement of Applied Sport Psychology, 1990).

Training stress is a reality for athletes at many competitive levels, and adapting to high training loads is a chronic concern for elite athletes. Helping athletes cope with training stress can be a critical step in reducing or preventing the ill effects of an overtraining syndrome or athlete burnout. The role of a sport psychologist presents a special opportunity to positively impact the bulk of an athlete's life, that portion spent in training.

REFERENCES

Ader, R. (1981). *Psychoneuroimmunology*. New York: Academic Press.

American Psychiatric Association. (1987). *Diagnostic and statistical manual of mental disorders* (3rd ed., rev.). Washington, DC: American Psychiatric Association.

American Psychological Association. (1992). Ethical principles of psychologists and code of conduct. *American Psychologist*, **47**, 1597-1611.

Andersen, M.B., & Williams, J.M. (1988). A model of stress and athletic injury: Prediction and prevention. *Journal of Sport and Exercise Psychology*, **10**, 294-306.

Association for the Advancement of Applied Sport Psychology (1990). Criteria for AAASP certification. *AAASP Newsletter*, **6**, p. 4.

Billings, A.G., & Moos, R.H. (1981). The role of coping responses and social resources in attenuating the stress of life events. *Journal of Behavioral Medicine*, **4**, 139-157.

Bompa, T.O. (1983). *Theory and methodology of training*. Dubuque, IA: Kendall/Hunt.

Borysenko, J. (1984). Stress, coping, and the immune system. In J.D. Matarazzo, S.M. Wiss, J.A. Herd, N.E. Miller, & S.H. Weiss (Eds.), *Behavioral health: A handbook of health enhancement and disease prevention* (pp. 241-260). New York: Wiley.

Caccese, T.M., & Mayerberg, C.K. (1984). Gender differences in perceived burnout of college coaches. *Journal of Sport Psychology*, **6**, 279-288.

Callister, R., Callister, R.J., Fleck, S.J., & Dudley, G.A. (1989). Physiological and performance responses to overtraining in elite judo athletes. *Medicine and Science in Sports and Exercise*, **22**, 816-824.

Capel, S.A. (1986). Psychological and organizational factors related to burnout in athletic trainers. *Research Quarterly for Exercise & Sport*, **57**, 321-328.

Carmichael, C. (1992). Yearly periodization training program for the elite level cyclist. *Cycling USA*, **4**(3), 8.

Costill, D.L. (1986). Detection of overtraining. *Sportsmedicine Digest*, **8**, 4-5.

Costill, D.L., Flynn, M.G., Kirwin, J.P., Houmard, J.A., Mitchell, J.B., Thomas, R., & Park, S.H. (1988). Effects of repeated days of intensified training on muscle glycogen and swimming performance. *Medicine and Science in Sports and Exercise*, **20**, 249-254.

Dale, J., & Weinberg, R. (1990). Burnout in sport: A review and critique. *Journal of Applied Sport Psychology*, **2**, 67-83.

Davis, J.O. (1991). Sports injuries and stress management: An opportunity for research. *The Sport Psychologist*, **5**, 175-182.

Dressendorfer, R.H., & Wade, C.E. (1983). The muscular overuse syndrome in long-distance runners. *Physician and Sportsmedicine*, **11**, 116-130.

Eysenck, H.J. (1979). Behavior therapy and the philosophers. *Behavior Research and Therapy*, **17**, 511-514.

Gieck, J., Brown, R.S., & Shank, R.H. (1982). The burnout syndrome among athletic trainers. *Athletic Training*, **17**(1), 36-41.

Hackney, A.C., Pearman, S.N., & Nowacki, J.M. (1990). Physiological profiles of overtrained and stale athletes: A review. *Applied Sport Psychology*, **2**, 21-33.

Hall, S.S. (1989). A molecular code links emotions, mind and health. *Science*, 62-71.

Hardy, C.J., Richman, J.M., & Rosenfeld, J.M. (1991). The role of social support in the life stress/injury relationship. *Sport Psychologist*, **5**, 128-139.

Heiby, E.M., & Campos, P.E. (1986). Measurement of individual differences in self-reinforcement. *Psychological Assessment*, **2**, 57-69.

Heil, J. (1993). Sport psychology, the athlete at risk, and the sports medicine team. In J. Heil (Ed.), *Psychology of sport injury* (pp. 1-15). Champaign, IL: Human Kinetics.

Henschen, K.P. (1986). Athletic staleness and burnout: Diagnosis, prevention, and treatment. In J.M. Williams (Ed.), *Applied sport psychology* (pp. 327-342). Palo Alto, CA: Mayfield.

Kirwin, J.P., Costill, D.L., Flynn, M.G., Mitchell, J.B., Fink, W.J., Neufer, P.D., & Houmard, J.A. (1988). Physiological responses to successive days of intense training in competitive swimmers. *Medicine and Science in Sports and Exercise*, **20**, 255-259.

Kuipers, H., & Keizer, H.A. (1988). Overtraining in elite athletes: Review and directions for the future. *Sports Medicine*, **6**, 79-92.

Lazarus, R.S., & Folkman, S. (1984). *Stress, appraisal and coping*. New York: Springer.

Levin, S. (1991). Overtraining causes Olympic-sized problems. *Physician and Sportsmedicine*, **19**, 112-118.

Maslach, C. (1976). Burned-out. *Human Behavior*, **5**, 16-22.

Matveyev, L. (1981). *Fundamentals of sports training*. USSR: Progress.

McNair, D.M., Lorr, M., & Droppleman, L.F. (1971). *Profile of Mood States manual*. Educational and Industrial Testing Service: San Diego, CA.

Meehl, P. (1954). *Clinical versus statistical procedures: A theoretical analysis and review of the evidence*. Minneapolis, MN: University of Minnesota Press.

Meichenbaum, D. (1985). *Stress inoculation training*. New York: Pergamon Press.

Morgan, W.P. (1985). Selected psychological factors limiting performance: A mental health model. In D.H. Clarke & H.M. Eckert (Eds.), *Limits of human performance* Champaign, IL: Human Kinetics.

Morgan, W.P. (October, 1991). *Monitoring and prevention of the staleness syndrome*. Invited lecture presented at the IOC World Congress on Sport Sciences, Barcelona.

(Sport Psychology Lab Report Number 150).

Morgan, W.P., Brown, D.R., Raglin, J.S., O'Connor, P.J., & Ellickson, K.A. (1987). Psychological monitoring of over-training and staleness. *British Journal of Sports Medicine, 21,* 107-114.

Morgan, W.P., Costill, D.L., Flynn, M.G., Rag-lin, J.S., & O'Connor, P.J. (1988). Mood disturbance following increased training in swimmers. *Medicine and Science in Sports and Exercise, 20,* 408-414.

Morgan, W.P., & Pollock, M. (1977). Psycho-logical characterization of the elite dis-tance runner. *Annals of the New York Academy of Science, 301,* 382-403.

Murphy, S.M. (1991, October). Intervention research, the good. In J.W. Whelan (chair), *Intervention research, the good the bad and the ugly.* Symposium presented to the Association for the Advancement of Applied Sport Psychology, Savan-nah, GA.

Murphy, S.M., Fleck, S.J., Dudley, G., & Callister, R. (1990). Psychological and performance concomitants of increased volume training in elite athletes. *Journal of Applied Sport Psychology, 2,* 34-50.

Pines, A.M., Aronson, E., & Kafry, D. (1981). *Burnout.* New York: Free Press.

Sarason, I.G., Sarason, B.R., & Pierce, G.R. (1990). Social support, personality, and performance. *Journal of Applied Sport Psy-chology, 2,* 117-127.

Selye, H. (1946). The general adaptation syn-drome and the disease process. *Journal of Clinical Endocrinology, 6,* 117-230.

Silva, J.M. (1990). An analysis of the training stress syndrome in competitive athletics. *Journal of Applied Sport Psychology, 2,* 5-20.

Smith, R.E. (1986). Toward a cognitive-affective model of athletic burnout. *Jour-nal of Sport Psychology, 8,* 36-50.

Smith, R.E., Smoll, F.J., & Ptacek, J.T. (1990). Conjunctive moderator variables in vul-nerability and resiliency research: Life stress, social support and coping skills, and adolescent sport injuries. *Journal of Personality and Social Psychology, 58,* 360-370.

Thibault, J.W., & Kelly, H.H. (1959). *The social psychology of groups.* New York: Wiley.

Wilson, V., & Bird, E. (1984). *Teacher-coach burnout.* Paper presented at the Annual Convention of the Northwest District Al-liance for Health, Physical Education, Recreation, and Dance, Eugene, OR.

Yukelson, D., & Murphy, S.M. (1993). Psycho-logical considerations in the prevention of sports injuries. In P. Renstrom (Ed.), *Sports injuries: Basic principles of preven-tion and care* (pp. 321-333). New York: Blackwell Scientific.

EPILOGUE

Looking back at the material in this book, I feel a great sense of enthusiasm at the new and exciting research and experiences described. To assemble the chapters in this book 10 years ago would not have been possible. The field has changed rapidly in the last decade, and we have learned much about sport psychology interventions. I would have wanted to read the chapters in this book if they had existed when I first studied sport psychology in the early 1980s. I'm glad and proud to have been able to assemble them here.

As I read this book as editor, I am impressed by the quantity and quality of research. As documented in chapter 1, it often has been difficult for researchers studying the psychology of sport and exercise to receive serious recognition for their work. Despite the fact that these pioneers have had to swim against the stream, they have accomplished a tremendous amount of varied, vigorous, and significant research. Today, when it is easy to specialize in only one or two areas, it is refreshing to read what has been accomplished in the diverse areas described by the chapter authors. The study of sport psychology has come of age and has reached a level of maturity that few of us might have realized it possessed.

Although a feeling of pride is justified, another strong impression is gained from reviewing the literature cited in this book. Much remains to be done. In many critical areas that demand understanding, little has been accomplished. In areas such as performance-enhancing drug use in sport, ethnicity and cultural issues, aggression in sport, and sexuality issues, little research exists. This emphasizes how critical is research to our understanding of such complex issues and how much can and should be done in understanding the impact of sport and athletic participation in our society. Perhaps we can publish a second edition of this book in the next few years and include chapters containing vigorous new research on these topics. I hope so and I look forward to it.

A book about interventions is a book about making a difference. Interventions promote change, and, guided by existing research, the potential exists for helping professionals to use sport psychology knowledge to promote positive change in sport. If we begin with the individual, change *is* possible. My hope is that the knowledge contained in this book will empower helping professionals to make a positive difference in the lives of the athletes they encounter.

Shane Murphy

CONTRIBUTORS

Throughout his career, **Shane M. Murphy, PhD**, has helped hundreds of elite athletes with performance and personal concerns. From 1987 to 1994 he served as the sport psychologist for the United States Olympic Committee (USOC). While with USOC, Dr. Murphy began a career-counseling program for elite athletes,

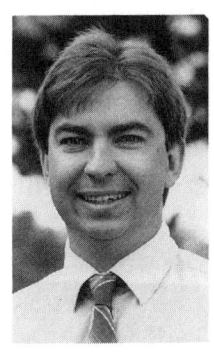

Shane Murphy, PhD, Editor

initiated a counseling program available to all athletes at the Olympic Training Center in Colorado Springs, organized a national conference on alcohol abuse education in sport, and produced a variety of educational programs in sport psychology for coaches and athletes. In 1992 he was appointed associate director of USOC's Division of Sport Science and Technology, a position he held until 1994, when he left the organization to pursue his writing and consulting interests.

Dr. Murphy was the U.S. team sport psychologist at the Olympic Games in Seoul and Albertville and at the 1987 U.S. Olympic Festival. He is a certified consultant of the Association for the Advancement of Applied Sport Psychology and has served on the editorial board of *The Sport Psychologist* since 1989. He has also published numerous articles and chapters on sport psychology.

Born and reared in Australia, Dr. Murphy earned his doctorate in clinical psychology from Rutgers University in 1985. He and his wife, Annemarie, have two children, Bryan and Theresa. He is an avid sports fan—baseball, football, soccer, rugby, cricket, and Australian football rank among his favorites—and participant, preferring a competitive game of tennis or golf.

Mark B. Andersen, PhD, is a licensed psychologist at the Victoria University of Technology in Melbourne, Australia. He has instructed in the psychology, sociology, and philosophy of sport. Dr. Andersen's recent work involves the psy-

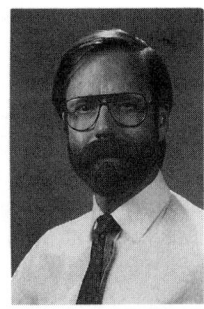

chosocial aspects of injury and inquiries into the delivery of psychological services to athletic populations. He has worked with high-school, college, professional, and Olympic athletes on a one-to-one basis for 9 years. He is an AAASP-certified consultant and is listed in the USOC sport psychology registry.

Chris M. Carr, PhD, is the psychologist for athletics at Washington State University. He coordinates and directs counseling and sport psychology services for student athletes, athletic trainers, and coaching staff at WSU. He also is a faculty member

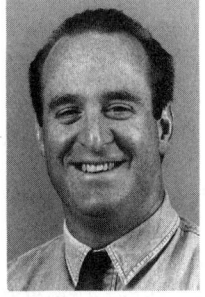

for the counseling services, provides supervision for graduate students, teaches courses in applied sport psychology, and coordinates the eating disorder education and drug education programs for the athletic department. Dr. Carr received his PhD in counseling psychology with a minor in sport psychology from Ball State University. He played football at Wabash College, was a graduate assistant football coach at Ball State, and spent a year in the U.S. Olympic Committee's sport psychology department as a clinical research assistant.

David B. Coppel, PhD, is a clinical psychologist and sport psychologist in private practice in Seattle, Washington. He is a clinical associate professor in the Department of Psychiatry and Behavioral Sciences at the University of Washington Medical 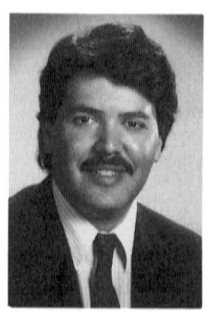 School, where he consults in neuropsychology. Dr. Coppel has been involved in clinical sport psychology consultation with athletes from numerous sports at all levels of competition, including high school, college, Olympic, and professional. He has consulted with numerous Olympic athletes and served as sport psychologist at the 1990 Goodwill Games. Currently he is the sport psychologist on the Sports Medicine Committee for the United States Figure Skating Association and is involved in elite-athlete and outreach training programs. Dr. Coppel has published more than 30 papers in scientific journals.

Steven J. Danish, PhD, is Director of the Life Skills Center and professor of psychology and preventive medicine at Virginia Commonwealth University. He is a licensed psychologist, a diplomate in counseling psychology, and a registered sport 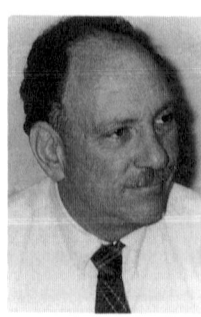 psychologist of the USOC. He is a Fellow of both the American Psychological Association and the Association for the Advancement of Applied Sport Psychology (AAASP). He is the author of more than 80 articles and eight books in the areas of counseling, community, and life span development psychology; health and nutrition; substance abuse prevention; and sport psychology. Dr. Danish has coached basketball at the high-school and college levels. He is the developer of the Going for the Goal Program, and was involved in the development and implementation of the Career Assistance Program for Athletes (CAPA) for the USOC and the Youth Education through Sports (YES) program for the National Collegiate Athletic Association (NCAA).

Charlene Donovan, MA graduated with honors from Rockhurst College in 1989 with a bachelor of arts in psychology and earned her master's degree in psychology from the University of Memphis, where she is now a doctoral student in clini- 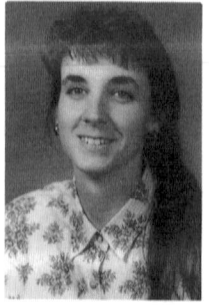 cal psychology. She has worked in a variety of clinical settings, including inpatient, chronic care, and outpatient. Her clinical interest centers on systemic therapies and health promotion. Ms. Donovan's research includes evaluations of therapy techniques, psychotherapy effectiveness, and the psychology of teaching. To apply her training as both a social scientist and a clinical psychologist, Ms. Donovan intends to pursue an academic position that involves research, teaching, and clinical psychology training.

Diane L. Gill, PhD is a professor in the Department of Exercise and Sport Science and associate dean of the School of Health and Human Performance at the University of North Carolina at Greensboro. She has published more than 50 research articles, several book chapters, and the book *Psychological Dynamics of Sport*. Her teaching and research focuses on the social psychological aspects of sport and exercise. She is former editor of the *Journal of Sport & Exercise Psychology*, past president of the North American Society for Psychology of Sport and Physical Activity (NASPSPA), and a Fellow of the AAASP, American Academy of Kinesiology and Physical Education, and Division 47 of the American Psychological Association (APA).

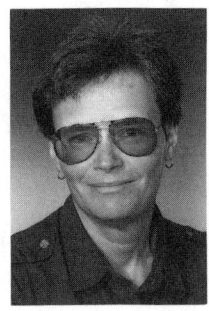

Frank Gardner, PhD, is in private practice in East Hills, NY.

Michael Greenspan, PhD, is a senior consultant with Kiddy and Partners, an organizational consulting firm in London, England. Prior to joining Kiddy and Partners, he spent four years as a licensed psychologist in the Arizona State University counseling center and was the head of Sport Psychology Services at ASU for three years. In addition to his work at the university, Dr. Greenspan provided outpatient psychological services, clinical sport psychology services, and performance enhancement services as a private practitioner. Most of his work was with student-athletes and amateur and professional golfers. Dr. Greenspan received his doctorate from Michigan State University in

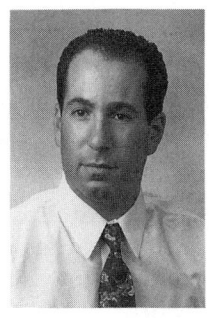

counseling psychology with a cognate in sport psychology.

Bruce D. Hale, PhD, is a principal lecturer in the Division of Sport, Health and Science at Staffordshire University in Stoke-on-Trent, UK. He contributed to this book while an affiliate assistant professor in exercise and sport science at The Pennsylvania State University. Dr. Hale received his doctorate from Penn State in physical education with an emphasis in sport psychology. He currently is registered as an educational sport psychologist with the Sports Medicine Committee of the USOC and is a certified consultant of the Association for the Advancement of Applied Sport Psychology and the British Association of Sport and Exercise Sciences. He has consulted with hundreds of college and elite athletes in performance-enhancement strategies and is a sport psychologist consultant for USAC Roller Skating, USA Wrestling, US Rugby, and the British Olympic Association.

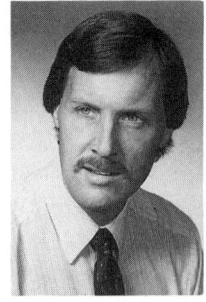

Jon C. Hellstedt, PhD, is professor of psychology at the University of Massachusetts-Lowell. In addition to teaching and conducting research, Dr. Hellstedt is a practicing psychotherapist who specializes in marital and family therapy. He is a frequent speaker and workshop leader and has conducted seminars for coaches and parents of young athletes sponsored by regional and national sport organizations. Dr. Hellstedt has coauthored the book *On the Sidelines: Decisions, Skills and Training in Youth Sport* and has written more than 13 articles

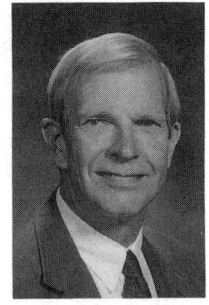

on parent involvement and young athletes' perceptions of parental pressure in the youth sport environment.

Sean McCann, PhD, is a sport psychologist with the Sport Science and Technology Division at the U.S. Olympic Training Center in Colorado Springs. He received his bachelor's degree in psychology from Brown University and his PhD in 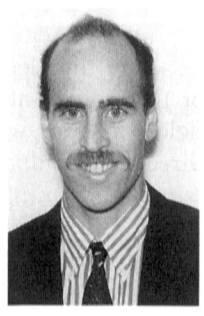 clinical psychology from the University of Hawaii; he completed his postdoctoral fellowship at the University of Washington. Dr. McCann works directly with Olympic athletes and coaches on stress management, performance enhancement, and counseling issues and supervises clinical research assistants working with resident athlete teams. Dr. McCann has published articles and presented papers on anxiety and performance, stress in athletes, and cognitive pain-management strategies in endurance sports.

Andrew W. Meyers, PhD, is professor of psychology and chairman of the Department of Psychology at The University of Memphis. Dr. Meyers received his doctorate from Pennsylvania State University in 1974. He has published extensively in the areas of 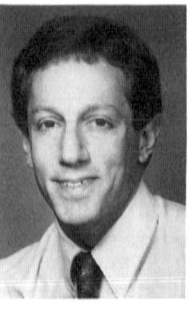 sport psychology, behavioral medicine, and children's problem solving. He is a Fellow of both the AAASP and Division 47 of the APA. Dr. Meyers is currently on the editorial boards of the *Sport Psychologist, Journal of Sport and Exercise Psychology*, and the *Journal of Applied Sport*.

Annemarie Infantino Murphy, PhD, is a licensed clinical psychologist in private practice with the AIM Care clinic in Colorado Springs, Colorado. She specializes in rehabilitation psychology and has an extensive background in neuro- 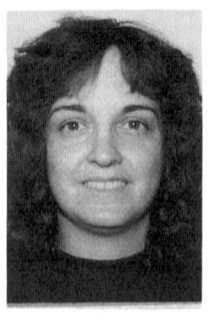 psychological testing. In her clinical practice Dr. Murphy has been involved with a number of athletes in their rehabilitation from injury. Dr. Murphy received her PhD in clinical psychology from Rutgers University with a focus on behavioral medicine and her undergraduate training at the State University of New York in Albany, where she worked with Dr. David Barlow. She completed her internship at the Medical University of South Carolina in Charleston.

Megan Neyer, PhD, is completing her doctoral work at the University of Florida in counselor education with an emphasis in sport and health psychology. She is the assistant director for the human performance lab at the U.S. Air 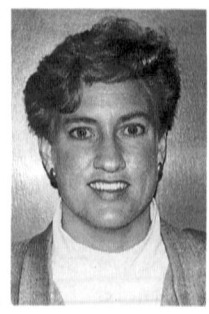 Force Academy, primarily in charge of sport psychology programs for the 27 intercollegiate teams. She is a former competitive elite athlete in diving, her accomplishments including being an Olympian, world champion, 15-time U.S. national diving champion, and 8-time NCAA champion. Her research interests include career and identity development, psychological aspects of injury rehabilitation, stress-injury relationship, eating disorders, and issues in psychoneuroimmunology.

Bruce C. Ogilvie, PhD, is a professor emeritus of psychology at San Jose State University and a member of the United States Olympic Committee's Sport Psychologist registry. His practice extends to professional, national, university, and 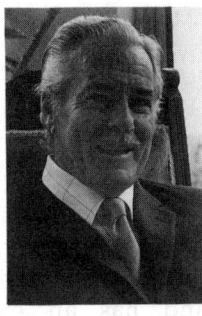 recreational athletes. Since 1954, his interest has been in the discovery and application of mental training methods for the enhancement of performance. His recent endeavors have been the dissemination of psychological principles and methods as means for reinforcing general wellness. Dr. Ogilvie is a team consultant to the U.S. Figure Skating Association, and a consultant to business and international medical health organizations. He also is a Fellow in the American College of Sports Medicine, the AAASP, the International Society for Sport Psychology (ISSP), and Division 47 of the APA.

Frank M. Perna, EdD, was a former clinical sport psychology fellow with the U.S. Olympic Training Center and health psychologist at Harvard University. Dr. Perna currently holds a research appointment in the Behavioral Medicine depart- 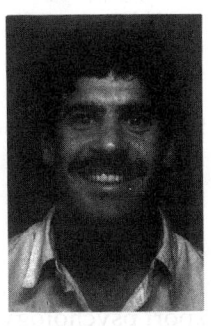 ment at the University of Miami, and he maintains a consulting practice with professional athletes and with the national governing body of several sports. Dr. Perna received his undergraduate psychology degree from East Stroudsburg State University, and a counseling psychology doctoral degree from Boston University. Dr. Perna's research has examined psychological variables affecting physiological recovery from exercise and athletic injury, transition out of sport, and the

adoption of health behavior (exercise, stress management, and smoking cessation) for chronically ill populations. He also is an avid runner who formerly competed at the national level.

Al Petitpas, EdD, is a professor in the Department of Psychology at Springfield College, where he directs the graduate training program in athletic counseling. He maintains a private practice at S.T.A.R.T. Sport Medicine Clinic in Springfield, Mas- 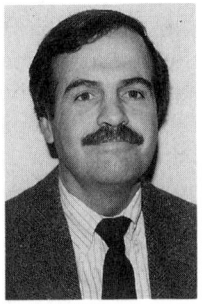 sachusetts, and served as consultant for the 1990 Olympic Festival and the USOC's Career Assistance Program for Athletes and Alcohol Education Program. His research interests include psychological concerns related to athletic injury and to career and personal development in athletes.

Robert A. Swoap, PhD, is a clinical associate and postdoctoral Fellow in Behavioral Medicine at Duke University, where he works in clinical psychology, conducts health psychology research, teaches, and consults with the athletic department. 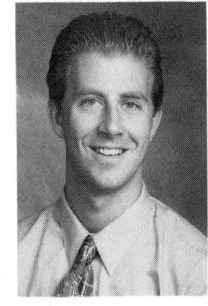 Dr. Swoap is a member of Division 47 of the APA, the AAASP, and the Society of Behavioral Medicine. He completed his doctorate degree in clinical and health psychology at the University of Florida, examining the effects of anxiety on swimming performance. His clinical and research interests include performance enhancement in athletics and in the workplace, developmental sport psychology, and health psychology. Earlier in his career, Dr. Swoap worked at the U.S. Olympic Training Center in the sport psychology department.

Maureen R. Weiss, PhD, is a professor in the Department of Exercise and Movement Science at the University of Oregon. Her research has focused primarily on the psychological and social development of children and adolescents through sport 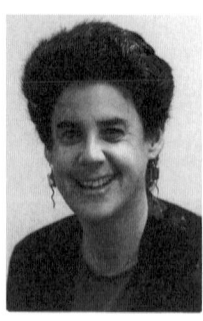 participation. She has published 56 journal articles, 8 book chapters, and coedited two Human Kinetics books, *Competitive Sport for Children and Youths and Advances in Pediatric Sport Sciences, Vol. 2: Behavioral Issues*. She also is editor for the *Research Quarterly for Exercise and Sport*. In addition, Dr. Weiss has given more than 110 professional or research presentations and 85 clinics and workshops for coaches, administrators, and teachers. In addition to her other responsibilities, Dr. Weiss directs the Children's Summer Sports program and has been an invited scholar and lecturer for numerous universities and professional organizations across the United States and in several other nations.

James P. Whelan, PhD, is an assistant professor and director of the psychological services center in the Department of Psychology at The University of Memphis, from which he received his PhD in 1989. The psychological services center is a training 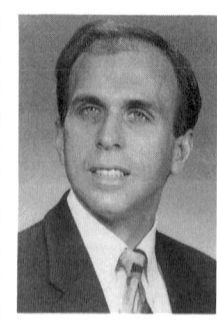 clinic for clinical psychology doctoral students and the setting for Dr. Whelan's psychotherapy-outcome research. His sport psychology interests focus on athletic performance-enhancement issues and the role of sport and exercise involvement on psychological well-being. He has published on the topics of treatment of child abuse and neglect, children's adjustment to disabilities, and health psychology. He also is actively involved with defining legal and professional practice standards for psychologists.

INDEX